Essentials of
Ophthalmology

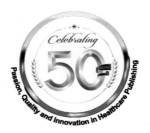

Essentials of
Ophthalmology

Seventh Edition

Samar K Basak
MBBS (Cal) MD (AIIMS) DNB FRCS (Glasgow)
Diplomate of National Board of Examiners in Ophthalmology, India
Director
Disha Eye Hospitals
Kolkata, West Bengal, India

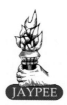

JAYPEE
JAYPEE BROTHERS MEDICAL PUBLISHERS
The Health Sciences Publisher
New Delhi | London | Panama

Jaypee Brothers Medical Publishers (P) Ltd

Headquarters

Jaypee Brothers Medical Publishers (P) Ltd
4838/24, Ansari Road, Daryaganj
New Delhi 110 002, India
Phone: +91-11-43574357
Fax: +91-11-43574314
Email: jaypee@jaypeebrothers.com

Overseas Offices

J.P. Medical Ltd
83 Victoria Street, London
SW1H 0HW (UK)
Phone: +44 20 3170 8910
Fax: +44 (0)20 3008 6180
Email: info@jpmedpub.com

Jaypee Brothers Medical Publishers (P) Ltd
Bhotahity, Kathmandu, Nepal
Phone: +977-9741283608
Email: kathmandu@jaypeebrothers.com

Jaypee-Highlights Medical Publishers Inc
City of Knowledge, Bld. 235, 2nd Floor,
Clayton, Panama City, Panama
Phone: +1 507-301-0496
Fax: +1 507-301-0499
Email: cservice@jphmedical.com

Website: www.jaypeebrothers.com
Website: www.jaypeedigital.com

Essentials of Ophthalmology

Sixth Edition : 2016

Seventh Edition : **2019**

ISBN 978-93-5270-988-5

Printed at: Samrat Offset Pvt. Ltd.

Dedicated to

Dr Bani Biswas

Who still loves me even after extensive hours with this book.

Dedicated to

Dr Asni Biswas

Preface to the Seventh Edition

The sixth edition of *Essentials of Ophthalmology* was published in January, 2016. Since then, much has changed in the landscape of medicine and health-care, and more specifically, in the field of ophthalmology. As our living environments and surrounding technologies change, so do the complications in the human body. Over the past three years, as a result of new studies and researches conducted and published, we have seen evolutions in disease management, diagnosis, surgical techniques, treatment patterns, hospital policies and so on. Therefore, it has become necessary to bring out this updated seventh edition of the book.

The highlights of this edition are—latest medical and surgical management of some diseases, and updates on newer investigations. The new look and the use of American spellings make the book reach out to a wider range of international readers. However, a few things have not changed in this edition, like its predecessors, plenty of diagrams and photographs are in four color. The bulleted format of the book, detailed illustrations, a selection of slit-lamp examination, and such features which facilitate revision have been retained.

The making of this edition has also been aided by the generous feedback from its readers, who are not just undergraduates, but also postgraduates and practising ophthalmologists from the Indian subcontinent. Thank all of you for your suggestions, thoughts and for pointing out the typos that were in the previous edition. Much appreciation also to the optometrists, who have written into tell that they have gained insight from the book. The sustained encouragement and engagement from readers is a great motivation to prepare a better edition.

I take this opportunity to thank all the doctors and staff members of Disha Eye Hospitals for their continued support and involvement. As usual, Dr Soham Basak has helped me polish this edition, and thanks to my wife Dr Bani and my daughter Sohini.

Finally, I do hope that this edition will encourage the readers to think critically about ophthalmology and ophthalmological practises. As always, I welcome all your suggestions, criticisms and comments.

Samar K Basak
E-mail: basak_sk@hotmail.com

Preface to the First Edition

Most medical colleges do not have a required undergraduate teaching course in ophthalmology. Consequently, the students are often sadly deficient in this subject, unless they are specially interested. In adition, an acute shortage of time, prevents the students from reading large textbooks on this subject. Many students complain that most of the available books are either too brief or too extensive. It is with the hope of bridging this gap that I have written this book.

This book focusses on the information in a concise, step-wise, outline format which is essential for getting a true picture of the subject. The arrangement of the subject matter is to-the-point, and up-to-date with plenty of line diagrams which are easily reproducible during examination. Though this book is essentially meant for the undergraduate students, I hope, it will be very useful to the postgraduate students as well as practising ophthalmologists, for a quick revision of the subject.

In conclusion, I shall be happy if this book proves itself to be a valuable guide both for the undergraduate and postgraduate students, especially during their examination. Any critical comment and suggestion from the students and teachers, regarding this effort, will be appreciated.

Samar K Basak

Acknowledgments

I am thankful to Prof BN Nag, Principal, NRS Medical College, Kolkata, West Bengal, India, for his support and encourgament. I am also thankful to the teachers, postgraduate and undergraduate students in the Department of Ophthalmology, for inspiring me during writing this book.

I am extremely grateful to my teacher, Prof VK Dada, Ex-Chief, RP Center for Ophthalmic Sciences, AIIMS, New Delhi, who had spent his valuable time reading the manuscript.

The material of this book is drawn from many sources—*Parsons' Diseases of the Eye, Kanski's Clinical Ophthalmology, Trevor-Roper's The Eye and its Disorders, Newell's Ophthalmology: Principles and Concepts, Wolff's Anatomy of the Eye and Orbit, Bruce-Shield's A Study Guide of Glaucoma, Abram's Practice of Refraction.* I express my sincere gratitude to all authors and respective publishers. For any instance, in which I have omitted to mention its source, it is hoped that the author will accept this blanket of acknowledgments.

I am greatly indebted to Dr Amitava Kundu, who has helped me to compile the manuscript. I gratefully thank my wife, Dr Bani Biswas and my children Soham and Sohini, for their cheerful acceptance of many evenings and holidays sacrificed, so that I could complete this book. Finally, I would like to convey my gratitude to Shri Jitendar P Vij (Group Chairman), Mr Ankit Vij (Managing Director), Mr MS Mani (Group President), Dr Madhu Choudhary (Publishing Head–Education), Dr Swapnil Shikha (Assistant Manager–Publishing) and all technical staff of M/s Jaypee Brothers Medical Publishers (P) Ltd, New Delhi, India.

Contents

Embryology and Anatomy

EMBRYOLOGY OF THE EYEBALL

The human eye originates from neuroectoderm, surface ectoderm and the extracellular mesenchyme which consists of both neural crest and mesoderm. Ocular development in the human embryo begins around 3rd week into embryonic life and continues through the 20th week of life (Table 1.1).

- Both the sensory and pigmentary layers of retina are developed from the neuroectoderm. These layers continue anteriorly to give rise to ciliary epithelium and the pigmented layer of the iris. The neuroglial and neural portions of the optic nerve are also originated from neuroectoderm.
- The surface ectoderm is the primordial of the crystalline lens (Table1.1), the conjunctiva, corneal epithelium and the eyelids with the epithelium of their glands.
- Neural crest cells are themselves derived from the ectoderm and lie close to the neural tube. They are responsible for development of sclera, cornea—

TABLE 1.1: Primordia of ocular structures

Surface ectoderm	Neuroectoderm	Mesoderm	Cranial neural crest cells
<ul><li>Conjunctival epithelium</li><li>Corneal epithelium</li><li>Eyelids—epithelium, glands, eyelash, skin</li><li>Caruncle</li><li>Lacrimal system</li><li>Lacrimal gland (also from neural crest)</li><li>Crystalline lens</li><li>Vitreous (also mesoderm)</li></ul>	<ul><li>Neurosensory retina</li><li>Optic nerve, axons, glia</li><li>Retinal pigment epithelium</li></ul>	<ul><li>Extraocular muscle</li><li>Fat (also neural crest)</li><li>Iris sphincter and dilated muscles</li><li>Iris stroma</li><li>Sclera (also neural crest)</li><li>Vascular endothelium</li><li>Vitreous (also surface ectoderm)</li></ul>	<ul><li>Bones—midline/ inferior orbital bones; parts of orbital roof and lateral rim</li><li>Orbital connective tissue</li><li>Choroidal stroma</li><li>Ciliary ganglion</li><li>Cornea-stroma and endothelium</li><li>Extraocular muscles sheath and tendon</li><li>Fat (also mesoderm)</li><li>Iris pigment epithelium</li><li>Melanocytes</li><li>Optic nerve sheath</li><li>Sclera (also mesoderm)</li><li>Trabecular meshwork</li></ul>

- ***Eyelids:*** Both from surface ectoderm and mesoderm
- ***Zonules (tertiary vitreous):*** Surface ectoderm and mesoderm
- ***Bruch's membrane:*** Neural ectoderm and mesoderm

Descemet's membrane and endothelium and connective tissue, and bony structure of the orbit.

- The mesoderm is the primordial of the extraocular muscles, endothelial lining of blood vessels of the eye, choroidal blood vessels, sclera and choroid, vitreous, zonular fibers, iris sphincter/dilated muscles, and iris stroma.
- Eye development is initiated by the master control gene *Pax6*. The *Pax6* gene locus is a transcription factor for the various genes and growth factors involved in eye formation.

THE EYE AT BIRTH

- Orbit is more divergent (50°) as compared to adult orbit.

- Eyeball is 70% of adult length, being almost fully developed at the age of 8 years.
- Cornea is 80% of its adult size, being fully developed at the age of 3 years.
- The newborn is hypermetropic by +2.5D.
- Pupil is small and does not dilate fully.
- Anterior chamber is shallow and the angle is narrow.

DEVELOPMENT (FIGS 1.1A TO E)

On either side of the cephalic end of forebrain, a lateral depression appears, known as *optic pit* (3rd week).

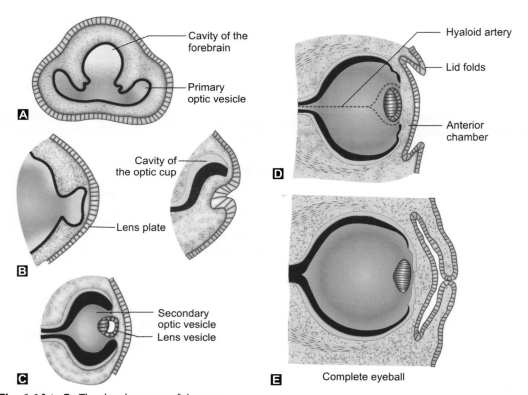

Figs 1.1A to E: The development of the eye
Solid red—neural ectoderm; *dotted area*—mesoderm; *hatched area*—surface ectoderm

Optic pit is thickened to form **optic plate**

↓

Optic plate changes into **primary optic vesicle**. **Lens plates** appear simultaneously (4th week). Optic vesicle invaginates to form optic cup. Pigment appears in outer layer of optic cup. Lens plate changes into **lens pit** and then into **lens vesicle** (end of 4th week)

↓

Fetal fissure closes. Lens separates from the surface, and primary lens fibers form. **Tunica vasculosa lentis** (to give nourishment) begins to develop (6th week)

↓

Sclera, cornea and extraocular muscles differentiate (9th week)

↓

Optic tracts are completed. Pars ciliaris and pars iridica retinae grow forward. **Lid folds** develop (10–12th week). Tunica vasculosa lentis begins to retrogress. Sphincter and dilator muscles, and ciliary muscles develop (4th month)

↓

Hyaloid artery disappears. Medullation of the optic nerve reaches lamina cribrosa (9th month). Macula leutea finally differentiates 4–6 months after birth.

GROSS ANATOMY OF THE EYEBALL (FIG. 1.2)

- It is not a true sphere, but consists of the segments of two modified spheres, one in front of the other.
- The cornea is more convex than the rest of the globe (7.8 mm radius as opposed to 12 mm).
- The anteroposterior diameter (*axial length*) is about 24 mm, while the vertical is 23 mm, and the horizontal is 23.5 mm.
- The eyeball is shorter in hypermetropes but longer in myopes.

THE GLOBE

- *Three concentric layers or tunics:*
  1. *Outer supporting layer:* It consists of transparent cornea, opaque sclera and their junction, the *limbus*.
  2. *Middle vascular layer:* It is called uvea, and consists of choroid, ciliary body and the iris.
  3. *Inner neural layer:* It is called retina, composed of two parts (1) a sensory portion and (2) a layer of pigment epithelium.
- *A crystalline lens:* The transparent structure is located immediately behind the iris, and is supported by fine fibers, called zonules.
- *Three chambers:*
  1. *Anterior chamber:* It is located between the iris and the posterior surface of the cornea. It communicates with the posterior chamber through the pupil.
  2. *Posterior chamber:* It is minute in size, bounded by the lens and zonules behind, and there is in front.
  3. *Vitreous cavity:* It is the largest and located behind the lens and zonules, and adjacent to the retina throughout.

THE CORNEA

Cornea (Fig. 1.3) is elliptical from front, being 12 mm horizontally, and 11 mm vertically. Posteriorly, it is circular with a diameter of 11.5 mm.

- *Thickness:* 500 micron at the center and 800–1000 micron at the periphery.
- *Radius of curvature:* Anterior surface 7.8 mm and of posterior surface 6.5 mm.
- *Refractive index:* 1.37.
- Cornea constitutes the anterior one-sixth of the eye.

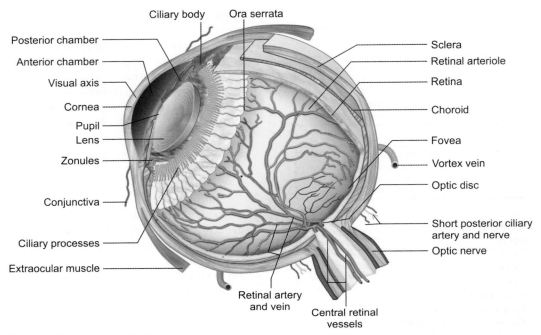

Fig. 1.2: The human eyeball

- It is the main refracting surface of the eye.
- *Dioptric power* is about +43.0 to +45.0D.

Structures

It consists of five layers:

1. *Stratified squamous epithelium*
   - 5–6 cells deep, continuous with the conjunctival epithelium.
   - The basal cells are tall with oval nuclei.
   - The intermediate layers (2–3 cells deep) are polyhedral wing cells.
   - The surface layers (about 2) are very flat, but not keratinized.
   - The corneal epithelium rests on a basement membrane, secreted by the basal cells.
2. *Bowman's layer (anterior elastic lamina)*
   - Anterior condensation of substantia propria.
   - Once eroded, it does not regenerate and leaves behind a superficial corneal scar.

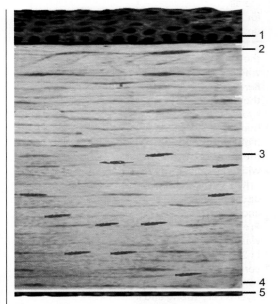

Fig. 1.3: Transverse section of the cornea

1—Epithelium; **2**—Bowman's membrane; **3**—Stroma; **4**—Descemet's membrane; **5**—Endothelium

3. *Substantia propria (stroma)*
   - Comprising 90% of corneal thickness.
   - Composed of collagen fibrils arranged in sets of lamellae, lying parallel to the surface.
   - They form a crystalline lattice, in a ground substance of glycoprotein and mucopolysaccharides.
   - Scattered between the lamellae are the *keratocytes*, and a few wandering leukocytes and macrophages.

> *Keratocytes (corneal fibroblasts)* are specialized fibroblasts residing mainly in the corneal stroma. They play the major role in keeping the cornea transparent, healing its wounds, and synthesizing its components. In a silent healthy cornea, keratocytes stay dormant, coming into action after any kind of injury or inflammation. Some keratocytes underlying the site of injury, even a light one, undergo apoptosis immediately after the injury. Other neighboring keratocytes, when acted upon by the same molecules, become active, proliferate and start synthesizing matrix metalloproteinases (MMPs) which is required for tissue remodeling. These activated cells are designated as 'active keratocytes'.
>
> Keratocytes are developmentally derived from the cranial population of *neural crest cells*, from where they migrate to settle in the mesenchyme. *Keratan sulfate* produced by keratocytes is thought to help maintain optimal corneal hydration. The average keratocyte density in the human stroma is about 20,500 cells per mm^3. The highest density is observed in the anterior 10% of the stroma. The number of keratocytes declines with age, at a rate approximately 0.45% per year.
>
> Keratocytes may play a role in ectatic corneal disorders. In keratoconus, excessive keratocyte apoptosis happens as a major pathological event.
>
> *Pre-Descemet's layer (Dua's layer):* A new layer was suggested by Harminder Singh Dua, et al. in 2013. It is hypothetically 15 μ thick, the fourth corneal layer from top, and located between the corneal stroma and Descemet's membrane. This layer is very strong and impervious to air, despite its thinness. This is still a controversial issue, as the existence of pre-Descemet stromal tissue remaining after pneumodissection is well known.

4. *Descemet's membrane (posterior elastic lamina)*
   - Strong, homogenous and very resistant membrane.
   - It readily regenerates after an injury.
   - It is secreted by endothelial cells and essentially their basement membrane.
   - In old age, it may bear some warty elevations called *Hassall-Henle's bodies* at its periphery.
5. *Endothelium*
   - A single layer of flattened polygonal endothelial cells.
   - Continuous with the endothelium over the anterior surface of the iris.
   - It does not regenerate in human being.

Nerve Supply

The corneal nerves are derived from the long and short ciliary nerves, branches of the ophthalmic division of trigeminal nerve.

They form the *pericorneal plexus* just outside the limbus, and then pass onto the cornea as 60–70 trunks. They loose their myelin sheaths after a millimeter or two, and reach the cornea. Cornea does not have proprioceptive sensation.

Blood Supply

Cornea is a vascular, but the corneoscleral limbus is supplied by the anterior conjunctival branches of anterior ciliary arteries and forms a perilimbal plexus of blood vessels.

▌THE SCLERA

It is a dense tough fibrous envelope that covers *posterior five-sixths* of the eye.
- Sclera has two large openings, the anterior (the corneal window) and the posterior (for optic nerve).
- Structures piercing the sclera are:
  - Four vortex veins (4 mm behind the equator).
  - Long and short ciliary nerves and vessels.

- Anterior ciliary nerves and vessels.
- Sclera is *thickest* posteriorly surrounding the optic nerve (1 mm), and is *thinnest* just posterior to the insertion of recti muscles (0.3 mm).

Structures

Sclera has three parts:
1. *Episclera:* It is the loose fibrous tissue, containing numerous fine capillaries.
2. *Sclera proper:* It is a dense network of collagen fibers. The sclera is white, because of variable diameter and irregular arrangement of collagen fibers of the stroma.
3. *Lamina fusca:* It is the inner layer, located adjacent to the choroid.

Blood Supply

It is from the episcleral and choroidal vessels. Anterior to the insertion of recti muscles, the anterior ciliary arteries form a dense episcleral plexus. These vessels become congested in ciliary congestion.

Nerve Supply

Short ciliary nerves posteriorly, and long ciliary nerves anteriorly, provide sensory innervation. Because of generous innervation, inflammation of the sclera is extremely painful.

▌THE LIMBUS

Transitional zone between the cornea and the sclera. It is 1–2 mm wide.
- Its internal boundaries are scleral spur posteriorly, and the Schwalbe's line.
- Its external boundaries are by sclerolimbal junction posteriorly, and corneolimbal junction anteriorly.
- Sclerolimbal junction (Fig. 1.4A) is the only consistent landmark of the limbus, used during cataract and glaucoma surgery.
- Limbus contains trabecular meshwork internally, through which the aqueous humor leaves the anterior chamber.

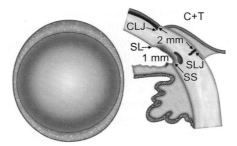

Fig. 1.4A: Surgical anatomy of the limbus

C+T—Conjunctiva and Tenon's capsule; **SL**—Schwalbe's line; **SS**—Scleral spur; **CLJ**—Corneolimbal junction (at the termination of the Bowman's membrane); **SLJ**—Sclerolimbal junction (junction of the white sclera and the translucent bluish limbus)

Limbal stem cells (Fig. 1.4B)
• The limbus contains multipotent stem cells which maintain epithelial cell turnover and plays an important role in corneal epithelial healing.
• The limbal stem cells (LSCs) transform to transient amplifying cells (TAC). The TACs migrate centripetally in the basal layer of epithelium and then multiply to replace the old or damaged cells.
• The LSC niche or locations are thought to be in the palisades of Vogt, limbal epithelial crypts, limbal crypts and focal stromal projections.

Angle of the Anterior Chamber

- Anterior chamber is bounded in front by the cornea, behind by the anterior surface of iris and part of the anterior surface of the lens which is exposed at the pupil (Figs 1.5A and B).
- The peripheral recess of the anterior chamber is known as *angle of the anterior chamber,* which is also known as the *cockpit of glaucoma.*
- It is bounded *anteriorly* by the corneosclera, and *posteriorly* by the root of the iris and the ciliary body.
- At this part in the inner layers of sclera, there is a circular venous sinus (sometimes broken up into more than one sinus) called

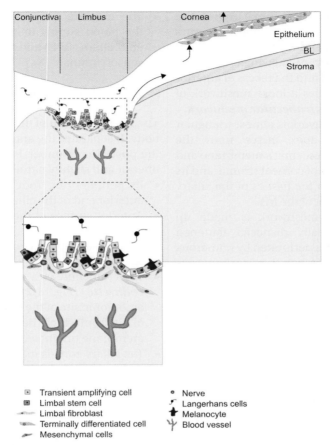

Fig. 1.4B: Limbal stem cells (LSCs) give rise to transient amplifying cells which divide and migrate towards the central cornea to replace the corneal epithelial cells

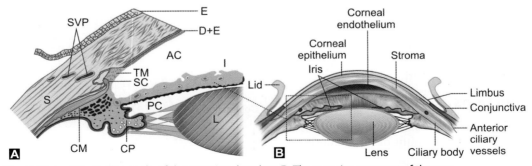

Figs 1.5A and B: A. The angle of the anterior chamber; **B.** The anterior segment of the eye

E—Corneal and conjunctival epithelium; **D+E**—Descemet's membrane + Endothelium; **TM**—Trabecular meshwork; **SC**—Schlemm's canal; **SVP**—Scleral venous plexus; **CM**—Ciliary muscle; **CP**—Ciliary processes; **L**—Lens; **I**—iris; **S**—Sclera; **CS**—Corneal stroma; **AC**—Anterior chamber; **PC**—Posterior chamber; **Z**—Zonules

canal of Schlemm. It is of great importance in the drainage of aqueous. The Schlemm's canal is lined by endothelial cells.

- At the periphery of the angle, between Schlemm's canal and the recess of anterior chamber, there lies a loose meshwork of tissues, known as *trabecular meshwork.*
- Trabecular meshwork is almost triangular in shape. Its apex arises from the termination of Descemet's membrane and the adjacent part of corneal stroma, and its base merges into the tissues of the ciliary body and the root of the iris.
- The trabecular meshwork is made up of circumferentially disposed flattened bands and each is perforated by numerous oval openings. Through these tortuous passages, communication exists between the Schlemm's canal and anterior chamber.
- The junctions between these cells are not 'tight', and the cells themselves have pores for aqueous drainage.
- Angle of the anterior chamber is best visualized by a gonioscope. Normally, the angle is wide open, and is about 20–45°. If the angle is less than 10°, there will be every chance of developing angle-closure glaucoma.

THE UVEA

The middle coat, or uvea means grape consists of three parts:
1. *Anterior:* Iris, a free circular diaphragm with a central opening called pupil.
2. *Intermediate:* Ciliary body
3. *Posterior:* Choroid.

Functions

- The iris with its central opening, pupil controls the amount of light entering the eye.
- The ciliary body secretes aqueous humor and contains smooth muscles responsible for changing the shape of the lens during accommodation.

- The choroid, a vascular layer, provides the blood supply to the retinal pigment epithelium (RPE) and the outer half of the sensory retina.

THE IRIS AND THE PUPIL

The iris lies in front of the lens and the ciliary body. It separates the anterior chamber from the posterior chamber. Pupil is situated just inferior and slightly nasal side of the center.

- Its periphery or 'root' is attached to the anterior end of the ciliary body.
- Anterior surface of the iris is divided into two zones (Fig. 1.6):
    1. Central papillary zone
    2. Peripheral ciliary zone.
- Their junction is a circular ridge called *collarette* (Fig. 1.7) which marks the embryonic site of the minor vascular circle of iris, from which the embryonic pupillary membrane originated.
- The ciliary zone is marked by many ridges and crypts, but the pupillary zone is relatively flat.

Structure

- *Anterior endothelium:* It is continuous with the corneal endothelium.

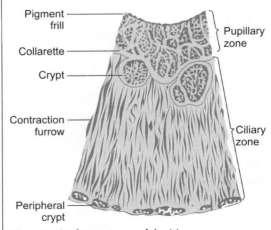

Pigment frill

Collarette

Crypt

Contraction furrow

Peripheral crypt

Pupillary zone

Ciliary zone

Fig. 1.6: Surface pattern of the iris

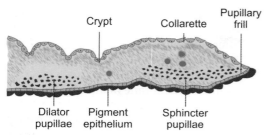
Fig. 1.7: Transverse section of the iris

- **Stroma:** It consists of spongy connective tissue with nerves, smooth muscles, and radial blood vessels forming the minor circle of iris.
- **Smooth muscles:** They are two in number:
  - **Sphincter pupillae:** A circular bundle of smooth muscles running around the pupillary margin causes constriction of the pupil.
  - **Dilator pupillae:** Arranged radially near the root of the iris, causes dilatation of the pupil.
- **Posterior two-layered epithelium:** Both layers are pigmented and developmentally derived from the retina. The anterior layer consists of flattened cells and the posterior layer consists of cuboidal cells.

Nerve Supply

- **Sensory:** Nasociliary nerve, branch of 1st division of 5th cranial nerve.
- **Sphincter pupillae:** Oculomotor nerve (3rd cranial).
- **Dilator pupillae:** Nerves derived from cervical sympathetic chain.

THE CILIARY BODY

The ciliary body is a ring of tissue about 6 mm wide that extends from the scleral spur to the ora serrata of the retina.

Structure

In anteroposterior section it is roughly an isosceles triangle, with base forwards. Iris is attached at the middle of its base.

- The chief mass of the ciliary body is composed of unstriped muscle fibers, called **ciliary muscle**. It has three parts, with a common origin circumferentially at the scleral spur:
  1. **Longitudinal:** The greater part, running antero-posteriorly.
  2. **Circular:** Concentrically with the root of the iris.
  3. **Radial**.
- The inner surface of ciliary body is divided into two regions:
  1. **Pars plicata:** Anterior part; about 70 plications are visible. Microscopically, they have ciliary processes responsible for the production of aqueous.
  2. **Pars plana:** Posterior smooth part; a relatively safe and a vascular zone for pars plana lensectomy and/or vitrectomy operation.
- They are covered by two layers of epithelium, continuous with the iris anteriorly, and retina posteriorly.

Ciliary body extends backward as far as the ora serrata. At this point the retina proper begins abruptly.

Nerve Supply

- **Sensory:** Via nasociliary branch of 5th cranial nerve.
- **Ciliary muscles:** Oculomotor (3rd cranial) and sympathetic nerves.

Blood Supply

By branches of **major circle** of iris which is formed by two long posterior ciliary arteries and seven anterior ciliary arteries (the **minor circle** lies within the iris stroma).

Functions

- Formation of aqueous humor by the ciliary processes.
- Ciliary muscles help in accommodation for near work.

- Ciliary muscles also help in opening up the Schlemm's canal, and thus facilitate in aqueous outflow.

THE CHOROID

- This vascular sheet separates the sclera from the retina. It is 0.25 mm thick at the posterior pole and 0.1 mm thick anteriorly.
- It is attached firmly to the sclera around the optic nerve and at the points of exit of the vortex veins.

Structures

It consists of three layers of blood vessels, having supporting structures on either side, i.e. suprachoroid (*lamina fusca*) on outer side and the basal lamina (*Bruch's membrane*) on the inner side.

Three vessel layers are (Fig. 1.8):

1. The *outer vessel layer (of Haller):* It is nearest to the sclera and consists of large veins that lead to the vortex veins.
2. The *middle vessel layer (of Sattler):* It consists of medium-size veins and arterioles, with fibrous tissues.
3. The *inner choriocapillaries:* It consists of large fenestrated capillaries.

Bruch's membrane: It is about 7 μ thick, and separates the choriocapillaries from the RPE. Electron microscopically, it consists of five layers (*from outside to inside*):

1. Basement membrane of the choriocapillaries
2. Outer collagen layer
3. Middle elastic layer
4. Inner collagen layer
5. Basement membrane of the RPE.

Bruch's membrane is important for blood-retinal barrier function.

Blood Supply (Fig. 1.9)

- *Short posterior ciliary arteries:* Originate from the ophthalmic artery as 2–3 branches. These branches are subdivided into 10–20 branches which perforate the sclera around the optic nerve, and directly communicate with the choriocapillaries.
- *Two long posterior ciliary arteries:* Perforate the sclera on either side of the optic nerve → via suprachoroidal space → to the ciliary body. There, each divides into two branches that extend circumferentially to form 'major arterial circle' of the iris, located in the ciliary body. Branches extend anteriorly to the iris.
- *Anterior ciliary arteries:* They are the terminal branches of two muscular arteries of each rectus muscle (except the lateral rectus, which has one muscular artery). The vessels provide supply to the ciliary body, and send branches to the major arterial circle of iris and also to the choriocapillaries.

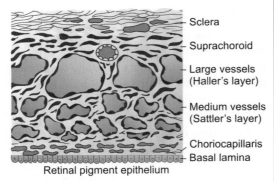

Sclera
Suprachoroid
Large vessels (Haller's layer)
Medium vessels (Sattler's layer)
Choriocapillaris
Basal lamina
Retinal pigment epithelium

Fig. 1.8: Transverse section of the choroid

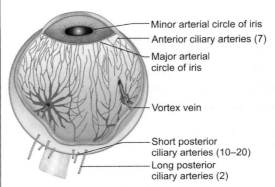

Minor arterial circle of iris
Anterior ciliary arteries (7)
Major arterial circle of iris
Vortex vein
Short posterior ciliary arteries (10–20)
Long posterior ciliary arteries (2)

Fig. 1.9: Blood supply of the uveal tract

Venous blood is collected from the iris, ciliary body and the choroid by a series of veins. These lead of four (or more) large ***vortex veins*** located behind the equator of the globe. The vortex veins drain into superior and inferior ophthalmic veins → cavernous sinus.

THE CRYSTALLINE LENS

The lens is a transparent biconvex body of crystalline structure.

- It is about 9 mm in diameter and 4 mm in thickness when the suspensory ligament is relaxed.
- Radius of curvature of anterior surface is 10 mm and that of posterior surface is 6 mm.
- The lens is held in its position by the suspensory ligament, called ***zonules*** of Zinn. They arise from the sides of the ciliary processes, and the valleys between them.
- The zonular fibers insert into the anterior and the posterior lens capsule near the equator, and extend further over the anterior surface more than the posterior surface.

Structures (Fig. 1.10)

- The ***lens capsule*** that envelops the entire lens.
- An anterior ***lens epithelium***.

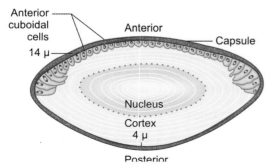

Fig. 1.10: Structure of the lens

- A ***lens substance***, consisting of the ***cortex*** (newly formed lens fibers) and the ***nucleus*** (a dense central area of old lens fibers).
- ***The capsule:*** It is a smooth, homogenous, a cellular highly elastic envelope, (but contains no true elastic tissue).
  The anterior capsule is the basement membrane of the anterior lens epithelium, and the thickest basement membrane of the body. The lens capsule is ***thickest*** on the anterior and posterior surface just central to the insertion of zonular fibers (14 μ) (i.e. pre-equator regions). It is ***thinnest*** at the posterior pole (3–4 μ).
- ***The lens epithelium:*** It consists of a single layer of cuboidal cells just deep to the capsule. There is no corresponding posterior epithelium. Towards the equator the anterior cuboidal cells gradually become columnar and elongated, and eventually converted into lens fibers. At the equator, the division of lens fibers is most active and mitosis is frequently observed.
- ***Lens substance:*** It consists of elongated lens cells (fibers). Mature lens fibers are cells which have lost their nuclei, and are no longer in contact with the posterior capsule. They form the greatest portion of the lens substance.
  - In the infantile lens, each lens fiber starts and finishes on the ***anterior and posterior Y sutures respectively*** in such a way, that the nearer the axis of the lens it commences, the farther away it ends (anterior Y is straight and the posterior Y is inverted).
  - Once this fetal nucleus is formed, these outlines become more irregular and more complicated.
  - In the beam of slit-lamp, various layers or ***zones of discontinuity*** may be seen and these represent the boundaries as follows (Fig. 1.11):
    - Embryonic nucleus (first 3 months of fetal life)
    - Fetal nucleus (3–8 months of fetal life)

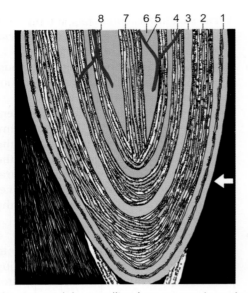

Fig. 1.11: Adult crystalline lens as seen in optical section of the slit lamp in higher magnification

1—Anterior capsule; **2**—Lens cortex; **3**—Adult nucleus; **4**—Infantile nucleus; **5**—Anterior Y suture; **6**—Fetal nucleus; **7**—Embryonic nucleus; **8**— Posterior Y suture

– Infantile nucleus (up to puberty).
– Adult nucleus (rest of life).

CHAMBERS OF THE EYE

The eye consists of three chambers—anterior chamber, posterior chamber, and vitreous cavity.
1. *Anterior chamber:* It is bounded anteriorly by the cornea, posteriorly by the front surface of the iris and lens, and peripherally by the anterior chamber angle. It is deepest at its central portion (2.5–3.0 mm), and its *volume* is 0.25 mL.
2. *Posterior chamber:* It consists of various boundaries are as follows:
   - *Anteriorly:* Iris,
   - *Laterally:* Ciliary processes,
   - *Medially:* Equator of the lens and
   - *Posteriorly:* Anterior surface of the lens. Its volume in adults is 0.06 mL.
3. *Vitreous cavity:* It contains vitreous humor which is a transparent gel-like structure. It is composed of a network of collagen fibers

suspended in a viscous liquid containing hyaluronic acid.

It has a saucer-like depression anteriorly, for the lens, called *patellar fossa*. Here, the vitreous humor is condensed, called *anterior hyaloids face*. The vitreous humor adheres firmly to the:
- Ciliary epithelium in the region of ora serrata (vitreous base),
- Peripheral retina,
- Margin of the optic disc, and
- Posterior capsule of the lens (Weigert's hyaloideocapsular ligament).

Running down the center of the vitreous, from the optic disc to the posterior pole of the lens—there is a canal, called *hyaloid canal of Cloquet*. Embryologically, the vitreous is divided into three parts:
1. *Primary* (mesenchymal, Cloquet's canal).
2. *Secondary* (most of the adult vitreous).
3. *Tertiary* (the lens zonules).

The vitreous contains a few cells, called *hyalocytes*, which are believed to be phagocytes (macrophage type).

Volume of the vitreous cavity is 4.5 mL.

THE RETINA

The retina is the membranous light sensitive coat of eyeball. It is transparent in life, and whitish after death.

The retina is derived from the inner and outer layers of the embryological optic cup. These two primary layers are loosely adherent across the potential space (representing the primary optic vesicle) so that they are readily separated by injury or disease. The *outer pigmented layer* remains as one-cell deep but the inner layer; the *sensory retina* becomes several layers by various visual relaying cells.

Structures

Retina apparently consists of *ten layers* (Fig. 1.12). From outside (choroid-side) inwards, they are:

1. Retinal pigment epithelium
2. Layer of rods and cones
3. External limiting membrane
4. Outer nuclear layer
5. Outer plexiform layer
6. Inner nuclear layer
7. Inner plexiform layer
8. Ganglion cell layer
9. Nerve-fiber layer
10. Internal limiting membrane.

- ***The retinal pigment epithelium:*** It is a single layer of flattened hexagonal cells with fine cytoplasmic villi, projecting for a short distance between the bases of rods and cones.

  The cells of RPE contain varying amount of melanin. The cells are taller at the fovea and contain more pigments (hence, the darker color in this region). Around

the optic disc they are heaped up as a ***choroidal ring***.

- ***Layer of rods and cones:*** They are the outer segments of photoreceptor cells, arranged in a palisade manner. The rods are about 125 million in number, but the cones are about 7 million. Each rod and cone may be divided into three parts (Fig. 1.13):

  1. ***An outer segment:*** It is cylindrical in shape, with its base related to the projecting villi of RPE. It consists of a dense vertical stack of 700 discs that originates from in folding of double layer of cell membrane. The infoldings contain the visual pigments.
  2. ***A cilium:*** It is a tubular connection with the inner segment that contains linear striations.
  3. ***An inner segment:*** It is divided into an ***outer ellipsoid*** and an ***inner myoid*** portion. The myoid part is densely packed with endoplasmic reticulum and Golgi bodies.

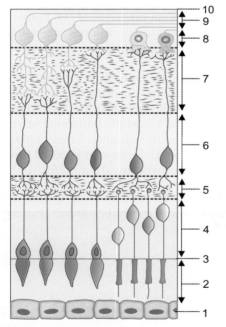

Fig. 1.12: Layers of the retina

1—Pigment epithelium; **2**—Layer of rods and cones; **3**—External limiting membrane; **4**—Outer nuclear layer; **5**—Outer plexiform layer; **6**—Inner nuclear layer; **7**—Inner plexiform layer; **8**—Ganglion cell layer; **9**—Nerve fiber layer; **10**—Internal limiting membrane

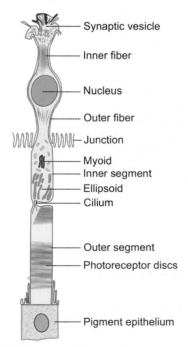

Synaptic vesicle

Inner fiber

Nucleus

Outer fiber

Junction

Myoid
Inner segment
Ellipsoid
Cilium

Outer segment
Photoreceptor discs

Pigment epithelium

Fig. 1.13: Diagram of the vertebrate visual cell

- **External limiting membrane:** It is a thin lamina, formed by the supporting fibers of Muller on which the rods and cones rest, and pierced by the fibers of these photoreceptors.
- **Outer nuclear layer:** It contains the rod and cone nuclei. Cone nuclei are larger and more oval than the rod nuclei, and carry a layer of cytoplasm.
- **Outer plexiform layer:** It is formed by the anastomoses of the photoreceptor cells, with bipolar and horizontal cells. The innermost portion of each rod and cone cell is swollen with several lateral processes, known as **rod spherules** and **cone pedicles**. Many photoreceptors converge onto one bipolar cell and interconnect with one another. But at the fovea, each 'midget' cone transmits to a single bipolar cell.
- **Inner nuclear layer:** It consists of the nuclei of bipolar, horizontal and amacrine cells. Amacrine cell processes pass inwards to synapse in the inner plexiform layer. The nuclei of Muller's fibers are also found here. Capillaries from the retinal vessels reach up to this layer, but the outer layers are a vascular, the rods and cones being nourished by the choriocapillaries.
- **Inner plexiform layer:** It consists of arborizations of the bipolar cells, with the ganglion cells and amacrine cells.
- **Ganglion cell layer:** It consists of large multipolar nerve cells, with clear round nuclei containing nucleoli, and have Nissl's granules in their cytoplasm. In the retinal periphery, a single ganglion cell may synapse up to a hundred bipolar cells, but in the macular region, there tends to be a single connection with the 'midget' bipolar cells.
- **Nerve fiber layer:** It consists of bundles of ganglion cell axons, running parallel to the retinal surface. The layer increases in depth as it converges towards the optic disc. These nerve fibers are fine and **non-medullated**. The macular fibers themselves pass directly to the disc as the **papillomacular bundle**.
- **Internal limiting membrane:** It is a thin lamina separating retina from the vitreous. It is formed by the union of terminal expansions of Muller's fibers, and essentially a basement membrane.

Regions

- **Ora serrata:** It is the anterior termination of retina, located about 8 mm from the limbus. Here, only two layers of primitive optic vesicle fuse, and continue forward as the ciliary epithelium.
- **Central retina (Fig. 1.14):** It is 4.5 mm in diameter. It extends from the fovea centralis—nasally, almost to the optic disc; same distance temporarily, and a similar distance above and below the fovea centralis. In this region, ganglion cell layer is more than one layer of cell bodies. The central part of this region is called **macula leutea** which contains a yellow pigment, xanthophyll.
  - The **fovea centralis** is a depressed area, located in the central retina, about 3 mm (2 dd) temporal to the optic disc and 0.8 mm below the horizontal meridian. It measures about 1.5 mm (1500 µm). Its central depression is called **foveola**, measuring about 0.5 mm (500 µm).

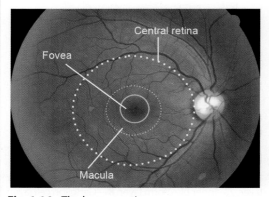

Fig. 1.14: The human retina

- The photoreceptors in the fovea are exclusively cones. All cell layers are displaced peripherally so that light falls directly on the cones' outer segment. The foveola is nourished solely by the choriocapillaries of the choroid and does not contain any vessels, hence, called *foveolar avascular zone (FAZ)*.
- *Peripheral retina:* The photoreceptors are mainly rods. The ganglion cells are larger, and their cell bodies are arranged in a single layer.
- *Functionally,* retina is divided into *temporal and nasal portion,* by a line drawn vertically through the center of the fovea. Nerve fibers originating from the cells temporal to this line pass to the lateral geniculate body of the same side and from nasal side, cross in the optic chiasma to reach the lateral geniculate body of the opposite side.
- *Ophthalmoscopically,* the ophthalmologist uses the optic nerve as a hub to divide the retina into superior and inferior temporal portions, superior and inferior nasal portions, and a central retina.

Blood Supply

Retina gets its nourishment from two sources:
1. *Outer portion:* It mainly by the choriocapillaries.
2. *Inner portion:* It mainly by the central retinal artery, the first branch of ophthalmic artery which enters the optic nerve about 10–12 mm posterior to the globe.

▌THE CONJUNCTIVA

It is a mucous membrane covering the inner surface of the eyelids and reflected to cover the anterior part of the eyeball over the sclera, up to the corneal margin.

Parts (Fig. 1.15)

- *Palpebral:* It consists of marginal, tarsal and orbital part. It is firmly adherent to the deeper tissue.
- *Bulbar:* It lies over the sclera and it is freely mobile.
- *Fornix:* It is the cul-de-sac at the junction of palpebral and bulbar conjunctiva.
- *Limbal:* It is the conjunctiva at the corneal junction which is adherent.

Structures

- *Epithelium:* There are two layers of epithelium over the palpebral conjunctiva, and transitional stratified squamous epithelium at the intermarginal strip.
  - From fornices to the limbus the epithelium is gradually thicker (4–6 layers).
  - Again, it is stratified epithelium at the limbus.
  - Goblet cells (mucin secreting cells) are present throughout the epithelium, especially more near the fornices.
- *Subepithelial layer:* It is an adenoid layer of loose connective tissue containing leukocytes.

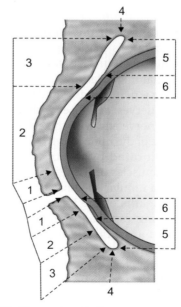

Fig. 1.15: The conjunctival areas
1—Marginal; **2**—Tarsal; **3**—Orbital; **4**—Fornicial;
5—Bulbar; **6**—Limbal

- *Fibrous layer:* It is much dense, and blended with the deeper structures (e.g. episclera or tarsus).

Nerve Supply

Ophthalmic division of trigeminal nerve (5th cranial).

Arterial Supply

- Anterior conjunctival artery from the anterior ciliary artery.
- Posterior conjunctival artery from the lacrimal artery.
- Palpebral branch of nasal artery.

▌TENON'S CAPSULE

Tenon's capsule is a thin membrane which envelops the eyeball from the optic nerve to the limbus, separating it from the orbital fat and forming a socket in which it moves.

Its inner surface is smooth, and is separated from the outer surface of the sclera. Its anterior part (anterior Tenon's capsule) adheres with the undersurface of the conjunctiva and attaches to sclera at the limbus. Posterior Tenon's capsule is made up of the fibrous sheath of the rectus muscles together with the intermuscular membrane.

The fascia is perforated behind by the ciliary vessels and nerves, and fuses with the sheath of the optic nerve and with the sclera around the entrance of the optic nerve.

It is perforated by the tendons of the extraocular muscles, and is reflected backward on each as a tubular sheath. The expansions from the sheaths of the lateral and medial recti are strong, especially that from the latter muscle, and are attached to the zygomatic bone and lacrimal bone respectively. They also check the actions of these two recti and are called the *medial and lateral check ligaments*.

There is thickening of the lower part of the Tenon's capsule, which is known as *suspensory ligament of the eye (of Lockwood)*. It is slung like a hammock below the eyeball, being expanded in the center, and narrow at its extremities which are attached to the zygomatic and lacrimal bones respectively.

Sub-Tenon's block for ocular surgery: Local anesthetic may be injected into the space between Tenon's capsule and the sclera to provide anesthesia for eye surgery, principally cataract surgery. After applying topical anesthetic drops to the conjunctiva, a small fold of conjunctiva is lifted off and a small nick made. A blunt, curved cannula is passed through the incision into the sub-Tenon's space and then 1.5 mL 2% lignocaine solution is injected. The advantages are a reduced risk of bleeding and of penetration of the globe, compared to peribulbar and retrobulbar blocks. However, the akinesia of the extraocular muscles may be less complete.

▌THE EXTRAOCULAR MUSCLES (FIG. 1.16)

They are six in number. Four rectus muscles and two oblique muscles.
- *Origin of rectus muscles:* Common origin from annular *tendon of Zinn* around the optic foramen at the apex of the orbit.
  - *Insertion:* They are inserted to the sclera as a spiral line *(spiral of Tillaux)* after piercing the Tenon's capsule. The distance from limbus are as follows:
    Superior rectus (S) = 7.7 mm
    Lateral rectus (L) = 6.9 mm
    Inferior rectus (I) = 6.6 mm
    Medial rectus (M) = 5.5 mm
- *Origin of superior oblique:* Common origin at the apex of the orbit from annular tendon of Zinn → runs to the trochlea, at upper and inner angle of orbit → becomes tendinous → reflected backwards under the superior rectus muscle.
  - *Insertion:* It is inserted in the sclera at superolateral part of the posterior pole of the globe.

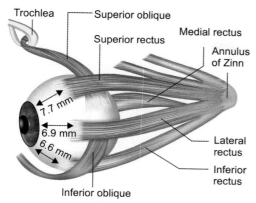

Trochlea — Superior oblique
Superior rectus — Medial rectus
Annulus of Zinn
7.7 mm
6.9 mm
6.6 mm
Lateral rectus
Inferior rectus
Inferior oblique

Fig. 1.16: Extraocular muscles of the eye

Note: Both oblique muscles insert behind the equator of the globe. The inferior oblique muscle passes inferior to the body of the inferior rectus muscle but beneath the lateral rectus muscle. The numbers indicate the distance of the insertion in mm from the corneoscleral limbus. Medial rectus (M) = 5.5 mm

- *Origin of inferior oblique:* Anteriorly from the lower and inner orbital walls near the lacrimal fossa. It is the only muscle, which does not arise from the apex of the orbit.
  - *Insertion:* It is inserted in the sclera at in ferolateral part of the posterior pole of the globe *(corresponds to the area near the macula).*
- *Nerve supply:* All the muscles are supplied by 3rd (oculomotor) cranial nerve except, lateral rectus—by 6th (abducens) nerve, and superior oblique—by 4th (trochlear) nerve.
- *Actions of extraocular muscles:* See Chapter 23.
  - *Medial rectus:* Adduction.
  - *Lateral rectus:* Abduction.
  - *Superior rectus:* Elevation on abduction and intorsion.
  - *Inferior rectus:* Depression on abduction and extorsion.
  - *Superior oblique:* Depression on adduction and intorsion.
  - *Inferior oblique:* Elevation on adduction and extorsion.

THE EYELIDS

The eyelids are thin curtains of skin, muscles, fibrous tissue and mucous membrane. The upper eyelid is limited above by the eyebrow, and the lower eyelid merges with the cheek. Each eyelid is divided by a horizontal furrow (sulcus) into an orbital and a tarsal part. The upper furrow is formed by skin—insertions of the levator palpebrae superior is muscle.

- *Palpebral aperture:* When the eyes are open, the eyelids form an elliptical opening, the *palpebral aperture (fissure)* which measures about 12 mm by 30 mm. The lateral canthus is about 2 mm higher than medial canthus (may be up to 5 mm in orientals). At the inner canthus, there is a small bay, the *lacus lacrimalis,* formed by the eminences (papillae) which bear the lacrimal puncta 6 mm lateral to the angle itself. There is a small separated knob of skin, *the caruncle,* bearing a few hairs or glands, contained in this bay. Just lateral to the edge of the caruncle, there is a crescentic fold of conjunctiva, the *plica semilunaris,* which is similar to the nictitating membrane in lower vertebrates.
- *Lid margin:* Located on the free margin of each eyelid are the openings of the lacrimal canaliculi (the puncta), the eyelashes and the openings of the glands. The medial one-sixth of the lid margin *(the lacrimal portion)* has no eyelash or gland openings, and is rounded. The lateral five-sixths *(the ciliary portion)* of the lid margin has square edges. The eyelashes on the upper eyelid margin curve upwards, and are more numerous than those of the lower eyelid margin, which curve downwards.

Structures

- *Cutaneous layer:* It is thin, smooth, delicate, elastic, having creases and without any long hair.

- *Subcutaneous tissue:* Loose areolar tissue devoid of fat.
- *Muscular layer*
  - Orbicular is oculi
  - Levator palpebrae superioris (LPS) in the upper lid only
  - Muller's muscle.
- *Fibrous layer*
  - Orbital septum in the upper part.
  - Tarsal plate in the lower part.
  Different glands of the eyelid (i.e. Meibomian glands, glands of Zeis, glands of Moll, glands of Krause and Woulfring) lie in this plane.
- *Palpebral conjunctival layer:* Inner most layer of the eyelid (Fig. 1.17).

Muscles of the Eyelid

- *Orbicular is oculi*
  - *Action:* Closure of lids, blinking, winking, squeezing and helps in the drainage of tears.
  - *Nerve supply:* Zygomatic branch of facial (7th cranial) nerve.
  - *In case of its paralysis:* There will be lagophthalmos (leading to exposure keratitis due to dryness of the cornea and conjunctiva).
- *Levator palpebrae superioris:* It is present only in the upper lid.

- *Origin:* From the apex of the orbit, above the annulus of Zinn.
- *Insertion:* It can be into five parts:
  1. The *main tendinous slip* is inserted into the upper margin and the anterior surface of the tarsal plate.
  2. *Anterior slip* to the skin of upper lid.
  3. *Posterior slip* to the conjunctiva of the upper fornix along with the sheath of superior rectus muscle.
  4. *Medial and*
  5. *Lateral slips* are attached to the medial and lateral palpebral ligaments respectively.
- *Action:* Elevates the upper eyelid including upper fornix, and helps in the formation of upper lid-fold.
- *Nerve supply:* Upper division of oculomotor nerve (3rd cranial nerve). Paralysis of LPS—causes ptosis.
- *Müller's muscle (unstriped)*
  - *Upper Müller's muscle:* Arises from the stripped fibers of levator muscle, passes downwards behind it, and is inserted into upper border of the tarsus.
  Action: It elevates the upper lid.
  - *Lower Müller's muscle:* It arises from inferior rectus muscle, lies below it, and is inserted into the lower tarsus.

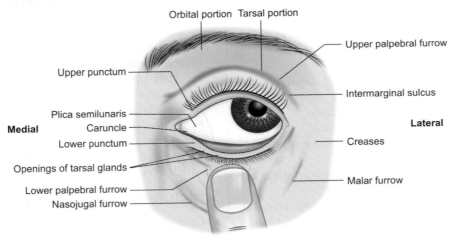

Fig. 1.17: The surface anatomy of the eyelids (left eye)

Action: It elevates the lower lid to some extent.

- *Nerve supply:* Cervical sympathetic nerve.
- *Paralysis of cervical sympathetic nerve* will cause Horner's syndrome (ptosis, miosis, enophthalmos and anhydrosis of the face).

Glands

- *Meibomian glands:* They are modified sebaceous glands (tubular) of larger size and responsible for oily secretion of the tear film. They are situated within the substance of tarsal plate, arranged vertically, and each opens by a single duct on the margin of the lid.
  - *Number:* 30–40 in the upper lid, and 20–30 in the lower lid.
- *Glands of Zeis:* They are sebaceous glands, lie in the lid margin, and open in the follicle of eyelashes.
- *Glands of Moll:* Modified sweat glands, situated immediately behind the hair follicles, and their ducts open into the ducts of Zeis' gland, or into the follicle, (not directly onto the skin surface as elsewhere).
- *Glands of Krause and Woulfring:* They are accessory lacrimal glands situated on the palpebral conjunctival side (Fig. 1.18).

Intermarginal Strip

It is the margin or free edge of the lid. It is covered with stratified epithelium which forms a transition between the skin and conjunctiva.
- *Structures* (from anterior to posterior):
  - Anterior round border
  - Eyelashes
  - Gray line
  - Orifices of the ducts of Meibomian glands and
  - Posterior sharp border.

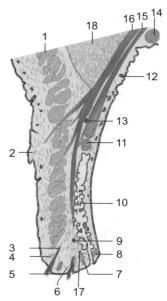

Fig. 1.18: Section through the upper eyelid

1—Orbicularis muscle; 2—Sweat gland; 3—Hair follicle; 4—Gland of Zeis; 5—Cilium; 6—Gland of Moll; 7—Marginal part of orbicularis muscle; 8—Subtarsalis part of orbicularis muscle; 9—Inferior arterial arcade, 10—Meibomian gland; 11—Gland of Wolfring; 12—Conjunctival crypts; 13—Superior arterial arcade; 14—Gland of Krause; 15—Muller's muscle; 16—Levator palpebrae superioris muscle; 17—Gray line; 18—Fat

- *Gray line* is an important landmark for operations in which the lid is splitted, since it indicates the position of the loose fibrous tissue between the orbicularis oculi and the tarsus.

Arterial Supply

- *In upper lid:* In the form of two arches:
  1. *Superior:* Lying between the upper border of tarsus and the orbicularis.
  2. *Inferior:* In front of tarsal plate, just above the hair follicle at the free edge.
- *In lower lid:* One arch near the free edge. The arteries are: (i) palpebral and lacrimal branch of ophthalmic artery, (ii) superficial temporal artery, (iii) infraorbital artery and (iv) facial artery.

Venous Drainage

Two plexuses in each lid—(i) post-tarsal, draining into the ophthalmic vein, and (ii) pre-tarsal, into the subcutaneous veins.

Lymphatic Drainage

- *From inner half:* Into the submandibular lymph node.
- *From outer half:* To the preauricular lymph node.

Functions

- Protection of eyeball proper, from external injuries, e.g. dust, fumes, foreign body, etc.
- Maintain the pre-corneal tear film (by sharp posterior borders of the lid margin).
- Interrupt and limit the amount of light entering the eye.
- Drainage of the tears by the lacrimal pump system.
- Emotional expressions.

THE LACRIMAL APPARATUS

The lacrimal apparatus consists of two parts:
1. *Secretory portion:* Lacrimal gland and accessory lacrimal glands of Krause and Woulfring.
2. *Drainage portion:* Via which the tears drain into the inferior meatus of the nose.

Secretory Portion

- *Lacrimal gland:* It is located in the anterolateral portion of the roof of the orbit in the lacrimal fossa. It has two parts—a large orbital portion and a small palpebral portion separated by lateral part of the aponeuroses of LPS muscle. It is a tubule alveolar type of gland. Their ducts open separately onto the superior temporal fornix (Fig. 1.19).
  Nerve supply: Via facial nerve, parasympathetic from lacrimal (salivary) nucleus.
- *Accessory lacrimal glands of Krause and Woulfring:* They are located deep in the

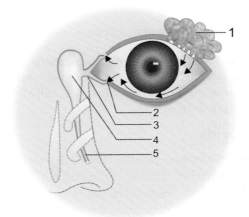

Fig. 1.19: Parts of the lacrimal apparatus
1—Lacrimal gland; **2**—Punctum; **3**—Common canaliculus; **4**—Lacrimal sac; **5**—Nasolacrimal duct

conjunctiva particularly in the fornices, mostly on the temporal side.

Drainage Portion

It is composed of the puncta, the canaliculi, the lacrimal sac and the nasolacrimal duct.
- *Two lacrimal puncta:* These are two small openings, situated near the posterior border of the free margins of the lid about 6 mm from the inner canthus. The punctum is situated upon a slight elevation (large in elderly people) called *lacrimal papilla*.
- *Two canaliculi:* It pass from the punctum to the lacrimal sac. They are first directed vertically for 1–2 mm, then horizontally for 6–7 mm. The canaliculi usually open separately into the outer wall of lacrimal sac. Sometimes, they join together to form a common canaliculus before opening into the sac.
- *Lacrimal sac:* It lies in the lacrimal fossa formed by the lacrimal bone. When distended it is about 15 mm long and 5–6 mm wide. The upper portion is called *fundus*, which lies slightly above the level of medial palpebral ligament. Sac itself is

covered by fibers of the orbicularis muscles and loose fibrous tissues.

- ***Nasolacrimal duct:*** It is the continuation of lacrimal sac. 12–24 mm long and 3–6 mm in diameter. The duct has two parts; intraosseous and intrameatal. It passes downwards, slightly outwards and backwards to open into anterior part of the outer wall of the inferior meatus of the nose. The upper end of the nasolacrimal duct is the narrowest part. The mucous lining forms an imperfect valve at the orifice into the nose ***(valve of Hasner).***

■ THE ORBIT

The orbits are pear-shaped cavities. Their medial walls are parallel, but lateral walls diverge at an angle of 45°. The orbit is roughly 40 mm in height, width and depth. Its ***volume*** is about 30 mL.

  Portions of seven bones (Fig. 1.20) form the orbit are—(1) frontal, (2) maxilla, (3) zygoma, (4) sphenoid, (5) palatine, (6) ethmoid and (7) lacrimal.

Contents

- The eyeball and intraorbital part of optic nerve
- Retrobulbar fat
- Extraocular muscles
- Ophthalmic arteries and veins
- 3rd, 4th and 6th nerve and first two divisions of 5th nerve
- Ciliary ganglion
- Sympathetic plexus
- Lymphatic vessels
- Tenon's capsule and orbital fascia
- Lacrimal gland and lacrimal sac.

Optic Foramina

It is located at the posteromedial portion of the orbit in the body of the sphenoid bone. It measures 4–10 mm in diameter.
Through it passes:

- The optic nerve with its sheaths,
- Ophthalmic artery and
- Sympathetic nerve from carotid plexus.

Superior Orbital Fissure

It is just lateral to the optic foramen, and is the gap between the greater and lesser wings of sphenoid. The fissure is divided into lateral and medial portions by the tendinous annulus of Zinn (Fig. 1.21).

- ***Passing through the annulus***
  - Two divisions of the oculomotor nerve (CNIII)
  - Abducens nerve (CNVI)
  - Branches of the ophthalmic division of trigeminal nerve (CNV), except the lacrimal and frontal branches.
- ***Passing through the lateral portion***
  - Lacrimal nerve
  - Frontal nerve
  - Trochlear nerve (CNIV)
  - Superior ophthalmic veins
  - Recurrent lacrimal artery

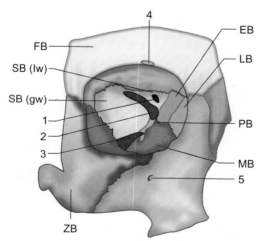

Fig. 1.20: The bony orbit
FB—Frontal bone; **MB**—Maxillary bone; **ZB**—Zygomatic bone; **SB**—Sphenoid bone-greater wing (gw); lesser wing (lw); **PB**—Palatine bone; **EB**—Ethmoid bone; **LB**—Lacrimal bone; **1**—Optic canal; **2**—Superior orbital fissure; **3**—Inferior orbital fissure; **4**—Supraorbital notch; **5**—Infraorbital foramen

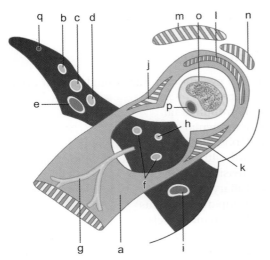

Fig. 1.21: Structures passing through the superior orbital fissure and the optic foramen

d—Trochlear nerve; **e**—Superior ophthalmic vein; **f**—Oculomotor nerve; **g**—Abducens nerve; **h**—Nasociliary nerve; **i**—Inferior ophthalmic vein; **j**—Superior rectus; **k**—Inferior rectus; **l**—Medial rectus; **m**—Levator palpebrae superioris; **n**—Superior oblique; **o**—Optic nerve; **p**—Ophthalmic artery; **q**—Recurrent lacrimal artery

- *Passing through the medial portion:* Inferior ophthalmic vein.

Inferior Orbital Fissure

It lies between the maxilla and the greater wing of sphenoid.

It transmits
- Maxillary division of trigeminal nerve
- Infraorbital artery
- Zygomatic nerve
- Branches of inferior ophthalmic vein draining into pterygoid venous plexus.

Surgical Spaces of the Orbit (Fig. 1.22)

From the surgical point of view, there are four spaces of the orbit. They are relatively self-contained, as the inflammatory processes are contained for a considerable period of

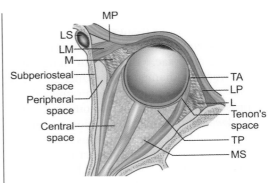

Fig. 1.22: Spaces of the orbit
L—Lateral check ligament; **LM**—Lacrimal portion of orbicularis muscle; **LP**—Lateral palpebral ligament; **LS**—Lacrimal sac; **M**—Medial check ligament; **MP**—Medial palpebral ligament dividing into a superficial and a deep band; **MS**—Muscle sheaths; **TA**—Anterior part of Tenon's capsule; **TP**—Posterior part of Tenon's

time and each of which must, if necessary, be opened separately.
- *The subperiosteal space:* Between the bones of the orbital wall and the periorbita (periosteum).
- *The peripheral orbital space:* Between the periorbita and the extraocular muscles which are joined together by fascial connections.
- *The central space:* A cone-shaped area enclosed by the muscles (the *muscle cone*).
- *Tenon's space:* Around the globe.

BLOOD SUPPLY OF THE EYE (FIG. 1.23)

ARTERIES (FIG. 1.24)

The eye and the orbital contents receive their main blood supply from the ophthalmic artery. The eyelids and conjunctiva have an anastomotic supply from the branches of both external carotid and ophthalmic artery.

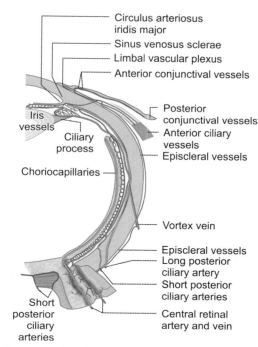

Fig. 1.23: The blood supply of the eye

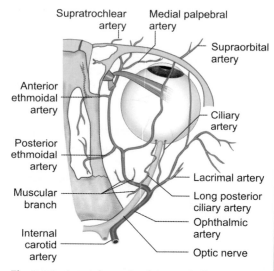

Fig. 1.24: Arterial supply of the eyeball

Ophthalmic Artery

It arises from the fifth bend of the internal carotid artery. It enters the orbit through the optic foramina, below and lateral to the optic nerve.

Branches

- The central retinal artery
- The short posterior ciliary arteries (10–20 in number)
- Two long posterior ciliary arteries
- Recurrent meningeal artery
- Lacrimal artery
- Variable number of recurrent arteries
- Muscular branches to each of the extraocular muscles.

The anterior ciliary arteries are the forward continuations of muscular arteries. Each rectus muscle has two muscular arteries *except the lateral rectus*, which has one.

External Carotid Artery

The blood supply to the eyelids and conjunctiva from the branches of the external carotid artery, originates from the external maxillary artery, the superficial temporal artery and the internal maxillary artery.

▌VEINS

Mainly through the superior and inferior orbital veins and they empty into the cavernous sinus (Fig. 1.25).

- *Superior orbital vein* communicates with the angular vein, and then to facial vein.

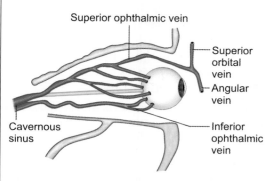

Fig. 1.25: Venous drainage of the eyeball

- **Inferior ophthalmic vein** communicates with the pterygoid venous plexus, and also to the cavernous sinus directly or via superior ophthalmic veins.
- Two or more **superior vortex veins** drain into the superior orbital vein and inferior vortex veins into the inferior orbital vein.
- The **central retinal vein** enters the cavernous sinus separately, or to the superior ophthalmic veins.

Cavernous Sinus

It is an irregular-shaped, endothelium lined venous space, situated on either side of the body of the sphenoid bone.

Connections (Figs 1.26A and B)

- The superior and inferior ophthalmic veins enter it from the front.
- The superior and inferior petrosal sinuses leave it from behind.
- It connects directly with pterygoid plexus, and indirectly via inferior ophthalmic veins.
- To the opposite sinus by two or three transverse sinuses which surround the pituitary stalk.

Structures passing through it (Fig. 1.27):
- Internal carotid artery with sympathetic plexus via medial wall.
- Abducens nerve is just lateral to the artery.
- Ophthalmic and maxillary divisions of the trigeminal nerve, are lateral and below the artery.
- Oculomotor and trochlear nerves are on its lateral wall, on the superior aspect.

One or more nerves may be affected by disease of the cavernous sinus, e.g. thrombosis of the sinus, rupture or aneurysm of the internal carotid artery.

▌ NERVES OF THE EYE

- **Visual optic nerve**
  The visual pathway—optic nerve → optic chiasma → optic tract → lateral geniculate body → optic radiation → visual cortex.
- **Motor**
  - **Oculomotor (NIII)**
    - **Superior division** → Superior rectus and LPS.
    - **Inferior division** → Medial rectus, inferior rectus, and inferior oblique.

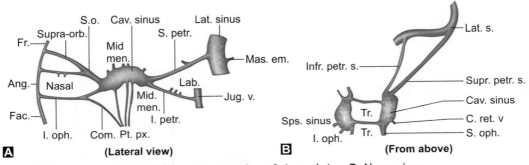

Figs 1.26A and B: Tributaries of the cavernous sinus. **A.** Lateral view. **B.** Above view
Ang.—Angular vein; **Cav. sinus**—Cavernous sinus; **Com.**—Communicating vein; **Fac.**—Facial vein; **Fr.**—Frontal vein; **I.oph.**—Inferior ophthalmic vein; **I.petr.,**—(infr. petr. s), Inferior petrosal sinus; **Jug. v.**—Jugular vein; **Lab.**—Labyrinthine veins; **Lat. sinus**—Lateral sinus; **Mas. Em.**—Mastoid emissary vein; **Mid. Men.**—Middle meningeal veins; **Nasal**—Nasal veins; **Pt. px.**—Pterygoid plexus; **S.o. (oph)**—Superior ophthalmic vein; **Supra-orb**—Supraorbital vein; **S. (Supr.) petr.**—Superior petrosal sinus; **Tr.**—Transverse sinus; **Sps. sinus**—Sphenoparietal; **C. ret. V**—Central retinal vein

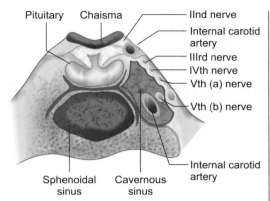

Pituitary Chaisma — IInd nerve
— Internal carotid artery
— IIIrd nerve
— IVth nerve
— Vth (a) nerve
— Vth (b) nerve

— Internal carotid artery

Sphenoidal Cavernous
sinus sinus

Fig. 1.27: Anatomy of the cavernous sinus and its relationship with the vital structures

- Short root to ciliary ganglion → ciliary and sphincter papillae muscle.
  - *Trochlear (NIV)* → Superior oblique.
  - *Abducens (NVI)* → Lateral rectus.
- *Mixed motor and secretory*
  Facial (NVII) → (i) Motor to face, especially to the orbicularis oculi; (ii) Secretory to the lacrimal gland.
- *Sensory*
  Trigeminal (NV) → Via ophthalmic and maxillary divisions.
- *Autonomic*
  - *Para sympathetic supply*
    - *Oculomotor nerve* (from the Edinger-Westphal nucleus) → inferior division → branch to inferior oblique → short root of ciliary ganglion → ciliary and sphincter papillae muscles
    - *Facial nerve* (from salivary nucleus) → lacrimal gland.

- *Sympathetic supply:* Postganglionic fibers from the superior cervical ganglion → around the internal carotid artery (carotid plexus) → cavernous plexus → via the ophthalmic division of 5th nerve → nasociliary nerve → long ciliary nerve avoiding the ciliary ganglion (some via ciliary ganglion without a relay → short ciliary nerves) → along with long ciliary arteries into the suprachoriodal space → enter ciliary body and iris, to supply dilator pupillae.

LYMPHATIC DRAINAGE (FIG. 1.28)

From the eyelids, conjunctiva and from the orbital tissues.
- *Medial group* drains into the submandibular lymph nodes.
- *Lateral group* drains into the preauricular lymph nodes and sometimes, into the postauricular lymph nodes.

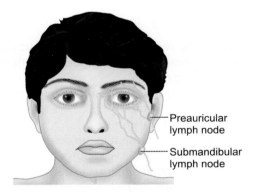

Preauricular lymph node

Submandibular lymph node

Fig. 1.28: Lymphatic drainage of the eyelids and conjunctiva

Physiology of the Eye

CORNEA

The cornea is a transparent tissue, anterior surface of which is bathed with tears, and endothelial surface is bathed in aqueous humor.

The stroma consists of type I collagen fibers of uniform diameter, arranged in a regular lattice work within a ground substance.

The ground substance consists of acid mucopolysaccharides, chondroitin sulfate (type A and type C), and keratin sulfate.

Transparency

In the visible range of spectrum (380 nm to 760 nm), the cornea transmits almost 100% of the light energy.

This transparency is due to following factors:
- *Anatomical factors:*
  - Avascularity of cornea
  - Absence of pigment in the cornea
  - Demyelinated nerve supply
  - Regular arrangement of the epithelial and endothelial cells
  - Regular arrangement of stromal collagen fibrils (lattice theory)
  - Paucity of cells in the stroma
  - Epithelial cells are non-keratinized
  - Anterior surface of the tear-film helps in forming a regular refracting surface.
- *Relative dehydration (deturgescence) of the stroma which is maintained by:*
  - Epithelium, which is largely impermeable to water

  - *Endothelial transport system:* The endothelial transport system pumps fluid from the corneal stroma to the aqueous by Na-K-ATPase mechanism.
  - Special intercellular junction in the endothelium is also responsible to control the fluid traffic.
- *Intraocular pressure (IOP):* It must be optimum to control fluid transport. An acute rise in IOP may result in corneal edema.

Nutrition and Permeability

- *The peripheral cornea* receives its nutrients via the blood stream of perilimbal plexus.
- *The central cornea* is avascular and the nutrition depends on substances that enter either via the endothelium or the epithelium.
- *Permeability:* The tear film is permeable to water-soluble substances.
  - The corneal epithelium is readily permeable to lipid-soluble substances, as the cell membrane is composed of lipoprotein.
  - The stroma and the endothelium are permeable to water-soluble substances.

Metabolism

Cornea gets its oxygen mostly from the atmosphere. Cornea requires energy to maintain its deturgescence, and also for epithelial cell renewal.

Energy in the form of adenosine triphosphate (ATP), is provided by the metabolism of glucose. The epithelium and the endothelium are the sites of most metabolism.

The metabolic pathways are:
- ***Glycolysis*** (Embden-Meyerhof pathway) which requires no oxygen.
- ***Tricarboxylic acid cycle*** (Kreb's cycle), in presence of oxygen, mainly in the epithelium.
- ***Hexose monophosphate (HMP) shunt:*** About 65% of corneal metabolism occurs via glycolysis and the remainder by way of Kreb's cycle and HMP shunt.

Wound Healing

- ***Epithelium*** regenerates rapidly, large abrasion is being covered within 24 hours. This involves both epithelial migration, and proliferation of the surviving epithelial cells. After 6 weeks, epithelium adheres to its underlying basement membrane firmly.
- ***Injury to the Bowman's membrane*** causes scar formation.
- ***Stromal healing:*** By multiplication of un-damaged keratocytes and migrated fibroblasts. New mucopolysaccharide synthesis begins after 24–48 hours, and established by 5th day. Stromal healing is not initiated until the defect is covered by epithelium.
- ***Endothelium:*** No multiplication occurs in human beings. The cells spread to cover the defect, by enlargement and migration.

▌LENS

The lens is a transparent crystalline structure, covered by a homogenous capsule, and has epithelium only beneath the anterior lens capsule.

Transparency

It transmits almost 80% of light energy. Its transparency is due to:
- Sparsity of cells
- Single layer of epithelial cells, which is not thick

- Close alignment of individual cells (the lens extracellular space is less than 5% of its total volume, so the ***zone of discontinuity*** is very small compared to the wavelength of light)
- Semipermeable character of the lens capsule
- Avascularity
- Its index of refraction ranges from about 1.406 at the center (nucleus) to about 1.386 in outer cortical layers, making it a gradient index lens.
- Pump mechanism of the lens fiber membranes, which maintains relative dehydration of the lens.
- ***Autoxidation:*** High concentration of reduced glutathione in the lens maintains the lens protein in a reduced state and ensures the integrity of the cell-membrane pump.

Metabolism

The lens fibers are composed entirely of soluble and insoluble proteins.
- ***Water-soluble proteins (85%)*** are αcrystalline, β heavy and β light crystalline, and γ crystalline; and they are found mainly in the lens cortex. Human lens protein is more labile than that of other species.
- ***Water-insoluble protein (15%):*** Albuminoid fraction and found mainly in the lens nucleus. With age insoluble protein increases. In strict physiological terms, the position of the lens within the eye is similar to a cell surrounded by extracellular fluid.
- ***The lens epithelium generates energy from carbohydrate metabolism:***
  - Anaerobic glycolysis by Embden-Meyerhof pathway—85%
  - Hexose monophosphate shunt
  - Kreb's cycle
  - Sorbitol pathway.

The lens epithelium maintains low concentration of sodium and water within the lens by active Na-K-ATPase pump system. Glycolysis provides the necessary ATP energy.

Pathogenesis of Cataract

Any opacity in the lens or its capsule is called a cataract. Three basic mechanisms cause a cataract:

1. Damage to the lens capsule that changes its membranous properties
2. Change in the lens-fiber protein synthesis
3. Increased lens hydration.

When a *cortical cataract* forms, the sodium-extruding mechanisms fail.

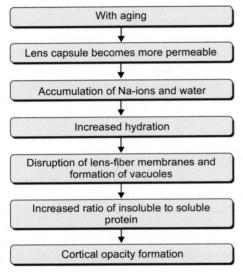

```
With aging
      ↓
Lens capsule becomes more permeable
      ↓
Accumulation of Na-ions and water
      ↓
Increased hydration
      ↓
Disruption of lens-fiber membranes and
formation of vacuoles
      ↓
Increased ratio of insoluble to soluble
protein
      ↓
Cortical opacity formation
```

In Nuclear Cataract

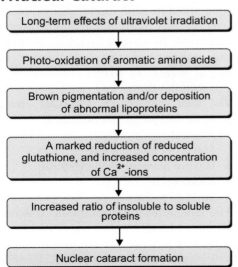

```
Long-term effects of ultraviolet irradiation
      ↓
Photo-oxidation of aromatic amino acids
      ↓
Brown pigmentation and/or deposition
of abnormal lipoproteins
      ↓
A marked reduction of reduced
glutathione, and increased concentration
of Ca²⁺-ions
      ↓
Increased ratio of insoluble to soluble
proteins
      ↓
Nuclear cataract formation
```

TEARS

Anterior surface of the eye is moistened by tears, secreted by the lacrimal gland and basic secretors, located in the margin of the eyelid and the conjunctiva. The basic secretors of the conjunctiva contribute 10% of the total mass of lacrimal gland.

Circulation of Tears

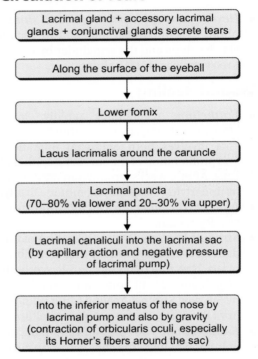

```
Lacrimal gland + accessory lacrimal
glands + conjunctival glands secrete tears
      ↓
Along the surface of the eyeball
      ↓
Lower fornix
      ↓
Lacus lacrimalis around the caruncle
      ↓
Lacrimal puncta
(70–80% via lower and 20–30% via upper)
      ↓
Lacrimal canaliculi into the lacrimal sac
(by capillary action and negative pressure
of lacrimal pump)
      ↓
Into the inferior meatus of the nose by
lacrimal pump and also by gravity
(contraction of orbicularis oculi, especially
its Horner's fibers around the sac)
```

Composition of Tears

- Very much similar to blood plasma, slightly more dilute (98.2% of water)
- Relative lack of protein (0.6%)
- pH of tear is 7.35, but it may vary with disease *(alkaline pH is found in vernal catarrh)*
- Osmotic pressure varies from that of blood (0.9% saline) to the equivalent of 1.4% saline (normal = 290–300 mOsmol)
- *Protective substances* present in tears are:
  - Immunoglobulins (IgA, IgG, and IgM)
  - Lymphocytes
  - Complements

- Lactoferrin
- *Lysozyme (muramidase):* A specific enzyme which is lethal to common bacteria, since it is mucolytic and dissolves the bacterial membrane.

Production

The average normal secretion of tears is 0.5–2.2 µL/min. The maximum capacity of conjunctival cul-de-sac is about 30 µL.

The lacrimal glands secrete continuously throughout the day, but not during sleep. Half of this secretion is lost from the surface by evaporation.

Reflex stimulation occurs in following situations:
- From irritative sensation of the cornea and the conjunctiva
- In yawning, coughing, sneezing or vomiting
- After psychic stimulation, as in weeping or laughing. This curious reflex is confined to human beings, and only develops in infants after 3–4 months.

- After exposure to bright lights
- Secretion can be stimulated by cholinergic drugs (e.g. pilocarpine) and inhibited by anticholinergic drugs (e.g. atropine).

Precorneal Tear Film (Figs 2.1 and 2.2) and its Functions

It is a relatively stagnant layer of tears that covers the corneal epithelium and consists of *three layers*, each of which has separate functions.

1. *The outer lipid layer:* It is secreted by the Meibomian glands, glands of Zeis, and glands of Moll.
   Functions
   - To retard the evaporation of the aqueous layer of the tear film
   - To increase surface tension and vertical stability of the tear film to prevent overflow of tears
   - To lubricate the eyelids.
2. *The middle aqueous layer:* It is the main bulk of the tear film and secreted by the lacrimal and accessory lacrimal glands.

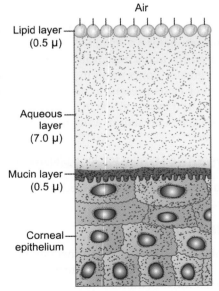

Fig. 2.1: Precorneal tear film (traditional view)

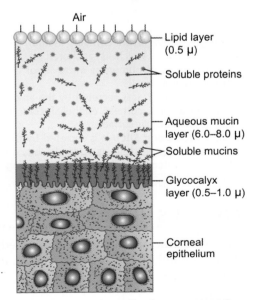

Fig. 2.2: Precorneal tear film (recent concept)

Functions

- To supply atmospheric oxygen to the corneal epithelium.
- It has antibacterial action due to presence of lysozyme and lactoferrin.
- To provide a smooth optical surface.
- To wash away dust and debris from the conjunctiva and cornea.

3. *The inner mucin layer:* It is secreted by the conjunctival goblet cells, glands of Manz, and crypts of Henle.

Functions

- To convert the corneal epithelium from a *hydrophobic* to a *hydrophilic* surface.
- To wet the microvilli of the corneal epithelium and thereby retains the precorneal tear film.

According to a recent concept

- *Outer lipid layer:* It contains both polar and nonpolar lipids. Polar lipids such as phospholipids and fatty acids lie adjacent to the aqueous mucin layer and *nonpolar lipids* such as cholesterol esters and triglycerides are present at the tear–air interface.
- *Middle aqueous–mucin layer:* Contains soluble mucins and proteins in additions to water and ions.
- *Inner glycocalyx layer:* Contains membrane-adherent mucin which is anchored at the cell membrane of numerous microvilli of the corneal epithelium.
- *Glycocalyx/MUC1:* It is secreted by the apical conjunctival and corneal epithelial cells. It provides hydrophilic surface.
- *Mucin (MUC4 and 5AC):* It is secreted by the conjunctival goblet cells. It adds viscosity to tears and protects the ocular surface during blinking.

▌AQUEOUS HUMOR

The internal structures of the eye are bathed and surrounded by the aqueous humor, a crystal clear fluid.

Functions

- It helps to maintain IOP
- It supplies nourishment to the cornea and the lens
- It maintains optical transparency
- It takes the place of the lymph that is absent within the eye.
  Refractive index = 1.336
  Composition
  Water content = 98.92%
  Solid = 1.08%

The composition of aqueous of the posterior chamber differs from the aqueous of the anterior chamber. Posterior chamber aqueous contains chloride and ascorbate in excess, than that of the anterior chamber aqueous. But there is deficiency of bicarbonates.

Solid Components

- *Proteins:* They are more dilute than plasma, due to blood–aqueous barrier. But when the protein concentration increased, a *plasmoid aqueous* results as in inflammation of anterior uvea (iridocyclitis), and also after surgery with newly-formed aqueous.
- *Non-electrolytes:* Examples, glucose, urea, uric acid, alcohol and creatinine (all are little less than those of plasma).
- *Electrolytes:* Na ions, K ions, chloride, and bicarbonates.
- *Organic acids:* Ascorbic acid is present in greater concentration than in plasma. Other acids present in aqueous are lactic acid and hyaluronic acid.
- *Oxygen* is present in aqueous in dissolved state.

Aqueous Humor Formation

Two mechanisms are involved: (1) Ultrafiltration and (2) Secretion.

Ultrafiltration

Capillary wall in the ciliary processes behaves as a crude semipermeable membrane. It retains most proteins, but allows smallest molecules to leave the bloodstream, and collects in the stroma of the ciliary processes, and then into the posterior chamber across the ciliary epithelium.

Secretion

By active secretion of the ciliary processes. Two mechanisms are involved:
1. *Bicarbonate system* mediated by carbonic anhydrase.
2. *Na-K-ATPase system* for electrolytes. Once formed, the aqueous is modified by metabolic processes of the cornea and lens, and this chiefly results in a fall in glucose and bicarbonate concentration, but a rise in lactate levels.

Circulation of Aqueous Humor

Circulation is necessary both for metabolic process and to regulate the IOP.

Aqueous formed in the ciliary region → flows from posterior chamber through the pupil into the anterior chamber → angle of the anterior chamber → trabecular meshwork → Schlemm's canal → aqueous veins → episcleral venous plexus.

Normal flow rate of aqueous—2 µL/ minute.

In addition, there is a second accessory exit *(uveoscleral outflow)* which may sometimes be of importance (as in *buphthalmos or in retinal detachment*). Aqueous formed in the ciliary body → suprachoroidal space → episcleral venous plexus.

Physiology of Vision

EFFECTS OF LIGHT ON THE EYE

When light falls upon the retina, it acts as a stimulus to rods and cones, which serve as the visual nerve endings. As there are no rods and cones in the region of optic disc, it has no visual sensation and this is called the **blind spot (of Mariotte).**

When light falls upon the retina, two essential reactions occur in the end-organs—**photochemical** and **electrical.**

Photochemical Changes (Fig. 3.1)

- The rods are the receptors for night (scotopic) vision and contain a pigment, visual purple or **rhodopsin.** The maximum absorption spectrum for **rhodopsin** is around 500 nm.
- Rhodopsin consists of a colorless protein, called **opsin** and is coupled with a chromophre, **11-cis retinal** (aldehyde of vitamin A).
- When light falls upon the rods, **11-cis retinal** component is converted into **all-trans retinal** through various stages.
- This reaction is reversible in the dark, i.e. **11-cis retinal** is regenerated from all-trans retinal and vitamin A (retinol) from the blood.
- **All-trans retinol** (an alcohol) is vitamin A and is transported in the blood to a specific retinal-binding protein.

The cones contain three different photo-pigments, with maximum absorption at 450, 535, and 570 nm, roughly corresponding to the blue, green, and red part of the visible spectrum. These pigments are called **iodopsin.** Cones not only respond to light of high intensities **(photopic vision),** but also act as receptors for color vision.

Electrical Changes

Visual transduction is the process by which light absorbed by the photoreceptors of the outer segment is converted into electrical energy. Though the process is complex, but a battery of **electrodiagnostic tests** are now in clinical uses for assessing the integrity of the retina and its central connections.

ELECTRO-OCULOGRAPHY (FIG. 3.2)

- The average electrical potential of the cornea is positive (about 6 mV) in relation to the retina
- When electro-oculography (EOG) is used, the increase in potential with light adaptation is measured, to evaluate the condition of retinal pigment epithelium (RPE).
- Electrodes are placed at each canthus and the changes in potential between these two electrodes are recorded as the eye moves.

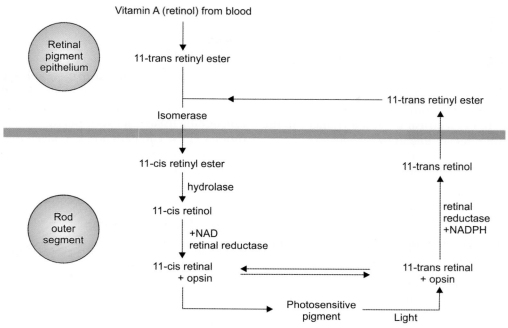

Fig. 3.1: Visual cycle

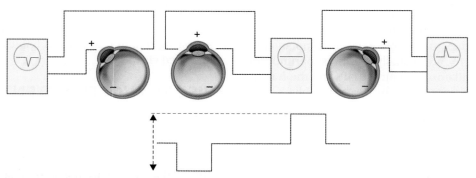

Fig. 3.2: Electro-oculography. The electrode closer to the cornea is positive, and when the eye turns, a deflection is induced in the recording system (below). The electro-oculography deflection is measured from the trough of the deflection on eyes left to the height of the deflection on eyes right

- The average amplitude of the resting potential in light and dark adaptation is measured.
- The ratio of *light peak (Lp)* to *dark trough (Dt)* is measured *(Arden ratio)*. (*Light peak* = maximum amplitude obtained in light and *dark trough* = minimum amplitude obtained in the dark).

- **Normal Arden ratio** is 1.80 (or 180%) or greater. 1.65 to 1.80 is borderline and less than 1.65 is significantly subnormal.

Subnormal Arden ratio implies a defect in photoreceptors or RPE. Like, Best vitelliform macular dystrophy, Stargart's macular dystrophy, retinitis pigmentosa and rod-cone dystrophies, choroideremia, gyrate atrophy, chloroquine or hydroxychloroquine toxicity, retained intraocular iron particles (siderosis bulbi), etc.

ELECTRORETINOGRAPHY (FIG. 3.3)

Electroretinography (ERG) means a gross record of electrical potential changes in the retina after stimulation with light.

A recorder is made by placing an active electrode on the cornea (via a contact lens) and the other is on the forehead. The small voltage is amplified and usually photographed from the face of the oscilloscope.

Electroretinography Waveforms

- An initial positive deflection R_1 (early receptor potential—ERP) is followed by a negative deflection R_2. These are due to photochemical reactions in the rod and cone outer segments.
- This is followed by a large negative wave called *a wave*, and this reflects photoreceptor activity.
- Then a large positive *b wave* follows. It is due to the response of bipolar cells. There are usually some superimposed oscillatory potentials (OPs) on the *b wave* as a response of the amacrine cells.
- Lastly, a small positive *c wave*, which is generated by RPE.

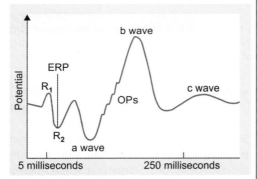

Fig. 3.3: Electroretinography

- The duration of entire response is less than 250 milliseconds.

Responses

The ERG is a mass response of the outer layers of the retina. A normal ERG implies a healthy retinal and choroidal circulation, and normally functioning tissues between the RPE and the bipolar cells. The ganglion cell layer, nerve fiber layer, and the optic nerve play no part in this response.

Pathologic responses may be supernormal, subnormal, negative or non-recordable.

Clinical Significances

- Electroretinography is a useful guide in diagnosis and prognosis of certain retinal disorders particularly in retinitis pigmentosa, chorioretinitis, rod-cone dystrophy, etc.
- In *siderosis bulbi* (earliest sign).
- Cortical blindness or hysterical blindness.
- Assessing retinal functions in presence of opacity in the media (e.g. cataract, corneal opacity, or in case of vitreous hemorrhage).
- Assessing retinal functions in babies with impaired vision.

VISUAL-EVOKED POTENTIAL (FIG. 3.4)

Stimulation of the retina with light changes the electrical activity of the cerebral cortex.

- The visual-evoked potential or response (VEP or VER) is the electroretinography (EEG), recorded at the occipital pole.
- Since the VEP is very small, and often indistinguishable from the background, other electrical activities, an averaging technique using a computer, are necessary to identify its waveforms.
- The only consistent recordable response is a large positive deflection occurring 120 milliseconds after stimulation when a pattern is used (pattern VEP) and 100

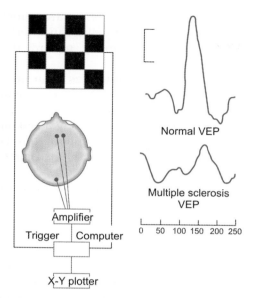

Fig. 3.4: Diagram of the system used to record the visual-evoked potential (VEP). The amplitude of the potential is shown to the right. In multiple sclerosis, the amplitude of the response is reduced, and there is a significant delay in the peak-time of the positive wave

milliseconds when a flash is used (flash VEP).
- Pattern VEP is related to visual acuity and is important to record the visual acuity in children.
- Flash VEP reflects the transmission of light from the entire retina, including the fast conducting axons.

Clinical Significances

- *In optic neuritis:* VEP amplitude is reduced and the latency is increased.
- It is also altered in macular disease or other optic nerve diseases.

So, VEP is important in assessing the macular or optic nerve functions in presence of opacities in the media.

VISUAL PERCEPTIONS (SENSATIONS)

Visual sensations result from stimulation of the retina with light. These are four types—(1) light sense, (2) form sense, (3) sense of contrast, and (4) color sense.

Light Sense

This is the faculty which permits us to perceive light in all its gradations of intensities.
- *Light minimum* is the minimum amount of light energy which, when falls upon the retina, causes a visual sensation. The light minimum for fovea is higher than parafoveal region. It is increased in diseases of rods and cones, e.g. retinitis pigmentosa.
- *Dark adaptation (Fig. 3.5):* The increase in sensitivity of the eye for detection of

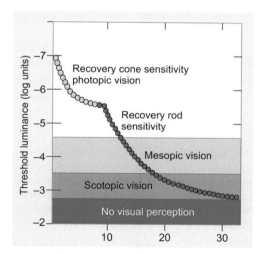

Fig. 3.5: The dark-adaptation curve. There is a plateau between 5 minutes and 9 minutes. The initial portion of the curve indicates the smallest light intensity that will stimulate cones. Rods attain their maximum sensitivity after 30 to 45 minutes. The luminance at −7 is that of sunlight. The luminance at −5 is that of good reading luminance for white paper. The luminance at −4 is that of city street lighting. The luminance at −3 is mean ground luminance in full moon

light that occurs in the dark is called **dark adaptation**.

- In the darkness, after the exposure of bright light, there is an initial increase in sensitivity following an exponential time course that reaches a plateau after 5 to 9 minutes. This initial phase is due to regeneration of photosensitive pigments in the cones.
- Then as lower exponential time course that reaches a plateau in 30–45 minutes. This second phase is attributed to rhodopsin regeneration.
- Dark adaptation is delayed by prolonged exposure to bright light.
- When fully dark-adapted, the retina is about 100,000 times more sensitive to light than when it is bleached.
- **Delayed dark-adaptation** occurs in diseases of rods, e.g. retinitis pigmentosa and in case of vitamin A deficiency.

- **Light adaptation:** It refers to the fall in the visual threshold on moving from darkness into a well lit room.

This decrease in sensitivity is involving two changes—(1) a neural process that is completed in about 0.05 seconds and (2) a slower process, apparently involving the uncoupling of retinal and opsin in rhodopsin, occurring in about 1 minute.

The rods are much more sensitive to low illumination than the cones, so that in the dusk we see with our rods **(scotopic vision)**; in bright light the cones, come into play **(photopic vision)**. Nocturnal animals (e.g. bat) have few or no cones, and diurnal animals (like squirrel) have no rods.

Mesopic vision: Is a combination of photopic and scotopic vision in low-light situations. Most of the night-time outdoor activities and traffic lighting are in the mesopic vision range.

Form Sense

This is the faculty which enables us to perceive the shape of the objects.

- Cone is responsible for **form sense** which is most accurate the fovea,

because here the cones are most closely set and highly differentiated.

- It falls off very rapidly toward the periphery.
- **Visual acuity** is defined as the ability to distinguish the shape of the objects and it applies to central vision.
- The form sense is not purely a retinal function for the perception of its composite form (e.g. letters)—is largely **psychological**.
- In order to discriminate the form of an object, its several parts must be differentiated.

So, for two point's discrimination, it is necessary that two individual cones should be stimulated by them, while the one, in between two cones remains unstimulated.

- Histologically, the diameter of a cone in the macular region is 0.004 mm and this, therefore, represents the smallest distance between two cones.
- It is found that in order to produce an image of minimum size of .004 mm **(resolving power of the eye)**, the object must subtend a visual angle of 1 minute at the nodal point. This is known as **minimum visual angle**.
- These principles have been embodied in Snellen's test type (Fig. 3.6), where each letter is perfectly placed in a square which is subdivided into small 25 squares. Each component part of the letter subtends an angle of 1 minute, and the entire letter subtends an angle of 5 minutes at the nodal point of the eye, from a given distance.

Sense of Contrast (Fig. 3.7)

It is the ability to perceive slight changes in luminance between regions which are not separated by definite borders. Of all the gratings, the two main variables are the degree of blackness to whiteness, and this is the contrast.

Contrast sensitivity is reduced in many ocular diseases, e.g. in glaucoma, macular

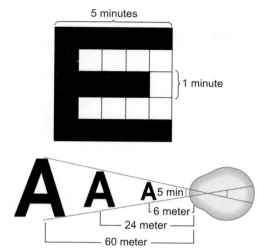

Fig. 3.6: Construction of the Snellen letter. Each part subtends an angle of 1 minute. Whole letter subtending an angle of 5 minutes at varying distance from the eye

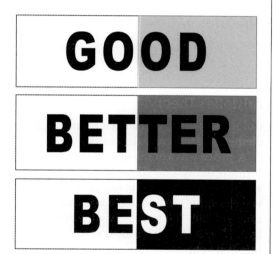

Fig. 3.7: Sense of contrast

disease or refractive errors, and sometimes, it is more important than the loss of visual acuity. It is especially important for screening the visual acuity in illiterates and young children.

Contrast sensitivity is also important in old age and after cataract surgery.

Contrast Sensitivity

In its simplest terms, contrast sensitivity means the ability of the visual system to distinguish between an object and its background. It indirectly assesses the quality of vision.

Contrast sensitivity is the reciprocal value of the contrast threshold. A patient who needs a lot of contrast to see a target has low contrast sensitivity and *vice versa*.

Blur is not the same as poor contrast sensitivity. People who have poor vision than 6/6 on Snellen's letter chart will experience blurred vision. On the other hand, a person who has poor contrast sensitivity (e.g. due to cataract) may still test well on the 6/6 letters on chart and he may still experience cloudy vision.

Contrast sensitivity is expressed using sine-wave gratings (Fig. 3.8). A sine-wave grating is a repetitive number of fuzzy dark and light bars, or cycle whose luminance profiles have the shape of simple mathematical function, sine. The number of cycles over a specified visual angle determines its spatial frequency.

Contrast sensitivity tests address the weakness of Snellen's high contrast acuity by varying two parameters—*grating size* and *contrast level*. It tests the functional vision, or how well individuals see everyday visual objects or scene (While driving or at work and play).

Contrast sensitivity changes with the age. As we get older, we lose contrast sensitivity, first at the higher spatial frequencies and then for all the spatial frequencies.

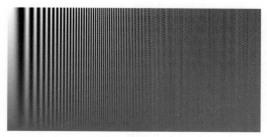

Fig. 3.8: Sinusoidal grating

Contrast Sensitivity Tests

Several test systems are available (both for distance and near)—the key difference is the target type:
- *Pelli-Robson chart (Fig. 3.9):* Low contrast letter charts with same size.
- *Regan chart:* Low contrast letter charts of variable size.
- *Functional acuity contrast test (FACT):* It measures the specific visual channel. It provides more informative *sine-wave grating curve.*
- *Cambridge contrast sensitivity test.*

Diseases and clinical applications

Contrast sensitivity testing provides early detection of eye diseases/conditions that a standard 6/6 letter acuity chart may not detect until the condition is more advanced. They are cataracts, glaucoma, amblyopia, age-related macular degeneration, optic neuritis, drug-induced maculopathy or neuropathy, diabetic retinopathy, etc.

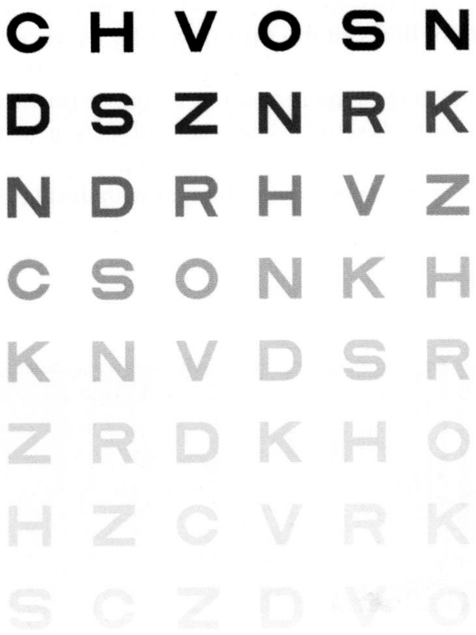

```
C H V O S N
D S Z N R K
N D R H V Z
C S O N K H
K N V D S R
Z R D K H O
H Z C V R K
S C Z D V O
```

Fig. 3.9: Pelli-Robson contrast sensitivity test chart

- With the advent of new technology such as *wave-front, aspheric intraocular lens (IOLs)* and refractive surgery—many intraocular lens ophthalmologists and ophthalmic companies are in favor of contrast sensitivity testing to monitor the progress of the patients.
- It is also recognized by the Food and Drug Administration (FDA) as a more comprehensive and accurate method of assessing vision in *clinical research trials.*

Color Sense

This is a faculty to distinguish between different colors as excited by light of different wavelengths. The appreciation of colors is a function of the cones and occurs only in photopic condition. In very low intensities of illumination, the dark-adapted eyes see no color and all objects are seen as gray, differing somewhat in brightness.

Theories of Color Vision

This is a complicated process that involves physical, biological, and psychological mechanisms.

Aristotle's Theory

Color vision derives from the intermingling of elements of light and darkness.

A more advanced eye of primates and human being can distinguish color which are just electromagnetic radiation of different wavelengths. We can see wavelengths in the range of 380–760 nm, the visible spectrum of light (Fig. 3.10). We *cannot see* ultraviolet or infrared light.

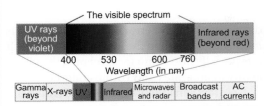

Fig. 3.10: The total range of electromagnetic spectrum and visible spectrum of light

We also do not perceive color in dim light (or in dark), because the light intensity is not enough to stimulate/bleach *iodopsin*. The threshold frequency of cones is high and requires more light for stimulation.

Trichromatic Theory (of Young-Helmholtz) (Fig. 3.11)

Trichromatic color vision is mediated by interactions among three types of color sensing cones in the retina. Each of the three types of cone contains a different type of photosensitive pigment which is composed of transmembrane protein, called *opsin,* and a light sensitive molecule, called *11 cis-retinal*.

The *three types of cone* are:
1. *Long wavelength (L):* Peak sensitivity at 570 nm (red-sensitive cones or *erythrolabe*).
2. *Medium wavelength (M):* Peak sensitivity at 535 nm (green-sensitive cones or *chlorolabe*).
3. *Short wavelength (S):* Peak sensitivity at 440 nm (blue-sensitive cones or *cyanolabe*). The peak sensitivity of rods (R) is 498 nm. Each different pigment is especially sensitive to certain wavelength of light (photon) to produce a cellular response. This response of a given cone varies not only with the *wavelength of light* that hits it, but also with its *intensity*. The brain would not be able to discriminate different colors if it had input from *only* one type of cone. Thus interaction between two types of cones is necessary to produce ability to perceive color and trichromatic color vision is accomplished by using combination of cell responses.

But trichromatic theory does not explain why red matched with green appears yellow, or why blue added to yellow appears white.

It also does not explain the phenomenon of complementary after images (if the eye is adapted to a yellow stimulus, the removal of stimulus leaves a blue sensation or after-image).

Opponent-process Theory (of Herring) (Fig. 3.12)

Opponent color theory states that the human visual system interprets information about color by processing signals from cones in an antagonist manner. The L, M, and S cones have some overlap in the wavelengths of light. So the visual system is more efficient to record differences between the responses of cones, rather than individual cone's response.

The opponent theory suggests that there are *three opponent channels*—red versus green, blue versus yellow, and white versus black. The last one is achromatic and detects dark-light variations, i.e. *luminance*. The responses to one color of an opponent channel are antagonistic to those of other color.

Although, *trichromatic* theory allows the visual system to *detect color* with L, M, and S cones (at the photoreceptor level); the *opponent theory* (Fig. 3.12) accounts for mechanisms that *receive and process* information from cones (inter-neurally). It is now accepted that *both the theories are important* to understand the mechanism of color vision (Fig. 3.12).

The recently proposed explanation seems to be more complex:
• L, M, and S cones respond best to long, medium, and short wavelength of light, respectively.

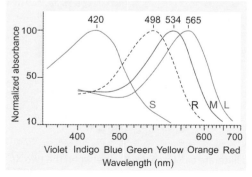

Fig. 3.11: Trichromatic theory of color vision

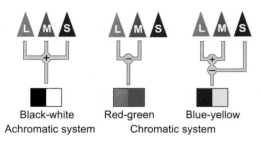

Black-white | Red-green | Blue-yellow
Achromatic system | Chromatic system

Fig. 3.12: Opponent color vision theory

- Information from cones is passed to the bipolar cells which may be cells in opponent process.
- This information is then passed to **two types** of ganglion cells—magnocellular (large cells) and parvocellular (small cells). **Parvocellular cells (P cells)** are the major cells **which handle information about color.** Two groups:
  1. One that processes information about difference between excitation of L and M cones and
  2. Other one that processes difference between S cones and a combined signal from both L and M cones.

  These two subtypes are responsible for **red-green** and **blue-yellow** processing, respectively.

Magnocellular cells are responsible for transmitting information about intensity of light in the receptive fields.

- Ultimately, these signals are decoded and processed in the brain. At this stage, color memory, context, and other factors modify the perception of color. After interpretation of these decoded signals, we **see** a color of an object we are looking at.

Color Blindness

Color blinds have defective color discrimination. It is of two type—(1) congenital and (2) acquired.

- **Congenital:** Most common, and inherited as an X-linked recessive anomaly. Male 7% and female only 0.7%, have congenitally defective color vision.

  Visual acuity is normal and ophthalmoscopically the fundi appear normal. The defect is present at birth and stationary.

  A **protanope** has (**protan** means first) the red sensation missing, a **deuteranope** (**deutan** means second) has the green, and **a tritanope** (**tritan** means third) has the blue sensation missing.

  Red-green blindness is more common in congenital type.

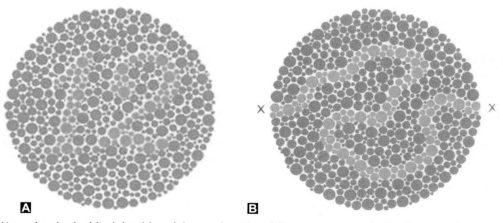

A   **B**

Normal and color blind should read the number 12 and illiterate can trace the line between the two Xs

Figs 3.13A and B

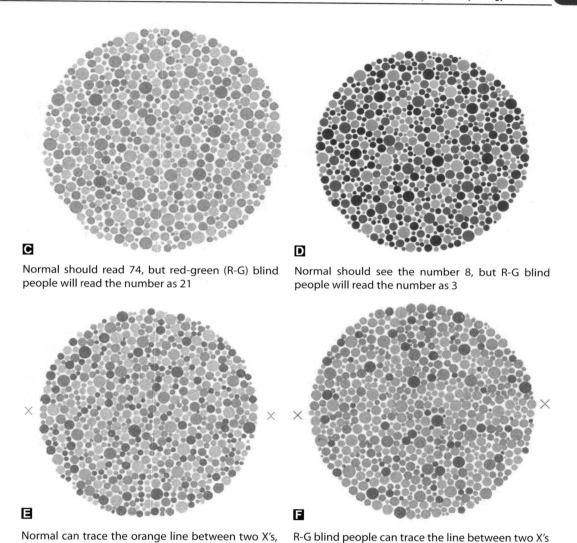

C

Normal should read 74, but red-green (R-G) blind people will read the number as 21

D

Normal should see the number 8, but R-G blind people will read the number as 3

E

Normal can trace the orange line between two X's, but R-G blind people cannot follow

F

R-G blind people can trace the line between two X's but normal people cannot follow

Figs 3.13C to F

Figs 3.13A to F: Ishihara's charts—for normal color vision and color blind people

The term ***achromatopsia*** means the individual borns with severely deficient color perception, where there is absence of all three cones, and thus visual acuity is also very much reduced, and nystagmus is present.

- ***Acquired color blindness:*** Occurs as a result of diseases of the cones, macular diseases, lental sclerosis, optic nerve disease, and drug-induced (e.g. ethambutol).

Importance: Social importance of color blindness is important particularly for drivers, pilots, chemists, biochemists, and also in higher education.

Tests for Color Blindness

- ***Pseudoisochromatic (Ishihara's) test (Figs 3.13A to F)*** is used for routine screening in most ophthalmologist's office. Here, a series of plates containing panels that are filled by colored dots in which bold numerical or different lines (for illiterates) are represented in dots of various tinted sets. This gives a fair assessment, especially for red-green (R-G) blindness.

- *Farnsworth-Munsell 100 hue test* is *scientifically accurate* and of academic interest.

- *Edridge-Green lantern test* is modified by various filters (e.g. to simulate mist, rain, fog, etc.). Mainly important for engine drivers.
- *Holmgren's wools test:* Color matches are done with different shades of colored wool.
- *Nagel's anamaloscope:* It is used to measure the qualitative and quantitative anomalies of color perception

Neurology of Vision

THE VISUAL PATHWAYS (FIG. 4.1)

- *The end-organ:* It is the neural epithelium of the rods and cones.
- *The first-order neuron:* It is the bipolar cell with its axons in the inner layers of the retina.
- *The second-order neuron:* It is the ganglion cell of the retina. Its axon passes into the nerve-fiber layer and along the optic nerve to the lateral geniculate body.
- *The third-order neuron:* It originates in the cells of lateral geniculate body, then travels by way of the optic radiations to the occipital cortex (visual center).

The visual pathways thus consist of:

- Two optic nerves
- An optic chiasma
- Two optic tracts
- Two lateral geniculate bodies
- Two optic radiations
- Visual cortex on each side.

In general, the fibers from the peripheral retina enter the periphery of the optic nerve, and the fibers near the optic disc enter the central part of the nerve.

The fibers from the macular area form the *papillomacular bundles*, which have a separate course. Partial decussation occurs where the nasal fibers cross at the chiasma.

The fibers of the peripheral retina have two distinct groups, corresponding to the nasal and temporal halves of the retina.

The fibers of the temporal half enter the chiasma and pass to the optic tract of same side, and then to the lateral geniculate body. The fibers from the nasal half enter the chiasma, decussate, and then pass to the optic tract of opposite side, then to the lateral geniculate body.

The third-order neurons pass by the optic radiation into the corresponding occipital lobe. It follows that a lesion of the optic radiation, optic tract, or occipital lobe will cause blindness of the temporal half of the retina of the same side and nasal half of the opposite side. Projecting this outward, such lesion will cause loss of vision in the opposite half of visual field a condition known as *hemianopia*.

Figure 4.1 describes the sites of lesions and the corresponding visual field defects in classical cases.

PUPILLARY PATHWAYS AND REACTIONS

Functions of the Pupil

- It regulates the amount of light that enters the eye depending on the state of retinal adaptation.
- It increases the depth of focus, particularly for near objects.
- It reduces the various optical aberrations, e.g. peripheral and chromatic aberrations, and also astigmatism.

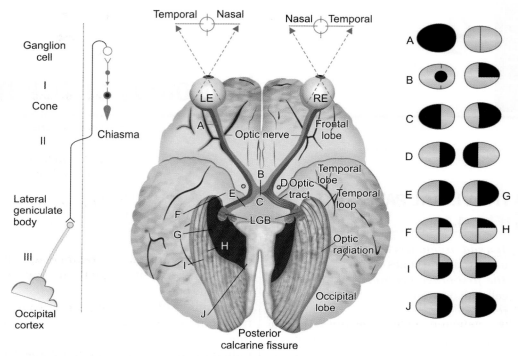

Fig. 4.1: Optic (visual) pathways—all the right and left nasal fibers decussate at the chiasma

The sites of lesions and corresponding visual field defect are **A**—Through optic nerve—ipsilateral blindness; **B**—At the proximal part of optic nerve at chiasmal junction—ipsilateral blindness with contralateral superior quadrantopia (Traquair's junctional scotoma); **C**—Middle of chiasma—bitemporal hemianopia; **D**—From lateral sides of chiasma—binasal hemianopia; **E**—Of optic tract—contralateral homonymous hemianopia; **F**—Of temporal lobe—contralateral quadrantic homonymous defects; **G**—Whole optic radiation—contralateral homonymous hemianopia; **H**—Anterior part of the optic radiations—contralateral inferior homonymous quadrantic defects; **I**—Posterior part of the optic radiations—contralateral superior homonymous quadrantic defects; **J**—Occipital cortex—contralateral homonymous hemianopia with macular sparing

The **sphincter pupillae** is supplied by the parasympathetic system through the third cranial nerve.

The **dilator pupillae** is supplied by the adrenergic fibers of the cervical sympathetic nerve.

The Pupillary Reflexes

Three reflexes are of clinical importance:
1. **Light reflex:** If light enters an eye, the pupil of this eye constricts (**direct light reflex**), and there is an equal constriction of the pupil of the other eye (**consensual light reflex**).

2. **Near reflex:** A constriction of pupil occurs on looking at a near object, a reflex largely determined by the reaction to convergence.
3. **Psychosensory reflex:** A dilatation of the pupil occurs on psychic or sensory stimuli.

Light Reflex

Rods and cones → optic nerve → optic chiasma (partially decussate) → optic tract → pretectal nucleus (instead of running to the lateral geniculate body) → partial decussation in the midbrain → Edinger-Westphal nucleus on each side → third nerve → inferior division

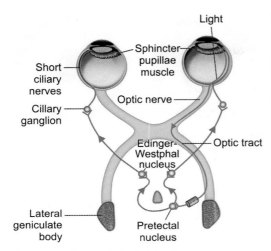

Fig. 4.2: Pathway of the light reflex

→ branch to inferior oblique → short root of ciliary ganglion → ciliary ganglion → short ciliary nerves → sphincter pupillae muscle (Fig. 4.2).

This decussation is important to explain the mechanism of consensual reaction, as well as direct reaction to light, and also for several pathological reactions.

Near Reflex

It initiates mainly by the fibers from the medial rectus muscle, which contracts on convergence.

Medial rectus muscle → via third nerve→ mesencephalic nucleus of fifth nerve → a presumptive center for convergence at pons → Edinger-Westphal nucleus → along the third nerve → accessory ciliary ganglion → sphincter pupillae muscle of the iris.

Sensory Reflex

It is a more complicated process, for both the dilator and constrictor centers play part in its production.

COMMON ANOMALIES OF PUPILLARY REFLEXES

Hippus

- Alternate rhythmic dilatation and constriction of the pupil.
- These oscillations are very large and often independent of the light.
- It is not a peripheral phenomenon, but depends upon the rhythmic activity of the central nervous system.
- It is found in ***multiple sclerosis***.

Marcus Gunn Pupil

- It is also known as ***relative afferent pupillary defect*** (RAPD) or pupillary escape phenomenon.
- It occurs in defect of the visual pathway anterior to the chiasma.
- ***It consists of:***
  - A diminished amplitude of pupillary reaction
  - A lengthened latent period
  - Pupillary dilatation (escape) with continuous light stimulation.
- ***Detection:*** The test for its detection is called ***swinging flash-light test***.
  Normally, if an illuminated pen light is alternately directed to each eye, the pupils constrict and do not vary as the light alternates between the eyes.
  In afferent pupillary defect, both pupils dilate when the light is moved from the unaffected eye to the affected eye. But they constrict when the light is directed to the normal eye.
- Afferent pupillary defect is most conspicuous in unilateral optic neuritis. It distinguishes the reduction of visual acuity caused by optic neuritis, from that caused by cystoid macular edema (CME) or central serous retinopathy (CSR).

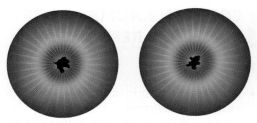

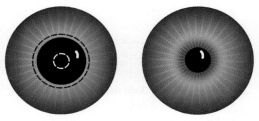

Fig. 4.3: Argyll Robertson's pupil
Miotic, irregular, non-reactive to light, but reacts on accommodation

Fig. 4.4A: Adie's pupil
Right pupil larger than fellow, reacts slowly to light and accommodation; redilatation occurs slowly

Argyll Robertson's Pupil (Fig. 4.3)

It is a bilateral abnormality characterized by failure of the pupils to constrict with light, but retention of constriction presents with accommodation.

- *The entire syndrome includes:*
  - Absence of light reaction
  - Presence of accommodation reaction
  - Pupils are miotic, irregular, eccentric, and unequal.
  - Atrophic depigmented patches on iris.
  - Pupils fail to dilate with mydriatic, but constrict further with eserine.
  - Presence of good vision in both eyes.
- *Causes*:
  - Tabes dorsalis (neurosyphilis), here all the signs are present.
  - *Non-syphilitic causes:* Diabetes, multiple sclerosis, hemorrhage, and tumors involving the pretectal region.

Here, pupils are not miotic, irregular or unequal, as seen in typical case.
- *Site of lesion:* Internuncial neurons between pretectal nucleus and Edinger-Westphal nucleus at the level of pretectum.

Adie's Pupil (Figs 4.4A and B) (Adie's Tonic Pupil)

It is a unilateral dilated but tonic pupil of unknown etiology, a common cause of anisocoria.
- *Etiology:* Mostly unknown.
  It may follow a viral illness and in some cases, associated idiopathically with reduced tendon reflexes (like, ankle jerks). There is an impairment of postganglionic parasympathetic innervations of the ciliary muscle or the sphincter pupillae, or both.
- *Clinical features:*
  - Mostly women than men of 3rd to 4th decade.

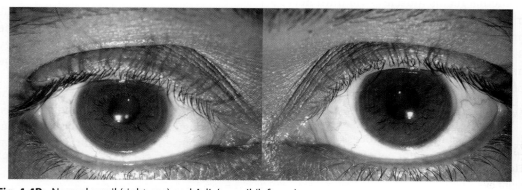

Fig. 4.4B: Normal pupil (right eye) and Adie's pupil (left eye)

- Initially uniocular, but later in many cases, second eye is also involved.
- Affected pupil is larger than the fellow.
- Poor pupillary reaction to light that may involve entire muscle or only a segment.
- Reaction to near is slow and tonic.
- Redilatation of pupil occurs slowly.
- Occasional paresis of accommodation and delay in focusing near object.
- *Vermiform movements* of the iris due to sector paralysis are appreciated during slit lamp examination.
- *Pharmacological diagnostic tests*
  - *With 0.125% pilocarpine:* The tonic pupil constricts rapidly, but with this concentration, the normal pupil (Fig. 4.4B) does not constrict. This is due to super-sensitivity of the cholinergic stimulation.
  - *With mydriatic (atropine):* The tonic pupil dilates with atropine, but the Argyll Robertson pupil does not.

> **Holmes-Adie's pupil:** It is the condition where Adie's pupil is associated with other signs of nervous system disease, such as absent knee jerks or ankle jerks.

Adie's pupil is a benign condition. Patient may have headache, or blurring of vision for near.

- *Treatment:* There is no effective treatment. Weak miotics may be helpful, or a near correction may be given for the affected eye.

Horner's Syndrome (Figs 4.5A and B)

It consists of *miosis, partial ptosis,* and *enophthalmos*, and sometimes, associated with unilateral absence of sweating of the face on the affected side (anhydrosis).

In congenital form, there may be associated heterochromia of the iris.

It arises from the damage of sympathetic innervation of the eye.

- *Etiology:*
  - In the cervical region—apical bronchial carcinoma, neck glands tumor, etc.
  - Centrally—as with multiple sclerosis, pontine tumor, syringomyelia, etc.
- *Clinical features:* The miosed pupil reacts normally to light and accommodation, but dilates poorly with cocaine drop.

If the lesion lies peripherally (post-ganglionic)—it dilates rapidly with 1 in 1,000 adrenaline drops. This is due to denervation supersensitivity, and this response enables to differentiate a pre- and postganglionic lesion of the sympathetic system.

- *Treatment:* If cosmetically unaccepted, ptosis may be corrected surgically (by mullerectomy).

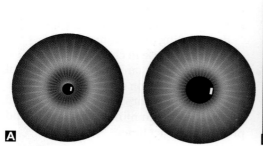 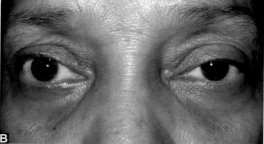

Figs 4.5A and B: A. Horner's syndrome pupil (right eye); **B.** Horner's syndrome pupil (left eye) (photograph)
Right eye—Miosis, ptosis, enophthalmos, and anhydrosis of the face on the side of lesion

Ocular Pharmacology

DRUG DELIVERY SYSTEM

Therapeutic substances may be introduced into the eye by two major routes—*systemic route* and *local route*.

1. **Systemic routes:** Here, the drug can be given by mouth or by injections, but it has its obvious limitations because of *two blood-ocular barriers*—the blood-aqueous barrier, and the blood-retinal barrier.
    i. **The blood-aqueous barrier:** It is formed by the nonpigmented layer of the ciliary epithelium, and by the endothelium of the iris vessels. Both of these tissues have tight junctions of the *leaky* type.
    ii. **The blood-retinal barrier:** It is located in the retinal pigment epithelium and the endothelium of the retinal blood vessels. Both of these tissues have tight junctions of *non-leaky* type.

    Drugs enter the eye in proportion to their lipid solubility and smaller molecule size, e.g. sulphonamides has much better penetration than penicillins.

    Severe inflammations and trauma damage the blood-ocular barriers and facilitate the penetration of the drugs in higher concentration.

2. **Local routes:** They are as follows:
    - Aqueous or viscous solutions, as drop
    - Ointments
    - Drug-impregnated contact lens
    - Membrane release system (ocusert)
    - Subconjunctival or subtenon injections
    - Retrobulbar or peribulbar injection
    - Injections directly into the eye.

- **Corneal penetration:** Compounds applied to the anterior globe surface, enter the anterior chamber mainly through the cornea. Epithelium is permeable to the lipid-soluble compounds and stroma to the water-soluble compounds. Thus, the highest intraocular concentrations following administration of compounds should be both water and lipid soluble. Since epithelium is the main barrier, permeability is much increased, if the epithelium is damaged or abraded.
- **Eye drops:** They are most popular and easy to instillate. One drop instillation is enough for each time, as the conjunctival sac cannot retain more than that.

  Disadvantages:
  - Shorter duration of action.
  - Dilution of the drug by tears.
  - Drainage through the nasolacrimal duct leading to systemic toxicity.
  - Difficult for use in children.
- **Ointments:** They are particularly useful for night application and also for children. Less systemic absorption via nasolacrimal duct. It also minimizes dilution and prolongs contact time.

  Disadvantages:
  - It cannot be used during day time as it causes blurring of vision.

- Allergic reaction to ointment or its base may occur.
- **Ocuserts** provide continuous release of a predetermined amount of drug over a period of 5–7 days. Ocusert (pilocarpine) was available earlier for glaucoma treatment and Lacrisert (polyvinyl alcohol) for dry eye management.
- **Drug-impregnated contact lens:** A soft contact lens is soaked in a compound, and when the lens is placed in contact with the cornea, it gradually releases the drug, e.g. pilocarpine for glaucoma treatment.
- **Subconjunctival or subtenon injections** are popular for administration of antibiotics, corticosteroids, or atropine. This is useful at the end of intraocular operation, or treatment of corneal ulcer, or iridocyclitis. A high tissue concentration is maintained for a long time. Here, the route of penetration of drug is mainly via the cornea, though the injection sites are different (*see* Chapter 28).
- **Injections into the eye**
  - Either into the **anterior chamber (intra-cameral)** or **vitreous (intravitreal)** is reserved for desperate cases, especially in endophthalmitis.
  - **Into the anterior chamber:** In intra-ocular lens implantation, e.g. **visco-elastic substance, adrenaline** to dilate pupil, preservative free lignocaine for iris anesthesia in topical phacoemulsific-ation, and **pilocarpine** to constrict the pupil.

Intravitreal Injections

Injecting drugs directly into the vitreous cavity is indicated in various posterior segment pathologies. Some patients may require multiple injections.

The various drugs given intravitreally are:

Drug group	Indications	Drugs
Antibiotics	Endophthalmitis	Vancomycin, Ceftazidime, Amikacin
Antifungals	Endophthalmitis	Amphotericin B, Voriconazole
Antivirals	Viral retinal necrosis or retinopathy	Ganciclovir, Foscarnet
Anti-VEGFs	Diabetic retinopathy, Wet ARMD, ROP	Ranibizumab, Bevacizumab, Aflibercept
Steroid	Macular edema in vascular retinal pathology or chronic uveitis	Triamcinolone acetonide

Steroids are sometimes administered as slow release implants for prolonged duration of action. The commonly used implants are: dexamethasone implant—Ozurdex, and fluocinolone implant Retisert and Iluvien.

ASTRINGENTS AND DECONGESTANT

Commonly used in ocular irritations or discomfort, and they are:

- **Zinc sulfate:** As drop, also used specifically in **Morax-Axenfeld bacillus** infection (angular conjunctivitis).
- **Silver nitrate (1%):** As antiseptic and astringent, useful in chronic conjunctivitis or to prevent *ophthalmia neonatorum* **(Crede's prophylaxis).**
- **Boric acid:** As an astringent.
- **Naphazoline:** As a decongestant.
- **Antihistamines:** As a milder alternative to steroids in allergic conjunctivitis.

ANTIBIOTICS

- *Topical antibiotics:* They are generally required to eliminate superficial bacterial infections.
  - Chloramphenicol (0.5%), tetracycline (1%), ciprofloxacin (0.3%), moxifloxacin (0.5%) or gatifloxacin (0.3% and 0.5%) have broad-spectrum effectivity.
  - Gentamycin (0.3%), ciprofloxacin (0.3%), tobramycin (1%), and ploymyxin-B are effective against Gram-negative bacilli.
  - Moxifloxacin, gatifloxacin, vancomycin, ceftazidime, and cefazoline has better sensitivity against Gram-positive organism.
  - Neomycin (0.5%) is also useful only in Gram '+ve' infections and causes local allergy in many cases.
  - Freshly prepared crystalline penicillin drops remain stable only for a week or 10 days, and is specifically used to treat gonococcal infections.
- *Systemic antibiotics:* Oral (intramuscular or intravenous) are required to eliminate intraocular infections, and in soft tissue infections. Newer penicillin preparations (like, cefazoline and other cephalosporins) are having higher penetration in intraocular tissues.
- *Subconjunctival antibiotics:* They are best for treating deep seated infections, as high concentrations are maintained in aqueous for a prolonged period, e.g. gentamycin, amikacin, vancomycin, etc.
- *Intraocular injections of antibiotics*: They either into the anterior chamber or the vitreous, may be necessary for intractable ocular suppuration, as in endophthalmitis. Gentamycin, ceftazidime, amikacin or vancomycin is usually used along with corticosteroids. But they may cause damage to the corneal endothelium or retina (macular damage or hemiretinal venous occlusion after vancomycin injection).
- Vancomycin has been recently reported to cause hemorrhagic occlusive retinal vasculitis (HORV).

ANTIVIRALS

Chemotherapy of ocular viral infections is concerned mainly with keratitis caused by *Herpes simplex virus (HSV)*, and also to some extent by *Herpes zoster virus.*

- *Acyclovir* is effective both topically and systemically. It is used as 3% ointment for 5 times daily, or oral tablets (200–400 mg) 4 times daily for 7–10 days in herpes simplex keratitis.
  - It is more potent (90%) than IDU and less toxic.
- *Ganciclovir ophthalmic gel (0.15%):* It is equally effective as acyclovir ointment in acute HSV keratitis. It is given 5 times daily for 7–14 days depending upon the response. Toxicity includes, irritation, blurring of vision, superficial punctate keratitis (SPKs), follicular reaction, etc.
- *TFT (Triflurothymidine or F3T)* is given as 3% drop for 5 times daily. It has less toxicity, greater potency and greater effectiveness in resistance cases.
- *Vidarabine (Ara-A)* as 3% ointment. Generally, it is more potent than IDU and active against IDU-resistant virus.
- *Idoxuridine (IDU) or 5-iodo-2-deoxyuridine* inhibits the synthesis of DNA.
  - It is used as 0.1% eye drop or 0.5% ointment. Eighty percent of dendritic keratitis is cured by two weeks. *Important side effects* are superficial punctate keratopathy and punctal stenosis.
  - It is applied 1 as drop, or 5 times daily as ointment.
- *Valaciclovir or valacyclovir:* It is an antiviral drug used in the management of severe HSV, herpes zoster opthalmicus (HZO) and CMV infection of the eye. It is a prodrug, being converted *in vivo* to acyclovir. It is given orally 500–1000 mg bid or tid doses.
- *Ganciclovir:* The first antiviral agent for the treatment of *cytomegalovirus (CMV)* retinitis. It is given as 5 mg/kg I/V bid for 14 days. Weekly intravitreal injections

of 400 micrograms of ganciclovir for maintenance therapy is also suggested. Myelosuppression is the main side-effect.

- **Generally oral valganciclovir** (combination of ganciclovir and valaciclovir) is the first line of treatment in CMV endotheliitis. It is given 900 mg bid for 21 days followed by 900 mg daily as maintenance dose.
- **Other drugs include:** Foscarnet or cidofovir intravenous and/or intravitreal injections in severe sight-threatening HSV, CMV infections in immunocompromised patients.

Note: Not all compounds are commercially available in India.

ANTIFUNGALS

The available antifungal drugs are fungistatic in nature. They are mainly used in **keratomycosis** and **fungal endophthalmitis**. Three groups of agents are used:
1. **Polyenes:** Natamycin, Amphotericin B, and nystatin.
2. **Imidazoles:** Voriconazole, ketoconazole, miconazole, econazole, fluconazole, itraconazole, etc.
3. **Flucytosine:** 5-fluorocytosine.

Natamycin is used topically as 5% suspension. It has fairly broad-spectrum effect against *Fusarium* and *Aspergillus*, and least against *Candida*. It is the most commonly used antifungal.

Amphotericin-B is too toxic for systemic use but may be used locally as 0.15–0.25% solution (made in 5% dextrose solution or in distilled water)—as eye drop at 1-hour interval. As this solution is preservative-free, it should be discarded after 4 days.

Nystatin is used topically (as 100,000 units/mL) in fungal keratitis—particularly effective against *Candida* species. It is less potent.

Voriconazole has very good broad-spectrum antifungal activity. It may be given orally (200 mg bid) or as a topical (1%) preparation. It is more effective against *Aspergillus* and *Candida*

than *Fusarium*. It may be used as adjunct therapy or monotherapy. It is expensive.

Ketoconazole is a well-tolerated oral antifungal drug. It is not effective against *Fusarium*.

Itraconazole (100 mg bid) orally and **econazole** as 2% topical preparation are sometimes used with other topical antifungals in resistance cases.

Fluconazole is also a well-tolerated oral drug and has broader spectrum of antifungal activity. It is used as 200 mg daily for 3–4 weeks. It is also available as 0.3% solution, as 1 hourly drop in fungal corneal ulcer.

Flucytosine is a less effective agent and used systemically. It is not much useful in oculomycosis.

AUTONOMIC DRUGS

Autonomic drugs act on sphincter and dilator pupillae muscles of the iris, and also on the ciliary muscles. They are **miotics** (pupil constricting), **mydriatics** (pupil dilating) or **cycloplegics** (drugs causing paralysis of accommodation).

Miotics

Miotics are the drugs which cause miosis or pupillary constriction.

Systemically used drug, e.g. morphine is a strong miotic.

Topical Miotics

- **Cholinergic drugs** are of three types:
  1. **Direct stimulant** at myoneural junction as acetylcholine, e.g. pilocarpine (1–4%), methacholine.
  2. **Indirect stimulant** by abolishing the effects of cholinesterase enzyme, i.e. **anticholinesterase,** e.g. eserine, (0.25–1%), neostigmine, demecarium bromide, diisopropylfluorophosphate (DFP) (0.1%), phospholine iodide (0.06–0.25%), etc.

3. **Combination** of direct and indirect actions—carbachol and urecholine.

- **Sympatholytic miotics:** They are rarely used topically, although thymoxamine (0.5%) solution is a powerful miotic, used as an antidote of phenylephrine.
- Miosis can be induced by direct stimulation with histamine.

All miotics stimulate the ciliary muscles to contract, so that the eye assumes a state of partial or complete accommodation. This is observed with long-acting anticholinesterases, e. g DFP, phospholine iodide, etc.

Uses of miotics

- Almost in all cases of glaucoma including primary angle-closure glaucoma (PACG) or primary open-angle glaucoma (POAG).
- In the treatment of accommodative convergent squint.
- May be useful in accommodation weakness.
- During cataract surgery, after placing a posterior chamber (PC) intraocular lense (IOL) or before placement of an anterior chamber (AC) IOL (with dilute pilocarpine directly into the anterior chamber).
- May be used to counteract the effect of mydriatics, used for ophthalmic examination.
- During different types of keratoplasty procedures: as in penetrating keratoplasty (PK in phakic cases), anterior lamellar and endothelial keratoplasty.

Mydriatics and Cycloplegics

Pupil dilating drugs are called **mydriatics**. All drugs which dilate the pupil also paralyze the accommodation in greater or lesser degree, due to paralysis of the ciliary muscles (cycloplegia).

Systemically used atropine causes pupillary dilatation.

Topical Mydriatics

- **Parasympatholytic mydriatics:** They abolish the action of acetylcholine and, thus, cause mydriasis by making it impossible for the sphincter muscle to contract, e.g. atropine (1%), homatropine (1–2%), hyoscine (0.1–1%), cyclopentolate (0.5–1%) and tropicamide (0.5–1%).

- **Sympathomimetic mydriatics:** Directly act on dilator pupillae to produce mydriasis, e.g. adrenaline (1 in 10,000) as intracameral injection (into AC)—add, phenylephrine drop (2.5–10%), and cocaine hydrochloride.

Phenylephrine has little effect on ciliary muscles and therefore, should not be considered as a cycloplegic. But other parasympatholytic drugs are all cycloplegics.

Among these, **atropine** is the strongest cycloplegic agent, and the effect lasts for 10–14 days. **Homatropine** is moderately effective and its effect lasts for 48–72 hours.

Cyclopentolate and **tropicamide** are very rapidly acting drug, the effect of which lasts only for 12–14 hours.

Uses of mydriatics

- Fundus examination.
- For preoperative assessment of cataract.
- During extracapsular cataract extraction (ECCE) or posterior segment surgery.
- To test any posterior synechia is present or not.
- To break posterior synechiae (along with cycloplegics).

Uses of cycloplegics:

- For perfect refraction in children, hypermetropic subject and in squints.
- Refraction in case where the pupil is very small.
- In cases of iridocyclitis, keratitis and endophthalmitis.
- In accommodative convergent squint.
- In case of accommodative spasm.
- With atropine as **penalization** treatment in amblyopia.

Indomethacin, flurbiprofen or diclofenac eye drop is used along with mydriatics for prolonging the mydriatic effect during intraocular surgery.

Combination of mydriatic cycloplegic is always better except in refraction, e.g. homatropine and phenylephrine, tropicamide and phenylephrine, etc.

Mydriatics should not be used in angle-closure glaucoma, or very shallow anterior chamber; and in case of operated anterior chamber or iris-fixation IOL. They should be used with caution.

LOCAL ANESTHETICS

The small size of the eye and the accessibility of its nerve supply permit most adult ocular surgeries to be done under local anesthesia.

They are of two types—*topical* and *infiltrative*.

Topical Anesthetics

They work by stabilizing the nerve membrane potential temporarily, so that it cannot be depolarized. They are:

- Lignocaine hydrochloride (4%). 2% may also be useful.
- Tetracaine (0.5%)
- Proparacaine (0.5%)
- Amethocaine (0.5%)
- Cocaine (2–4%): Also causes mydriasis.

Among these amethocaine and proparacaine, although less potent, are less damaging to the corneal epithelium. They are especially useful in tonometry or gonioscopy.

Nowadays, most of the adult cataract surgery, refractive surgeries and other small surface procedures done under topical anesthesia—using lignocaine, proparacaine or with tetracaine drops 3 times 5 minutes before surgery.

Infiltrative Anesthetics

Simultaneous motor and sensory block are obtained by infiltration of anesthetic agents in and around the eyeball.

They may be *facial block* (to paralyze orbicularis oculi muscle,) *retrobulbar block, peribulbar block, regional block of the eyelids* (to excise local lesion), etc.

For infiltration, lignocaine (2%) is normally used. *Bupivacaine* (0.5%), a long-acting local anesthetic agent is usually mixed with lignocaine (50:50) to achieve better and prolonged anesthetic effect.

Adrenaline (1 in 100,000) prolongs the effect of anesthesia by inducing vasospasm in the injected area, but with slower action.

It also reduces the chance of bleeding during surgery, especially in oculoplast procedures.

Hyaluronidase enhances the dispersion and absorption of local infiltrative anesthetic agents. The increased dispersion makes possible, a more effective motor block. But it limits the duration of anesthetic effect.

OCULAR HYPOTENSIVE

The drugs causing lowering of intraocular pressure is called *ocular hypotensives*. Two types—systemic and local.

Systemic Ocular Hypotensive

- *Carbonic anhydrase inhibitors*, e.g. acetazolamide 250 mg tab, 1–2 tabs 4 times daily. As there is chance of hypokalemia, a potassium supplement is necessary along with it, in the form of tablet or syrup. Other carbonic anhydrase inhibitors, e.g. ethoxzolamide, methazolamide and dichlorphenamide may also be used.
- *Hyperosmotic agents:* (1) Inj. mannitol: 20% solution is used intravenously and (2) Oral glycerine: 30 mL with 30 mL of lemon or orange juice is given 3 times daily (*see* also Chapter 16).

Local Ocular Hypotensive

- *Parasympathomimetic:* Pilocarpine (1–4%) eye drop, 3–4 times daily. 2% solution is commonly used.
- *Beta-blockers:* (1) Timolol maleate (0.25–0.5%) twice daily and (2) betaxolol (0.50%) twice daily.

- *Sympathomimetics:* Epinephrine (0.5–2%) twice daily.
- *Topical carbonic anhydrase inhibitor:* 2% solution of dorzolamide hydrochloride—3 times daily, and 1% brinzolamide eye drop—3 times daily in open angle glaucoma and ocular hypertension.

Prostaglandin analogs (PGA): Like, latanoprost, bimatoprost, travatoprost, etc. are more commonly used nowadays.

Ocular hypotensive may be used alone or in combination (local and systemic; or two local drops) depending upon the height of intraocular pressure (*see* also Chapter 16).

Ocular hypotensive effect can also be achieved by retrobulbar injection of 1 mL of 70% alcohol, especially in case of absolute glaucoma with pain.

CORTICOSTEROIDS

The corticosteroids reduce the inflammatory responses of the ocular tissues by:

- Decreasing capillary permeability,
- Limiting exudation and
- Inhibiting the formation of new vessels and granulation tissue.

They inhibit the cyclooxygenase and lipoxygenase pathways by inhibiting phospholipase A2, thereby inhibiting the release of arachidonic acid.

All corticosteroids are prepared as ketone-based formulation except loteprednol which is prepared as ester-based formulation. They stay within the tissue more with good therapeutic effects and the same time with more toxicity. Whereas, enzymatic degradation occurs quickly with loteprednol; and it is less potent with less toxicity.

Indications

- *Sterile ocular inflammations*, e.g. disciform keratitis, episcleritis, scleritis, uveitis, optic neuritis, chemical injury, etc.
- *Allergic problems*, e.g. phlycten, seasonal allergic conjunctivitis, contact dermatitis, vernal keratoconjunctivitis, allergic blepharoconjunctivitis, etc.
- *Postoperative*, e.g. following cataract surgery, keratoplasty, vitrectomy, trabeculectomy, etc.
- *Miscellaneous*, e.g. pseudotumor of the orbit, graft rejection, endocrine exophthalmos, temporal arteritis, post-herpetic neuralgia, etc.

Preparation and Mode of Administration

Local

Three types—topical, periocular, and intraocular.

Topical Preparation:

Mostly available as drops and also as ointment, sometimes with some antibiotic combination in India.

- Hydrocortisone acetate: 0.5%
- Prednisolone acetate: 1.0%
- Dexamethasone phosphate: 0.1%
- Betamethasone: 0.5%
- Fluorometholone: 0.1%
- Loteprednol etabonate: 0.5% and 0.2%
- Difluprednate: 0.05% (a precursor of prednisolone).

Periocular:

- *Subconjunctival:* Mainly, injection dexamethasone and in combination with gentamycin—after intraocular surgeries—like cataract, keratoplasty, etc.; in anterior uveitis—only dexamethasone.
- *Posterior sub-Tenon's:* Inj. triamcinolone as in postoperative cystoid macular edema (CME); chronic uveitis, etc.
- *Peribulbar:* As in optic neuritis; thyroid ophthalmopathy, cornea graft rejection.

Intraocular:

- *Intravitreal injection:* Triamcinolone acetonide 4 mg/0.1 mL is useful in uveitic CME, exudative AMD, DME, and PDR.

- *Sustained-release intravitreal drug-delivery:* Fluocinolone, dexamethasone, combination of dexamethasone and cyclosporine, e.g. Ozurdex 0.7 mg dexamethasone intravitreal implant.

Systemic

Two types—oral and intravenous.

Oral:

- Prednisolone is the most commonly used oral corticosteroid.
- Initial dose is 1–1.5 mg/kg/day and maximum adult dose is 60–90 mg/kg/day. Maintenance dose is 10 mg/kg/day. Tapering is done based on the response by every 1–2 weeks.

  Blood glucose level, weight, and BP should be regularly monitored. Bone density should be checked within first 3 months and annually thereafter. Calcium and vitamin D supplements may be needed.
- Oral methylprednisolone or betamethasone: May be used in some cases.

Intravenous:

- *Methylprednisolone:* If an immediate response is needed then intravenous bolus injection of methylprednisolone can be given 500–1000 mg/day for 2–3 days followed by oral prednisone. This is expensive. This is given in optic neuritis, acute graft rejection, Vogt-Koyanagi-Harada syndrome, sympathetic ophthalmia, thyroid ophthalmopathy, etc.
- *Injection dexamethasone:* In anaphylactic shock, and also as bolus doses in graft rejection where the patient cannot afford intravenous methyl prednisolone.
  - High dose steroids should not be given for more than 1 month. Disease worsening/no response after 2–4 weeks is an indication for addition of immunosuppressive agents.

- Side effects of systemic steroids must be kept in mind.

Complications and Side Effects

Local

- Increased risk of superinfection, either with fungus, bacteria or HSV.
- *Steroid-induced glaucoma:* It is due to reduced aqueous outflow and occurs more with dexamethasone followed by difluprednate. Fluorometholone and loteprednol have little effect on intraocular pressure, although they are less potent.
- *Steroid-induced cataract:* It is mainly posterior subcapsular cataract (more often following systemic use of steroids).
  - Delayed wound healing
- Corneal melting due to increased collagenase activity
- Mydriasis
- Transient ptosis and occasionally transient myopia
- Papilledema due to pseudotumor cerebri.

Systemic

- Peptic ulceration
- Generalized edema due to sodium and electrolyte imbalance
- Cushing appearance
- Increased severity of diabetes
- Osteoporosis
- Mental changes
- Benign intracranial hypertension.

TRIAMCINOLONE ACETONIDE

Triamcinolone acetonide (TA) is an intermediate acting, relatively powerful steroid. It blocks the breakdown of the blood-ocular barrier by modifying the vascular endothelial growth factor (VEGF) receptor. It is used in both anterior as well as posterior segment disorders.

- *Giant papillae and venal kerato-conjunctivitis (VKC):* A supratarsal injection of triamcinolone is useful in VKC presenting with giant cobble-stone papillae and which is refractory to conventional treatment. Usually 0.5 mL (20 mg) is injected bilaterally. It results in a dramatic improvement in the size of the papillae, limbal involvement, itching and size of shield ulcers.
- *Sub-tenon injection of triamcinolone:* A posterior sub-Tenon injection of 20 mg TA is useful in resolving CME due to posterior segment inflammation, e.g. uveitis, diabetes, post-cataract surgery, post-venous occlusion. However, IOP must be carefully monitored post injection.
- *Intravitreal triamcinolone acitonide:* It is useful in the management of postuveitic macular edema, pseudophakic macular edema, post-branch retinal vein occlusion central retinal vein occlusion (post-BRVO/CRVO) macular edema and in choroidal neovascularization. This injection must be preservative free TA preparation. Post-injection endophthalmitis and secondary glaucoma are serious complications.
- *Chromovitrectomy:* Triamcinolone aceta-mide has the ability to adhere to and stain the vitreous. Thus it is a helpful tool in visualizing the vitreous during vitrectomy, both in the anterior and posterior segment. This injection should also be preservative free.
- *Triamcinolone (0.1%) eye ointment:* Used in cases of atopic keratoconjunctivitis or other allergic disorders of conjunctiva or lids.

NONSTEROIDAL ANTI-INFLAMMATORY DRUGS

As the corticosteroids have many complications, some nonsteroidal anti-inflammatory agents are being used recently. They are as follows:
- Flurbiprofen sodium
- Diclofenac sodium
- Ketorolac tromethamine
- Indomethacin
- Bromfenac
- *Nepafenac:* It has the best corneal and intraocular penetration.

They are mainly used as eye drops except indomethacin which is commonly used as oral medicine.

> They are mainly anti-prostaglandins. They compete with the arachidonic acid for cyclo-oxygenase binding, thereby prevent conversion of arachidonic acid to prostaglandins.

Uses

- Prevent intraoperative miosis during intraocular surgery. It is used with mydriatics in routine practice just before surgery.
- As prophylactic and therapeutic agent in cystoid macular edema (CME).
- Reduce ocular inflammation when steroids are contraindicated; as in vernal conjunc-tivitis; scleritis, allergic conjunctivitis, mild iridocyclitis and postoperative cases.

VISCOELASTIC SUBSTANCES

These are tissue-protective viscoelastic liquids with molecular weights ranging from 30,000 million Daltons to 4 million Daltons. They are non-toxic, non-antigenic, and they do not interfere with normal wound healing.

The substances are as follows:
- Sodium hyaluronate (1% and 1.4%)
- Methyl cellulose (2%)
- Chondroitin sulphate
- Hydroxypropyl methylcellulose (HPMC).
  Among these, methylcellulose is cheaper and most widely used, though sodium hyaluronate has the most favorable viscoelastic properties (but, the cost is much higher).

Roles of viscoelastics in intraocular surgeries:
- It creates and maintains depth of the anterior chamber during surgery.

- It *protects corneal endothelial cells* from mechanical trauma.
- *It provides a highly viscous environment* to control a circular capsulorhexis.
- It fully *reforms the capsular bag* to facilitate easy 'in-the-bag' IOL fixation.
- It acts as an internal tamponade in vitreoretinal surgery.
- Overall, it *acts as a soft instrument* to maneuver intraocular tissue gently.
- It may also be used as *an artificial tear, or for gonioscpic examination*.

Indications

- Cataract extraction and IOL implantation
- Penetrating and endothelial keratoplasties
- Glaucoma filtering surgery
- Vitreoretinal surgery.

Complications

Early postoperative secondary glaucoma is common with viscoelastic substance which blocks the angle of the anterior chamber. So, after completion of surgery, it should be thoroughly aspirated from the anterior chamber by diluting with irrigating solution.

IMMUNOSUPPRESSIVE AGENTS IN OPHTHALMOLOGY

Classification

- *Antimetabolites:* Azathioprine, methotrexate, mycophenolate mofetil.
- *Alkylating agents:* Cyclophosphamide and chlorambucil.
- *T-cell inhibitors:* Cyclosporine A, tacrolimus, sirolimus.
- *Biologic response modifiers:* Infliximab, adalimumab, daclizumab, rituximab, etc.

Antimetabolites

- *Azathioprine:* It is a purine nucleoside analogue and interferes with deoxyribonucleic acid (DNA) replication and ribonucleic acid (RNA) transcription.
- *Indications:* Given in chronic uveitis, Behcet's disease, and sarcoidosis.
- *Dose:* 1–3 mg/kg/day for months to years.
- *Side effects:* Bone marrow suppression is the most serious side effect and hence a total blood count should be done every 4–6 weeks. Liver function test (LFT) should be done every 12 weeks. The drug is stopped if total white blood cells (WBC) less than 3000/mm^3 or platelets less than 100,000/mm^3.
- *Methotrexate:* It is a folic acid analogue and it inhibits dihydrofolate reductase and interferes with DNA replication.
  - *Indications*: Given in panuveitis, intermediate uveitis, vasculitis, scleritis and orbital pseudotumor.
  - *Dose:* 7.5–25 mg/week (single dose) and folate 1 mg/day is given concurrently.
  - *Side effects:* Bone marrow suppression, hepatotoxicity, nausea, anorexia are the side effects.
  - Complete blood count and LFT should be done every 1–2 months.
- *Mycophenolate mofetil:* It metabolizes to mycophenolic acid which reversibly inhibits inosine monophosphate dehydrogenase that inhibits guanosine nucleotide synthesis without incorporating into DNA. Major effects are on T and B lymphocytes.
  - *Indications:* It is use in Stevens-Johnson syndrome (SJS), ocular cicatricial pemphigoid (OCP), and high-risk corneal transplants.
  - *Dose:* It has good oral bioavailability and should be given on an empty stomach at the dose of 1–1.5 g twice daily.
  - *Side effects:* Gastrointestinal distress and diarrhea are the most common side effects. Bone marrow suppression is serious problem in some patients.
  - Complete blood counts should be performed every week for 1 month, then every 2 weeks for 2 months and then monthly.

Essentials of Ophthalmology

Alkylating Agents

- **Cyclophosphamide:** There is alkylation of DNA and RNA resulting in cross-linking and cell death. It decreases the number of activated T lymphocytes.
  - **Indications:** Given in severe bilateral sight threatening uveitis, Behcet's, progressive systemic sclerosis, Wegener's granulomatosis, intermediate uveitis, sympathetic ophthalmitis and necrotizing scleritis.
  - **Dose:** Starting dose is 150–200 mg/day and then 2 mg/kg/day in intermittent pulses. Dose is adjusted to maintain the leukocyte counts between 3,000/mm^3 and 4,000/mm^3.
  - **Side effects:** Increased risk of malignancy, bone marrow suppression, teratogenicity, hemorrhagic cystitis, ovarian suppression, and azoospermia are the side effects.
- **Chlorambucil:** DNA-DNA cross-linking and DNA-protein cross-linking occurs leading to interference in DNA replication and nucleic acid function.
  - **Indications:** Given in Behcet's and sympathetic ophthalmitis.
  - **Dose:** 0.1–0.2 mg/kg/day.
  - **Side effects:** Reversible bone marrow suppression, opportunistic infections, permanent sterility in men, amenorrhea and teratogenicity are the side effects.

T-cell Inhibitors

- **Cyclosporine:** Obtained from the fungus *Beauveria nivea*. It is a calcineurin inhibitor that eliminates T-cell receptor signal transduction and down-regulate IL-2 gene transcription and receptor expression of CD4$^+$ T-lymphocytes.
  - **Indications:** Oral cyclosporine A is used in VKH, sympathetic ophthalmitis and high-risk cornea transplants cases.
  - **Doses:** It is available in two oral emulsions—neoral (microemulsion) and sandimmune. These two formulations are not bioequivalent. Neoral is begun at 2 mg/kg/day and sandimmune at 2.5 mg/kg/day. Dose is adjusted to 1–5 mg/kg/day.
  - **Side effects:** Most serious side effect is nephrotoxicity. Monthly monitoring of blood pressure, serum creatinine and complete blood counts is a must.
  - Topical cyclosporine (0.05%) is used in dry eye diseases. Topical cyclosporine (2%) may be helpful in VKC, high-risk corneal transplants where oral and topical steroids are contraindicated.
- **Tacrolimus:** Obtained from *Streptomyces tsukubaensis*.
  - **Indications:** Same as cyclosporine.
  - **Dose:** Given orally at 0.1–0.15 mg/kg/day.
  - **Side effects:** Nephrotoxicity is less than cyclosporine. Serum creatinine and complete blood counts should be monitored monthly.
- **Tacrolimus ointment (0.01% or 0.03%):** It is used in recalcitrant cases of VKC, in various types of ocular surface inflammation (as in SJS, OCP, etc.).

Biologic Response Modifiers

- **Infliximab:** It is a chimeric, monoclonal IgG1κ antibody against tumor necrosis factor-α (TNF-α) and thus decreases pro-inflammatory cytokines.
  - **Indications:** Given in human leukocyte antigen B27 (HLA-B27) associated uveitis and Behcet's disease.
  - **Dose:** Initial dose—5 mg/kg. 1st dose is on 1st day of therapy; 2nd dose is at the end of 2 weeks and 3rd dose is at the end of 6 weeks.
  - **Side effects:** Major side effect is increased risk of infections like tuberculosis. It may enhance brain lesions associated with multiple sclerosis.

Cyclosporine in Ophthalmology

Cyclosporine A (CsA) is a neutral, hydrophobic, cyclic peptide of amino acids which can be isolated from several species of fungi. The unusual structure of CsA is responsible for very low water solubility, causing highly variable and incomplete absorption from its conventional oral or topical formulations.

- It acts as a selective inhibitor of interleukin-2 (IL-2) release during the activation of T-cells and causes cell-mediated immune response suppression.
- *In dry eye:* CsA's inhibits subconjunctival and lacrimal gland inflammation, resulting in an increase in tear production and conjunctival goblet-cell density in moderate-to-severe dry eye patients.

Indications and Doses

Systemic:

- Along with oral corticosteroids or as corticosteroids-sparing agents in non-infectious ocular inflammations. As in autoimmune uveitis, Bechets' disease, VKH syndrome, sympathetic ophthalmia, severe scleritis, etc.
- High-risk penetrating keratoplasty: To prevent graft rejection.
- May be in Stevens Johnson syndrome and mucous membrane pemphigoid.
- *Dose:* 2–3.5 mg/kg/day of cyclosporine is effective and has a low-risk of side effects.

Topical:

- Topical CsA emulsion (0.05%) (Restasis) is approved by the USFDA for dry eye syndrome.
- *Dose:* One drop twice daily for 3–6 months or more. The drug is to be kept in refrigerator.
- *The other indications of 0.05% emulsion:* Superior limbic keratoconjunctivitis, adenoviral keratoconjunctivitis, Meibomian gland dysfunctions, etc.
- *Topical CsA (2%) in various oil:* It may be useful in severe VKC, in high-risk grafts where steroids are contraindicated.

Side Effects

- *For systemic use:* It includes gingival hyperplasia, pancreatitis, hirsutism, hypertension, renal and hepatic dysfunctions and an increased vulnerability to opportunistic fungal and viral infections.
- *For topical use:* Burning and stinging sensation are most common.
- Cyclosporine A, both oral and topical preparations are very expensive.

ANTI VASCULAR ENDOTHELIAL GROWTH FACTOR AGENTS

- VEGF means vascular endothelial growth factor, is a naturally occurring signal protein which is responsible for angiogenesis or growth of blood vessels.
- Besides having a role in normal vascular growth, VEGF is also responsible for new vessels growth in various parts of the eye especially in the retina. VEGF is primarily responsible for many retinal diseases by increasing leakage from these new vessels, causing retinal hemorrhage and macular edema.
- VEGF-A is a chemical signal that also stimulates angiogenesis in a variety of diseases, especially in carcinoma. Bevacizumab is the first clinically available angiogenesis inhibitor to treat colorectal carcinoma in the USA.
- The anti-VEGF agents block the VEGF molecules and thus benefit the patients by decreasing the abnormal and harmful new blood vessels formation, and by decreasing the leakage and macular edema. This leads to stabilization of vision and even improvement in vision in many cases.

The available anti-VEGF agents are:
- *Monoclonal antibody:* Bevacizumab (avastin).

- *Antibody derivative:* Ranibizuab (lucentis).
- *Aptamer:* Pegaptanib (macugen).
- *Fusion proteins-VEGF trap:* Aflibercept (eylea).
- *Oral molecules:* Lapatinib, sunitinib, sorafenib.
- *Miscellaneous:* Bevasiranib.

Indications

- Wet age-related macular degeneration (AMD)
- Choroidal neovascular membrane (CNM)
- CRVO/BRVO and macular edema
- Proliferative diabetic retinopathy (PDR)
- Diabetic macular edema (DME)
- Preoperative in vitreoretinal (VR) surgery for PDR and vitreous hemorrhage
- Eales disease and Coats' disease
- Refractory post-surgical CME
- Neovascular glaucoma (NVG) and/or neovascular iris (NVI)
- To treat corneal neovascularization, e.g. in lipid keratopathy or prior to penetrating keratoplasty (PK).
- In early pterygium recurrence to prevent further progression.

Contraindications

- Fibrovascular epiretinal proliferation (FVP) threatening the macula.
- Patients with active ocular or periocular inflammation.
- Uncontrolled hypertension.
- Cardiovascular diseases.

Complications

- Raise in IOP
- Cataract formation
- Infective endophthalmitis
- Risk of arterial thromboembolic events; like, cerebrovascular accidents, increasing myocardial infarction
- Rebound macular edema

- Immunoreactivity
- Retinal detachment.

Bevacizumab (avastin): Humanized monoclonal antibody that blocks VEGF having an off-label use in ophthalmology. Available as a 4 mL vial (100 mg) and dose is 1.25 mg/0.05 mL. Nonocular uses of avastin include metastatic colorectal cancer, non-small cell lung cancer, metastatic breast cancer, metastatic renal cell carcinoma and glioblastoma multiforme.

Ranibizumab (lucentis/accentrix): Binds and inactivates all isoforms of VEGF. It penetrates the internal limiting membrane (ILM) and can gain access to the subretinal space. Available as a single use glass vial (2 cc) and dose is 0.5 mg/0.05 mL.

Pegaptanib (macugen): It is a pegylated aptamer and selectively binds VEGF-165 with a high affinity. Available as a single dose prefilled syringe 0.3 mg/90 µL.

Aflibercept (eylea): It is indicated for the treatment of patients with—neovascular wet age-related macular degeneration and macular edema following CRVO. It may also be helpful in patients that do not completely respond to lucentis and avastin. It has the potential of lasting effect longer than lucentis and avastin.

SYSTEMIC REACTIONS TO LOCAL INSTILLATION OF MEDICINES

After instillation, the drug may be absorbed through the conjunctiva or by nasal mucous membrane via lacrimal passages. Some drugs really cause systemic toxic reactions even after local instillation.

Among these, 1% atropine and 10% phenylephrine, may cause characteristic systemic reactions because a single eye drop (1 mL = 15 drops) may exceed the systemic therapeutic dose.

Drug	1 drop	Systemic dose
1% atropine	0.67 mg	0.6 mg
10% phenylephrine (i.e. adrenaline)	6.67 mg	5.0 mg

- **Atropine intoxication:** Dry mouth, difficulty in swallowing, the skin is dry, red and hot; the body temperature is raised; tachycardia, and there may be behavioral changes.
- **Pilocarpine:** Gastrointestinal overactivity, sweating, tremor, bradycardia and decreased blood pressure.
- **10% phenylephrine:** It may increase blood pressure dangerously in old age. Cerebrovascular accidents, and cardiac arrhythmia with extrasystole may also occur.
- **Cyclopentolate:** It may cause hallucination, ataxia, vertigo, behavioral changes, and at times syncopal attack.
- **Timolol maleate:** It cause respiratory distress specially in bronchial asthma patients, and cardiac arrhythmia in patients with heart block.

Eye drops should be prevented from entering the nasolacrimal duct by maintaining pressure over the inner corners of the closed eyelids for 2 minutes after instillation. An ointment or an oily suspension is better to minimize systemic absorption.

OCULAR REACTIONS TO SYSTEMIC MEDICATION

Ocular side effects may occur from the systemic administration of the drugs. Some of them are as follows:

- **Corticosteroids:** Posterior subcapsular cataract and glaucoma are most important. Others are myopia, exophthalmos, papilledema (due to benign intracranial hypertension).
- **Chloroquine:** It is usually dose dependent (a regime of 200 mg/day for more than one year), and **three important effects** are:
  1. **Keratopathy:** Whitish dots in a whorl pattern in the cornea, usually reversible on discontinuation of the drug.
  2. **Myopathy:** Failure of accommodation (reversible).
  3. **Retinopathy:** A severe pigmentary degeneration of the retina that may progress into blindness. The typical lesion is **Bull's eye maculopathy** (concentric rings of pigment loss and hyperplasia around the fovea), leading to central scotoma. The first sign of retinal toxicity is the demonstration of an arcuate scotoma with a red target (decreased color sensation). Retinopathy may not be reversible at late stage.
- **Quinine:** Irreversible constriction of visual fields, impaired dark adaptation, and loss of vision (quinine amblyopia).
- **Ethambutol: Optic neuritis** in 2% of those treated, leading to reduced visual acuity and color vision, and a central scotoma. This optic neuritis is reversible.
- **Phenothiazines (chlorpromazine):** conjunctival pigmentation (light-brown), anterior subcapsular cataract and pigmentary retinopathy.
- **Digitalis:** Photopsia (flash), xanthopsia (yellow vision) and central scotoma.
- **Oral contraceptives:** Retinal vascular thrombosis, papilledema due to benign intracranial hypertension in susceptible individuals. **Contact lens** wearers develop an **intolerance** with discomfort and irritation due to corneal edema.
- **Vitamin A:** Papilledema due to benign intracranial hypertension, and retinal hemorrhage.
- **Rifampicin:** Orange-colored tears, which may stain a soft contact lens; painful purulent conjunctivitis.
- **Sulphonamides including acetazolamide:** They induce myopia either through

spasm of accommodation, or by increased refractive index of the lens. Severe dry eye due to SJS may result blindness.

- **Amiodarone**: Vortex keratopathy, visual disturbances, optic neuritis,
- **Amantadine:** Visual hallucination, blurring of vision, reduced endothelial cell count and corneal edema,

OCULAR PRESERVATIVES

Ocular medications (eye drops) are composed of unique mixtures of:
- The active drug
- A preservative
- The drug delivery system
- Viscosity-increasing agents
- An aqueous buffered vehicle.

All multidose topical ophthalmic preparations uses preservatives. In fact, it is mandatory by drug regulation by all countries.

Preservative Benefits

- Plays the key role in maintaining the sterility of ophthalmic solutions through multiple uses.
- Protects against bacterial, fungal or viral contamination that can occur when the dropper tip touches the skin, eyelids, fingers or other non-sterile surfaces. Once the tip is contaminated, the offending agent may be aspirated back into the bottle; or it may blend into the solution with the next use as the medication collects on the tip before dropping into the eye.
- But the ophthalmic ointments are often supplied non-preserved, presumably because they are not as susceptible to contamination from retrograde flow back into the tube.
- Also prolongs the shelf life of the formulation by preventing biodegradation and maintaining drug potency.

Preservative Toxicity

- Primary concern with many preservatives is not their value or efficacy, but rather their recognized cytotoxic side effects.
- Although intermittent use of preserved multidose eye drops in normal individuals is probably not harmful, but high concentration (or prolonged and frequent use) of some preservatives can cause damage and irritation to the ocular tissue, particularly in patient with dry eye or glaucoma.
- Preservative-induced toxicity does not have distinct signs or symptomatology. So, damage due to ophthalmic preservatives often goes undiagnosed.
- But nowadays, it is most often considered the culprit in damaging the corneal epithelium leading to disruption of the corneal apical glycocalyx.
- Awareness of the potential effects of preservatives on overall ocular surface health is relatively low among the physician.

Types and Mechanism of Action

Ocular preservatives can be classified into **two main categories** detergents and oxidative preservatives.

1. **Detergent preservatives**
   - They act upon microorganisms by altering cell membrane permeability and lysing the cytoplasmic content, e.g. benzalkonium chloride (BAK), Polyquad, chlorobutanol and thimerosal.
   - Ocular toxicity can occur because some detergent preservatives can affect eukaryotic cells and thus, cause ocular damage.
2. **Oxidative preservatives**
   - They are usually smaller molecules that penetrate the cell membranes and interfere with the cellular function.

- Stabilized oxychloro complex (SOC) and sodium perborate are *two examples* of oxidative preservatives.

> Oxidative preservatives have an advantage over detergent preservatives because they can provide enough activity against microorganisms while having negligible toxicity on eukaryotic cells.

Common Ocular Preservatives

Benzalkonium Chloride

- Benzalkonium chloride is a quaternary ammonium compound and is often used in conjunction with disodium ethylenediaminetetraacetic acid (EDTA).
- Edetate sodium is an additive which augments the preservative activity of BAK. However, it is not a true preservative by itself. This is just to lower the concentration of primary preservatives.
- Benzalkonium chloride is the *most common* and *gold standard* preservative used in topical multidose vials for many years. It is chemically stable, does not degrade easily, even at a higher temperature. It is usually used at a concentration of 0.01% to 0.02%. BAK acts upon microorganisms by altering cell membrane permeability and lysing cytoplasmic contents.
- Benzalkonium chloride does not appear to have significant adverse effects unless its frequency exceeds four to six times per day. This becomes a concern when patients use other drops on top of chronic medications, such as glaucoma drops or tears substitutes.
- We need to be careful with its use in patients when they are using several medications; are overdoses or have a history of compromised corneal epithelium.

Polyquad (Polyquaternium-1)

- It is a new polymeric quaternary ammonium preservative and it has less toxic effect on corneal epithelial cells than BAK.

- It does not go into deep level and only cause superficial epithelial damage compared to BAK. It is used as 0.001% in ophthalmic solution.

Chlorobutanol

- It is an alcohol-based preservative; so it does not have surfactant action. It works by disorganizing the lipid structure of the cell membrane which increases cell permeability and leads to cell lysis.
- Chlorobutanol has broad-spectrum antimicrobial activity. It is used as 0.5% in ophthalmic preparation and in human corneal epithelial cells, the cytotoxic effects are less severe.

Thimerosal

It is used as 0.001–0.004% in ophthalmic drops. It causes cellular retraction, cessation of mitotic activity, and superficial corneal epithelial cell loss.

Phenylmercuric Nitrate, Methylparaben and Propylparaben

They have similar antimicrobial activities as chlorobutanol, but they are relatively *more epitheliotoxic* than chlorobutanol or thimerosal.

Noble Preservatives

Stabilized Oxychloro Complex or Purite

- Stabilized oxychloro complex (SOC) is a relatively new preservative and consists of an equilibrium mixture of oxychloro compounds—99.5% chlorite (ClO_2^-), 0.5% chlorate (ClO_3^-) and trace amount of chlorine dioxide (ClO_2).
- It has bactericidal, fungicidal and viricidal activity.
- Stabilized oxychloro complex dissipates by converting into component normally

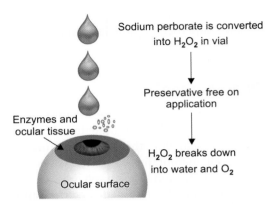

Fig. 5.1: Sodium perborate—mechanism of action

found in tears, such as sodium ion (Na^+), chloride-ion (Cl^-), oxygen and water. Due to oxidation potential of chlorite and possibly from the generation of chlorine dioxide in presence of acidic environments of the microbes, it leads to disruption of the protein synthesis and thereby kill them.

- Sodium chlorite, the key component of SOC, has been used in water purification plant since 1944. It is also used in toothpaste, mouthwash and some antacids. SOC has wide spectrum of antimicrobial activities at a low concentration of 0.005% w/v.

Sodium Perborate (Fig. 5.1)

- It works by oxidizing cell walls or membranes and thereby disrupting the cellular functions. It destroys most bacteria, and can also destroy some viruses and most of the fungi.
- When sodium perborate is combined with water it is converted into hydrogen peroxide, an effective antimicrobial agent. Once sodium perborate enters the eye, it is decomposed to water and oxygen by catalase and other enzymes present in the tear film. It is much gentler than any other preservatives.

Both sodium perborate and purite are noble preservatives and offer attractive options as multidose drugs for patients who either require more than 6 doses/day or for those who use more than one type of drop to treat concomitant diseases (e.g. glaucoma and dry eye).

Refraction of the Normal Eye

THE OPTICAL SYSTEM OF THE EYE

The Roles of the Cornea and Lens

Light that enters the eye is refracted at each of the refractive surfaces that lie in its pathway between the air and the retina. But for all practical purposes, refraction by t e eye, takes place at two structures—***the anterior corneal surface*** and ***the lens***.

- ***Refraction at anterior corneal surface:*** Here the major part of ocular refraction takes place, because of:
  - Radius of curvature is 8 mm (approximately).
  - Big difference in the refractive indices of the air (1) and the cornea (1.37).
  - Optical power of cornea = + 43D (40–45D).
- ***Refraction by the lens:*** This is complicated by the lack of optical homogenecity of the lens substance:
  - The nucleus has a greater optical density.
  - Greater curvature of its surfaces.

Both of these effects enhance its converging power.

Optical power of the lens = +17D (16–20D) (in non-accommodative state).

SCHEMATIC EYE (FIGS 6.1A AND B)

From the above discussion, it is clear that the optical system of the eye reduces itself into two elements only. This simplified optical system

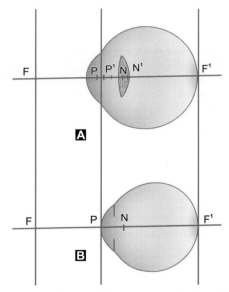

Figs 6.1A and B: A. Schematic eye; **B.** Reduced eye Upper figure represents schematic eye, with the two focal points at F and F[1], the two principal points at P and P[1], and the nodal points at N and N[1]. The reduced eye, drawn in scale to correspond, is shown below, with the two principal foci at F and F[1], the single refracting, surface at P corresponding to the mean of P and P[1], and the nodal point at N, corresponding to the mean of N and N[1]

in the eye is the *schematic eye* which has three pairs of cardinal points:

1. Two principal points (P and P^1)
2. Two nodal points (N and N^1)
3. Two focal points (F and F^1).

REDUCED EYE

In schematic eye, the two principal points and the two nodal points are very close together, so close, indeed, it is better to consider an intermediate point in between them.

Thus, the optical system of the eye is being treated as a single ideal refracting surface. This is the *reduced eye (of Donder)*.

It has following features (Table 6.1):

- Radius of curvature = 5.73, which separates two media of refractive indices 1 and 1.336.
- One principal point (P)—lies about 1.35 mm behind the anterior corneal surface.

TABLE 6.1: Refractive index for substances of interest in ophthalmology

Substances	Refractive Index
Air	1.00
Water	1.33
Aqueous humor	1.34
Vitreous humor	1.33
Cornea	1.37
Crystalline lens	1.39
PMMA (IOL)	1.49
Hydrophilic acrylic (IOL)	1.43
Hydrphobic acrylic (IOL)	1.47–1.54
Silicone (IOL)	1.41
Crown glass	1.52
Flint glass	1.65
CR-39 plastic lens	1.498
Other plastic lenses	1.54 to 1.75
Silicone oil (used in vitreoretina surgeries)	1.405

Abbreviations: **PMMA**—Polymethyl methacrylate; **IOL**—Intraocular lens

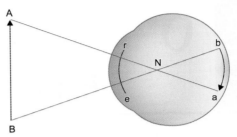

Fig. 6.2: Formation of retinal images

The image 'ab' of an object 'AB' is formed, by drawing lines from A and B through nodal point N. 're' is the position of the refracting surface of the reduced eye. 'ANB' or 'aNb' represents the visual angle

- One nodal point (N) (optical center)—lies 7.08 mm behind the anterior corneal surface, i.e. just in front of the posterior pole of the lens.
- *Two principal foci:*
  - Anterior = 15.7 mm in front of the cornea.
  - Posterior = 24.13 mm behind the cornea, i.e. in an average eye, on the retina.

Refractive index for substances of interest in ophthalmology is described in Table 6.1.

The Formation of Retinal Images (Fig. 6.2)

Since the nodal point (N) acts as the optical center of the reduced eye, rays which pass through it will not be appreciably refracted. It is evident that the image thus formed is inverted and diminished (just as an image formed by a convex lens). It is reinverted psychologically at its accustomed size in the cerebral cortex.

The angle, subtended by the object at the nodal point is called *visual angle* and it is, of course, equal to the angle, subtended by the retinal image at the nodal point.

PHYSIOLOGICAL OPTICAL DEFECTS

There are certain inherent limitations in the eye as a perfect refracting system.

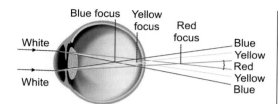

Fig. 6.3: Chromatic aberration in the eye. The blue rays being normally focused in front of the retina and the red rays behind it

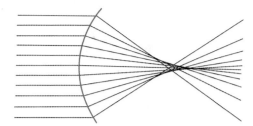

Fig. 6.4: Spherical aberration

- ***Diffraction of light:*** Light brought to a focus does not come to a point, but gives rise to a blurred disc of light surrounded by several dark and light bands. In human eye, diffraction is of little consequence unless the pupil diameter is less than 2 mm.
- ***Chromatic aberration (Fig. 6.3):*** There is a tendency of white light to be split up into its components after refraction, and the image will have a colored edge.
  After refraction of white light:
  - A yellow light is focused on the retina.
  - A blue (short wavelength) light is slightly pre-retinal (eye is myopic for blue).
  - A red (longer wavelength) light is slightly post-retinal (eye is hypermetropic for red). This property is used for testing refraction by the duochrome ***(Duochrome test).***
  - Chromatic aberration can be neutralized by ***achromatic lens.*** A convex lens of crown glass (refractive index = 1.52) combined with a concave lens of half the strength of flint glass (refractive index = 1.65) is used for this purpose.
- ***Spherical aberration (Fig. 6.4):*** As the periphery of a spherical lens has a higher refracting power than the central part, the peripheral rays are focused nearer to the lens than the central ones.

  This error can be eliminated by making the anterior surface greater than that of the posterior ***(aplanatic lens).***

- ***Decentration:*** The center of curvature of the separate lens systems of the eye are never exactly placed on the optic axis (Fig. 6.5).
  - ***Optic axis (AB)*** is the axis through the centers of the various media of the eye.
  - ***Visual axis (OM)*** is the line passing through the macula and nodal point.
    The angle between these two axes is called ***angle alpha*** (α). Normally visual axis cuts the cornea on nasal side of the optic axis. It is "positive-α" (about 5°), and causing an "apparent squint". It may be "negative" when the visual axis cuts the cornea on the temporal side.
  - ***Pupillary line*** is the line which passes perpendicularly through the central point of the pupil. The optic axis is difficult to determine, but it virtually corresponds to the central pupillary line.

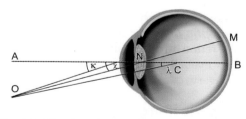

Fig. 6.5: Visual angles: 'Angle χ' = between optical and visual axis; 'Angle κ' = between pupillary line and visual axis; 'Angle λ' = between optic and fixation axis

AB—Optical axis; **OM**—Visual axis; **OC**—Fixation axis

Angle kappa (κ), the angle between the visual axis and the pupillary line, thus, roughly corresponds with angle alpha (α).

■ *Fixation axis (OC)* is the line joining the point of fixation with center of rotation of the eyeball.

Angle gamma (γ) is the angle between optic axis and fixation axis. When optic axis of a lens does not coincide with that of the eye, the lens is not centered and induces a prismatic effect.

In general, each cm of decentration of 1D lens induces an image displacement equivalent to 1 prism diopter.

- *Peripheral aberrations:* The clarity of the image at retinal periphery is impaired by a number of optical aberrations. These include *comma, radial astigmatism, image distortion*, etc.

EXTRANEOUS IMAGERY IN NORMAL EYE

- *Dioptric imagery:* When light falls on the eye, the major part of it passes through the ocular media to reach the retina and the imagery that forms is called dioptric imagery.
- *Catoptric imagery:* A part of the light will always be reflected from the media of the eye, and will be apparent to the observer as catoptric imagery.
- *Entoptic imagery:* Some light may reach the retina by reflection of structures within the eyeball and they produce entoptic imagery.

Catoptric Imagery

The light that is reflected by the ocular media back to the observer may be either regularly reflected light, or diffusely reflected light. They are appreciated because of the zones of optical discontinuity.

Purkinje-Sanson Images (Fig. 6.6)

There are four types of images:

- *1st image:* It derives from the anterior corneal surface. It is the *brightest* and erect image, and moves in the same direction.
- *2nd image:* It derives from the posterior corneal surface; it lies adjacent to 1st image. It is faint but erect image.
- *3rd image:* It derives from the anterior lens surface. It is *largest*, dim, and erect image.
- *4th image:* It derives from the posterior lens surface. It is small, dim and *inverted*, as the posterior lens surface is concave. The image lies at the pupillary plane and moves in the *opposite direction*.

Purkinje-Sanson images are important to diagnose corneal pathology, different types of cataract, and presence or absence of lens. If the patient is taken in a dark room, or the pupil is dilated, the images will be better appreciated.

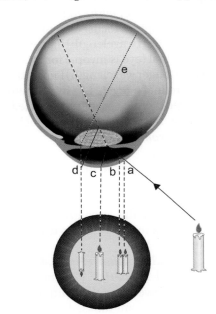

Fig. 6.6: Purkinje-Sanson images

a—anterior corneal reflection; **b**—posterior corneal reflection; **c**—anterior lens reflection; **d**—posterior lens reflection; **e**—second order reflection

Entoptic Imagery

An entoptic image arises, when light from any structures within the eye reaches the retina, so as to excite visual sensation.

Any structure in front of rods and cones, and less transparent, can be made visible entoptically. They may be normal structures (in connection with retinal circulation), anatomic anomalies, or normal response to an abnormal stimulus.

- *Opacities in the media* as (1) in the cornea or lens, gives a fixed black spot; (2) in the vitreous—as floaters, like flies to a large floating black spots, as spider web or soot.
- *Retinal vessels* as branching black lines or corpuscular movements (*flying corpuscles*) are better appreciated in blue field.
- *Phosphene are* the visual sensations that can result from abnormal stimuli, e.g. prolonged pressure on the globe with finger.

CHAPTER 7

Refractive Errors

DEFINITIONS AND CLASSIFICATIONS

Emmetropia (no refractive error): It is the ideal condition in which the incident parallel rays come to a perfect focus upon the light sensitive layer of the retina, when accommodation is at rest (Fig. 7.1).

Ametropia (refractive error): It is the opposite condition, wherein the parallel rays of light are not focused exactly upon the retina, when the accommodation is at rest.

Anisometropia (unequal error): When the refractive condition of the two eyes are unequal.

Ametropia or ***refractive errors*** may be of three main types:

1. ***Hypermetropia*** principal focus is formed behind the retina (Fig. 7.1).
2. ***Myopia*** principal focus is formed in front of the retina (Fig. 7.1).
3. ***Astigmatism;*** the refractive system is unequal in different meridians, and no single point focus is formed upon the retina.

Ametropia may be due to one or more of the following conditions:

- ***Abnormal length of the globe (axial ametropia):*** The anteroposterior diameter of the eye is too short in hypermetropia or too long in myopia. ***1 mm shortening will cause +3.0D hypermetropia, similarly 1 mm enlargement will cause –3.0D myopia.***

- ***Abnormal curvature of the refractive surfaces of the cornea or lens (curvature ametropia):***
  - Too weak or flat curvature of the cornea or lens results in hypermetropia and too strong or steep curvature results in myopia. ***1 mm flattening will cause +6.0D hypermetropia, similarly 1 mm steepening causes –6.0D myopia.***
  - Irregular or unequal curvature, in different meridians, gives rise to astigmatism.

- ***Abnormal refractive indices of the media (index ametropia):*** This is clinically evident in case of lenticular changes.
  - If the index of the lens cortex is increased, as in early cortical cataract—there is hypermetropia.
  - Conversely, if the index of the nucleus increases, as in nuclear sclerosis (early nuclear cataract)—myopia is produced.

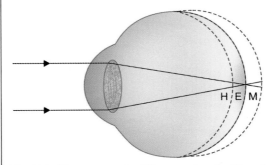

Fig. 7.1: Hypermetropia (H), emmetropia (E) and myopia (M)

- If the increase in the refractive index of the nucleus is very marked—a 'false lenticonus' may be produced. Here, the central part of the lens is myopic, but the peripheral part is hypermetropic.
- If the index of any part varies irregularly (as in developing cataract)—an 'index astigmatism' is produced.

- *Abnormal position of the lens:* If the crystalline lens is displaced backward—*hypermetropia* will result, and if forward—*myopia*.
- *Obliquity of the media:* As in lenticular obliquity [subluxated lens or oblique placement of intraocular lens (IOL)]—*astigmatism* will result.
- *Absence of an element of the system:* Absence of the lens (aphakia) produces high *hypermetropia*.

HYPERMETROPIA (LONG-SIGHTEDNESS)

It is the refractive error, in which the incident parallel rays of light are brought to a focus posterior to the light-sensitive layer of the retina, when the accommodation is at rest.

Etiology

- *Axial hypermetropia* is by far the most common.
  - In fact, all the newborns are almost invariably hypermetropic (approximately + 2.5D). This is due to shortness of the globe and is physiological.
  - It may also occur pathologically, when retina is displaced forward [retinal detachment, central serous retinopathy (CSR), orbital tumors, retinal tumor, etc.].
  - In microphthalmos or nanophthalmos ('*nano*' means '*dwarf*'—where the axial length is less than 20.0 mm), there is high hypermetropia.

- *Curvature hypermetropia* as in cornea plana, following a corneal injury, lens plana, etc.
- *Index hypermetropia* due to increase in refractive index of the lens-cortex in old age.
- *Removal of the lens* (aphakia).

Clinical Types

Depending upon the act of accommodation, *total hypermetropia (tH)* may be divided into:

- *Latent hypermetropia (lH):* Which is corrected physiologically by the tone of the ciliary muscle. As a rule, latent hypermetropia amounts to only one diopter. It can be revealed only after atropine cycloplegia.
- *Manifest hypermetropia (mH):* It is made up of two components:
  1. *Facultative hypermetropia (fH)* is that part of hypermetropia which can be corrected by the effort of accommodation.
  2. *Absolute hypermetropia (aH)* which cannot be overcome by the effort of accommodation.
     tH = lH + mH (fH + aH)
     - As the tone of the ciliary muscle decreases with age, some of the lH become manifest.
     - As the range of accommodation gets reduced with age more of the fH becomes absolute.
     - In early life (unless the error is unusually large), the accommodative power can correct it all, and none of the hypermetropia is absolute.
     - But after age of 60 years, all of hypermetropia becomes absolute (as the accommodation is minimum).
     - Total hypermetropia is usually elicited after complete paralysis of accommodation, i.e. by atropinization.

Optics

Theoretically, far point *(punctum remotum)* of the emmetropic eye is at infinity. But in hypermetropia, far point of the eye is a virtual point behind the eye.

- In hypermetropia, rays coming from a point on the retina will be divergent than the corresponding rays of the emmetropic eye (Fig. 7.2A).
- So, in hypermetropia the formation of a clear image is impossible, unless the converging power of the optical system is increased (Fig. 7.2B).
- This may be done in two ways:
  1. By the eye itself, i.e. by the effort of accommodation (Fig. 7.2C).
  2. By artificial means, i.e. by a convex lens placed in front of the eye (Fig. 7.2D).

Symptoms

They vary with the amount of hypermetropia and the age of the patient (accommodative effort).

- Blurred vision—more for near than for the distant.
- Eye strain (accommodative asthenopia).
- Artificial myopia—due to excessive accommodation → spasm of the ciliary muscle.
- Convergent squint—due to continuous efforts of accommodation → excess of convergence → dissociation of muscle balance → a convergent squint.
- Early onset of presbyopia.

Signs

- **Small eyeball** (in all directions)
- **Smaller cornea**
- **Shallow anterior chamber:** It predisposes to angle-closure glaucoma since the size of the lens is normal.
- **Apparent divergent squint:** It is due to a large positive **angle alpha** (α), as the macula is relatively far from the disc.
- **Ophthalmoscopy:** Optic disc is smaller, hyperemic, with less defined edges, even

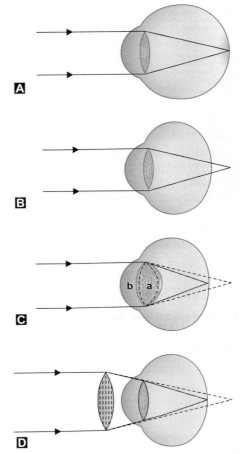

Figs 7.2A to D: Optics of hypermetropia. **A.** Parallel rays come to a focus upon the retina in emmetropic eye; **B.** Parallel rays come to a focus 'behind' the retina (hypermetropia); **C.** Parallel rays are brought to a focus upon the retina by increasing the refractivity of the lens (a) normal lens (b) more convex in accommodation; **D.** Parallel rays are brought to a focus upon the retina by a convex spectacle lens

simulating a papillitis *(pseudoneuritis)* (Fig. 7.3).

- **Shot-silk retina:** A peculiar sheen is a reflex effect of the retina (Fig. 7.3).
- **Blood vessels:** Undue tortuosity and abnormal branching.

Problems with hypermetropic eye

- Amblyopia—more with unilateral high hypermetropia

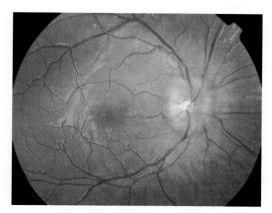

Fig. 7.3: Hypermetropic fundus—pseudo-neuritis and shot-silk appearance

- Accommodative convergent squint
- Angle-closure glaucoma
- Early onset of presbyopia.

Clinical test to find out different types of hypermetropia:
- The ***strongest convex*** lens with which the patient can still maintain full distant vision (6/6)—indicates manifest hypermetropia.
- While, if the patient cannot normally see 6/6 without a lens—then the ***weakest convex lens*** that will allow him to read this line indicates his absolute hypermetropia.
- Facultative hypermetropia is the manifest hypermetropia minus absolute hypermetropia (fH = mH − aH).

Treatment

Mild hypermetropia without any definite symptom does not require any treatment especially for young individual.

Treatment is required in middle-aged patient, in high hypermetropia and if the patient is having symptoms. Treatment may be ***optical, surgical,*** and ***laser***.

Optical

Glasses and contact lens.
- ***Glasses:*** Convex lenses are prescribed after full cycloplegic correction, particularly in children. Refraction under atropine is obligatory for small children.
  - A child with convergent squint may require ***full atropine correction***. But such glasses often make the distant vision blurred.
  - So a fair compromise ***(rule)*** may be manifest hypermetropia plus a quarter of latent hypermetropia for final prescription.
  - ***Contact lens:*** The power is little more than spectacle power. It is useful for high hypermetropia.

Surgical

- Clear lens extraction with IOL implantation (monofocal or multifocal)—may be a choice for hypermetropic patients above 40 years of age.
- Intraocular lens implantation—most popular in aphakic hypermetropia.

Laser

Photorefractive keratoplasty (PRK) with excimer laser or hyperopic LASIK. Here, peripheral cornea is made thinner with laser, thereby cornea becomes more convex.

MYOPIA (SHORT-SIGHTEDNESS)

It is that dioptric condition of the eye in which, incident parallel rays come to a focus anterior to the light sensitive part of the retina, when accommodation is at rest.

Myopia means ***I shut the eye***; the term was introduced from the habit of half-shutting the eye (gaining the advantage of stenopeic slit vision) to improve distant vision.

Etiology

- ***Axial myopia:*** When the axial length is more.
- ***Curvature myopia:*** When the curvature of the cornea or lens is more, e.g. kerato-

conus, keratoglobus or megalocornea, and lenticonus.

- *Index myopia:* Nuclear sclerosis and in diabetes (as the index of nucleus is more).
- *Forward displacement of the lens.*

The progressive myopia is largely hereditary (recessive) and frequently racial. Here, the characteristic changes of distension and degeneration at the posterior pole of the eye is genetically determined.

There are few reports which state that myopia is aggravated by close work, watching TV, computer game or any other *exactions* of the civilized world.

Clinical Types

It is of three types—*congenital*, *simple*, and *pathological*.

1. *Congenital or developmental myopia*
   - The child is born with elongated eyes.
   - The refraction may be up to –10D.
   - Typical fundus changes are seen.
   - Progression is rare.
2. *Simple myopia*
   - Most common clinical type.
   - Does not progress much after the adolescence.
   - May be up to –5D or –6D.
   - No degenerative changes are seen in the fundus, although peripheral retinal degeneration may be seen in later life.
   - Associated with good vision with a good prognosis.
3. *Pathological myopia*
   - It is also called *progressive* or *degenerative myopia*.
   - Myopia appears in childhood (5–10 years of age), and increasing steadily with age up to 25 years or beyond.
   - The final amount of myopia may be –15D to –25D or more.
   - There are typical degenerative changes in the fundus.
   - Strongly hereditary and more common in female.

- More in Japanese, Chinese or Jews.
- Prognosis is usually poor.

If the myopia is more than –6D, it is called high myopia.

Optics

- Far point of the emmetropic eye is at infinity. But in myopia, the far point is at a finite distance in front of the eye (Figs 7.4A to C).
- In myopia, the rays coming from a point on the retina are less divergent than the corresponding rays in emmetropic eye.
- So, in myopic eye, the clear image is only possible when the diverging power of optical system is increased, i.e. by means of a concave lens (Fig. 7.4D).
- Since the nodal point is farther away from the retina, the image is larger, but blurred.

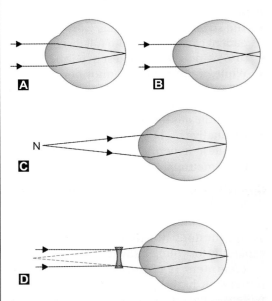

Figs 7.4A to D: Optics of myopia. **A.** Parallel rays are being focused upon the retina (emmetropia); **B.** Parallel rays being focused 'in front' of the retina (myopia); **C.** When looking at a near object, the divergent rays are focused upon the retina. N is the near point; **D.** Parallel rays are brought to focus upon the retina by a concave spectacle lens

- There may be an apparent convergent squint due to the presence of large negative *angle alpha*.

Symptoms

- ***Impaired distant vision:*** This is the most prominent symptom. Greater the degree of myopia, greater is the blurring for distant vision.

  Serious visual loss with loss of central vision may be seen in progressive myopia.
- ***Eye strain:*** It is only with small degree of error, but not so obvious as in case of hypermetropia.
- ***Exophoria*** or ***divergent squint:*** Myope exerts less accommodation → converge to a lesser extent → leading to exophoria, or even a manifest divergent squint. (Accommodation will worsen rather than to improve vision, in myopic eye).
- ***Black floaters*** (due to vitreous degeneration), and sometimes ***flashes of light*** are noticed.
- ***Delayed dark adaptation*** or even night blindness seen in progressive myopia.
- ***Sudden loss of vision*** due to retinal detachment which may lead to ultimate blindness (especially in pathological myopia).

Signs

Opposite of those found in hypermetropia:
- Prominent eyeball (pseudo-proptosis)

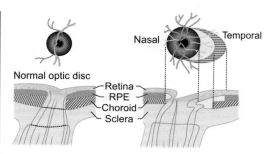

Fig. 7.5: The myopic crescent and super traction crescent

RPE—Retinal pigment epithelium

Note: Retina and choroid become separated from the disc on the temporal side, forming a myopic crescent. They encroach over the disc on the nasal side forming the supertraction crescent, thus blurring the disc margin

- Larger cornea, deep anterior chamber and a large pupil
- Apparent convergent squint
- Degeneration (liquefaction) of the vitreous.
- ***Ophthalmoscopically (Figs 7.5 and 7.6):***
  - ***In simple myopia:*** It is almost normal, with only a large disc. Temporal crescent may be seen. There may be peripheral retinal degenerations.
  - ***In pathological myopia***
    - ***Optic disc:*** Large disc with mild pallor. Large physiological cup. Temporal crescent (Fig. 7.6A), or sometimes annular crescent (Fig. 7.6B). There

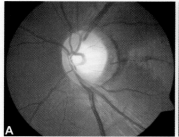 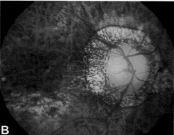 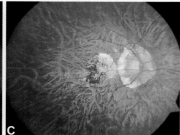

Figs 7.6A to C: Fundoscopic findings in myopia. **A.** Temporal crescent; **B.** Annular crescent; **C.** Retinal degeneration

may be supertraction crescent on nasal side. Posterior staphyloma.
- *Macula: Dull, **Foster-Fuchs fleck*** (spot) and degeneration (Fig. 7.6C).
- *General fundus:* Pale and tessellated appearance. There may be choroidal sclerosis and patches of choroidal atrophy.
- *Peripheral retina:* Cystoid degeneration is common, other degenerations are also seen.
- *Incidence of open-angle glaucoma* is more (applanation tonometry is mandatory as the scleral rigidity is low in myopia).

Complications

These are mainly with progressive myopia.
- Retinal tear → vitreous hemorrhage
- Retinal detachment
- Degeneration of the vitreous
- Primary open-angle glaucoma (higher incidence).
- Posterior cortical and nuclear cataract.

Treatment

Optical

Glasses and contact lens.
- *Glasses:* By appropriate concave lenses. *Myopia must never be overcorrected*
  - *In cases of low myopia (up to –6D):* A full correction is given for constant use, especially for children. In adults, weaker lenses for near work are essential.
  - *In high myopia (more than –6D):* Slight undercorrection is always done, and same, or weaker lenses are prescribed for the near work.

  Problems of high minus glasses
  - Minification of the object and the image appears very bright and clear, which is uncomfortable.
  - Image distortion ('barrel' distortion) due to spherical aberration.

- Reduced peripheral field of vision.
- Cosmetically, the eyes appear smaller behind the glasses.
- *Contact lenses:* It have most important role in myopic correction.

Advantages
- Less magnification of image
- Image distortion can be eliminated
- Field of vision is increased
- May arrest myopia to-some-extent.

Disadvantages
- Not tolerated by all patients
- Needs extreme accuracy and hygiene
- Costly
- Corneal problems, like infection, abrasions, etc. are dangerous.

Surgery

- *Keratorefractive surgeries*
  - *Radial keratotomy (RK) (Figs 7.7 and 7.8):* Here, the myopia is reduced completely or partially by flattening the

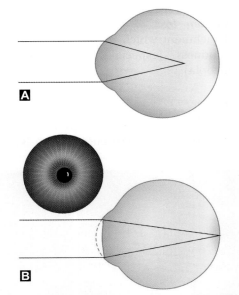

Figs 7.7A and B: Radial keratotomy. **A.** Parallel rays in front of retina in myopia; **B.** Parallel rays being focused upon the retina after radial keratotomy

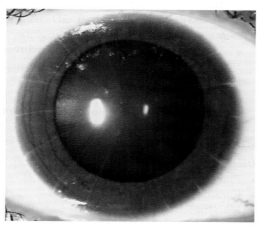

Fig. 7.8: Radial keratotomy—16 radial cuts

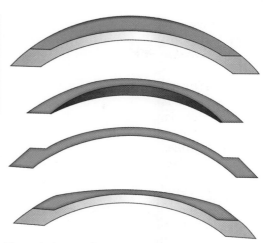

Fig. 7.9: Myopic keratomileusis

cornea, by giving a series (4–16) of deep radial incisions. Obsolete procedure nowadays.

- *Keratomileusis (Fig. 7.9):* A lenticule is prepared from removed anterior part of the cornea of the patient and re-shaped. This is also an obsolete procedure.
- *Fukala's operation:* Removal of clear crystalline lens if the myopia is –21D or near, and make the patient aphakic.
- *Clear lens extraction (CLE):* Extracapsular cataract extraction with posterior chamber intraocular lens (PCIOL) implantation may be a good choice in high myopia. Here, the lens may be clear without any cataractous change.

Minus phakic intraocular lens: A minus anterior chamber intraocular lens (ACIOL) or PCIOL implantation is done, even in presence of clear crystalline lens.

Among these, removal of clear crystalline lens with PCIOL implantation and phakic IOL implantation are becoming popular nowadays throughout the world.

Intracorneal rings (ICR): Two rings are inserted intrastromal corneal ring segments (INTACS) in the paracentral area to flatten the central cornea. This is especially useful in keratoconus.

Laser

- *Photorefractive keratoplasty:* Here, the cornea is re-shaped by photoablation of superficial corneal tissue by excimer laser. Photorefractive keratoplasty (PRK) is now replaced by laser-assisted stromal *in situ* keratomileusis (LASIK) procedure.
- *LASIK*: Here, the superficial corneal flap is lifted first, and then central corneal stromal bed is ablated by excimer laser to correct myopia. It is the most popular method nowadays. But it is a very costly procedure (Figs 7.10A to D).

General Hygiene

It is important in case of children like, good nutritional diet, exercise, fresh environment, proper position for reading in good illumination, etc. *But exercise of the extraocular muscles cannot cure myopia, or other refractive errors*.

Note: Femtosecond laser assisted surgeries for myopia are described in Chapter 28 (Page 559).

Genetic Counselling

There need be no restraint on marriage and procreation among simple myopes.

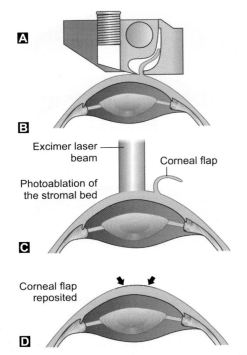

Figs 7.10A to D: LASIK procedure. **A.** Lamellar corneal flap by microkeratome; **B.** Corneal flap being lifted; **C.** Excimer laser photoablation; **D.** Flap re-posited. Cornea is thinner and flatter

- A parent with degenerative myopia should be warned that any offspring may have same disability.
- Two highly myopic adults with degenerative changes should never, from the medical point of view, have children.

ASTIGMATISM

It is the type of refractive error, in which the incident parallel rays do not come to a point focus upon the retina, due to refraction varies in different meridians of the eye.

Etiology

Curvature astigmatism

- **Corneal**
  - Astigmatism 'with the rule' (direct astigmatism)—theoretically, no eye is 'stigmatic' as the vertical meridian is more curved than horizontal by 0.25D owing to pressure of the upper lid over the globe.
  - Astigmatism 'against the rule' (indirect astigmatism) when the horizontal curvature is greater than vertical.
    - It may be seen as normal variation.
    - Postoperative following cataract surgery or trabeculectomy.
- **Lenticular:** As in lenticonus.

Diseases of the cornea
- Pterygium
- Keratoconus
- Marginal degeneration
- Corneal scar.

Index astigmatism: In early cataract, due to inequalities of refractive index in different sectors (cause of polyopia).

Decentration of the lens
- Subluxation of the crystalline lens
- Decentration or tilting of the IOL.

Types
Regular Astigmatism

The two principal meridians of greatest and least curvature are at right-angle to each other.
1. **Oblique:** The two meridians do not lie in the principal planes but remain at right angle to each other.
2. **Bi-oblique:** The axes are not right-angled but crossed obliquely.

It is of following types (Figs 7.11A to E):
- **Simple:** Where one of the principal meridian is emmetropic and the other is myopic or hypermetropic (**simple myopic or simple hypermetropic astigmatism**).
- **Compound:** Where both the principal meridians are either myopic or hypermetropic (**compound myopic or compound hypermetropic astigmatism**).
- **Mixed:** Where one principal meridian is myopic, and the other one is hypermetropic. Visual acuity is relatively less impaired in mixed astigmatism.

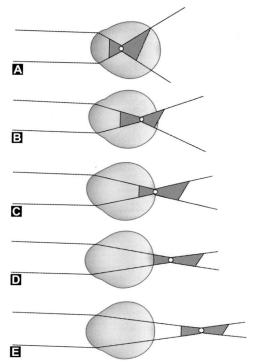

Figs 7.11 A to E: Classification of regular astigmatism (o: circle of least diffusion). **A.** Compound myopic astigmatism; **B.** Simple myopic astigmatism; **C.** Mixed astigmatism; **D.** Simple hypermetropic astigmatism; **E.** Compound hypermetropic astigmatism

Irregular Astigmatism

Here, the surface is so distorted that it admits no geometrical analysis, and it cannot be corrected adequately with glasses.
- Scarring of the cornea
- Keratoconus
- Incipient cataract
- Lenticonus
- After penetrating keratoplasty.

Optics

A regularly astigmatic surface is said to have a *toric curvature*.
- The more curved meridian will have more convergent power, than the less curved.

- If parallel rays fall upon such a surface, the vertical rays will come to a focus sooner than the horizontal.
- The rays after refraction will be symmetrical when referred to the vertical and horizontal planes, but they will have two foci.
  - The whole bundle of rays is called *Strum's conoid*, and the distance between the two foci, is called *focal interval of Strum*.
  - Refractive properties of such astigmatic surface are described in Figure 7.12.
The surface is having different curvatures in two meridians—the vertical meridians (VV) being more curved than horizontal (HH). The appearances of the bundle of rays at different points are illustrated in the Figure 7.12.
- *Point A* is a horizontal oval ellipse, since vertical rays are converging more rapidly than the horizontal.
  If the retina is placed at A: Compound hypermetropic astigmatism results.
- *Point B* will be horizontal straight line, as the vertical rays have come to a focus, while the horizontal rays are still converging.
  If the retina is placed at B: Vertical meridian is emmetropic, whereas the horizontal meridian is still hypermetropic, resulting in simple hypermetropic astigmatism.
- *Point C, D and E:* The vertical meridian will be in the condition of a myopic, and the horizontal still in that of a hypermetropic eye—this is mixed astigmatism.

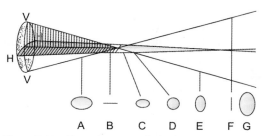

Fig. 7.12: 'Strum's conoid'—refraction by an astigmatic lens

- *Point D:* The two opposing tendencies are equal and the section becomes a circle—this is called *the circle of least diffusion*.
- *Point F:* The vertical meridian is still myopic (divergent) and the horizontal rays have come to a focus (emmetropic)—the section will be a vertical line. This is simple myopic astigmatism.
- *Point G:* Section is vertically oval, since both the rays are diverging.

  If the retina is placed at G: Both meridians are myopic, and it is compound myopic astigmatism.

Importance of circle of least diffusion: Distant vision is often found to be surprisingly good with relatively high degree of mixed astigmatism. This is because, the circle of least diffusion falls upon or near the retina, and there is least amount of distortion of the images at this point.

Symptoms

- Decrease in visual acuity.
- *Asthenopia or eye strain*: It is often worse in low degree of astigmatism than in higher, because of endeavors to accommodate so as to produce a circle of least diffusion upon the retina. This is more in hypermetropic astigmatism.
- Eye ache and headache
- *Running together* of the letters while reading, and the eyes quickly become fatigued.

Signs

- Head tilt in children, especially in oblique astigmatism.
- Half-closure of the lids (as in myope) to achieve greater clarity of stenopeic vision.
- Signs of causative factor (e.g. scarring of the cornea, decentration of the lens, etc.).
- Ophthalmoscopically, the disc appears oval or tilted in high degree of astigmatism.

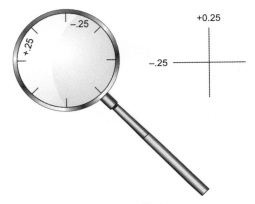

Fig. 7.13: Jackson's cross cylinder

Investigations

- *Retinoscopy:* For determination of its power and axis.
- *Keratometry:* To measure the corneal curvatures. It is useful to measure the power and axis of corneal astigmatism, and to find out irregular corneal surfaces.
- *Jackson's cross cylinder (Fig. 7.13):* The most convenient form is a combination of a −0.25D sphere with + 0.50 D cylinders.

  It is to check the power and axis of the cylinder in the optical correction.
- *Astigmatic fan (Fig. 7.14):* It is also to measure the amount and axis of the astigmatism.

  The cylinder which renders the outline of the whole fan equally clear, is a measure of astigmatism. And the axis of the cylinder is at right angle to the line, which was initially most clearly defined.
- *Astigmatic dial:* It measures the degree of astigmatism in relation to the cornea (Fig. 7.15).
- *Placido's disc:* To find out irregular corneal surfaces.
- *Photokeratoscope:* Illuminated Placido's disc with photographic facility. This is for permanent record.
- *Computerized corneal topography.*

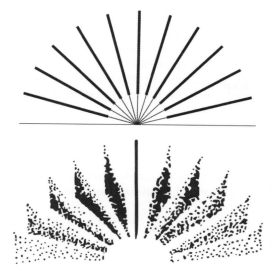

Fig. 7.14: (Above) Astigmatic fan. (Below) As seen by a patient with astigmatism at a horizontal axis. The vertical lines appear most clear and the others are progressively less well-defined

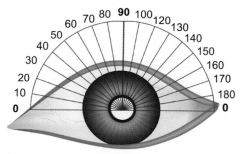

Fig. 7.15: Degree of astigmatism in relation to the cornea

Treatment
Regular Astigmatism

- *Spectacles:* Full cylindrical correction with perfect axis. It should be used both for the distant and near vision.
- *Contact lenses:* Rigid lenses are useful. Soft contact lens can correct only little astigmatism.
- *Surgery*
  - Astigmatic correction by giving cuts in the direction of more curved or steep axis called limbal relaxing incision (LRI).
  - Removal of sutures—in astigmatism following cataract surgery or keratoplasty.
- *Laser:* Excimer laser (by LASIK or PRK) is used to re-shape the cornea in a particular meridian.

Irregular Astigmatism

Best treatment is by contact lens. Excimer laser may be helpful phototherapeutic keratectomy (PTK) for superficial corneal scar responsible for irregular astigmatism.

APHAKIA

Literally, "aphakia" means absence of the crystalline lens from the eyeball. *Optically,* it means absence of the crystalline lens from its normal anatomical position in the pupillary area (patellar fossa).

Etiology

- *Congenital:* Rare
  - *Primary:* It is resulting from failure of the development of the lens in fetal life.
  - *Secondary:* The lens forms but gets absorbed *in utero* due to some factors.
- *Acquired*
  - *Postoperative (most common):* Following cataract surgery [needling, intracapsular cataract extraction (ICCE) or extracapsular cataract extraction (ECCE)].
  - *Post-traumatic:* Following blunt or penetrating injury of the eye. It includes subluxation or dislocation of the lens.
  - *Post-inflammatory:* Following large perforated corneal ulcer.
  - *Couching:* An ancient surgery (still practiced by some quacks), where the lens is forcibly dislocated into the vitreous by a needle via limbus.

Optics

The optical condition of the aphakic eye is very simple. It consists of a curved surface, the cornea, separating two media of different refractive indices—air (1.00) and aqueous plus vitreous (1.33).

- As the radius of curvature of cornea is 8 mm, the:
  - Anterior focal distance—23 mm (15 mm in the normal eye)
  - Posterior focal distance—31 mm (24 mm in the normal eye)
  So parallel rays of light brought to a focus 31 mm behind the cornea (Fig. 7.16).
- The dioptric system must, therefore, be supplemented by a strong converging (convex) lens, and usually, if the eye were originally emmetropic, of about +10D.
- The nodal point of the eye is thus moved forward.
- If the aphakic eye is 31 mm long, the rays will focus upon the retina and no correcting lens would be required for the distant vision. The axial myopia of a phakic eye which is 31 mm long—equals to –21D.

Optical Defects

- *Acquired high hypermetropia:* Crystalline lens contributes +15D to +20D in the normal eye.
- *Astigmatism against the rule:* Since, the cornea is flatter in vertical meridian, and it is due to contracture or fibrosis of the limbal scar. The amount of astigmatism is +1.0 to +3.0D initially, but gradually diminishes.
- *Absence of accommodation.*
- *Change in color vision:* Due to increased entry of infrared or ultraviolet rays into the eye, which are normally absorbed by the crystalline lens.

Clinical Features

- *History*
  - Blurred vision for distance and near.
  - History of cataract operation in most cases.
- *Signs:* Following a standard cataract surgery.
  - *Vision* (unaided)—only finger counting at 2–3 ft. Patient may have thick convex glasses, or if recently operated, using dark glasses.
  - *Sutures* may be visible at the upper limbus.
  - *Linear scar* at the upper limbus.
  - *Anterior chamber:* Deep (as the iris recedes back in absence of the lens).
  - *Iris:* (1) Iridodonesis or tremulousness of iris due to loss of support from the lens. (2) Peripheral buttonhole iridectomy (PI) mark (Fig. 7.17).

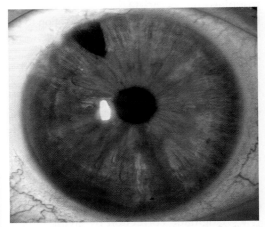

Fig. 7.17: Very good aphakia with peripheral button-hole iridectomy (PI) mark

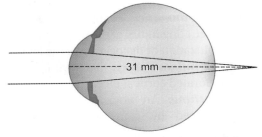

31 mm

Fig. 7.16: Hypermetropia in aphakia. Parallel rays are brought to a focus, 31 mm behind the cornea

- **Pupil:** Jet black reflex (due to loss of reflection of light rays from the anterior surface of the lens).
- Absence of 3rd and 4th Purkinje images (in ICCE) and only absence of 3rd image (in ECCE).
- **Retinoscopy:** Reveals high hypermetropia and astigmatism.
- **Ophthalmoscopy:** As in hypermetropic fundus with a small optic disc.

In **congenital aphakia** or in **dislocation of lens,** the clinical pictures are different, as there is:

- No history of operation
- No limbal scar mark
- No astigmatism
- Poor vision even with glasses because of amblyopia or other complications.

Treatment (Fig. 7.18)

Spectacle Correction

If the eye is previously emmetropic the power will be approximately:

Distant vision: +10.0 DSph with +2.0 DCyl × 180°.

Near vision: +13.0 DSph with + 2.0 DCyl × 180°.

Two separate glasses are given for distant and near vision. Bifocal glasses are usually troublesome, as most of the patients cannot tolerate them.

A +3.0 DSph addition is given for near vision, as there is loss of accommodation due to absence of lens, and the comfortable reading distance is 33 cm (i.e. 100/33 = +3.0D).

Glasses are prescribed usually 4 to 6 weeks after the surgery, as by this time wound healing is nearly completed.

Disadvantages of aphakic glasses

- **Image magnification (Fig. 7.19)** of about 25–30%.
- **Spherical aberration (Fig. 7.20):** Producing 'pin-cushion distortion'. Patient finds himself in a 'parabolic world'.
- **Lack of physical coordination,** particularly for finer movements.
- **Roving-ring scotoma (Fig. 7.21)** or **Jack-in-the-box** phenomenon—due to prismatic aberration at the edge of the thick lens.
  The scotoma extends from 50–65° from central fixation. It is not fixed, and its movements are initiated by the movements of the eyeball.
- Restriction of the visual field, and **poor eccentric visual acuity.**
- In monocular cases—there will be **high aniseikonia,** resulting in binocular diplopia. So, the normal eye must be blocked by a frosted or a balanced (+10.0D) glass.
- **Colored vision**—due to absence of natural filter of the crystalline lens, and due to chromatic aberration.
- Inaccurate spectacle correction because of erroneous vertex distance.
- The glasses are very thick, heavy, and cumbersome.

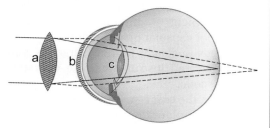

Fig. 7.18 Correction of aphakia
a—Spectacle; **b**—Contact lens; **c**—Intraocular lens

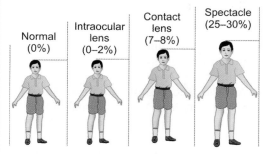

Fig. 7.19: Image magnification

Normal (0%)
Intraocular lens (0–2%)
Contact lens (7–8%)
Spectacle (25–30%)

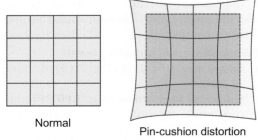

Normal

Pin-cushion distortion

Fig. 7.20: Spherical aberration in a high-power convex lens

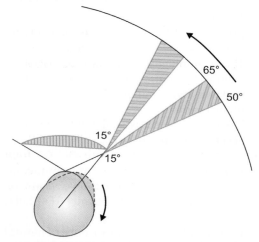

Fig. 7.21: Roving-ring scotoma in spectacle-corrected aphakia. Depending on the position of the eye, objects tend to appear and disappear

- Cosmetically embarrassing—as the eyes appear larger behind the glasses.

Contact Lens

Advantages

- Image magnification is 7–8%, and this magnification is usually tolerated by the patient.
- All the aberrations are less, so there is (1) increase in the visual field, (2) improvement of physical coordination, and (3) better eccentric visual acuity.
- In monocular cases, diplopia is usually absent with retention of binocularity.

- *In traumatic cases*, contact lens is the only mean to correct aphakia, where IOL implantation may not be possible.
- Cosmetically, it is well accepted.

Disadvantages

- Lack of dexterity in old patients.
- Foreign body sensation.
- Lens spoilage (due to loss, breakage, dislodgement, etc.) leading to high recurrent expenditure.
- Corneal complications—like erosions, ulceration, edema, vascularization, etc. may be troublesome.
- Light spectacles are required for reading, and/or for distant vision.

Secondary Intraocular Lens Implantation

Advantages

- Image magnification is only 0–1%.
- No spherical and prismatic aberrations.
- Minimum or no aniseikonia, with rapid return of binocularity.
- Normal peripheral field of vision and eccentric vision.
- Good hand-eye coordination and spatial sensation.
- Freedom from handling of the optical devices (e.g. contact lens or heavy spectacles).
- Cosmetically, it is best accepted.

Disadvantages

- Risks and complications may be more, e.g. corneal decompensation, lens displacement, chronic iridocyclitis, posterior capsular opacification, etc.
- It needs specially trained surgeons and sophisticated instruments, like operative microscope.
- Initially, the cost is more.

An IOL implantation may be done in an aphakic eye after careful examination. This may be:

- *Secondary anterior chamber IOL* in aphakia following ICCE.
- *Secondary posterior chamber IOL* in aphakia following ECCE.
- *Secondary scleral fixation IOL (SFIOL)* in aphakia following ICCE.

The best optical correction is, of course, a primary PCIOL implantation, which is the *most current concept in the surgical management of cataract.* Intraocular lens details are discussed in Chapter 25.

ANISOMETROPIA

This is a condition in which the refractions of the two eyes are unequal.

It is extremely common in small amount, and may be found in every possible variety.

Etiology

- Usually congenital
- Unequal rates of change in refraction between the two eyes.
- Corneal diseases and cataract.
- Following surgical and nonsurgical trauma.

Vision

- *Binocular vision:* It is the rule with smaller degrees of defect.
  Each 0.25D difference between the two eyes causes 0.5% difference in size between the two retinal images.
  A difference of 5% of the image size can be tolerated well (i.e. 2.50D difference of refraction between two eyes). If it is more, the effort of fusion may give rise to the symptom of eye strain or diplopia.
- *Alternating vision:* Each of the two eyes is used one at a time, e.g. one eye is emmetropic or mild hypermetropic, but the other eye is myopic.

- *Exclusively uniocular:* If the defect in one eye is high with poor visual acuity, the other and better eye will then be used exclusively. In this case, the worse eye will soon become amblyopic.

Problems with Anisometropia

- *Imperfect binocular vision*—an effort to fuse the images leads to symptom of eyestrain.
- *Amblyopia (anisometropic)*, especially in children.
- *Development of squint*—convergent squint in children and divergent in adult.
- *Diplopia*—due to unequal image sizes.

Treatment

- *Contact lenses*—are most suitable.
- *Iseikonic lenses*—correct the difeerence by their optical construction, but their clinical results are often disappointing.
- If the patient is amblyopic—treatment for amblyopia.
- Excimer laser PRK or LASIK.

Monovision
It is used in patients needing correction for both reading and distance. It is the practice of prescribing a corrective prescription for one eye for distant vision and the other eye for near vision. The idea is that a person will always be able to see both near and far. Unfortunately, acuity is only one aspect of vision. The eyes need to work together to produce a three-dimensional image in the brain. On using this type of correction, the person disrupts this ability which interferes with depth perception. Since one eye is corrected for near and one for far, one eye will always be in visual somatic dysfunction, causing very large and noticeable visual strains. These strains will eventually manifest as other symptoms.

Accommodation and its Disturbances

ACCOMMODATION (FIG. 8.1)

It is the ability to see the near object clearly, by increasing the converging power of the eye. This is by increasing the refractivity of the lens by increasing the curvature of its anterior surface.

At rest, the radius of curvature of the anterior surface of the lens is 10 mm and that of the posterior surface is 6 mm.

In accommodation, the curvature of the posterior surface remains almost the same, but the anterior surface changes, so that in strong accommodation, its radius of curvature becomes 6 mm. The refraction of the eye in this condition is called its *dynamic refraction*.

Mechanism of Accommodation

In unaccommodative state of the eye, the suspensory ligament is in tension, so the lens remains flat (Fig. 8.2).

In accommodation: There is contraction of the ciliary muscles → reduction of the circle formed by the ciliary processes → suspensory ligament relaxes → elastic capsule of the lens acts unrestrainedly to deform the lens substance → lens then alters its shape to become more spherical (perhaps conoidal).

This conoidal shape assumes by the lens, may be due to configuration of the capsule, which is thicker behind the iris than in the center.

The shape of the lens is thus the result of a balance between its own elasticity and that of its capsule *(modern version of von Helmholtz theory)*.

Accommodation Pathway

It initiates mainly by the fibers from the medial rectus muscle, which contracts on convergence.

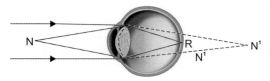

Fig. 8.1: Accommodation in an emmetropic eye parallel rays being focused upon the retina at R. When a near object N, is looked at, focus behind the retina at N[1]. In order to bring this upon at R (N[1]), the lens increases its convexity

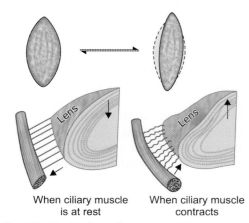

When ciliary muscle is at rest   When ciliary muscle contracts

Fig. 8.2: Mechanism of accommodation

Medial rectus muscle → via third nerve→ mesencephalic nucleus of fifth nerve → a presumptive center for convergence at pons → Edinger-Westphal nucleus → along the third nerve → accessory ciliary ganglion → sphincter pupillae muscle of the iris.

Range of Accommodation

- Far point (**punctum remotum**) is the farthest point at which object can be focused on the retina with ciliary muscle relaxed, and it varies with the emmetropia, myopia or hypermetropia.
- Near point (**punctum proximum**) is the nearest point at which small objects can be seen clearly after full accommodation.

Range of accommodation is the difference between these two distances.

Amplitude of accommodation (Fig. 8.3) is the difference in refractive power of the eye between these two points. It gradually diminishes throughout the life.

Physical and Physiological Accommodation

Two factors are responsible for the act of accommodation:

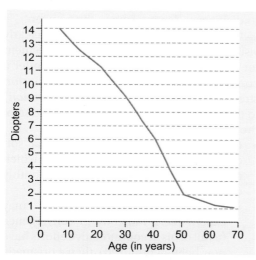

Fig. 8.3: Amplitude of accommodation with age

1. The ability of the lens to alter its shape (**physical accommodation**) and it is measured in diopter.
2. The power of the ciliary muscle to contract (**physiological accommodation**).

The physiological accommodation is the cause, and the physical accommodation is the effect.

There are two other phenomena which occur with accommodation—(1) pupils become smaller and (2) convergence of the eyes.

Age changes: As the age advances, the amplitude of accommodation progressively decreases—from 14D at the age of 10, to 4D at 45 years, and by 60 years it is only 1D years (near point then being one meter away). This is due to a progressive sclerosis of the lens so that it becomes less malleable, tending to set in unaccommodative shape.

Presbyopia

It means *the eye sight of old age*. This is a physiological aging process, in which the near point gradually recedes beyond the normal reading or working distance.

Causes

Diminution of accommodative power with age, and the factors are:
- Lens matrix is harder and less easily moulded.
- Lens capsule is less elastic.
- Progressive increase in size of the lens.
- Weakening of the ciliary muscle.

Symptoms

- Gradual difficulty in reading small prints, particularly in the evening or in dim illumination.
- Inability to perform near work meticulously, e.g. sewing, threading a needle, etc.
- Fatigue or headache while doing near work.

- ***Arms are not long enough*** is a common experience.

Treatment

To provide the patient with appropriate convex lens so that his accommodation is reinforced, and his near point is brought within a useful and workable distance.

Methods of prescription

- Knowledge of patient's **static refraction** (for distance).
- To know the distance at which the patient is accustomed to carry out his close work.
- Subjective test of near vision for each eye with addition of appropriate convex lenses to the distant correction.
- It is customary to start with an addition of +0.75 or +1.00 DSph.
- It is always better to under-correct than to over-correct. Since, if the lenses tend to be strong, the normal relation of accommodation and convergence will be disturbed.

Benjamin Franklin first invented the bifocal lens for his own presbyopia in 1783.

The glasses may be:

- ***Unifocal or monofocal lenses:*** It is in the form of rim (half-eye spectacles).
- ***Bifocals lenses (Figs 8.4A and B)***
  - ***Kryptok bifocals (Fig. 8.4A):*** These are crescent-shaped lenses for near vision. In kryptok bifocal, the near-field becomes smaller.
  - ***Executive bifocals (Fig. 8.4B):*** It has wider field, but cosmetically does not look nice and heavier.

Usual Rule (*Though Not Always Fixed*)	
Age	**Near addition**
40 years	+ 1.0 DSph
45 years	+ 1.5 DSph
50 years	+ 2.0 DSph
55 years	+ 2.5 DSph
60 years	+ 3.0 DSph
Above 60 years	+ 3.0 to + 3.5 DSph

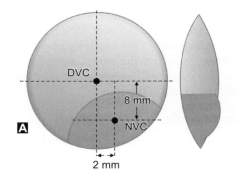

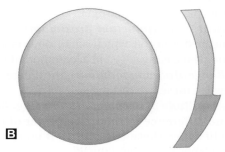

Figs 8.4A and B: Bifocal lenses. **A.** Kryptok; **B.** Executive **DVC**—Distant visual center; **NVC**—Near visual center.

- ***Trifocal*** or multifocal (omnifocal) lenses may also be given.
- ***Progressive multifocal lenses (Fig. 8.5) (no-line bifocals)*** correct vision for all distances—far, intermediate and near.

  Unlike bifocal lenses that have one clearly visible segment for near vision and one segment for distant vision; progressive lenses offer a continuous, gradual change in prescription strength from the lower (***reading correction***) to the upper (***distance correction***) portion of the spectacle's lens.
- ***Contact lenses:*** Usually, multifocal soft contact lenses. It is daily wear lens which may be daily disposable or monthly disposable.
  - ***Prisms:*** Sometimes patient may experience a difficulty in convergence (as all of his accommodative efforts have now been neutralized), then a prismatic addition is helpful.
  - ***Surgery:*** Various surgical methods have been proposed to treat presbyopia.

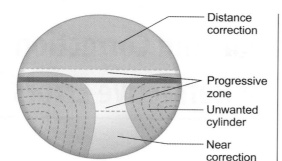

Fig. 8.5: Schematic representation of progressive lens demonstrating different zones of focus

These include—monovision LASIK, conductive keratoplasty (CK), presbyopic LASIK, and more recently, the corneal inlay. Beside these, presbyopic clear lens extraction with multifocal or accommodative intraocular lens (IOL) implantation. Anterior ciliary sclerotomy is another procedure proposed earlier.

Insufficiency of Accommodation

In this condition, the accommodative power is below the lower limit of normal for the patient's age.

Causes

- Early presbyopia.
- Weakness of the ciliary muscle due to general debility, anemia or toxemia.
- Open-angle glaucoma due to impairment of effectivity of the ciliary muscle by the increased intraocular pressure.

Symptoms

- Eye strain
- Difficulty with near work.

Treatment

- Treatment of the cause
- Reading spectacles (near addition)
- Accommodation exercises.

Paralysis of Accommodation

Causes

- **Unilateral**
  - Cycloplegics (e.g. atropine)
  - Contusion of the eye
  - Paralysis of the third cranial nerve.
- **Bilateral** (Paresis is more common)
  - Diphtheria
  - Syphilis
  - Diabetes
  - Alcoholism.

  Mydriasis usually accompanies the paralysis of accommodation. The prognosis is good in cases due to drugs or diphtheria. In trauma the condition may be permanent.

Treatment

- Treatment of the cause
- If the paralysis is permanent—suitable convex glasses may be prescribed
- Miotics are seldom useful.

Spasm of Accommodation

Causes

- Found mainly in children, who attempt to compensate his refractive error.
- Myopes are more affected than hypermetropes.
- May occur artificially by instillation of miotics (e.g. with pilocarpine in young glaucoma patients).
- Neurotic individuals who converge excessively.

Symptoms

- Asthenopia
- Blurring for distant vision (due to variable degrees of artificial myopia).

Treatment

- Atropinization for a few days or weeks.
- Assurance; if necessary, psychotherapy.

Estimation and Correction of Refractive Errors

In estimating the refraction of the eye the best routine is, first to estimate the condition *objectively*, and then to verify and adjust this finding by *subjective tests*.

Objective methods are:
- Retinoscopy (skiascopy or shadow test)
- Refractometry
- Keratometry.

OBJECTIVE METHODS

RETINOSCOPY

It is the most practical method of estimating the condition of refraction objectively, *with accommodation at rest*.

Optics: It entails a study of the movements of the retinal image produced by a beam of light that sweeps across the pupil.

The observer then watches this illuminated retinal image by looking down the path of incident light, through a hole in the center of a mirror (retinoscope) (Figs 9.1A and B).

- *If the eye is emmetropic:* Parallel rays of light come to a point focus on retina, so they are emerging in the same pathway.
- *If the eye is hypermetropic:* Parallel rays converge behind the retina and hence, the emerging rays are divergent.

The principle of retinoscopy is to make every observing eye emmetropic, so that the emerging rays should form a parallel beam.

Procedure

Cycloplegia

It is required in children and young patients. In adults and old patients, it is usually not necessary.

- *If the patient is less than 5 years:* Atropine eye ointment (1%) is to be applied three times daily for 3 days.
- *If the patient is between 5 and 15 years:* 1% cyclopentolate, or 2% homatropine eye drop is instilled for 3 times, about 1 hour before examination.
- *If the patient is between 15 and 20 years:* The same procedure may be undertaken.

The refraction under cycloplegia is always pathological because the shape of the lens has been altered. A *postcycloplegic test (PCT)* is therefore advisable.

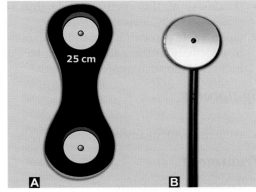

Figs 9.1A and B: Retinoscopic mirror. **A.** Double mirror. **B.** Single plane mirror

Dark-room Test

Retinoscopy should preferably be conducted in a darkroom.

- Examiner sits at 1 meter away from the patient (point of reversal will then be 1.5D). It is even more convenient to sit at arm's length, i.e. two-thirds meter away, so that the trial lenses can be held in the other hand while the light beam is passed. The point of reversal is then 1.5D.
- The patient is normally seated and looking toward the far end of the room (relaxed eye).
- Source of light is from behind the patient.
- The surgeon looks through a *plane mirror* with central perforation, and light is reflected into the patient's eye.
- The mirror is slowly moved from side to side in different meridians, and movement of the shadow is noted.
- In hypermetropia, emmetropia and myopia of less than 1.0D the reflex moves in the same direction, in myopia of 1.0D there is no shadow, in myopia of greater than 1D the shadow moves in the opposite direction.
- Increasing convex (if the movement is on the same side) or concave (if on the opposite side) lenses are placed before the eye until the *point of reversal* is reached. *At this point there will be no movement of the shadow, and pupil will be brightly illuminated.*
- The procedure is done for each meridians separately.
  - In simple spherical refractive error—the movement and the point of reversal will be same in both meridians.
  - In astigmatism, they are different. If the axes are oblique, the shadow themselves will seem to move obliquely and the mirror is then tilted accordingly.

Calculation

Refraction of patient's eye = lens required to reach end point = –1D (myopia).

Since the surgeon is sitting at 1 meter distance, and if he is at two-thirds meter, it will be –1.5D (myopic).

So the refraction of the eye = –1.0D + lens.

Examples

- If the end-point is with + 4.0 D lens:
  Refraction = –1.0D + 4.0D = +3.0D.
- Similarly with – 4.0D lens:
  Refraction = –1.0D – 4.0D = –5.0D
- If the end-point is with + 1.0D lens:
  Refraction = –1.0D + 1.0D = 0, i.e. the patient is emmetropic.
- In case of astigmatism, each meridian is to be calculated separately.

> **Streak retinoscopy (Figs 9.2A and B):** Instead of circular light as obtained by a plain mirror, a self-illuminated streak of light is used. Here, the appearances of the shadow are more dramatic. Axis of the astigmatism is easily determined. It has certain other advantages:
> - It can be done in any position of the patient.
> - It can be done in difficult patients, e.g. in children or non-cooperative patient or for the patient under general anesthesia.
> - It can be used preoperatively.

REFRACTOMETRY (OBJECTIVE OPTOMETRY)

It is a method to determine the degree of ametropia by special instrument called *refractometer*.

In it, a clear retinal image of a test object is formed by an optical system, and the degree of adjustment required, gives a measurement of the ametropia.

Recently, electronic refractometry (auto-refractometer) (Fig. 9.3) is popularly used in clinical practice. Apart from regular use, this instrument is excellent for quick screening of refractive errors in a given population.

KERATOMETRY (FIG. 9.4)

It measures the astigmatism of the anterior surface of the cornea at two points about 1.25 mm on either side of the center.

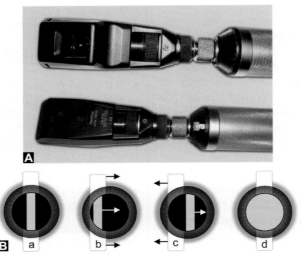

Figs 9.2A and B: A. Streak retinoscope. **B.** Reflexes taken by streak retinoscope at different point (a. Reflex parallel to retinoscopic streak; b. Reflex and streak in a "with" movement in hypermetropia; c. Reflex and streak in an against movement in myopia; d. Reflex at the point of neutralization)

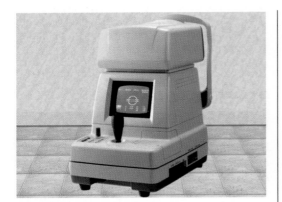

Fig. 9.3: Auto-refractometer

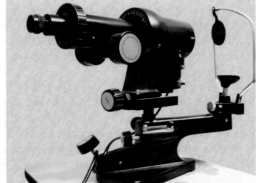

Fig. 9.4: Keratometer

Types of keratometry: manual and automated. Automated keratometry are more accurate, e.g., with simple auto-keratometry, with optical biometry devices; and by different corneal topography and tomography instruments.

Since lenticular astigmatism may coexist, *this technique is not reliable except in aphakia.* It is useful in measuring the curvature of the cornea:

- In contact lens practice.
- For diagnosis of certain corneal conditions, e.g. keratoconus, pellucid marginal degeneration, etc.

- Before cataract operation for measuring intraocular lens (IOL) power (biometry) and for planning of incision in cataract surgery to reduce astigmatism.

SUBJECTIVE METHODS

SUBJECTIVE VERIFICATION OF REFRACTION

After objective test, it should always be verified subjectively by testing the visual acuity. If a cycloplegic has been used, the process should be repeated in a *post-cycloplegic test*.

Procedures

- Each eye is to be tested separately, the other eye being blocked, and then finally tested together.
- Appropriate lenses as found by objective test are inserted in the trial frame.
- Slight modification of the inserted lens gives a maximum visual acuity.
- Verification may be needed with a *cross cylinder*, or *astigmatic fan* in case of astigmatism.
- Sometimes, *fogging method* is necessary to induce a relaxation of accommodation especially in hypermetropia.

> Here, the eyes are made artificially myopic by addition of convex lenses (e.g. + 4.0D). This is then gradually lessened by a small fraction (0.5D) until the maximum acuity is just reached. The first lens is not removed until the next is in position, to prevent from accommodation becoming active.

As a rule, the patient is given the strongest hypermetropic, or weakest myopic correction with normal visual acuity.

- The addition of the correction for near work (if necessary), and testing of the acuity with near-types, uniocularly and then binocularly.
- Then the spectacles are ordered with necessary comments (e.g. for constant wear, or near works only, etc).

EXAMINATION OF THE FUNDUS

Adequate ophthalmoscopic examination of the ocular fundus requires dilation of the pupil. *Caution is required in dilating the pupils of patients with shallow anterior chambers to avoid precipitation of an acute attack of angle closure glaucoma*. The methods of fundus examination should be as follows:

- *With a retinoscopic plain mirror from 1 meter distance:* This is to know the fundal glow and refractive status.
- *With an ophthalmoscope or a plain mirror at a distance of 22 cm (distant direct ophthalmoscopy):* This is:
  - To know the opacities in the media.
  - To discover the edge of a subluxated or dislocated lens.
  - To recognize a retinal detachment or a tumor.
  - To confirm the results found by external examination.
- *By direct ophthalmoscopy:* The details of central retina up to the equator are examined uniocularly. The image is erect and virtual. The magnification is about 15 times.
- *By indirect ophthalmoscopy:* The details of the retina up to the periphery (ora serrata) are examined binocularly.
- *By slit lamp with special lenses* (by eliminating refractive influence of the corneal curvature): (i) Hruby lens (–58.6D), (ii) fundus contact lens, (iii) Goldmann three-mirror contact lens and (iv) more popularly with the help of +90 D or +78 D lens.

Fundus examination includes (Fig. 9.5):
- *Fundal glow:* Good, poor or absent.
- *Optic disc:* Margin, color, shape, cup/disc ratio, neural rim, venous pulsation and any abnormal vessels.

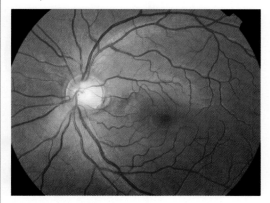

Fig. 9.5: Normal fundus

- *Retinal vessels:* Vascular reflexes, arterio-venous (AV) crossing, any abnormal or new vessels.
- *General fundus:* Any abnormality, e.g. exudates, hemorrhage, pigment patch, tumor, new vessels, etc.
- *Macula and foveal reflex:* The fovea centralis is situated about 2dd temporal to the optic disc (dd = disc diameter; 1 dd = 1.5 mm). Any abnormality, e.g. cyst, hole, scar, edema, hemorrhage, etc. should be looked for.
- *Choroidal blood vessels:* Normally they are not visible, but in case of sclerosis they appear as ribbons.

METHODS OF OPHTHALMOSCOPY

There are two forms of ophthalmoscopy—direct and indirect.

Direct Ophthalmoscopy (Figs 9.6A and B)

The hand-held direct ophthalmoscope is designed to provide a direct magnified (X15) view of the fundus. The source of illumination is projected by means of a mirror or prism coinciding with the observer's line of vision through the aperture.

Procedure

- The ophthalmoscope is held close to the observer's eye and approximately 15 cm from the patient's eye.
- It is held in the right hand and observer uses his/her right eye to examine patient's right eye. Similarly to examine the patient's left eye, it is held in the left hand and the observer uses his/her left eye.
- The patient should fix on a distant target with the eye as steady as possible.
- The observer has to adjust ophthalmoscope power setting to accommodate for the patient's refractive error and/or his/her own.
- If both patient and observer are emmetropic, the lens is set at 0. A red reflex will be seen and is considered normal.
- Moving the ophthalmoscope as close to the patient's eye as possible and using the 'plus' or 'minus' lens, the observer will able to see central retina in details up to the equator.
- Lens setting at more 'plus' power will focus the ophthalmoscope in the vitreous or more anterior.

Indirect Ophthalmoscopy (Figs 9.7A and B)

This technique is generally used by retina specialist and involves the use of ahead

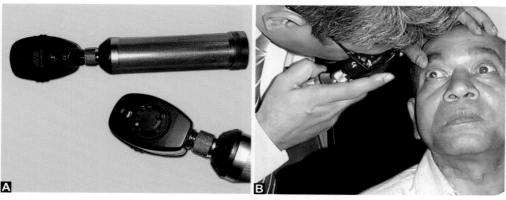

Figs 9.6A and B: **A.** Direct ophthalmoscope; **B.** Procedure of direct ophthalmoscopy

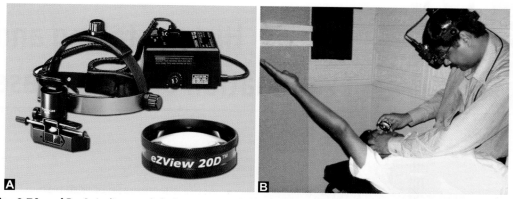

Figs 9.7A and B: A. Indirect ophthalmoscope with lens; **B.** Procedure of indirect ophthalmoscopy

mounted; prism directed light source coupled with use of a high condensing lens (+14, +20 or +30D) to see the retinal image. A +20D condensing lens is most commonly used.

The retinal image formed by the indirect ophthalmoscopy *is inverted, real and capable of being seen at the focal plane of the lens*.

The image is brilliantly illuminated, binocular stereoscopic one that covers approximately 10 times of the area compare to direct ophthalmoscope. The image is, however, smaller (X 3 times). It is essential to see retinal periphery to locate different types of lesions.

Because of its stronger illumination, it allows light to pass through moderate opacities in the media which are obstructive to direct ophthalmoscope.

History-taking and Examination of an Eye Case

HISTORY-TAKING

Before examining the patient's eye, a careful history of ocular complaints should be taken.

- Name, age, gender, address and occupation of the patient.
- Date of admission and/or date of examination.
- Chief presenting complaints of the patient, its duration and mode of presentation Common eye complaints are asfollows:
  - Painless progressive dimness of vision
  - Pain ⎫ may be together as
  - Redness ⎬ acute pain, redness
    ⎭ and watering
  - Watering and discharge
  - Itchiness of the eyes
  - Foreign body sensation
  - Sudden loss of vision
  - Dimness of vision at night
  - Stickiness of the eyelids
  - Small swelling on the eyelids
  - Abnormal fleshly mass in the eye
  - Disfigurement of the eyeball
  - White opacity over the black of the eye
  - Smallness of the eyeball
  - Abnormal deviation of the eyeball
  - Headache
  - History of any injury.
- *Past history*
  - Acute pain, redness and watering in the same eye or other eye
  - Ocular trauma
  - Wearing of spectacle
  - Acute infectious fever with rash
  - Similar problem in the other eye.
- *Operative history*
  - Any operation on the same eye or opposite eye with date of operation
  - Duration of hospital stay at that time
  - Any known operative complication.
- *Medical history including medication*
  - Diabetes, hypertension
  - Bronchial asthma
  - Tuberculosis
  - Tobacco, alcohol
  - Acidity, heart burn
  - Drug history including drug allergy
  - Straining factors (e.g. chronic cough, enlarged prostate or bleeding piles, etc.).

EXAMINATION OF AN EYE CASE

- *General examination:* Pallor, jaundice, pulse, respiration, blood pressure (BP), any obvious abnormalities (e.g. malnutrition in case of Bitot's spot or keratomalacia; Rickets in case of congenital cataract, pock marks on the face in leukoma, etc.).
  Heart, lungs, central nervous system (CNS), and gastrointestinal track (GIT).
- *Ocular examination:* Examination of the anterior segment of the eye (up to the lens–iris diaphragm) can be done by three methods:
  1. Diffuse illumination with a good torch light.

2. Focal/oblique illumination using a pencil torch and loupe (uniocular or binocular).
3. Focal/oblique illumination with the help of a slit-lamp biomicroscope.

METHOD OF EXAMINATION BY TORCH AND UNIOCULAR LOUPE

Patient is placed in a dark room and examined with a pencil torch light focused about 2 feet away from the patient's side.

The surgeon holds the loupe by thumb and index finger while lifting the upper lid by middle finger and two other fingers rest on eyebrow. Surgeon moves very close to the loupe to see the enlarged image of the cornea, iris or lens in details.

It is useful to search for *superficial punctate keratitis (SPK), keratic precipitates (KPs), minute foreign body, caterpillar hairs,* etc.

Uniocular Loupe

Its power is +40.0D (Fig. 10.1).
- *Advantages:*
  - 10 times magnified image
  - Small and handy instrument.
- *Disadvantages:*
  - Both hands are engaged during examination

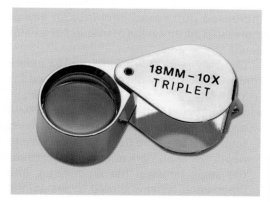

Fig. 10.1: Uniocular loupe

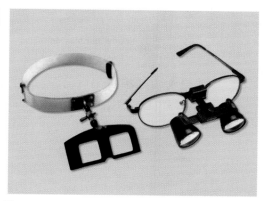

Fig. 10.2: Binocular loupe

- Inconvenience due to closeness to the patient
- No depth perception.

Binocular Loupe (Fig. 10.2)

It is kept fixed before the surgeon's eyes by an elastic band or a belt at forehead.
- *Advantages*
  - Both hands remain free during ocular examination
  - Depth of lesion is better judged
  - Convenient, as surgeon is away from the patient.
- *Disadvantages*
  - Low magnification (3–4 times)
  - Interpupillary distance may be difficult to adjust.

EXAMINATION WITH A SLIT LAMP

It is the best method as bright illumination and various grades of magnification are used.

A slit-lamp biomicroscope has three parts (Fig. 10.3):
1. Illumination system
2. Viewing system
3. Mechanical devices to adjust the slit lamp.

It is binocular, so depth perception is accurate. In fact, one can cut a cross section (optical

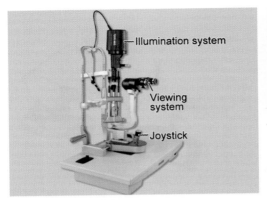

Fig. 10.3: Slit-lamp biomicroscope

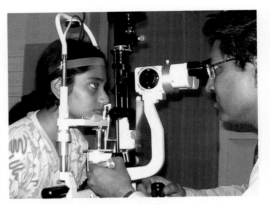

Fig. 10.4: Slit-lamp examination

section) of the anterior segment of the living eye for detailed microscopic examination (Fig. 10.4).

Uses

- Detailed microscopic examination of the anterior segment of the eye layer by layer.
- For fundus examination by Hruby (spell as Ruby) lens (–58.6D) or + 90D lens.
- For examination of angle of the anterior chamber by gonioscope.
- To measure intraocular pressure (IOP) by applanation tonometer.
- For fluorescein staining with blue filter.
- For anterior segment photography.
- As a delivery system for argon and yttrium aluminium garnet (YAG) laser.

Slit-lamp Examination of the Anterior Segment (Fig. 10.4)

Slit lamp offers a variety of illuminating and observing methods:

- Diffuse illumination
- Direct (focal) illumination
  - Broad beam (parallelepiped)
  - Narrow beam (optical section)
- Indirect illumination
- Retroillumination
  - Direct
  - Indirect
- Specular reflection
- Sclerotic scatter
- Oscillatory illumination.

Direct Diffuse Illumination (Figs 10.5A to C)

It is a good method of observing the eye and adnexa in general. Diffusers are generally ground glass plates that cover the light source. The slit should be opened wide and the magnification should be set as low as possible to enable a large field of view.

Direct Focal Illumination

This is the most common method of viewing all tissues of the anterior eye, the focused slit is viewed directly by the observer through the microscope. The magnification can be increased quite markedly (10x to 40x or more) to view any areas of interest in greater detail.

Generally a very wide beam is used for surface study, whilst a very narrow one is used for sections.

- ***Narrow beam (optical section) (Figs 10.6A and B):*** Once an abnormality has been found it is easier to determine the precise depth using an optical section. Generally the angle between the illuminating and observation systems should be set around 45–60°.

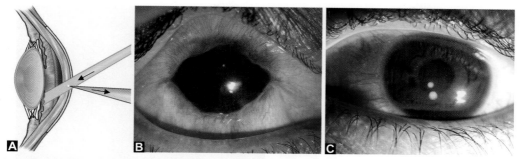

Figs 10.5A to C: Direct diffuse illumination. **A.** Schematic representation; **B and C.** Photograph

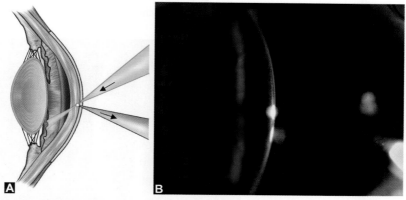

Figs 10.6A and B: Direct focal (narrow beam). **A.** Schematic representation; **B.** Photograph

A good corneal section will allow at least four layers to be seen—tears (outer), epithelium (and Bowman's membrane), stroma seen as the central gray granular area and the fainter back line which is the endothelium (and Descemet's membrane).

- *Broad beam (parallelepiped) (Figs 10.7A and B):* A useful combination of the two is the parallelepiped section of the cornea, which uses a 2 mm slit width enabling corneal surface as well as stroma to be studied. This allows us to ascertain the depth of any interesting feature, e.g. foreign body, corneal abrasion. Direct illumination on the front surface of the crystalline lens reveals the ***orange peel effect*** and on the iris allows observation of iris pattern.

Indirect Illumination (Figs 10.8A and B)

Structures are often easier to see under indirect illumination as glare is reduced, e.g. opacities, corneal nerves and limbal vessels.

When using the slit lamp, direct and indirect illumination are viewed simultaneously, structures viewed in the illuminated field are seen under direct illumination, but as this does not fill the whole of the field of view, anything which reflects or scatters light from outside the illuminated area is being viewed by indirect.

To view certain features by indirect illumination, first locate it by direct illumination and keeping the viewing system unchanged swing the lamp to oneside.

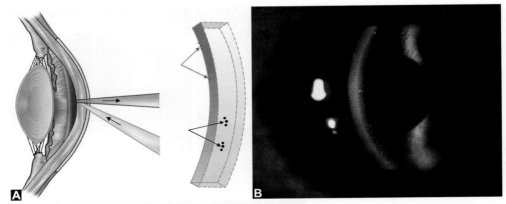

Figs 10.7A and B: Direct focal (broad-beam illumination). **A.** Schematic representation; **B.** Photograph

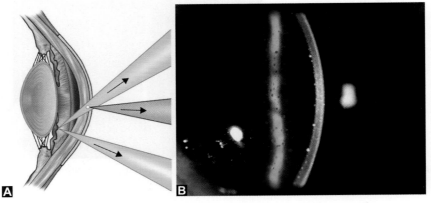

Figs 10.8A and B: Indirect illumination. **A.** Schematic representation; **B.** Photograph

Retroillumination

The light is reflected off the deeper structures, such as the iris or retina, while the microscope is focused to study the cornea in the reflected light. Features that are opaque to light appear dark against a light background (e.g. scars, pigment, and vessels containing blood).

- *Direct retroillumination (Figs 10.9A and B):* The observed feature on the cornea is viewed in the direct pathway of reflected light. The angle between the microscope and the illuminating arm is about 60°.
- *Indirect retroillumination (Figs 10.10A and B):* The angle between the microscope and slit lamp arms is greatly reduced or increased so that the feature on the cornea is viewed against a dark background.

Specular Reflection (Figs 10.11A to C)

This type of viewing is achieved by positioning the beam of light and microscope such that the angle of incidence is equal to the angle of reflection. The light can be reflected from either the anterior (i.e. tears and epithelium) or posterior (i.e. endothelium) corneal surface.

Note that the reflected light should pass through only one eyepiece and therefore this method is monocular.

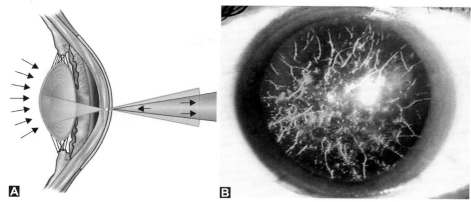

Figs 10.9A and B: Direct retroillumination. **A.** Schematic representation; **B.** Photograph

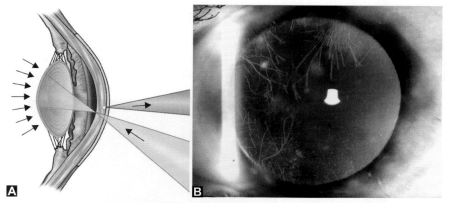

Figs 10.10A and B: Indirect retroillumination. **A.** Schematic representation; **B.** Photograph

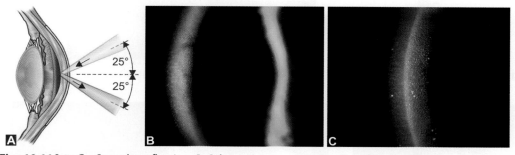

Figs 10.11A to C: Specular reflection. **A.** Schematic representation; **B and C.** Photograph

- *Method for viewing the posterior surface:* The angle between the light and microscope arms should be about 50–60°.

A 2 mm wide parallelepiped and magnification of 20x–25x is used.

Find the image of the illuminating bulb, then move the light beam until the image of the bulb is just behind the posterior surface of the parallelepiped (Incidence = reflection when the dazzle from the precorneal fluid is seen).

Focus on the back of the parallelepiped. A mosaic of hexagonal endothelial cells will appear. The posterior endothelium and keratic precipitates may thus be studied.

This method of illumination is particularly useful to examine the endothelium layer of the cornea (e.g. blebs, polymegathism), although very high magnification is necessary, at least 40x is required and to see individual cells at 80x.

Sclerotic Scatter (Figs 10.12A and B)

This method uses the principle of total internal reflection. A narrow vertical slit (1–1.5 mm in width) is directed in line with the temporal (or nasal) limbus. A halo of light will be observed around the limbus as light is internally reflected within the cornea, but scattered by the sclera.

Any corneal opacities, edema or foreign bodies will be made visible by the scattering light, appearing as bright patches against the dark background of the iris and pupil. It is important that the room illumination is as dark as possible.

Oscillatory Illumination

A beam of light is rocked back and forth by moving the illuminating arm or rotating the prism or mirror. Occasional aqueous floaters and glass foreign body in the anterior chamber are easier to observe.

Special Stains for Epithelial Lesions

- *Fluorescein staining (Fig. 10.13A):* To stain various corneal pathologies in the epithelium level, e.g. corneal abrasion,

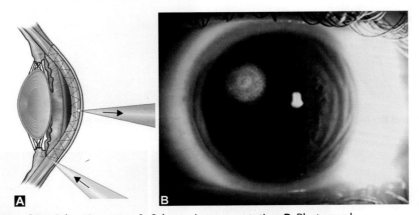

Figs 10.12A and B: Sclerotic scatter. **A.** Schematic representation; **B.** Photograph

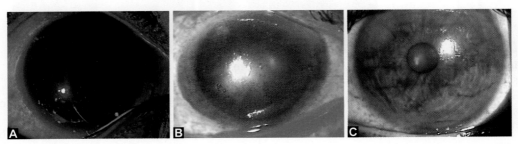

Figs 10.13A to C: Special stains. **A.** Fluorescein staining; **B.** Rose Bengal staining; **C.** Lissamine green staining

erosions, filaments, epithelial defects, dendrite in herpes simplex virus (HSV) keratitis, superficial punctate keratopathies (SPKs), Seidel's test, tear film break up time (TFBUT), etc.

- **Rose Bengal staining (Fig. 10.13B):** It is useful for devitalized tissue, e.g. dendrite in HSV keratitis, punctate epithelial erosions (PEE) in dry eye and other lesions, conjunctival stain in dry eyes. It causes mild to moderate irritations of the eyes.
- **Lissamine green staining (Fig. 10.13C):** It is same as rose Bengal, except it does not cause much irritation.

Ocular examination proforma

At the undergraduate level only anterior segment of the eye is to be examined. A good torch and loupe are necessary for this. Examination of each eye should be done separately. Always examine the right eye first.

Right eye   Left eye
- Visual acuity
- Ocular movement
- Lids: Lid margins, eyelashes, lid proper, palpebral aperture
- Conjunctiva
- Sclera
- Cornea
- Anterior chamber
- Iris
- Pupil: Size, shape, appearance
- Light reflex: Direct and consensual
- Lens
- Lacrimal apparatus
- Digital intraocular tension
- Palpation: Preauricular and submandibular lymph nodes, any swelling related to the eye
- Transillumination (only if there is a largemass)
- Head posture, visual axis, facial symmetry

In undergraduate examination, in some centers, examiner may ask to examine one eye only. In that case write your findings for that eye only. For the other eye, just have a look with the torch light, and keep the findings in your mind. This is for better correlation with your diagnosis and management during crossing by the examiners.

CLINICAL EXAMINATION OF THE EYE

Visual Acuity

It is the ability or power of the eye by which objects are distinguished one from the other.

It also measures the smallest retinal image, formed at the foveal region which can be appreciated regarding shape and size (central vision).

Visual acuity (VA) is tested for distant and near objects called **distant vision** and **near vision**. Each eye is to be tested separately without spectacle **[uncorrected visual acuity (UCVA)]** with spectacle **[best spectacle corrected visual acuity (BSCVA)]** and with pinhole for distant vision only.

Principle of Normal Visual Acuity

It means when two distinct points can be only recognizable as separate when they subtend an angle of 1 minute of an arc at the nodal point of the eye.

Nodal point is an imaginary optical center or point which lies just in front of the posterior pole of the crystalline lens in the schematic eye.

Distant Vision

In case of Snellen's chart, each letter is perfectly placed in a square which is divided into 25 small squares. Each single letter subtends an angle of 5 minute and each component part of the letter subtends an angle of 1 minute at the nodal point of the eye, from a given distance in meters.

Snellen's distant vision chart (Fig. 10.14)

Various charts are available in different languages, for illiterate (E chart or Landolt's broken ring) and for children (toys or picture chart).

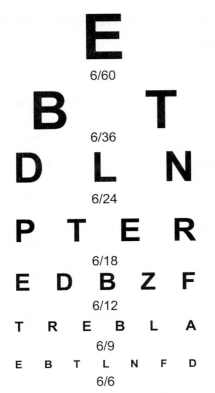

Fig. 10.14: Snellen's distant vision chart

The Snellen's chart should be read at a distance of 6 meters or 20 feet. If the room is 3 meters, with the help of a plane mirror and reverse chart this 6 meter distance is achieved. Rays coming from 6 meters or more are parallel for all practical purposes, hence accommodation does not come to play.

Visual acuity is written as numerator/denominator. **Numerator** is the distance of the patient from the chart and usually it is 6 meters or 20 feet. **Denominator** is the distance at which a normal person or the distance at which patient should be able to read.

As for example, 6/36 means that the patient reads from a distance of 6 meters what a normal person can read from a distance of 36 meters, or the patient reads from a distance of 6 meters what the patient should read from 36 meters. The normal distant visual acuity is recorded as 6/6 or 20/20.

Procedures of recording distant vision (Fig. 10.15)

The patient is asked to sit or stand at 6 meters distance (i.e. 20 feet). Patient is asked to close his left eye with the cup of the palm, little bit obliquely to cross the opposite forehead. Patient is asked to read with his right eye from the top line to downward. The last line that patient reads, is recorded as the visual acuity of the right eye, e.g. top letter is 6/60, 2nd line is 6/36, 3rd line is 6/24 and so on. If patient can read some letters (not all letters) of a line, in that case visual acuity is recorded as part (e.g. 6/9p, 6/12p, etc.).

- If the patient cannot read the first line (i.e. her visual acuity is less than 6/60), then she is brought nearer to the chart at a distance of 5 meters, 4 meters, 3 meters, and so on, till he is able to read the top letter of the chart. The vision is then recorded as 5/60, 4/60, 3/60, respectively.
- If the patient cannot read the top letter at 1 meter distance, he is then asked to count the examiner's finger against an illuminated background. The rough distance at which he can count finger is recorded, e.g. VA:FC (finger counting) at half meter.
- If vision is still less, the examiner will move his hand in front of the patient's eye. If he

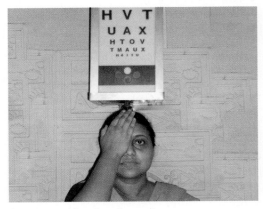

Fig. 10.15: Visual acuity testing

can appreciate the movements of the hand, then vision is recorded as hand movement (HM) close to face.

- If the patient cannot perceive hand movements—he is then taken to a dark room (ideally) and asked to close one eye firmly with the palm and look straight or look at his thumb of the other hand held in front of the eye to be tested and advised not to move that eye.

  The light is thrown on the open eye from all direction, i.e. up, down, nasal and temporal. If the patient can recognize the light and indicate its direction correctly, his visual acuity is perception of light (PL) and projection of Rays (PR) present.

  This vision is recorded as PL + PR⊠ in the right eye or left eye.

- If the patient is not able to perceive light from a particular quadrant, then a negative sign is put against that quadrant, e.g. VA = PL + PR⊠, i.e. patient is having inaccurate PR.

- If the patient can see the glow of light only, but cannot indicate the side of the projected rays, his VA is recorded as **only PL** with **inaccurate PR**.

> When light is thrown from one quadrant—the retina of the opposite quadrant is stimulated. "PL present" indicates the optic nerve is healthy with normal functioning nerve fiber layer of retina. PL is absent in optic atrophy.
>
> **PR accurate** indicates the normal function of peripheral four quadrants of the retina. PR may be defective in detachment of retina, big patch of chorioretinal atrophy, advanced open angle glaucoma, etc.

- Last of all, if the patient cannot see or perceive the glow of the torch light—his vision is recorded as VA = No PL.

  (Ideally, the illumination in the Snellen's chart is 100 foot candles, but it should not be less than 20 foot candles.)

  The other eye, i.e. left eye is to be tested in a similar manner.

Lastly, one should record the distant visual acuity with both eyes open, i.e. binocular distant visual acuity.

LogMAR Visual Acuity (Fig. 10.16)

LogMAR stands for logarithm of the minimum angle of resolution.

The chart was designed by Bailey and Lovie for the 'early treatment diabetic retinopathy study' (ETDRS) which is designed to be used at a distance of 4 meters.

At this distance the top lines will give a score of 1.0. Each line below will give a score 0.1 less than the line above.

Five letters are chosen for each line (using a balanced distribution). Each of the five letters, in each line, count for a score of 0.1/5 = 0.02.

Therefore, if a patient reads the 0.4 line in its entirety, he will have a score of 0.4.

If patient reads the 0.4 line plus three letters of the 0.3 line, then he will have a score of 0.34, which results from the five letters of line 0.4 minus the score for each letter read from the 0.3 line, i.e. $0.40 - (0.02 \times 3) = 0.34$.

Principle of LogMAR Chart

Ten Sloan/Snellen letters have been chosen for their equality of readability and the letters are S, D, K, H, N, O, C, V, R and Z. All of these letters have been allocated at a difficulty level.

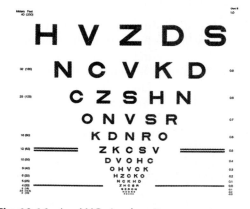

Fig. 10.16: LogMAR visual acuity

These have been arranged on the charts in equal lines of 5.

The progression of letter height is that any line is 1.2589 times greater than the line below. This multiplier is the root of ten or 0.1 log unit.

Therefore, a three line worsening of visual acuity is equal to a doubling of the visual angle regardless of the initial acuity.

The charts are designed for use at 4 meters which helps with smaller examining rooms and, of course, the size of the chart.

Steps of visual acuity testing with LogMAR chart:
- Set the patient/chart distance to 4 meters.
- Cover one eye. If the patient cannot read any letters, move the chart to a distance of 1 meter from the patient and add 0.6 to the LogMAR score for the for each line.
- Repeat for the second eye.
- If the patient is still unable to read any letters proceed to another means of assessment of their acuity.

LogMAR scale is more important than the traditional Snellen's notation:
- Use of LogMAR scale allows analysis of visual acuity scores more effectively and comparisons of results more precisely.
- It offers this because the equal linear steps of the LogMAR scale represent equal ratios in the standard size sequence.

Visual Acuity Expression

Visual acuity depends upon—(1) how accurately light is focused on the macula, (2) the integrity of neural elements of the eye, and (3) the interpretative faculty of the brain.

It is often measured according to the size of the letters viewed in a Snellen's chart. In some countries, VA is expressed as a ***LogMAR fraction*** and in some as a ***decimal notation*** (Table 10.1).

Using the ***meter*** as a unit of measurement, VA is expressed relative to 6/6. Otherwise, using the foot, visual acuity is expressed relative to 20/20. For all practical purposes 6/6 vision is

TABLE 10.1: Visual acuity notation in different scales

Meter	Foot	Decimal	LogMAR
6/60	20/200	0.10	1.0
6/48	20/160	0.13	0.9
6/37	20/125	0.16	0.8
6/30	20/100	0.20	0.7
6/24	20/80	0.25	0.6
6/18	20/63	0.32	0.5
6/15	20/50	0.40	0.4
6/12	20/40	0.50	0.3
6/9	20/32	0.63	0.2
6/7	20/25	0.80	0.1
6/6	20/20	1.00	0.0
6/4	20/16	1.25	−0.1
6/3.75	20/12.5	1.60	−0.2
6/3	20/10	2.00	−0.3

equivalent to 20/20. In the decimal system a value of 1.0 is equal to 6/6 or 20/20.

LogMAR scale is rarely used clinically. It is more frequently used in statistical calculations because it provides more scientific equivalent for the traditional clinical statement of ***line lost*** or ***line gained***.

Normal VA is frequently considered to be what was defined by Snellen as—***the ability to recognize a letter when it subtends 5 minute of an arc***. That is Snellen's chart 6/6 meter, 20/20 feet, 1.00 decimal or 0.0 logMAR. It is possible to have vision superior to 6/6 or 20/20.

Recent developments in refractive technology (surgery or corrective lens) have resulted in conferring a vision up to 6/3 or 20/10. Some birds (e.g. Hawk) are believed to have an acuity of around 6/1 or 20/3, which is much better than human eyesight.

Near Vision

It is always tested and corrected after correcting the distant vision. Different charts are used to record near vision.

N6

Various conditions may cause cataract. Heredity is the determining factor in congenital and juvenile cataracts. Toxic substances, certain eye injuries, chronic systemic diseases (such as diabetes) or other specific eye diseases - all may cause cataract. But, by far the

N8

most common cause is simply the aging process. As we grow older, the crystalline lens gradually loses its

N10

water content and increase in density. This natural process may set the stage for the

N12

cataract formation. Some kind of cataract

N18

formation is expected in

N24

virtually everyone

N36

over the age of

N48

seventy.

Fig. 10.17: Near vision 'N' chart

- Jaeger's chart—J_1, J_2, J_3, J_4, etc.
- The 'N' chart—N_6, N_8, N_{10}, N_{12}, N_{18}, etc. (Fig. 10.17).
- Snellen's near chart—It is 1/17th times photographic reduction of the original Snellen's chart for distance.

Procedure

The patient is asked to sit in a brilliantly illuminated place. Near vision chart is held at a distance of 25–33 cm depending upon the patient's nature of near work. The patient is asked to read the chart from bigger print size to smaller prints. The line that he reads up to, is recorded, e.g. N_{12}, N_6, etc. Each eye should be tested separately first, and then binocularly. Normal near acuity is N_6 in 'N' chart.

Ocular Movements

Any imbalance, uniocular and binocular is to be noted.

The sign used for ocular movement is *union Jack position*, i.e. in 6 cardinal gazes.

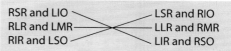

RMR: Right medial rectus
RSO: Right superior oblique
RIR: Right inferior rectus
LMR: Left medial rectus
LSR: Left superior rectus
LSO: Left superior oblique

RLR: Right lateral rectus
RSR: Right superior rectus
RIO: Right inferior oblique
LLR: Left lateral rectus
LIR: Left inferior rectus
LIO: Left inferior oblique

Any underaction or overaction is noted with '–' (minus) or '+' (plus) sign. Normally, a person has orthophoria. Any abnormality in the ocular movements is noted down.

Lids

Normally upper lid covers about 1–2 mm of cornea at 12 o'clock position and the lower lid just touches the limbus at 6 o'clock position. Eyelids are examined for congenital or acquired lesion.

Lid Margin

- Thickened—multiple chalazion, blepharitis.
- Inverted (entropion) or everted (ectropion).
- Any ulcer or scales (blepharitis).

Eyelashes

- Misdirected and touching the globe (trichiasis).
- Loss or scantiness of eyelashes—(madarosis) in blepharitis.
- *Matting of the eyelashes:* Due to mucopurulent discharge (Fig. 10.18A).

Lid Proper

- Thickened—multiple chalazion, blepharitis
- Redness—blepharitis, stye
- Edema—hordeolum, allergic conjunctivitis, insect bite, corneal ulcer, lid abscess
- Localized swelling—chalazion, cyst, growth.

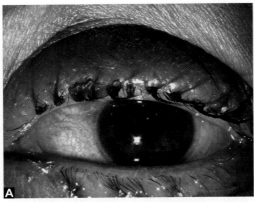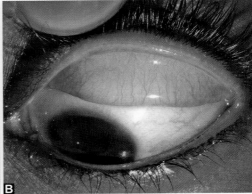

Figs 10.18A and B: **A.** Lid edema with matting of eyelashes; **B.** Eversion of the upper eyelid

Palpebral aperture: 8–9 mm vertically and 20–25 mm horizontally.

- Narrow—phthisis bulbi, ptosis, lid edema, Horner's syndrome, enophthalmos, microphthalmos
- Wide—Lid retraction (thyroid ophthalmopathy), proptosis, other eye in unilateral ptosis

Any other specific lid sign: Lid lag, lagophthalmos, black eye, coloboma or pigmentation is to be noted.

Conjunctiva

Conjunctiva is a mucous membrane covering the sclera and inner side of the eyelids. It is to be examined for any type of congestion, inflammatory or allergic reactions, degenerative lesions and foreign bodies.

Bulbar conjunctiva, palpebral conjunctiva (lower and upper), limbal conjunctiva and fornices—all are to be examined.

- *Examination of the lower palpebral conjunctiva, lower fornix and lower part of bulbar conjunctiva* can be easily done by pulling down the lower lid by the thumb or index finger, while the patient is asked to look upwards.
- *Examination of upper palpebral conjunctiva* is done by everting the upper lid (Fig. 10.18B).

- *Examination of upper fornix* requires double eversion, with the help of a lid retractor.
- *Examination of bulbar conjunctiva and limbal conjunctiva* are done by separating both lids while the patient is asked to move his eyeball in different directions.

Bulbar conjunctiva:
- Luster
- Congestion
- Discharge
- Edema or chemosis
- Subconjunctival hemorrhage
- Pterygium
- Pinguecula
- Bitot's spot
- Symblepharon and
- Cyst, nodule, nevus or growth

Palpebral conjunctiva:
- Papillae
- Follicles
- Concretions
- Scarring (as in trachoma)
- Foreign body
- Any tumor mass and
- Arrangement of blood vessels

Limbal conjunctiva:
- Circumcorneal congestion (CCC) or ciliary congestion
- Phlycten
- Nodules

- Follicles and
- Scar or bleb of previous surgery. Differences between conjunctival congestion and ciliary congestion (*see* Chapter 12, page 146).

Sclera

It is dense tough fibrous envelope that covers 5/6th of the eyeball. Normally, the sclera is whitish in adult and bluish in children, and is covered by the conjunctiva.

- Nodule—episcleritis, scleritis
- Congestion—dusky ciliary congestion in scleritis
- Ectasia—ciliary or equatorial staphyloma
- Thinning—long standing scleritis
- Blue sclera—buphthalmos, *osteogenesis imperfecta*.

Cornea

It is avascular, transparent structure forming the anterior one-sixth of the eyeball, It is examined for its size, shape, surface, curvature, transparency, opacity, staining, vascularization, sensation and keratic precipitates (KPs).

Size

Horizontally 12 mm, vertically 10–11 mm.
- *Size increased:* Megalocornea, buphthalmos.
- *Size decreased:* Microcornea, microphthalmos.

Shape

Normally, it is like a part of a sphere. It may be flat, conical or globular.
- Flat—cornea plana, phthisis bulbi
- Conical—keratoconus, pellucid marginal degeneration
- Globular—keratoglobus, buphthalmos.

Surface

Normally, it is smooth, shiny and regularly curved. Surface and curvature are tested with:
- Window reflex
- Slit lamp
- Placido's disc
- Photokeratoscope
- Keratometer
- Corneal topography or tomography.
  There will be distortion of the image or window reflex in case of keratoconus, corneal edema, corneal ulcer or opacity, etc.

Corneal Staining

Not necessary in all cases.
- *Fluorescein staining:* It is used for denuded epithelium (corneal abrasion, erosions or ulcers) (Figs 10.19A and B).
- *Rose Bengal staining:* It is used for devitalized cells. Useful in xerosis of the conjunctiva and cornea (dry eye).
- *Alcian blue:* It stains mucus selectively.

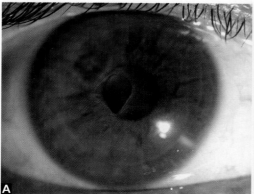 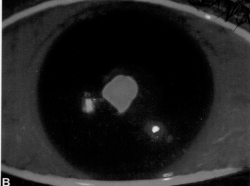

Figs 10.19A and B: Corneal abrasion. **A.** Normal view; **B.** Fluorescein staining

Transparency

The cornea is optically transparent. This transparency is due to certain anatomical and physiological factors. They are as follows:

- Avascularity of the cornea
- Demyelinated nerve supply
- Regular arrangement of the stromal collagen fibrils (lattice theory)
- Active endothelial pump mechanism
- Optimum intraocular pressure.

Any interference with these factors affects the corneal transparency. Thus the cornea becomes hazy in corneal edema, ulcers, scars, vascularization, mucopolysaccharidosis (MPS), acute attack of angle-closure glaucoma, absolute glaucoma, etc.

Opacity

For development of a corneal opacity at least the Bowman's membrane must have to be damaged.

Grades of opacity (Figs 10.20A to D)

- **Nebula:** Only Bowman's membrane is involved.
- **Macula:** Bowman's membrane and part of the anterior stroma are involved.
- **Leukoma:** Full thickness cornea is involved.
- **Adherent leukoma:** A full thickness corneal opacity with iris inclusion. It indicates corneal perforation or a penetrating injury in the past.

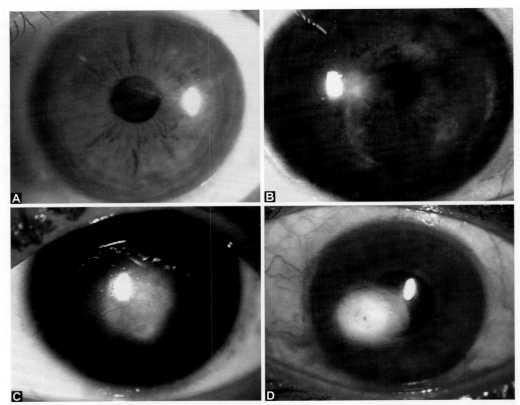

Figs 10.20 A to D: Grades of opacity. **A.** Nebular corneal opacity; **B.** Macular corneal opacity; **C.** Leukomatous corneal opacity; **D.** Adherent leukoma

In case of corneal opacity look for:
- Its density (grade)
- Situation and extent in relation to the pupillary axis and limbus
- Any pigmentation
- Any vascularization—superficial or deep
- Adherent or not
- Its sensation.

Causes of corneal opacity
- Degeneration
- Dystrophy
- Trauma (surgical/nonsurgical)
- Healed infection (keratitis or corneal ulcer) and
- Congenital (MPS)

Corneal Sensation

Method of examination: Patient is asked to look straight with both eyes wide open. A wisp of cotton is brought close to the patient's eye from the temporal side (to avoid optical blinking reflex) and the lower part of cornea is touched with it. The blinking reflex of the lids is observed. Avoid any accidental touch to the eyelashes (a false blinking will result).

Cornea is supplied by ophthalmic division of 5th cranial nerve and it has no kinesthetic sensation.

Causes of loss of corneal sensation:
- Herpetic keratitis
- Acute attack of angle closure glaucoma
- Keratomalacia
- Leprosy
- 5th nerve damage
- After corneal surgery
- Neuroparalytic keratitis
- Long standing corneal edema, etc.

Vascularization (Fig. 10.21 and Table 10.2)
- Is it localized or circumferential?
- How much area is involved?
- Is it superficial or deep?

Causes of corneal vascularization:
- Corneal ulcers

TABLE 10.2: Differences between superficial vascularization and deep vascularization	
Superficial vascularization	**Deep vascularization**
• It can be traced over the limbus into the conjunctiva	• Its seem to come from an abrupt end at the limbus
• Bright red and well-defined	• Greyish red (red blush) and ill-defined
• Branches in an arborescent fashion, and fans dichotomously	• Branches at acute angles and runs in a radial fashion
• It may raise the epithelium over them and corneal surface is uneven	• Deep inside the stroma and corneal surface remains smooth

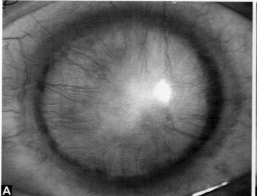 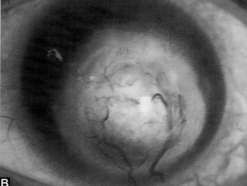

Figs 10.21A and B: Vascularization. **A.** Superficial; **B.** Deep

- HSV stromal keratitis
- Interstitial keratitis
- Leprosy
- Diabetes
- After penetrating keratoplasty, etc.

Keratic precipitates (KPs): These are deposits of inflammatory cells on the lower part of corneal endothelium and best seen by a slit lamp. They may be: Fine, Medium, Mutton fat, Pigmented, and Fresh or old.

This is due to inflammation of the anterior uveal tract (anterior uveitis or iridocyclitis).

Ulcer or abrasions: Details of ulcer, e.g. size, shape, extent, margin, floor, central or peripheral, etc. are to be noted. Also note the staining pattern with fluorescein dye if necessary.

Anterior Chamber

It is the space between the cornea and the iris. Normally, it contains aqueous humor. It is approximately 25 mm in depth at its center.

- ***Depth:*** Normal, shallow, deep and irregular (Figs 10.22 and 10.23).
- ***Causes of shallow anterior chamber***
  - Hypermetropia
  - Hypermature cataract (Morgagnian)
  - Intumescent cataract
  - Angle-closure glaucoma
  - Choroidal detachment
  - Pupillary block
  - Wound leak after intraocular surgery
  - Perforating injury or perforating corneal ulcer, etc.

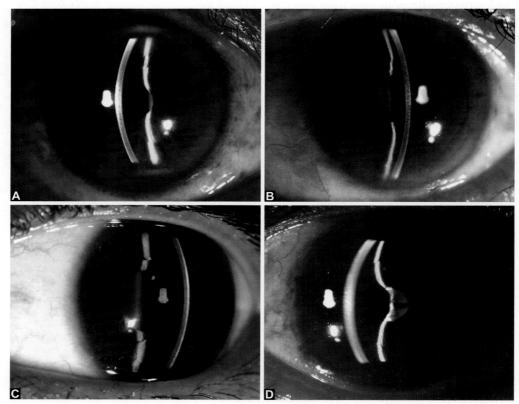

Figs 10.22A to D: Anterior chamber depth. **A.** Normal depth; **B.** Shallow; **C.** Deep; **D.** Funnel-shaped

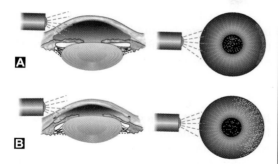

Figs 10.23A and B: Oblique illumination by torch light. A screening measure to estimate the anterior chamber depth; **A.** With a deep chamber, nearly the entire iris is illuminated; **B.** When the iris is bowed forward, only the proximal portion is illuminated, but a shadow is seen in the distal half

- *Causes of deep anterior chamber*
  - Myopia
  - Aphakia
  - Keratoconus/keratoglobus
  - Buphthalmos
  - Posterior dislocation of the lens, etc.
- *Causes of irregular anterior chamber*
  - Subluxation of the lens
  - *Iris bombe* (funnel shaped anterior chamber)
  - Adherent leukoma
  - Iris cyst
  - Angle recession, etc.
- *Abnormal contents of the anterior chamber (Figs 10.24A to D)*

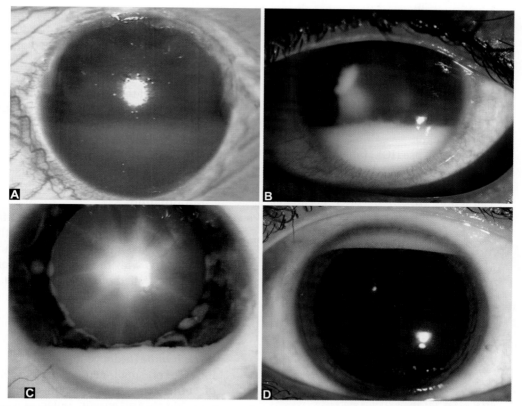

Figs 10.24A to D: Abnormal contents of anterior chamber. **A.** Hyphema-blood; **B.** Hypopyon-pus; **C.** Pseudohypopyon in retinoblastoma; **D.** Inverse hypopyon—emulsified silicone oil

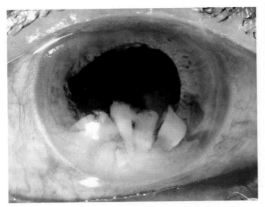

Fig. 10.25: Lens fragment in anterior chamber

- Blood (*hyphema*), e.g. traumatic, postoperative, herpetic iridocyclitis, spontaneous.
- Pus (*hypopyon*), e.g. in corneal ulcer, acute iridocyclitis, endophthalmitis.
- Malignant cells (*pseudohypopyon*), e.g. in retinoblastoma.
- Lens matter [after extracapsular cataract extraction (ECCE)] (Fig. 10.25).
- Albuminous material (aqueous flare) as in iridocyclitis.
- Intraocular lense (IOL) (anterior chamber IOL or irisclaw IOL) (Fig. 10.26).
- Vitreous [after intracapsular cataract extraction (ICCE) or after accidental rupture of posterior capsule in ECCE].

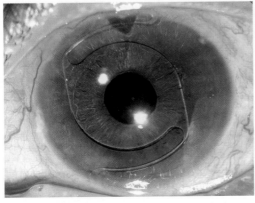

Fig. 10.26: Anterior chamber intraocular lens

Angle of the anterior chamber is examined by *gonioscope*. Normally, it is not possible to see angle structure due to high corneal refractive power and iriscorneal interface.

Iris

It is a brown or black diaphragm hanging in front of the lens, and is perforated centrally which is known as *pupil*.
- *Color:* Difference in color of iris between two eyes is called *heterochromia*.
- *Causes of heterochromia*
  - Congenital
  - Iris atrophy
  - Heterochromic cyclitis of Fuchs
  - Pigmented tumor of the iris
  - Siderosis bulbi, etc.
- *Pattern:* 'Muddy iris' in iridocyclitis where the pattern is lost. Here, the iris becomes edematous, swollen, water-logged and shows impaired mobility.
- *Iridodonesis:* Tremulousness of iris (due to loss of support of the lens). This is elicited by asking the patient to move the eyeball in different directions.
  - *Causes of iridodonesis*
    - Aphakia
    - Dislocation or subluxation of lens
    - Sometimes in pseudophakia and
    - Buphthalmos.
- *Synechia:* Abnormal adhesions of the iris are called *synechiae*. Adhesion of iris with the cornea is called anterior synechia, and adhesion of iris with the lens capsule, or vitreous face is called *posterior synechia*.
  - *Causes of anterior synechia*
    - Perforated corneal ulcer
    - Penetrating injury
    - Angle closure glaucoma and
    - *Iris bombe* (iridocyclitis).
    In case of small central perforation of cornea, one may not find anterior synechia, instead anterior polar cataract is found.
  - *Causes of posterior synechia:* Iridocyclitis.

- ***Vascularization*** of iris is called ***rubeosis iridis***, found in diabetes, central retinal venous thrombosis, heterochromic cyclitis of Fuchs, etc.

- ***Any gap in iris:*** Congenital gap (***coloboma*** of the iris found at the inferonasal region) or marks of iridectomy (peripheral or complete) is to be noted (Figs 10.27A and B).

  Peripheral button hole iridectomy is done in cataract surgery (11 and/or 1 o'clock position), in angle-closure glaucoma or trabeculectomy operation.

  YAG laser peripheral iridectomy (PI) is done in angle-closure glaucoma. Inferior PI is done in vitreoretinal surgery and endothelial keratoplasty. The goal of PI is to prevent secondary pupillary glaucoma.

  Complete iridectomy marking may be found in aphakic patient (if there is any vitreous loss during ICCE or in presence of extensive posterior synechiae or in case of small pupil with hard cataract during ECCE as in pseudoexfoliation).

Pupil

It is a circular aperture at the center of the iris diaphragm (Fig. 10.28A). It regulates the amount of light entering the eye, and helps in maintaining the depth of focus. Pupil is examined for its position, size, shape, reactions and color of its reflex.

- ***Position:*** The pupil is situated just inferior and nasal to the center of the iris. It may be eccentric, known as *corectopia,* as seen in congenital corectopia, after penetrating injury or after vitreous loss in cataract surgery (updrawn pupil).

- ***Size:*** Normally, it varies between 2 and 4 mm. It may be smaller (miosis) or larger (mydriasis).

- ***Causes of miosis (pupil size less than 2 mm) (Fig. 10.28B)***
  - Extreme of ages
  - In bright light
  - Opium addict
  - Morphine intoxication
  - Pontine hemorrhage
  - Acute iritis
  - During sleep
  - Use of miotics (e.g. pilocarpine).

- ***Causes of mydriasis (pupil size more than 6 mm)***
  - In dark
  - Optic atrophy (Fig. 10.28C)
  - Acute attack in angle-closure glaucoma
  - Absolute glaucoma
  - Comatose patient
  - Head injury
  - 3rd nerve palsy and

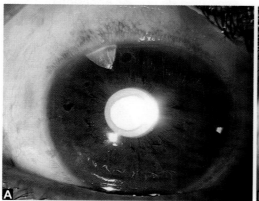 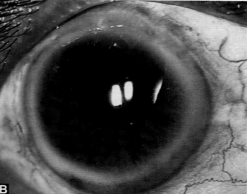

Figs 10.27A and B: **A.** Peripheral iridectomy mark; **B.** Pupil after complete iridectomy in aphakia

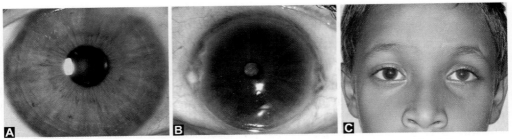

Figs 10.28A to C: A. Normal pupil; **B.** Miotic pupil in aging; **C.** Mydriasis in optic atrophy right eye

- Use of mydriatics (e.g. atropine, homatropine, phenylephrine, etc.).
- *Shape (Fig. 10.29):* Normally, it is perfectly circular. It may be of following types:
  - *Irregular:* Iritis, post-traumatic
  - *D-shaped:* Iridodialysis
  - *Boat or hammock-shaped:* Vitreous loss in cataract surgery. Optic capture after IOL implantation
  - *Pear-shaped and updrawn:* Incarceration of iris with corneal wound
  - *Festooned:* Iridocyclitis
  - *Mid-dilated and oval:* Acute attack in angleclosure glaucoma
  - *Oval and inferonasal:* Coloboma of the iris
  - *Key-hole appearance:* After optical iridectomy.

- *Light reactions:* The pupil constricts briskly on exposure to bright light and dilates in the dark. The afferent pathway is via the optic nerve and the efferent, via the 3rd cranial nerve. Light reactions are direct and consensual.
  - *Direct light reaction:* The patient is asked to cover one eye with his own palm, and the beam of pencil light is thrown on the pupil of uncovered eye from one side, noting the nature of pupillary constriction. Normally, the reaction is brisk and sustained.
  - *Consensual light reaction:* Pupil of the contralateral eye constricts when the light beam is thrown on the ipsilateral eye.

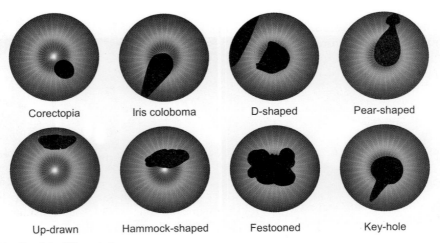

Corectopia · Iris coloboma · D-shaped · Pear-shaped

Up-drawn · Hammock-shaped · Festooned · Key-hole

Fig. 10.29: Pupil in different shapes

Ill sustained papillary reaction is a sign of optic neuritis. In *optic atrophy*, direct light reaction is absent but consensual reaction is present.

In relative afferent pupillary defect (RAPD) or Marcus-Gunn pupil, both pupils dilate when the light is moved from the unaffected eye to the affected eye. RAPD is mostly seen in unilateral optic neuritis.

- *Color reflex of the papillary area:*
  - Jet black papillary reflex—aphakia
  - White papillary reflex—cataract
  - Glassy papillary reflex—pseudophakia
  - Amaurotic cat's eye reflex—retinoblastoma, congenital cataract, persistent hyperplastic primary vitreous (PHPV) endophthalmitis, coloboma of choroid, etc. (*see* page 382).

Lens

The crystalline lens is a transparent biconvex structure with a nucleus, cortex and the capsule.

It is supported by suspensory ligaments, called zonules, attached to the ciliary processes and the valleys between them.

Color of the Lens

Normally, it is transparent.
- *Grayish-white:* Immature cortical cataract
- *White or pearly white:* Mature cataract
- *Milky white:* Hypermature cataract
- *Shrunken and white with calcified spots on the anterior capsule:* Hypermature sclerotic cataract
- *Amber:* Early nuclear cataract
- *Brown:* Cataracta brunescens (nuclear cataract)
- *Black:* Cataracta nigra (nuclear cataract).

Position

Normally, it is in the pupillary area. Note for any subluxation or dislocation.

- *Phacodonesis* or *tremulousness* of the crystalline lens is a sign of lens subluxation.
- *Opacity* or any subluxation is better judged with dilated pupil.
- *Aphakia* means absence of crystalline lens from its normal anatomical position (i.e. from the papillary area).
- *Ectopia lentis* is the congenital malposition of the lens, due to faulty development of the lens zonules, as seen in Marfan's syndrome, homocystinuria, Weill Marchesani's syndrome, etc.
- *Pseudophakia* means the presence of an IOL in the eye after cataract operation with IOL implantation.

Iris Shadow (Figs 10.30A and B)

It is a concave shadow of the papillary margin of the iris, cast upon the lens when light is thrown obliquely.

It signifies that some clear cortical fibers are still present beneath the lens capsule (i.e. between there is margin and the actual opacity of the lens). It is present in immature cataract. But it is absent in mature or hypermature cataract. In case of mature cataract all the

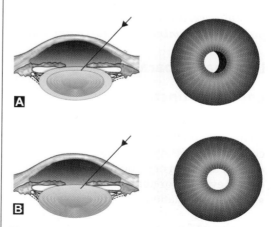

Figs 10.30A and B: Iris shadow. **A.** Present—immature cataract; **B.** Absent—mature or hypermature cataract

substance of lens becomes opaque, so iris margin lies almost in contact with the opaque lens surface—so no iris shadow will form if light is thrown obliquely.

Pigmentation on the Anterior Lens Surface

- A sign of posterior synechiae in old irido-cyclitis
- In traumatic cataract (Vossius's ring)
- Sometimes, in case of persistent pupillary membrane.

Purkinje's images: Note the 3rd and 4th Purkinje's images in a dark room. 3rd image is formed by the anterior convex surface of the lens and it moves in the same direction, and is erect. 4th image is formed by the posterior concave lens surface. It is inverted and moves in the opposite direction.

In *aphakia*; both the 3rd and 4th images are absent.

In *mature or hypermature cataract*; 3rd image is present but the 4th image is absent.

In *immature cataract*; 3rd image is present, but 4th image may be absent or distorted.

The structures beyond the lens like the vitreous, retina and optic nerve are not possible to examine with a torch and loupe.

Lacrimal Apparatus

Lacrimal Puncta

They are situated on the medial side of the lid margins on the papilla. They are always in contact with the eyeball. Note:
- They are open or stenosed.
- Any eversion or noncontact with globe
- Any inflammation.

Lacrimal Sac

- *Skin over the sac area:* Swollen, inflamed, any excoriation, fistula or scar mark.

- *Pressure over the sac region* (by pressing with the thumb just below the medial canthus):
    - Regurgitation of mucoid material (mucocele), pus (pyocele) through the puncta.
    - Swelling is present but no regurgitation via puncta—encysted mucocele.
    - Sometimes regurgitates may go into the nasopharynx, i.e. there is block in common canaliculus.
- *Acute signs of inflammation* (i.e. swelling, redness, raised temperature and tenderness)—acute dacryocystitis.

Note: Nasal cavity is better examined grossly for DNS, polyps, hypertrophied inferior turbinate, etc. in case of chronic dacryocystitis.

Digital Tonometry

Technique

As everything is digital in modern era—so, it is better to be termed as "finger tension".

Rough assessment of IOP by eliciting the fluctuation of the eyeball. The patient is asked to look downwards at his feet. Examiner places both index fingers side by side above the upper border of the tarsal plate on the upper lid, resting the other fingers lightly on the forehead (Figs 10.31A and B). One index finger is stationary and the other one presses the globe, there by conveying the amount of fluctuation to the stationary finger. Fluctuation can be appreciated well by regular practice. The intraocular tension is graded as normal, high or low.

The eyeball is hard in all primary and secondary glaucomas. It is *stony hard* (the fluctuation is absent) in absolute glaucoma.

The eyeball is soft in chronic uveitis, recent penetrating injury, wound leak, choroidal detachment and retinal detachment. In phthisis bulbi, it is soft as water bag.

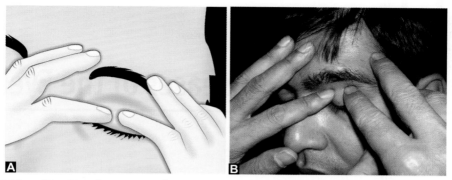

Figs 10.31A and B: Digital tonometry (finger tension); **A.** Schematic representation; **B.** Photograph

Other means of recording IOP:
- *Schiøtz tonometer:* By indentation of the cornea with this instrument, IOP can be recorded from a chart after getting the scale reading.
- *Applanation tonometer:* Greatest accuracy of IOP is determined by this method by applanating the central portion of the cornea. This instrument is an optional attachment to the slit lamp.
- Non-contact air-puff tonometer (NCT): is popular as a screening device for IOP measurement in busy clinic or OPD.
Normal IOP is about 14–21 mm of Hg.

Diseases of the Eyelids

SOME CONGENITAL ABNORMALITIES

Symblepharon, ankyloblepharon, ectropion, entropion, trichiasis, coloboma, epicanthus, blepharophimosis, ptosis—all may occur as congenital malformation (Table 11.1).

Epicanthus (Figs 11.1A and B)

- Most common congenital condition.
- A semilunar skin fold, situated above and sometimes covering the inner canthus.

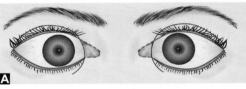

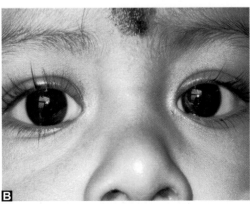

Figs 11.1A and B: Epicanthus, note the appearance of pseudo-convergent squint. **A.** Schematic representation; **B.** Photograph

TABLE 11.1: Some abnormalities of the eyelids	
Ankyloblepharon	Adhesion between upper and lower eyelid margins
Ablepharon	Absence of the eyelid
Blepharophimosis	Decreased dimensions of the palpebral fissure
Blepharospasm	Tonic spasm of orbicularis oculi muscle
Coloboma	Absence of some ocular tissue
Distichiasis	Accessory row of eyelashes
Ectropion	Outward turning of the lid margin
Entropion	Inward turning of the lid margin
Epiblepharon	Extra fold of skin in the lower lid
Epicanthus	Extra fold of skin on medial side of the lower lid (palpebronasal fold)
Euryblepharon	Enlarged palpebral aperture
Floppy eyelid syndrome	Floppy, easily eversible upper lid with papillary conjunctivitis at the upper tarsus
Lagophthalmos	Inability to close the eyelid completely
Myokymia	Fascicular tremor of the orbicularis oculi muscle
Ptosis	Drooping of upper eyelid
Symblepharon	Adhesion between the palpebral and bulbar conjunctiva
Telecanthus	Widely separated nose and eye (medial canthi)
Trichiasis	Misdirected eyelashes

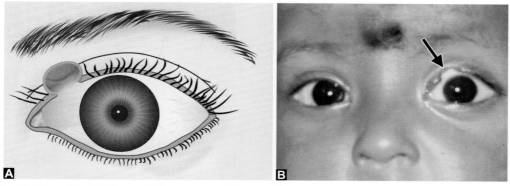

Figs 11.2A and B: Coloboma of the upper eyelid. **A.** Schematic representation; **B.** Photograph (arrow)

- Usually bilateral, and simulate the appearance of pseudoconvergent squint.
- It is normal in Mongolian races.
- Easily treated by plastic repair.

Coloboma of the Eyelid

- A notch at the edge of the lid.
- Most commonly in the middle of the upper lid (Figs 11.2A and B).
- Often associated with underlying dermoid cyst.
- *Treatment* is by plastic repair at a very early age to prevent exposure keratitis.

Blepharophimosis (Fig. 11.3)

- *It is a syndrome consists of following clinical features:*
  - Narrowing of the vertical and horizontal palpebral apertures
  - Telecanthus
  - Inverse epicanthus fold and
  - Ptosis.
- Autosomal dominant inheritance.
- *Treatment:* Plastic reconstruction of the lids, along with bilateral brow suspension for the ptosis in stages.

Distichiasis (Figs 11.4A and B)

Extra posterior row of cilia, occasionally present in all four lids:

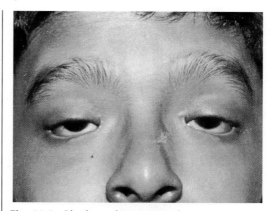

Fig. 11.3: Blepharophimosis syndrome

- This posterior row occupies the position of meibomian glands.
- Meibomian glands change to ordinary sebaceous glands in this condition.
- The eyelashes may irritate the cornea.
- *Treatment* is done by cryotherapy or excision with grafting.

ABNORMALITIES OF SHAPE AND POSITION (FIG. 11.5)

Entropion

Entropion is an inward turning of the eyelid with rubbing of the eyelashes on the conjunctiva and/or cornea.

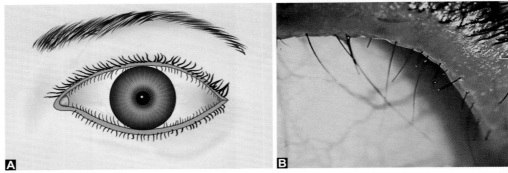

Figs 11.4A and B: Distichiasis of the upper lid. **A.** Schematic representation; **B.** Photograph

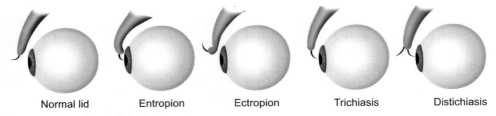

Normal lid   Entropion   Ectropion   Trichiasis   Distichiasis

Fig. 11.5: Abnormalities of the lid margin

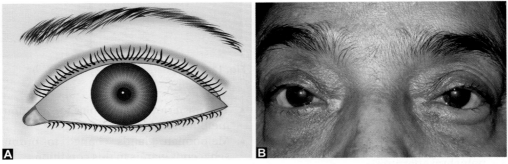

Figs 11.6A and B: **A.** Entropion of the lower eyelid (schematic representation); **B.** Senile entropion—left lower lid (photograph)

Classification

Involutional (Figs 11.6A and B)

Most common type and affects the lower lid only.

Etiopathology: Due to four changes:

1. Upward movement of preseptal part of orbicularis oculi of the lower lid.

2. A thinning of the tarsal plate with subsequent atrophy—leading to horizontal lid laxity.
3. Thinning of the orbital septum and weakening of the lower lid retractors—lead to decrease in vertical lid stability.
4. A relative disparity between lid and globe (enophthalmos) from atrophy of the adipose tissue.

Symptoms
- Foreign body sensation
- Pain
- Lacrimation and discharge.

Signs
- In turning of the lower eyelid
- Conjunctival congestion
- Discharge with matting of the eyelashes
- Blepharospasm
- Superficial corneal opacities and distortion of the window reflex
- Sometimes, corneal ulceration.

Treatment: Two types of procedures are:

1. **Temporary procedures**
   - **Adhesive tape**—pulling the skin outward with a strip of adhesive tape.
   - **Cautery**—over the skin below the lashes.
   - Transverse lid everting suture.
   - **Alcohol injection**—along the edge of the lid.

2. **Permanent procedures**
   - **Weis' procedure:** A full-thickness horizontal lid splitting with marginal rotation.
   - **Horizontal lid shortening:** An excision of full-thickness trapezoid-shaped area of the lid at the lateral canthus and then suturing the margins, to treat horizontal lid laxity.
   - **Tucking of inferior lid retractors (Fig. 11.7):** It may be done as a primary procedure, or in recurrent cases.
   - **Fox procedure (Fig. 11.8):** Excising a base-down triangle of the tarsus and conjunctiva, and then sutured together.

Cicatricial

It is due to scarring of the palpebral conjunctiva. It may involve both the upper and lower lids. Frequently, the tarsus is deformed and thickened.

Causes
- Chemical injuries
- Lacerated injuries

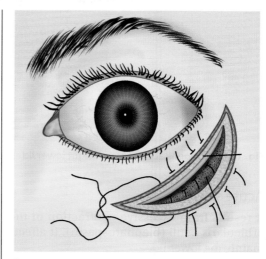

Fig. 11.7: Tucking of inferior lid retractors

- Trachoma
- Radiation
- Stevens-Johnson syndrome
- Ocular cicatricial pemphigoid.

Treatment: Aim of the treatment, is to keep the eyelashes away from the globe.
- Soft contact lens.
- Various plastic operations, and the ideas are:
  - To alter the direction of the lashes
  - To transplant the lashes
  - To straighten the distorted tarsus.
- Mucous membrane grafting (from buccal mucosa) to replace the scarred conjunctiva.

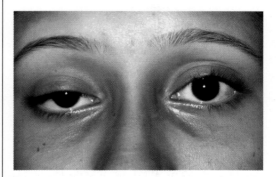

Fig. 11.8: Fox procedure

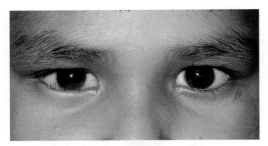

Fig. 11.9: Congenital entropion—right lower lid

Acute spastic

It results from excessive contraction of the orbicularis oculi (blepharospasm). It affects mainly the lower lid.

Causes
- Chronic conjunctivitis
- Keratitis
- Postoperative.

Treatment
- Removal of the cause and it resolves spontaneously
- Removal of bandage in postoperative cases
- *Temporary relief by:*
  - Lid everting suture
  - Adhesive tape (lid taping).

Congenital (Fig. 11.9)

It is rare and usually caused by deformity of the tarsal plate. It may be associated with microphthalmos or anophthalmos.

Sometimes, epiblepharon may occur with congenital entropion. It is an abnormal skin fold usually at the medial one-third of lower lid, and turns the lid margin inward.

Treatment
- Resection of the abnormal portion of the tarsus.
- Excess skin may be excised if there is epiblepharon.

Ectropion

It is an outward turning of the eyelid away from the globe.

Clinical Features

- In case of lower lid involvement → inferior punctum is not in contact with the globe → epiphora and excoriation of the skin around the lid.
- Chronic exposure of the conjunctiva → secondary infection and keratinization → keratitis or frank corneal ulcer.

Classification

Involutional (Senile) (Figs 11.10A and B)

It is the most common form, which affects the lower lid in elderly. It is due to excessive horizontal lid-length with weakness of the preseptal portion of the orbicularis.

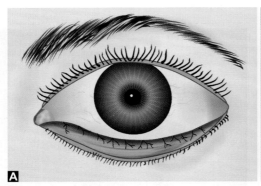
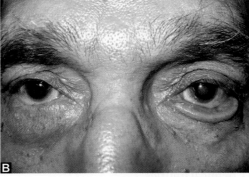

Figs 11.10A and B: A. Ectropion of the lower eyelid (schematic representation); **B.** Senile ectropion—left lower lid (photograph)

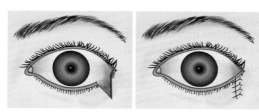

Fig. 11.11: Bick's procedure

The lid laxity can be assessed with the *snap test*. Pull the lower eyelid downward and assess how long it takes to return to a normal position. A return of less than 1 second (without blinking) is normal.

Treatment: It is corrected by reducing the horizontal lid laxity:

- *Zeigler's cautery* to correct the medial lid laxity with punctual eversion.
- *Medial conjunctivoplasty* for mild cases of medial ectropion.
- *Horizontal lid shortening* to correct ectropion involving the whole lid.
- *Bick's procedure (Fig. 11.11)* excision of a full-thickness triangular wedge of lid at the outer canthus and then suture vertically.
- *Byron-Smith modification of Kuhnt-Szymanowski procedure (Fig. 11.12):* Pentagonal wedge resection of the lid margin, along with excision of a triangular skin flap laterally.

Cicatricial

It is caused by contracture of the skin and underlying tissues.

Causes
- Burns (chemical/thermal) (Fig. 11.13)
- Trauma
- Inflammation.

It affects either the upper or lower lid.

Treatment
- Excision of the scar with a skin-graft to the raw area. Skin of the opposite upper eyelid is ideal for this purpose.
- Lengthening of the vertical-shortening of the lid—by Z-plasty.

Paralytic

It follows the paralysis of the orbicularis and is also associated lagophthalmos.

Treatment: The main aim is to prevent exposure keratitis.

- *In mild cases*
  - Frequent instillation of artificial tears—to prevent corneal drying.
  - Antibiotic ointment, or an adhesive tape to close the lid at night to prevent corneal exposure.
- *In severe cases*
  - *Tarsorrhaphy:* Shortening of the palpebral aperture by lateral tarsorrhaphy, while awaiting any spontaneous recovery.
  - *Lateral canthoplasty* is more acceptable cosmetically.
  - Correction by silicone-slings.

Congenital

Rare, and may be associated with blepharophimosis. In severe cases—surgery is necessary.

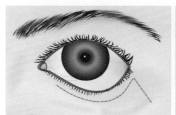
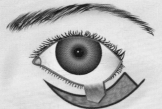
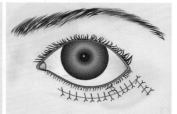

Fig. 11.12: Modified Kuhnt-Szymanowski's procedure

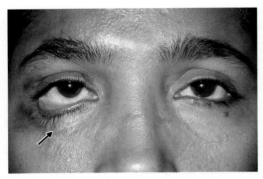

Fig. 11.13: Cicatricial ectropion of the right lower lid after chemical injury (arrow)

Mechanical

Just the sequel to a swelling of the lower lid, e.g. a large chalazion, a tumor, or even lid edema. It can be easily rectified.

Trichiasis (Figs 11.14A and B)

Trichiasis is the inward misdirection of the eyelash(es) which irritate the cornea and/or the conjunctiva.

Pseudotrichiasis: When the misdirection is secondary to entropion.

Etiology
- **Congenital**—known as **distichiasis**.
- **Acquired**—due to diseases those causes carring of the eyelid margin, e.g. stye, ulcerative blepharitis, membranous conjunctivitis, trachoma and post-traumatic.

Symptoms
- Foreign body sensation
- Lacrimation and pain.

Signs
- Conjunctival congestion
- Reflex blepharospasm
- Ciliary congestion
- Recurrent erosions of the cornea
- Superficial corneal opacities
- Vascularization of the cornea.

Treatment
- **Epilation:** Removal of the offending eyelashes with cilia forceps. This must be repeated every 6–8 weeks.
- **Soft bandage contact lens:** To protect the cornea temporarily.
- **Permanent procedures:** By destroying the hair roots.
  - **Electrolysis** (under local anesthesia): A fine needle (negative pole) is introduced into the hair follicle, and a current of 2 mA is passed. End point is judged by the appearance of foam, and the eyelash with bulbus root can be easily lifted out.
  - **Electrodiathermy:** A current of 30 mA is used for 10 seconds.
  - **Cryotherapy:** Very effective for a row of ingrowing eyelashes. Under local anesthesia, the cryoprobe is applied to lid margin and then freeze at –20°C → prolonged thawing → refreeze. Depigmentation of the skin is a problem.

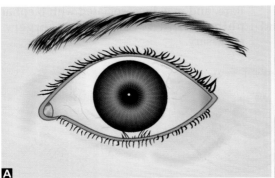
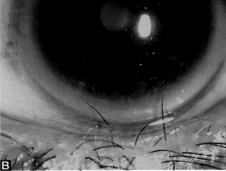

Figs 11.14A and B: Trichiasis. **A.** Schematic representation; **B.** Photograph

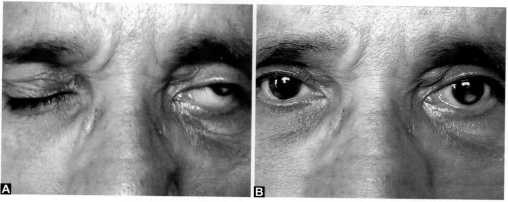

Figs 11.15A and B: Lagophthalmos with healed exposure keratitis in the left eye

- *Irradiation* is effective in severe cases, but it produces conjunctival keratinization.
- *Argon laser cilia ablation* is also effective.
- *Plastic repair:* If many cilia are misdirected, operative procedure as entropion is most effective.

Lagophthalmos (Figs 11.15A and B)

This is the condition of inadequate closure of the eyelids, resulting in exposure of the eye.

Literally *lagos* is a Greek word for hare, an animal which always sleeps with its eyes open.

Etiology nocturnal lagophthalmos: It is found in children, in Mongolian races, and terminal ill patient. It causes no trouble, since the eyes roll upwards (Bell's phenomenon) spontaneously during sleep.

Pathological
- Facial palsy
- Proptosis and thyroid exophthalmos
- Comatose patient
- Cicatricial deformity of the upper lid.

Sequelae
- Eye is red, irritable and watery
- Dryness of the lower part of the bulbar conjunctiva and cornea.

- Exposure keratitis → corneal ulceration → corneal perforation.

Treatment
- *Nocturnal lagophthalmos* does not require any treatment.
- Instillation of artificial tear at day time, and antibiotic ointment at night are required to prevent corneal drying.
- Closure of the lids by adhesive tapes.
- Soft bandage contact lens along with artificial tears to prevent exposure keratitis.
- *Tarsorrhaphy:* A temporary or permanent adhesion is created between upper and lower lids which may be lateral or paracentral.
- *Lid (upper) load operation* with gold plate—useful in facial palsy.
- Treatment of the cause—as in proptosis due to orbital tumor or thyroid exophthalmos.

Symblepharon (Figs 11.16A to C)

This is a condition of adhesion of the lid to the globe, as a result of adhesion between the bulbar and palpebral conjunctiva.

Etiology: Any cause which produces raw surfaces upon two opposed areas of bulbar and palpebral conjunctiva will lead to adhesion during the healing process.
- Chemical burns (mostly alkali)
- Thermal burns

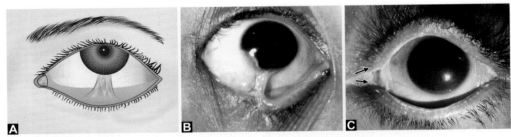

Figs 11.16A to C: Symblepharon. **A.** Schematic representation; **B and C.** Photographs (arrows)

- Membranous conjunctivitis
- Ocular cicatricial pemphigoid (OCP)
- Stevens-Johnson syndrome
- Postoperative
- Trachoma.

Pathology
- Bands of fibrous tissue are formed, and stretching between the lid and the globe.
- The bands may be narrow or broad.
- Cornea is also involved in severe cases.

Types: There are three types of symblepharon are as follows:
1. *Anterior symblepharon:* Bands are limited to the anterior parts and not involving the fornix.
2. *Posterior symblepharon:* Bands are obliterating the fornix only.
3. *Total symblepharon:* The lids are completely plastered against the globe and leaving a small fixed palpebral aperture.

Symptoms
- *Pain and redness*—due to exposure.
- *Watering*—due to inadequate lacrimal drainage.
- *Diplopia*—due to limitation of the ocular movements resulting from pronounced adhesion.
- Cosmetic disfigurement.

Signs
- Signs of exposure
- Restriction of ocular movement

- Visible fibrotic band
- Obliteration of the fornix at places.

Treatment
- *Prevention*—most important
  - *Sweeping a glass rod*—well coated with ointment, around the upper and lower fornices, so that they are well packed with ointment. This procedure is to be repeated several times each day according to severity.
  - *Scleral contact lens/shell fitting*—to separate the two mucosal surfaces to prevent their adhesions.
- *When established*
  - *If there is a small band*—just excise the band
  - *If it is extensive*
    - Radical excision of the scarred conjunctival tissues
    - Mucous membrane graft to cover the bare area (mucous membrane is taken from upper fornix of opposite eye, or from the buccal mucosa).
- *Prevention of recurrence of adhesion*
  - By therapeutic contact lens
  - By scleral shell atleast for 6 weeks.
  - High dose of steroids (local and systemic) is helpful to prevent formation of excessive granulation tissues).

Blepharochalasis and dermatochalasis

Blepharochalasis (Fig. 11.17A)
- Usually bilateral
- May be unilateral or individuals (around 20 years)
- Both sexes are equally affected
- Usually starts at puberty with an intermittent, painless angioneurotic edema and redness of the lid
- Aggravated by crying and menstruation
- Initially, there is loss of skin elasticity with subcutaneous atrophy
- Ultimately, skin hangs down over the lid margin
- Orbital fat and lacrimal gland may prolapse
- Cosmetic surgery may be helpful.

Dermatochalasis (Figs 11.17B and C)
- Usually bilateral
- Mostly senile; in younger individual a familial tendency is noted
- Loss of skin elasticity
- Skin atrophy is seen with prolapse of fat, mainly nasally in the upper lid
- Later, lower lid is also involved with bagginess and sac-like bulging of fat (herniation) in the whole lid
- This is due to relaxation and defect in orbital fascia
- Cosmetic surgery is useful, but a recurrence is common.

Floppy Eyelid Syndrome

It is a condition characterized by floppy, easily eversible upper eyelid with papillary conjunctivitis at the upper tarsus.

Symptoms

- Chronically red and irritable eye, often worse on a waking from sleep.
- A mild mucus discharge.
- The patients are typically obese and often with sleep apnea syndrome.

The symptoms are thought to be result from spontaneous eversion of upper eyelid during sleep. This allows the superior palpebral conjunctiva to rub against a pillow or bedsheet.

Signs

- Upper eye lid can be easily everted without an accessory device (finger or cotton tip applicator).
- Soft and rubbery superior tarsal plate.
- Papillary reaction of superior tarsal conjunctiva.
- Superficial punctate keratitis (SPKs).

Differential Diagnosis

The following conditions may produce superior tarsal papillary conjunctivitis, but in all cases, the upper lid is not easily eversible.
- **Vernal conjunctivitis** seasonal, itching, ropy discharge and papillary reaction of upper tarsal conjunctiva.
- **Giant papillary conjunctivitis** most often related to soft contact lens wear and exposed nylon suture.
- **Superior limbic keratoconjunctivitis** hyperemia and thickening of upper bulbar conjunctiva, often with filaments and corneal pannus.

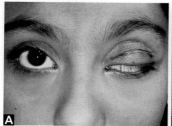 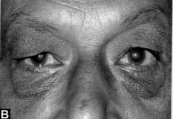 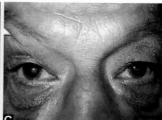

Figs 11.17A to C: A. Blepharochalasis in left upper eye lid; **B and C.** Dermatochalasis in both upper eye lids

- *Toxic keratoconjunctivitis* follicles and/or papillae are more prominent in lower tarsal conjunctiva in a patient using eye drops.

Treatment

- Topical antibiotics, e.g. ciprofloxacin eye drop—4 times daily.
- Artificial tears—1–2 hourly in presence of SPKs.
- Antibiotic ointment at bed time.
- The eyelids are taped during sleep, or alternately an eye shield is worn to protect eyelids from rubbing against a pillow/bedsheet. The patient is advised to refrain from sleeping face down.
- An eyelid tightening surgical procedure is often helpful.

Ptosis (Blepharoptosis) (Fig. 11.18)

It signifies a drooping of the upper eyelid, which may be unilateral or bilateral, and partial or complete.

Etiology

Congenital ptosis

- Due to imperfect differentiation of the levator muscle.

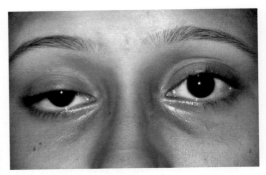

Fig. 11.18: Right sided ptosis

- Often associated with weakness of underlying superior rectus muscle (as levator muscle together with superior rectus, is the last extraocular muscle to be differentiated).
- Often hereditary (dominant).
- May be associated with epicanthus or blepharophimosis.
- May be associated with synkinesis (synkinetic ptosis).
- *Marcus-Gunn jaw-winking phenomenon (Figs 11.19A and B):* There is retraction of the ptotic eyelid, with stimulation of ipsilateral pterygoid muscle (jaw-movement).
- *Misdirected third nerve:* Retraction of the upper lid with various ocular movements.

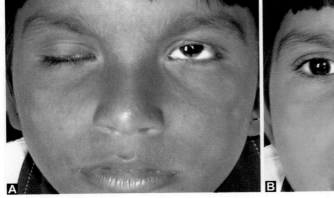
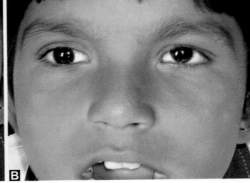

Figs 11.19A and B: Ptosis with Marcus-Gunn jaw-winking phenomenon

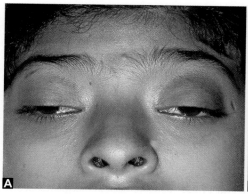 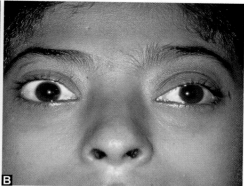

Figs 11.20A and B: Myasthenia gravis. **A.** Before prostigmin test; **B.** After prostigmin test

Acquired ptosis

- *Neurogenic*
  - Partial or complete third nerve palsy
  - Horner's syndrome.
- *Myogenic*
  - Myasthenia gravis (Figs 11.20A and B)
  - Ocular myopathy
  - Bilateral senile ptosis (Fig. 11.21).
- *Mechanical*
  - Excess of weight due to edema, tumors, large chalazion, etc.
  - Conjunctival scarring
  - Symblepharon of the upper lid.
- *Traumatic:*
  - Trauma to the levator muscle
  - Post-surgical (e.g. after cataract surgery).

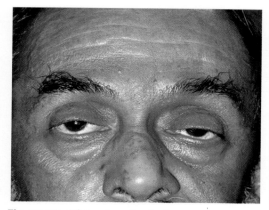

Fig. 11.21: Bilateral senile ptosis

Pseudoptosis

- Due to surgical anophthalmos, microphthalmos and phthisis bulbi
- Due to hypotropia
- Due to dermatochalasis.

Clinical Evaluation of Ptosis

History
- Age of onset
- Family history
- Presence of diplopia
- Variability of ptosis
- Symptoms of systemic problems
- Any contributing factor.

Examination
- *Amount of ptosis:* By noting the ptotic lid margin with respect to the limbus and pupil (Fig. 11.22).
  - Mild ptosis = 2 mm
  - Moderate ptosis = 3 mm
  - Severe ptosis = 4 mm or more.
- *Ptosis measurements*
  - *Margin reflex distance (Fig. 11.23):* Margin reflex distance 1 (MRD1) is the distance in mm from the light reflex on the patient's cornea to the level of the center of the upper lid margin with the patient seeing in primary gaze.
    - Eyes of examiner and patient are at the same level. Light held in examiner's hand is directed toward the glabella of the patient

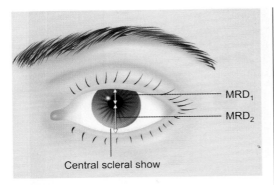

Fig. 11.22: Measurement of ptosis
MRD—Marginal reflex distance

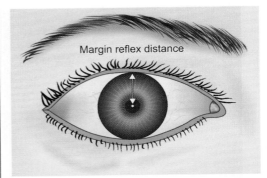

Fig. 11.23: Measurement of margin reflex distance

- If the reflex is not seen, then the number of mm of eyelid raised is then recorded as MRD 1 (negative value)
- The amount of ptosis in unilateral cases is the difference between MRD 1 on ptotic side and that of normal side
- In bilateral cases, the MRD 1 is subtracted from normal MRD 1 of 4–4.5.

■ **MRD 2** is the measurement of the corneal light reflex to the center of the lower lid with the patient seeing in primary gaze. A measurement greater than 5 mm is considered normal. Sum of MRD 1 and MRD 2 is equal to the palpebral fissure width.

■ **MRD 3** is the distance of the ocular light reflex to the center of the upper lid margin when the patient looks in extreme up gaze. Generally MRD 3 is equal to MRD 1. But in associated superior rectus weakness/palsy—MRD 3 is more than MRD 1.

- *Margin limbal distance or MLD* is the distance from the 6 o'clock limbus to the center of the upper lid margin when the patient looks in extreme up gaze. It is about 9.0 mm. The difference in MLD between two sides in unilateral cases, or the

difference with normal in bilateral cases multiplied by 3 would give the amount of levator resection required.

■ *Margin crease distance or MCD* is the distance from the upper eyelid margin to the lid crease measured in down gaze. In women, a normal central MCD measurement is about 8–10 mm, and in men it is about 5–7 mm. It helps in planning the surgical incision. When more than one lid creases are present, the most prominent one is to be considered (Fig. 11.24).

■ *Palpebral fissure height or PFH*—the distance between the upper and lower eyelid in vertical alignment with the pupillary center.

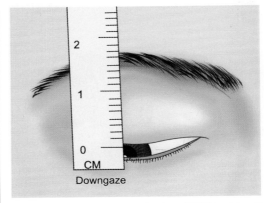

Fig. 11.24: Margin crease distance (MCD)

- Normal = women: 9–10 mm and in men: 7–10 mm in primary gaze
- Upper lid: 2 mm below superior limbus. Lower lid: 1 mm above the inferior limbus
- Should be examined in primary gaze, upgaze and downgaze
- Amount of ptosis = difference in palpebral apertures in unilateral ptosis or difference from normal in bilateral ptosis
- Ptotic lid in congenital unilateral ptosis is usually higher in downgaze due to failure of levator to relax
- Ptotic lid in acquired ptosis is invariably lower than normal lid in downgaze.

- *Assessment of levator function*
  - The brow is immobilized by pressure with the thumb (to negate the action of frontalis).
  - Patient is asked to look down and then to look up.
  - Amount of excursion of the upper lid margin is then measured with a ruler (2 mm of movement is contributed by the superior rectus muscle).
    - Normal = 15 mm
    - Good = 8 mm or more
    - Fair = 5–7 mm
    - Poor = 4 mm or less
- *Ocular motility testing*

- *Jaw-winking phenomenon*
- *Bell's phenomenon*
- *Corneal sensitivity in neurogenic ptosis*
  - *Photograph:* As preoperative record
  - *Tensilon test* is to exclude *myasthenia gravis.* Improvement of ptosis with intravenous injection of edrophonium (Tensilon), or prostigmin if the ptosis is due to myasthenia (Fig. 11.20)
  - *Neurological evaluation* if the ptosis is neurogenic.

Treatment

- *Fasanella-Servat operation (Figs 11.25A to C)*
  - It is simple tarso-conjunctival resection.
  - Useful in mild ptosis with good levator function (e.g. Horner's syndrome).
- *Levator resection*
  - Useful in congenital unilateral ptosis with fair to good levator function.
  - It may be via
    - *Skin approach (Everbusch's)* especially where larger resection is necessary
    - *Conjunctival approach (Blaskowics')* particularly useful for moderate resection of superioris (LPS).
- *Brow (frontalis) suspension (Fig. 11.26)*
  - In bilateral cases where the levator action is poor.

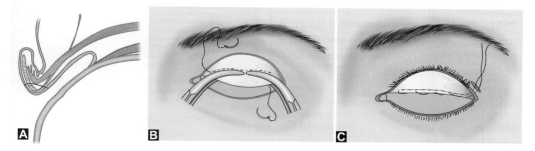

Figs 11.25 A to C: Fasanella-Servat operation. **A.** Resection of upper tarsal border with its attached Muller's muscle and conjunctiva; **B.** Upper tarsal border is caught between two mosquito forceps; **C.** Wound closure after resection of lid tissues within the forceps

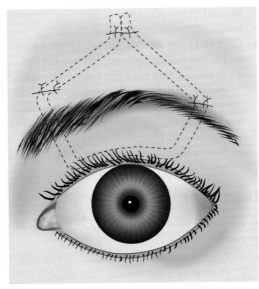

Fig. 11.26: Frontalis (brow) suspension

- Here, the tarsus is fixed to the frontalis muscle via a sling of fascia lata or non-absorbable materials.
- *Aponeurosis strengthening*
  - Useful for acquired ptosis with good levator function.
  - Performed either by advancement or by tucking.
  - Advancement may be combined with levator resection in severe ptosis.

Timing of surgery in congenital ptosis
- *Severe ptosis:* Early intervention is necessary due to danger of stimulus deprivation amblyopia.
- *Mild to moderate ptosis:* Surgical correction is done between 3 years and 4 years of age, when accurate measurement can be obtained.

Blinking

Blinking spreads tears over the surface of the eye, and limits the amount of light entering the eye. It may be:
- *Involuntary:* Once in every 5 seconds and lasts about 0.3 second. It is absent in neonates.
- *Voluntary (winking):* It is generally uniocular, and used to illustrate a variety of emotions.
- *Reflex:* It may follow with the peripheral stimulation of trigeminal (sensory blinking), optic (optical blinking) or auditory nerve.

Blepharospasm

It is an involuntary, tonic, spasmodic, bilateral contraction of the orbicularis oculi muscles. It lasts for few seconds to several minutes.

Causes

- *Essential blepharospasm:* It may occur spontaneously in old age. Other muscles of the face may be simultaneously involved.
- *Reflex blepharospasm (Fig. 11.27)* is precipitated by sensory stimuli, e.g.
  - Corneal abrasions
  - Keratitis or corneal ulcer
  - Dust, fumes, or chemical irritation.

Reflex blepharospasm can be abolished by topical anesthesia.

Treatment

- *Essential blepharospasm* is difficult to treat.
  - Alcohol injection to the facial nerve may be helpful.

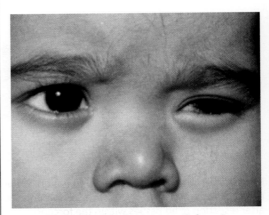

Fig. 11.27: Reflex blepharospasm (left eye)

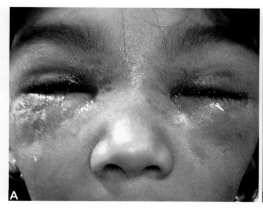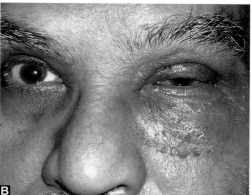

Figs 11.28A and B: A. Contact dermatitis—atropine induced; **B.** Left-sided contact dermatitis

- Botulinum toxin (Botox) injection into the orbicularis muscle around the eyelid in severe cases.
- ***Reflex blepharospasm:*** Treatment of the cause.

Contact (Irritant) Dermatitis (Figs 11.28A and B)

It is characterized by a frequently recurrent, weeping eczematous lesion of the skin, associated with severe itching and swelling of the lids.

Mostly allergic in nature, and principally dependent on external irritants, e.g.
- Cosmetics (most important), hair dye
- Topical drugs, e.g. neomycin, penicillin, and atropine are most important (Figs 11.28A and B)
- Industrial chemicals
- ***Spectacle dermatitis*** caused by nickel or plastic frame.

Treatment

- Removal of all possible external allergens.
- Antihistamine tablet.
- Local application of corticosteroids ointment.

Blepharitis

Blepharitis is the subacute or chronic inflammation of the eyelid.

Etiological factors are complex:
- Age—mostly in children
- Usually bilateral
- Irritation—from cosmetics, dust, smoke
- Uncorrected refractive errors (rubbing of the eyes to gain clear vision → chronic infection)
- Seborrhea (dandruff) of the scalp—mainly in squamous variety
- Chronic conjunctivitis
- ***Parasitic infestation:*** 'Blepharitis acarica' due to *Demodex folliculorum,* and 'phthiriasis palpebrum' (Fig. 11.29) due to crablouse, *Phthirus pubis.*

Types of Blepharitis

Two types of blepharitis are as follows:
1. ***Squamous blepharitis (Fig. 11.30):*** It is characterized by hyperemia, usually limited to the eyelid margins. It is not an infective condition.

    Symptoms
    - Redness of the eyelid margins
    - Burning and discomfort of the eyes
    - Epiphora.

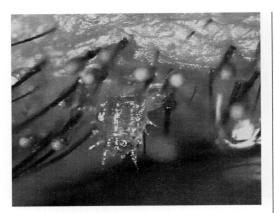

Fig. 11.29: Phthiriasis palpebrum

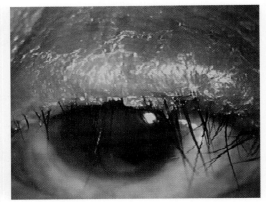

Fig. 11.31: Ulcerative blepharitis

Signs

- White dandruff-like scales on the lid margins
- On removal of scales, underlying surface is found hyperemic, but no ulceration
- Falling of the eyelashes (madarosis)
- Thickening of the lid margins (tylosis)
- Associated seborrheic dermatitis of the scalp.

2. ***Ulcerative blepharitis (Fig. 11.31):*** It is caused by acute or chronic suppurative inflammation of the follicles of the eyelashes and glands of Zeis and Moll. *Staphylococcus aureus* is usually the causative agent superimposed on predisposing conditions.

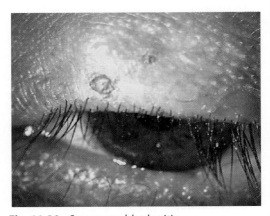

Fig. 11.30: Squamous blepharitis

Symptoms

- Itching, lacrimation and redness
- Soreness of the lid margins
- Loss of eyelashes.

Signs

- Yellow crusts are deposited at the roots of the eyelashes with matting.
- The crusts are removed with difficulty, and bring eyelashes with it. On removing the crusts, small ulcers are seen around the bases of the eyelash, which bleed easily.
- Loss of cilia with distortion of the eyelid margins, or misdirected cilia.

Sequelae of blepharitis: These are mainly seen in ulcerative form of blepharitis, and often serious.

- Chronic conjunctivitis
- ***Madarosis:*** Loss of eyelashes due to destruction of the follicles by deep ulceration.
- ***Trichiasis:*** When the ulcer heals, the cicatricial tissue contracts with misdirection of the remaining cilia.
- ***Tylosis:*** Hypertrophy of the lid margins with consequent drooping.
- ***Ectropion*** of the lower lid with epiphora.
- ***Marginal keratitis***—particularly seen in lower third of the cornea.
- ***Instability of the tear-film*** with consequent dry eye.

Treatment

Squamous blepharitis

- Mainly, treatment of seborrheic dermatitis of the scalp by means of specific shampoo
- **Lid hygiene:** Scales on eyelid margins is removed by a moistened cotton-tip applicator twice daily
- Antibiotic-steroid eye ointment is applied locally, twice daily for 2–4 weeks.

Ulcerative blepharitis

- **Local treatment**
  - **Lid scrub:** Warm sodium bicarbonate lotion (3%) is applied to the lid margin to soak the crusts. Alternately, a baby shampoo or 0.1% selenium sulfide solution may be used. Then removal of the crusts by a cotton-tip applicator.
  - Epilation of loose and diseased eyelashes.
  - Antibiotic-steroid ointment is to be applied by rubbing the lid margins 3 times daily.
  - Antibiotic drop or ointment is to be added. Chloramphenicol and ciprofloxacin are most effective against *Staphylococcus aureus*. Neomycin is best avoided because of high incidence of allergic reaction. If associated with dry eyes, use artificial tears 4–8 times daily.
- **Systemic therapy:** Systemic tetracycline or doxycycline for two weeks is useful in severe form of ulcerative blepharitis. It is better avoided in children due to dental complications.
- **General treatment:** Ocular hygiene and hand washing
  - Avoid hair oil, kajal or other ocular cosmetics
  - Correction of refractive errors
  - Treatment of seborrheic capitis by antidandruff shampoo
  - Treatment of louse infestation.

Meibomianitis (Figs 11.32A and B)

It is a chronic infection of the meibomian glands, especially occurs in the middle-age.

It is mostly due to staphylococcal infection, but may also occur in trachoma.

Symptoms

- Watering
- Frothy discharge—mainly at the canthi
- Foreign body sensation.

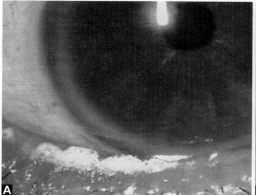 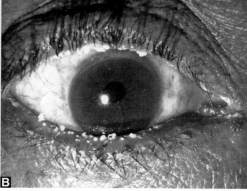

Figs 11.32A and B: A. Meibomian seborrhea; **B.** Meibomianitis (tooth paste sign)

Signs

- A white, frothy secretion (seborrhea) (Fig. 11.32A) on the eyelid margins and at the canthi.
- On pressing the lid margin—meibomian secretion is expressed as tooth paste (tooth paste sign) (Fig. 11.32B).
- On eversion of the eyelids—vertical yellowish streaks shining through the conjunctiva are seen.
- Associated features of blepharitis or chalazion may be seen.

Meibomian gland dysfunction (MGD)

In this condition the meibomian glands are not secreting enough lipid layer or it is of poor quality lipid. Often, the gland openings get plugged up so that less lipid secretion comes out of the glands.

The MGD is very common, and a highly complex disease condition that is caused by several host, microbial, hormonal, metabolic and environmental factors.

In early stages, the patients are often asymptomatic, but if left untreated, MGD can cause or exacerbate dry eye symptoms and blepharitis. Symptoms include: dryness, burning, itching, stickiness or crustiness; watering, chronic red eyes, photophobia, recurrent chalazion or styes and ultimately intermittent blurring of vision. There are different grading system for MGDs.

For asymptomatic patients, performing gland expression with digital pressure to the central lower lid followed by assessing ocular surface damage is useful. Other sophisticated instruments (including meibography) are available to diagnose the condition.

Treatment:
- Eyelid/eyelash hygiene—by warm compresses, lid massage and lid scrubbing with soft soap or baby shampoo.
- Topical lubricants—to relieve symptoms, reduce tear film evaporation, and stabilize lipid layer
- Topical or systemic antibiotics (oral doxycycline or azithromycin)—to control infections
- Treatment of Demodex infestation with tea tree oil.

Oral omega-3 fatty acids (flaxseed oil)—to improve the quality and consistency of the meibomian glands secretion.

Treatment

- Hot compress
- Tarsal massage (vertical lid massage), and removal of secretion with a moist cotton applicator
- Systemic doxycycline; and steroid-antibiotic ointment 2–4 times daily.

External Hordeolum (Stye) (Figs 11.33A and B)

It is an acute suppurative inflammation of the follicle of an eyelash, or associated gland of Zeis or Moll.

Etiology

- Causative organism is usually *Staphylococcus aureus.*
- Common in children and young adults, but may occur at any age.
- Low general resistance as in debility or diabetes.
- Uncorrected refractive errors.
- Associated with boils, acne of the face or neck (stye in crops).

Symptoms

- Acute pain and swelling of the lid margin.
- Sense of heaviness and discharge.

Signs

- Redness and edema of the affected lid.
- Local temperature is raised.
- A swollen area at the lid margin, and it has a whitish, round, raised pus point in relation to the root of a cilium.
- The swelling is tender.
- Matting of eyelashes may be present.
- Enlargement of the preauricular or submandibular lymph node.

Complications

- Ulcerative blepharitis

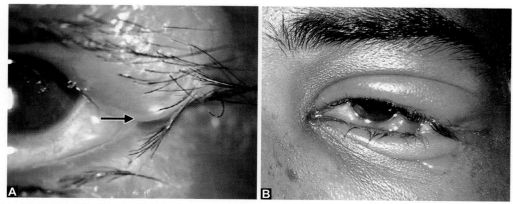

Figs 11.33A and B: External hordeolum. **A.** Stye (arrow); **B.** Preseptal cellulitis

- Cellulitis and lid abscess
- Rarely orbital cellulitis
- Very rarely cavernous sinus thrombosis.

Treatment

- Hot compress—3–4 times daily
- Evacuation of pus—by pulling out the affected eyelash (epilation)
- Alternately, a tiny horizontal incision may be given to drain out the pus
- Continue hot compress—3–4 times daily
- Systemic analgesics (like, ibuprofen or aspirin) 2–3 times daily with antacids
- Local antibiotic drop (chloramphenicol or ciprofloxacin) 4–6 times daily and ointment at night
- In case of 'stye in crops'
  - Postprandial blood sugar to exclude diabetes
  - In addition to local treatment, a course of systemic tetracycline or doxycycline is needed for 7–14 days
- Correction of refractive errors if any
- Improvement of nutrition and general hygiene, especially in children.

Chalazion (Figs 11.34A and B)

It means a *hail stone*. It is a chronic nonspecific inflammatory granuloma of the meibomian gland.

Etiology

- Children and young adults
- Blepharitis
- Chronic conjunctivitis, e.g. trachoma
- Diabetes mellitus in adults
- *Errors of refraction* (excessive rubbing of eyes to gain clear vision → chronic inflammation → obstruction of the meibomian ducts).

Pathogenesis

Chronic inflammation of the gland by a low virulence organism → blockage of the duct of the meibomian gland → accumulation of lipid secretion → break down of lipids into components of oleic acid → mucosal irritation → cellular infiltration with formation of giant cells → proliferation of fibroblasts → 'granuloma' formation.

Histology

- Centrally, cheesy sebaceous material.
- Surrounded by granulation tissue—having lymphocytes, epithelioid cells and foreign body type of giant cells, and fine blood vessels.
- Whole thing is enclosed by a fibrous capsule.

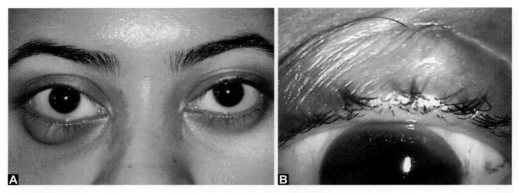

Figs 11.34A and B: Chalazion. **A.** Right lower lid; **B.** Upper lid (magnified view)

Symptoms

- Painless nodular swelling of the eyelid
- Drooping of the eyelid (in case of a large, or multiple chalazion).

Signs

- A small pea-size nodular swelling, away from the lid margin.
- It is firm, tense and non-tender.
- No signs of inflammation.
- Skin over the swelling is normal and free from it.
- On eversion, the tarsal conjunctiva underneath the nodule is velvety-red or purple, and slightly elevated.
- Regional lymph nodes are not involved.

Course (fate) of a chalazion

- Spontaneous resolution (if it is small)
- May remain as such
- Increases in size leading to mechanical ptosis
- Secondarily infected, called **internal hordeolum (Fig. 11.35A)**
- It can turn into **marginal chalazion (Fig. 11.35B)**—the granulation tissue formed in the duct of the gland, projects as a reddish-gray nodule on the intermarginal strip
- It may burst either through the conjunctiva (as a fungating mass of granulation tissue), or through the skin
- It may be calcified
- Very rarely, a malignant change may occur (meibomian carcinoma), especially in

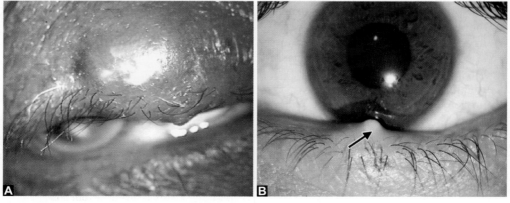

Figs 11.35A and B: **A.** Internal hordeolum; **B.** Marginal chalazion (arrow)

old age with a history of recurrence. So, a histopathological examination is a must in such cases.

Treatment

- **In case of small chalazion**
  - Hot fomentation
  - Steroid-antibiotic ointment with lid massage for a few days.
  - Intralesional (intrachalazion) injection of depot steroids (e.g. 0.1–0.2 mL of triamcinolone, 40 mg/mL) may be helpful, especially if the chalazion is near the lacrimal punctum. A steroid injection may lead to permanent depigmentation of the skin at the injection site.
- **In moderate to large chalazion:** Incision and thorough curettage under local anesthesia is done as an OPD procedure.
- **In marginal chalazion (Fig. 11.35B):** Under local anesthesia
  - Press out the material with thumb and index finger
  - Electrocoagulation by passing 20–30 mA current for few seconds.
- **In case of internal hordeolum (Fig. 11.35A):**
  First, treat the acute inflammation by:
  - Hot fomentation 3–4 times daily
  - Systemic analgesics with antacids
  - Local antibiotic like chloramphenicol or ciprofloxacin drop or ointment
  - Rarely, a systemic antibiotic. After the acute phase subsides, treatment is done by incision and curettage.
- **Correction of refractive errors (if any).**

IMPORTANT LID TUMORS

Xanthelesma

- This is slightly raised, yellow plaque, most commonly found at the inner portion of the upper or lower eyelid (Fig. 11.36)
- They are often symmetrical in the two lids, and on both sides
- Most common in elderly female
- They grow slowly, and produce only a cosmetic defect
- **Predisposing factors**
  - More commonly, it is spontaneous
  - Sometimes, associated with diabetes and excess serum cholesterol
- **Histologically**, it is the cutaneous deposition of lipid material, being engulfed by histocytes (foam cells).

Treatment

- Surgical excision
- Destruction by chemicals (trichloroacetic acid), diathermy or photocoagulation
- Recurrence is very common.

Hemangiomas

Cavernous hemangiomas are common in children (Fig. 11.37).
- Hemangioma often follows the distribution of the first and second divisions of the fifth nerve.
- Sometimes, it is associated with hemangioma of the choroid (may be with glaucoma), and hemangioma of the lep-

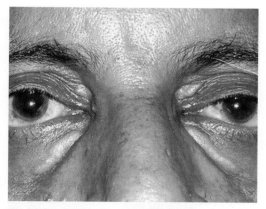

Fig. 11.36: Xanthelasma of all four lids

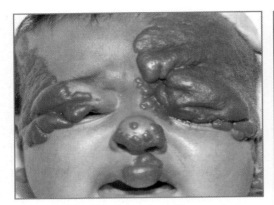

Fig. 11.37: Capillary (strawberry) hemangioma

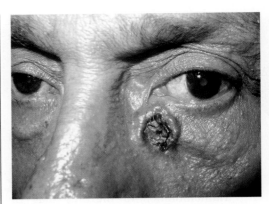

Fig. 11.39: Basal cell carcinoma of the lower lid

tomeninges, called Sturge-Weber syndrome (Fig. 11.38).
- Hemangiomas appear bluish when seen through skin, and form swellings which increase in size on crying, or lowering the head.

Treatment

- Small hemangiomas may well be left alone.
- But, large hemangiomas require treatment by intralesional steroid injection, or by superficial radiotherapy.

Basal Cell Carcinoma (Rodent Ulcer)

Basal cell carcinoma is the most common malignant tumor of the eyelid, occurring

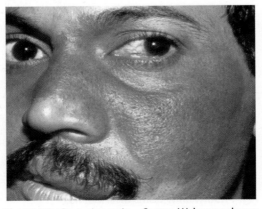

Fig. 11.38: Port wine stain—Sturge-Weber syndrome

almost twenty times more often than squamous cell carcinoma
- Lower lid is more commonly involved, especially near the inner canthus (Fig. 11.39).
- It starts as a small pimple which ulcerates, and if the scab is removed, it is found that the edges are raised (rolled out edges) and indurated.
- The ulcer spreads very slowly, and the growth extends under the skin in all directions and penetrates deeply.
- It does not metastasize.
- The tumor arises from the basal cell of the epidermis and consists of islands of neoplastic cells (cell nests).

Treatment

- **Surgical excision** with a 3 mm margin outside the obvious tumor
- **Radiotherapy:** It is radiosensitive
- **Cryotherapy**—for small and superficial tumors
- **Exenteration**—if the tumor invades the globe or orbit in neglected cases.

Squamous Cell Carcinoma (Fig. 11.40)

It is the second most common malignancy of the eyelid, usually arising from preexisting senile keratosis.

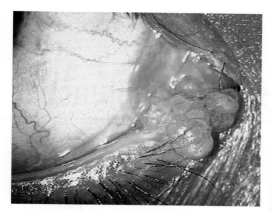

Fig. 11.40: Squamous cell carcinoma

- It appears as a nodule, an ulcerative lesion, or a papilloma.
- The growth rate is faster than the rodent ulcer, and it metastasizes into the regional lymph nodes.
- The diagnosis is confirmed by biopsy.

Treatment

Radical surgery with postoperative radio-therapy.

Meibomian Gland Carcinoma (Figs 11.41A and B)

It is a rare tumor arising from the meibomian glands:
- The tumor appears as a discrete, yellow, firm nodule which is sometimes incorrectly diagnosed as *recurrent chalazion*
- Sometimes, diffuse tumor along the lid margin may be mistaken as 'chronic blepharitis'
- Widespread metastasis is common
- Prognosis is poor in comparison to previous two tumors.

Treatment

- Radical excision with reconstruction of the lid
- Recurrence after radiotherapy is common.

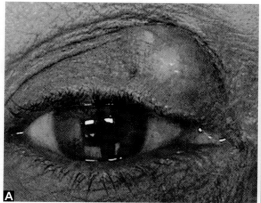
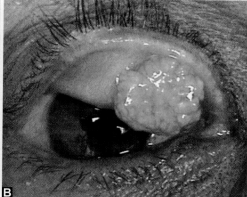

Figs 11.41A and B: A. Meibomian carcinoma—mimicking a chalazion; **B.** After everting the lid (same patient)

Diseases of the Conjunctiva

CONJUNCTIVAL DISEASES

Symptoms

- Discomfort or burning sensation
- Discharge from the eyes
- Stickiness of the lids during sleep
- Itching
- Blurring of vision, or colored halos as the mucus flakes floats across the cornea
- Severe pain suggests corneal involvement
- Dryness of the eyes
- Abnormal mass or pigmentation.

Signs

- Abnormality in appearance
- Variety of discharge
- Vascular changes
- Edema (chemosis)
- Pigmentation
- Keratinization
- Hemorrhage
- Follicle formation
- Papillary hyperplasia
- Symblepharon
- Fleshy mass
- Conjunctival scarring
- Associated involvement of the lids or cornea.

HYPEREMIA OF THE CONJUNCTIVA

It is the passive dilatation of the conjunctival blood vessels that occur without exudation or cellular infiltration.

Causes

- Conjunctival irritation by smoke, dust or fumes
- Exposure to wind and sun
- Following bath or swimming
- Prolonged wakefulness and is aggravated by near work.

Symptoms

- May be absent
- A gritty foreign body sensation
- Many patients are distressed because of the redness only.

Signs

- Only redness; otherwise conjunctiva is normal
- Temporary blanching is noted with 1 in 1000 epinephrine solution.

Treatment

- No treatment is necessary except the removal of the cause.
- Temporary relief is obtained by topical instillation of decongestant drop, containing either *phenylephrine* or *naphazoline*.

CONJUNCTIVITIS

Conjunctivitis is an inflammation of the conjunctiva characterized by cellular infiltration and exudation.

Classification

Conjunctivitis can be classified as infective and allergic.

Infective Conjunctivitis

Acute
- Catarrhal
- Serous
- Mucopurulent
- Purulent
- Membranous.

Subacute or chronic
- **Nonspecific**
  - Simple chronic
  - Angular
  - Follicular.
- **Specific**
  - Trachoma
  - Tuberculosis
  - Syphilis
  - Tularemia.

Allergic Conjunctivitis

- Simple allergic
- Phlyctenular
- Vernal (spring catarrh)
- Giant papillary.

Diagnosis

It is based on—history, clinical examination and laboratory investigations.

History

- Unilateral or bilateral
- Involvement of the other members of the family or community
- Exposure to toxins, or chemicals
- Associated symptoms—e.g. fever, pharyngitis, rhinitis, urethritis, etc.

Clinical Features

Three main features which should be considered are as follows:

1. Type of discharge,
2. Characteristics of conjunctival reaction, and
3. Preauricular lymphadenopathy.

Types of discharge

- **Watery discharge:** Viral and toxic inflammation.
- **Mucinous discharge:** Vernal conjunctivitis and keratoconjunctivitis sicca.
- **Purulent discharge:** Severe acute bacterial infection.
- **Mucopurulent discharge:** Mild bacterial as well as chlamydial infection. It typically, gives rise to glueing up of the eyelids in the morning.
- **Serosanguineous discharge:** Sometimes in adenoviral keratoconjunctivitis.

Conjunctival reaction

It requires a good illumination and magnification. A slit-lamp examination is better.
- **Congestion (injection):** It is conjunctival congestion (Figs 12.1A and B) is characterized by bright red superficial vessels which are most intense in the fornices and least at the limbus. It should be differentiated from the ciliary congestion or injection (Figs 12.2A and B) (circumcorneal) which is due to deeper diseases of the anterior segment (Table 12.1).
- **Subconjunctival hemorrhage** occurs in:
  - Acute hemorrhagic conjunctivitis (picornavirus) (Fig. 12.3)
  - Adenoviral conjunctivitis
  - Bacterial conjunctivitis—especially in *Pneumococcus* and *Hemophilus* species.
- **Edema (chemosis):** The exudation of fibrin and protein rich fluid, through the permeable capillaries produces a translucent swelling of the conjunctiva.

In the bulbar conjunctiva, where the attachments to the globe are lax, large quantity of the exudates cause ballooning of the conjunctiva. The palpebral conjunctiva is little affected, but the lids are often edematous.

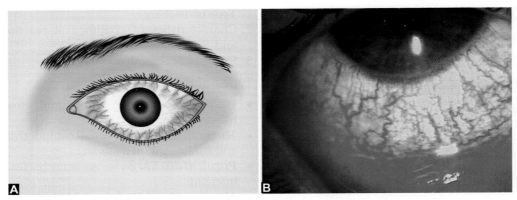

Figs 12.1A and B: Conjunctival congestion. **A.** Schematic representation; **B.** Photograph

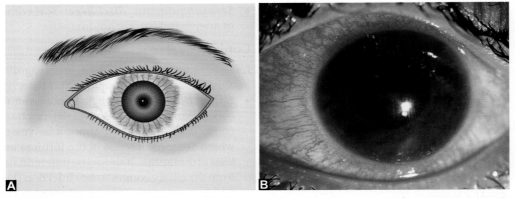

Figs 12.2A and B: Ciliary congestion—acute attack in angle closure glaucoma. **A.** Schematic representation; **B.** Photograph

TABLE 12.1: Difference between conjunctival and ciliary congestions		
Features	**Conjunctival congestion**	**Ciliary congestion**
Appearance	Vessels superficial; bright red; mostly in the fornices and fade towards the limbus; branched dichotomously	Vessels deep: violet or dusky-red mostly at the limbus, and fade towards the fornices; branched radially
Blood vessels	• Vessels fill up from the fornix • Branches of posterior conjunctival vessels	• Vessels fill up from the limbus • Branches of anterior ciliary vessels
Epinephrine test (1:1000)	Constricts vessels, "whitens" the conjunctiva	No effect
Disease	Conjunctivitis	Keratitis, iridocyclitis or angle closure glaucoma

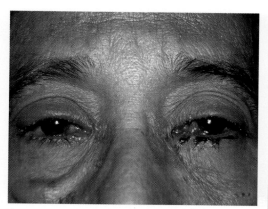

Fig. 12.3: Acute hemorrhagic conjunctivitis

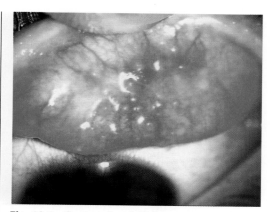

Fig. 12.5: Conjunctival follicles

Chemosis (Fig. 12.4) is mainly seen in severe bacterial infection (e.g. *Gonococcus*), allergic conjunctivitis and associated orbital inflammations.

- *Follicles (Fig. 12.5):* They are round swellings (0.5–2 mm in diameter) and are due to localized aggregations of lymphocytes in the subepithelial adenoid layer. Each follicle is encircled by tiny blood vessels. *Conjunctiva of the newborn is unable to produce follicles before 2–3 months of age, due to lack of adenoid layer.*

Follicles are seen in follicular conjunctivitis, trachoma, toxins or with drugs (brimonidine or with other antiglaucoma drugs).

- *Papillae:* These are essentially vascular structures invaded by inflammatory cells. In papilla, there is hyperplasia of the normal system of vascularization with glomerulus like bunches of new capillaries, growing into the epithelium (Fig. 12.6). *A papillary reaction is more nonspecific, being of less diagnostic importance than a follicle.*

It is mostly seen in vernal conjunctivitis, trachoma and giant papillary conjunctivitis.

- *Membranes*
  - *True membranes (Fig. 12.7A):* They form when the inflammatory exudates permeate the superficial layers of the conjunctival epithelium.

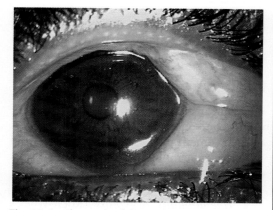

Fig. 12.4: Chemosis of the conjunctiva

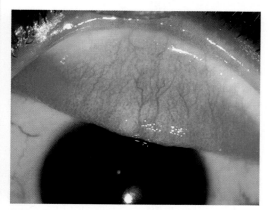

Fig. 12.6: Conjunctival papillae

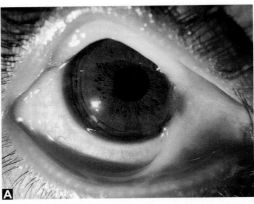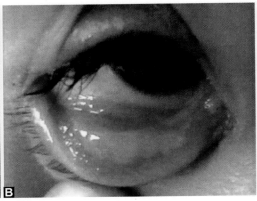

Figs 12.7A and B: A. True membrane; **B.** Pseudomembrane

- **Pseudomembranes (Fig. 12.7B):** They consist of coagulated exudates loosely adherent to the inflamed conjunctival epithelium. They can be easily peeled off, leaving the epithelium intact without or with some bleeding. Pseudomembrane forms in adenoviral, vernal, pneumococcal and gonococcal conjunctivitis.

Preauricular lymphadenopathy

Preauricular lymph node enlargement is a feature of viral and chlamydial infections but is seldom found in bacterial conjunctivitis except in *Neisseria gonorrhoeae.*

Laboratory Investigations

The main indications are as follows:
- Severe purulent conjunctivitis—to identify the pathogens and sensitivity pattern
- Follicular conjunctivitis—to differentiate viral from chlamydial infection
- Chronic or recurrent conjunctivitis—to find out etiological diagnosis
- Ophthalmia neonatorum.

Conjunctival scraping and staining

Scraping is taken from the site of maximal disease with a sterile spatula. The materials are then spread on a glass slide for Gram and Giemsa stains.

- **Gram staining:** It is used to identify the bacteria and to some extent fungus. It is not useful to detect the cellular response.
- **Giemsa staining:** It is used to identify the cellular response. It also demonstrates the inclusion bodies.

Culture

The materials taken from exudates and lid margins with sterile cotton swab are placed in blood agar or chocolate agar medium. Later, sensitivity pattern is to be determined.

ACUTE MUCOPURULENT CONJUNCTIVITIS (FIGS 12.8A TO C)

It is a common type of acute conjunctival inflammation, characterized by marked hyperemia and a mucopurulent discharge.

Etiology

- Occurs at any age
- Poor personal hygiene
- Involvement of the other members of the family or schoolmates.
- **Causative organisms:**
  - *Staphylococcus aureus* (most common),
  - *Haemophilus aegyptius* (Koch-Week's bacillus)—a Gram-negative bacillus

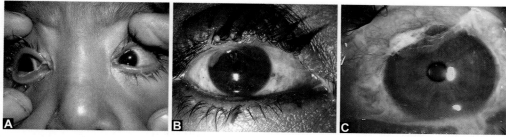

Figs 12.8A to C: Acute mucopurulent conjunctivitis

- *Pneumococcus*
- *Streptococcus,* etc.

Clinical Features

The disease is usually bilateral, but one eye may be affected earlier, or more severe, than the other.

Symptoms

- Redness of the eyes
- Mucopurulent discharge
- Grittiness or foreign body sensation
- Stickiness of the eyelids
- Photophobia
- Colored halos around the light.

Signs

- One eye may be more affected than the other
- Lid edema
- Matting of the eyelashes
- Conjunctival congestion and chemosis
- Mucopurulent discharge or flakes of mucopus
- Subconjunctival petechial hemorrhage (Fig. 12.9).

Composition of the discharge: Tears, mucus, epithelial cells, bacteria, leukocytes, fibrin and rarely red blood cells.

Complications if not treated properly:
- It may subside spontaneously by 10–15 days.
- It may pass into less intense, chronic conjunctivitis.

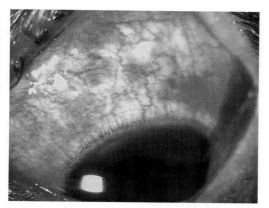

Fig. 12.9: Subconjunctival petechial hemorrhage

- Abrasion of the cornea → corneal ulcer.
  - Marginal corneal ulcer → pseudopterygium formation
  - Chronic dacryocystitis (very rarely).

Treatment

- Frequent eye wash with lukewarm saline solution to clean crusts and discharge. Use dark glasses to prevent photophobia.
- A broad-spectrum antibiotic eye drop, e.g. moxifloxacin, gatifloxacin or ciprofloxacin is used frequently. Depending upon the severity, it may be four times daily to 1 hourly.
- An antibiotic eye ointment like tetracycline, gentamicin or chloramphenicol at bed time.
- Neomycin is better avoided, as it causes ocular allergy in 8% of the cases.
- Other family members are to be treated simultaneously.

- ***To prevent spread or cross infection***
  - The patient must keep his hands clean.
  - The patient should lie on the affected side (to prevent its spread to the unaffected eye).
  - Personal belongings of the patient like towel, handkerchief, pillow, etc. should be kept separately.

PURULENT CONJUNCTIVITIS

This is a severe, acute conjunctivitis with purulent discharge mainly caused by *Neisseria gonorrhoeae.*

- Sometimes, the same clinical picture may be found in staphylococcal, streptococcal and with mixed infections.
- This is rare nowadays.
- ***Types:*** It occurs in two forms—(1) ***purulent conjunctivitis*** in adults, *(2)* ***ophthalmia neonatorum*** in newborns.

Adult Purulent Conjunctivitis (Fig. 12.10)

- ***Incubation period:*** Few hours to 3 days.
- Males are usually affected.
- Right eye is more commonly involved.

Clinical Features

- Massive swelling of the lids.

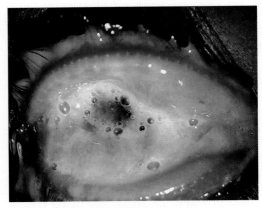

Fig. 12.10: Purulent conjunctivitis

- Copious purulent discharge.
- Conjunctival chemosis with or without membrane formation.
  - Corneal involvement → leading to central corneal ulcer → perforation.
  - Preauricular lymphadenopathy with tenderness.
  - Rise in body temperature and mental depression.

Diagnosis

- The most important diagnostic point is the ***coincidence of urethritis.***
- Conjunctival scraping and exudate show Gram '–ve' intracellular organisms.

Complications

- Corneal edema
- Central corneal ulceration
- Perforated corneal ulcer and its sequela
- Iridocyclitis (may be with hypopyon)
- Ultimately, leading to blindness.

Treatment

Patient should be kept in isolation.

- Frequent irrigation of the eyes with warm normal saline.
- Penicillin eye drop (freshly prepared in distilled water 10,000 units/mL) every minute for half an hour, then every 5 minutes for 1 hour, then hourly for 3–5 days.
- Alternately, newer antibiotics like—norfloxacin or ciprofloxacin eye drop may be used in the same doses.
- Tetracycline eye ointment at bed time.
- Systemic antibiotic—like crystalline penicillin or ciprofloxacin should be given intravenously for 3–5 days. Intramuscular injection of ceftriaxone—1.0 g/daily for 5 days, if the patient is allergic to penicillin.
- Atropine (1%) eye ointment is added, if there is corneal involvement.
- Every precaution is to be taken to prevent the spread of infection.

Ophthalmia Neonatorum (Fig. 12.11)

It is a conjunctivitis occurring during the first month of life as a result of carelessness at the time of birth.

Etiology (Table 12.2)

- Gonococcal infection is rare nowadays, but it is most serious.
- *Chlamydia oculogenitalis* is the most common cause of ophthalmia neonatorum nowadays.

Clinical Features

- In gonococcus, usual presentation is between 1 and 3 days after birth with a *hyperacute purulent conjunctivitis*.
- In other cases, it is a catarrhal or mucopurulent conjunctivitis.
- In chlamydial infection, the conjunctival reaction is *papillary only*, without any follicular response.
- Cornea is frequently involved in gonococcal infection and may be perforated with its sequelae.

Treatment

Curative

- Staining of smear and culture of the exudate to know the sensitivity pattern.

TABLE 12.2: Etiology and manifestations of ophthalmia neonatorum

Etiology	Manifestations
Chemicals	In hours (antibiotic, detergent)
Gonococcal	1–3 days
(Other) Bacterial	4–5 days
Chlamydial	5–10 days

- Penicillin eye drop (freshly prepared, 5,000 IU/mL in distilled water)—is instilled as 1 minute interval for half an hour, then 5 minutes interval for 1 hour, and then hourly 3–5 days.
- Ciprofloxacin or norfloxacin eye drop may be given in same manner.
- *For chlamydia*
  - 10% sulphacetamide drop—4 times daily.
  - 1% tetracycline ointment—2 times daily.
  - Systemic erythromycin 50 mg/kg in four divided doses for 3 weeks.
- Systemic penicillin, 50,000 units/kg intramuscularly in two divided doses daily for 7 days.
- Atropine (1%) eye ointment, if there is any corneal involvement.

Prophylaxis

Proper antenatal care of the mother, and any vaginal discharge should be treated meticulously.

- Asepsis and care are to be maintained to protect the eyes during delivery.
- Sulphacetamide (10%), ciprofloxacin or norfloxacin eye drop—four times daily for 7–10 days, is advised following birth.

    Alternately, tetracycline (1%) eye ointment twice daily for few days.

> **Crede's prophylaxis:** One drop of 1% silver nitrate is instilled into the eyes of the baby, just after the birth. It should never be stronger than 1%—otherwise corneal opacity may result.
>   Crede's prophylaxis was used earlier to prevent gonococcal ophthalmia, which is rare nowadays.

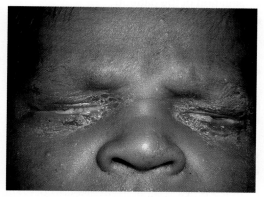

Fig. 12.11: Ophthalmia neonatorum (gonococcal)

MEMBRANOUS CONJUNCTIVITIS (FIG. 12.12)

It is a type of acute conjunctivitis, associated with membrane formation on the inflamed conjunctiva.

Etiology

- Membranous conjunctivitis is mostly caused by *Corynebacterium diphtheriae*.
- Sometimes, it is caused by *Pneumococcus* or *Streptococcus*, especially in weak children with eruptive fever.
- Chemical irritants (e.g. alkali) may be the cause in adults.

Clinical Features

Usually in children between 2 years and 8 years. It occurs in two forms—(1) Mild and (2) Severe.

1. ***In mild cases***
   - Edema of the lids
   - Mucopurulent or sanious discharge
   - Conjunctival congestion
   - White membrane on the palpebral conjunctiva
   - This membrane peels off rapidly without much bleeding.

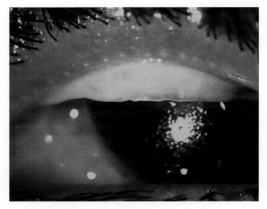

Fig. 12.12: Membranous conjunctivitis

2. ***In severe cases***
   - Lids are more edematous, red, hot and tense
   - Scanty, thick conjunctival discharge
   - Pain and tenderness
   - Thick white or grayish-yellow membrane on the palpebral conjunctiva.
   - This membrane is difficult to separate, and ***after removal, bleeding is very common***.
   - Preauricular lymphadenopathy
   - Later, the membrane sloughs off, leaving a red, raw granulating surface
   - Then, there is danger of adhesions, forming between the bulbar and palpebral parts of conjunctiva (symblepharon).

> ***Ligneous conjunctivitis:*** It is a type of membranous conjunctivitis where the woody-type of membrane is cast off but recurs again and again.

Complications

- Corneal ulcer, which may slough out
- Symblepharon
- Trichiasis and entropion
- Xerosis of the conjunctiva.

Treatment

Every case should be treated as diphtherial, unless there is good negative evidence.

- Isolation of the patient.
- Intramuscular injection of crystalline penicillin 50,000 units/kg, twice daily for 7 days.
- Antidiphthericum serum (40,000–60,000 units) intravenously, and to be repeated after 24 hours if necessary.
- Penicillin drop (freshly prepared 10,000 units/mL) every half an hour.
- Erythromycin eye ointment at bed time.
- Atropine (1%) eye ointment if the cornea is involved.
- Prevention of symblepharon formation.

SIMPLE CHRONIC CONJUNCTIVITIS

It is a chronic simple or catarrhal inflammation of the conjunctiva.

Etiology

- As a continuation of simple acute conjunctivitis.
- Continuous irritation of the eyes, due to smoke, dust, heat, bad air, late hours, abuse of alcohol, etc.
- Permanent local irritation by trichiasis, concretions in the palpebral conjunctiva, retained foreign body, chronic dacryocystitis, chronic rhinitis, etc.
- Seborrhea of the scalp (dandruff) is a common factor.

Symptoms

- Burning and grittiness of the eyes
- Redness more in the evening
- Difficulty in keeping the eyes open
- Slight frothy discharge
- Lids may or may not be stuck together.

Signs

- Apparently, the eyes may look normal
- Lower fornix is congested
- Upper and lower palpebral conjunctiva may be congested with a velvety papilli form roughness
- Thin sticky discharge.

Treatment

- Elimination of the cause of irritation.
- Culture and sensitivity of the conjunctival swab and accordingly local antibiotic drop, and ointment are given.
- Astringent and decongestant eye drop, e.g. zinc sulfate, boric acid, naphazoline, etc. four times daily.
- In difficult cases, conjunctival sac is painted with 1% solution of silver nitrate.

- Repeated lid massage, if there is excessive Meibomian gland activity.

ANGULAR CONJUNCTIVITIS (FIGS 12.13A AND B)

It is a chronic conjunctivitis, where the conjunctival inflammation is limited to intermarginal strip, especially at the outer and inner canthi.

Etiology

- Typically, caused by *Moraxella*, a Gram-negative diplobacillus (thick rods placed endtoend). They produce a proteolytic ferment which acts by maceration of the epithelium.
- Rarely by *Staphylococcus*.

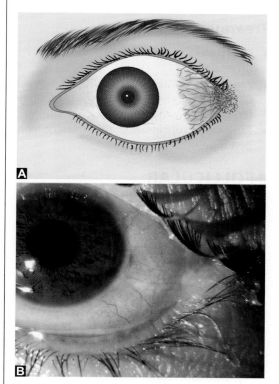

Figs 12.13A and B: Angular conjunctivitis. **A.** Schematic representation; **B.** Photograph

Symptoms

- Discomfort, with slight mucopurulent discharge.
- Itching and excoriation of the skin near the outer or inner canthus of eyes.
- Frequent blinking.

Signs

- Congestion of the conjunctiva, limited to the intermarginal strip, near the outer and inner canthi.
- Congestion of the adjacent bulbar conjunctiva.
- Excoriation of the skin at the outer and inner canthi.
- If untreated, the condition becomes chronic and may give rise to blepharitis. Sometimes, a shallow marginal corneal ulcer or central ulcer with hypopyon may form.

Treatment

- Oxytetracycline (1%) eye ointment, 2–3 times daily.
- Zinc oxide containing eye drop, 4–6 times daily (this acts by inhibiting the proteolytic ferment of the organism).
- Zinc oxide ointment to the lidmargins at bed time.

FOLLICULAR CONJUNCTIVITIS

These are acute, subacute or chronic inflammation of the conjunctiva with the appearance of the follicles.

Causes

- *Acute follicular conjunctivitis:*
  - Inclusion conjunctivitis
  - Epidemic keratoconjunctivitis
  - Pharyngoconjunctival fever
  - Newcastle conjunctivitis
  - Herpetic keratoconjunctivitis

- Trachoma (chlamydial)
- Due to chemicals and toxins
- Drug toxicity, e.g. brimonidine, pilocarpine, eserine, idoxyuridine (IDU), diisopropylfluorophosphate (DFP), etc.
- Associated with tonsillitis or adenoids in children.

Acute Follicular Conjunctivitis (Figs 12.14A to C)

There is always a tendency of corneal involvement in acute follicular conjunctivitis. So, the typical lesion is most of the time a keratoconjunctivitis.

Inclusion Conjunctivitis

Causative agent: *Chlamydia oculogenitalis.* The primary source of infection is mild urethritis in male and cervicitis in female.

Mode of infection
- *In neonates*—during birth.
- *In adults*—by the fingers and through the water of the swimming pool (*swimmingbath conjunctivitis*).

Though, the most common cause of swimming-bath conjunctivitis is adenoviral infection. Incubation period: 5–10 days.
- Follicular hypertrophy more in lower lid.
- Papillary hypertrophy may be present.
- Superficial punctate keratitis and pannus formation.

Epidemic Keratoconjunctivitis

Causative agent: Adenovirus (type 8 and 19).

Clinical features
- Very much contagious and often occurs in epidemic form.
- Marked conjunctival inflammation with scanty discharge.
- After 7–10 days—superficial punctate keratitis (Fig. 12.15) and subepithelial infiltrates develop with photophobia.
- Preauricular lymphadenopathy.

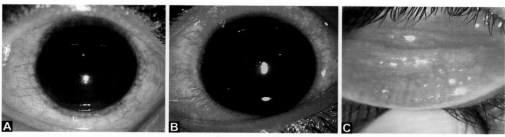

Figs 12.14A to C: Acute follicular conjunctivitis—note the limbal follicles in figure 'A'

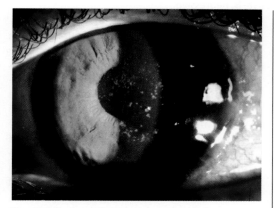

Fig. 12.15: Superficial punctate keratitis

- Subepithelial corneal opacities may persist for months.

Pharyngoconjunctival Fever

Causative agent: Adenovirus (type 3 and 7)

Clinical features
- Usually children are affected
- Acute follicular conjunctivitis
- Pharyngitis and fever
- Preauricular lymphadenopathy
- Superficial punctate keratitis is rare.
- It subsides quickly.

Newcastle Conjunctivitis

Causative agent: Newcastle virus derived from contact with diseased fowls. Clinically, it is similar to pharyngoconjunctival fever.

Acute Herpetic Keratoconjunctivitis

Causative agent: Herpes simplex virus.

Clinical features
- Usually seen in young children
- Follicles are usually large
- Small dendritic lesion on the cornea
- Pannus formation
- Corneal sensation is reduced
- Preauricular lymphadenopathy.

Treatment

- *In inclusion conjunctivitis:* 10–20% sulfacetamide drop and systemic tetracycline (250 mg 4 times for 14 days) are useful.
- *In other cases*
  - Mild astringent and decongestant drop.
  - Antivirals like IDU or acyclovir may be helpful in herpetic lesions.
- Antibiotic drop may be added to prevent secondary infection, especially in children.
- When the cornea is involved—mild cycloplegic (like tropicamide or cyclopentolate) is to be added.

Trachoma

Trachoma means *rough* and *swelling*. It is a chronic inflammation of the conjunctiva and the cornea characterized by the presence of follicles and papillary hypertrophy of the conjunctiva, and by growth of blood vessels over the cornea.

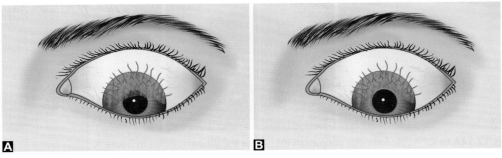

Figs 12.16A and B: Trachomatous pannus. **A.** Progressive; **B.** Regressive

The specific agent is *C. trachomatis*, a Bedsonian group of organism. Trachoma was previously known as **Egyptian ophthalmia**.

Etiological Factors

- Any age
- Agent: *C. trachomatis* and other pathogenic microorganisms also aggravate the disease process
- Dry, dirty and sandy weather
- Poor, unhygienic conditions
- **Eye-seeking flies** (Musca sorbens)
- Use of kajal or surma by the same family members from the same container
- Close person-to-person contacts.

Symptoms

- Foreign body sensation or grittiness
- Itching
- Watering, photophobia and redness
- Discharge is usually scanty but may be more due to secondary infections.

Acute trachoma: When a secondary infection like mucopurulent or purulent conjunctivitis is superimposed on a relatively mild chronic trachoma, it is called acute trachoma.

Signs

- Bulbar congestion
- Velvety papillary hypertrophy
- **Follicles:** Mostly seen in upper tarsal conjunctiva; on the limbus (leading to **Herbert's pits—pathognomonic**) or on the bulbar conjunctiva.
- **Pannus:** It is a characteristic sign. It is defined as fine subepithelial neovascularization, arranged vertically with round cell infiltration mainly seen at the upper limbus and upper part of cornea.

It is of two types—progressive and regressive (Figs 12.16 and 12.17). In **progressive pannus,** the cellular infiltration extends beyond the terminal ends of neovascularization. In **regressive pannus**, the vessels extend a short distance beyond and area of cellular infiltration.

The above-mentioned signs are seen in active trachoma. Further signs are described later in the healed stage or stage of sequelae.

Classification

- McCallan's classification
- Jone's classification
- WHO classification.

McCallan's classification

Stage-I:	*Incipient trachoma*: Immature follicles on upper palpebral conjunctiva with no scarring	
Stage-II:	Established trachoma	
IIA:	*Follicular hypertrophy predominant (Fig. 12.18A)*	
IIB:	*Papillary hypertrophy predominant (Fig. 12.18B)*	
Stage-III:	*Cicatrizing trachoma*: Follicles and scarring at upper tarsal conjunctiva	
Stage-IV:	*Healed trachoma*	

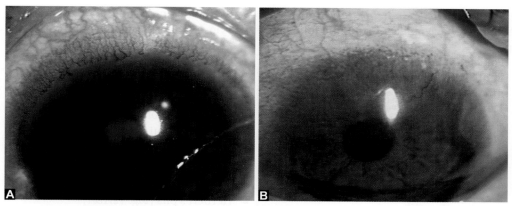

Figs 12.17A and B: A. Trachomatous pannus; **B.** Healed pannus

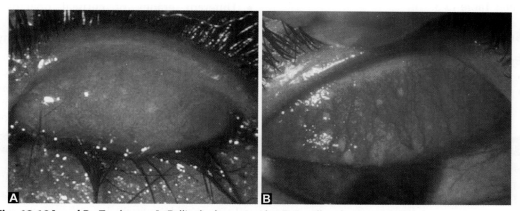

Figs 12.18A and B: Trachoma: **A.** Follicular hypertrophy; **B.** Papillary hypertrophy

Pitfalls of McCallan's classification

- It is only based on conjunctival findings. Degrees of corneal involvement are not mentioned.
- It fails to grade the severity of the disease and visual disability.
- It only tells about the evolution of the disease, but not the prognosis.

Jone's classification

Class 1: Blinding trachoma: Hyperendemic (or endemic) trachoma caused by *C. trachomatis*—serotypes A, B, Ba and C. It spreads from eyetoeye by transfer of ocular discharge by eyeseeking' flies and is associated with secondary bacterial infections.

Class 2: Non-blinding trachoma: It is by serotypes, A, B, Ba or C in mesoendemic or hypoendemic area, with better socioeconomic conditions of the victims. It is generally mild with limited transmission because of improved hygiene. Very low incidence of secondary bacterial infection.

Class 3: Para-trachoma: It is caused by serotypes—D, E, F, G, H, I, J, or K mostly seen in urban population.

It is an eye disease by *C. trachomatis*, where the organisms spread via sexual transmission from a genital reservoir with sporadic transfer to the eye, e.g. inclusion conjunctivitis in adult or ophthalmia neonatorum.

Diagnostic criteria in field study: Individual cases must have at least two of the following signs:
- Follicles at the upper tarsal conjunctiva
- Limbal follicles or their sequelae, *Herbert's pits* (Fig. 12.19A)
- Typical conjunctival scarring (stellate shaped scar) (Fig. 12.19B)
- Vascular pannus, mostly at the upper limbus. Herbert's pits are the only clinical signs unique to trachoma, but they do not occur in every case.

WHO classification

Refer Table 12.3.

Sequelae of Trachoma

Eyelids
- Ptosis (sleepy eyes)
- Scaphoid or boat-shaped lid

- Entropion and trichiasis
- Tylosis (rounding of the lid borders)
- Madarosis (loss of eyelashes)
- Chalazion.

Conjunctiva
- Loss of fornices
- Parenchymatous xerosis
- Symblepharon
- Pigmentation
- Pseudopterygium.

Cornea
- Herbert's pits (Fig. 12.19A)
- Healed pannus leading to hazy cornea
- Different grades of corneal opacity—nebula, macula or leukoma
- Trachomatous nodular keratopathy (Salzmann's nodular degeneration)
- Loss of sensation.

Lacrimal sac: Chronic dacryocystis.

TABLE 12.3: WHO classifications of trachoma		
Recent WHO classification of trachoma (FISTO)		
Trachomatous **F**ollicles (TF)	Implies active disease which needs treatment.	***Trachomatous inflammation, follicular:*** • Five or more follicles of at least 0.5 mm diameter on the upper tarsal plate should be present • Some papillae may be present in addition, but the palpebral conjunctival blood vessels are visible • This stage implies that the patient, if properly treated, should recover with no scarring or minimal scarring
Trachoma **I**ntense (TI)	Severe disease which needs urgent treatment	***Trachomatous inflammation, intense:*** • The follicles and papillae are so numerous and inflamed that more than 50% of the palpebral conjunctival blood vessels cannot be seen clearly • This stage indicates a severe infection with high-risk of serious complications
Trachomatous **S**carring (TS)	Old, now inactive infection	***Trachomatous scarring:*** Tarsal conjunctival cicatrization with white fibrous bands
Trachomatous **T**richiasis (TT)	Needs corrective surgery	Presence of at least one trichiatic eyelash
Trachomatous **O**pacities (TO)	Corneal opacities from previous trachoma cause visual loss	Presence of a corneal opacity covering part of the papillary region

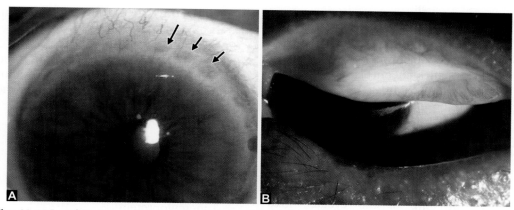

Figs 12.19A and B: A. Herbert's pits at the limbus (black arrows); **B.** Trachoma scar

Treatment

Therapeutic

Chlamydia is sensitive to erythromycin, tetracycline, sulfonamides and rifampicin.

Systemic:
1. The antibiotic of choice for treating active trachoma is oral azithromycin. The dose for children is 20 mg/kg in a single dose; adults receive a single dose of 1 g.
2. Oral doxycycline—100 mg/day for 3–4 weeks (except children below 14 years of age).

Local:
- Tetracycline (1%) eye ointment is the second drug of choice: twice daily for 6 weeks. Alternately, sulfacetamide eye drop (20% or 30%) if available can be given 4 times daily for 6 weeks.

This is followed by *intermittent treatment* with tetracycline eye ointment—twice daily for 5 consecutive days, or once daily for 10 consecutive days in each month for 6 months. This is especially important in epidemic or hyperendemic zone.

Prophylactic

- Improvement of personal hygiene and environmental sanitation.
- Avoid kajal, surma, etc.
- Avoid person-to-person close contacts.
- Periodic treatment with tetracycline (1%) eye ointment as *intermittent therapy*.
- Health education.

Treatment of complications

- Excision of the fornix
- Tarsectomy
- Surgery for the trichiasis and entropion
- Pannus may be treated by cryo-application or peritomy
- Corneal ulcers—on general line
- Mechanical expression of the follicles by roller (Knapp's) forceps, silver nitrate painting or diathermy (may cause more scar formation).

SAFE strategy for trachoma in 'Vision-2020 programme' (*see* Chapter 26, pages 515–516):
  S = Surgery for trichiasis/entropion
  A = Antibiotics
  F = Facial cleanliness
  E = Environmental sanitation.

ALLERGIC CONJUNCTIVITIS

Simple Allergic Conjunctivitis

This is an acute or subacute nonspecific urticarial reaction, due to a large amount allergen reaching the conjunctival sac.

Causes

- Hay fever
- Pollens of certain flowers
- Dust, cosmetics, chemicals, etc.
- Contact with pet animals
- Certain local drugs, e.g. neomycin, atropine, IDU, etc.

Clinical Features

- *Symptoms*: Itching, redness and lacrimation
- *Signs:* Swelling of the eyelids, mild chemosis with diffuse papillary responses. Cornea is rarely involved.

Treatment

- Removal of the allergens.
- Combination of a vasoconstrictor (naphazoline) with an antihistamine (antazoline or xylometazoline)—four times daily.
- Corticosteroids drop in severe cases.
- Antihistamine tablets are often helpful to suppress other symptoms like running nose.
- Topical use of 2–4% sodium cromoglycate to prevent remissions or olopatadine eye drop twice daily.

PHLYCTENULAR CONJUNCTIVITIS

It is an allergic reaction of the conjunctiva caused by endogenous bacterial toxins and characterized by bleb or nodule formation near the limbus.

- Phlycten means a *bleb*.
- Histopathologically, the bleb is composed of compact mass of mononuclear lymphocytes and polymorphs underneath the epithelium.

Etiology

- *Age:* Children of 4–14 years
- Unhygienic condition and malnutrition
- *Endogenous toxins*, like:
  - Tuberculoprotein
  - Toxins from *Staphylococcus/Streptococcus* (from tonsillitis or adenoids)
  - Toxins from intestinal parasites.

Clinical Types

- *Phlyctenular conjunctivitis (Figs 12.20A and 12.21A):* When the conjunctiva alone is involved.
- *Phlyctenular keratoconjunctivitis (Figs 12.20B and 12.21B):* When at the limbus and involves both the conjunctiva and cornea.
- *Phlyctenular keratitis:* When cornea alone is involved (rare).

Symptoms

- Redness with formation of bleb
- Irritation and lacrimation
- Pain and photophobia in the presence of corneal involvement.

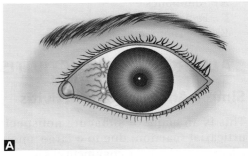 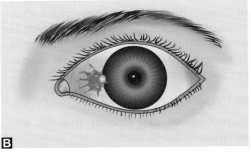

Figs 12.20A and B: Phlyctenular; **A.** Conjunctivitis and **B.** Keratoconjunctivitis

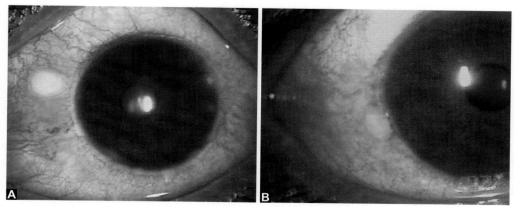

Figs 12.21A and B: A. Phlyctenular conjunctivitis; **B.** Limbal phlycten

Signs

- One or more, small, round and raised nodule at, or near the limbus. They are gray or pinkish-white in color and 1–3 mm in diameter.
- Localized bulbar congestion surrounding the nodule.
- No conjunctival discharge.
- In the presence of secondary infection, whole conjunctiva is congested with mucopurulent discharge.
- May be associated with enlarged neck glands, tonsillitis or adenoids.

Course

Firstly, there is a true vesicular stage → epithelium becomes necrotic → small ulcers are formed → healing occurs without any scar.

Complications

They are mainly due to involvement of the cornea which is rather infrequent.
- Phlyctenular keratitis
- Fascicular ulcer
- Superficial phlyctenular pannus
- Ring ulcer (an allergic ulcer usually does not perforate, unless secondarily infected).

Investigations

They are only indicated when the phlyctens are multiple or recurrent.
- ***To detect tuberculosis***
  - Sputum for acid-fast bacilli (AFB)
  - Blood for total leukocyte count (TLC), differential leukocyte count (DLC), erythrocyte sedimentation rate (ESR)
  - X-ray chest
  - Mantoux test.
- ENT consultation to exclude chronic tonsillitis or adenoids.
- Stool for ova, parasite and cysts (OPC).
- Conjunctival swab and corneal scraping when the cornea is involved.

Treatment

- Corticosteroid eye drops (like, dexamethasone or fluorometholone) 4–6 times daily.
- In case of secondary infection, first treat bacterial conjunctivitis by local antibiotic drops (like, chloramphenicol or ciprofloxacin) and then treat with local corticosteroid drops.
- When cornea is involved—atropine (1%) eye ointment, or homatropine eye drop 2–3 times daily.
- Improvement of the nutritional status.

- Treatment of the causal factor, e.g.
  - Treatment of tuberculosis
  - Treatment of tonsillitis or adenoids
  - Anthelmintic for intestinal parasites.

VERNAL CONJUNCTIVITIS (FIG. 12.22)

Vernal conjunctivitis (*spring catarrh*) is a bilateral, recurrent, seasonal allergic conjunctivitis in children caused by exogenous allergens.

Etiological Factors

- *Age:* 5–14 years.
- Boys are more affected than girls.
- Prevalent in summer months in India and subsides during winter.
- External allergens like dust, pollens and molds in presence of dry, hot weather.
- Family history of allergy.
- Self-limiting course [in majority of the cases (around 11–14 years of age)].
- Immunoglobulin E (IgE) mediated mechanism plays an important role.

Symptoms

- *Intense itching* (due to alkaline nature of the discharge).

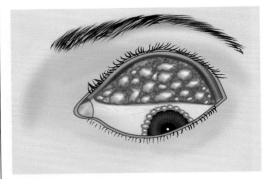

Fig. 12.22: Vernal conjunctivitis

- *Ropy discharge* (due to fibrinous nature of the discharge).
- *Photophobia* burning and foreign body sensation.

Signs

Three types of vernal conjunctivitis— (1) palpebral, (2) bulbar and (3) mixed.

Palpebral type is the most common but bulbar type is more common among blacks.

- *Palpebral type (Fig. 12.23A)*
  - Cobble-stone appearance of papillary hypertrophy of the palpebral conjunctiva (due to dense fibrous tissue and pressure exerted by the adjacent hard papillae).

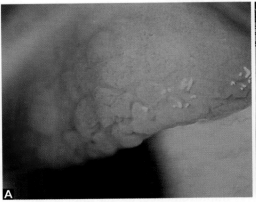
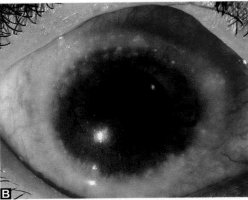

Figs 12.23A and B: Vernal conjunctivitis. **A.** Palpebral type; **B.** Bulbar type with Horner-Tranta's dots

- ■ The color of the papillae is bluish-white (milky-hue) due to hyaline degeneration.
- ■ In severe cases, the connective tissue septae rupture, giving rise to giant papillae.
- ● *Bulbar type*
  - ■ Multiple, small, nodule-like gelatinous thickening around the limbus, mostly at the upper.
  - ■ Discrete superficial spots (*Horner-Trantas dots*) are found scattered around the limbus (Fig. 12.23B).
- ● *Mixed type:* It has the picture of both types.

Histopathology of Papillae

- ● Tufts of capillaries
- ● Dense fibrous tissue
- ● Large numbers of eosinophils with plasma cells and histocytes
- ● Covering epithelium is hypertrophied and at places there are hyaline degenerations.

Course and Complications

Seasonal recurrences with exacerbation and remission are common. Ultimately in majority of the cases, the disease is self-limiting around the puberty. Complications are mainly due to corneal involvement (vernal keratoconjunctivitis).

The keratopathy changes are as follows:
- ● Punctate epithelial keratitis.
- ● Epithelial microerosions—leading to corneal ulceration (shield ulcer) (Fig. 12.24).
- ● Corneal plaque.
- ● Subepithelial scarring—usually in the form of a ring scar.
- ● *Pseudogerontoxon* resembles an arcus senilis with appearance of *cupid's bow*.
- ● Limbal stem cell deficiency (LSCD).
- ● Patients with vernal catarrh also have a *higher incidence of keratoconus*.

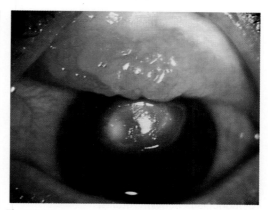

Fig. 12.24: Vernal keratoconjunctivitis—shield ulcer

Treatment

- ● Cold compress which is soothing.
- ● *Topical steroids*, like dexamethasone or prednisolone, 4–8 times daily depending upon the severity. Steroid-antibiotic mixture is not preferred.
- ● Long-term use of topical steroids has problems like cataract and glaucoma. *Dilute steroid preparations* (1:10) can be used rather safely.
- ● Alternately, soft steroids like, fluoro-metholone or loteprednol eye drop is more preferable.
- ● *Disodium cromoglycate* (2–4%)—four times daily as drops. It can be used safely for a prolonged period. It mainly, prevents the fresh attack, as it is a mastcell stabilizer.
- ● *Topical antihistaminics* like azelastine, epinastine, olopatadine, are helpful to give relief from severe itching.
- ● *Topical nonsteroidal anti-inflammatory drugs*—like ketorolac, flurbiprofen, or diclofenac may be useful.
- ● Tab Montelukast (5 mg)—daily may be used for few weeks in case of intense itching.
- ● For giant papillae—cryoapplication, β-irradiation or excision may be done.
- ● Acetylcysteine (10–20%) drop—to prevent excessive mucus production.
- ● Protection from external allergens.

Giant papillary conjunctivitis (Fig. 12.25)

It is a foreign body associated allergic conjunctivitis characterized by formation of giant papillae on the palpebral conjunctiva.

Originally, the papillae were thought to be at least 1 mm to diagnose giant papillary conjunctivitis. Now, it is accepted that the papillae are at least 0.3 mm in diameter on the upper palpebral conjunctiva in association with classic symptoms. Three groups of patients are affected:
1. Soft contact lens wearer
2. Artificial eye wearer
3. Postoperative patients with protruding ends of monofilament nylon sutures.

Clinical features are almost similar to palpebral type of vernal catarrh except the presence of giant papillae which are characteristic.

Treatment
- Discontinuation of contact lenses for 3 months and then re-fitted with rigid gas permeable contact lenses.
- Removal of the sutures.
- Topical steroids and sodium cromoglycate as in vernal catarrh.

CONJUNCTIVAL DEGENERATIONS

Concretions (Lithiasis)

- These are minute hard yellow/white spots in the palpebral conjunctiva.

- They are due to the accumulation of degenerated epithelial cells and inspissated mucus in the depression, called *Henle's glands*.
- They never become calcareous, so the term is a misnomer.
- They are common in elderly and usually symptomless. But sometimes, they may project and irritate the cornea.
- They may be easily evacuated with a sharp needle.

Pinguecula (Fig. 12.26)

- This is a yellowish, triangular deposit on the conjunctiva near the limbus at the palpebral aperture.
- They are found in elderly people who are exposed to strong sunlight, dust and wind.
- The apex of the triangle is away from the cornea, and it affects the nasal side first, then the temporal.
- Though it looks like fat (*Pinguecula* means *fat*), but is due to hyaline infiltration and elastotic degeneration of the submucosal conjunctival tissue.
- Normally, it is symptomless and does not require any treatment. But when inflamed, it is treated with topical steroids.

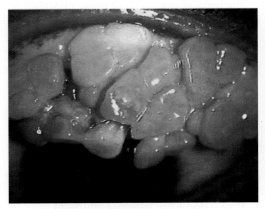

Fig. 12.25: Giant papillary conjunctivitis

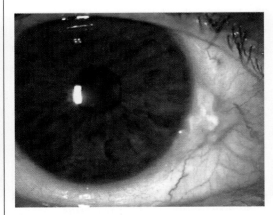

Fig. 12.26: Pinguecula

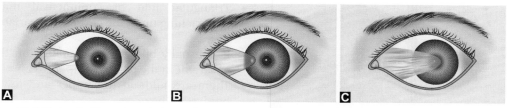

Figs 12.27A to C: Pterygium (schematic representation). **A.** Atrophic; **B.** Progressive; **C.** Crossing the papillary area

Pterygium

It is a degenerative condition of the sub-conjunctival tissue which proliferates as a triangular fold of tissue mass to invade the cornea, involving the Bowman's membrane and the superficial stroma, the whole thing being covered by conjunctival epithelium.

Literally, *pterygium* means a *wing*.

Etiology

Not precisely known, but a few factors are responsible:

- Ultraviolet irradiation (more among farmers and outdoor workers).
- Exposure to hot, sandy and dusty weather.
- Pinguecula may act as a precursor.

Stages

There are two types of stages—progressive and atrophic stages (Figs 12.27 and 12.28).

1. *Progressive*
   - It is thick, fleshy with prominent vascularity.
   - It is gradually increasing in size and encroaching towards the center of cornea.
   - Opaque infiltrative spot (cap) is seen just in front of the apex of the ptery-gium.
   - Deposition of iron as a line (Stocker's line) is seen in corneal epithelium in front of the apex.
2. *Atrophic (stationary)*
   - It is thin, attenuated with poor vascularity.
   - No opaque spot (cap) is seen.
   - It is stationary.

Parts (Fig. 12.29)

- *Apex or head:* It is the apex of the triangular mass.
- *Neck:* It is the constricted portion at the limbus.
- *Body:* It is the remaining bulky part.
- *Cap:* It is a semilunar infiltrative opaque spot just in front of the apex. This is due to cellular infiltration.

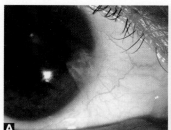
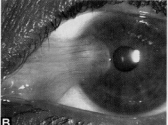
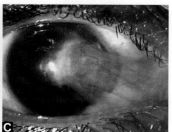

Figs 12.28A to C: Types of pterygium (photographs); **A.** Atrophic; **B.** Progressive; **C.** Covering the pupillary area

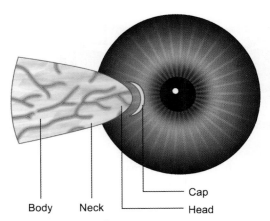

Fig. 12.29: Parts of a pterygium

Body   Neck   Cap   Head

Symptoms

- ***Appearance of a mass*** on nasal, or rarely on temporal side of the cornea. Sometimes, both nasal and temporal sides are involved (doubleheaded pterygium).
- ***Dimness of vision*** due to corneal astigmatism or obstruction of the visual axis.
- Rarely, ***diplopia*** due to limitation of ocular movements, especially in recurrent pterygium with symblepharon.

Signs

- Decreased visual acuity.

- Triangular fold of conjunctival mass encroaching upon the cornea in a variable degree.
- It is usually bilateral, and mainly on the nasal side at the palpebral aperture.
- There are folds at the upper and lower borders of the mass.
- Limitation of movements in few cases.

Pseudopterygium (Figs 12.30A and B)
• It is the adhesion of a fold of conjunctiva to a peripheral cornea, due to some inflammation. • It is seen at any age; usually unilateral, stationary, and at any meridian. • Causes are chemical burns, peripheral corneal ulcer, foreign body, etc. • As it is fixed to the cornea only at its apex, a probe can be passed easily beneath the neck of the pterygium (probe test). • Treatment is only by excision.

Treatment

Treatment is done on the basis of types of pterygium.

- ***Atrophic pterygium, and if just on the cornea:*** It is best left alone with periodic follow-up.
- ***Progressive pterygium:***
  - Excision of the pterygium with the conjunctiva and keeping the limbus and adjacent scleral area bare (bare sclera technique).

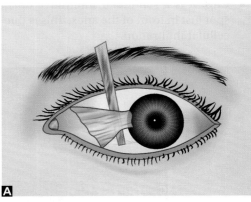

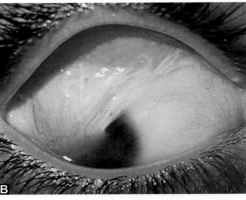

Figs 12.30A and B: Pseudopterygium. A probe can be passed beneath the neck of the pseudopterygium.
A. Schematic representation; **B.** Photograph

- Subconjunctival dissection of the pterygium and then excision with bare sclera. Then cover the bare area with conjunctival autograft (*see* Chapter 25, page 496).
- ***Transposition operation (Mc Reynolds):*** The apex is freed and turned down under the bulbar conjunctiva and sutured in this position.

  A pterygium cannot be removed without leaving a scar on the cornea as it involves the Bowman's membrane and superficial stroma.
- ***Recurrent pterygium (and also to prevent recurrence):***
  - After excision, the bare scleral area is treated with:
    - ***Beta-irradiation*** (by strontium-90), not more than 2,000 rads during the first week of surgery.
    - Thiotepa solution as drop (1 in 2,000)—4 times daily for 6 weeks.
    - Mitomycin C (0.02%) solution— locally during operation or as drop postoperatively.
  - ***Conjunctival limbal autograft:*** The current standard treatment is to cover the bare scleral area with conjunctival autograft or limbal autograft (CAG) or (CLAU). This graft is fixed with fibrin glue or 8-0 vicryl or 10-0 nylon sutures. The recurrence rate is lowest in this procedure.
  - ***Lamellar keratoplasty*** of the affected part, along with excision of pterygium.
- ***Pterygium involving the pupillary area:*** Resection of the pterygium with anterior lamellar keratoplasty is the treatment of choice (*see* Figs 12.27C and 12.28C).

CONJUNCTIVAL CYSTS

- ***Lymphangiectasis (lymphatic cysts):*** They are very common and arise as the dilatation of the lymph spaces.
- ***Retention cysts:*** They occur due to the obstruction of the ducts of accessory

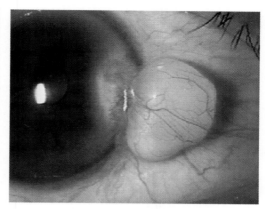

Fig. 12.31: Conjunctival implantation cyst

lacrimal gland of Krause in the upper fornix.
- ***Implantation cyst:*** This occurs due to implantation of conjunctival epithelial cells, following an injury or after an operation (e.g. squint, pterygium, etc.) (Fig. 12.31).
- ***Parasitic cyst:*** This is due to subconjunctival ***cysticercus*** or ***hydatid*** cyst. This is rare.

CONJUNCTIVAL TUMORS

Classification
1. Nonpigmented tumors

– Congenital (choristomas)

Dermolipoma	Epibulbar dermoid

– ***Acquired***

Benign	Malignant
Papilloma	Carcinoma-in-situ
Angioma	Squamous cell carcinoma

2. Pigmented tumors
- ***Simple nevus***
- ***Precancerous***
  Junctional nevus
  Precancerous melanosis
  Lentigo malignum
- ***Malignant melanoma***

Dermoids

They appear as solid white masses, most frequently at the limbus, especially in lower outer quadrant (Fig. 12.32).

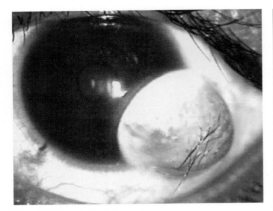

Fig. 12.32: Limbal dermoid

- They consist of skin with sebaceous glands and hair.
- Surgical excision with a lamellar sclerocorneal patch graft is the treatment.

Dermolipomas (Lipodermoids)

- They appear as soft, yellow, movable subconjunctival masses, located at the outer canthus or at the limbus.
- They consist of fibrous tissue and fat, and sometimes, with dermoid tissue on their surface.
- In some cases, they are associated with **Goldenhar's syndrome (Figs 12.33A and B)** (preauricular tags, vertebral anomalies and hemifacial hypoplasia).

- **Treatment:** Surgical excision; though sometimes, it is seen that the fat is continuous with that of the orbit.

Carcinoma In Situ (Intraepithelial Epithelioma) (Fig. 12.34)

- It is sometimes called **Bowen's disease**.
- It appears as a slightly elevated, fleshy mass with tuft of blood vessels at the limbus in an elderly subject.
- The lesion is superficial to the basement membrane and conjunctiva is freely mobile.
- Treatment is by surgical local excision followed by cryoapplication.
- Alternately, chemotherapy may be tried with: Mitomycin C drop; fluorouracil (5-FU) drop or interferon drops for few months.

Squamous Cell Carcinoma (Fig. 12.35)

- It appears as a reddish-gray fleshy mass with broad base and characterized by deep invasion into the stroma with fixation to the underlying structure.
- It is mainly seen at the limbus.
- It arises from a papilloma or carcinoma *in situ.*

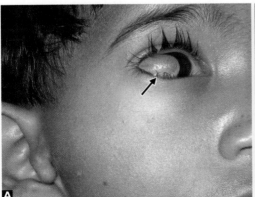
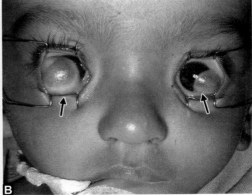

Figs 12.33A and B: Goldenhar's syndrome. **A.** Unilateral; **B.** Bilateral dermolipoma (arrows)

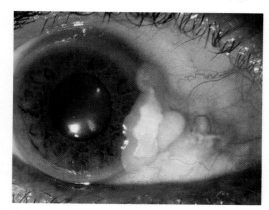

Fig. 12.34: Intraepithelial epithelioma

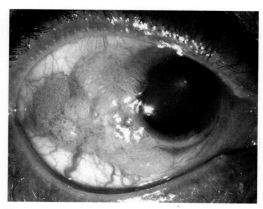

Fig. 12.35: Squamous cell carcinoma

- Distant metastasis may occur in advance cases.
- Treatment is by radical excision, enucleation or exenteration of the orbit.

Ocular Surface Squamous Neoplasia (OSSN)

It encompasses a wide spectrum of disease involving abnormal growth of dysplastic squamous epithelial cells on the ocular surface.

Subtypes

- ***Conjunctival intraepithelial neoplasia (CIN):*** It is a slow-growing tumor that arises from a single mutated cell on the ocular surface. The other names of CIN includes—Bowen's disease, conjunctival squamous dysplasia, intraepithelial epithelioma and epithelial dyskeratosis.

- ***Corneal intraepithelial neoplasia:*** It refers to same lesions of the cornea with minimum involvement of the conjunctiva.
- ***Squamous cell carcinoma (SCC):*** It is a malignant lesion which tactually penetrates the cornea or conjunctival basement membrane, with metastatic potential.
- ***Mucoepidermoid carcinoma:*** It represents a rare aggressive, and more invasive variant of SCC.

In western world, it mainly occurs in men in their 60s and 70s. However, in Africa and Asia, OSSN is more common in younger patients and clinically more aggressive. Risk factors include UV light, HIV infection, human papillomavirus (HPV), xeroderma pigmentosa and mutations of p53—a tumor suppressor gene. Patients are often asymptomatic, and diagnosis is made only on careful, routine eye examination. Some patients complain of redness and ocular irritation secondary to inflammation.

Clinical Examination

- Typically, patients present with a gelatinous or plaque like interpalpebral slow-growing conjunctival gray/white lesion.
- About 95% of CIN lesions occur at the limbus. The lesion may be flat or elevated and may be associated with feeder vessels. Rose Bengal stain is often used to highlight the lesion.
- SCC presents similarly to CIN; but usually immobile and more raised from surface. The feeder vessel is large, suggestive of epithelial basement membrane breach. The lesions are typically keratinized and papillary in appearance.
- Ultrahigh resolution optical coherence tomography (OCT) has important role in diagnosis.

Treatment

- ***Topical chemotherapy:*** Interferon-α2b (1 million IU/mL); mitomycin C (MMC—0.02 to 0.04%); and 5-FU as eye drop has the advantage of treating the entire ocular surface and avoiding surgical complications. Interferon is costly and requires refrigeration. These drops are toxic, requires punctal occlusion. Treatment is continued for 3–5 months or more with on- and off-cycles. Effective in 60–100% cases.

- *Intralesional/subconjunctival* interferon or antivascular endothelial growth factor (VEGF), (bevacizumab) may be useful as an adjunct.
- *Surgery:* Total excision (no touch technique) with at least a 3–4 mm uninvolved conjunctival margin. Additional double or triple cryofreeze-thaw is applied to the conjunctival edges, limbal zone, and bare scleral bed to kill any remaining dysplastic cells. The bare area may be covered by amniotic membrane grafting.

  More extensive surgeries (like, lamellar sclerectomy or exenteration) may be required with scleral or deeper involvement.
- *Recurrence:* It may occur in one-third cases after surgical excision.

Simple Nevus (Fig. 12.36)

- This appears as a single, sharply demarcated, flat or slightly elevated lesion, most commonly near the limbus.
- It is congenital and tends to enlarge or darken during pregnancy or puberty.
- Excision is only indicated for cosmetic reason.

Precancerous Melanosis (Fig. 12.37)

- This is a small pigmented tumor of the conjunctiva which spreads as a diffuse patch of pigmented lesion.
- It occurs in elderly people.

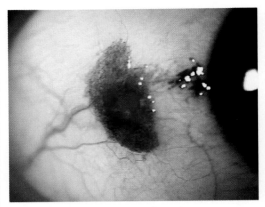

Fig. 12.37: Precancerous melanosis

- In 20% cases, it proceeds to frank malignant changes.
- It is radiosensitive at the precancerous stage.
- Local excision with postoperative radiotherapy may limit the disease.

Malignant Melanoma (Fig. 12.38)

- It is typically seen at the limbus in elderly patient.
- Pigmented melanomas are more common than nonpigmented melanomas.
- It may arise *de novo,* or from a precancerous lesion, e.g. junctional nevus, precancerous melanosis or lentigo malignum.

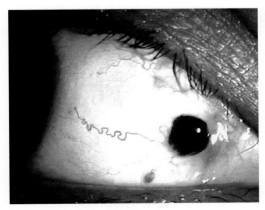

Fig. 12.36: Conjunctival simple nevus

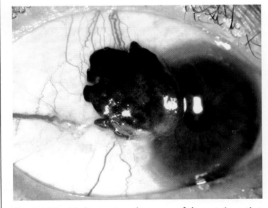

Fig. 12.38: Malignant melanoma of the conjunctiva

- It spreads over the surface of the globe, but rarely penetrates it.
- Metastasis is common.
- **Treatment** is by radical excision of the mass, enucleation or exenteration of the orbit.

SYMPTOMATIC CONDITIONS OF THE CONJUNCTIVA

Subconjunctival Hemorrhage (Figs 12.39A and B)

Subconjunctival hemorrhage is common, since the vessels are loosely supported. Rupture of a conjunctival blood vessel causes a bright red, sharply delineated area surrounded by the normal appearing conjunctiva.

Etiology

- **Traumatic**
  - **Direct trauma to the eyeball:** Posterior limit of the hemorrhage is visible.
  - **Head injury or injury to the orbit:** Blood usually seeps under the conjunctiva 12–24 hours after the head injury. Posterior limit of the hemorrhage is not visible.
- **Infective:** In some conjunctivitis, e.g. due to *Pneumococcus*, Koch-Week's bacillus, adenovirus or picornavirus.

- **Mechanical:** Due to venous congestion and consequent rupture of the small vessels, e.g. bronchitis, whooping cough, compression of the neck or chest, etc. (Fig. 12.40A). May be associated with retrobulbar hemorrhage and ecchymosis of lids called **Panda bear** or **Raccoon eyes sign** (Fig. 12.40B).
- **Arteriosclerosis and hypertension.**
- **Blood dyscrasias:** Leukemia, purpura, hemophilia, etc.
- **Vicarious menstruation:** Leading to periodic hemorrhage.
- **Idiopathic.**

Fate of Subconjunctival Hemorrhage

- At first, it is bright red in color. This is due to **oxyhemoglobin**, as it is in constant contact with the atmospheric oxygen.
- Subsequently, it changes to orange-yellow or blackish-red, then to yellow discoloration; this is due to breakdown of oxyhemoglobin.
- Ultimately, it gets absorbed within 2–3 weeks, depending upon the amount of hemorrhage.

Treatment

- No treatment is necessary in most of the cases, as it is absorbed automatically.

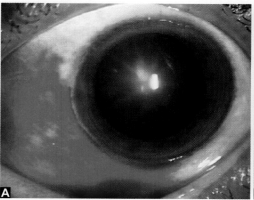 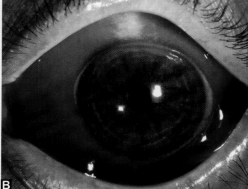

Figs 12.39A and B: Subconjunctival hemorrhage

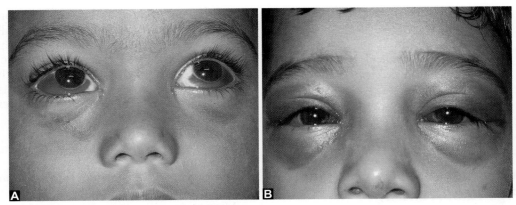

Figs 12.40A and B: A. Bilateral subconjunctival hemorrhage in a child with whooping cough; **B.** With ecchymosis of lids (Panda bear or Raccoon eyes sign)

- Initially, cold compress is helpful as it constricts the blood vessels.
- In severe cases, if the extravasated blood causes prolapse of the conjunctiva through the interpalpebral fissure, subconjunctival space may be punctured to drain the blood.
- Treatment of the cause.

Conjunctival Xerosis (Figs 12.41A and B)

This is a dry, lustreless condition of the conjunctiva.

Types

Two types of xerosis are described as follows:
1. *Xerosis epithelialis:* Due to vitamin A deficiency with associated protein–energy malnutrition (PEM).
2. *Xerosis parenchymatous:* Following cicatricial changes of the conjunctiva, e.g. trachoma, chemical burns, pemphigoid, diphtheria, prolong use of β-blocker, etc.

Following prolonged exposure of the eye, e.g. proptosis, ectropion, lagophthalmos, comatose patients, etc.

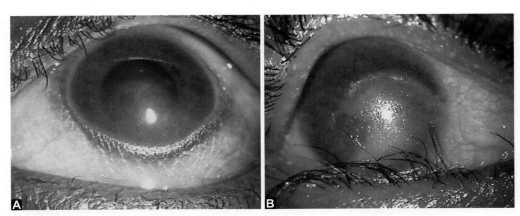

Figs 12.41A and B: A. Severe conjunctival xerosis; **B.** Severe xerosis in ocular pemphigus

Pathology

- Epithelium becomes epidermoid, like that of the skin with granular and horny layer.
- There is destruction of goblet cells of the conjunctiva.
- Profuse growth of *Corynebacterium xerosis*.

Pathogenesis

Goblet cells cease to secrete mucus → vicarious activity of the Meibomian glands → fatty secretion covers the dry surface → watery tears fail to moisten the conjunctiva.

It must be noted that xerosis has nothing to do with any failure of function on the part of the lacrimal gland. The conjunctiva can be quite efficiently moistened by its own secretion alone, and if the lacrimal gland is removed, xerosis usually does not follow.

On the other hand, xerosis may follow in spite of normal or increased lacrimal secretion, if the secretory activity of the conjunctiva itself is impaired.

Treatment

- ***Local treatment***
  - Use dark glasses.
  - Artificial tears eye drop to relief dryness, like methylcellulose, carboxymethyl cellulose (CMC); hydroxypropyl methyl cellulose (HPMC); sodium hyaluronate, polyvinyl alcohol, etc. 1–2 hourly depending upon the severity. Teargel may be used at night.
  - Treatment of the ocular conditions responsible for dry eye, e.g. treatment of trachoma, ectropion correction, tarsorrhaphy, etc.
- ***General treatment*** (*see* Chapter 26)
  - Administration of vitamin A [in case of vitamin A deficiency showing Bitot's spot (Fig. 12.42)].
  - Correction of nutritional status.

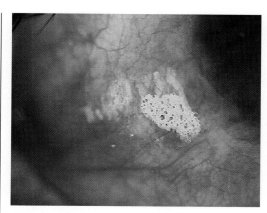

Fig. 12.42: Bitot's spot

Stevens-Johnson Syndrome (Fig. 12.43)

It is a mucocutaneous vesiculobullous disease caused by a hypersensitivity to antibiotics (penicillins), sulfonamides (including acetazolamide), phenylbutazone, allopurinol, phenytoin sodium, etc.

The basic lesion is thought to be an acute vasculitis affecting the conjunctiva and other mucous membranes.

Clinical Features

- ***Systemic***
  - Fever, sore throat, cough
  - Symmetrical erythematous and vesiculobullous reaction affecting the skin (scalp is spared) and mucous membrane of the body.
- ***Ocular***
  - Conjunctiva is involved in 50% of cases.
  - Mucopurulent conjunctivitis with membrane or pseudomembrane formation.
  - Keratinization of posterior lid margins (sand paper appearance) is the main cause of total limbal stem cell deficiency (LSCD).
  - Scarring of the conjunctiva and lid margins—with trichiasis (acquired

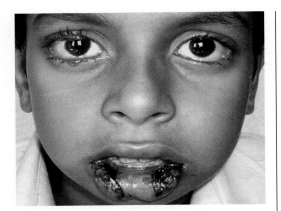

Fig. 12.43: Stevens-Johnson syndrome—conjunctival and oral lesion

distichiasis), symblepharon and obliteration of the fornices.

Treatment

- Discontinuation of the offending drugs.
- Systemic antibiotics and corticosteroids.
- Topical antibiotics, topical steroids and artificial tears as long-term treatment.
- Surgical correction of entropion, lid margin deformity, symblepharon, trichiasis, etc.

CHAPTER 13

Diseases of the Cornea and Sclera

EVALUATION OF CORNEAL DISEASES

Symptoms

- **Pain:** The cornea is richly supplied by sensory nerve endings. In corneal abrasions or bullous keratopathy, the direct stimulation of bare nerve endings causes severe pain.
- **Decreased visual acuity:** It is caused by loss of central corneal transparency.
- **Halos:** They are due to diffraction of light by epithelial and subepithelial edema.
- **Photophobia.**
- **Lacrimation:** It is due to reflex stimulation of the corneal nerve.

Signs

The precise localization of corneal defects is best done by slit-lamp biomicroscopy.

- **Epithelium:** Punctate erosions, edema, filaments, superficial punctate keratitis, and staining with fluorescein and Rose-Bengal.
- **Stroma:** Infiltrates, edema, vascularization, deposits, and scarring (opacities).
- **Descemet's membrane:** Breaks, folds, localized thickening (excrescences), etc.
- **Deposition of pigments:** Corneal pigment deposition is associated with a variety of disorders (Table 13.1).
- **Corneal thickness (by pachymetry)** either by the optical or ultrasonic pachymeter.

TABLE 13.1: Pigment deposition in the cornea

Types of pigment	Sign (Disorders)	Corneal location
Iron	• Fleischer's ring (keratoconus)	• Epithelium
	• Hudson-Stahli's line (old opacity) (Fig. 13.1)	• Epithelium
	• Stocker's line (pterygium)	• Epithelium
	• Ferry's line (filtering bleb)	• Epithelium
	• Siderosis	• Mainly stroma
	• Blood staining of the cornea	• Mainly stroma
Copper	Kayser-Fleischer's ring (Fig. 13.2) • Wilson's disease • Chalcosis	Descemet's membrane
Melanin	Krukenberg's spindle (pigment dispersion syndrome)	Endothelium

- It indicates the functional integrity of the corneal endothelium.
- Ultrasonic or topographic pachymetry is useful before laser-assisted in situ keratomileusis (LASIK) and other keratorefractive operations.
- **Corneal sensation:** Loss of corneal sensation is an important sign to diagnose viral keratitis and neuroparalytic keratitis.

Laboratory diagnosis: Material for laboratory analysis is obtained by scraping of the ulcer, from its base and margin.

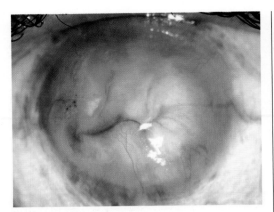

Fig. 13.1: Hudson-Stahli's line

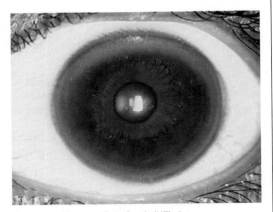

Fig. 13.2: Kayser-Fleischer's (KF) ring

It is then plated onto the glass slides for Gram-staining and potassium hydroxide (KOH) preparation to identify the bacteria and fungus respectively. Part of the material is inoculated onto the following culture media.

- *Blood agar* mainly for aerobic bacteria.
- *Sabouraud's media* for fungus.

CONGENITAL ANOMALIES

Microcornea (Fig. 13.3)

- Corneal diameter is less than 10 mm with decreased radius of curvature.
- There is hypermetropia, and chance of narrow angle glaucoma in later years.

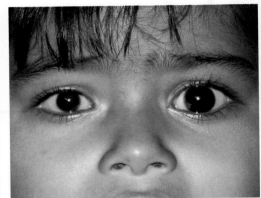

Fig. 13.3: Microcornea with microphthalmos (right eye)

- This term is reserved for corneal affection alone. But when the entire eyeball is small, it is called *microphthalmos* which is more common.
- *Systemic association:* Ehler-Danlos syndrome, Weill-Marchesani syndrome, Waardenburg's syndrome.

Megalocornea (Fig. 13.4)

- It is a bilateral condition, in which the corneal diameter is more than 14 mm.
- The patient is myopic.
- There are deep anterior chamber, tremulousness of iris and subluxation of the lens with or without cataract formation.

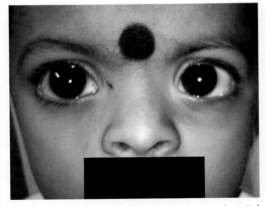

Fig. 13.4: Megalocornea (right eye more than left eye)

- Megalocornea must be differentiated from congenital glaucoma by tonometry and gonioscopy.

Congenital Corneal Opacities

- Central corneal opacity (Peter's anomaly) is due to defect in embryogenesis, due to incomplete separation of the lens from the surface ectoderm.
- It is usually associated with other anomalies in the iris or angle of the anterior chamber, with glaucoma.

Posterior Embryotoxon

- An unusual prominence of Schwalbe's line which is the peripheral termination of Descemet's membrane.
- It appears as a ring opacity in the deeper layer of the cornea.

CORNEAL EDEMA (FIGS 13.5A AND B)

- The integrity of both epithelium and the endothelium is necessary to maintain cornea in its relatively dehydrated state.
- It is associated with increased corneal thickness, and a variable decrease in corneal transparency.

- Source of fluid is either the aqueous humor (via endothelium) or the tears (via epithelium).

Pathology

- Fluid accumulates between the basal epithelial cells → then, in between the lamella and around the nerve fibers of the stroma → total haziness.
- In long-standing cases, the epithelium tends to be raised into large vesicles or bullae, leading to **bullous keratopathy** (Fig. 13.6).

Etiology

- **Inflammatory:** Corneal ulcer, erosions, acute iridocyclitis (due to endothelial damage).
- **Traumatic:** Mechanical trauma and post-surgical—due to endothelial damage, particularly when vitreous remains adherent to it.
- **Increased intraocular pressure:** Acute edema in angle-closure glaucoma and epidemic dropsy glaucoma. Chronic edema in long-standing cases—as in absolute glaucoma and buphthalmos.
- **Dystrophic condition of the cornea,** e.g. Fuchs' endothelial dystrophy and

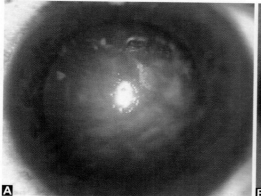
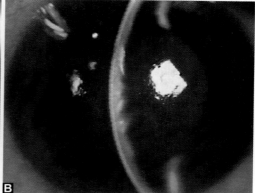

Figs 13.5A and B: Corneal edema. **A.** Diffuse illumination; **B.** Slit section

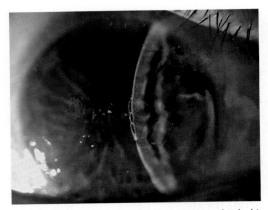

Fig. 13.6: Bullous keratopathy in pseudophakic eye in slit section

congenital hereditary endothelial dystrophy (CHED).
- *Hypoxia of the cornea:* As in contact lens wearer due to epithelial edema, as a result of prolonged deprivation of atmospheric oxygen.

Symptoms

- *Colored halos* around the light with red color being outside, and blue inside.
- *Decreased visual acuity*—due to corneal haziness and irregular astigmatism.

Treatment

- Use of hot air (by hair dryer).
- Frequent instillation of concentrated sodium chloride (5%) solution, or ointment containing 6% or 15% sodium chloride.
- Glycerine drop (to clear edema quickly and temporarily), but it is irritant.
- Bandage soft contact lenses, especially in case of ruptured bullae.
- Epithelium is stripped off, and is to be replaced with a thin conjunctival flap.
- Endothelial keratoplasty (DSEK or DMEK) or penetrating keratoplasty to improve visual status.

INFLAMMATION OF THE CORNEA (KERATITIS)

Modes of Infection

- *Exogenous infections:* Most common; and cornea is primarily affected by virulent organisms.
- *From the ocular tissues:* Owing to direct anatomical continuity, the diseases of:
  - Conjunctiva—spread to the corneal epithelium.
  - Sclera—to the stroma.
  - Uveal tract—to the endothelium.
- *Endogenous infections:* Rare, as the cornea is avascular. They are typically allergic in nature.

Keratitis or inflammation of the cornea may be classified as follows:

Superficial keratitis
- Infective keratitis
  - Bacterial
  - Fungal
  - Viral
  - Acanthamoebal.
- Non-infective keratitis
  - Central
    - Exposure keratitis
    - Neurotrophic keratitis
    - Atheromatous keratitis.
  - Peripheral
    - Marginal keratitis
    - Phlyctenular keratitis
    - Mooren's ulcer
    - Terrien's degeneration
    - Rosacea keratitis
    - Keratitis associated with collagen vascular diseases.

Deep keratitis
- Interstitial keratitis
- Disciform keratitis
- Sclerosing keratitis.

In strict sense, keratitis and corneal ulcer are not always synonymous.

A *corneal ulcer is defined* as a loss of corneal epithelium with underlying stromal infiltration and suppuration associated with signs of inflammation with or without hypopyon.

BACTERIAL KERATITIS

Predisposing Factors

Intact corneal epithelium cannot be penetrated by any organism except, *Neisseria gonorrhoeae, Neisseria meningitidis,* and *Corynebacterium diphtheriae.* In these cases, suppurative keratitis is always associated with a purulent conjunctivitis.

With the other bacteria, keratitis is invariably associated with one or more of the following predisposing factors:

- ***Trauma to the corneal epithelium:*** By injury, foreign body, trichiasis, entropion, contact lens wear, etc.
- ***Underlying corneal diseases:*** Herpetic keratitis, corneal erosions, bullous keratopathy, keratomalacia, etc.
- Neurotrophic or exposure keratopathy
- Dry eyes
- Chronic dacryocystitis or blepharitis
- Use of topical steroids
- Lowering of general body resistance, e.g. malnutrition, diabetes, systemic immunosuppressive therapy, etc.

Pathology

Uncomplicated, localized corneal ulcer is having four stages—stages of infiltration, progression, regression, and cicatrization (Figs 13.7A to D).

Stage of Infiltration and Progression

- Edema and localized necrosis of the anterior part of the corneal stroma.
- Necrotic tissue is cast off leaving a saucer-shaped defect, known as ulcer.
- Epithelium is sloughed off simultaneously with an involvement of larger area.
- Dense infiltration of polymorphs followed by macrophages. This infiltration extends for some distance around the ulcer.
- There is an associated iritis due to toxin being absorbed into the anterior chamber.
- This reaction is so toxic that leukocytosis takes place, and polymorphs poured out of the blood vessels pass into the aqueous, and gravitate at the bottom of anterior chamber. This is hypopyon and this pus remains sterile, so long as the Descemet's membrane is intact.

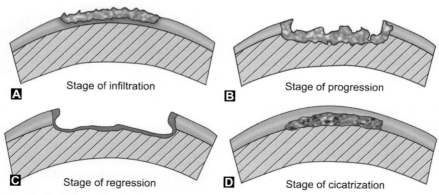

A Stage of infiltration
B Stage of progression
C Stage of regression
D Stage of cicatrization

Figs 13.7A to D: Pathological stages of corneal ulcer

Stage of Regression

- The defect becomes larger, as there is digestion of the necrotic tissue by the polymorphs.
- Line of demarcation appears surrounding the ulcer.
- Infiltrations at the edges and the base start to disappear, and polymorphs are replaced by mononuclear cells.
- The ulcerated area becomes smooth and relatively clear.

Stage of Cicatrization

- Healing of the defect occurs by formation of the fibrous tissue.
- The fibrous tissue is derived from:
  - Invading mononuclear cells
  - Keratocytes
  - Endothelial cells of the new vessels.
  - The epithelium grows from the edges of the defect to form a permanent covering.

Clinical Features

Symptoms

- Acute pain, redness, and lacrimation
- Photophobia
- Decreased visual acuity
- White spot on the cornea.

Signs

- Marked blepharospasm
- Lid edema
- Ciliary congestion of the conjunctiva
- Ulcer usually starts as a grayish-white, circumscribed infiltration, with edema of the surrounding tissue. There is absence of window reflex. The margins of the ulcer are overhanging, and the floor is covered by necrotic material. The extent of the ulcer may be detected by fluorescein staining and seen with blue filter. Ulcer area stains as brilliant green.

Later, the ulcer becomes gradually smooth in the regressive stage, and ultimately, scar tissue begins to appear the edges and the floor of the ulcer.
- Some degree of features of iritis.
- Hypopyon may be present (Fig. 13.8).
- Intraocular pressure (IOP) may be raised in presence of hypopyon. But if the ulcer perforates, IOP decreases.

Certain bacteria produce characteristic response:
- *Staphylococcus aureus* and *Streptococcus pneumoniae*—produce oval, yellowish-white, dense, opaque, stromal ulcer surrounded by relatively clear cornea.
- *Pseudomonas*—mucopurulent sticky and greenish exudate, irregular deep ulcer with "ground-glass" appearance of surrounding stroma. Ulcer progresses very rapidly, and results in corneal melting and perforation within 48 hours.
- *Enterobacteriaceae* (*E. coli, Proteus, Klebsiella*, etc.) produce a shallow ulcer with pleomorphic grayish-white necrotic area. Sometimes, they produce ring-shaped corneal infiltrates.

Healing of a Corneal Ulcer

- Healing of the corneal ulcer is taken place by the formation of fibrous tissue.
- The new fibers are not arranged regularly as in normal lamellae, and they refract the light irregularly. Therefore, the scar is more or less opaque.

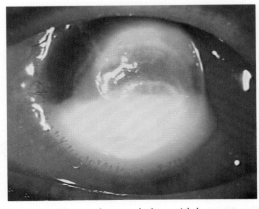

Fig. 13.8: Bacterial corneal ulcer with hypopyon

- Bowman's membrane is never regenerated, and once it has been damaged, it leaves some degree of permanent corneal opacity.
- Scar tissue may not fill the gap exactly as level of surface, which is then little flattened—leading to the formation of *corneal facets*.
- If the corneal scar is thin, the resulting opacity is slight, it is called *nebular*. If rather more dense—it is called *macular*, and if still more dense and white—it is called a *leukomatous* (Figs 13.9A to C).

Old central leukoma, sometimes shows a horizontal pigmented line (Hudson-Stahli's line) at the palpebral aperture.

- A thin, diffuse nebula on the pupillary area, interferes more with the vision than a strictly localized dense leukoma, so long as the latter does not block the whole papillary area. The reason is, leukoma stops all the light which falls upon it, whereas the nebula refracts the light irregularly causing an irregular astigmatism.

Complications

- *Ectatic cicatrix:* Thinned, scarred cornea bulges under the influence of normal IOP.
- *Descemetocele (Figs 13.10A and B):* Herniation of the elastic Descemet's membrane through the ulcer as a transparent vesicle. It may persist,

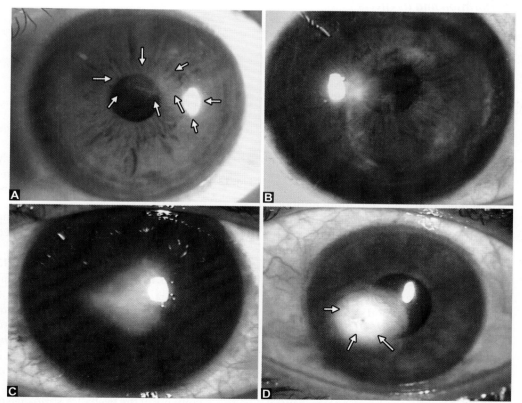

Figs 13.9A to D: Corneal opacity. **A.** Nebular (arrows); **B.** Macular; **C.** Leukomatous; **D.** Adherent leukoma (arrows)

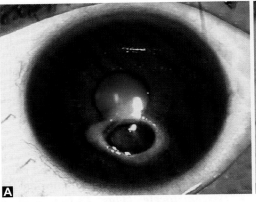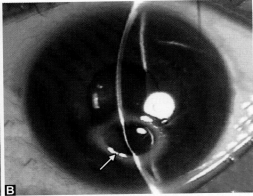

Figs 13.10A and B: Descemetocele (arrow)

surrounded by a white cicatricial ring, or it may eventually rupture.

- **Perforation and its effects**
    - It is caused by sudden exertion (sneezing, coughing, etc.) → acute rise in IOP → weak floor of the ulcer is unable to support this pressure → gives way.
    - Once the ulcer perforates → sudden escape of aqueous → sudden fall in IOP → iris-lens diaphragm moves forward and comes in contact with the back of the cornea.
    - **The advantages of perforation**
        - Pain is alleviated due to lowering of IOP.
        - Better nutrition, and more antibody or antibiotics will reach the ulcer area due to diffusion of fluid.
        - Rapid healing of the ulcer in some eyes.
    - **Complications of perforation:** They vary according to the location and the size of the perforation.
        - **Anterior synechia:** If the perforation is very small, the iris becomes gummed down the opening, and the adhesion organizes.
        - **Iris prolapse:** If the perforation is large and peripheral or paracentral (Figs 13.11 and 13.12).

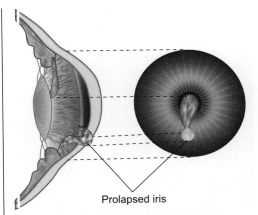
Prolapsed iris

Fig. 13.11: Corneal ulcer with perforation

- **Adherent leukoma:** Due to healing of *the perforated ulcer* with prolapsed iris (Fig. 13.9D).
- **Anterior staphyloma (Figs 13.13 and 13.14):** In case of large perforation → total prolapse of the iris → pseudocornea formation → organization to form cicatrix in which the iris remains incarcerated → whole thing bulge out due to high IOP.
- **Phthisis bulbi (Fig. 13.15):** In case of large perforation → extrusion of the contents of the eyeball → shrinkage of the globe with low IOP.

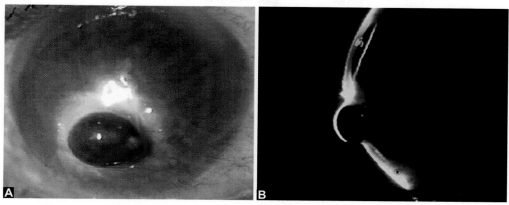

Figs 13.12A and B: Perforated corneal ulcer with iris prolapse

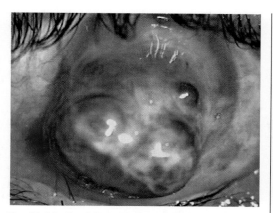

Fig. 13.13: Partial anterior staphyloma

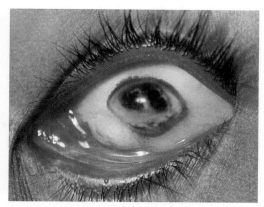

Fig. 13.15: Phthisis bulbi

- *Subluxation or dislocation of the lens:* Due to sudden forward movement of the lens.
  - *Anterior capsular cataract:* When the perforation is at the center and small, the lens remains long in contact with the ulcer.
  - *Corneal fistula (Figs 13.16A and B):* Due to repeated perforation → sealing of perforation by the exudate → re-opening due to strain → fistula formation.
  - *Expulsive hemorrhage:* Due to sudden lowering of IOP → sudden dilatation of the choroidal vessels.

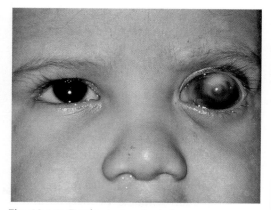

Fig. 13.14: Total anterior staphyloma

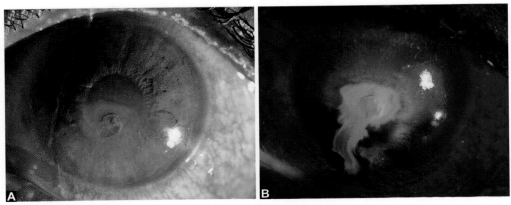

Figs 13.16A and B: A. Corneal fistula; **B.** With positive Seidel's test

- *Purulent acute iridocyclitis* and its complications.
- *Panophthalmitis (Fig.13.17)*: Due to spread of infection into the vitreous cavity.

Management

A bacterial ulcer is a sight-threatening disease that demands urgent identification and eradication of the causative organism.

This is best performed with hospitalization of the patient.

- *Identification of the organisms:* This is done by smear preparation, and culture and sensitivity test of the scrapings, taken from the base and margin of the ulcer as described earlier.

Meanwhile, the aggressive treatment with antibiotics is started, till the reports are available, when it may be changed accordingly.

- *Antibiotics*
  - Gram "positive" organisms usually respond to cephazolin, vancomycin, gatifloxacin , and moxifloxacin.
  - Gram "negative" organisms are sensitive to gentamicin, tobramycin, polymyxin B, amikacin, ciprofloxacin, etc.
  - *Route of administration*
    - *Topical commercial preparation:* The drops are instilled at half hourly intervals round the clock for the first few days. Then, depending upon the response, the frequency of instillation may be reduced.
    - *Topical fortified drop (concentrated) preparation:* It is the most effective way to maintain a high and sustained level of antibiotics at the site of infection, e.g. 5% fortified cefazolin, fortified tobramycin. Fortified tobramycin = 2 mL of parenteral tobramycin (80 mg) + 5 mL bottle of commercially available tobramycin eye drop. The resultant solution contains 14 mg/mL, and is stable for up to 30 days.

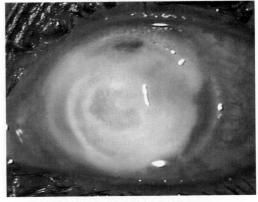

Fig. 13.17: Corneal ulcer—panophthalmitis

– *Subconjunctival injections* are for moderate to severe cases. It may be mixed with injection atropine. Gentamicin (20–40 mg) is usually preferred.

– *Systemic antibiotics:* It is usually not necessary except, marginal bacterial ulcer, perforating corneal ulcer, one-eyed cases and if the sclera is involved.

There is no need to change the initial antibiotics, if the response is good. But, if it is not so, the subsequent therapy is depended upon the sensitivity pattern.

- *Atropine sulfate (1%)* eye drops, 3 times daily to prevent ciliary spasm, and to control iritis.
- *Hot fomentation* is to improve circulation and to relieve pain.
- *Analgesics with antacids* for pain.
- *Removal of local predisposing factor* if any, like trichiasis, foreign body, chronic dacryocystitis, etc.
- *Tab acetazolamide* or *timolol maleate eye drop (0.5%)* to control IOP in selected cases.
- If the ulcer does not respond with these treatment, *debridement* and *cauterization* of the ulcer under topical anesthesia may be done.
  - *Debridement* means removal of necrotic material by scraping the floor with a spatula or no. 15 Bard-Parker blade.
  - *Cauterization* is done by pure carbolic acid or by iodine (1% iodine in potassium iodide solution).
  - Carbolic acid penetrates more deeply, and extends its antibacterial property more widely.
- If the ulcer still does not respond, and if there is a threat of perforation—*therapeutic penetrating keratoplasty* is the best choice. Alternately, a temporary tarsorrhaphy may be useful to save these eyes.

- *Treatment of complications*
  - *Descemetocele:* Rest and pressure bandage, followed by therapeutic keratoplasty.
  - *If the ulcer perforates:* Alternate pressure bandage and medical treatment, or temporary tarsorrhaphy.
  - *In case of small or impending perforation*—tissue adhesive (cyano-acrylate glue) with bandage contact lens (BCL).
  - *In leukoma or adherent leukoma:* Penetrating keratoplasty.
  - *For superficial opacities in pupillary axis:* Deep anterior lamellar keratoplasty.
  - *A leukoma with no perception of light (PL):* Treated either by tattooing of cornea or cosmetic contact lens.
  - *Anterior staphyloma:* Staphylectomy or enucleation, then artificial eye.
  - *Panophthalmitis:* Evisceration and then artificial eye.
  - *Corneal fistula:* (i) Cyanoacrylate glue (tissue adhesive) application with BCL; (ii) Penetrating keratoplasty.

Corneal abscess (Fig. 13.18): It is localized collection of pus in the cornea. Here, the epithelium is usually intact.

It is similar to corneal ulcer. But in the treatment—evacuation of pus is done first, by a fine needle or knife, before starting the topical antibiotic therapy. The response of treatment will then be appreciated.

HYPOPYON CORNEAL ULCER (ULCUS SERPENS) (FIG. 13.19)

It is a typical bacterial ulcer which has a tendency to creep over the cornea in a serpiginous fashion, and associated with hypopyon and violent iridocyclitis.

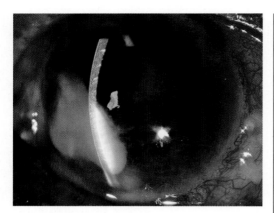

Fig. 13.18: Corneal abscess

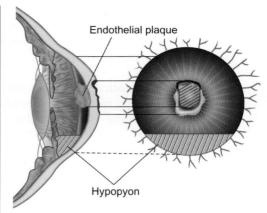

Fig. 13.19: Hypopyon corneal ulcer

Etiology

- It occurs commonly in old debilitated persons or the alcoholics.
- *Causative agent*—*Pneumococcus* in most of the cases.
- Source of infection—mostly chronic dacryocystitis.

Symptoms

Same as the bacterial corneal ulcer, but there is remarkably little pain during the initial stage, hence, the treatment is often unduly delayed.

Signs

- Grayish-white, disc-shaped ulcer near the center of the cornea.
- The ulcer is more at the edges than at the center, and is particularly well-marked in one specific direction.
- A cloudy-gray area surrounds the ulcer area and again, more marked in the same direction.
- On one side the ulcer spreads, while on the other side it may undergo simultaneous cicatrization, and the edges may be covered by fresh epithelium.
- The whole cornea may be come hazy.
- Violent iridocyclitis with a definite hypopyon.
- Conjunctival and ciliary congestion.
- Lids are edematous.

It must be noted that any corneal ulcer may be associated with hypopyon. But a corneal ulcer with hypopyon (due to other cause) is not equivalent to hypopyon corneal ulcer or ulcus serpens which has the above typical features (Fig. 13.20).

Corneal ulcer with hypopyon is found in:
- Pneumococcal infection
- *Pseudomonas pyocyanea*
- Gonococcal, staphylococcal, streptococcal, *Moraxella*, etc. infection
- Mycotic hypopyon corneal ulcer, as with *Aspergillus*, *Fusarium* or *Candida* species.

Course

- Great tendency for early perforation of the cornea with its sequelae.
- Hypopyon increases in size very rapidly. Leading to secondary glaucoma.
- Ultimately, panophthalmitis may occur.

Treatment

Treatment is almost same as the treatment of a corneal ulcer. Special points are:
- Overhanging edges of the ulcer are due to be excised, and the floor is to be scraped with aspatula.
- Paracentesis to evacuate the pus if the hypopyon is massive.
- Secondary glaucoma is treated with anti-glaucoma agent like tablet acetazolamide and/or timolol maleate (0.5%) eye drop.

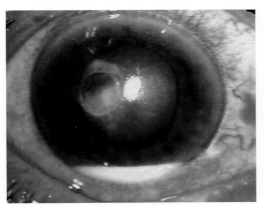

Fig. 13.20: Hypopyon corneal ulcer—bacterial

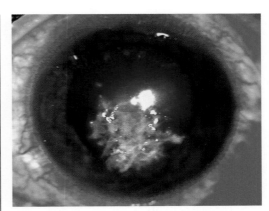

Fig. 13.21: Fungal keratitis by filamentous fungus

- If there is any evidence of chronic dacryocystitis:
  - Temporary punctal cautery
  - Dacryocystectomy.

MYCOTIC KERATITIS, KERATOMYCOSIS OR FUNGAL CORNEAL ULCER

Causative Agents

- *Filamentous fungus:* Aspergillus and *Fusarium* are common in our country. They are most prevalent among agricultural workers.
- *Yeast: Candida albicans,* frequently affects the immunocompromised host.

Predisposing Factors

- Same as bacterial keratitis.
- Indiscriminate use of topical steroids.
- Immunocompromised subjects.

Mode of Infection

Mycotic keratitis is typically preceded by ocular trauma (often trivial in nature), mainly by agricultural and vegetable matters.

Symptoms

Same as for the bacterial ulcer, but the symptoms are less prominent than an equal-sized bacterial ulcer.

Signs

- Dry looking, yellowish-white lesion with indistinct margin.
- Filamentous fungus keratitis has delicate, feathery, finger-like projection into the adjacent stroma (Fig. 13.21). It may be surrounded by grayish-halo and multiple satellite lesions (Fig. 13.22). Sometimes, it may be ring-shaped (Fig. 13.23).

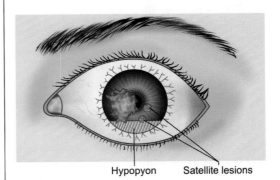

Hypopyon   Satellite lesions

Fig. 13.22: Fungal corneal ulcer

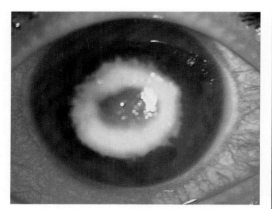

Fig. 13.23: Ring-shaped fungal corneal ulcer

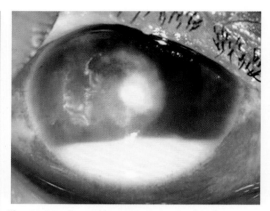

Fig. 13.25: Fungal keratitis—convex hypopyon

- Candida keratitis—typically appears as collar-button abscess without any feathery edge (Fig.13. 24).
- The overlying epithelium is elevated and may be intact.
- Some degree of iridocyclitis and massive dense hypopyon are common. This hypopyon is immobile with upper convex border (Fig. 13.25).

  Unlike bacterial ulcer, the hypopyon may not be sterile, as the fungi can penetrate the Descemet's membrane into the anterior chamber even without perforation.
- Vascularization usually does not occur.

Investigations

- 10% potassium hydroxide (KOH) mount preparation of the smear to demonstrate causative fungus microscopically (Fig. 13.26).
- Culture in Sabouraud's media.

Treatment

- Scraping and debridement of the ulcer.
- Atropine eye ointment—3 times daily.
- *Antifungal drugs*
  - *Topical*
    - Natamycin (5%) eye drop, 1 hourly. It is effective against most common

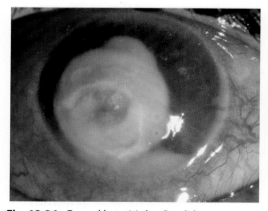

Fig. 13.24: Fungal keratitis by *Candida*

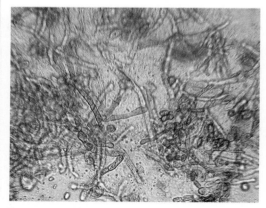

Fig. 13.26: Filamentous fungus in KOH mount preparation

fungi mainly *Fusarium* and *Aspergillus* spp.
- Topical amphotericin B (0.15–0.25%), 1 hourly, effective against *Aspergillus* and *Candida*.
- Voriconazole eye drop—1–2 hourly. It is more effective against *Aspergillus.*
- Nystatin eye ointment, 5 times daily. It is only effective against *Candida*, but less potent.

Topical antifungals are to be instilled for a long time, as the response is often delayed.
- **Systemic:** If the ulcer is deep, or marginal, or if it is perforated, tablet ketoconazole or tablet fluconazole may also be tried for 2–3 weeks.
- Cauterization of the ulcer may be done in non-responsive cases.
- Therapeutic penetrating keratoplasty (TPK) is the last choice in non-responsive cases.

ACANTHAMOEBA KERATITIS (FIG. 13.27)

Acanthamoeba is a free-living protozoa which has a trophozoite and a cystic form. It is found in stagnant water (pond, swimming pool, bath tub, etc.) and contact lens solution and contact lens cases.

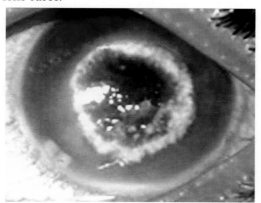

Fig. 13.27: Acanthamoeba keratitis

Modes of Infection

- ***Contact lens wearer*—**via contaminated solution.
- ***Noncontact lens wearer*—**direct contamination after a minor trauma.

Clinical Features

- Frequently misdiagnosed as herpetic or fungal keratitis for many weeks.
- Severe pain, and it is out of proportion to the degree of inflammation (radial keratoneuritis).
- Progressive chronic stromal keratitis with recurrent breakdown of corneal epithelium.
- Frequent development of paracentral ring-shaped ulcer or abscess which may perforate.
- A nodular scleritis is a frequent finding.
- It may be associated with limbal inflammation (limbitis).
- It does not respond to conventional antimicrobial treatment.

Diagnosis by KOH mount preparation or by calcofluor white staining of the smear for amoebic cyst. Acanthamoeba is cultured in special media—*E. coli* enriched nutrient agar plate.

Treatment

- Propamidine isethionate (Brolene) (0.02%) drops and ointment
- Neomycin drops and ointment
- Polyhexamethylene biguanide (PHMB) (0.001%) drops is also helpful
- Chlorhexidine (0.02%) eye drop (prepared from mouthwash)—1 hourly
- In resistant cases, a therapeutic penetrating keratoplasty may be required.

VIRAL KERATITIS

Herpes Simplex Viral Keratitis

Infection with herpes simplex virus (HSV) is extremely common, and in the majority of the cases, it is subclinical.

Herpes simplex virus (HSV) is of two types:
1. **HSV1** causes infection above the waist (lips and eyes), and is acquired by kissing.
2. **HSV-2** causes infection below the waist (genital herpes), and is acquired venereally. Primary infection may be subclinical or correct indentation cause mild ocular problems.

Following the primary infection, the virus travels up to the trigeminal ganglion, and lies there in a latent state.

During recurrences, the virus travels down along the sensory nerve to its target tissues, and causes recurrent lesions.

Predisposing factors for recurrence
- Poor general health
- Common cold and fever
- Menstruation
- Mild trauma
- Topical and systemic corticosteroids
- Immunosuppressive agents, etc.

Primary Herpetic Keratitis

- Typically it occurs between 6 months to 5 years of age.
- The typical lesion is an acute follicular conjunctivitis.
- Fine epithelial keratitis may be present, which sometimes progresses into dendritic figure.
- Vesicular eruptions and edema of the lids.
- It seldom causes serious problem and is treated by acyclovir eye ointment, five times a day for 2 weeks.

▌RECURRENT HSV KERATITIS

Dendritic Keratitis (Fig. 13.28)

Symptoms

- Acute pain, redness, and lacrimation
- Photophobia and blurring of vision.

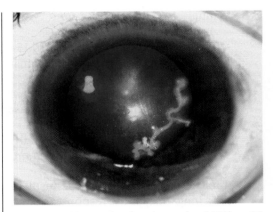

Fig. 13.28: Herpes simplex virus—dendritic keratitis

Signs

- Circumciliary congestion
- Initially, numerous whitish plaques of epithelial keratitis appear on the cornea known as superficial punctate keratitis (SPK), and they quickly desquamate to form erosions.
- These erosions coalesce with each other and spread in all directions, and send out lateral branches with knobbed ends, to form "dendritic" or "tree-like" figure and this is pathognomonic.
- The bed of the ulcer stains with fluorescein, and diseased cell at the margin takes up Rose-Bengal stain.
- Corneal sensation is diminished or absent.

Geographical Keratitis (Ulcer) (Fig. 13.29)

This is much larger epithelial lesion with typical "geographical" or "amoeboid" configuration which occurs as a continued enlargement of dendritic ulcer.

This is likely to occur following inadvertent use of topical steroids.

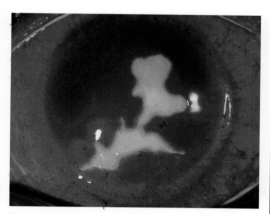

Fig. 13.29: Herpes simplex virus—geographical keratitis

Treatment

- Debridement of the ulcer.
- *Antiviral agents (anyone)*
  - Acyclovir (3%) eye ointment, 5 times daily for 14 days.
    - It is the drug of choice.
    - Prolong use of acyclovir ointment causes superficial punctate keratopathy.
  - Ganciclovir ointment
  - Trifluorothymidine (TFT) (1%) drop, every 2 hours during the day. It is more toxic than acyclovir.
  - Adenine arabinoside (Ara-A) (3%) ointment, 5 times daily.
  - Oral acyclovir (200–400 mg), 1 tablet 4 times daily for 15–10 days may be added.
  - Oral valaciclovir (500–1,000 mg): 1 tablet twice daily for 7 days, then 1 tablet daily for 3 weeks.
- Atropine (1%) or homatropine (2%) eye drop, 2–3 times daily.
- Improvement of general health.
- Cryocautery or iodine cautery of the ulcer in resistance cases.

Stromal Necrotic Keratitis

- Caused by active viral invasion and destruction.
- Cheesy and necrotic appearance of the stroma.
- Associated with anterior uveitis, called herpetic keratouveitis.
- Vascularization, scarring, and even perforation may occur.
- *Treatment* by oral acyclovir, topical antiviral, atropine, and judicious use of corticosteroids.

Metaherpetic Keratitis (Trophic Ulcer)

- It is due to persistent defects in the basement membrane of the corneal epithelium.
- It is not an active viral disease.
- The margin is gray and thickened due to heaped-up epithelium.
- *Treatment* by artificial tears, patching or bandage contact lens.

Disciform Keratitis or HSV Endotheliitis (Figs 13.30A and B)

Disciform keratitis or HSV endotheliitis is a deep keratitis with disc-like edema, mainly caused by herpes virus (and sometimes due to vaccinia and herpes zoster virus).

Pathogenesis

A delayed type of hypersensitivity reaction to HSV-antigen → low grade stromal inflammation with damage to the underlying endothelium → passage of aqueous into the corneal stroma.

Clinical Features

- *In mild form*, only focal disc-shaped stromal edema with fine keratic precipitates (KPs). There is no necrosis or no neovascularization.
- *In severe form*
  - Stromal edema is more diffuse
  - Presence of Descemet's folds
  - Deep vascularization
  - Focal bullous keratopathy

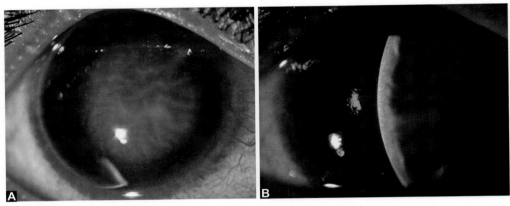

Figs 13.30A and B: Herpes simplex virus—disciform keratitis (slit section)

- Wessely's immune ring surrounding the edema
- Marked anterior uveitis
- Absent or diminished corneal sensation.

Treatment

- The first aim is to heal any associated epithelial lesion.
- Topical corticosteroid drops (4–5 times daily) under antiviral cover (acyclovir ointment 2–5 times daily) are given. The use of diluted steroid drops reduces the incidence of any steroid-related complication.
- Cycloplegic, like atropine eye ointment.
- In majority of the cases, it resolves over a period of several weeks.

Prophylaxis for HSV Keratitis Recurrence

Herpetic eye disease, especially stromal keratitis and endotheliitis, is notorious for recurrence episodes. The chance of recurrence, without continued treatment, ranges from 25% to 30% over 1-year period.

Indications for oral antiviral prophylaxis: Multiple recurrences, postoperatively in any ocular surgery especially keratoplasty, vascularization or scar approaching visual axis.

Recommended prophylaxis with oral acyclovir (400 mg twice daily) or oral valaciclovir (500 mg once daily) for 12-month period which reduces recurrence to 9–14%.

HERPES ZOSTER OPHTHALMICUS

- Herpes zoster ophthalmicus (HZO) is a common infection caused by the varicella-zoster virus.
- The infection mainly affects the elderly patients.
- It is more common in immunocompromised hosts (as in HIV).

Pathogenesis

- After initial exposure, the virus remains latent in the trigeminal ganglion.
- Under the stress, it becomes reactivated, replicates, and migrates down the ophthalmic division of the trigeminal nerve to develop ocular complications.

Hutchinson's sign (rule) (Fig. 13.31): When the tip of the nose is involved, the eye will also be involved, since both are supplied by the nasociliary nerve.

Symptoms

- Vesicular eruptions around the eye, forehead, and scalp.

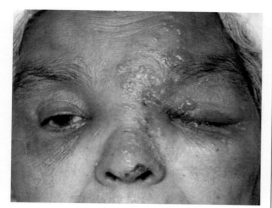

Fig. 13.31: Herpes zoster ophthalmicus—Hutchinson's sign

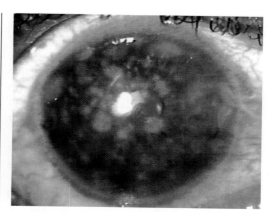

Fig. 13.32: Nummular keratitis

- Severe pain along the distribution of the ophthalmic division of 5th nerve.
- Photophobia and lacrimation.

Signs

There are three stages:

Stage I: Acute lesions—which develop within 3 weeks.

Stage II: Chronic lesions—may persist for up to 10 years.

Stage III: Recurrent lesions—which may reappear after 10 years.

Stage I: Acute Ocular Lesions

- **Lids:** Redness, edema, and vesicular eruptions.
- **Conjunctiva:** Acute mucopurulent conjunctivitis.
- **Sclera:** Episcleritis and scleritis.
- **Cornea**
  - Punctate epithelial keratitis.
  - **Microdendrites:** Small, fine, multiple dendritic or stellate lesions

> **Differential diagnosis from HSV dendrite**—in herpes zoster, the dendrites are peripheral, broader, plaque-like, raised from the surface, more frequently stellate-shaped, and without any terminal knobs.

- **Nummular keratitis (Fig. 13.32):** Multiple granular lesions, surrounded by a halo of stromal haze.
- **Disciform keratitis.**
- Sensation is diminished or absent.
- **Iris:** Acute iridocyclitis with hyphema (hyperacute iritis) and patches of iris atrophy.
- **Intraocular pressure may be raised.**
- **Retina:** Acute retinal necrosis.
- **Neuro-ophthalmological:** Optic neuritis and cranial nerve palsies—affecting the 3rd (most common), 4th, and 6th nerves.

Stage II: Chronic Ocular Lesions

- Ptosis, due to scarring of the lid
- Trichiasis, entropion, and lid notching may also occur
- Mucus-secreting conjunctivitis
- Scleritis
- Nummular and disciform keratitis
- 7% of the patients present with postherpetic neuralgia, which is worse at night and aggravated by touch and heat.

Stage III: Recurrent Ocular Lesions

Like episcleritis, scleritis, mucus-plaque keratitis, nummular keratitis, iritis and secondary glaucoma.

Treatment

- *Oral acyclovir:* 800 mg 5 times daily for 7 days. It reduces pain, accelerates healing, and curtails vesiculation. It is also effective in anterior uveitis. It has no benefit on postherpetic neuralgia.
- Pain is relieved by *strong analgesics*, or even by injection pethidine.
- *Antibiotic corticosteroid preparation* for skin lesions. Calamine lotion promotes crust formation and is better avoided.
- *Topical steroids* in presence of corneal involvement, and anterior uveitis or scleritis.
- *Topical antibiotics* to prevent secondary infection.
- *Cycloplegic for iritis or severe keratitis.*
- *Systemic steroids*—indications:
  - To reduce the severity of postherpetic neuralgia
  - Optic neuritis
  - Cranial nerve palsy.
- *Artificial tears and bandage soft contact lens* for persistent epithelial defects.
- *Penetrating keratoplasty* in case of dense scarring of the cornea.

LAGOPHTHALMIC KERATITIS EXPOSURE KERATITIS

This is due to exposure of the cornea when it remains insufficiently covered by the lids.
- The epithelium of the exposed cornea becomes dessicated and the stroma becomes hazy.
- Finally, owing to drying, the epithelium is cast off, and the raw area may be invaded by the microorganisms.

Clinical Features

- It ranges from minimum epithelial erosions to severe ulceration, secondary infection and even perforation.

- The lower-third of the cornea is commonly affected, as this part remains more exposed (Figs 13.33A and B).

Other features and treatment have already been described earlier (*see* Chapter 11, page 127).

NEUROTROPHIC KERATITIS

- It occurs in an anesthetic cornea.
- It appears that corneal sensation is very important to maintain the health of the corneal epithelium.
- The loss of sensory influence alters the metabolic activity of the epithelium, thereby causing edema and exfoliation of the epithelial cells.

Etiology

- *Congenital:* Very rare. Riley-Day syndrome, anhidrotic ectodermal dysplasia, congenital insensitivity to pain may be the cause.
- *Acquired*
  - Section or affection of the 5th nerve
  - Herpes simplex virus and varicella zoster virus keratitis
  - Diabetes mellitus
  - Leprosy.

Neuroparalytic keratitis: It is due to paralysis of the motor nerve that closes the eyelids, and is normally a sequel to facial palsy. The picture is similar to "exposure keratitis".

Clinical Features

- Punctate epithelial erosions involving the interpalpebral area.
- Exfoliation of the epithelial cells followed by central ulceration.
- Corneal sensation is absent.

Treatment

- Routine treatment of corneal ulcer
- Ointments and patching
- Amniotic membrane transplantation

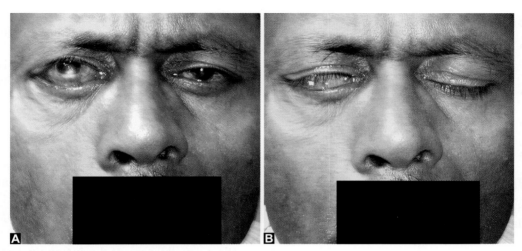

Figs 13.33A and B: Bell's palsy with corneal ulcer—right eye

- Tarsorrhaphy for several months. No anesthesia is required during tarsorrhaphy, as the sensation of the lids and conjunctiva are absent.

ATHEROMATOUS ULCER

- It develops over an old leukoma with degenerative changes.
- It may start spontaneously or after a minor trauma.
- The degenerated tissue breaks away from the surface, and an ulcer develops.
- The ulcer progresses rapidly with a little tendency to heal.
- It gets easily infected and perforation may occur.

Treatment

- Ointments and patching
- Bandage contact lens and tear substitutes
- If the eye is blind and painful—enucleation or evisceration is better.

PERIPHERAL ULCERATIVE KERATITIS (PUK)

This is a group of diseases, characterized by keratitis and/or melting of the corneal periphery.

Marginal Keratitis (Catarrhal Ulcer) (Fig. 13.34)

It is caused by hypersensitivity reaction to staphylococcal exotoxins, and prevalent in patients having chronic staphylococcal blepharitis.

Symptoms

- Mild ocular irritation
- Lacrimation and photophobia.

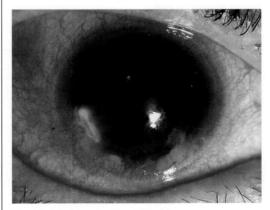

Fig. 13.34: Marginal keratitis

Signs

- Subepithelial infiltrates at the periphery, mostly at 4–8 o'clock position, or at 10–2 o'clock position.
- They are separated from the limbus by a clear zone of cornea.
- The lesions spread circumferentially and form a ring ulcer.
- Corneal sensation is unaffected.

Treatment

Broad-spectrum antibiotic drops—4 times daily.

- Topical corticosteroids, 3–4 times daily for a few days.
- Mild cycloplegic, like cyclopentolate or tropicamide.
- Simultaneous treatment of blepharitis to prevent recurrence.

Mooren's Ulcer (Chronic Serpiginous Ulcer) (Fig. 13.35)

It is a chronic progressive peripheral ulcer of unknown etiology.

It may be due to an ischemic necrosis resulting from vasculitis of the perilimbal vessels.

Very rarely, it occurs following cataract surgery and hookworm infestation.

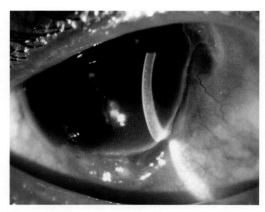

Fig. 13.35: Mooren's ulcer

There are two types of Mooren's ulcer.
1. *A limited form:* Unilateral and usually affects the elderly people.
2. *A progressive form:* Bilateral, relentlessly progressive and affects the younger people.

Symptoms

- Severe pain
- Photophobia and lacrimation
- Decreased vision due to irregular astigmatism and involvement of the visual axis in late stage.

Signs

- Ulcer usually starts at the *interpalpebral area* as patches of gray infiltrates at the margin.
- It spreads slowly undermining the epithelium and superficial stroma.
- Advancing border of the ulcer is having an overhanging edge.
- Later, it involves the entire circumference of the cornea.
- It also spreads towards center of the cornea, and also invades the sclera.
- Healing takes places from the periphery, and the healed area becomes vascularized, thinned, and opaque.
- Perforation may occur with minor trauma.

Treatment

- *Topical corticosteroids*—at hourly intervals.
- *Cycloplegics* like atropine drops.
- *Conjunctival excision (peritomy):* A 3 mm collar of conjunctiva is excised from the limbus and parallel to the ulcer.
- Tissue adhesive (cyanoacrylate glue) with bandage contact lens (TA BCL) along with peritomy if the ulcer is deep.
- *Immunosuppressive therapy:* Especially in bilateral cases—where the prognosis is worse.
  - Systemic corticosteroids

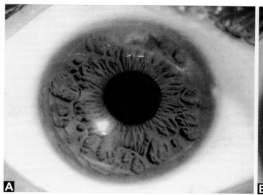 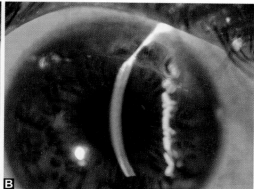

Figs 13.36A and B: Terrien's marginal degeneration. **A.** Upper limbus; **B.** Thinning

- Cytotoxic drugs, like cyclophosphamide, azathioprine, or methotrexate.
- Lamellar sclerocorneal patch graft, if there is a threat or frank perforation.

Terrien's Degeneration (Figs 13.36A and B)

It is a rare, slowly progressive, bilateral marginal degeneration of the cornea, affecting the adults and elderly people.

Clinical Features

- 75% of the patients are male.
- The lesion starts as fine yellow-white punctate stromal opacities at the *upper part of the cornea*.
- It is separated from limbus by a clear zone.
- Eventually, thinning leads to the formation of a peripheral gutter.
- The sharp-edge toward the center becomes demarcated by yellow-white lipid deposits.
- Overlying epithelium is intact, and does not stain with fluorescein.
- Thinning slowly spreads circumferentially, and vascularization is prominent.
- Vision gradually falls due to increasing corneal astigmatism.
- A few patients develop recurrent episodes of pain.
- Perforation occurs in 15% of cases.

Treatment

- Contact lens may be helpful to correct astigmatism.
- Steroid drops in case of inflammation.
- Penetrating keratoplasty or deep lamellar sector keratoplasty is required in case of perforation.

PHLYCTENULAR KERATITIS (FIG. 13.37)

Although phlyctens are commonly found at the limbus, they may also occur within the corneal margin. Like phlyctenular conjunctivitis, it predominantly affects the children.

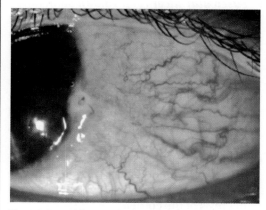

Fig. 13.37: Phlyctenular keratitis

Etiology: As already discussed in conjunctival disease.

Pathology

- A typical nodule is formed on the Bowman's membrane with adjacent epithelium, as localized lymphocytic infiltrations.
- The epithelium is readily destroyed and a phlyctenular ulcer is formed.
- The denuded surface easily becomes infected, usually by *Staphylococci.*
- When multiple phlyctens develop at the corneal margin, blood vessels from the limbus grow toward the nodules, thus producing phlyctenular pannus.

Clinical Features

- *Symptoms* include—pain, photophobia, lacrimation and blepharospasm.
- Mucopurulent discharge in presence of secondary infection.
- The corneal phlycten is a gray nodule, slightly raised above the surface, and an ulcer is yellow in color.
- It may resolve spontaneously, or may extend radially onto the cornea.
- Very rarely, it may give rise to severe ulceration and perforation.

Complications

- *Fascicular ulcer (Fig. 13.38):* Sometimes, phlyctenular ulcer slowly migrates from the limbus toward the center of the cornea in a serpiginous way. It carries a leash of blood vessels which lie in a shallow gutter formed by the ulcer. It is a superficial allergic type of ulcer, which never perforates. When the ulcer heals, the vessels become attenuated with formation of corneal opacity which is densest at its apex.
- *Ring ulcer:* It is formed by multiple phlyctens which coalesce together at the corneal periphery. It may lead to total necrosis of the cornea.

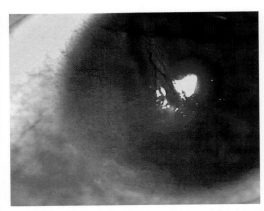

Fig. 13.38: Fascicular ulcer (note the blood vessels)

- *Phlyctenular pannus:* It is usually associated with multiple phlyctens.
- *Perforation of the cornea:* It may occur especially when secondarily infected.

Treatment

- Topical corticosteroids, 4 times daily.
- Atropine (1%) eye drop, 2 times daily.
- Topical antibiotic, if secondarily infected, 4–6 times daily.
- If the fascicular ulcer has reached the pupillary area, it is better to allow it to progress further, as the corneal opacity left by the ulcer tract, is less dense than the site at which the ulcer stops.

Marginal Corneal Ulcer Associated with Systemic Collagen Vascular Diseases

Marginal corneal ulceration and thinning may occur in four main diseases:
1. Rheumatoid arthritis
2. Systemic lupus erythematosus
3. Polyarteritis nodosa
4. Wegener's granulomatosis.

The peripheral corneal changes are:
- Peripheral keratitis
- *Peripheral corneal guttering (contact lens cornea):* Thinning or guttering occurs along the entire corneal periphery. As the central part of the cornea remains of normal thickness, the appearance resembles a hard contact lens placed on the eye—hence, the term

Contd...

Contd...

- Peripheral keratolysis, resulting in descemetocele formation and even perforation
- Sclerosing keratitis
- Variable degree of corneal scarring and vascularization
- Other ocular manifestations include—scleritis, choroidal vasculitis, retinal vasculitis, keratoconjunctivitis sicca, anterior ischemic optic neuropathy, etc.

Treatment
- Systemic and topical corticosteroids
- Immunosuppressive agents
- Conjunctival excision (peritomy)
- Peripheral tectonic keratoplasty.

INTERSTITIAL KERATITIS

Interstitial keratitis (IK) is an inflammation affecting chiefly the corneal stroma, without primary involvement of the epithelium or endothelium.

Causes: Three causes are congenital syphilis, tuberculosis, Cogan's syndrome.

Syphilitic Interstitial Keratitis

Pathology

The disease is fundamentally a uveitis, and the keratitis, which clinically masks the uveitis, is secondary. These reactions are largely allergic, since the *spirochetes* have never been detected in the cornea or uvea.

Clinical Features

It is a late manifestation of congenital syphilis developing between 5 years and 15 years. It is usually bilateral, and unilateral cases occur in delayed type, after the age of thirty, particularly in acquired syphilis.

Symptoms

- Initially, irritation and haziness of the cornea.
- Later pain, lacrimation, photophobia and severe blepharospasm with increased haziness of the cornea.
- Profound loss of vision.

Signs

Ocular signs
- Circumcorneal congestion.
- The lesion starts as one or more hazy patches in deeper cornea from the margin toward the center (Fig. 13.39A).
- They fuse together in 2–4 weeks, and the whole cornea becomes hazy with a steamy surface, giving rise to **ground-glass appearance**.
- Meanwhile, deep vascularization develops, and the vessels meet in the center of the cornea. Since, the vessels are covered by a layer of hazy cornea, they appear as a dull, reddish-pink patch, known as **salmon patch of Hutchinson**.
- As a rule, there is always an associated iridocyclitis.
- After 2–4 months, the cornea begins to clear from periphery toward the center, and the vessels become nonperfused (only remain as fine lines of ghost vessels) (Fig. 13.39B). If there is re-inflammation of the cornea, the vessels may refill with blood.
- The clearing of the cornea takes many weeks or months, but little improvement can be expected after 18 months. Ultimately, majority of the patients regain some useful vision.

General signs
- **Hutchinson's triad**
  - Interstitial keratitis (IK)
  - Permanent deafness
  - Hutchinson's teeth (notching of the two upper permanent incisors).
- Prominent frontal eminences
- Flatness of the nasal bridge
- Rhagades at the angle of the mouth
- Shotty cervical lymph nodes
- Periosteal nodules on the tibia.

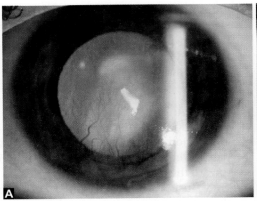 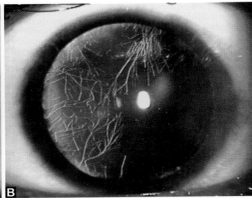

Figs 13.39A and B: Interstitial keratitis. **A.** Lesion at the center; **B.** Ghost vessels

Treatment

- *Systemic penicillin:* Its role is doubtful. It may shorten the course of the disease.
- *Topical corticosteroids* as drops or ointment, 4–6 times daily.
- *Atropine (1%)* ointment, 2 times daily.
- *Penetrating keratoplasty*, if there is any permanent dense corneal opacity.

Tuberculous Interstitial Keratitis

This is similar to the syphilitic interstitial keratitis, but is more often unilateral and sectorial.

Treatment is with antitubercular drugs, topical steroids and cycloplegics.

Cogan's Syndrome

It is very rare, non-syphilitic interstitial keratitis associated with vestibule cochlear disturbances (tinnitus, vertigo, and deafness). It typically affects middle-aged patients.

Treatment is with systemic steroids (to prevent permanent deafness), topical steroids and cycloplegics.

CORNEAL DEGENERATIONS AND DYSTROPHIES

Degeneration and dystrophy are not synonymous. Degeneration means, that the normal cells of a tissue undergo some pathological changes under the influences of some abnormal circumstances. Dystrophy means, the cells have some in born defects which may cause pathological changes with passage of time (Table 13.2).

TABLE 13.2: Difference between corneal degeneration and corneal dystrophy

Corneal degeneration	Corneal dystrophy
Usually unilateral and asymmetrical	Usually bilateral and symmetrical
Located peripherally	Located centrally
Accompanied by vascularization	No vascularization
No inheritance pattern	Hereditary (usually autosomal dominant)
Onset in middle life or later	Relatively early in onset
Secondary to some compromising factors, e.g. aging, inflammation, chemicals, trauma or systemic diseases	Unrelated to any systemic or local disease, or condition

DEGENERATIONS

- Arcus senilis
- Band-shaped keratopathy
- Pellucid marginal
- Salzmann's nodular
- Arcus juvenilis
- Lipid keratopathy
- Terrien's marginal
- Limbal girdle of Vogt

Arcus Senilis (Gerontoxon) (Fig. 13.40)

- It is bilateral lipid degeneration of the peripheral cornea, affecting the most elderly persons.
- It starts in the superior and inferior perilimbal cornea, and then progresses circumferentially to form a band.
- The band is about 1 mm wide and its central border is diffuse, whereas the peripheral edge is sharp.
- The peripheral sharp-edge is separated from the limbus by a clear zone of cornea, which may become thinned *(senile furrow)*.
- *Histologically:* The lipid is first deposited anterior to the Descemet's membrane and then in the anterior stroma, just beneath the Bowman's layer.
- It does not affect the vision.

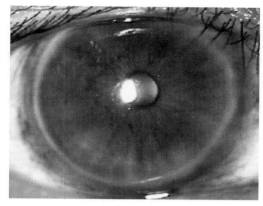

Fig. 13.41: Arcus juvenilis

Arcus Juvenilis (Anterior Embryotoxon) (Fig. 13.41)

It is similar to arcus senilis, except it occurs under the age of 40 years. The condition is usually associated with systemic hyperlipidemias with raised serum cholesterol. So, a serum lipid profile is indicated in these patients.

Band-shaped Keratopathy (BSK) (Fig. 13.42)

- It is caused by deposition of calcium salts in the subepithelial layer of the cornea, and characterized by a horizontal band-shaped opacity.

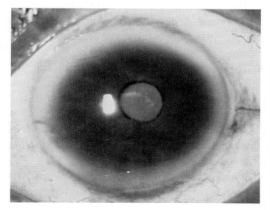

Fig. 13.40: Arcus senilis with mature cataract

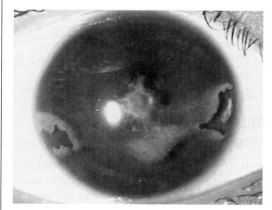

Fig. 13.42: Band-shaped keratopathy

- The calcific band is largely at the palpebral fissure, and separated from the limbus by a clear zone.
- The band begins in the periphery at 3 and 9 o'clock position and affects the central area later on.
- There are numerous holes, where the corneal nerves penetrate the Bowman's layer.
- As the band progresses, the epithelium becomes irregular and subsequently, its breakdown may be very painful.
- ***Pathologically:*** The calcium (mainly hydroxyapatite) is deposited in the Bowman's layer, in the epithelial basement membrane, and most superficial part of the stroma. The remaining layers of the cornea are clear.

Etiology

- Childhood chronic iridocyclitis, especially with juvenile rheumatoid arthritis (JRA)
- ***Other ocular conditions:*** Phthisis bulbi absolute glaucoma, interstitial keratitis
- Systemic hypercalcemia
- Idiopathic—in the elderly.

Treatment

- Scraping of the epithelium overlying the opacity, and application of 0.01 M solution of disodium EDTA (ethylene diamine-tetraacetic acid) for 10 minutes. Then the eye is patched with antibiotics and cycloplegics till the cornea is re-epithelialized.
- Phototherapeutic keratectomy (PTK) by excimer laser may be useful.
- Lamellar keratoplasty for optical reason.

Salzmann's Nodular Degeneration (Fig. 13.43)

- It is characterized by elevated subepithelial bluish-gray nodules (number one to nine), in either scarred cornea or at the edge of transparent cornea.

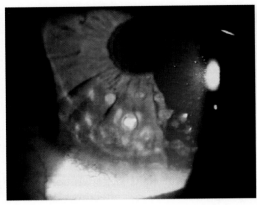

Fig. 13.43: Salzmann's nodular degeneration

- The degeneration is unilateral in 80% cases and occurs more often in females.
- It occurs as a late sequel of corneal diseases like phlyctenulosis, trachoma, chronic keratitis, or vernal keratoconjunctivitis.
- Bowman's layer is missing over the nodules and the epithelium is irregular. The nodules represent excessive secretion of basement membrane-like material.
- Usually, there is no need of treatment. Lamellar keratoplasty may be required to improve vision when the nodules are central inlocation.

Pellucid Marginal Degeneration (Fig. 13.44)

- This is a rare, bilateral, slowly progressive marginal degeneration (thinning) of the cornea between 20 years and 40 years of age.
- The thinning involves only in the inferior cornea, and the ectasia occurs just above the thinned area, giving rise to the appearance like keratoconus.
  But in keratoconus the thinning involves at the center and the maximum ectasias within the area of thinning.
- Fleischer's ring does not occur, but this condition may be complicated by acute hydrops.

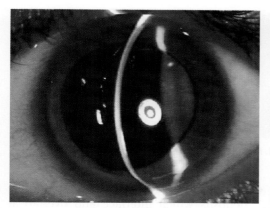

Fig. 13.44: Pellucid marginal degeneration

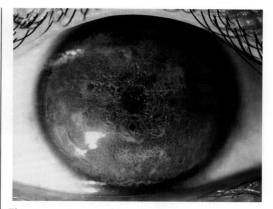

Fig. 13.45: Reis-Buckler's dystrophy

- There is no vascularization (unlike Mooren's or Terrien's degeneration) or lipid deposition (unlike Terrien's degeneration).
- *Treatment* is usually not required, except correction of astigmatism by rigid gas permeable contact lenses.

DYSTROPHIES

Classification

Anterior dystrophies
Epithelium and Bowman's membrane
- Cogan's microcystic
- Recurrent corneal erosion syndrome
- Reis-Bucklers (Fig. 13.45)
- Meesmann
- Map-dot-fingerprint.

Stromal dystrophies
- Granular
- Macular
- Lattice
- Central crystalline
- Congenital hereditary stromal.

Posterior dystrophies
- Descemet's membrane and endothelium
- Cornea guttata
- Fuchs' endothelial
- Posterior polymorphous
- Congenital hereditary endothelial.

Ectatic dystrophies
- Keratoconus
- Posterior keratoconus
- Keratoglobus.

Anterior Dystrophies

- These are probably the more common dystrophies, frequently misdiagnosed, mainly due to their variable presentation.
- Most of the patients remain asymptomatic, but the others develop recurrent corneal erosions with photophobia and lacrimation.
- All are autosomal dominant inheritance.
- Visual loss usually occurs due to irregular astigmatism.

Treatment

- Most of them do not require treatment.
- Recurrent erosions are treated with artificial tears, antibiotic ointment, mild cycloplegic, and patching of the eyes.
- Only a few cases may require lamellar keratoplasty.

Stromal Dystrophies

Granular Dystrophy (13.46A)

- Autosomal dominant inheritance.
- Usually starts around puberty and progresses very slowly.
- The lesions appear as discrete, crumb-like white granules within the anterior stroma of the central cornea.
- The peripheral cornea remains always clear.

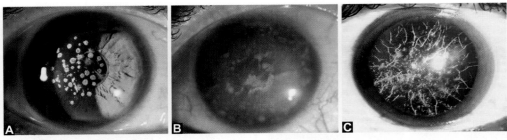

Figs 13.46A to C: Stromal dystrophies. **A.** Granular; **B.** Macular; **C.** Lattice

- The lesions spread into the deeper stroma, and the stroma in between the lesions remains clear.
- The patient remains asymptomatic for many years, although a few patients complain of light scattering.
- *Histochemically*, the deposits are hyaline, and stain bright red with *Masson Trichrome.* Visual acuity, however, remains good and penetrating keratoplasty or deep anterior lamellar keratoplasty is required in some cases with dense lesions.

Macular (Fig. 13.46B)

- Autosomal recessive inheritance.
- The disease starts during early life with *significant impairment of vision.*
- The lesions are focal, gray-white, poorly defined opacities in cloudy stroma.
- With time the lesions spread to the entire corneal stroma *including the peripheral cornea.*
- *Histochemically,* the deposits are glycosaminoglycans (acid mucopolysaccharide) and stain with *alcian blue.*
- Most patients require penetrating keratoplasty during early life to improve visual acuity.

Lattice (Fig. 13.46C)

- Inheritance is autosomal dominant.
- Usually presents during early life with recurrent corneal erosions.

- The lesions are branching spider-like deposits which interlace and overlap at different levels within the stroma.
- With time, a diffuse corneal haze develops, and corneal sensation is diminished.
- *Histochemically*, the deposits are amyloid, and stain with *Congo red.*
- Visual acuity may be significantly impaired by the age of 30–40 years.
- Penetrating keratoplasty is then required to improve the vision. *Recurrence of the dystrophy in the graft is common.*

Posterior Dystrophies

Cornea Guttata (Fig. 13.47)

- This is a common aging process, resulting in focal accumulation of collagen on the posterior surface of the Descemet's membrane.

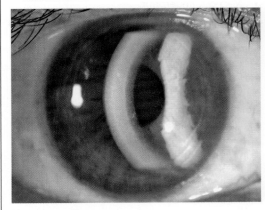

Fig. 13.47: Cornea guttata

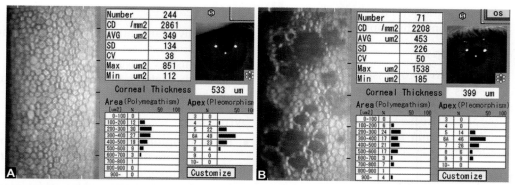

Figs 13.48A and B: Specular microscopic photography. **A.** Normal endothelial cells; **B.** Cornea guttata with low endothelial cell density

- They appear as excrescences or warts of Descemet's membrane, formed by the stressed endothelium.
- They disrupt the normal endothelial mosaic, and appear as dark spots *(beaten metal appearance)*.
- The corresponding peripheral lesions (Hassal-Henle bodies) are of no significance, but the central corneal lesions (guttata) may occur as a part of early stage of Fuchs' endothelial dystrophy.
- Specular microscopy often helps in arriving at a diagnosis (Figs 13.48A and B).

Fuchs' Endothelial Dystrophy (Figs 13.49A and B)

- Usually autosomal dominant inheritance.
- Slowly progressive, bilateral disease affects elderly people, and is more common in females.

- *Early change—corneal guttata* without any symptom. They gradually become more numerous and begin to spread toward the periphery.
- *Endothelial decompensation* soon starts causing the stroma to become edematous. This gradually increases due to malfunction of the endothelial pump.
- *Epithelial edema* gradually develops with increased stromal thickness. Visual acuity is grossly impaired at this stage.
- *Bullous keratopathy (Fig. 13.49C)* develops due to persistence of epithelial edema. When the bullae rupture, it causes severe pain, photophobia, and lacrimation.
  The other causes of bullous keratopathy:
  - Postsurgical—aphakic bullous keratopathy, pseudophakic bullous keratopathy
  - Absolute glaucoma

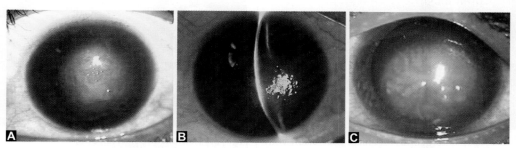

Figs 13.49A to C: A and B. Fuchs's dystrophy with corneal edema; **C.** Bullous keratopathy

- Chronic iridocyclitis, disciform keratitis
- Keratoconus (hydrops).

Complications

- As the disease progresses, stromal opacity develops with vascularization. Bowman's layer is replaced by degenerative pannus.
- There is increased prevalence of open-angle glaucoma in patients with Fuchs' dystrophy.

Treatment

- For early epithelial edema—5% sodium chloride drop (hypertonic saline) for 4–6 times daily and 6% sodium chloride eye ointment at night.
- *Reduction of IOP* by timolol maleate (0.5%) drop—2 times daily.
- *Therapeutic (bandage) soft contact lens* is effective to control pain by protecting the exposed corneal nerves, and also by flattening the bullae.
- *Keratoplasty* is the ultimate choice.

Ectatic Dystrophies

Keratoconus

It is a bilateral conical protrusion of the central part of the cornea with thinning of its central and inferior paracentral areas (Fig. 13.50).

Clinical features

- It usually starts at around puberty and slowly progressive.
- Family history is usually negative.
- Although bilateral, most of the times, the involvement is largely asymmetrical.

Symptoms

- Initial symptom is impaired vision (in one eye it is more than the fellow eye), *due to irregular myopic astigmatism*. This visual loss can only be improved by rigid contact lenses.
- Later on, there is further impairment of vision, and contact lens can no longer correct this visual loss.

Signs

- Irregular retinoscopic reflex.
- Distortion of mires in Placido's disc or keratometer.
- Vertical folds at the level of deep stroma and Descemet's membrane (*Vogt's striae*).
- Prominent corneal nerves.
- Thinning of the central cornea with protrusion just below and nasal to the center.
- *Munson's sign* make it "bulging" or "tenting" of the lower lids when the patient looks down (Fig. 13.51).

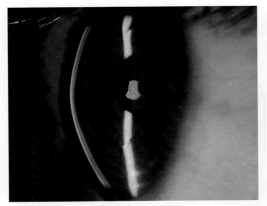

Fig. 13.50: Keratoconus—conical protrusion with thinning

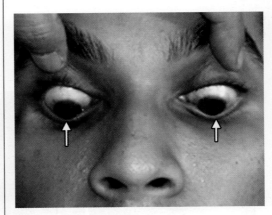

Fig. 13.51: Munson's sign (arrows)

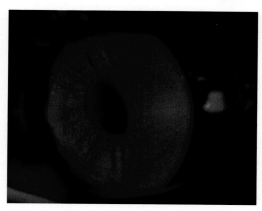

Fig. 13.52: Fleischer's ring under cobalt blue light

- *Fleischer's ring:* Epithelial iron deposition at the base of the cone (Fig. 13.52).

Associations

The systemic and ocular associations of keratoconus include—Down's syndrome, Marfan's syndrome, Turner's syndrome, atopic dermatitis, blue sclera, vernal conjunctivitis, retinitis pigmentosa, and ectopia lentis.

Complications

- *Acute hydrops (Fig. 13.53)*—due to sudden rupture of the Descemet's membrane, and acute see page of the aqueous into the corneal stroma and epithelium. These breaks usually heal within 6–10 weeks,

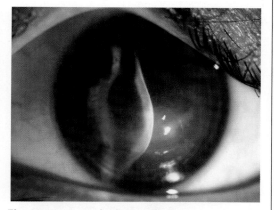

Fig. 13.53: Acute hydrops in keratoconus

and the edema gradually clears. But a variable amount of apical stromal scarring is developed.
- Intolerance to contact lens after few years.

Keratoconus does not rupture spontaneously even if there is extreme thinning of the cornea.

Treatment of Keratoconus

- *Not to rub the eyes:* Always advice patients to avoid rubbing of the eyes, as this causes progression of keratoconus.
- *Glasses:* Usually effective in milder form of keratoconus. But, as the disease progresses, it causes more progressive myopia and irregular astigmatism; and spectacles correction does not work.
- *Contact lenses:* A variety of contact lenses are available for keratoconus. They are: rigid gas permeable (RGP) contact lens, custom soft contact lens, toric soft contact lens, "Rose-K" contact lens, "piggybacking" contact lens; scleral and semi-scleral lenses, prosthetic contact lens (PROSE), etc.
- *Collagen cross-linking (CXL):* This procedure, also called corneal collagen cross-linking with riboflavin (C3R), strengthens cornea to arrest the progression of keratoconus. It is relatively a noninvasive procedure that uses topical riboflavin (vitamin B$_2$) and then UV light to strengthen chemical bonds of collagen fibers in the cornea. It is effective in young adults and children with keratoconus up to 90% of cases.
- *INTACS:* Are corneal segment rings those are placed within the stroma to reshape (flatten) the cornea in keratoconus. INTACS may delay but cannot prevent a corneal transplant.
- *CXL combined with other procedure:* Like, INTACS, or PRK in early keratoconus.

- *Corneal transplantation:* Intolerance to contact lens; nonfitting of contact lens; very advanced keratoconus with apical scarring or after healed hydrops. Deep anterior lamellar keratoplasty (DALK) is the procedure of choice. But penetrating keratoplasty (PK) is also a good option with scarring. Prognosis of graft is excellent in keratoconus.
- *Treatment of acute hydrops:* Topical steroids; 5% hypertonic saline drop; soft bandage contact lens; intracameral injection of 14.6% (isoexpansile) C3F8 gas with compression sutures. In majority case, they healed with minimal scarring with surprisingly good vision.

Posterior Keratoconus

It is a rare disorder, in which the posterior cornea is having excavation, and the anterior cornea does not protrude. The condition gives rise to mild irregular astigmatism and is nonprogressive.

Keratoglobus

This is a very rare condition, characterized by thinning and protrusion of the entire cornea. Astigmatism is usually not very irregular, unless scarring has occurred following acute hydrops.

OTHER CORNEAL DISORDERS

Superficial Punctate Keratitis (Figs 13.54 to 13.56)

This is punctuate epithelial keratitis, scattered all over the cornea, usually due to a viral infection.

Etiology

- *Viral infections:* Herpes simplex, herpes zoster, vaccinia, adenovirus (as a part of epidemic keratoconjunctivitis or pharyngoconjunctival fever), molluscum contagiosum, etc.
- Keratoconjunctivitis sicca (KCS)
- Staphylococcal exotoxin (associated with blepharitis) and Meibomianitis
- Contact lens wearer
- Foreign body in the upper palpebral conjunctiva, e.g. minute iron/dust particle, caterpillar hair, etc.
- Unknown (Thygeson's superficial punctate keratitis).

Pathology: It occurs in the deeper layers of corneal epithelium. Sometimes, it extends into Bowman's membrane and superficial parts of the stroma (*subepithelial punctate keratitis*).

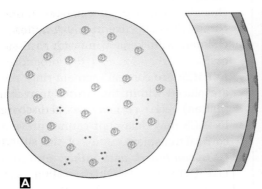
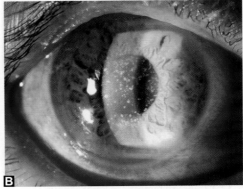

Figs 13.54A and B: Superficial punctate epithelial keratitis. **A.** Schematic representation; **B.** Photograph

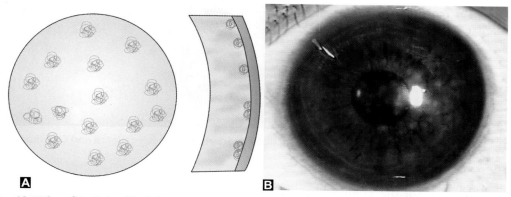

Figs 13.55A and B: Subepithelial punctate keratitis. **A.** Schematic representation; **B.** Photograph

Symptoms: Irritation, photophobia, and lacrimation.

Signs

- The epithelial opacities appear as raised gray dots, scattered all over the cornea.
- The lesions sometimes stain with fluorescein (Fig. 13.56), and always turn bright-red with Rose-Bengal.
- Sensation may be diminished (*herpetic*).
- Ciliary congestion.
- Preauricular lymphadenopathy may be present (*adenoviral*).

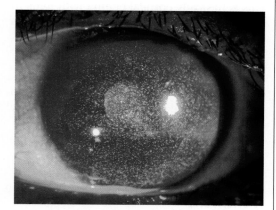

Fig. 13.56: Fluorescein staining in diffuse superficial punctate keratitis

Treatment

- Antibiotic ointment and cycloplegics in most cases.
- Antiviral drugs, if corneal sensation is diminished.
- Topical steroids, if associated with staphylococcal blepharitis.
- Artificial tears frequently.
- Removal of foreign body, if any.

Superior Limbic Keratoconjunctivitis (Figs 13.57A to C)

- This is a bilateral chronic inflammation of the superior tarsal and bulbar conjunctiva, with edema of the superior limbal conjunctiva.
- The disease is usually bilateral, more in females and with *thyroid dysfunction*.
- It follows a chronic course with remissions and exacerbations, but the prognosis is ultimately good.
- *Symptoms* include, foreign body sensation, photophobia, pain and mucoid discharge.
- *Signs* include:
  - Papillary hypertrophy of the superior tarsus.
  - Hyperemia and keratinization of the superior bulbar conjunctiva.

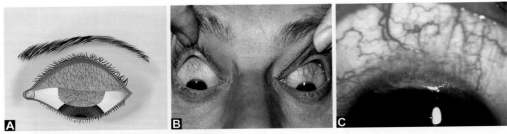

Figs 13.57A to C: Superior limbic keratoconjunctivitis. **A.** Schematic representation; **B and C.** Photographs

- Thickening of the conjunctiva at the superior limbus.
- Superior cornea shows punctate epithelial erosions (stains with fluorescein and Rose-Bengal) and filaments.

Treatment

- Artificial tears and soft bandage contact lens.
- Silver nitrate (1%) is applied to the affected conjunctival area.
- Resection of a block of superior bulbar conjunctival tissue.
- Thermocauterization of the superior bulbar conjunctiva.

Photophthalmia (Photokeratitis)

It is a condition characterized by acute multiple erosions of the corneal epithelium after exposure to ultraviolet (UV) rays.

Causes

- Exposure to bright flash of a short-circuit.
- Exposure to welding arc with naked eyes (*welding keratitis*).
- Exposure to UV rays, reflected from snow surfaces *(snow blindness)*.

Clinical Features

- There is a **latent period of 4–5 hours** between the exposure and the onset of symptoms.

- *Symptoms* include, extreme burning pain, lacrimation, and photophobia.
- There is swelling of the lids, conjunctival chemosis and congestion, and multiple erosions of the corneal epithelium.

Treatment

- Cold compress
- Antibiotic ointment and mild cycloplegics, and patching the eyes for 24 hours
- *Prevention:* Wearing protective glasses when such exposure is to be anticipated. Crooke's glass, which cuts off UV rays and infrared rays, is very useful in this situation.

Striate Keratopathy (Keratitis) (Figs 13.58A and B)

This is basically corneal edema with folds in the Descemet's membrane, which appear as delicate gray lines in the cornea.

Causes

- Following cataract operation—due to endothelial damage by instruments, by IOL, and also by tight suturing.
- Corneal ulcers or wounds—as radial striae around the lesion.
- After tight bandaging of the eye.

Treatment

- They disappear spontaneously within 12 weeks as the wound heals.

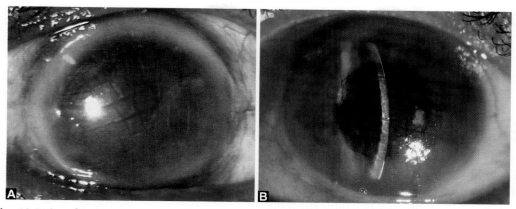

Figs 13.58A and B: Mild and severe striate keratopathy after cataract surgery

- Sometimes, they persist and may cause endothelial decompensation.

Filamentary Keratopathy (Keratitis) (Figs 13.59A and B)

- This is disease with the formation of epithelial threads (filaments) on the cornea.
- The filaments (2 mm or less in length) adhere to the cornea by one end, while the other, moves about freely.

Causes

- Keratoconjunctivitis sicca
- Superior limbic keratoconjunctivitis

- Following cataract surgery
- Herpes simplex keratitis
- Recurrent erosions
- Diabetes mellitus.

Clinical Features

- Patient presents with foreign body sensation, photophobia and lacrimation.
- As the filaments are anchored to the epithelial cells, pulling on them is very painful.
- It is beautifully stained by Rose-Bengal and fluorescein.

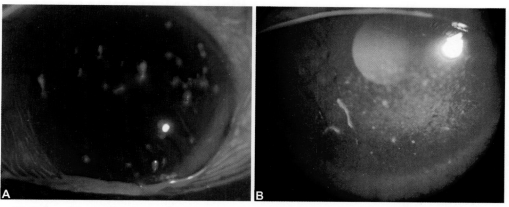

Figs 13.59A and B: **A.** Filamentary keratopathy; **B.** Superficial punctate keratitis and filaments in dry eye

Treatment

- Removal of the filaments, by scraping them from the underlying epithelium, and then patching
- Bandage contact lens
- Artificial tears eye drop frequently.

Keratomalacia

This is characterized by a desiccation and subsequent necrosis of the cornea due to lack of vitamin A. The characteristic feature is the absence of inflammatory reaction. For more details, *see* Chapter 26.

CONTACT LENSES (FIG. 13. 60)

Contact lenses are worn directly over the cornea and beneath the eye lids.

There are three main types of contact lens:
1. ***Hard:*** It is made of PMMA (polymethylmethacrylate) or perspex.
2. ***Rigid gas permeable (RGP):*** It is made of mixture of a hard and a soft material (Fig. 13.61A).
3. ***Soft (hydrophilic):*** It is made of HEMA (hydroxyethyl methacrylate) and hybrid materials (Fig. 13.61B).

Hard Lenses

These lenses cover the part of the cornea and have a diameter of 7–10.5 mm.

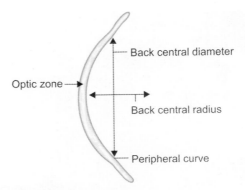

Fig. 13.60: Contact lens

Advantages

- Most durable and cheap.
- Cleaning and maintenance are easy.
- It can correct the astigmatism in a greater extent.
- Less chance of corneal infection.

Disadvantages

- Only suitable for daily wear for short duration.
- Not permeable to atmospheric oxygen. Cornea suffers from quick hypoxia leading to epithelial edema ***(Sattler's veil)***.
- Most uncomfortable, and requires adaptation by progressive increase in wearing time.
- May give rise to annoying glare at night.

Rigid Gas Permeable Lenses

They also cover the part of the cornea.

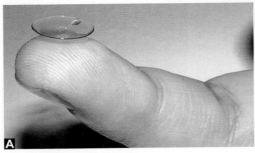
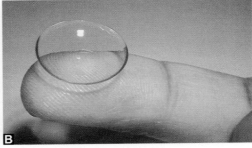

Figs 13.61A and B: A. Rigid gas permeable; **B.** Soft contact lens

Advantages

- Permeable to atmospheric oxygen in variable amount. So, the cornea does not suffer much from hypoxia.
- Suitable for daily wear, and for a longer duration than hard lens.
- Others are same as hard lens.

Disadvantages

- Less durable and costly.
- Less comfortable (though little better than hard lens) and requires slow adaptation.
- Tend to scratch and fracture more easily.

Soft (Hydrophilic) Lenses

They cover the entire cornea and extend 1–2 mm over the sclera. They have a diameter of 13–14.5 mm. The amount of oxygen passing through the lens is directly related to its water content.

They are used as **daily-wear, extended-wear** (more than 24 hours) and as **therapeutic bandage lenses**.

Advantages

- It can be used both in day and at night.
- Most comfortable and does not require adaptation time.
- Lens loss is less.

Disadvantages

- More delicate, more easily damaged and have a shorter life.
- It cannot correct astigmatism more than 0.5–1.0D.
- Cleaning and maintenance of the lenses are difficult.
- Associated with higher incidence of corneal infection.

Indications of Contact Lenses (Fig. 13.62)

Optical

About 95% of the contact lenses are worn as an alternative to glasses.

- **Myopia** is the most common indication.
- **Aphakia** especially in unilateral aphakia, and aphakia following congenital cataract operation.
- **Astigmatism** irregular astigmatism, as in fine nebular opacity, keratoconus, etc.
- **Anisometropia**
- **High hypermetropia.**

Therapeutic

By soft bandage contact lenses and the indications are:

- Bullous keratopathy
- Recurrent corneal erosion syndrome
- Filamentary keratopathy
- Persistent epithelial healing defects
- Dry eye syndrome
- Metaherpetic keratitis
- Chemical burns—to prevent symblepharon formation
- Wound leaks, along with tissue adhesives.

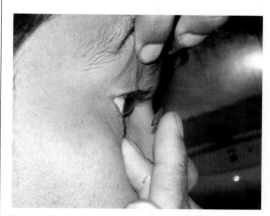

Fig. 13.62: Contact lens wearing

Diagnostic

- Fundus contact lens
- Goldmann's three-mirror contact lens
- Radio-opaque contact lens for diagnosis of intraocular foreign body
- Gonio lens
- Lenses for laser therapy.

Miscellaneous

- *Cosmetic*—to hide an unsightly corneal scar with no visual potential.
- *Vehicle for drug delivery*, e.g. contact lens soaked in pilocarpine.
- *Protective*—as in aniridia or albinism with painted iris and a central clear pupillary area.
- *Occluders*—for treatment of amblyopia in children who cannot tolerate conventional occlusion.
- *Occupational:* Practically useful among sportsmen, salesgirls, actor, models, etc.

Complications of Contact Lenses

They are more common with soft lenses, especially with the extended-wear type.

Conjunctival Complications

- *Allergic conjunctivitis*—mainly related to allergy to the preservatives (e.g. thimerosal) present in contact lens cleaning solution.
- *Giant papillary conjunctivitis (GPC):* It has an immunologic origin in which contact lens deposits, especially the proteins act as allergens.

Corneal Complications

- *Epithelial edema* mainly due to hypoxia (*Sattler's veil*).
- Peripheral corneal *vascularization*.
- *Sterile corneal ulceration* which usually heals, once the contact lens wear has been discontinued.

- *Infection*, particularly *Pseudomonas* keratitis and *Acanthamoeba* keratitis are the most serious.
- *Warpage of the cornea*—resulting in severe and permanent astigmatism.

Problems with the Contact Lens

- *Lens deposits*—mucoproteins, calcium, lipid or even micro-organisms can adhere to the lens surface.
- *Lens digestion*—organisms, particularly fungi can digest lens material while growing intoit.
- *Lens spoilage*—due to aging, loss of lens shape, discoloration, and by manual or mechanical trauma.

DISEASES OF THE SCLERA

Diseases of the sclera are relatively rare. The reasons are: (i) relative avascularity of the sclera and (ii) lack of reaction of its dense fibrous tissue to any insult.

For the same reasons, when they do occur, the diseases tend to be chronic and sluggish.

Blue Sclera (Fig. 13.63)

The sclera appears more blue than white. This is due to visibility of the underlying uveal pigment through the thinned sclera.

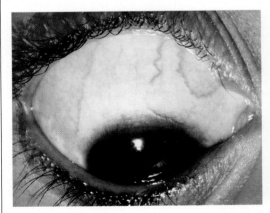

Fig. 13.63: Blue sclera

Causes

- Normally in babies
- *Osteogenesis imperfect* (blue sclera, *fragilitas ossium,* and deafness)
- Buphthalmos
- High myopia
- Following scleritis
- Ciliary staphyloma
- Marfan's syndrome
- Ehler-Danlos syndrome.

INFLAMMATION OF THE SCLERA

Classification

Episcleritis
- Simple
- Nodular

Anterior scleritis
- Diffuse
- Nodular
- Necrotizing
  - With inflammation
  - Without inflammation (scleromalacia perforans)

Posterior scleritis

Episcleritis

This is a benign inflammatory process affecting the deep subconjunctival connective tissue (episclera), and sometimes, including the superficial sclera lamella.

Etiopathology

- Young adults, more in female.
- Idiopathic (most common).
- Allergic reaction to endogenous toxins, e.g. streptococcal or tubercular.
- Infectious, e.g. herpes zoster, herpes simplex, syphilis, etc.
- Other collagen—vascular diseases.

Pathologically, there are dense lymphocytic infiltrations in the subconjunctival and episcleral tissue.

Symptoms

- Mild pain or irritation of the eye.
- Localized redness.

Signs

Two clinical types—simple and nodular.
1. *Simple episcleritis:* There is sectorial redness with mild tenderness.
2. *Nodular episcleritis:* A small purple nodule with surrounding injection, is situated 2–3 mm away from the limbus (usually on the temporal side). The nodule is immobile and tender (Fig. 13.64).

Complications

Normally, the condition is transient with spontaneous remission within a few days. But sometimes, it gives rise to following complications:
- *Recurrent attacks:* When the attacks are fleeting but frequently repeated, it is called *episcleritis periodica fugax.*
- Chronic episcleritis
- Deeper extension into the sclera, leading to scleritis
- Sclerokeratitis
- Adherence of the conjunctiva with the sclera after repeated attacks.

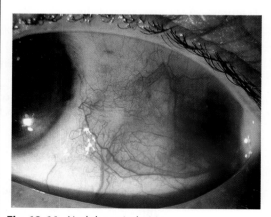

Fig. 13.64: Nodular episcleritis

Treatment

- Cold artificial tears—4 times daily are helpful in many cases of simple episcleritis.
- Corticosteroids drops—4 times daily, and ointment at night.
- Oral anti-inflammatory agents, like ibuprofen, indomethacin or diclofenac.
- Nonsteroidal anti-inflammatory drops, e.g. flurbiprofen, nepafenac or diclofenac drop, when steroids are contraindicated.
- Tablet aspirin or indomethacin for a prolonged period to prevent recurrences, even when no history of "rheumatism" can be elicited.

Scleritis

Scleritis (inflammation of the sclera) is a more serious disease than episcleritis.

Etiology

- Usually bilateral and occurs most frequently in women.
- Associated with *connective tissue disorders* in 50% of the cases, e.g. rheumatoid arthritis, polyarteritis nodosa, systemic lupus erythematosus, Wegener's granulomatosis, relapsing polychondritis, etc.

- Herpes zoster as a local cause.
- Miscellaneous systemic conditions, like tuberculosis, sarcoidosis, syphilis, leprosy, etc.

Pathology

Deposition of immune-complex in the sclera leading to inflammation → marked infiltration of lymphocytes in the sclera lamellae with edema → breakdown of swollen lamellae with necrosis → scleral thinning → simultaneous inflammation of the uveal tract, causing uveitis.

Symptoms

- Intense deep-seated pain with radiation toward the forehead.
- Redness and lacrimation.

Signs

- *Diffuse anterior scleritis:* The inflammation is more widespread involving either a segment of the globe, or the entire anterior sclera with intense deep seated vascularization *(brawny scleritis)*.
- *Nodular anterior scleritis (Fig. 13.65)*
  - An extremely tender, firm immobile nodule separated from the overlying

Differences between episcleritis and scleritis

Features	Episcleritis	Scleritis
Definition	A superficial disease of episcleral tissue, a mild condition	A deep severe destructive disease of sclera; not a mild condition
Symptoms	Redness is the main presentation	Severe boring pain is the main presentation
Signs	Less tender. Bright red in color. Only superficial edema. No KPs, no feature of uveitis	More tender nodule. Purplish in color. Sclera appears thickened. Presence of keratic precapitates (KPs), feature of uveitis
Drug test with 10% phenylephrine	Quick blanching of blood vessels	No such blanching of blood vessels
Prognosis	Favorable, complications usually do not occur	Poor, complications like dimness of vision, scleral thinning, staphyloma and sometimes perforation may occur

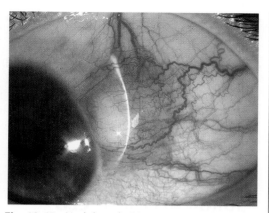

Fig. 13.65: Nodular scleritis

congested episcleral tissue. Sclera is edematous over the nodule.

- Multiple nodules may extend around the limbus causing *annular scleritis*.
- *Anterior necrotizing scleritis with inflammation (Figs 13.66A and B)*
  - Avascular patches appearing in the episcleral tissue.
  - Marked thinning of the sclera with increased visibility of underlying uvea.
  - Associated anterior uveitis.
  - Complications like, cataract, keratitis, keratolysis and secondary glaucoma may develop with severe visual loss.
  - Avascular patch may perforate acutely.

- *Anterior necrotizing scleritis without inflammation [scleromalacia perforans (Fig. 13.67)]*
  - Typically occurs in female patients, with long-standing seropositive rheumatoid arthritis.
  - The condition is *painless*, and starts as a necrotic patch in the normal sclera.
  - Eventually, extreme sclera thinning occurs, and the underlying uvea bulges through it.
  - Spontaneous perforation is extremely rare.
- *Posterior scleritis*
  - It is usually not associated with specific systemic diseases.
  - Inward extension (toward choroid) of the inflammatory process may give rise to *uveal effusion syndrome*—choroiditis, choroidal effusion, exudative retinal detachment, macular edema, etc.
  - Outward extension onto the orbit may give rise to proptosis and extraocular muscles involvement.

Investigations

- Total hemogram, serum uric acid
- X-ray chest and sacroiliac joints
- Mantoux test

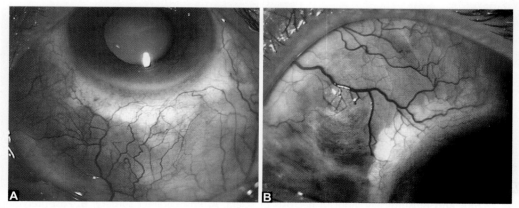

Figs 13.66A and B: Necrotizing scleritis with inflammation. **A.** Thinning; **B.** Bluish discoloration

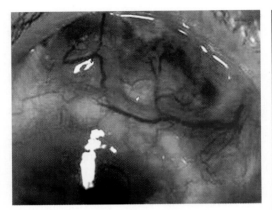

Fig. 13.67: Scleromalacia perforans

- Venereal disease research laboratory (VDRL) and fluorescent treponemal antibody absorption (FTA-ABS) for syphilis.
- Full immunological evaluation for tissue antibodies for collagen vascular diseases, e.g. rheumatoid factor, antinuclear factor, soluble immune-complex, lupus erythematosus (LE) cells, etc.
- B-scan ultrasonography to detect posterior scleritis.

Treatment

- Tablet indomethacin—100 mg daily for 4 days, reducing to 75 mg daily until the inflammation resolves.

- Oral prednisolone—60–80 mg daily, then the dose can be tapered accordingly, as the inflammation subsides.
- Local corticosteroids are less effective, and subconjunctival injection is contraindicated for fear of perforation of the globe.
- Systemic immunosuppressant-like, alkylating agents, or oral azathioprine in severe and unresponsive cases.
- Atropine (1%) eye ointment—2 times daily for associated uveitis.

SURGICALLY INDUCED NECROSIS OF SCLERA (FIGS 13.68A AND B)

It is a rare postoperative immune-mediated necrosis of the sclera. It may be triggered by excessive use of cautery, use of antimetabolites during pterygium or glaucoma surgery, etc.

It may be seen after cataract surgery, pterygium surgery, trabeculectomy or vitreoretinal surgery.

Treatment

- Topical and systemic steroids
- Systemic immunosuppressive therapy
- Scleral patch graft in extreme situation.

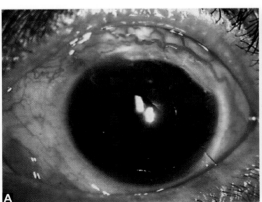
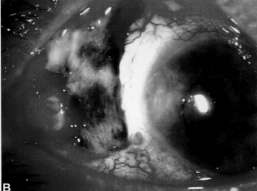

Figs 13.68A and B: Surgically induced necrosis of sclera. **A.** Post-cataract surgery; **B.** Post-pterygium surgery

Diseases of the Uvea

UVEAL DISEASES

The symptoms and signs vary considerably with the portion of the uvea affected.

Symptoms

- *Pain:* Severe, deep, boring, aching pain associated with diseases of the iris and ciliary body. Pain is absent in choroidal involvement.
- *Redness:* Inflammation of the iris and ciliary body causes red eye which is absent in choroidal inflammation.
- *Visual loss:* It is more in choroidal disease as it affects the overlying retina.
- *Floaters:* It is again more in choroidal disease due to exudation of inflammatory cells and protein into the vitreous.

Signs

- *Ciliary congestion:* It is present in inflammation of the iris and ciliary body, but absent in choroiditis.
- *Distortion of the pupil:* It is due to abnormalities in the iris.
- *Accommodation:* It is disturbed in ciliary body involvement.
- *Release of cells and protein* occurs in anterior chamber in iris inflammation, in vitreous in choroidal inflammation; and both in the anterior chamber and vitreous cavity in ciliary body inflammation.
- *Keratic precipitates (KPs):* They are seen in inflammation of the iris and ciliary body.

- *Ophthalmoscopic* abnormal signs are found in choroidal involvement, with associated retinal signs due to chorioretinal involvement.

CONGENITAL ANOMALIES

Anomalies of the Pupil

- *Corectopia:* Displacement of the pupil from its normal position, usually to the nasal side (normally, the pupil is situated just nasal to the center of the cornea).
- *Polycoria:* Multiple pupils—(a) true polycoria—multiple pupils, each having a sphincter muscle, are extremely rare, (b) pseudopolycoria—multiple pupils without sphincters, are common.
- *Pear-shaped pupil:* It is due to coloboma of the iris.

Aniridia

It is usually a bilateral condition in which the whole of the iris is appeared to be missing on external examination (Figs 14.1A and B).

- The rudimentary iris, concealed behind the corneoscleral limbus, is only visible by gonioscopy.
- It is due to failure of anterior growth and differentiation of the optic cup.

Symptoms

They are photophobia, nystagmus and low visual acuity (6/60 or less).

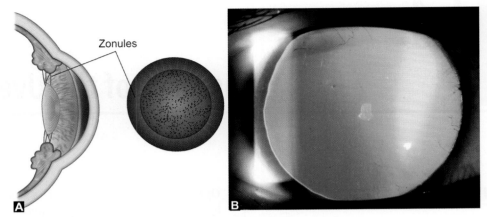

Figs 14.1A and B: Aniridia. **A.** Schematic representation; **B.** Photograph

Signs

- Ciliary processes and suspensory ligaments of the lens are visible.
- Associated secondary glaucoma with glaucomatous optic atrophy in 25% of the cases. Associated foveal hypoplasia.
- Total or 360-degree limbal stem cell deficiency (LSCD) is present in half of the cases.
- Mental retardation and congenital cataract in some cases.
- Aniridia and Wilms' tumor are associated with deletion of the short arm of chromosome 11 (Miller's syndrome).

Treatment

- Provision of an artificial pupil by means of an iris-painted soft contact lens. This reduces photophobia, but does not improve vision.
- The glaucoma responds poorly to medical and surgical treatment.

Persistent Pupillary Membrane

Pupillary membrane is the anterior vascular sheath of the lens, a fetal structure, which normally disappears shortly before birth (Figs 14.2A and B).

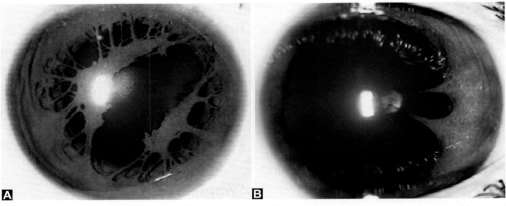

Figs 14.2A and B: A. Persistent pupillary membrane; **B.** Persistent pupillary membrane with anterior polar cataract

- Persistent pupillary membrane is due to continued existence of part of this membrane.
- This appears as fine strands of membrane, running inward from the collarette and sometimes, inserting into the anterior lens capsule or spanning the pupil.
- *It is never at the pupillary margin* (a point to differentiate it from the posterior synechiae which are formed at the pupillary margin).
- It usually does not interfere with vision.

Colobomas

Colobomas are developmental imperfect closure of the fetal fissure.

Consequently, they show an absence of any or all the structures of inner two layers which lie along the corresponding inferonasal sector of the eye.

Coloboma may be *typical* or *atypical*.

- *Typical:* It is always found along the lower nasal sector of the eye due to imperfect closure of the fetal fissure.
- *Atypical:* It is seen in other position and mainly confined to the iris (Figs 14.3A and B).

Typical Coloboma

Genesis: Overgrowth of the inner layer of the optic cup → eversion of the lips of the fetal fissure → obstruction of the natural union between the lips → failure of development of the retina and underlying structures.

Typical coloboma may be complete or incomplete:

- *Complete:* It extends from the pupil to the optic nerve, with a sector shaped gap, occupying about one-eighth of the circumference of the retina and choroid, ciliary body and iris, and causing a corresponding indentation of the lens where the zonular fibers are missing (Figs 14.3 and 14.4).

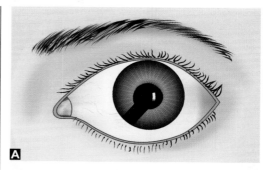

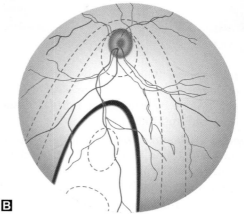

Figs 14.3A and B: Coloboma of the uveal tract. **A.** Iris coloboma; **B.** Choroidal coloboma

Complete coloboma is usually bilateral, often hereditary, and may be associated with a congenital cyst or microphthalmos.

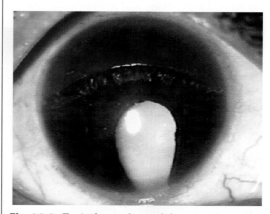

Fig. 14.4: Typical complete coloboma with cataract

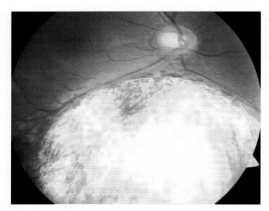

Fig. 14.5: Incomplete choroidal coloboma

- *Incomplete:* When it stops short of the optic nerve, or of the iris, or else, or even partitioned by islands of normal tissue (Figs 14.5 and 14.6A).

Typical coloboma of the iris: The pupil is pear shaped with broad base toward the pupillary margin. Isolated typical coloboma of the iris is rare. It usually extends up to the ciliary body.

Atypical coloboma of the iris: Isolated coloboma of the iris (Fig. 14.6B) is usually atypical, since the fetal fissure normally closes before the iris if formed, and it occurs at any meridian.

This is probably due to obstruction in the anterior growth of the optic cup by a large vessel of the fibrovascular sheath of the lens.

Albinism

This is a hereditary disorder in which there is absence or reduction of melanin pigmentation throughout the body.

- Albinism may be divided into two main types—*oculocutaneous (Fig. 14.7)* and *ocular*.
- *Clinically*, the patient suffers from dazzling. There is associated photophobia, nystagmus, defective vision and occasionally strabismus.
  Visual acuity is further lowered by high myopia and astigmatism.
- *On examination*, the iris looks pink and translucent (Fig. 14.8), owing to lack of pigment.
- *Ophthalmoscopically*, the fundus (Fig. 14.9) appears orange-pink in color. The retinal and choroidal vessels are seen with great clarity and glistening white sclera is visible in between them. Macula is also involved.
- *Partial albinism* is more common, where the absence of pigment is limited to the choroid and retina. Here, the iris is brown or blue colored, and macular region may also be pigmented and looks normal. Visual acuity is much better in partial albinism.

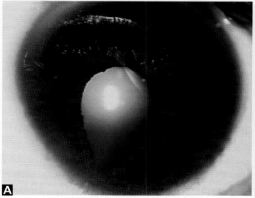
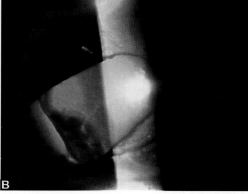

Figs 14.6A and B: A. Incomplete iris coloboma; **B.** Atypical iris coloboma

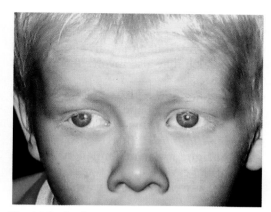

Fig. 14.7: Oculocutaneous albinism

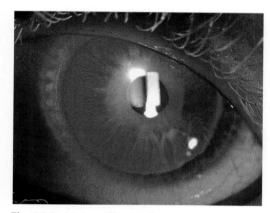

Fig. 14.8: Iris transillumination

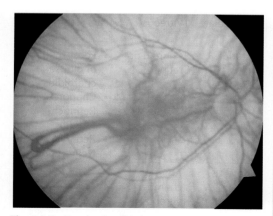

Fig. 14.9: Fundus in albinism

Treatment

- As photophobia is the main symptom, dark glasses may be helpful.
- Alternately, a soft contact lens with painted iris is very useful.

Heterochromia Iridum

Heterochromia iridum means the two irides show a significant difference in color (Fig. 14.10).

Heterochromia iridis means part of the same iris, usually a sector, shows difference in color from the remainder.

> The *blue iris* is due to absence of pigment in the iris stroma, the pigment in the retinal epithelium being seen through the translucent stroma.

Heterochromic iridum may be *hypochromic* or *hyperchromic*:

- *Hypochromic heterochromia:* The eye with lighter colored iris is abnormal (Fig. 14.11)

  Causes
  - Simple congenital heterochromia
  - Horner's syndrome
  - Heterochromic cyclitis of Fuchs
  - Glaucomatocyclitic crisis
  - Amelanotic tumors of the iris
  - Iris atrophy.

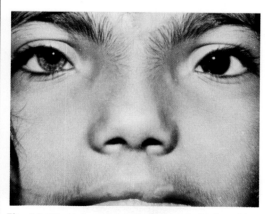

Fig. 14.10: Heterochromia of the iris (right—blue, left—deep brown)

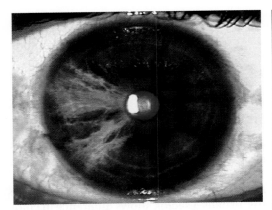

Fig. 14.11: Hypochromic heterochromia

- *Hyperchromic heterochromia:* The iris on the side of the disease is darker than its fellow (Fig. 14.12).

  Causes
  - Retained intraocular iron foreign body (siderosis bulbi)
  - Malignant melanoma of the iris
  - Ocular hemosiderosis (e.g. following long standing hyphema)
  - Microcornea with heterochromia.

Heterochromic iridis—may be congenital or acquired (iris atrophy due to herpetic uveitis, trauma, acute attack of angleclosure glaucoma, after cataract surgery, etc.).

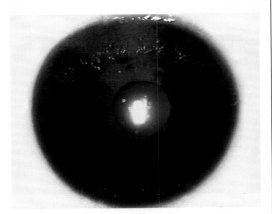

Fig. 14.12: Hyperchromic heterochromia

UVEITIS

- *Uveitis:* An inflammation of the uveal tract which may also involve the adjacent structures.
- *Endophthalmitis:* This is a severe form of intraocular inflammation involving the ocular cavities and inner coats of the eyeball.
- *Panophthalmitis:* This is also a severe form of intraocular inflammation involving the ocular cavities and all three coats of the eyeball as well as Tenon's capsule.

Classifications

The useful classifications are as follows:

Standardization of Uveitis Nomenclature Classification

In an effort to better organize the classification and grading of different uveitic entities, the (Table 14.1). Standardization of uveitis

TABLE 14.1: Anatomical classification of Standardization of Uveitis Nomenclature (SUN)

Type	Primary site of inflammation	Includes
Anterior uveitis	Anterior	• Iritis chamber • Anterior cyclitis • Iridocyclitis
Intermediate uveitis	Vitreous	Pars planitis
Posterior uveitis	Choroid or retina	• Focal, multifocal or diffuse choroiditis • Chorioretinitis • Retinochoroiditis • Retinitis • Neuroretinitis
Panuveitis	Anterior chamber, vitreous, and retina or choroid	

nomenclature (SUN) Working Group developed a process to standardize the approach to reporting clinical data for improving the consistency.

Onset
- Sudden
- Insidious.

Duration
- *Limited:* Less than 3 months duration
- *Persistent:* More than 3 months duration.

Course
- *Acute:* Sudden onset and limited duration.
- *Recurrent:* Repeated episode separated by periods of inactivity without treatment more than 3 months duration.
- *Chronic:* Persistent uveitis with relapse in less than 3 months, after discontinuing treatment.

Activity of Uveitis Terminology

Term	Definition
Inactive	Grade 0 cells
Worsening activity	Twostep increase in level of inflammation (e.g. anterior chamber cells, vitreous haze) or increase from grade 3+ to 4+
Improved activity	Two-step decrease in level of inflammation (e.g. anterior chamber cells, vitreous haze) or decrease to grade 0.
Remission	Inactive disease for more than 3 months after discontinuing all treatment for eye disease

Etiological Classification

- *Idiopathic:* 25–30% of all cases.
- *Exogenous:* After external injury, either by microorganisms or by other agents from outside.
- *Endogenous:* Either caused by micro-organisms or other agents (immune complex) from within the patient. The causes of endogenous uveitis are:

- *Secondary to systemic diseases*
  - Seronegative arthritis
  - Tuberculosis, syphilis and leprosy
  - Sarcoidosis
  - Ulcerative colitis.
- *Secondary to infections*
  - Viral, e.g. herpetic
  - Fungal, e.g. candidiasis
  - Parasitic, e.g. toxoplasmosis.
- *Lens-induced uveitis*
- *Idiopathic specific uveitis*
  - Pars planitis
  - Fuchs' heterochromic cyclitis
  - Sympathetic ophthalmitis.
- *Others*
  - Malignant tumors (Masquerade syndrome)
  - Associated with septic infection, e.g. sinusitis, otitis media, tonsillitis, etc.
  - Direct spread from the adjacent structures, e.g.
    - Cornea (deep keratitis)
    - Sclera (scleritis)
    - Retina (retinitis), etc.

A number of diseases associated with uveitis occur much more frequently in those persons with certain specific HLA types, e.g.
- HLA–B 27—in acute anterior uveitis
- HLA–B 5—in Behcet's disease
- HLA–DR4—in VKH syndrome.

Pathological Classification

- Granulomatous
- Nongranulomatous

The main clinical differences between the two are summarized in Table 14.2.

Basic pathomechanisms in uveitis
- Vasodilatation
- Increased capillary permeability
- Migration of inflammatory cells into the ocular cavities.

TABLE 14.2: Clinical difference between granulomatous uveitis and nongranulomatous uveitis

Granulomatous uveitis	Nongranulomatous uveitis
Insidious onset and chronic course	Acute onset and short course
Relatively mild and white eye	Severe and red eye
Nodules (Keoppe's and Bussaca's) on the iris	No such nodules on the iris
Medium to large KPs (often mutton-fat type)	Fine keratic precipitates (KPs)
Mild flare	Intense flare, often with heavy fibrinous exudates
Anterior uvea and retina choroid are equally involved	Mainly limited to the anterior uvea
Tuberculosis, sarcoidosis, leprosy, etc. are usually responsible	Mainly idiopathic and allergic in nature

ANTERIOR UVEITIS (IRIDOCYCLITIS)

Symptoms

- **Pain:** Acute, severe with radiation along the branches of the 5th nerve. It is typically worse at night
- **Redness:** It is due to vasodilatation
- **Photophobia**
- **Lacrimation**
- **Dimness of vision:** It is due to:
  - Plasmoid (turbid) aqueous
  - Vitreous exudates
  - Exudates in the pupillary area
  - Cystoid macular edema
  - Secondary glaucoma
  - Ciliary muscle spasm
  - Complicated cataract.

Ocular Signs (Fig. 14.13)

Circumcorneal ciliary congestion (CCC): It is one of the hallmarks of acute anterior uveitis.

Keratic Precipitates (Fig. 14.14)

They are cellular deposits on the corneal endothelium.

- **Distribution:** The inflammatory cells are wandering in the aqueous by convection current and stick to the edematous endothelial cells of the cornea. They arrange in a basedown triangular area at the lower part of the cornea *(Arlt's triangle)* (Fig. 14.15) due to gravitation. The smaller ones are above and the larger ones are below. However, in Fuchs' cyclitis, they are scattered throughout the endothelium.
- **Size:** The KPs may be small (fine), medium and large *mutton-fat* types.
- **The small and medium-size KPs** are due to deposition of lymphocytes and plasma cells, and they are seen in non-granulomatous or acute uveitis.
- **The large KPs** are due to deposition of macrophage and epithelioid cells, and they are seen in granulomatous uveitis (as in tuberculosis or sarcoidosis).
- **Age:** The KPs may be fresh or old.
- **Fresh** KPs are round, white, fluffy and hydrated in appearance.
- **Old KPs** are shrunken, faded and become pigmented with crenated edge, and halos are seen surrounding them. Old *mutton-fat* KPs have **ground-glass** appearance.

Anterior Chamber

- **Aqueous flare:** It is due to leakage of proteins into the aqueous through the damaged capillaries, causing a Tyndall effect. It is not necessarily a sign of active uveitis, particularly in absence of aqueous cells. The flare is graded (Table 14.3 and Fig. 14.16) (from 0 to 4+) depending upon the degree of obstruction of iris details under slit lamp.

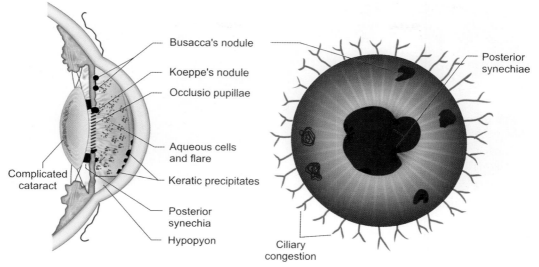

Fig. 14.13: Signs of iridocyclitis

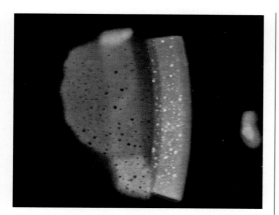

Fig. 14.14: Fine to medium keratic precipitate in acute iridocyclitis

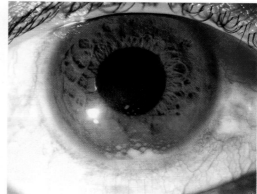

Fig. 14.15: Mutton fat keratic precipitates (within the Arlt's triangle)

TABLE 14.3: Grading of anterior chamber, flare	
Grades	**Description**
0	None
1+	Faint
2+	Moderate (iris and lens details clear)
3+	Marked (iris and lens details hazy)
4+	Intense (fibrin or plastic aqueous)

- **Aqueous cells:** It is due to exudation of inflammatory cells into the aqueous presence of cells in aqueous always indicates active inflammation.

  The cells should be counted and (Table 14.4) graded (from 0 to 4+) under oblique slit lamp beam (1 mm long and 1 mm wide) (Figs 14.16 and 14.17).

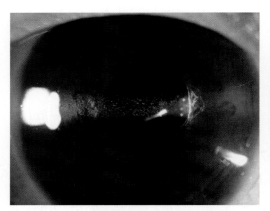

Fig. 14.16: Aqueous flare and cells

TABLE 14.4: Grading of anterior chamber cells	
Grades	**Cells in field***
0	<1
0.5+	1–5
1+	6–15
2+	16–25
3+	26–50
4+	50+

*Field size is 1 x 1 mm slitbeam

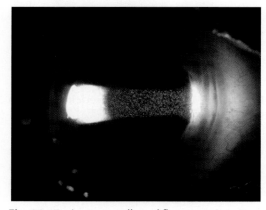

Fig. 14.17: Aqueous cells and flare more intense

- **Hypopyon:** It is classically seen in Behcet's syndrome or infectious cases (herpetic uveitis).

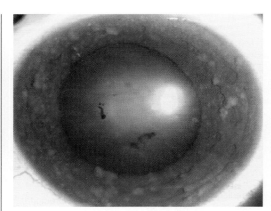

Fig. 14.18: Busacca's nodule

- **Hyphema:** Herpetic uveitis and in traumatic uveitis.
- **Depth**
  - Deep and irregular—in posterior synechiae
  - Funnel shaped—in iris bombe.

Iris

- **Muddy iris or loss of iris pattern:** This is due to accumulation of fluid and exudates over the surface of the iris.
- **Iris nodules:** It is seen in granulomatous uveitis.
  - **Koeppe's nodule:** At the pupillary border, and smaller in size.
  - **Busacca's nodule (Fig. 14.18):** On the surface of the iris, away from the pupil.
- **Iris atrophy and heterochromia:** It is seen in Fuchs' heterochromic cyclitis and herpetic uveitis.
- **Rubeosis iridis:** Iris neovascularization develops in chronic anterior uveitis and in Fuchs' heterochromic cyclitis.
- **Synechiae**
  - **Posterior synechia:** It is the adhesion between the anterior lens surface and the iris. This is due to organization of fibrinous exudate between the pupillary margin and the lens surface. This adhesion may be localized or diffuse.

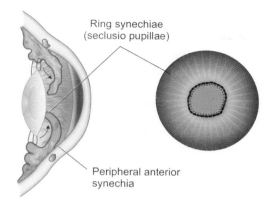

Fig. 14.19: Iris bombe

– *Ring (annular) synechiae:* Posterior synechiae extending for 3600 around the pupil (seclusio pupillae), prevent the passage of aqueous from the posterior to the anterior chamber. This gives rise to forward bowing of the peripheral iris causing an *iris bombe* (Fig. 14.19). This may lead to elevation of intraocular pressure due to secondary angle closure by the peripheral iris (Fig. 14.20).

– *Total posterior synechiae:* Adhesion of entire iris with the anterior lens capsule.

▪ *Anterior synechiae:* Adhesion of iris with the corneal endothelium. It is usually peripheral and secondary to iris bombe.

● Ectropion of the uveal pigment at the pupillary margin.

Pupil

● *Sluggish or non-reacting pupil:* This is due to edema of the iris and also due to posterior synechiae.

● *Miotic pupil:* It is due to (i) water logging of the iris, (ii) toxins act on powerful sphincter pupillae, and (iii) ring synechiae.

● *Irregular or festooned pupil:* Irregular dilatation of the pupil with mydriatic, and it is due to posterior synechiae (Fig. 14.21).

● *Occlusio pupillae:* Pupil is blocked or occluded by the organized fibrinous exudates.

Lens

Changes are mostly seen in chronic or healed anterior uveitis.

● *Pigmentation* on the anterior surface of the lens.

● *Complicated cataract:* Polychromatic luster and bread-crumb appearance at the posterior cortex.

● *Cyclitic membrane:* It forms behind the lens, due to organization of the fibrinous exudates.

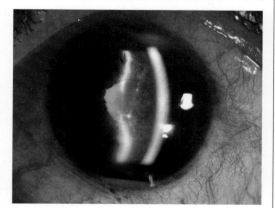

Fig. 14.20: Ring synechia with iris bombe in acute iridocyclitis with hypopyon

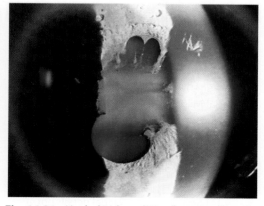

Fig. 14.21: Healed iridocyclitis—festooned pupil

Tension

- May be normal.
- *Decreased*—in acute iridocyclitis (due to acute ciliary shock).
- *Increased*—in long standing anterior uveitis (due to secondary angle-closure or may be steroid induced).

Posterior Segment

- *Vitreous opacities:* Due to exudation and inflammatory cells in the vitreous. It is more common in cyclitis (Table 14.5).
- *Fundus changes:* Cystoid macular edema due to liberation of toxins. It is more with chronic anterior uveitis.

Systemic Signs

General examination is important to find out the etiological factor, e.g. examination of skin (rash, vitiligo, psoriasis), hair (poliosis, alopecia), genitourinary tract (urethritis), respiratory tract (tuberculosis), buccal mucosa (ulceration), etc.

Sequelae and Complications of Anterior Uveitis

- Posterior synechiae
- Ring synechiae → *seclusio pupillae* → iris bombe → peripheral anterior synechiae → secondary angle-closure glaucoma

TABLE 14.5: Grading of vitreous opacities

Grades	Description	Clinical findings
0	Nil	None
1	Minimal	Posterior pole clearly visible
2	Mild	Posterior pole details slightly hazy
3	Moderate	Posterior pole details very hazy
4	Marked	Posterior pole details barely visible
5	Severe	Fundal details not visible

- Total posterior synechiae
- Occlusio pupillae
- Secondary glaucoma: It is due to:
  - Albuminous aqueous blocking the angle.
  - Associated trabeculitis and trabecular edema.
  - Ring synechiae → iris bombe → peripheral anterior synechiae → secondary angle-closure glaucoma.
  - *Occlusio pupillae* →anterior synechiae → secondary angle-closure glaucoma.
  - Steroid-induced (due to prolonged steroid therapy).
- *Cyclitic membrane:* It occurs more in cyclitis and forms behind the lens
- Complicated cataract
- Pseudoglioma, due to vitreous exudation
- Cystoid macular edema
- *Phthisis (atrophic) bulbi:* It prolonged cyclitis → ciliary body atrophy → less secretion of aqueous → atrophic bulbi
- *Tractional retinal detachment:* It is due to traction by the cyclitic membrane
- Bandshaped keratopathy (BSK); more common in children with juvenile (idiopathic) rheumatoid arthritis, and chronic iridocyclitis.

Investigations

- Routine hemogram
- *Serological tests:* Antinuclear antibody (ANA); rheumatoid factor (RF); HLAtyping; venereal disease research laboratory (VDRL) and fluorescent treponemal antibody absorption (FTAABS) (for syphilis); ELISA, etc.
- *Skin tests:* (a) Mantoux test (tuberculosis) (b) Kveim test (sarcoidosis)
- *X-ray* (a) chest—for tuberculosis and sarcoidosis (b) joints—arthritis group
- *Gallium scan:* For sarcoidosis
- *Urine culture:* Urethritis
- *Anterior chamber paracentesis* for polymerase chain reaction (PCR) to diagnose organisms and cellular analysis.

Treatment

Local

- Hot compress—3–4 times daily
- Use dark glasses
- *Atropine (1%) eye drop or ointment—3* times daily.

Atropine acts in three ways:
1. By keeping the iris and ciliary body at rest.
2. By reducing hyperemia.
3. By preventing the formation of posterior synechiae and breaking down, if any already formed.

Combined mydriatic-cycloplegics (like phenylephrine and homatropine, or phenylephrine and tropicamide) are sometimes better in place of atropine.

Atropine or any other cycloplegic should be continued for at least 10–14 days after the eyes appear to be quiet (or the aqueous cells disappear), otherwise a relapse is likely to occur.

A powerful mydriatic effect can be obtained by subconjunctival injection of 0.3 mL mydricaine (a mixture of atropine, procaine and adrenaline) often called a *dynamite mixture* to break the recently formed synechiae.

- *Corticosteroids:* They are used as topical drops or ointment, or as subconjunctival or sub-Tenon injection.
  - Betamethasone, dexamethasone, or prednisolone drops—6 hourly to 1 hourly, depending upon the severity of the inflammation.
  - Corticosteroid ointment—at bed time.
  - Subconjunctival injection of dexamethasone (may be mixed with injection atropine)—daily (if required).
  - Sub-Tenon injection of long-acting steroid (methyl prednisolone or triamcinolone)—every 2–3 weeks.

Topical steroids are gradually tapered off with the response.
- *Nonsteroidal anti-inflammatory drops:* Diclofenac, indomethacin, nepafenac or flurbiprofen, 4–6 times daily when topical steroid is contraindicated.

Systemic

- *Systemic corticosteroids:* If the response to topical steroid is poor, oral prednisolone—1–1.5 mg/kg body weight day, is given in a tapering dose.
- *Anti-inflammatory (nonsteroidal) drugs:* Like aspirin, indomethacin, diclofenac to reduce the pain and inflammation.
- Systemic antibiotic or antituberculous drugs in selective cases.
- Very rarely, *immunosuppressive* agents, e.g. in rheumatoid sclerouveitis.

Treatment of Complications

- *Secondary glaucoma:* Tab acetazolamide—250 mg 3–4 times daily, and/or timolol maleate (0.5%) drops twice daily.
- *Annular synechiae:* Laser iridotomy.
- *Iris bombe:* Laser iridotomy or 4-point iridotomy *(quadri-puncture)* with a von Graefe's cataract knife.
- *Cataract extraction:* Extracapsular extraction is done under cover of systemic steroids which are also to be continued in the post operative and atropine periods.
  A hydrophobic foldable intraocular lens implantation is preferable in post-uveitic cataract after ECCE.
- *Band-shaped keratopathy:* Epithelial scraping and application of 0.1 M solution of disodium EDTA.

INTERMEDIATE UVEITIS (PARS PLANITIS)

Etiology

The exact cause is still not clear. It is thought to be due to some immunological reactions at the pars plana and outer layers of the peripheral retina.

Clinical Features

- **Age:** Second to fourth decade.
- **Sex:** It can affect either sex.
- **Laterality:** It usually bilateral (80%).
- **Incidence:** In 5–15% of all uveitic patients.
- **Symptoms:** Floaters and blurring of vision.

Signs

- **Posterior segment**
  - Inflammatory cells in the anterior vitreous.
  - Snow-ball opacities in the vitreous cavity.
  - Snow-bank exudates over the pars plana which is best seen with an indirect ophthalmoscope.
  - Absence of focal inflammatory lesions in the fundus.
- **Anterior segment:** It is due to spillover anterior uveitis:
  - Moderate aqueous cells and flare.
  - Posterior synechiae.

Complications (Causes of Visual Loss)

- Complicated cataract
- Cystoid macular edema (CME)
- Vitreous hemorrhage
- Retinal detachment (tractional).

Treatment

- Mild cases are self-limiting, and do not require any treatment except periodic observation.
- But, in moderate to severe cases (vision less than 6/12) or in the evidence of CME, the treatment is:
  - **Sub-Tenon injection of depot steroid every 2–3 weeks.**

- **Systemic corticosteroids**—oral prednisolone (60 mg/day) for two weeks—then tapered off slowly.
- **Cryotherapy**—if above treatment fails.
- **Pars plana vitrectomy**—if cryotherapy is ineffective.
- **Immunosuppressive agents**, very rarely.

POSTERIOR UVEITIS

Etiology

- **Infectious:** Toxoplasmosis, tuberculosis, syphilis, etc.
- Autoimmune
- Idiopathic.

Symptoms

- **Floaters:** More with peripheral lesions.
- **Impaired vision:** Mainly with lesions involving the fovea and papillomacular bundle.

Signs

- **Anterior segment:** Usually normal.
- **Posterior segment**
  - **Vitreous**
    - **Opacities:** Various types of vitreous opacities, caused by inflammatory cells and exudates are:
      - **Fine opacities:** They are composed of individual inflammatory cells.
      - **Coarse opacities:** They are result of severe tissue destruction.
      - **Stringy opacities:** They are caused by alterations in the vitreous gel itself.
      - **Snow-ball opacities:** They are the large opacities seen in pars planitis, sarcoidosis and candidiasis.

Grading of vitreous opacities (0 to 4+) is done by assessing the density of the opacity, of the fundus with direct or indirect (better) ophthalmoscope (see Table 14.5).

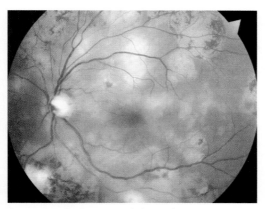

Fig. 14.22: Disseminated choroiditis

- **Fundus:** The lesion may be central, focal, multifocal, geographical or diffuse.
  - **Choroiditis (Figs 14.22 and 14.23):**
    - **Active lesions:** They are white, yellow or grayish patches with reasonably well demarcated margins (Fig. 14.23).
    - **Inactive lesions:** They are well-defined white patches of chorioretinal atrophy with pigmented margins.
    Retinal blood vessels pass over the choroiditis patch without interruption.
  - **Retinitis:** They appears as white, cloudy areas with indistinct margins, sometimes difficult to differentiate from healthy retina.
  - **Vasculitis:** Periphlebitis is more common than periarteritis. Cellular infiltrates around the blood vessels cause perivascular cuffing.
    In severe periphlebitis, there is perivascular accumulation of granulomatous materials—called **candle-wax dripping** (Fig. 14.24), seen in sarcoidosis.
  - **Neovascularization:** It may be seen in pars planitis or sarcoidosis.
  - **Exudative retinal detachment:** It is in severe choroiditis, e.g. toxoplasmosis.
  - **Optic nerve findings:** It includes optic neuritis (from contagious foci) or optic atrophy (secondary to retinal damage).

Investigations

- Investigations for tuberculosis
- Investigations for sarcoidosis
- Venereal disease research laboratory (VDRL) and FTAABS for syphilis
- Toxoplasma serology (Sabin-Feldman dye test, ELISA)
- Enzyme-linked immunosorbent assay (ELISA) for toxocariasis.

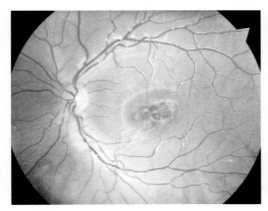

Fig. 14.23: Central choroiditis

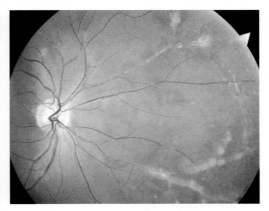

Fig. 14.24: Perivasculitis—candle-wax dripping

Treatment

- *For specific infective etiology*
  - Treatment for toxoplasmosis
  - Treatment for toxocariasis
  - AT drugs, etc. with systemic steroids if necessary.
- *Idiopathic posterior uveitis*
  - *Systemic corticosteroids:* Oral prednisolone—1–1.5 mg/kg body weight/day, then in tapering doses.
  - Posterior sub-Tenon injections of depot steroid.
  - Rarely, immunosuppressive agents.

Panuveitis

It is the severe form of uveitis which involves the whole uveal tract.

Common causes are as follows:
- Sympathetic ophthalmitis
- Vogt-Koyanagi-Harada syndrome
- Sarcoidosis
- Behcet's disease.

SPECIFIC UVEITIC ENTITIES

Fuchs' Heterochromic Cyclitis

It is a chronic, nongranulomatous anterior uveitis with insidious onset.

It is usually unilateral and affects middle-aged adult.

Symptoms

Most of the patients are asymptomatic until the development of complicated cataract.

Signs

- Fine KPs are scattered throughout the entire endothelium.
- A faint aqueous flare and cells.
- Posterior synechiae are typically absent.
- Diffuse iris stromal atrophy.
- *Heterochromia* affected eye is usually hypochromic.

- *Mydriasis:* It is due to atrophy of sphincter pupillae.
- Fine neovascularization of the iris and at the angle (*Amsler's sign:* Bleeding from these new fine vessels following anterior chamber paracentesis).
- Vitreous may have cells.

Complications: Two main complications—(i) cataract and (ii) glaucoma.

Treatment

- Topical corticosteroids in active stage.
- Mydriatics are unnecessary.
- Extracapsular cataract extraction (ECCE) with intraocular lens (IOL) implantation can be done safely for cataract with good prognosis.

UVEITIS IN JUVENILE RHEUMATOID ARTHRITIS

Juvenile (idiopathic) rheumatoid arthritis (JRA) is a seronegative idiopathic inflammatory arthritis developing in children below 16 years of age.

It is classified as:
- Systemic onset JRA *(Still's disease):* Uveitis is extremely rare.
- *Polyarticular JRA:* Uveitis is fairly rare.
- *Pauciarticular JRA:* Uveitis develops in about 20% of the cases.

Anterior uveitis in JRA is chronic (Fig. 14.25), nongranulomatous, usually bilateral and mostly affecting the girls.

Symptoms: Asymptomatic at the onset, but later, vision is impaired due to complications.

Signs

- Eye is typically white (*white iritis*) even in presence of severe inflammation.
- Small to medium size KPs.
- Posterior synechiae are very common.
- Pigment deposition on the lens surface.

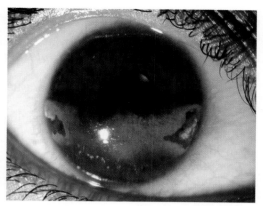

Fig. 14.25: Chronic uveitis in idiopathic rheumatoid arthritis with band-shaped keratopathy (BSK) and complicated cataract after surgery

Complications

- Complicated cataract
- Secondary glaucoma
- Band-shaped keratopathy (common)
- Ultimately, phthisis bulbi.

Treatment

- Topical steroids and cycloplegics.
- Sub-Tenon injection of depot steroids.
- *Oral prednisolone in selected cases:* They are as this can affect the growth and bone formation of the young patients.
- Cataract surgery is best done by pars plana lensectomy with vitrectomy.

Reiter's Syndrome
• It consists of a triad of urethritis, conjunctivitis and seronegative arthritis.
• Uveitis is typically unilateral, acute and non-granulomatous.
• *Treatment:* Topical steroids and cycloplegics.

UVEITIS IN HERPES ZOSTER

- The iridocyclitis is (hyper) acute, non-granulomatous with small KPs.
- Associated severe iris ischemia causes hypopyon which may be mixed with blood.

- Sectorial iris atrophy with distortion of the pupil in 20% cases.
- *Complications:* Secondary glaucoma, complicated cataract and very rarely phthisis bulbi (due to ciliary body ischemia) may occur.
- *Treatment:* Vigorously with topical steroids, cycloplegics and if necessary with systemic steroids.

TUBERCULAR UVEITIS

It is usually a chronic, granulomatous uveitis. It may be non-granulomatous anterior or posterior uveitis (choroiditis), or vasculitis (Eales' disease) depending upon the immunological status of the patient.

- *Anterior uveitis:* Classically, it is a granulomatous type of uveitis with large mutton-fat KPs. It is usually bilateral, through the second eye may be affected after a few months.
- *Posterior uveitis:* Commonly, it occurs as a focal or multifocal choroiditis. Rarely, a large choroidal granuloma may be seen in the fundus.

Investigations

- X-ray chest, erythrocyte sedimentation rate (ESR) and Mantoux test
- *Therapeutic (Isoniazid) test:* A therapeutic trial of 300 mg/day isoniazid for 3 weeks is reliable. If this causes a dramatic improvement the diagnosis of tuberculosis is highly likely.

Treatment

- Topical steroids and cycloplegics.
- Full course of AT drugs.

SARCOID UVEITIS

Sarcoid is a multisystem disorder of unknown etiology, commonly affecting young adults, and usually presents with bilateral hilar lymphadenopathy and oculocutaneous lesions.

- *Ocular findings are*—keratoconjunctivitis sicca, conjunctival granuloma and uveitis.
- *Uveitis:* It may be anterior, posterior or panuveitis.
  - *Anterior uveitis*
    - *Acute granulomatous:* It is seen in young patients with acute sarcoidosis.
    - *Chronic granulomatous:* It usually bilateral and seen among old patients. Busacca's nodules are more frequently seen than Koeppe's nodules, with typical 'muttonfat' KPs. Band-shaped keratopathy, complicated cataract and glaucoma are frequent complications.
  - *Posterior uveitis*
    - *Snow-ball* opacities in the vitreous.
    - Peripheral retinal periphlebitis with candle-wax drippings.
    - Retinal neovascularization at the periphery.
    - Pre-retinal nodules (sarcoid nodules), mostly located inferiorly and anterior to the equator (*Lander's sign*).
    - Papillitis, optic nerve granuloma, optic disc neovascularization may also be seen.

Investigations

- X-ray chest—hilar lymphadenopathy
- Serum angiotensin converting enzyme (ACE) usually elevated
- Serum calcium—raised
- Kveim test
- Gallium-67 scan of the head and neck.

Treatment

- *Anterior uveitis:* Topical steroids and cycloplegics.
- *Posterior uveitis:* Systemic steroids and posterior sub-Tenon injection of depot steroids.

TOXOPLASMOSIS

Toxoplasmosis is an infestation by an intracellular protozoan parasite, *Toxoplasma gondii.*

The cat is the definitive host of the parasite, and human can be infested by three ways:
1. *Ingestion of under-cooked meat* by eating the flesh of intermediate host like pig, sheep, cattle, etc.
2. *Ingestion of oocyte* via feces of pet cat.
3. *Transplacental* from infested pregnant mother to the fetus.

Toxoplasmic uveitis may be:
- Congenital posterior toxoplasmic lesions.
- Recurrent toxoplasmic retinochoroiditis.

Acquired toxoplasmosis: It does not cause any ocular lesion, and usually remains subclinical. All the cases of toxoplasmic uveitis in adults are due to recurrence of an old healed congenital chorioretinitis.

Congenital Toxoplasmosis

- Transplacental transmission occurs only when the mother is infested during the pregnancy. But if the mother is infested before pregnancy the fetus will not be affected.
- The 'three Cs' of congenital toxoplasmosis are *chorioretinitis, convulsions and calcification*.
- Most cases are subclinical. In these children, bilateral (Figs 14.26A and B) healed chorioretinal scars are usually detected in later life.

Recurrent Toxoplasmosis

- The recurrence usually takes place between the age of 10–35 years.
- The primary lesion is a retinitis, and the inflammatory reaction seen in choroid, iris and retinal vessels is believed to be immunological in origin.
- *Clinical features of recurrent lesions: Symptoms:* Visual loss, and due to:
  - Opacities in the media.

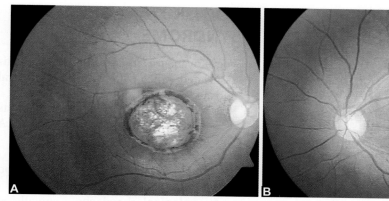

Figs 14.26A and B: Bilateral congenital toxoplasmosis

- Direct involvement of the fovea.
- Involvement of the papillomacular bundle and rarely the optic nerve head.
- Cystoid macular edema.

Signs

- **Severe vitritis** resulting in inflammatory cells in the vitreous.
- **Focal necrotizing retinitis** is a satellite lesion adjacent to the edge of the old scar. Active retinitis is a white or yellowish white lesion with fluffy indistinct edges at the postequatorial fundus.
- **Deep retinitis** is less common.
- **Papillitis** sometimes, the active retinitis is located adjacent to the optic nerve (juxtapapillary choroiditis of Jensen), or occasionally on the optic nerve head itself.
- Occasionally, there is an associated anterior uveitis.

Complications

- Cystoid macular edema
- Subretinal neovascularization
- Tractional retinal detachment.

Diagnosis

- Sabin dye test
- Fluorescent antibody (FA) test
- ELISA for toxoplasma antibody.

Management

Treatment is indicated only when the retinitis is severe and threatening the macula or optic nerve head.

- **Steroids:** They should not be given (in any form) alone, and it should be combined with anti-toxoplasmic drugs.
  - **Topical:** In associated anterior uveitis.
  - **Posterior sub-Tenon injection:** In retinochoroiditis.
  - **Systemic (oral):** In presence of severe vitritis or in vision-threatening lesions.
- **Systemic anti-toxoplasmic drugs**
  - **Sulphonamides:** Sulfadiazine or triple sulfa (sulfadiazine/sulfamerazine/sulfamethazine)—2.0 g loading dose, then 1 g 4 times daily for 3–4 weeks.
  - **Clindamycin:** Orally 300 mg, 4 times daily for 3 weeks.
  - **Pyrimethamine:** 75–100 mg loading dose, followed by 25 mg daily for 3–4 weeks.

    If it is combined with clindamycin, only a 1 week course will then be necessary. Pyrimethamine is a **folic acid antagonist**, which may cause thrombocytopenia and leucopenia. So, **folinic acid**, 10 mg/day, orally (mixed with orange juice) is to be added with pyrimethamine.

- *Minocycline:* 100 mg once or twice daily for 4 weeks.

TOXOCARIASIS

Toxocara is an intestinal round worm of cats *(Toxocara cati)* and dogs *(Toxocara canis)*. Human ocular toxocariasis is caused by accidental ingestion of food contaminated by feces of pet cat or dog.

- It usually presents between the age of 2 and 9 years with leukocoria, squinting or unilateral loss of vision.
- *Signs include* chronic endophthalmitis, vitreous clouding and severe cyclitic membrane formation.
- Toxacara endophthalmitis is considered in differential diagnosis of retinoblastoma where there is an associated secondary glaucoma.
- Diagnosis is confirmed by ELISA.
- *Treatment:* (a) Anthelminthic drugs (thiabendazole); (b) Pars plana vitrectomy in case of pseudoglioma formation.

BEHÇET'S DISEASE

It is accompanied by recurrent oral ulceration, genital ulceration, skin lesions together with neurological and articular manifestations.

- Conjunctivitis, episcleritis and keratitis are seen in a few patients.
- *Fundus shows:* Vitritis, retinal vasculitis, focal area of retinal necrosis, macular edema and optic neuropathy.
- Visual prognosis is poor, and is due to phthisis bulbi or secondary optic atrophy.
- *Treatment*
- Topical and systemic steroids
- Oral chlorambucil for prolonged period.

VOGT-KOYANAGI-HARADA SYNDROME

- Vogt-Koyanagi-Harada is a severe panuveitis associated with cutaneous, neurological and auditory involvement.
- It is more common in Japanese patients who have an increased prevalence of HLA DR4 and HLADR53 (Fig. 14.27).
- *Extraocular lesions*
  - *Cutaneous*—alopecia, vitiligo and poliosis (Fig. 14.28).
  - *Neurological*—headache, convulsion and cranial nerve palsy.
  - *Auditory*—tinnitus, vertigo and deafness.
- *Ocular lesions*
  - A granulomatous iridocyclitis
  - Multifocal exudative choroiditis
  - Exudative retinal detachment
  - Optic neuritis in some cases.
- *Treatment*
  - Anterior uveitis—topical steroids and cycloplegics.
  - Exudative retinal detachment—usually subsides after systemic corticosteroid therapy.

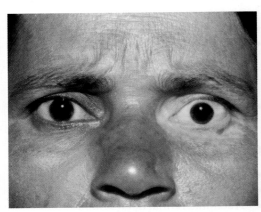

Fig. 14.27: Vogt-Koyanagi-Harada syndrome (left eye)

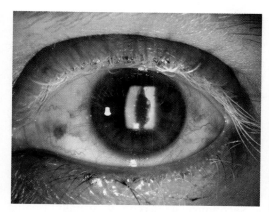

Fig. 14.28: Uveitis in Vogt-Koyanagi-Harada syndrome—note poliosis of the eyelashes

SYMPATHETIC OPHTHALMITIS

It is a rare, **bilateral** granulomatous panuveitis that occurs following a penetrating injury or surgical trauma.
- The traumatized eye is called **exciting eye**, and the fellow eye which also develops uveitis is called **sympathizing eye**.
- Eighty percent cases of sympathetic ophthalmitis occur within 3 months, and 90% of cases occur within 1 year after trauma.

Symptoms (Insidious Onset)

Initial symptoms in the **sympathizing eye** are pain, photophobia, and difficulty in near vision due to loss of accommodation. In the **exciting eye** there is also pain, irritation and redness.

Signs

- In the **exciting eye** there is ciliary congestion and evidence of initial insult.
- In the **sympathizing eye**
  - Earliest feature is **retrolental flare**.
  - Typical granulomatous uveitis with mutton-fat KPs, iris nodules, posterior synechiae and secondary glaucoma.

- **Posterior segment shows:** (i) Small, deep, yellow-white spots (Dalen-Fuchs' nodules) scattered throughout the fundus, and (ii) perivasculitis and retinal edema.

Complications

Cataract, secondary glaucoma, and eventual blindness from phthisis bulbi may occur in many cases.

Etiopathogenesis

Sympathetic ophthalmitis almost always results from a penetrating injury. Wounds in the ciliary region (**dangerous zone** of the eye) involving the ciliary body, and its incarceration in the scar, are considered especially dangerous. It very rarely occurs if actual suppuration has taken place in the **exciting eye**.

It is an autoimmune reaction to antigens in uveal tissue, uveal pigments or retinal antigen (retinal-S antigen).

Pathology

Histopathology is similar in both the exciting and sympathizing eye.
- Nodular aggregation of lymphocytes and plasma cells scattered throughout the uveal tract.
- Pigment epithelium of the iris, ciliary body and choroid proliferates, and along with epithelioid cells and macrophages, they form the nodules called **Dalen-Fuchs'** nodules.
- Retina also becomes heavily infiltrated with lymphocytes and plasma cells.

Treatment

Therapeutic

- Intensive therapy with topical, sub-Tenon injections and systemic corticosteroids. Systemic steroids are given in high doses (80–100 mg/day) and are gradually tapered, once the uveitis is controlled.

- Immunosuppressive agents in steroid-resistant cases.

Preventive

- Prompt and meticulous closure of all penetrating injury.
- If the injured eye is unsalvageable, enucleation should be done within 2 weeks following injury.
- Beneficial effect of enucleation of the exciting eye, after the development of sympathetic ophthalmitis is controversial.
- Many surgeons prefer enucleation of the exciting eye within 2 weeks of the onset of sympathetic ophthalmia, as it favorably affects the eventual prognosis of the sympathizing eye.

GLAUCOMATOCYCLITIC CRISIS (POSNER-SCHLOSSMAN SYNDROME)

Glaucomatocyclitic crisis is characterized by acute or subacute attacks of secondary open-angle glaucoma associated with mild anterior uveitis.

The disease affects the young adults and usually unilateral. During an attack, the intra-ocular pressure is usually severely elevated (40–60 mm of Hg), and lasts for few hours to few days.

Symptoms

- Colored halos around the light
- Diminution of vision
- Mild headache, but pain is rare.

Signs

- Corneal epithelial edema
- Fine nonpigmented KPs
- Normal anterior chamber depth
- Aqueous cells and flare
- Posterior synechiae formation are rare.

Differential Diagnosis

The condition is to be differentiated from acute attack of angle-closure glaucoma, as the treatment with atropine would be disastrous in a case of angle-closure glaucoma.

A normal depth of anterior chamber and presence of few KPs establish the diagnosis of glaucomatocyclitic crisis.

Treatment

- Topical steroids and cycloplegics
- Secondary glaucoma is usually treated with tablet acetazolamide, and timolol maleate drops.

CYTOMEGALOVIRUS RETINITIS (FIG. 14.29)

It is a rare chronic diffuse exudative lesion of the retina caused by cytomegalovirus (CMV) which occurs in patients with an impaired immune system, e.g.

- Acquired immunodeficiency syndrome (AIDS)
- Cytotoxic chemotherapy
- Long-term immunosuppression following renal transplantation.

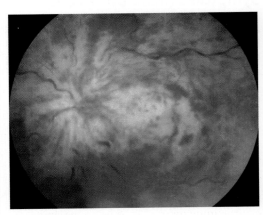

Fig. 14.29: Cytomegalovirus retinitis—central retinal venous occlusion

Signs

- Scattered white patches with perivascular sheathing.
- Full thickness hemorrhagic retinal necrosis with edema sometimes described as ketchup (tomato sauce) on cottage cheese appearance at the posterior pole.
- Ultimately, whole retina is involved with subsequent retinal atrophy.

Treatment

Intravenous injection of gancyclovir or foscarnet may cause regression in some cases.

ONCHOCERCIASIS (RIVER BLINDNESS)

- It is caused by a filarial worm *Onchocerca volvulus*.
- The vector is the blood-sucking black fly *Simulium*.
- Onchocerciasis is mainly seen in endemic areas of African countries.
- *Ocular lesions* are sclerosing keratitis, retinitis and anterior uveitis.
- Iridocyclitis and chorioretinitis are the *cause of blindness* due to onchocerciasis.
- *Specific therapy* of onchocerciasis is diethylcarbamazine (for microfilaria) and suramin (for adult worm).
- *Ivermectin is now the drug of choice* for the treatment.
- Onchocerciasis is now included in Vision-2020 programme (*see* Chapter 26).

PRESUMED OCULAR HISTOPLASMOSIS SYNDROME

This syndrome has been related to *Histoplasma capsulatum* infection. It is presumed because:
- Presumed ocular histoplasmosis syndrome (POHS) has never been reported in patients with active systemic histoplasmosis.
- The organism, *H. capsulatum* has not been recovered from an eye with POHS.
- Histoplasmin skin test is positive in 90% of patients with POHS.
- Increased prevalence of POHS, where histoplasmosis is endemic, e.g. Mississippi-Ohio-Missouri river valley.

Symptoms

It is asymptomatic unless it involves the macula, and the earliest symptom of macular involvement is metamorphopsia.

Signs

- Atrophic mid-peripheral spots called *histospots*.
- Peripapillary atrophy.
- Linear chorioretinal atrophy.
- Subretinal choroidal neovascularization, resulting in hemorrhagic disciform lesion at the macula.
- The vitreous is never involved.

Treatment

Argon-laser photocoagulation of subretinal neovascular membranes is advised to prevent the formation of disciform macular scar.

ACUTE RETINAL NECROSIS

Acute retinal necrosis (ARN) is an extremely rare devastating necrotizing retinitis, affecting the otherwise healthy individuals.
- *Symptoms* are periorbital pain followed by blurring of vision.
- *Signs* are noticed either at the posterior pole or at the periphery of the fundus:
  - Deep, multifocal, yellowish white patches with sheathing of the vessels.
  - The lesions gradually become confluent and represent a full thickness necrotizing retinitis.
  - Most of the eyes develop retinal holes, with rhegmatogenous retinal detachment.

- It usually resolves within 4–12 weeks, leaving behind atrophic retinal areas. In some eyes, visual acuity remains fairly good despite severe necrosis.
- **Treatment:** Systemic antibiotics, steroids, and cytotoxic agents may be beneficial.

ACQUIRED IMMUNODEFICIENCY SYNDROME (AIDS)

Human immunodeficiency virus (HIV) is the causative organism of this invariably fatal disease.

Ocular complications occur in about 75% of AIDS patients and almost all ocular structures are affected.

The lesions are due to retinal micro-vasculopathy, occurrence of Kaposi's sarcoma and opportunistic super-infections by *Pneumocystis carinii*, *Toxoplasma*, CMV, herpes zoster virus (HZV), *Candida*, molluscum contagiosum, etc.

- **Retinal microvasculopathy**
  - Cotton wool spots are the most common ocular lesion and are seen in 50% of the patients (Fig. 14.30).
  - They are probably due to immune complex deposits in the precapillary arterioles.
  - They appear as discrete fluffy opacities and are transient.
  - Superficial and deep hemorrhages are seen in some patients.
- **Kaposi's sarcoma**
  - It involves the eyelids and conjunctiva.
  - It appears as a bright-red mass, most frequently in the lower fornix of the conjunctiva.
  - When it affects the lid, it can lead to entropion, trichiasis, blepharoconjun-ctivitis, etc.
- **Opportunistic infections**
  - Cytomegalovirus retinitis is the most common opportunistic infection and the major cause of visual loss in AIDS patients. Its appearance is a grave prognostic sign as most of the patients will die within 6–8 weeks
  - Herpes zoster ophthalmicus
  - Candida endophthalmitis
  - Toxoplasma retinochoroiditis
  - Herpes simplex infection
  - Molluscum contagiosum of lids (Fig. 14.31).

Management

- Zidovudine (azidothymidine) is seen to be effective in HIV retinitis.

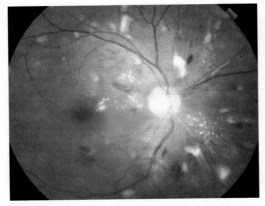

Fig. 14.30: Cotton wool spots in retinal micro-vasculopathies in AIDS

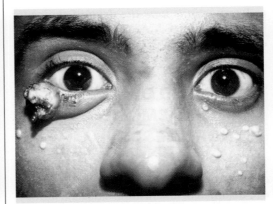

Fig. 14.31: Molluscum contagiosum in AIDS

- In CMV retinitis—intravascular injection of **Gancyclovir** or **Foscarnet** may be effective.
- Kaposi's sarcoma is sensitive to radiotherapy.

ENDOPHTHALMITIS

It is a severe form of intraocular inflammation involving the ocular cavities and inner coats of the eyeball.

Etiology

Infective

Most of the cases are infective in nature, which may be:

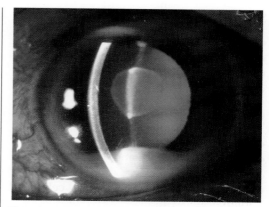

Fig. 14.33: Endogenous bacterial endophthalmitis

- **Exogenous**
  - Following penetrating injury.
  - Following intraocular surgery (Fig. 14.32).
  - Following wound leak or bleb infection (after glaucoma surgery).
  - Spread from the adjacent structures, e.g. perforating corneal ulcer.
- **Endogenous:** Septic emboli from bacterial endocarditis (Fig. 14.33), otitis media, meningitis, following urologic surgery, etc. (metastatic endophthalmitis). They are mainly seen in immune-compromized subjects.

Common organisms include:
- **Bacteria:** *Staphylococci, Streptococci, Pneumococci, Pseudomonas, Bacillus subtilis, E. coli,* etc.

- **Fungus:** *Candida, Aspergillus, Fusarium,* etc. (Fig. 14.34).
- **Parasitic:** Toxocara.

Toxic (Sterile)

- Retained intraocular foreign body, e.g. pure copper.
- Following IOL implantation (due to chemicals adherent to the implant).
- Toxic reaction to the chemicals, adherent to the instruments (following chemical sterilization).
- Necrosis of intraocular tumors.
- Phacoanaphylactic uveitis leading to endophthalmitis.

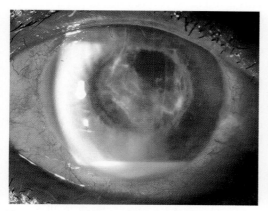

Fig. 14.32: Endophthalmitis after cataract surgery

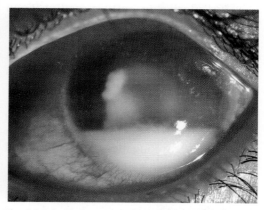

Fig. 14.34: Endogenous fungal endophthalmitis

Symptoms

- Usually unilateral with subacute onset.
- Moderate pain and redness of the eye.
- Photophobia and lacrimation.
- Gross impairment of vision.

Signs

- Lid edema.
- Ciliary congestion and chemosis of the conjunctiva.
- Keratic precipitates, aqueous cells and flare.
- Vitreous is somewhat hazy which prevents clear view of the fundus.
- Later, a yellowish-white reflex appears at the pupillary area indicating massive exudation in the vitreous.
- Intraocular pressure is low and eyeball gradually shrinks to phthisis bulbi.
- Sometimes, it may progress into panophthalmitis.
- Ultimately, vision reduces to 'no PL.'

Management

It should be very energetic and prompt.

- *Aqueous or vitreous tap:* A vitreous tap gives a better yield than aqueous tap.
  - Smear preparation for Gram-stain, Gimsa stain and potassium hydroxide mount.
  - *Inoculation in culture media:* Blood agar, chocolate agar and Sabouraud's media.
- *Intravitreal injections:* It is to be given within 6 hours to achieve maximum intra ocular concentration of antibiotics.
  - *Antibiotics:* Gentamicin (400 µg), cephazoline (2.25 mg), vancomycin (1.0 mg), ceftazidime (0.2 mg), amikacin (0.2 mg). Among these ceftazidime and vancomycin are mostly preferred.
  - *Antifungal:* Amphotericin B (5 µg) in case of suspected proved fungal endophthalmitis.
  - *Steroids:* Dexamethasone (360 µg) may be added to antibacterial agent.
- *Antibiotic therapy:* Systemic (intravenous or intramuscular), topical, and sub-conjunctival or sub-Tenon injection, are employed.
  - *Systemic:* (i) *Oral:* Ciprofloxacin—750 mg—1 g twice daily for 7 days, (ii) *Intravenous:* Cephazoline—1 g 4 times daily.
  - *Topical:* Fortified tobramycin and moxifloxacin drops every 30 minutes.
  - *Sub-Tenon:* Gentamicin (40 mg) and cephazoline (125 mg) daily for 5–7 days.
- *Antifungal:* (i) *Systemic:* Oral ketoconazole or fluconazole is given for 4–6 weeks. (ii) *Topical:* Natamycin or amphotericin B (0.15%) drop is given every 30 minutes.
- *Steroids:* They are indicated only in suspected bacterial endophthalmitis. Systemic (prednisolone—60 mg/day) and topical (dexamethasone 1 hourly).
- *Subsequent therapy:* It is governed by the culture results.
- *Vitrectomy:* Early vitrectomy is considered if the intravitreal injection fails to control endophthalmitis within 48–72 hours, and the vision is considerably reduce.

PANOPHTHALMITIS (FIGS 14.35A AND B)

This is the most severe form of inflammation of the ocular cavities which involves all three coats of the eyeball as well as the Tenon's capsule.

Etiology

Same as endophthalmitis except the toxic causes. Panophthalmitis is mostly caused by bacterial infections.

Symptoms

- Severe pain with radiation
- Swelling of the eyelids

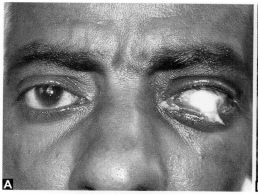 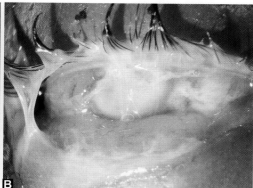

Figs 14.35A and B: Panophthalmitis

- Complete loss of vision
- Fever, malaise, headache, etc.

Signs

- No perception of light (no PL).
- Marked lid edema.
- Conjunctival chemosis and congestions.
- Slight proptosis, and there may be limitation of movements.
- Cornea is hazy and necrotic.
- Anterior chamber is full of pus.
- Intraocular tension is raised initially.
- Globe may rupture at the limbus or at the pre-existing wound, and pus will come out at those places.
- The signs may gradually subside, and the eye becomes a shrunken mass of fibrotic tissue (phthisis bulbi).

Complications

- Orbital and facial cellulitis
- Cavernous sinus thrombosis
- Meningitis or encephalitis.

Treatment

- Medical treatment with intensive antibiotics is very rarely successful.
- Evisceration of the eyeball is finally the treatment of choice (*see* chapter 25).
- Enucleation is contraindicated.

DEGENERATIONS OF UVEAL TRACT

Iridocorneal Endothelial Syndromes

This is a spectrum of diseases of unknown etiology, essentially due to abnormalities in the corneal endothelium.

After metaplasia, the ***corneal endothelium proliferates***, and ***Descemet's membrane***-like material covers the anterior iris surface and angle of the anterior chamber, causing iris anomalies and secondary glaucoma.

These disorders are slowly progressive over a period of 10 years or more. Women are more commonly affected than men.

The spectrum includes three conditions:
1. ***Progressive essential iris atrophy (Figs 14.36A and B)***
   - It is a ***unilateral*** condition characterized by ***patchy iris atrophy*** with partial or complete hole formation.
   - There is distorted and displaced pupil (***corectopia***).
   - ***Holes in the iris*** get are gradually enlarged and coalesce together.
   - ***Glaucoma*** then ensues from peripheral anterior synechiae and from damage to the trabecular meshwork.

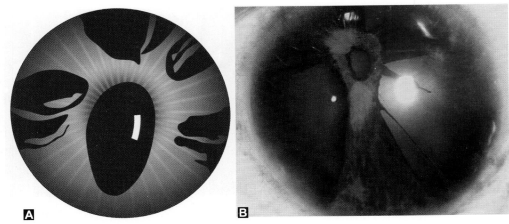

Figs 14.36A and B: Essential iris atrophy—polycoria; corectopia and PAS

- *Treatment* is directed toward secondary glaucoma, and is often, not effective either by medical or surgical means.
2. *Iris nevus syndrome (Cogan-Reese)*
   - Characteristic feature is dark brown pigmented nodules in the iris stroma (as small woolen spherules) (Fig. 14.37A).

Iridoschisis

- It is a rare, diffuse, bilateral, senile degenerative condition of the iris. It may also be precipitated by trauma.
- Large dehiscences appear on the anterior mesodermal layer of the iris and strands of tissue may float into the anterior chamber.
- Treatment is not necessary.

- Peripheral anterior synechiae and secondary glaucoma may also occur.
- *Treatment* is directed toward the control of secondary glaucoma.
3. *Chandler's syndrome (Fig. 14.37B)*
   - It is mainly associated with *endothelial disturbances and corneal edema*.
   - *Iris atrophy is minimal* and without a tendency to hole formation.
   - Peripheral anterior synechiae and *secondary glaucoma are less common*, and the control of glaucoma is easier.
   - *Penetrating or endothelial keratoplasty* may be considered for corneal edema.

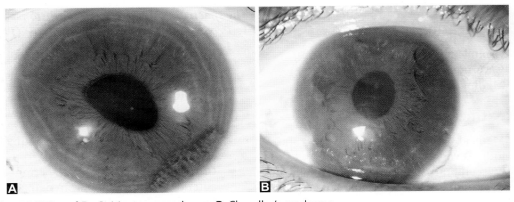

Figs 14.37A and B: **A.** Iris nevus syndrome; **B.** Chandler's syndrome

RUBEOSIS IRIDIS (FIG. 14.38)

It means neovascularization of the iris. It occurs as an irregularly distributed network of new vessels on the iris surface and the stroma.

Causes

- Diabetes mellitus
- Central retinal venous occlusion
- Heterochromic cyclitis of Fuchs
- Carotid artery occlusive diseases
- Intraocular tumors
- Anterior segment ischemia
- Following vitrectomy in aphakic eyes.

The new blood vessels and associated fibrous tissue may cover the trabecular meshwork and cause peripheral anterior synechiae. These ultimately close the angle of the anterior chamber and cause an intractable neovascular glaucoma.

Treatment

Neovascular glaucoma is difficult to treat.

- *Panretinal photocoagulation* is the treatment of choice in most cases. Photoablation of the neovascularized retina is followed by involution of iris vessels.
- *Panretinal cryocoagulation* helps similarly, especially in presence of opacity in the media (e.g. cataract or vitreous hemorrhage).
- *Cyclocryotherapy* in resistant cases.

CHOROIDAL DEGENERATIONS

As the outer layers of the retina receive their nourishment from the choriocapillaries, degeneration of the choroid is often associated with atrophy of the retina, and migration of pigments in the superficial retinal layers. Secondary degenerations occur following inflammatory lesions, myopia, or in late stages of glaucoma.

Primary Choroidal Sclerosis (Fig. 14.39)

It is a degenerative vascular sclerosis of the choroid associated with secondary degeneration of the retina. It occurs as an isolated lesion and is not associated with generalized vascular sclerosis.

Pathologically, the sclerosis is limited to the choriocapillaries and precapillary arterioles, and the veins are being less affected.

Ophthalmoscopy shows diffuse atrophy of the retinal pigment epithelial (RPE) and choriocapillaries, and a tessellated appearance of the fundus. The larger sclerosed choroidal vessels are more visible as white lines against the irregular pigmented areas.

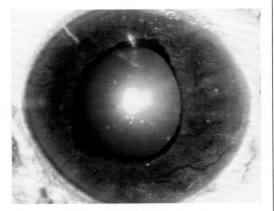

Fig. 14.38: Rubeosis iridis with ectropion uveae

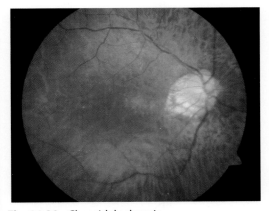

Fig. 14.39: Choroidal sclerosis

It occurs in two forms:

1. ***Diffuse or generalized sclerosis:*** It affects the whole fundus. It may cause bilateral progressive diminution of vision, particularly at night.

2. ***Localized sclerosis:*** It affects the central area or circumpapillary region and is also known as central areolar choroidal dystrophy. Central vision is gradually reduced with development of central scotoma.

Gyrate Atrophy of Choroid (Fig. 14.40)

This is an inherited (autosomal recessive), inborn error of amino acid metabolism due to defective activity of ornithine ketoacid amino transferase enzyme resulting in hyperornithinemia.

- The ***symptoms*** include progressive dimness of vision with night blindness in young adults.
- ***Ophthalmoscopy*** shows, scalloped to circular patches of chorioretinal atrophy in the far and mid-retinal periphery. The patches increase in size and coalesce together, and finally, whole fundus is affected, with preservation only of the macula.
- ***Perimetry*** shows, constriction of the peripheral visual field corresponding to the extent of fundus lesion.

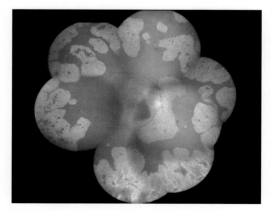

Fig. 14.40: Gyrate atrophy of the choroid

- ***Treatment:*** A diet low in proteins and arginine (precursor of ornithine) may be beneficial.

Massive doses of pyridoxine (vitamin B_6) normalize the hyperornithinemia and may have beneficial effect on the ocular lesion.

Choroideremia

It is an inherited (X-linked recessive) choroidal atrophy with secondary atrophy of the retina, resulting in night blindness.

- The disease characteristically affects only males and starts within 5–10 years of age with defective night vision.
- ***Ophthalmoscopy*** shows, diffuse mottled depigmentation of the RPE. Eventually, large patches of chorioretinal atrophy develop in the equatorial region. The atrophy then spreads centrally and peripherally, with annular scotoma and progressive constriction of the visual field. Central vision is last to be affected.

The retinal vessels are characteristically normal.

- Female carriers often clinically show mild fundus changes (patchy atrophy and mottling of the RPE at the equator), though they are asymptomatic.
- No treatment is available.

Angioid Streaks (Fig. 14.41)

Angioid streaks are irregular and jagged network of red to brown lines, mainly seen in the central fundus.

- They are produced by cracklike dehiscences in the collagenous and elastic portion of the Bruch's membrane.
- The streaks or lines typically radiate outward in a tapering fashion from the peri papillary area.
- The lesions are approximately the width of a retinal vessel, which may thus resemble (angioid). But the streaks are darker, have an irregular contour with serrated edges, and tend to terminate abruptly.

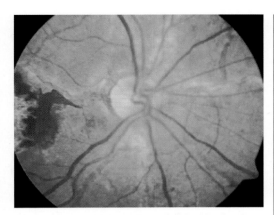

Fig. 14.41: Angioid streak

- *Systemic associations*
  - Pseudoxanthoma elasticum (Grönblad–Strandberg syndrome)—most common.
  - Paget's disease
  - Ehlers–Danlos syndrome
  - Sickle cell disease
  - Rarely, acromegaly, hypercalcemia and lead poisoning.
- Ocular changes are normally asymptomatic. The causes of visual impairment may be due to:
  - Involvement of the fovea by a streak,
  - Choroidal neovascularization, or
  - Choroidal rupture.

Acute Posterior Multifocal Placoid Pigment Epitheliopathy

- It is a rare, bilateral, idiopathic disease affecting the young adults.
- The *primary site of lesion* is at the level of RPE, although it has also been suggested as a *vasculopathy* of the choriocapillaries.
- Initially, the *patient presents* with a subacute loss of central vision, and within a few days the fellow eye is usually affected.
- *Ophthalmoscopy* shows, the typical deep, cream colored placoid lesions, involving the posterior pole within the equatorial region.

- *Fundus fluorescein angiography* shows patchy irregular choroidal filling with late staining.
- Spontaneous resolution with good visual recovery is usual, within a few weeks.
- There is no *effective treatment*.

Serpiginous (Geographical) Choroidopathy

It is a rare, idiopathic, recurrent disease of the RPE and choriocapillaries affecting the middle-aged patient.
- Initially, the patient remains asymptomatic.
- The chorioretinal lesion usually starts around the optic disc, and spreads outwards in all directions.
- *Acute lesions* are cream colored opacities with hazy border without any inflammatory cells in the vitreous.
- With healing, they become inactive, leaving scalloped 'punched out' areas of chorioretinal atrophy.
- Fresh acute lesions usually arise as extensions from old scars, and successive attacks result in serpiginous extension of the destruction process peripherally from the peripapillary area.
- Involvement of the fovea causes a permanent loss of central vision.
- Fluorescein angiography confirms the diagnosis.
- There is no *effective treatment*.

CHOROIDAL DETACHMENT (FIG. 14.42)

It means separation of the choroid from the sclera which occurs frequently.

Causes

- *Following intraocular operations:* Sudden lowering of intraocular pressure → vasodilatation of the choroidal vessels

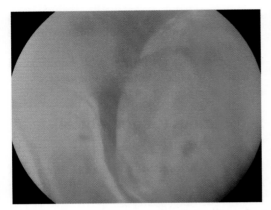

Fig. 14.42: Choroidal detachment with retinal detachment (Kissing choroidals)

→ exudation on to the outer lamella of the choroid → detachment
- Following intraocular hemorrhage
- Choroidal tumors
- Exudative choroiditis.
  Photopsia and floaters (as seen in retinal detachment) are absent.

Signs

- Shallow anterior chamber.
- Intraocular pressure is very low as a result of hyposecretion of aqueous due to a concomitant ciliary body detachment.
- It may be visible as dark brown mass by oblique illumination after mydriasis.
- *Ophthalmoscopy* shows smooth, elevated, darkbrown bullous lesions, which are more prominent on the temporal and nasal sides.
  The elevations do not extend to the posterior pole because they are limited by the adhesions, where the vortex veins enter their scleral tunnels.

Treatment

The prognosis is usually good. The choroid is reattached, and anterior chamber is reformed, without any treatment. However, in some persistent cases, it requires treatment.

- Corticosteroids drop and posterior sub-Tenon injection of triamcinolone may be useful in some eyes. Tablet acetazolamide, 250 mg 4 times daily.
- To look for 'wound leak' and if it is there—treatment is done by regular patching or conjunctival flap or resuturing.
- In recalcitrant cases, drainage of the sub-choroidal fluid through a diathermy puncture at the most prominent site of detachment has been suggested.

IRIS CYSTS

Iris cysts are not very uncommon, and they may be *primary* or *secondary*.

Primary Iris Cysts (Figs 14.43A and B)

- They usually arise from the iris pigment epithelium and very rarely, from the iris stroma.
- Those arising from the pigment epithelial layer, are stationary and asymptomatic.
- They are globular, dark brown structures which transilluminate.
- Treatment is required in selected cases if it touches the cornea.

Secondary Iris Cysts (Figs 14.44A and B)

- *Implantation cysts:* They develop from implantation of epithelial cells on to the iris following intraocular surgery or penetrating injury.
  - The cysts lie on the anterior surface of the iris, and grayish white in color.
  - They frequently enlarge and lead to complications, like anterior uveitis and glaucoma.
  - *Surgical excision* is the treatment of choice.

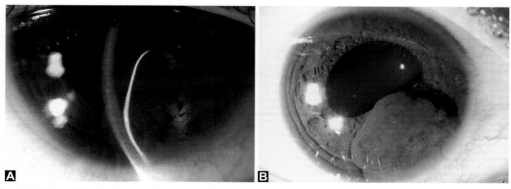

Figs 14.43A and B: A. Primary iris cysts; **B.** Same in slit section

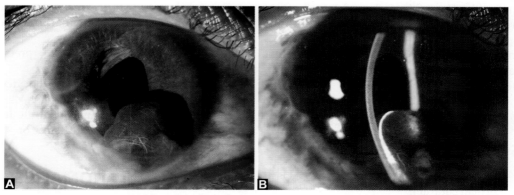

Figs 14.44A and B: Secondary iris cyst. **A.** Post-cataract surgery; **B.** Translucent in slit section

- *Drug-induced iris cysts:* They occur following prolonged use of long-acting miotics, such as phospholine iodide.
  - *Treatment:* Withdrawal of the drug and simultaneous use of phenylephrine (2.5%) with long-acting miotic, prevents formation of the iris cysts.

TUMORS OF THE UVEAL TRACT

See Chapter 20.

Diseases of the Lens

Being avascular and composed entirely of epithelium surrounded by a capsule, the lens is incapable of becoming inflamed. Its cells, apart from those at the equator and the anterior epithelium, are incapable of proliferation. Its major function is to transmit and refract light rays. Its only way of responding to insults is to become opaque.

DISEASES OF THE LENS

Symptoms

- *Decrease of vision for far and near:* It is in cortical cataract.
- *Dimness of vision for distance with good near vision without glasses:* It is in nuclear sclerosis.
- *Monocular diplopia or polyopia, and colored halos:* It is in early immature cortical cataract.
- *Acute pain, redness and watering in an eye with cataract:* It is in lens-induced secondary glaucoma or uveitis.
- *White pupillary reflex (leukokoria):* As noticed by the parents or relatives.

Signs

- *Color* of the crystalline lens.
- *Presence of iris shadow:* It is indicates immature cataract.
- *Presence of Purkinje's 3rd and 4th images:* It is indicates normal transparent lens as they are formed by the *anterior*

convex and *posterior concave* surfaces of the lens respectively.

- *Fundal glow on distant direct ophthalmoscopy shows:* The cataracts as dark opacities against the red background.
- *Slit-lamp examination* for precise location and details of the opacity.
- *Absence of the lens:* It is indicated by deep anterior chamber and tremulousness of the iris, due to loss of support of the iris, and by the absence of 3rd and/or 4th Purkinje's images.

CONGENITAL ANOMALIES OF THE LENS

Anomalies of the Lens Shape

Coloboma (Fig. 15.1)

There is a defect usually in the lower margin, and it may be associated with similar defects involving the iris, ciliary body and choroid. The notching or indentation in the lens is simply due to a localized defect in the zonule, allowing the lens equator to retract. Giant retinal tear may occur in these eyes. Restoration of defective zonule is not possible (Fig. 15.1).

Anterior Lenticonus

This is an anterior conical projection of the center of the lens. It interferes with vision as the central part of the lens becomes highly myopic. Ophthalmoscopically, a dark disc-like

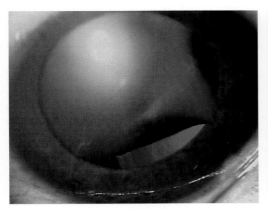

Fig. 15.1: Coloboma of the lens

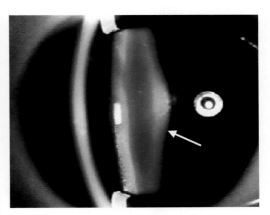

Fig. 15.3: Posterior lenticonus (arrow)

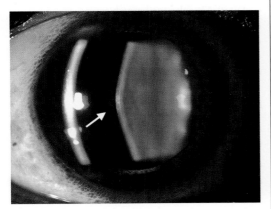

Fig. 15.2: Anterior lenticonus (arrow)

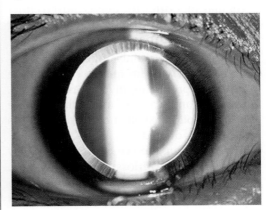

Fig. 15.4: Spherophakia

(oil globule) reflex is visible in the center of the red-reflex, which distorts the fundus view (Fig. 15.2).

It occurs in some patients with **Alport's syndrome** with familial hemorrhagic nephritis and sensorineural deafness.

Posterior Lenticonus (Fig. 15.3)

It is more common than anterior lenticonus with a posterior conical or globular (lentiglobus) bulge in the axial zone of the lens.

The posterior bulge increases progressively with age, and the lens cortex in the cone may become opaque and obscure the lenticonus. It also gives *oil globule* appearance in ophthalmoscopy.

Spherophakia (Microspherophakia) (Fig. 15.4)

- In spherophakia, the lens is small and spherical (increased anterior and posterior curvatures of the lens).
- The zonular fibers are easily visible with papillary dilatation. Subluxation of the lens is common, because the stretched zonules become weak and breakable.
- Angle-closure glaucoma occurs when the small, round lens blocks the flow of aqueous through the pupil. As this glaucoma is aggravated by miotics and relieved by mydriatics, it is called *inverse glaucoma*.

- The causes of spherophakia are:
  - Familial microspherophakia
  - Weill-Marchesani syndrome (WMS)
  - Marfan's syndrome
  - Hyperlysinemia.

ECTOPIA LENTIS

Ectopia lentis is a congenital, bilateral, subluxation or dislocation of the lens.
- In **subluxation** (due to partial zonular defect), the lens is displaced sideways, but remains behind the pupil.
- But in **dislocation** (when the lens loses all zonular supports), the lens is moved either forwards into the anterior chamber, or backwards into the vitreous.

The symptoms are mainly optical.
- In **subluxation**, the lens becomes more spherical producing myopic astigmatism. The division of 'phakic' and 'aphakic' zone of the pupil is usually not evident, unless the pupil is dilated.
- In **dislocation**, the eye becomes markedly hypermetropic with loss of accommodation. Migration of the dislocated lens into the anterior chamber or vitreous causes secondary glaucoma.
  A subluxated lens usually, but not inevitably becomes dislocated with increasing age.

Signs

- An irregular, deep anterior chamber with tremulousness of the iris.
- Diagnosis should be confirmed after full dilatation of the pupil. The edge of the displaced lens appears in the papillary area as a dark crescent in oblique illumination **(subluxation)**.

Causes

They are mainly hereditary in nature.
- Marfan's syndrome
- Homocystinuria
- Weill-Marchesani syndrome
- Ehlers-Danlos syndrome
- Hyperlysinemia
- Familial ectopia lentis
- Sulfite oxidase deficiency.

Marfan's Syndrome

Autosomal dominant, a multisystem mesodermal dysplasia.

Ocular features
- The lens is typically displaced upward and inward (Fig. 15.5A)
- Hypoplasia of the iris causes poor dilatation of the pupil
- Axial myopia

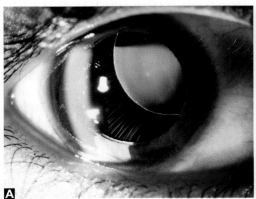 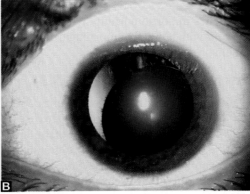

Figs 15.5A and B: A. Marfan's syndrome—lens displacement upward and inward; **B.** Homocystinurea—lens displacement downward and outward

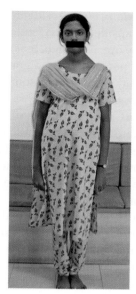

Fig. 15.6: Marfan's syndrome—long extremities

- Secondary glaucoma
- Retinal detachment due to high incidence of peripheral retinal degeneration.

Systemic features
- Arachnodactyly (spider fingers)
- Long extremities (Fig. 15.6)
- Hyperextensibility of the joints
- High-arched palate
- Dissecting aortic aneurysm
- High incidence of hernias.

Homocystinuria

- Autosomal recessive; an inborn error of metabolism.
- Inability of convert methionine to cystine.
- Deficiency of enzyme cystathionine synthatase.

Ocular features
- The lens is subluxated downward and outward (Fig. 15.5B).
- Secondary glaucoma, due to pupillary block.

Systemic features
- Fair complexion with malar flush

- Mental retardation
- Poor motor control
- Increased thromboembolic manifestation due to an excessive platelet adhesiveness.
- General anesthesia is hazardous
- Diagnosis is confirmed by urine test with sodium nitroprusside.

Weill-Marchesani Syndrome

- Autosomal recessive; a mesodermal dysplasia
- Short stature, stubby fingers
- Microspherophakia, which may be subluxated
- Secondary papillary block glaucoma
- Retinal detachment.

Familial Ectopia Lentis

- Autosomal recessive
- Unassociated with any systemic defect
- May be associated with ectopic pupil—*ectopia lentis et pupillae.*

Treatment

- Spectacles or contact lenses are used to correct the optical defects, preferably through the phakic part.
- Lens extraction is difficult, complications are common and visual results are often poor.
- Pars plana lensectomy with vitrectomy is better than other surgical means.
- A scleral fixation posterior chamber intraocular lens (IOL) may be for visual rehabilitation.

LENS-INDUCED OCULAR DISEASES

In addition to the glaucoma resulting from displacement of the lens, the other lens-induced ocular problems are:
- *Phacolytic glaucoma (Fig. 15.7):* In some eyes with hypermature cataract when

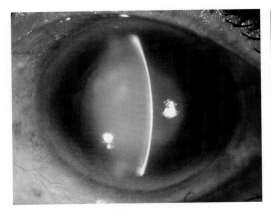

Fig. 15.7: Phacolytic glaucoma

the capsule leaks, large phagocytes filled with lens material obstruct the trabecular meshwork, causing a secondary open-angle glaucoma.

Treatment: First, urgent medical control of glaucoma followed by lens extraction with IOL implantation at early as possible.

- **Phacogenic (phacomorphic) glaucoma (Fig. 15.8A):** A rapid swelling of the lens (as in senile intumescent cataract, or following trauma to the lens capsule) may cause a secondary angle-closure glaucoma (Fig. 15.8B), if the anterior chamber is already shallow.

Treatment is almost same as the phacolytic glaucoma.

- **Phacotoxic uveitis:** Accidental trauma to the lens capsule liberates lenticular protein within the eye. Although, lens proteins are relatively poor antigens, a granulomatous uveitis may develop and sometimes with secondary glaucoma.

Treatment consists of administration of corticosteroids and lens extraction.

- **Phacoanaphylactic uveitis:** Rarely, after extracapsular cataract extraction, the immune system appears to be sensitized to lens protein.
  - Extracapsular extraction with retention of cortical material in the second eye, then may sometimes cause an endophthalmitis.
  - Dislocation of lens nucleus or nuclear fragments in the vitreous cavity during an extracapsular extraction or phacoemulsification, also causes severe uveitis.
  - The lens material must be removed from the eye by means of vitrectomy and lensectomy.

CATARACT

Literally, cataract means **waterfall**. Any opacity of the lens or its capsule causing visual impairment is called cataract.

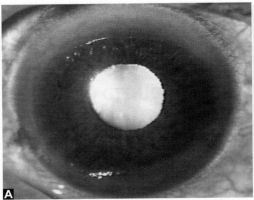
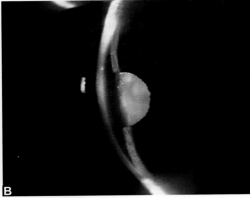

Figs 15.8A and B: A. Phacomorphic glaucoma; **B.** Secondary angle-closure

Care must be taken in using the term 'cataract' clinically, since, it often excites anxiety which may be entirely unjustified. It is to be remembered that many congenital opacities are stationary, and even in senile cataract the opacities may remain localized for many years without causing serious visual impairment.

So, it is often wise to tell such patient that he has lental opacity and to suggest that the development of cataract may be long delayed and will be dealt with according to the need.

Classification of Cataract

No classification of cataract is entirely satisfactory. It may be classified as follows:
- Congenital or developmental cataract
- Acquired cataract
  - Senile
  - Traumatic
    - Mechanical
    - Irradiation
    - Electric shock
  - Complicated (due to some other ocular disease)
    - Anterior uveitis
    - High myopia
    - Retinal detachment
    - Retinitis
    - Glaukomflecken
  - Secondary (due to some systemic disease)
    - Diabetes mellitus
    - Hypocalcemia
    - Myotonic dystrophy
    - Atopic dermatitis
  - Toxic (due to drugs)
    - Corticosteroids
    - Chlorpromazine
    - Miotics (long-acting)
    - Busulfan
    - Amiodarone
    - Gold
  - Syndromes associate with cataract
    - Down's
    - Lowe's
    - Treacher Collins
    - Wilson's disease
    - Fabry's disease
- After cataract: Posterior capsule opacification.

CONGENITAL OR DEVELOPMENTAL CATARACT

It means cataract that presents at birth, or develops soon after the birth.

The lens is formed in layers, the central or fetal nucleus being the earliest formation, around which the concentric zones are subsequently laid down and the process is continuing until the late age of life.

Congenital or developmental cataract (Fig. 15.9) has therefore, a tendency to affect a particular zone, which was being formed when this process is disturbed. The lens fibers laid down previously and subsequently are often normally formed, and remain clear.

As times goes on, such an opacity is usually deeply buried into the substance of the lens by subsequent formation of normal fibers.

Developmental cataract has a tendency to follow the architectural pattern of the lens, and from its location, an estimate can be made about the stage of development at which the opacity occurred.

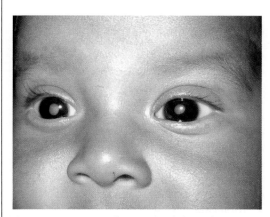

Fig. 15.9: Congenital cataract—bilateral

In strict sense, congenital and developmental cataract are not synonymous. In widest sense, most forms of cataract (even the senile cataract) may be considered as developmental, for the human lens grows until late in life, until the age of 80–90 years. The criteria of congenital cataract are:
- Any lens opacity present at birth.
- Such opacities must be situated within the fetal nucleus, or at the most within the inner-most part of the infantile nucleus.
- Diameter of the opacity (partial cataract) must be less than 5.75 mm (i.e. the frontal diameter of newborn lens). If the size of the opacity is more than 5.75 mm, the cataract must be postnatal.

Causes

- Mostly unknown
- Hereditary
- Chromosomal abnormalities, e.g. Down's syndrome
- Maternal malnutrition (vitamin D deficiency and hypocalcemia as in zonular cataract)
- Maternal infections, as in rubella
- Fetal hypoxia owing to placental hemorrhages
- Drug intake during the pregnancy, e.g. corticosteroids.

Morphologically, several types of congenital cataract (lens opacities) are recognized with the slit-lamp biomicroscope.

Morphological Types (Fig. 15.10)

- Punctate (blue-dot) cataract
- Anterior polar cataract—pyramidal reduplicated
- Posterior polar cataract
- Nuclear cataract
- Coronary cataract
- Coralliform/floriform cataract
- Christmas tree cataract (in myotonic dystrophy)
- Zonular (lamellar) cataract
- Total cataract.

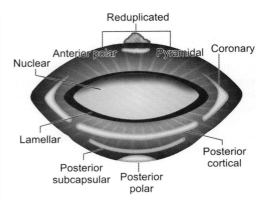

Fig. 15.10: Morphological types of cataract

Punctate (Blue-dot) Cataract (Fig. 15.11)

Perhaps, this is the most common type of congenital cataract.
- It appears as multiple, tiny blue spots, scattered all over the lens, especially in the cortex by oblique illumination with the slit-lamp
- The bluish color is due to the effects of dispersion of light in the same way that the sky appears blue
- The visual acuity is not affected.

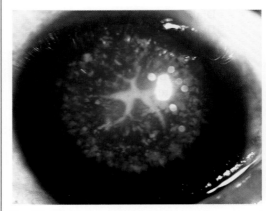

Fig. 15.11: Blue-dot and sutural cataract

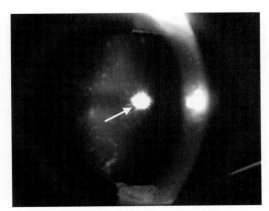

Fig. 15.12: Anterior polar cataract (arrow)

Anterior Polar Cataract (Fig. 15.12)

- It is sharply demarcated opacity at the anterior lens capsule, and usually the size of a pin's head.
- It may project forward into the anterior chamber like a pyramid (*pyramidal cataract*); or subsequently, a subcapsular cataract may develop, just behind it with a clear zone in between (*reduplicated cataract*).
- This is due to delayed formation of the anterior chamber during development of the lens.

- These opacities are stationary and rarely interfere with vision.

Posterior Polar Cataract (Figs 15.13A and B)

- This is due to residue of the attachment of hyaloids artery on the posterior lens capsule.
- This is usually dot-like (*Mitendorf's dot*) and in significant.
- However, in few cases, the lens may be invaded by fibrous tissue and a *total cataract* is formed.

Coronary Cataract (Fig. 15.14)

- This is the type of developmental cataract occurring *at puberty.*
- It is situated in the deep layer of the cortex and the most superficial layer of the nucleus.
- It appears as a *corona* or club-shaped opacities, near the periphery of the lens, while the axial region and the extreme periphery remain clear.
- As they are hidden by the iris, dilatation of the pupil is essential to recognize these opacities.
- It does not interfere with vision.

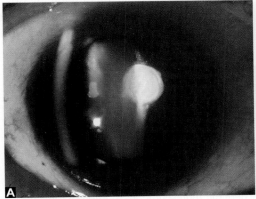
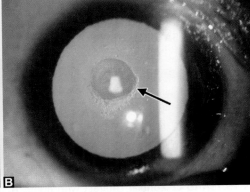

Figs 15.13A and B: Posterior polar cataract. **A.** Slit section; **B.** Retroillumination (arrow)

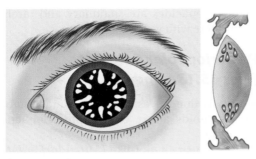

Fig. 15.14: Coronary cataract

Zonular (Lamellar) Cataract (Figs 15.15A to C)

- It is probably the most common type of developmental cataract presenting with visual impairment.
- It may be congenital or occurs within the first year after birth.
- It is usually bilateral and often hereditary (*autosomal dominant*) without any other ocular anomaly.
- It is associated with *hypovitaminosis-D* (may be with evidences of ricket), or *hypocalcemia* (may be with tetany or defective tooth enamel) and *maternal malnutrition*.
- A unilateral cataract may follow blunt trauma of the eye.
- *Characteristics*
  - It consists of concentric, sharply demarcated zones (lamellae) of opacities surrounding a core that is clear and enveloped by the clear cortex externally (Figs 15.15A to C).

- There may be linear opacities, like spokes of a wheel (called *riders*) that extends outward toward the equator, and when present, it is *pathognomonic*.
- Child with zonular cataract may present with photophobia due to light scattering.
- Surgery is considered when the visual acuity is less than 6/18.

Rubella Cataract (Fig. 15.16)

- Rubella infection during pregnancy may cause widespread ocular and systemic defects.
- Incidence of cataract is more, if the infection is contracted in the second month of pregnancy; and sometimes in the third month.
- The cataract is originally nuclear and progresses to become total (pearly-white in color) (Fig. 15.16).
- It is associated with microphthalmos, nystagmus, strabismus, glaucoma, iris hypoplasia and change to *salt-and-pepper retinopathy.*
- The systemic associations are congenital heart disease—patent ductus arteriosus (PDA) microencephaly, mental retardation, deafness and dental anomalies.
- *Pathologically,* the nucleus is found to be necrotic and it may harbor the virus for up to 2 years following birth.
- Removal of such cataract frequently provokes an intense uveitis or endophthalmitis (probably by liberation of retained virus) with disappointing visual result.

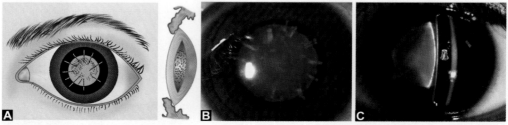

Figs 15.15A to C: Zonular cataract with riders. **A.** Schematic representation; **B.** Photograph—note the spoke-like riders; **C.** Zonular cataract in slit section

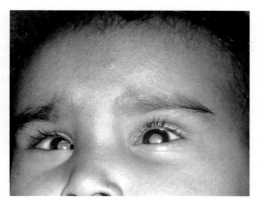

Fig. 15.16: Congenital rubella cataract

- However, in view of total bilateral cataract, complete aspiration, should usually be attempted with a complete iridectomy (as the pupils dilate poorly) and high dose of corticosteroids.
- All the congenital anomalies associated with maternal rubella in the first trimester can be avoided by vaccination of the mother.
- The rubella-vaccine is itself toxic to the fetus, and it must therefore be administered at least 3 months before the pregnancy.

Management of Pediatric Cataract

Prognostic Factors

The prognosis of pediatric cataracts depends on few factors:
- Unilateral or bilateral
- Density of cataract during presentation
- Degree of visual impairment
- Associated ocular defects
- Associated systemic defects
- Probable cause of the cataract
- Commitment of the parents.

Investigations

- Ocular examination, especially
  - Assessment of the visual function by:
    - Fixation reflex
    - Optokinetic nystagmus (OKN)
    - Catford drum test
    - Visual evoke potential (VEP)
    - Forced preferential looking (FPL)
  - Look for associated nystagmus and strabismus
  - Density of the cataract
  - Fundus examination with dilated pupils.
- Thorough systemic examination including the study of the family.

Laboratory Investigations

- **TORCH test:** Patient and maternal serum are studied for antibodies against toxoplasma (TO), rubella (R), cytomegalovirus (C) and herpes simplex virus (H).
- Test for galactosemia (reducing substances in urine).
- Test for Lowe's syndrome (urine chromatography for amino acids).
- Test for hypoglycemia (blood glucose).
- Tests for hypocalcemia (serum calcium, phosphate and X-ray skull).

Indications of Surgery

- About 50% of the opacities do not progress or interfere with vision and can safely be ignored.
- If the opacity is partial with useful vision, surgery should better not to be considered. The vision of 6/12 or 6/18 with accommodation is more valuable than a vision of 6/9 without accommodation, after operation.
- All dense cataracts (unilateral or bilateral) and partial cataracts with vision less than 6/18, are to be operated as early as possible.

Other modes of treatment
• **Mydriatics:** For axial cataract, and with convex glasses to maintain near vision.
• **Optical iridectomy** for axial cataract and if the opacity is stationary. It is obsolete nowadays.

Timing of Surgery

- The critical period for development of fixation reflex is between 6 weeks and 6 months of age. So, the best time for surgery is before this period to prevent stimulus-deprivation amblyopia.
- In dense monocular cataract, the surgery should be done as early as possible, may be on the next day after birth.

Surgical Techniques

- **Simple discussion or needling** operation is becoming obsolete nowadays, because of more complications (after cataract occurs in almost all cases → needs repeated surgeries → retinal detachment in future).
- **Pars plana lensectomy with vitrectomy** perhaps, is the most suitable surgery for congenital cataracts.
- **Planned extracapsular cataract extraction (ECCE)** as in adult ECCE; by phacoemusification technique as in a posterior chamber IOL may be considered with ECCE if the child is older than 3 years of age.

The incidence of posterior capsule opacity (PCO) after ECCE with posterior chamber intraocular lens (PCIOL) is very high (may be up to 100%) in young children. A primary posterior curvilinear capsulorhexis (PCCC) with or without vitrectomy is helpful to prevent PCO in this group. It is based on the theory that removing the scaffold for the migration of lens epithelial cells will provide a permanently clear optical zone.

Visual Rehabilitation

- **Conventional aphakic glasses:** It is only useful for bilateral aphakia, but technical difficulties in wearing heavy spectacles (+15D or more) in young children should be kept in mind.
- **Extended-wear soft contact lens:** It is especially for uniocular aphakia. Extreme

cooperation and commitment of the parents are very important.
- **Posterior chamber IOL implantation:** It should certainly, not to be considered before the age of 3 years because at that age the growth of the eye has leveled off.
- **Amblyopia therapy:** It should be started as soon as possible in the form of occlusion or **atropine penalization** in the other eye. This is a must for unilateral cataract.

▌ SENILE CATARACT

The aging lens tends to become opaque after the age of 50 years and by the age of 70 over 90% of the population show some evidence of cataract.

It occurs equally in men and women, and is usually bilateral, but often develops earlier in one eye than the other (Fig. 15.17).

There is a considerable genetic influence in its occurrence, and in hereditary cases, it may appear at an earlier age (even before the age of 50) in successive generations (*presenile cataract*).

Senile cataract may be broadly divided into two types (though they may occur concurrently).

1. **Cortical or soft cataract (75–80%):** The classical features of hydration followed by coagulation of lens proteins, appear primarily in the cortex.

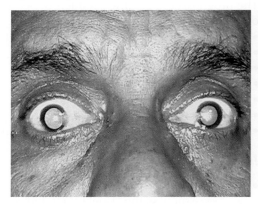

Fig. 15.17: Bilateral senile mature cataract

2. ***Nuclear or hard cataract (20–25%):*** The essential feature is as low progressive sclerosis in the lens nucleus.

Cortical (Soft) Cataract (Fig. 15.18)

- ***Cuneiform:*** It starts as wedge-shaped spokes of opacity at the periphery and gradually encroaches toward center.
- ***Cupuliform cataract:*** It is also known as posterior cortical cataract and starts as a saucer-shaped opacity in the posterior cortex just beneath the capsule.

Cuneiform Cataract (Fig. 15.19)

Symptoms

- Painless, progressive loss of vision
- ***Uniocular diplopia or polyopia:*** It is due to irregular refractions by different sectors of the lens producing multiple images.
- ***Coloredhalos:*** It is due to accumulation of fluid droplets in between the lens fibers.
- ***Black spots in front of the eyes:*** The spots are fixed.
- ***Glare***, particularly at night, during facing head-lights.
- Progressive decrease in peripheral visual field.
- ***White opacity inside the black of the eye*** (as noticed by the friends or relatives).

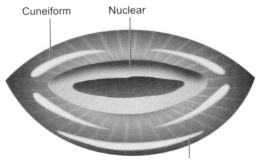

Fig. 15.18: Types of senile cataract

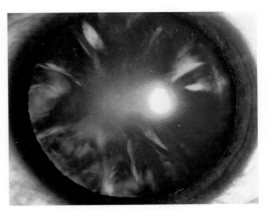

Fig. 15.19: Cuneiform cortical cataract

Stages and signs

- ***Stage of lamellar separation:*** A demarcation of the cortical fibers is due to their separation by fluid, and can only be seen with the slit-lamp.
- ***Stage of incipient cataract***
  - Cuneiform opacities with clear area in between them, appear in the periphery of the lens.
  - The bases of the wedge-shaped opacities are peripheral, and they are most common in ***lower nasal quadrant.***
  - They appear as gray opacities with oblique illumination, but appear black against the red fundal glow with the ophthalmoscope or retinoscopic mirror.
  - They gradually encroach to the axial area and vision becomes impaired.
- ***Immature stage (Fig. 15.20A):*** As time goes on, opacification becomes more diffuse, and the deeper layers of the cortex become cloudy.
  - ***Vision:*** It may be reduced to finger counting.
  - ***Lens:*** Grayish or grayish-white.
  - ***Iris shadow:*** Present.

Painless Progressive Loss of Vision

The common causes of painless progressive loss of vision are:
- Senile cataract
- Open angle glaucoma
- Presbyopia
- Degenerative myopia
- Retinitis pigmentosa
- Diabetic retinopathy
- Age-related macular degeneration (ARMD)
- Papilledema [due to intracranial space-occupying lesions (SOL)].

Differential Diagnosis

- **Senile cataract:** Aged patient; grayish-white or white pupillary reflex; iris shadow—present in immature type; normal IOP; and poor or absent fundal glow.
- **Open angle glaucoma:** Aged patient; high IOP; typical glaucomatous field defects and cupping of the optic disc.
- **Presbyopia:** Aging process—gradual dimness of vision in near only; no lental opacity; normal IOP; no cupping of the disc and near vision is regained by simple 'plus-power' glasses.
- **Degenerative myopia:** Younger subject; increasing high 'minus-power' glasses; normal IOP; typical myopic degenerative changes in the fundus.
- **Retinitis pigmentosa:** Middle-aged patient; positive family history; night blindness; tubular field defect; normal IOP; typical fundus changes—bone-corpuscle pigments, arteriolar attenuation and waxy pallor of the disc.
- **Diabetic retinopathy:** Young adult or aged; history of long standing diabetes, often uncontrolled; with or without cataract; typical fundus picture—dot and blot hemorrhage, hard exudates, macular edema, neovascularization, vitreous hemorrhage, tractional retinal detachment (RD); fundus fluorescein angiography (FFA) is diagnostic.
- **Age-related macular degeneration:** Aged patients; progressive central loss of vision; anterior segment and IOP are essentially normal; retinal pigment epithelium (RPE) atrophy; detachment of RPE with subretinal neovascular membranes (SRNVMs) formation; FFA is diagnostic.

Contd...

Contd...

- **Papilloedema:** Any age; bilateral onset; associated headache and vomiting; normal reacting pupil; normal IOP, bilateral optic disc swelling and may be with superficial hemorrhage, soft exudates and macular star; CT scan or MRI may detect intracranial SOL.

Iris shadow is a concave shadow of the papillary margin of the iris, cast upon the grayish lens, when light is thrown upon the eye from the same side.

It implies that some clear cortical fibers are still present beneath the lens capsule, i.e. between the papillary margin of the iris and the actual opacity. Therefore, it is present in immature cataract.

- **Fundal glow:** It is faint, as the pupillary area is becoming more occupied by the dark shadow.
- **Purkinje's image:** It is the 4th image may be present (but distorted), or absent in advance cases.

Intumescent Cataract

It is seen in some cases of immature cataract, in which the lens becomes swollen due to progressive hydration of the cortical layers. The anterior chamber is shallow, and there may be chance of secondary angle-closure glaucoma.

- **Mature stage (Fig. 15.20B):** The lens is completely opaque.
  - **Vision:** The hand movement to perception of light (PL).
  - **Lens:** White or pearly-white in color.
  - **Iris shadow:** Absent—as the cortex is completely opaque, the papillary margin lies almost in contact with the opacity, separated only by the capsule, the iris then casts no shadow.
  - **Fundal glow:** Absent
  - **Purkinje's images:** Fourth image is absent.
- **Hypermature stage:** If the process is allowed to go on without any intervention, the cortex becomes disintegrated and then

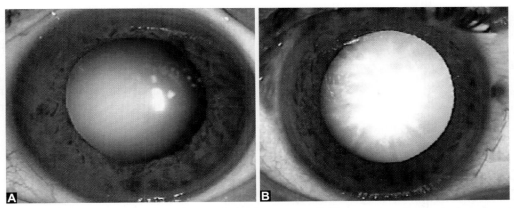

Figs 15.20A and B: A. Immature cataract—iris shadow present; **B.** Mature cataract—iris shadow absent

liquefied, or transformed into a pultaceous mass. It is of two types:

1. ***Morgagnian cataract (Fig. 15.21):*** Here, the cortex liquefies and the nucleus may sink at the bottom within the lens capsule.
   - The cortex appears milky-white and the nucleus appears as a brown mass, limited above by a semicircular line, which may change its position.
   - Anterior chamber may be shallow and may give rise to secondary angle-closure glaucoma.

2. ***Sclerotic cataract (Fig. 15.22):*** The lens becomes more and more inspissated, and shrunken in appearance, due to loss of fluid from the lens.
   - The lens is more flat and yellowish-white in appearance.
   - The anterior capsule becomes thickened due to proliferation of the anterior cuboidal cells, and there may be calcium or cholesterol crystals on it.
- Owing to shrunken lens, the iris becomes tremulous with deep anterior chamber, and finally the lens may be

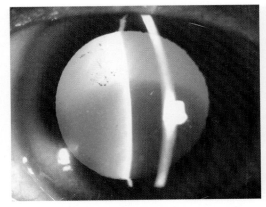

Fig. 15.21: Hypermature cataract—morgagnian

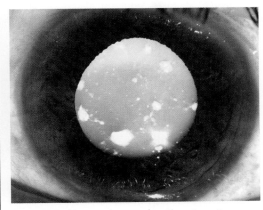

Fig. 15.22: Hypermature sclerotic cataract

subluxated due to degeneration of the zonules.

A long-standing hypermature cataract may give rise to the following complications:

- Subluxation or dislocation of the lens
- Lens-induced glaucoma
- Lens-induced uveitis
- Ultimately, there will be absolute glaucoma with 'no PL.'

Cupuliform Cataract (Posterior Cortical Cataract) (Fig. 15.23A)

The opacity starts in the axial region of the posterior cortex, and slowly progresses to involve the entire posterior cortex. Other types of cataract may supervene on it.

Symptoms

- Marked diminution of vision, as the opacity is near the nodal point of the eye.
- Vision is poor in bright light, especially during the day time (as the pupil becomes constricted in bright light and the opacity is axial). Patients with posterior cortical cataract always see better in darkness (dawn or dusk).

Signs

- It is difficult to see with a torch light in undilated pupil.

- The exact position of the opacity is best judged by a slit-lamp and with ***dilated pupil***. It appears as yellowish-white layer in the posterior cortex.
- In distant direct ophthalmoscopy (with a retinoscope in the dark room)—it appears as a central dark spot against red fundal glow.
- Forth Purkinje's image is blurred.

Nuclear (Hard) Cataract (Fig. 15.23B)

Nuclear cataract tends to occur earlier than the cortical variety, often soon after 40 years of age. At first, the nucleus appears more refractile and as time progresses, it becomes diffusely cloudy and often yellowish in color.

The cloudiness gradually spreads toward the cortex and the lens becomes tinted dark-brown called brown cataract (***cataracta brunescens***). Ultimately, it becomes black, and called black cataract (***cataracta nigra***) (Figs 15.24A to D). The discoloration of the lens in nuclear cataract, is due to deposition of melanin and other pigments derived from photo-oxidation of aromatic amino acids present in the lens.

At maturity, the sclerotic process may extend almost to the capsule, so that, the entire lens functions as a nucleus, but hypermaturity does not occur.

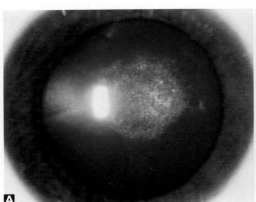
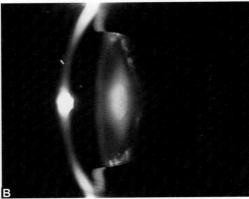

Figs 15.23A and B: A. Cupuliform cortical cataract; **B.** Cupuliform and nuclear cataract

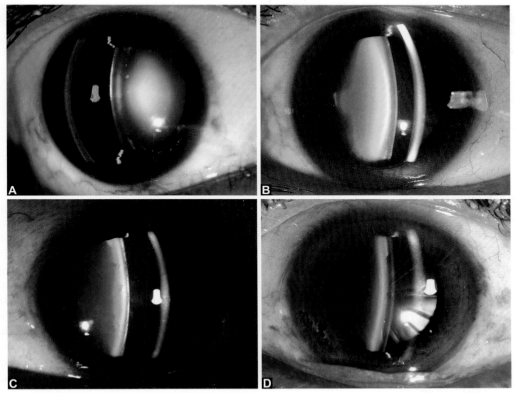

Figs 15.24A to D: Nuclear cataract. **A.** Grade NS II; **B.** Grade NS III: Amber color; **C.** Grade NS IV: Brown cataract; **D.** Grade NS IV+: Black cataract

Symptoms

- *Gradual impairment of vision for distance:* It is initially due to a progressive myopia owing to increased refractive index of the nucleus *(index myopia)*. This myopia neutralizes the plus power of presbyopia. Hence, a patient who was using presbyopic glasses for reading, is able to read better without any glasses when nuclear sclerosis sets in. This is felt as an improvement of vision by the patient, and is termed as *second sight*.
- *Change in color values:* Particularly, with the blue end of the spectrum (as the lens is yellow-brown in color).
- Ultimately, very slowly there will be considerable loss of vision, due to increasing cloudiness of the nucleus.

Signs

- *Vision:* It may be reduced to hand movements in dense opacity.
- *Color of the lens:* It is yellow, brown or black (better appreciated in dilated pupil).
- *Iris shadow:* Usually present.
- *Slit-lamp grading* of the hardness of the nucleus can be judged by the pigmentation of the nucleus. This is essential for phacoemulsification.

Grading of hardness	Appearance of nucleus
Grade 1+ (soft) ↓	Gray or greenish-yellow
Grade2+ ↓	Yellow nucleus
Grade3+ ↓	Amber
Grade 4+ (rock hard)	Brown to black

Difference between immature and mature cataract		
Features	Immature cataract	Mature cataract
Symptoms	• Partial loss of vision • Diplopia/polyopia • Rainbow halos	• Total loss of vision • White opacity noticed by the patients or relatives
Signs • Visual acuity • Color of the lens • Iris shadow • Purkinje's images • Fundal glow • Retinoscopy • Spectacles correction	• Vision reduced to varying degree • Gray/grayish-white • Present • Third image is seen, fourth image may be distorted • Present • Possible • May improve vision	• Vision reduced to hand movement or perception of light (PL) • White/pearly-white • Absent • Only third image is seen, fourth image is absent • Absent • Not possible • Does not improve vision

- **Ophthalmoscopy:** Initially, little change of the fundal glow may be seen with ophthalmoscope, except that the fundus details are hazy. Later, the fundal glow may be entirely blackened.
- **Retinoscopy:** May reveal false lenticonus where the central part of the pupil is myopic and the peripheral part is hypermetropic.

Lens Opacities Classification System III (Fig. 15.25)

The most popular grading system is lens opacities classification system III (LOCS III). LOCS III uses a reference set of standard photographs that defines the extent of opacities in cortical and subcapsular zones and the color/grade of the nuclear opacity. By using LOCS III, the cataract can be classified as: Nuclear color/opalescence = NC/NO: 1–6, cortical opacities = C: 1–5 and posterior subcapsular opacities = P: 1–5.

MANAGEMENT OF CATARACT

Medical Treatment

No treatment can restore the cataractous lens to its original transparent state. Similarly, there is no known method of preventing its progression. The only way is to disperse the lens opacities is to remove the lens.

The medical treatment of cataract is, thus purely symptomatic.
- Frequent and accurate refraction to maintain vision at the best possible level.
- Using optimum illumination and magnifying glasses.
- Weak mydriatics, e.g. phenylephrine (2.5%) for axial opacities to provide visual improvement.

Surgical Treatment

Indications of Surgery

- **For optical reason:** This is by far the most common indication and varies from patient-to-patient. The opacity has progressed to such an extent that the patient can no longer be able to carry out his day-to-day activity efficiently, with best visual correction.
- **For medical reasons:** When the presence of a cataract is adversely affecting the health of the eye, as in:
  - Phacolytic glaucoma.
  - Secondary angle-closure glaucoma due to intumescent cataract.
  - **Vitreoretinal diseases:** Examples are vitreous hemorrhage, diabetic retinopathy or retinal detachment, treatment of which is being hampered by the presence of lens opacities.

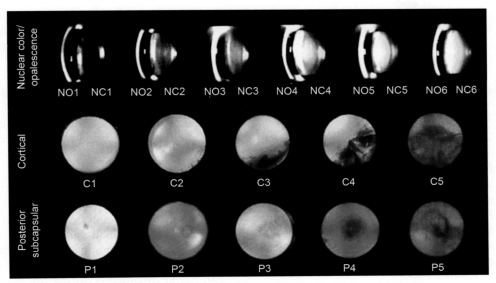

Fig. 15.25: Cataract classification system—lens opacities classification system (LOCS) III

Difference between cortical and nuclear cataract	
Cortical cataract	**Nuclear cataract**
• Usually starts at late 50s • Starts with uniocular diplopia/polyopia or colored halos	• Tends to occur earlier than cortical • No such symptoms
• Give rise to index hypermetropia able spectacles	• Gives rise to index myopia. This myopia neutralizes the plus power of presbyopia and the patient is to see small prints without
• Appears grayish, white to milky-white with the maturity of the cataract	• Appears yellow, brown or black with progression of cataract
• Progress is gradual and ultimately progress into hypermature stage with liquefaction of the cortex	• Progress is very slow and ultimately the entire lens functions as a nucleus, but hypermaturity does not occur
• More chance of lens-induced glaucoma	• Little chance of lens-induced glaucoma

- *For cosmetic reasons:* Rarely, this is an indication in order to obtain a black pupil.

Investigations Prior to Surgery

The main aims of the investigations are:
- To detect underlying local or systemic pathology, which can affect the management adversely.
- To prevent intraoperative or postoperative complications.

- To calculate the power of IOL.
- To predict the visual outcome after surgery.

History

- Any trauma or inflammation of the eye.
- Any posterior segment disease, like macular lesions, venous thrombosis, vitreous hemorrhage, etc. in the past.
- Nature of glasses using in the past.

- Diabetes, hypertension, cardiac problems, bronchial asthma, dental and aural problems, urinary problems, etc.
- Drug allergy.

Local Investigations

Ocular examination

- Vision and refraction of the eye to be operated.
- *Perception of light (PL):* If the eye has 'no PL'—a favorable prognosis for visual improvement is nil.
- *Projection of rays (PR):* It indicates the gross function of the peripheral retina. It tells nothing about the condition of the macula.
- *Importance*
  - An 'accurate PR' excludes the possibility of a large retinal detachment, or an absolute field defect.
  - 'Inaccurate PR' may be seen in retinal detachment, big patch of chorioretinal atrophy, or in advanced stage of glaucoma.
  - 'Inaccurate PR' does not necessarily indicate an inoperable situation, as the opaque media can diffuse light so much that all directional quality may be lost.
- *Pupil:* To examine the light reactions and to estimate the ability of the pupil to dilate before surgery.
- *Slit-lamp examination*
  - To evaluate the type and extent of cataract.
  - To evaluate the health of the cornea, e.g. presence of guttata or frank Fuchs' endothelial dystrophy
  - To find out the evidences of old iridocyclitis, e.g. old keratic precipitates, posterior synechiae or pigments over anterior lens surface.
  - To find out any pathology of anterior segment of the other eye.
- *Intraocular pressure:* It is preferably by applanation tonometer.

- *Patency of the lacrimal passage:* It is to find out any pathology of the lacrimal drainage system and treat accordingly before cataract operation.
- *Fundoscopy*
  - *Eye to be operated* in case of immature cataracts.
  - *Fellow eye* for bilateral lesions like diabetic retinopathy, age-related macular degeneration, etc.

Conjunctival swab for culture and sensitivity tests

- Operation should not be performed in presence of any pathogenic organism. The value of conjunctival swab culture is doubtful, since the conjunctival sac can harbor organisms during the period, between the reporting time and day of operation.
- Most of the surgeons do not advise conjunctival swab culture, and as a routine, advise to use antibiotic drops and ointment into the conjunctival sac for a few days prior to operation.

Calculation of intraocular lens power

There are three ways to decide the power of IOL to be implanted:

1. *Using standard power (+19D):* This is generally no longer acceptable.
2. *Based on basic refraction:* It means the refractive error prior to the onset of cataract. The formula for posterior chamber IOL is:

$$P = 19D + (R \times 1.25)$$
(P = implant power and R = basic refractive error)

Accordingly, a patient with –2.00D myopia will need an implant power of:

$$P = +19D + (-2.00 \times 1.25) = +16.50D$$

It is useful where ultrasound biometry facility is not **available.**

3. ***Using SRK regression formula:*** It requires:
- ***Keratometry*** is to determine the corneal power.
- ***USG-A scan*** is to determine the axial length of the eyeball.

'*SRK*' stands for '*Sanders, Retzlaff* and *Kraff*' and the ***formula is:***

$$P = A - 2.5 \times L - 0.9 \times K$$

Where, **P** = implant power, to achieve emmetropia, **L** = axial length in mm and **K** = corneal power in diopter. **A** = specific constant, which varies with the implant type, design and the manufacturer, e.g. typical A constant for PCIOL = 116.5 or 118.0 or 118.7 and for ACIOL = 115.0, etc.

Formulas for intraocular lens power calculation:
- ***First generation:*** SRK formula (regression)
- ***Second generation:*** SRK II formula (regression)
- ***Third generation:*** SRK/T; Hoffer Q; Holladay 1 formulas (theoretical)
- ***Fourth generation:*** Holladay 2; Haigis formula (regression and theoretical).

Most common regression formulas are the SRK and SRK II. They are popular because of simplicity. SRK formula is best to use when the axial length (AL) is between 22 and 24.5 mm.

Subsequently, SRK II formula is attempted to optimize axial length for short and long eyes. In this formula, a correction factor is added— to increase the lens power in short eyes and decrease it in long eyes.

P = A1 – 0.9K – 2.5L. Where A1 = (A–0.5 greater than 24.5; A1 = A for axial length (AL) between 22 and 24.5; A1 = (A+1) for AL between 21 and 22; A1 = (A+2) for AL between 20 and 21; and A1 = (A+3) for AL less than 20.

Even more customized formulas are required today to calculate anterior chamber depth (ACD) based on AL and corneal curvature. ***SRK/T (T for theoretical)*** is one such formula, representing a combination of linear regression method with a theoretical eye model. The SRK/T and other third generation formulas work best for near-schematic eye measurements; specifically, the SRK/T is best for eyes longer than 26.00 mm. SRK/T calculation, however, does not account for effective lens position (ELP).

Modern theoretical formulas are based on schematic optics and the eye is considered as dual lens system (i.e. IOL and cornea). The predicted distance between them is called ELP, which is used to calculate IOL power. ELP correlates well with IOL placement inside the eye, whether it is in anterior chamber, in-the-sulcus or in-the-bag. It also varies with IOL configuration and the location of its optical center.

In the ***original theoretical formula*** the ELP was considered a constant value of 4 mm for every lens in every patient. Better results are obtained by relating the expected ELP to the axial length, anterior chamber depth, corneal curvature and IOL itself.

Optical biometry is now becoming the gold standard for measuring the eye for IOL power calculations. The two popular optical biometers are:
1. IOL Master—uses partial coherence interferometry (PCI) technology
2. Lenstar—uses low-coherence optical reflectometry (LCOR) technology

Advantages:
- These highly sophisticated machines combine keratometry reading, non-contact axial length measurement and IOL power calculation based on the IOL type
- The newer formulae are built into the system, so everything is done at a single machine
- The machines measure other parameters like—anterior chamber depth, lens thickness, white-to-white diameter which are needed in the newer formulae
- Also, multiple readings are taken for each patient which improves the accuracy.

Disadvantage:
- Expensive
- Technicians need more training to use the system
- Not accurate in mature cataracts or dense posterior subcapsular cataracts
- Patient with poor fixation.

When the AL is between 22.5mm and 26.0 mm, and K value is between 41D and 46D—any modern formula can be used. Outside this range—Holladay 2 and Haigis formula is better. These formulas are programmed into the IOL Master, Lenstar and most modern optical biometry machine, thus eliminating any need for regression formulas.

There are special cases, like postrefractive [radial keratotomy (RK), laser-assisted *in situ* keratomileusis (LASIK) or photorefractive keratectomy (PRK)] cases, post-vitreoretinal surgery cases, especially the silicone-filled eyes—where IOL power calculation for each eye is differently calculated.

> **AL (axial length)**: Distance between the center of the anterior corneal surface and the fovea. It is usually measured by ultrasonography (USG) A-scan or optical coherence biometry. The axial length (AL) is the most important factor in IOL power calculation. 1 mm error in AL measurement results in a refractive error of approximately 3.0D error of IOL power.
>
> Two types of A-scan ultrasound biometry are currently in use—contact applanation biometry and immersion A-scan biometry. Immersion A-scan gives accurate measurement. A mean shortening of 0.25–0.33 mm may be possible with applanation AL measurements, which translates into an error of approximately 1D IOL power.

Macular function tests

These tests are important to predict the visual potential of the eyes with opaque media such as cataract, total leukoma or vitreous hemorrhage.

- *Two-point discrimination test:* This is performed in a dark room. The patient is asked to look through an opaque disc perforated with two pin-holes close together, behind which a light is held. If he can appreciate the presence of two lights— macular function is probably good.
- *Maddox rod test:* The patient is asked to look at a distant light through a Maddox rod. If the red-line of light is continuous and unbroken, macular function is probably good.
- *Color vision test:* If the patient can identify red, green or blue light in presence of an opaque medium—his macular function is good.
- *Pupillary light reflex:* This should be brisk even in presence of a mature cataract. This indicates good optic nerve function.
- *Purkinje's entoptic view of retina:* Patient can see his whole retinal vessels, after pressing the lower lid with an illuminated bulb. An intelligent patient may be able to detect a patch of choroiditis or macular degeneration.
- *Blue-field entoptoscopy:* It allows the observation of one's own leukocytes (flying corpuscles) flowing in macular retinal capillaries.
- *Illuminated Amsler's grid test:* This is useful in assessing macular function in eyes with visual acuity of 6/60 or less.
- *Modified photo stress test:* This is with the help of an indirect ophthalmoscope with at least 6 volts of illumination. A prolonged recovery time indicates a maculopathy.
- *Laser interferometry and potential acuity meter (PAM):* Both the methods are used to estimate the potential visual acuity in terms of Snellen's equivalent. They are helpful in immature cataracts.
- *Foveal electroretinogram (ERG).*
- *Visual evoked response (VER):* It comments on integrity of the macula and optic nerve.
- *USG B-scan*: It gives the valuable anatomical in formations concerning the vitreous and entire retina.

Specular microscopy

It is necessary to count, and to study the morphology of the corneal endothelial cells. It is especially important in cataract with suspected endothelial dystrophy. Normal cell count in elderly subject is 2,000–2,500 cells/ sq.mm. Special precautions are to be taken before an IOL implantation, if the cell count is less than 1,500 cells/sq.mm.

Systemic Investigations

- *Blood pressure:* Any systemic hypertension should be controlled prior to surgery to avoid complications like retrobulbar hemorrhage, hyphema, expulsive hemorrhage, etc. Pre-existing hypertensive retinopathy may be responsible for poor visual prognosis after surgery.
- *Blood sugar postprandial:* Presence of diabetes mellitus increases the risk of infection, delayed wound healing and intraocular hemorrhage. Pre-existing diabetic retinopathy is also responsible for poor vision after surgery.
- Dental and ENT checkup for septic foci.
- Urine for routine and microscopic examination particularly for albumin, sugar and pus cells.
- X-ray chest, electrocardiogram (ECG) and cardiological consultation for selective patients with heart disease.
- Preoperative anesthetic check-up for complicated patients and for children, if general anesthesia (GA) is needed.

Surgical Techniques in Senile Cataract

An increasing variety of cataract extraction methods are being employed depending on the:
- Needs of the patient,
- Availability of the changing technology, and
- Training of the surgeon.

Extracapsular cataract extraction (ECCE)
- Conventional ECCE
- Manual small incision cataract surgery (MSICS)
- Phacoemulsification
- Femtolaser cataract surgery.
  Posterior chamber IOL implantation with any of the above techniques.

Intracapsular cataract extraction (ICCE): It is very rarely done (in grossly subluxated or dislocated lens), resulting aphakia (Figs 15.26A and B).

Lensectomy with vitrectomy: It is in children or in grossly subluxated/dislocated lens.
  Intraocular lens implantation may or may not be possible in ICCE or lensectomy cases.

Glaucoma surgery: It is combined with any types of ECCE with IOL implantation.

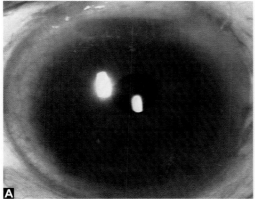 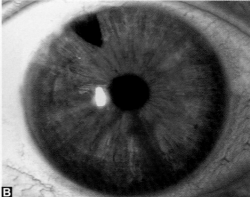

Figs 15.26A and B: A. Pseudophakia; **B.** Aphakia

Vitreoretinal surgery: It is combined with any types of ECCE with IOL implantation.

Keratoplasty: It is combined with lens extraction with or without IOL implantation. Keratoplasty with ECCE with IOL implantation is conventionally called ***triple procedure.***

Each of these techniques have an endless number of variations.

Extracapsular Cataract Extraction

It involves excision of central part of the anterior capsule (anterior capsulotomy), followed by expression of the nucleus and cortical cleaning. The posterior capsule, equatorial region and peripheral part of the anterior capsule are being left intact.

Merits

- Chances of vitreous loss is very minimal.
- The occurrence of vitreous-related anterior segment complication is negligible.
- Less chance of cystoid macular edema (CME) due to intact posterior capsule.
- Less chance of retinal detachment.
- A posterior chamber IOL in-the-bag is usually implanted along with ECCE, which is an ideal IOL (Figs 15.27A and B).
- An intact posterior capsule guards against infection (like endophthalmitis) for a prolonged period.

Demerits

- A difficult microsurgical technique, costly and takes time to master.
- Iridocyclitis and glaucoma due to lens particles are common.
- Opacification of the posterior capsule (after cataract) occurs in a significant number of cases, requiring yttrium aluminum garnet (YAG) laser capsulotomy or needling.
- Extracapsular cataract extraction cannot be done in dislocation and is difficult in subluxation of the lens.

Manual Small Incision Cataract Surgery

Manual small incision cataract surgery (SICS) (or more commonly called SICS) is a low-cost, small-incision form of ECCE that is popular in the developing countries. Compared to conventional ECCE, manual SICS has the advantages of stitchless self-sealing wound with much faster rehabilitation.

In presence poor-resource settings, manual SICS also has several other advantages over phacoemulsification; like—shorter operative time, no need for high technology and also lower cost. Recent studies have shown that, outcomes and complication rates between patients undergoing phaco and manual SICS with PCIOL implantation are comparable.

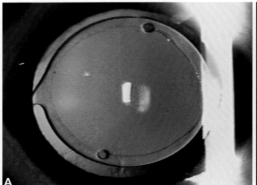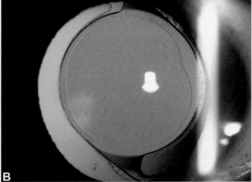

Figs 15.27A and B: Pseudophakia: **A.** Rigid PMMA PCIOL in-the-bag; **B.** Single piece foldable PCIOL in-the-bag

There are several techniques and modifications of performing manual SICS with comparable visual and surgical outcomes.

Phacoemulsification

It is basically an ECCE with the help of a highly sophisticated instrument called *phacoemulsifier*. Here the lens nucleus and cortical matter are emulsified by ultrasonic vibration (using a hollow 1 mm titanium needle vibrating 40,000 times/sec), and then removed by simultaneous controlled irrigation and aspiration. Finally, the whole posterior capsule and part of the anterior capsule are left intact as a *capsular bag*.

It is a safe method of performing ECCE with in-the-bag PCIOL implantation in almost all types of cataracts.

Merits

- Small incision cataract surgery—most of the times suture is not required called *suture less cataract surgery*
- More rapid wound healing
- Shorter convalescence
- Early stabilization of refraction with minimum or no astigmatism.

Demerits

- The equipment is expensive.
- Most difficult technique.
- High incidence of complications by the beginners, like iris damage, wound burn, corneal decompensation, posterior capsular rent or nucleus drop into the vitreous.
- It is difficult to perform in white mature cataract and grade 4+ nuclear cataract. *Operative details* (*see* Chapter 25).

Rehabilitation

A successfully performed cataract extraction is only the first step in the visual rehabilitation of the patient. The optical correction following cataract extraction is dealt elsewhere (*see* Aphakia, Chapter 7).

Intracapsular cataract extraction

In this technique the whole crystalline lens including the capsule is removed by various means, leaving a clear pupillary area.

Merits
- Relatively simple, quick, cheap and suitable for camp surgery.
- No chance of after cataract, since there is no posterior capsule and no need for treatment of after cataract.
- No possibility of developing uveitis and secondary glaucoma due to lens particle.

Demerits
- It cannot be performed safely on patients under 35 years of age.
- Posterior chamber IOL implantation is impossible.
- The incidence of vitreous-related anterior chamber problem is higher, e.g. pupillary block, delayed wound healing, endothelial decompensation, glaucoma, or lately, infection by vitreous-wick syndrome.
- The incidence of postoperative CME is higher.
- The incidence of postoperative (aphakic) retinal detachment is higher.
- Corneal astigmatism is more as the limbal section is larger.

SPECIFIC CATARACT ENTITIES

Complicated Cataract

- Complicated cataract results from a disturbance of the lens-metabolism due to inflammatory or degenerative diseases of the eye, such as iridocyclitis, choroiditis, high myopia, retinitis pigmentosa, retinal detachment, etc.
- The opacity usually commences in the posterior cortex in the axial region (*posterior cortical cataract*). The opacity appears grayish-white with irregular border extending toward the equator and the nucleus in oblique illumination (*bread-crumbs appearance*).

- With slit-lamp examination, the opacity shows a characteristic rainbow display of colors, the *polychromatic luster* (Fig. 15.28).
- The opacity may remain stationary for many years, or it may gradually spread peripherally and toward the nucleus until the entire lens is involved.
- Vision is much impaired even in early stage, owing to the position of the opacity near the nodal point of the eye.

Treatment

- *For inflammatory causes:* ECCE with or without PCIOL under local and systemic steroids.
- *For degenerative causes:* Extracapsular extraction with PCIOL implantation is considered.

Operative and visual prognosis in complicated cataract are usually poor.

Diabetic Cataract

Diabetes mellitus is associated with two types of cataract.

1. *Early onset senile cataract*
2. *True diabetic cataract:* This occurs in poorly controlled juvenile diabetic patients with gross disturbances in water balance.

The opacities are bilateral (Fig. 15.29) and cortical, predominantly involve the anterior and posterior subcapsular region.

- They consist of minute white dots of varying size, like snowflakes (Fig. 15.30) and are usually called *snow-storm cataract*. A true diabetic cataract may progress to complete maturity in less than 72 hours.
- *Mechanism:* Excess glucose in the lens → metabolizes to sorbitol (glucose alcohol) → increase osmolality of the lens → imbibitions of water into the lens → formation of vacuoles in the cortex → opacification.
- During early stage (during water vacuolation) the cataract is reversible, but once the lens proteins undergo coagulation, the opacities become irreversible.
- *Surgery* is usually uncomplicated in diabetic cataract, but associated retinopathy often reduces the visual outcome.

Galactose Cataract

Galactose is the metabolic product of lactose which is the main carbohydrate of milk.

Galactose cataract is associated with two kinds of *recessively inherited* galactosemic enzyme deficiencies:

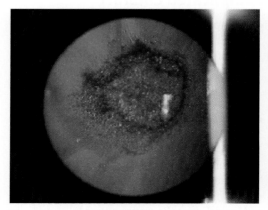

Fig. 15.28: Polychromatic luster in complicated cataract

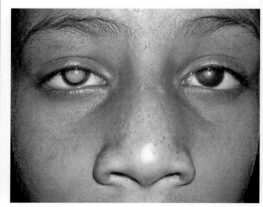

Fig. 15.29: Bilateral cataract in juvenile diabetes

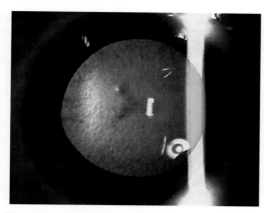

Fig. 15.30: True diabetic cataract—snow flakes

1. ***Classical galactosemia:*** It is caused by the absence of enzyme galactose-1-phosphate-uridyl-transferase (GPUT).
   - ***Ocular features:*** About 75% of the infants with classical galactosemia develop bilateral oil-droplet subcapsular lental opacities which may progress to maturity within a few months unless treated promptly.
   - ***Systemic features:*** It includes diarrhea, vomiting, hepatosplenomegaly, nutritional failure and mental retardation.
2. ***Galactokinase (GK) deficiency:*** It is a milder form and only associated with infantile cataract in an apparently ***healthy child***.
   - ***Mechanism:*** Metabolic pathway from galactose to glucose derivatives is blocked by deficiency of GPUT and GK enzymes → thus blocking the normal metabolic pathway of lens metabolism—instead, shunting of metabolism by aldose reductase to produce dulcitol, a sugar-alcohol similar to sorbitol → increased osmotic pressure causes swelling of the lens → disruption of lens fibers with vacuolation → opacification of the lens.
   - Reducing sugar in urine and red blood cell enzyme assay confirm the diagnosis.

- ***Treatment*** includes removing all lactose and galactose from the diet. This will prevent the development of cataract and even in early stage, it may reverse the lental changes.

Traumatic Cataract

It may be either due to a concussion or penetrating injury (*see* Chapter 24).

Heat Cataract

It is produced by prolonged exposure to infrared rays, and occurs in industry. It is seen among glass-blowers in glass factories (***glass-blower's cataract***) and also among ***iron workers,*** especially tin-plate mill-men and chain-makers.
- The cataract appears as a small disc-like opacity in the posterior cortex which is sharply demarcated.
- There is an associated ***exfoliation*** (true exfoliation) of the lens capsule, in which the lamella of the capsule may be curled up in the papillary area as large sheets.
- ***Mechanism:*** The heat (infrared) rays act not directly on the lens, but are absorbed by the pigment of the iris and ciliary body, and thus influence the lens fibers indirectly.

Posterior Capsular Opacification After-cataract

It is a membranous, white opacity formed by the remnants of anterior and posterior capsules of the lens, following extracapsular cataract extraction and discussion of the congenital or traumatic cataract.

Incidence

In adults, it is about 5–35%, within 1–5 years after the surgery, and more common in children (may be up to 100%).

Mechanisms

- When the cataract is not mature, some soft, clear cortex, sticks to the capsule which may be difficult to remove during operation.
- This gets partially absorbed by the action of aqueous, but, often gets entrapped by adhesion of the remnants of anterior capsule with the posterior capsule.
- In such cases, the cuboidal cells which line the anterior capsule, continue to fulfill their function of formation new lens fibers. These lens fibers under the abnormal condition are abortive and opaque.
- Along with it, organized inflammatory exudates (from iridocyclitis), or fibrin (from hyphema)—may also contribute to the formation of after-cataract.

The after-cataract may be:
- Capsular,
- Capsulolenticular, and
- Pigmentary or hemorrhagic.

Again it may be *Elschnig's pearl type* (Fig. 15.31A) or *fibrous type* (Fig. 15.31B). Elschnig's type causes more visual disability than fibrous type.

- *Elschnig's pearl:* The subcapsular cubical cells proliferate and instead of forming lens fibers, they sometimes, develop into large balloon-like cells which fill the pupillary aperture. This balloon lens-cell looks like pearl, and is known as Elschnig's pearl.
- *Soemerring's ring:* It is ring behind the iris, formed by the lens fibers enclosed between the two layers of lens capsule and found in some cases of after-cataract. It may dislocate into the anterior chamber and causes secondary glaucoma (Fig. 15.32).

Treatment

- *YAG-laser capsulotomy (Fig. 15.33):* This modern technique is especially useful in after-cataract following ECCE with PCIOL implantation.
  YAG-laser acts by photodisruption of the tissue. It is safe, non-invasive (no chance of infection) and a quick OPD procedure.
- *Discission or needling:* When the membrane is thin, then with the help of a Bowman's needle or Zeigler's knife, a gap is made in the central papillary area.
  Repeated needling disturbs the anterior face of the vitreous and subsequently, vitreous gets organized at places which may ultimately lead to retinal detachment in future.
- *Capsulectomy, membranectomy or capsulo-iridectomy:* It is done by using fine scissors, when the after-cataract is dense and adherent to the iris.

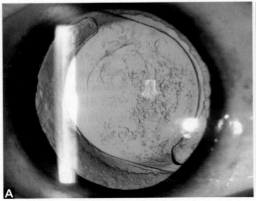 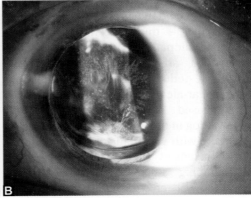

Figs 15.31A and B: Posterior capsular opacification. **A.** Elschnig's pearl type; **B.** Fibrous type

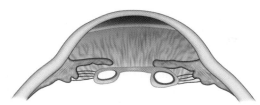

Fig. 15.32: Soemerring's ring in after-cataract

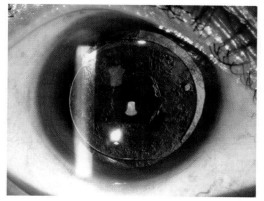

Fig. 15.33: Nd-YAG-laser capsulotomy in posterior capsular opacification

Prevention of PCO formation
• Continuous curvilinear capsulotomy (CCC).
• Good cortical cleaning including the peripheral and equatorial parts.
• Polishing of the posterior capsule.
• Polishing of the under-surface of the remaining anterior capsular ring.
• Insertion of PCIOL in-the-bag.
• Use biconvex PCIOL or plano-convex with convexity towards the posterior capsule.
• In case of capsulorhexis, the margin of the capsular opening must overlap 0.5–1 mm within the margin of the optic of IOL. That means, if the IOL-optic is 6.0 mm, the rhexis diameter should be 5.0–5.5 mm.
• Hydrophobic acrylic IOL has least incidence of PCO.
• Lastly, square-edge optic designed IOL.

SUBLUXATION OF THE LENS (FIGS 15.34 AND 15.35)

This is a condition of the lens in which a portion of the supporting zonule is absent and the lens lacks support in that quadrant.

In subluxation, the lens usually remains in the papillary area, though there may be tilting or displacement in any meridian.

Etiology

- *Congenital ectopia lentis* (discussed)
- *Acquired*

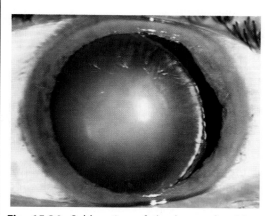

Fig. 15.34: Subluxation of the lens—after blunt trauma

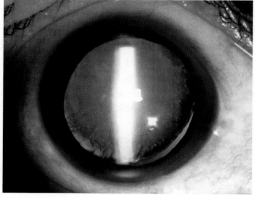

Fig. 15.35: Subluxation of the lens—high myopia

- **Spontaneous**: It is due to:
  - Excessive stretching of the zonules, as in buphthalmos, high myopia or perforation of corneal ulcer.
  - **Degeneration of the zonules**, as in hypermature cataract and patient with latent syphilis.
- **Traumatic:** It is due to tear of the zonules following blunt or penetrating injury.

Symptoms

- Monocular diplopia
- Dimness of vision due to myopic astigmatism.

Signs

- Unequal depth of the anterior chamber.
- Tremulousness of the iris (**iridodonesis**) and the lens (**phacodonesis**).
- Diagnosis should be confirmed after full dilatation of the pupil. The edge of the lens is visible as a dark crescentic line in oblique illumination.
- Indirect ophthalmoscopy may show two images of the disc due to phakic and aphakic zones in the pupil.
- Secondary glaucoma may be present in some cases.

Treatment

- If the lens remains clear and there is no irritative symptom—glasses are prescribed against phakic part to correct lenticular myopic astigmatism.
- Alternately, if the aphakic zone in the pupil is more—aphakic correction may be considered.
- In presence of cataract or irritative symptoms are:
  - **For small zonular tear:** ECCE with PCIOL may be considered. A capsular tension ring (CTR) is helpful in some cases of subluxation. Here, a fine PMMA

(poly methyl methacrylate) made ring is placed within the capsule bag to give support to zonule.
- **If the zonular tear is more:** Intra-capsular cataract extraction with vectis is the treatment of choice. This is then followed by anterior vitrectomy with or without ACIOL implantation.
- Sometimes, a scleral fixation PCIOL may be considered, when the other eye is normal or pseudophakic.

DISLOCATION OF THE LENS (FIGS 15.36A AND B)

This is the condition, in which the crystalline lens is completely unsupported by the zonular fibers, so that the lens is completely displaced from the papillary area.

Etiology

- Same as subluxation of the lens.
- Deliberate dislocation of the cataractous lens in the vitreous cavity (by forcible backward pushing)—an ancient (and unwise) surgical procedure, called couching or reclination. It is still sometimes practiced in rural India by the quacks.

Symptoms

- Marked dimness of vision for distance and near, due to high hypermetropia and loss of accommodation.
- Slight improvement of vision in dislocated hypermature cataract.
- Migration of the dislocated lens into the anterior chamber or vitreous, gives rise the symptoms of uveitis and glaucoma.

Signs

- **Signs of aphakia:** Like, deep anterior chamber, jet black pupil, iridodonesis and absence of third and fourth Purkinje

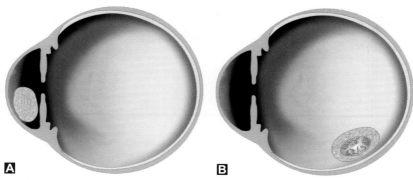

Figs 15.36A and B: Dislocation of the lens. A. Anterior; B. Posterior

images but without an iridectomy, or a limbal scar mark.

- When the lens is dislocated into the anterior chamber and clear—it appears as an ***oil-globule*** due to total internal reflection.
- In posterior dislocation—after dilation of the pupil, the lens can be seen as translucent or opaque mass, lying at the bottom of the vitreous cavity.
- In traumatic cases, associated ocular pathology may also be seen.

Complications

It is more with dislocation of lens than with subluxation:

- Secondary glaucoma
- Severe iridocyclitis
- Low-grade cyclitis due to irritation of the ciliary body region by the lens
- Vitreoretinal degeneration.

Treatment

- ***Anterior dislocation (Fig. 15.37):*** Immediate intracapsular extraction of the lens and vitrectomy with or without implantation of ACIOL.
- ***Posterior dislocation (Fig. 15.38)***
  - No inflammatory signs—dislocated lens may be kept as such, and only aphakic glasses are prescribed.
  - In presence of complication—the lens has to be extracted (lensectomy) along with vitrectomy and then ACIOL may be implanted.

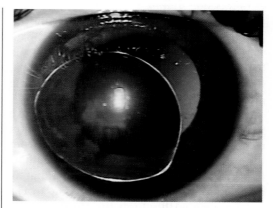

Fig. 15.37: Anterior dislocation of the lens

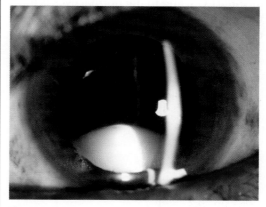

Fig. 15.38: Posterior dislocation of the lens with intact vitreous face

A scleral fixation (SF) PCIOL can be implanted by the experts in this situation. The haptic of the IOL is fixed with sclera with prolene sutures or tissue-glue (called, ***glued IOL***).

Glaucoma

INTRAOCULAR PRESSURE

It is the internal pressure exerted by the intraocular fluids on the coats of the eyeball. The normal intraocular pressure (IOP) is between 10 mm Hg and 20 mm Hg (in contrast, the normal tissue pressure is about 2 mm Hg and intracranial pressure is 7 mm Hg).

Two main factors, concerned with the maintenance of IOP are the rate of secretion of aqueous humor and its rate of outflow from the eye. Most (75%) of the resistance to outflow is in the trabecular meshwork immediately adjacent to the canal of Schlemm (Fig. 16.1).

The ease with which the fluid exits, is indicated as the **coefficient of the facility of outflow** ('C'), and in the normal eyes is more than 0.2 µL/min/mm Hg of pressure within the eye. It is measured clinically by tonography.

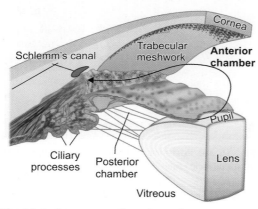

Fig. 16.1: Aqueous outflow channels

Under normal conditions, the rate of aqueous production is relatively constant, so that, in clinical practice, the main determinants of IOP are the **resistance of exit channels,** and the **outflow pressure** (IOP minus episcleral venous pressure).

Factors Modifying Intraocular Pressure

Physiological Variations

The IOP normally fluctuates 2–5 mm Hg throughout the day.

- **With respiration and heart beat:** The pressure fluctuates up to 5 mm Hg with each breath and 1–2 mm Hg with each heartbeat.
- **With time of the day:** A characteristic diurnal variation is seen, with a minimum around 6.00 PM, and a peak on waking in the morning. In normal eyes, this difference seldom exceeds 3–4 mm, but in glaucoma it is often much higher.
- **With the venous pressure:** The Valsalva maneuver causes a rise in episcleral venous pressure, reduces aqueous outflow, and temporarily elevates the IOP.
- **With the arterial pressure:** Transient rise in IOP with the rise of systemic blood pressure.
- **With the osmotic pressure of blood:** When plasma osmolarity rises (as with intravenous mannitol, or oral glycerol), the IOP falls, whereas, reduced osmolarity

(as with water drinking provocative test) raises IOP.

Local Mechanical Factors

- **Dilatation of the pupil:** The IOP may rise if the anterior chamber is shallow, owing to a relative obstruction of the drainage angle by the iris.
- **Changes in the solid content of the eye:** A rise in IOP may result from rapid increase in size of the lens (intumescent cataract) or from the rapid growth of an intraocular neoplasm.
- **Pressure from outside:** IOP rises whenever the lids are closed, and forcible blepharospasm may cause rise of 5 mm or more; while contraction of rectus muscles may equally provoke a significant increase.

Pharmacological Factors

The ciliary muscle is inserted into the trabeculum, so the contraction of the ciliary muscle makes the trabecular meshwork more porous increases the facility of outflow reduces IOP.

- **Outflow facility:** Pilocarpine acts directly on the ciliary muscle to contract, and the coincident miosis is also important in relieving the pupillary block and obstruction of the drain-age angle in acute glaucoma.
- **Outflow facility** is also increased by adrenaline and other β-blockers, and decreased by topical steroids.
- **Reduction of the aqueous production:** Adrenaline and carbonic anhydrase inhibitors are most important.
- **Atropine** produces a slight fall in IOP, possibly by facilitating the drainage of aqueous via uveoscleral route.

Measurement of Intraocular Pressure

- **Manometry:** It is measured by inserting a cannula, directly into the anterior chamber

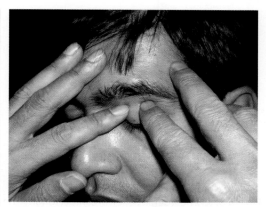

Fig. 16.2: Digital tonometry (finger tension)

which is connected with a manometer. This is the most accurate method, but impossible in clinical practice, and only useful in experimental animals.

- **Digital tonometry (finger tension):** Intraocular tension is roughly assessed by digital palpation, fluctuating the down-turned eye between the two index fingers through the upper lid (above the tarsal plate) (Fig. 16.2).

  This is a routine clinical method and yields a fairly accurate assessment to experienced fingers. It is sometimes recorded as '+', '++', '+++', if increasingly high, or '-', '--', '---', if increasingly soft. In very high IOP—this fluctuation is absent (**stony hard**) and in very low IOP (**phthisis bulbi**)—it is **soft like a water bag.**
- **Instrumental tonometry:** Intraocular tension is measured by two types of tono-meter:
  1. **Contact tonometer (Fig. 16.3)**
     i. **Indentation tonometer:**
        - Schiotz (manual type)
        - Mackay-Marg (electronic type)
     ii. **Applanation tonometer (AT):**
        - Goldmann AT (slit-lamp mounted)
        - Perkins' AT (hand-held)

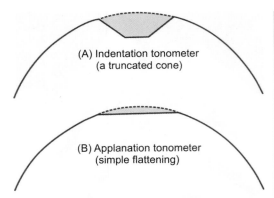

(A) Indentation tonometer
(a truncated cone)

(B) Applanation tonometer
(simple flattening)

Fig. 16.3: Corneal deformation in contact tonometry

2. *Noncontact tonometer (NCT)*

Schiotz (indentation) tonometry (Fig. 16.4A): This is based on the principle, that a plunger will indent a soft eye more than a hard eye. It is constructed in such a way that, when placed on the eye, the plunger together with a present weight, indents the cornea.

The amount of indentation is measured on a scale, and then the corresponding intraocular tension (Fig. 16.4B) (in mm Hg) can be calculated from an accompanying table. The normal IOP in Schiotz tonometer is 14–20 mm Hg.

- *Advantages:* It is cheap, easy to use, convenient to carry and does not require a slit-lamp for measurement.
- *Disadvantage:* Schiotz tonometer (Fig. 16.5) is not so accurate, since the intra-ocular tension recorded, is influenced by ocular (scleral) rigidity.

Scleral rigidity means resistance to distensibility of the outer coats of the eyeball, especially the sclera. Increased elasticity of the outer coats of the eye, is called *low scleral rigidity*. It may occur in high myopia, thyroid exophthalmos, miotic therapy and postoperative eyes. In these cases, Schiotz tonometer may record a falsely low reading of IOP when compared with an applanation tonometer.

Similarly, if the eye has an abnormally **high scleral rigidity** (as in hypermetropic eyes, microphthalmos) a falsely high level of IOP may be recorded.

Abnormalities of scleral rigidity can be detected with a Schiotz tonometer by using two different weights (e.g. 5.5 g and 10 g). If the two measurements are identical, then the scleral rigidity is normal. If there is a discrepancy, then the scleral rigidity is abnormal and the value can be determined by consulting *Friedenwald's nomogram.* The average normal coefficient of scleral rigidity is 0.0215.

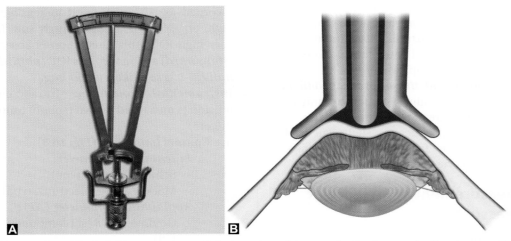

Figs 16.4A and B: A. Schiotz tonometer; **B.** Indentation of the anesthetized cornea by the plunger of the tonometer in order to measure intraocular tension

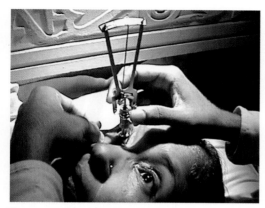

Fig. 16.5: Schiotz tonometry

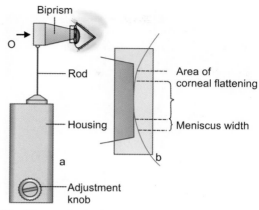

(O = Observer's view)

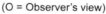

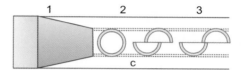

Fig. 16.6: Goldmann-type applanation tonometry. **a**—basic features of tonometer, shown in contact with patient's cornea, **b**—shows tear film meniscus created by contact of biprism and cornea, **c**—view through biprism (1) reveals circular meniscus (2) which is converted into semicircles (3) by prisms

Applanation tonometer: This is based on the principle of *Imbert-Fick's law*. It states that for an ideal, thin-walled sphere, the pressure inside the sphere (p) equals to the force necessary to flatten its surface (F) divided by the area of flattening (A), i.e. P = F/A.

An applanation tonometer measures the IOP by flattening (rather than indent) the cornea over a specific area (applanation of circle with a diameter at 3.06 mm). This is more accurate since the pressure values recorded are not influenced by scleral rigidity.

- *Goldmann applanation tonometer (Fig. 16.6)* is mounted on a slit-lamp and a special plastic prism rests on the cornea, the pressure being adjusted until it achieves a standard disc of contact as outlined by a pre-instilled drop of fluorescein (Fig. 16.7).
- *Perkins' (hand-held) applanation tonometer (Fig. 16.8)* is similar except, that it does not require a slit-lamp, and it can be used even in supine position.

The normal IOP in applanation tonometry (ATn) is 15.5 ± 2.5 mm of Hg. The normal IOP

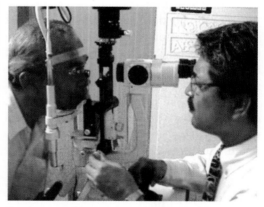

Fig. 16.7: Goldmann's applanation tonometry

ranges from 10 to 21 mm of Hg. If a value is more than 21 mm of Hg, it is considered high IOP.

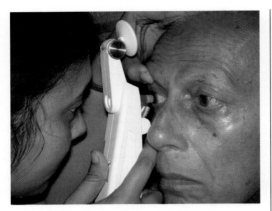

Fig. 16.8: Perkins' applanation tonometry

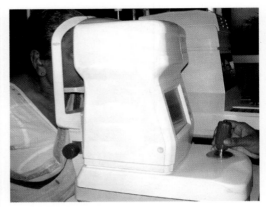

Fig. 16.9: Noncontact tonometry

CORNEAL THICKNESS AND GLAUCOMA

Central corneal thickness (CCT) variations affect the apparent IOP as measured by applanation tonometer. Thinner corneas tend to give a reading of lower IOP whereas thicker corneas tend to overestimate the IOP value falsely. A CCT lower than 555 microns is an independent risk factor for the development of primary open angle glaucoma. When originally devised, it was believed that significant variations in corneal thickness were uncommon and a CCT of 520 μ was assumed in calibration of the Goldmann applanation tonometer.

In each case of suspected glaucoma, especially for the open angle type, it is necessary to measure the CCT by pachymetry. Again, the ultrasonic pachymeter is currently the gold standard.

Different nomograms (Ehler's, Dresdner's, or Doudhty's) are used to correct IOP with CCT variations. But, no nomograms have been identified to this day to be full proof. One may use 15 μ corneal thickness as being equivalent to 1 mm of Hg as a rough average to arrive at the corrected IOP reading.

Other Types of Tonometer

- **Pneumotonometer:** It is an electronic tonometer. It is useful for patient's with corneal scarring or altered corneal shape.
- **Air-puff noncontact tonometry:** No local pediatric is required. No chance of cross infection. Ideal for use in mass glaucoma screening program. Its accuracy is also satisfactory (Fig. 16.9).

DEFINITIONS OF GLAUCOMA

- **Glaucoma** is a symptomatic condition where the functional integrity of the eye is disturbed, resulting in characteristic irreversible loss of visual field due to persistent raised IOP.

> **Glaucoma** is a multifactorial optic neuropathy in which there is a characteristic loss of retinal ganglion cells and atrophy of the optic nerve. Though controversial, this definition of American Academy of Ophthalmology excludes IOP as a criterion and says this is a risk factor.

- **Ocular hypertension:** The patient is having bilateral, high intraocular tension (i.e. above 21 mm Hg) without any field defect, or cupping of the disc. These patients should be kept under observation as some of them may develop open-angle glaucoma in future.

- *Low-tension glaucoma (LTG):* This is also called ***normal-tension glaucoma (NTG),*** in which a few patients develop characteristic field defects and cupping of the optic disc, in spite of normal IOP.

This is a variety of open-angle glaucoma, and may be associated with some cardiovascular abnormality which is responsible for reduced optic nerve head perfusion.

Classification of Glaucoma

Congenital or developmental
- *Primary:* Due to primary developmental anomaly at the angle.
- *Secondary:* Associated with other ocular or systemic disorders.

Acquired
- *Primary*
  - Angle-closure glaucoma (PACG)
  - Open-angle glaucoma (POAG)
- *Secondary:* Associated with some ocular or systemic diseases.

CONGENITAL OR INFANTILE GLAUCOMA (BUPHTHALMOS)

It is a congenital or infantile glaucoma due to aqueous outflow obstruction, as a result of failure of the development of tissue at the angle of the anterior chamber.

ETIOPATHOGENESIS

- ***Primary congenital glaucoma*** (Fig. 16.10) is inherited as autosomal recessive trait.
- Boys are more affected than girls.
- It is usually bilateral.
- Forty percent cases are true congenital, and in 50% of cases, the disease manifest within one year of birth ***(infantile glaucoma) (Figs 16.11 and 16.12).***

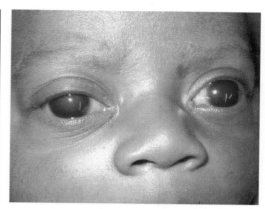
Fig. 16.10: Primary congenital glaucoma—bilateral

- ***Pathogenesis:*** (a) Presence of a cellular membrane ***(called Barkan's membrane),*** obstructs the aqueous outflow. (b) Abnormal cleavage of the anterior chamber angle is responsible.
- ***Associated factors:*** A developmental anomaly, elsewhere in the eye is responsible for obstruction of the aqueous outflow (secondary congenital glaucoma), e.g.
  - Aniridia,
  - Neurofibromatosis,
  - Sturge-Weber syndrome,
  - Rubella syndrome,
  - Mesodermal dysgenesis (Rieger's anomaly and Peter's anomaly), etc.

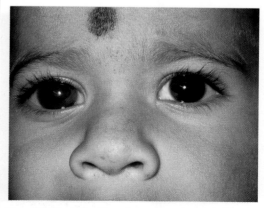
Fig. 16.11: Infantile glaucoma—buphthalmos—right eye

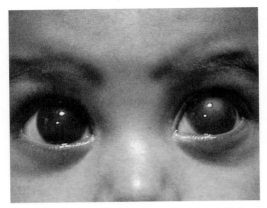

Fig. 16.12: Infantile glaucoma—buphthalmos (both eyes)

SYMPTOMS

- Marked photophobia
- Blepharospasm
- Watering.

SIGNS

- *Eyeball:* It becomes enlarged, if the IOP becomes elevated prior to age of 3 years. This enlarged eyeball due to glaucoma, is known as buphthalmos (means ox-eye).
- *Sclera:* Bluish discoloration.
- *Cornea:* It is enlarged, globular and steamy. Horizontal curvilinear lines are seen on the back of the cornea, known as *Haab's striae* (Fig. 16.13A), and they represent healed breaks of Descemet's membrane (Fig. 16.13B). Corneal sensation is diminished.
- *Anterior chamber:* Deep.
- *Iris:* Tremulousness of the iris with patches of atrophy.
- *Lens:* Flattened, and displaced backward. There may be subluxation.
- *Fundus:* Shows cupping of the disc, but it may regress when the IOP is normalized quickly.
- *Intraocular tension:* High, but it is usually neither marked, nor acute.
- *Refractive error:* The patient becomes myopic. But the amount of myopia is less than anticipated from the increased axial length, owing to flattening and backward displacement of the crystalline lens.

MANAGEMENT

- *Evaluation under anesthesia:* Examination should be performed under general anesthesia. It includes:
  - *Measurement of corneal diameter:* In infant, the mean horizontal corneal diameter is 10.0 mm. If a corneal diameter is more than 12 mm within first year, it is always pathological.

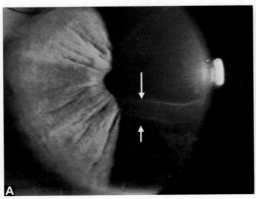
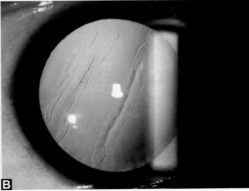

Figs 16.13A and B: A. Haab striae—congenital glaucoma (horizontal curvilinear line) (arrows); **B.** Descemet tear—birth trauma (vertical curvilinear line)

- **Intraocular tension:** It is preferably measured with Parkin's (hand-held) applanation tonometer, as the scleral rigidity is very low in children. The normal IOP in an infant under **Halothane** anesthesia is approximately 9–10 mm Hg, and a pressure of 20 mm Hg or more should arouse suspicion.
- **Gonioscopy:** To study the angle with the help of gonio lens.
- **Treatment**
  - **Medical:** It is of no value. Miotics or β-blocker is given only for temporary period prior to surgery.
  - **Surgical:** Treatment of congenital glaucoma is essentially surgical.
    - **Goniotomy:** An arcuate incision is made with a special knife, halfway between the iris and the Schwalbe's line.
    - **Goniopuncture:** A puncture is made through the whole thickness of the trabecular region into the subconjunctival space.
    - **Trabeculotomy:** A fine metal probe is passed into the Schlemm's canal, and is then swept into the anterior chamber, thus exposing the Schlemm's canal directly to the aqueous humor.
    - **Combined trabeculectomy and trabeculotomy:** It may give the best surgical result amongst all types of surgery.
  - **Rehabilitation:** It is extremely important to detect and treat any refractive error and amblyopia. Corneal opacity may be treated by penetrating keratoplasty.

ACQUIRED GLAUCOMA

PRIMARY ANGLE-CLOSURE GLAUCOMA

Primary angle-closure glaucoma (Fig. 16.14) (PACG) is an acute, subacute or chronic

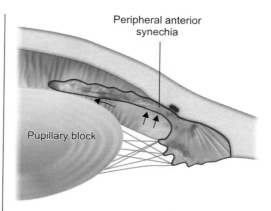

Fig. 16.14: Angle-closure glaucoma

glaucoma, due to obstruction of the aqueous outflow, solely caused by closure of the angle by the peripheral iris.

Etiology

- **Age:** 4th to 5th decade
- **Sex:** Female: male = 4:1
- **Personality:** Emotional, nervous people with unstable vasomotor system.
- **Type of the eye affected:**
  - Small hypermetropic eye
  - Shallow anterior chamber
  - Narrow anterior chamber angle, due to:
    - Smaller cornea,
    - Bigger size of the lens, and
    - Bigger size of the ciliary body.
- **Laterality:** Initially unilateral, but frequently becomes bilateral.

Mechanisms of Angle-closure (Figs 16.15A and B)

- **Pupillary block mechanism:** The initiating event is thought to be a **functional pupillary block** (between the pupillary portion of the iris and the anterior lens surface) in mid-dilated position.

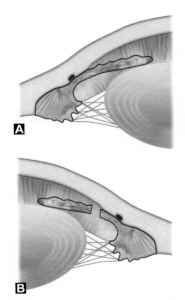

Figs 16.15A and B: Mechanisms of angle-closure. **A.** Pupillary block mechanism; **B.** Plateau iris mechanism. In the second mechanism **(B)**, note the deep central anterior chamber, the flat iris plane, patent iridectomy, and infolding of the peripheral iris at the angle

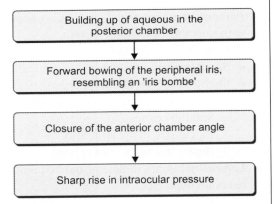

- **Plateau iris mechanism:** It is due to an abnormal anatomical configuration of the anterior chamber angle. The angle is closed by infolding of the iris into the angle in association with pupillary dilatation, but without a significant pupillary block component. Peripheral iridectomy does not help to control IOP in this situation.

Pilocarpine is the only drug which controls this situation. Otherwise, surgery is required.

Stages

It is divided into *five stages*—(1) Prodromal stage, (2) Stage of constant instability, (3) Acute congestive attack, (4) Chronic congestive stage and (5) Stage of absolute glaucoma.

Prodromal Stage

Symptoms
- Colored halos around the light
- Blurring of vision
- Occasional headache.

Signs: Eye remains white and without congestion, even-though, there may be transient sudden rise in IOP up to 40 or 60 mm Hg.

Stage of Constant Instability

This second phase is reached, when intermittency of prodromal attacks is replaced by regularity.

The IOP may rise in the late afternoon and evening, but reduces spontaneously during sleep (as the pupil becomes constricted).

Acute Congestive Attack

An acute congestive attack occurs sooner or later, and is always associated with closure of the angle, and a severe elevation of IOP.

Pathology

The crisis in acute attack is due to acute ischemia, perhaps, associated with the liberation of prostaglandin-like substances. If the attack lasts for several hours or days, irreversible damage may occur to the ocular tissues.

The effects on different ocular structures during and following an acute attack are:
- **Accumulation of the fluid occurs** in all the layers of cornea. This is due to imbibition of fluid in the cornea caused by dysfunction of 'endothelial pump' owing to sharp rise in IOP.

Contd...

Contd...

- *Circumcorneal congestion and chemosis* of the conjunctiva, are due to stasis with increased permeability of the capillaries.
- *Peripheral anterior synechiae* occur as a result of prolonged or repeated acute congestive attacks. Initially, there is iridocorneal contact and later on, the contact becomes iridotrabecular.
- *Pupil is mid-dilated* and oval. Iris shows atrophic changes adjacent to the sphincter muscle. This is due to ischemia of the sphincter pupillae.
- *Glaucom-fleckens* (Fig. 16.16) are small grayish-white anterior subcapsular opacities occur in the pupillary zone. They are diagnostic of previous attack of angle-closure glaucoma, and due to atrophy of the newly formed lens fibers.
- *Optic nerve head* is usually edematous and hyperemic, and is due to anterior ischemic optic neuropathy. Cupping of the optic disc is usually evident after 2 weeks, if the disease passes into chronic congestive phase.

Clinical features of an acute attack

Symptoms

- Acute, intense, unbearable pain, radiating along the distribution of 5th cranial nerve.
- Severe headache often with nausea and vomiting, often mistaken for an acute abdomen.

- Marked dimness of vision, is mainly due to ischemic optic neuropathy, and partly due to corneal edema.
- Redness, lacrimation and photophobia.

Signs

- *Eyeball:* Tenderness present.
- *Eyelids:* Marked edema with narrowing of the palpebral aperture.
- *Conjunctiva:* Both ciliary and conjuntival congestion with chemosis.
- *Cornea:* Steamy and insensitive.
- *Anterior chamber:* Very shallow, cells and flare may be present [but no keratic precipitates (KPs)].
- *Iris:* Pattern is lost and discolored.
- *Pupil:* Mid-dilated and vertically oval (Fig. 16.17). Reaction to light and accommodation are absent.
- *IOP:* Markedly elevated.
- *Visual acuity:* It may be reduced to perception of light (PL) and projection of rays (PR).
- *Fundus:* It cannot be visualized due to hazy cornea.
- But after instillation of glycerin drop (it clears the cornea temporarily), the fundus may be visible with hyperemic optic disc with small hemorrhages, and with spontaneous pulsation of the central retinal artery. There is no cupping.

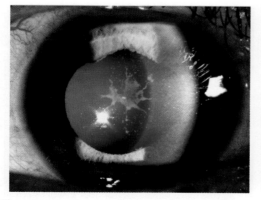

Fig. 16.16: Glaucom-fleckens (spilled-milk appearance)

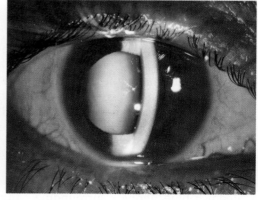

Fig. 16.17: Acute attack of primary angle-closure glaucoma—fixed mid-dilated, vertically oval pupil

- Similarly, after instillation of glycerin drop, gonioscopy shows marked narrowing of the angle, with or without peripheral anterior synechiae.
- The fellow eye, usually has a shallow anterior chamber, and a narrow angle.

Termination of an acute attack

- Spontaneous improvement with lowering of IOP.
- It may pass into chronic congestive stage.
- Recurrence of attacks which may lead to:
  - Marked impairment of vision due to acute-ischemic optic neuropathy, followed by cupping.
  - Irregular constriction of the visual field.
  - Permanent peripheral anterior synechiae when three-fourth part of the iris is attached to the cornea, a 'false angle' is formed. Ultimately, all lead to the chronic congestive stage.
- Rarely, it passes into the absolute glaucoma stage, with total loss of vision (no PL).

Chronic Congestive Stage

This is sometimes called creeping angle closure or chronic angle closure glaucoma, as the angle becomes slowly and progressively closed.

Clinical features

- Visual acuity is always impaired.
- Congested and irritable eye.
- IOP remains permanently elevated.
- Cupping of the disc appears.
- Peripheral anterior synechiae develop, mostly in the upper part of the angle, but gradually spread around the whole circumference.
- Typical glaucomatous field defects become evident. The chronic congestive phase, if untreated, gradually passes into the final stage of absolute glaucoma.

Stage of Absolute Glaucoma

- Painful blind eye with no PL.
- Reddish-blue zone surrounding the limbus, due to dilated anterior ciliary vein.

- **Cornea:** Cloudy and insensitive; there may be associated bullous keratopathy or filamentary keratopathy.
- **Anterior chamber:** Very shallow.
- **Iris:** Patches of atrophy, ectropion of the uveal pigments.
- **Pupil:** Dilated and grayish in appearance. There is no light reaction.
- **Optic disc:** Large and deep cupping with atrophic changes.
- **Tension:** Extremely high (stony hard).

Absolute glaucoma (Fig. 16.18): It is the end stage of any glaucoma, whether congenital or acquired, primary or secondary; and characterized by extremely high IOP (stony hard) with no PL. *Ultimately, the sequelae may be:*
- *Staphyloma formation,* due to continued high IOP → thinning of the sclera.
- *Increased danger of rupture,* from slight injury.
- *Atrophic bulbi:* Continued pressure on the ciliary body → atrophy of the ciliary body → decreased aqueous production → eyeball shrinks atrophic bulbi.

Diagnosis

In the acute and chronic congestive stages, the nature of the condition is usually obvious. But the diagnosis of angle-closure glaucoma, is really difficult in the prodromal stage, and is of immense importance.

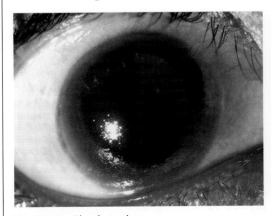

Fig. 16.18: Absolute glaucoma

Diagnostic criteria in early stages are:
- The history of seeing *colored halos,*
- The presence of a *narrow angle* of the anterior chamber, and
- The inducement of a rise of tension *(positive provocative tests).*

Colored Halos

The colored halos are due to accumulation of fluid in the corneal epithelium and alterations in the refractive condition of the corneal lamellae. They are seen around the lighted bulb. The colors are distributed as in the spectrum of rainbow, with red being outside and violet innermost.

Similar colored halos may be seen in early immature cataract. These two can be differentiated by *Fincham's stenopeic slit test,* where a stenopeic slit is passed before the eye, across the line of vision. As it passes, a glaucomatous halo remains intact, but diminished in intensity, whereas a lenticular halo is broken up in segments which revolve as the slit is moved.

If the patient gives a vague history, the halo can be demonstrated to him, by his looking through a thin layer of lycopodium powder enclosed between two glass plates made up as a trial lens.

Gonioscopy

Before gonioscopy, narrow angle may be suspected in presence of shallow anterior chamber by routine torch light oblique illumination (Figs 16.19A and B).

The purpose of gonioscopy (Fig. 16.20) is to identify abnormal angle structures, and to estimate the width of the chamber angle.

Optics

Normally, the angle cannot be visualized directly through an intact cornea, because light rays emitted from angle structures undergo *total internal reflection* (Figs 16.20A to C). A gonioscope eliminates total internal reflection by replacing the cornea-air interface by a new lens-air interface that has a greater refractive index than that of the cornea and tears.

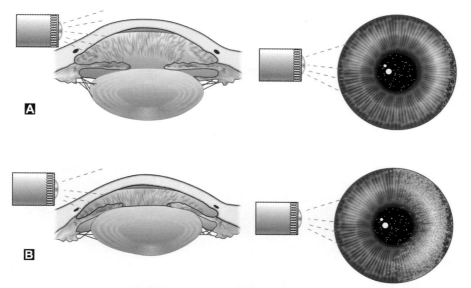

Figs 16.19A and B: Oblique illumination by torch light—a screening measure to estimate the anterior chamber depth. **A.** With a deep chamber, nearly the entire iris is illuminated; **B.** When the iris is bowed forward, only the proximal portion is illuminated, but a shadow is seen in the distal half

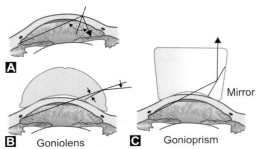

A

B Goniolens   **C** Gonioprism

Figs 16.20A to C: Optical principle of gonioscopy. **A.** As the light from anterior chamber angle exceeds the critical angle at the 'cornea-air interface', it is reflected back in the eye; **B and C.** Contact lenses eliminate total internal reflection and allow light to enter the lens and then be refracted (goniolens) or reflected (gonioprism) beyond the 'lens-air interface'

Mirror

Types of gonioscopy

- *Direct gonioscopy with gonio lenses:* They provide a direct view of the angle. They are used both as diagnostic and operative purposes, e.g. Koeppe, Barkan, Thorpe gonio lens, etc.
- *Indirect gonioscopy with gonioprisms:* They provide a mirror image of the opposite angle, and can only be used under a slit-lamp, e.g. Goldmann single-mirror or three-mirror gonioscope, Zeiss four-mirror gonioscope, etc.

- *Normal angle structures (Fig. 16.21)*
  From anterior to posterior
  - *Schwalbe's line,* is an opaque line which represents the peripheral termination of the Descemet's membrane.
  - *Trabecular meshwork* (degree of pigmentation varies), with occasional visibility of the Schlemm's canal.
  - *Scleral spur* is the prominent white line which represents the most anterior projection of the sclera.
  - *Ciliary band,* a gray or dull-brown band of ciliary body, at the insertion of iris root.

When a gonioscope is not available, *slit-lamp technique of van Herick* may be used with a fair accuracy. Here, the depth of the peripheral anterior chamber (PAC) is estimated by comparing it to the adjacent corneal thickness (CT) 1 mm inside the limbus.

The presence of a narrow-angle of the anterior chamber, as evident from gonioscopy (Figs 16.22 and 16.23), is invaluable in the diagnosis of the disease.

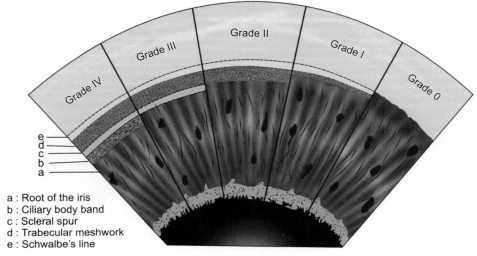

a : Root of the iris
b : Ciliary body band
c : Scleral spur
d : Trabecular meshwork
e : Schwalbe's line

Fig. 16.21: Grading of the anterior chamber angle (Table 16.1)

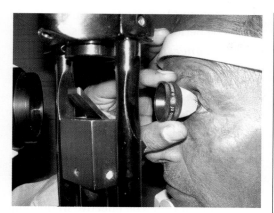

Fig. 16.22: Gonioscopy

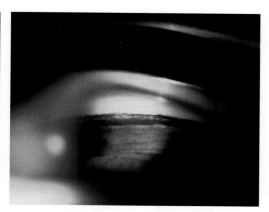

Fig. 16.23: Normal gonioscopic appearance of the angle of the anterior chamber

> ***Van Herick slit-lamp grading of the angle,***
> ***(Figs 16.24 and 16.25)***
> Grade 4 : PAC >1 CT-wide open angle
> Grade 3 : PAC = ¼ – ½ CT-mild narrow angle
> Grade 2 : PAC = ¼ CT-moderately narrow angle
> Grade 1 : PAC <¼ CT-extremely narrow angle

Provocative Tests

These are a variety of tests for ACG suspects and have been designed to precipitate an attack of angle-closure glaucoma in the ophthalmologist's office (where it can be treated promptly).
Physiological provocative tests: Before the test is started, the IOP is recorded.
- ***Dark room test:*** The patient is left in a dark room for 1 hour. He must remain awake so that pupils remain dilated.
- ***Prone test:*** The patient lies in prone position for 1 hour.

- ***Prone-dark room test:*** The patient lies prone in a dark room (awake) for 1 hour. This appears to be the most popular and best physiologic provocative test.
  After one hour, the IOP is measured, and gonioscopy is performed. A pressure rise of 8 mm Hg or more, in presence of a closed angle, is taken as a positive response.
- ***Mydriatic (pharmacological) provocative test:*** A short-acting topical mydriatic (e.g. 0.5% tropicamide) is instilled, and a pressure rise of 8 mm Hg or more, is considered to be positive.
- ***Mapstone's (pilocarpine-phenylephrine) test:*** 2% pilocarpine and 10% phenylephrine are instilled simultaneously every minute for three applications, to achieve a mid-dilated pupil. A pressure rises greater than 8 mm Hg, is considered as a positive response.

TABLE 16.1: Grading of the angle of the anterior chamber (Schaffer's rading)

Grade	Angle	Gonioscopic view	Clinical interpretation
IV	Wide open (35–450)	All structures visible	Closure improbable
III	Open (20–350)	Scleral spur visible	Closure improbable
II	Moderately narrow (10–200)	Trabecular meshwork visible	Closure possible
I	Extremely narrow (<100)	Schwalbe's line visible	Closure imminent
0	Completely closed (00)	Nothing visible	Closure present

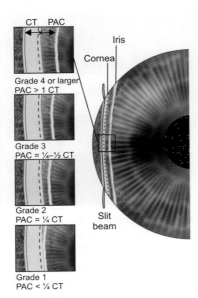

Fig. 16.24: Van Herick slit-lamp grading for estimating the depth of the peripheral anterior chamber (PAC) by comparing it to the peripheral corneal thickness (CT)

- *If the provocative test is negative*, this does not necessarily mean that the angle is incapable of closure in near future. The patient should be warned of possible symptoms of angle-closure and followed up periodically.
- *A positive provocative test* means that the angle is capable of spontaneous closure, but it does not mean that closure is imminent or inevitable. So, the possible complications of iridectomy or Laser iridotomy have to be weighed against the risk of frank ACG.

Management

In early stages (intermittent attacks)

- *Miotic therapy:* Instillation of pilocarpine 2% every 5 minutes, is usually effective in pulling the iris from the angle and aborting the attack. The fellow eye should be treated with 2% pilocarpine, 3 times daily.
- *Yttrium aluminum garnet laser peripheral iridotomy* (YAG PI) or surgical peripheral iridectomy (surgical PI) should then be performed in both eyes.

In acute congestive attack: Although, the treatment of acute PACG is essentially surgical, the initial treatment is medical.

- *Medical therapy*
  - *Tablet acetazolamide (250 mg):* 2 tabs stat, and then followed by 1 tablet 4 times daily, with potassium supplement.
  - *Corneal indentation*: Simple repeated indentations of the central part of the cornea with asquint hook or a sterile swab-stick may be effective in opening the angle. By this maneuver, aqueous will exit from the anterior chamber and the IOP will drop. This is only effective in absence of significant synechial closure of the angle.
  - *Hyperosmotic agents:* They act by drawing water out of the eye and reduce the IOP.
    - *Intravascular injection of mannitol (20%):* The dose is 1–2 g/kg body weight, i.e. 300–500 mL is given intravenously over a period of 30–45 minutes.
    - *Oral glycerol (50% solution):* 30 mL (1 oz) of pure glycerol with equal amount of fruit (lemon) juice stat, and then 3 times daily. Cannot be used in diabetics.
    - *Isosorbide:* It is used orally, and it does not cause nausea. It can be used safely in diabetic patients.
  - *Pilocarpine* (2% or 4%) eye drop is instilled every 5 minutes till the pupil gets constricted, then 3–4 times daily. The *fellow eye* should be treated simultaneously with pilocarpine 2%, 3 times daily.
  - *Strong analgesics* (even injection pethidine) and antiemetic may be needed to reduce pain and vomiting.
  - *Steroid-antibiotic drops* are instilled frequently to reduce congestion.

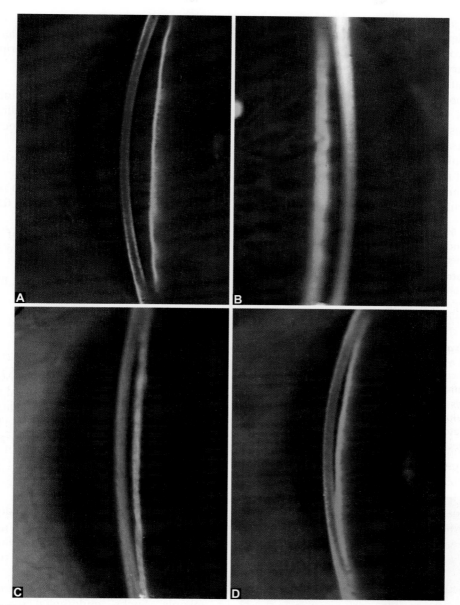

Figs 16.25A to D: Van Herick slit-lamp grading of the angle (see also schematic representation in Fig. 16.24): **A.** Grade 4; **B.** Grade 3; **C.** Grade 2; **D.** Grade 1

Once the IOP has been reduced medically and eye becomes quiet, the further management is:

■ *Continue medical treatment* with pilocarpine 2% drop 3–4 times daily. This is only indicated in old patient with poor general health, and where a laser is not available.

■ *Surgery:* (i) Laser iridotomy or surgical peripheral iridectomy and if necessary, (ii) Filtration surgery.

- **Surgical therapy:** A careful gonioscopy (indentation gonioscopy with Zeiss four-mirror gonioscope is much better) is necessary in deciding the percentage of angle closure by peripheral anterior synechiae, before considering the type of surgery.
  - If the angle-closure (by synechiae) is less than 50%, then laser iridotomy or a surgical peripheral iridectomy should suffice.
  - If the angle-closure is more than 50%, then a filtration operation (e.g. trabeculectomy) is indicated.

Laser iridotomy: In general, Nd:YAG or argon laser iridotomy (Fig. 16.26) has replaced surgical peripheral iridectomy in most cases.

Advantages
- A noninvasive procedure without any chance of infection.
- A painless, OPD procedure.
- It is cheap for the patient.

Disadvantages
- Not widely available, as the instrument is costly.
- Difficult to perform in presence of corneal edema and flat anterior chamber.
- May cause corneal endothelial burns and localized lental opacity.
- Iridotomy hole may be blocked by scar tissue, especially in black individuals.

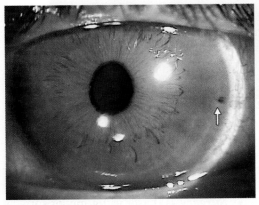

Fig. 16.26: Nd:YAG peripheral iridectomy opening (arrow)

- **Treatment of the fellow eye:** The 'fellow' or second eye is also to be treated by Laser iridotomy or a surgical peripheral iridectomy, as soon as possible.
  - **In chronic congestive stage**
    - Laser iridotomy may be tried initially. If this is unsuccessful, a filtration operation (e.g. trabeculectomy) should be performed.
    - Miotics are not useful at this stage.
  - **In absolute glaucoma stage**
    - **Cyclocryotherapy:** This is to reduce the aqueous secretion and thereby the IOP will reduce.
    - **Retrobulbar injection of 70% alcohol:** This is to destroy the ciliary ganglion.
    - If the pain is still unbearable, the eye may be enucleated.

PRIMARY OPEN-ANGLE GLAUCOMA

Primary open-angle glaucoma (POAG) is a chronic, slowly progressive, bilateral raised IOP with an open angle and associated with glaucomatous cupping and visual field loss. It was previously referred to as **chronic simple glaucoma**.

Etiology

- **Age:** Common in 5th and 6th decade.
- **Sex:** Equal in both sexes.
- **Inheritance:** Probably in a multifactorial manner. In 5–20% cases, POAG runs in family.
- **Ocular association:** Examples are high myopia, Fuchs' endothelial dystrophy, retinal venous occlusion, retinal detachment, retinitis pigmentosa, etc.
- **Systemic association:** Examples are diabetes mellitus, thyroid disorders, cardiovascular abnormalities, etc.
- **Corticosteroid responsiveness:** Individual with POAG or a family history of the disease,

are more likely to respond to chronic steroid therapy with a significant rise in IOP.

Pathogenesis

The elevation of the IOP in POAG is due to obstruction of the aqueous outflow. However, the precise mechanism of outflow obstruction is not known.
- **Electron microscopic picture shows**
  - **Changes in the trabecular meshwork**
    » Faulty collagen of the trabecular tissues.
    » Proliferation of endothelial lining with thickening of basement membrane.
    » Narrowing of intertrabecular spaces, amorphous material in the juxtacanalicular tissue.
  - **Collapse of the canal of Schlemm.**
  - **Sclerosis** of the intrascleral channels.

All lead to increased resistance to aqueous outflow.
- **Immunologically,** there is increased γ-globulin and plasma cells in the trabecular meshwork. In some patients, positive antinuclear antibody reactions have been reported. These findings support an immunogenic mechanism in POAG.

Symptoms

Because of its insidious onset and silent nature, POAG is usually asymptomatic until it has caused a significant loss of visual field. However, the patient may present with:
- Painless, progressive loss of vision.
- Mild headache or eye ache.
- Increasing difficulty in near works, and frequent change of presbyopic glasses. This is due to accommodative failure owing to pressure upon the ciliary muscle and its nerve supply.
- A defect in the visual field (by an intelligent patient).

Signs

- Visual acuity may remain good till the late stage.
- Cornea is usually clear.
- Anterior chamber depth is normal.

- Pupillary reaction remains normal until the late stage.
- Increased IOP with a large diurnal variation.
- Cupping of the optic disc.

The diagnosis of POAG, therefore, depends on classical triad of:
- Raised IOP,
- Cupping of the optic disc, and
- Classical visual field defects.

Raised Intraocular Pressure

Patients with POAG frequently show a wider variation in IOP than normal individuals. A single pressure reading of 21 mm Hg or less does not exclude the diagnosis. So, it is necessary to measure the IOP at different times of the day.

Initially, there is a rhythmic swing in IOP, which is an exaggeration of normal diurnal variation. In most patients, the IOP falls during evening (contrary to what happens in angle-closure glaucoma).
- **Morning rise of tension**—20% of cases.
- **Afternoon rise of tension**—25% of cases.
- **Biphasic rise of tension**—55% of cases.

The difference between the 'peak pressure' and the 'base pressure' gradually diminishes, and a permanent elevation is then occurred above 21 mm Hg.

A variation of IOP over 5 mm Hg should always excite suspicion of glaucoma, even, although the whole reading lies under the limit of 21 mm Hg.

Cupping of the Optic Disc (Figs 16.27A and B)

POAG is usually suspected by finding an abnormal optic disc on routine fundus examination. Documentation of progression or arrest of cupping, together with perimetry, plays a vital role in assessing the efficacy of treatment.

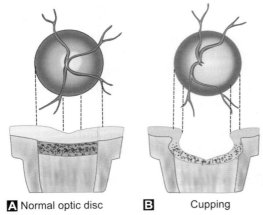

A Normal optic disc **B** Cupping

Figs 16.27A and B: Cupping of the optic disc in compare to the normal optic disc

Ophthalmoscopic appearance of normal disc

- Optic nerve head is vertically oval.
- The central portion of the disc contains a depression, the cup and the area of pallor.
- The tissue between the cup-margin and the disc margin is called as **neural rim**.
- Retinal vessels ride up the nasal wall of the cup often with kinking at the cup margin.
- Most normal eyes have a horizontal **cup disc ratio (C:D)** of 0.3 or less (cup-disc ratio is determined by a ratio between the width of the scleral canal and the volume of glial supporting tissues).
- Large physiological cups (e.g. in myopia or normal subjects) are shallower and do not progress.
- Normal optic nerve heads are characterized by symmetry of the cups and an evenness of the neural rim.

- **Glaucomatous disc changes:** The disc changes of glaucoma are typically progressive and asymmetric, and present in characteristic clinical patterns.
  - ■ **Early glaucomatous changes (Fig. 16.28):**
    - Cupping usually starts as **focal enlargement** at the inferotemporal quadrant, but it may enlarge in concentric circles.

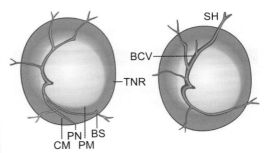

Fig. 16.28: Early disc changes in glaucoma **BS**—Bayonetting sign; **CM**—Cup margin; **PM**—Pallor margin; **BCV**—Baring of circum linear vessels; **SH**—Splinter hemorrhage; **TNR**—Temporal neural rim; **PN**—Polar notching

- **Bayonetting sign:** It is the double angulation of the blood vessels, as they pass sharply backward, and then turn along the steep wall of the excavation before angling again onto the floor of the cup.
- Area of cupping may progress ahead of the area of pallor.
- **Thinning of the neural rim:** It is mostly on the temporal side. It is actually alterations in the neural rim of an eye with glaucoma that leads to changes in the cup as well as to loss of visual field.
- **Nasal shifting** (Figs 16.29A to H) of retinal blood vessels.
- **Splinter hemorrhages** at the disc margin.
- **Baring of circumlinear vessels** may be seen at the disc margin.
- **Progressive enlargement and deepening of the cup** with loss of neural tissue.
- ■ **Advanced glaucomatous changes**
  - **Total cupping (Fig. 16.30):** It appears as a white disc with loss of all neural rim, and bending of all retinal vessels at the margin of the disc. This is also called **bean-pot cupping**, as seen in cross-section (Figs 16.31A and B).

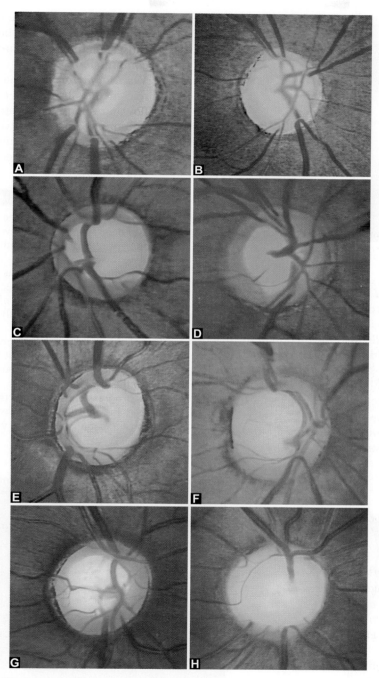

Figs 16.29A to H: Cupping of the disc. **A and B.** Normal and asymmetry of the cup size; **C.** Nasal shifting of blood vessels; **D.** Inferior notching; **E.** Bayonetting sign; **F.** Baring of the blood vessels; **G.** Over-passing phenomena, **H.** Thinning of neuroretinal rim

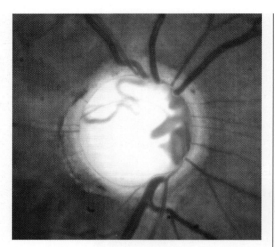

Fig. 16.30: Total cupping of the optic disc

- **Total pallor of the disc,** as there is glaucomatous optic atrophy.
- Openings of the lamina cribrosa are visible up to the margin of the disc—**laminar dot sign.**
- **Pathogenesis of cupping and optic atrophy:** The present evidence suggests that obstruction of the axoplasmic flow with ultimate loss of axons, is involved in the pathogenesis. **Two factors** are responsible for this obstruction:

1. **Mechanical factor:** The elevated IOP forces lamina cribrosa backward and causes death of the neurons by direct compression.
2. **Vascular factor:** Ischemia plays a major role in the obstruction of axoplasmic flow in response of elevated. This leads to atrophy of axons without corresponding increase of supporting glial tissue. Lamina cribrosa becomes weaker and bulges backward.

Retinal nerve fiber layer (RNFL) defects:

In some eyes, in early stages, the retinal nerve fiber layer defects are detected, even prior to the development of cupping and detectable loss of visual field.

The normal RNFL appear as fine parallel striations that cross over the larger blood vessels and enter the disc. Visualization of this striation is best by as ophthalmoscope with red-free light. The changes are:
- **In early glaucomatous damage:** Some of the striations will be replaced by slit-like defects or grooves, mostly one disc-diameter above and below the disc.
- **With progression:** The defects are wedge-shaped and mostly in the lower peripapillary region and baring of the blood vessels.

Contd...

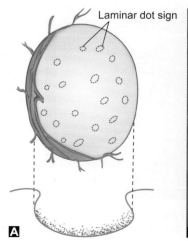

Laminar dot sign

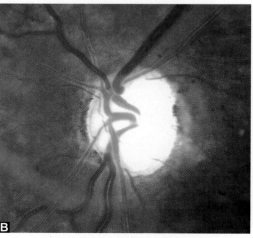

A   **B**

Figs 16.31A and B: A. Bean-pot cupping in cross-section; **B.** Bean-pot cupping of the optic disc

Contd...

- ***In late stage:*** There is total atrophy of the nerve fiber layer and complete baring of the large retinal vessels.

These signs may have prognostic value, since it has been shown to correlate highly with visual field changes, and may precede visual field loss.

Classical Visual Field Defects

Normal visual field

The normal visual field is described by Traquair as ***island of vision surrounded by a sea of blindness***.

- ***Boundary:*** The peripheral limits of the visual field, which normally measures from the fixation points are approximately—60° above and nasally, 70–75° below, and 100–110° temporally.
- ***Point of fixation:*** The area of maximum visual acuity in the normal field, and it corresponds to the foveola of the retina.
- ***Blind spot:*** This is an area of absolute scotoma (***non-seeing area***) within the boundaries of normal visual field, and it corresponds to the region of optic nerve head. It is located approximately 15° temporal to the fixation point.

Testing the visual field

There are several techniques of testing the field of vision.

- ***Confrontation technique:*** It is a rough, but very useful clinical test which should be applied in every case, if there is any suspicion of a defect in visual field.
  It is useful in advanced glaucoma (not in early cases) and in neuro-ophthalmological lesions. If any defect is indicated by this method, it must be accurately mapped out and recorded with the perimeter.
- ***Kinetic techniques:*** This involves moving the test object from a non-seeing area, and recording the point at which it is first seen, in relation to fixation. ***Two basic types*** of screen are used for kinetic visual field testing.

- ***Perimeters:*** The screen may be either an arc or a bowl of a radius of 330 mm.
  - ***Lister's perimeter:*** A rotable arc, capable of being revolved round a pivot, and along which a test object can be moved.
  - ***Goldmann's perimeter:*** A hemispherical bowl, over which a target (a spot of light of adjustable size and illumination) can be directed.

  The Goldmann's perimeter is more standardized, and is preferable for glaucoma examinations, as with this, both the central and peripheral visual fields can be recorded.
  The targets of perimeter consist of circular white disc (or a spot of light) of diameters ranging from 1–10 mm. The ***isopters*** represent the limits of the field of vision with each target, and are accordingly labelled 1/330 (1 mm target at 330 mm distance the radius of perimeter), 2/330, 10/330, etc.
  Colored discs or colored spots of light are exceptionally used for estimation of a differential field loss to color. In normal conditions, ***the blue field is largest***, slightly smaller than the white; then follows the yellow, red, and green. The field for blue and yellow is roughly 10° less in each direction than that for white, that for red and green another 10° less.
- ***Tangent screen (Bjerrum screen):*** It is a black felt or flannel, on which central 30° of the visual field can be studied. Estimation of defects of the central field (scotometry or campimetry) is performed with this screen.
  The screen is normally 1 m square or 2 m square, with the patient is seated at 1 m or 2 m from the screen. With the patient fixing on a white button at the center of the screen, the examiner moves a target

from the periphery toward fixation until the patient indicates recognition of the target. After plotting the blind spot, the procedure is repeated at various directions around the fixation point until the isopter has been mapped (and labelled as 1/1000, 2/1000, 3/1000, etc.). The blind spot normally covers an area, vertically oval, between 12°–18° temporal to the fixation point, and its edges are sharp and abrupt with any target (small or large).

Lister perimetry and Bjerrum screen scotometry have the advantages of low cost and simplicity of operation. They can elicit 80% of field defect, especially in advanced glaucoma. However, their values are limited in glaucoma investigation, as they cannot detect early glaucomatous field defect and are non-reproducible (which is essential for glaucoma management).

- *Static techniques:* In static perimetry, the visual field can be plotted by using a stationary light target of variable brightness against a background whose luminance may be similarly adjusted (either in photopic or scotopic condition).

In general, the static perimetry is superior to kinetic methods for glaucoma patients, as it is more accurate and reproducible.

Automated perimeters

Examples for automated printery are Fieldmaster, Ocuplot, Autofield, Humphrey or Octopus (Fig. 16.32) they are currently being developed which utilize computers to program visual field sequences. They provide exact repeatable tests through a selection of visual field testing procedure. Each of them has an electronic fixation control and an automatic recording of missed points. They are more sensitive than manual perimetry, and always reproducible.

The primary value of automated perimetry at present is to screen the glaucoma patients to

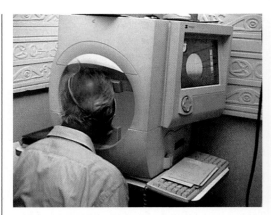

Fig. 16.32: Automated perimetry—Humphrey analyzer

detect early field loss, and also for management. It is to be remembered that field loss cannot be detected before 35% neuronal loss due to glaucoma.

Anatomical Basis of Field Defects (Figs 16.33A and B)

Retinal nerve fibers are distributed in a characteristic pattern. Most fibers reach the nerve head by a direct route, except those are temporal to the macula, which arch above and below the fovea. These *arcuate nerve fibers* do not cross the horizontal line temporal to the fovea. Nasal nerve fibers follow a direct path to the optic nerve head.

The arcuate nerve fibers, related to superior and inferior temporal portion of the optic nerve head, are *most sensitive* to glaucomatous damage.

Macular fibers follow as straight course into the optic nerve head, and get affected last with retention of central vision until the advanced stage of the disease.

The Glaucomatous Field Defects

Isopter contraction: Peripheral isopter contraction may be significantly smaller prior to any field loss.

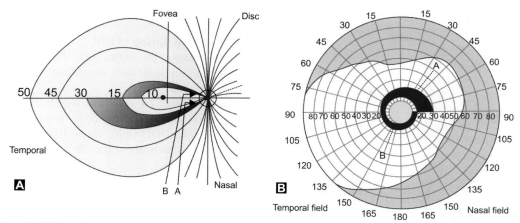

Figs 16.33A and B: A. The course of the nerve fibers in the retina—showing the fibers involved in field defects A and B, in Figure 16.33B; **B.** Arcuate scotomata in the field of vision corresponding with lesions A and B in Figure 16.33A

- **Baring of the blind spot:** It (exclusion of the blind spot) is also considered to be an early field defect in glaucoma.
- **Angioscotomata:** They are long, branching scotomata, above or below the blind spot, which are presumed to be resulted from shadows created by large retinal vessels, and are felt to be an early change.
- **Isolated paracentral scotomata:** One or more isolated paracentral scotomata develop in the Bjerrum or arcuate area (Figs 16.34A to H).

Arcuate or Bjerrum area: An arcuate area above and below the fixation from the blind spot to the median raphe, and corresponds to arcuate nerve fibers.

The nasal extreme may come within 1° of fixation, along the median raphe and extend nasally for 10°–20°.

Defects in superior arcuate area usually occur before those in the inferior area, because of the greater tendency for early glaucomatous cupping in the inferior temporal pole of the optic nerve head.

- **Seidel's scotoma:** A sickle-shaped defect arises from the blind spot and tapers to a point in a curved course with concavity toward the fixation point.

- **Bjerrum's or arcuate scotoma:** A relatively larger area of defect in the form of arching scotoma, which eventually fills the entire arcuate area, from blind spot to the median raphe. With further progression, a double arcuate (ring or annular) scotomata will develop (Figs 16.35A to D).

Other causes of ring scotoma: High myopia, aphakic spectacle correction, retinitis pigmentosa and panretinal photocoagulation.

- **Roenne's nasal step:** The arcuate defects may not proceed at the same rate in the upper and lower portion of the eye. Consequently, a step-like defect is frequently created where the arcuate defects meet at the median raphe. This is called **Roenne's nasal step** and it is mostly superior nasal step, as superior field is involved somewhat more frequently.
- **Generalized constriction of the peripheral field** along with double arcuate scotoma leads to tubular field of vision **(tubular vision)** in which only central vision remains clear.

Causes of tubular vision other than glaucoma: Retinitis pigmentosa, high myopia, central retinal artery occlusion with sparing of cilioretinal artery.

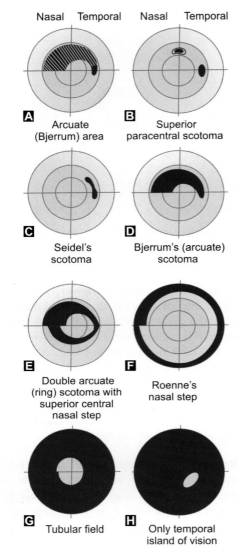

Figs 16.34A to H: Glaucomatous field defects

- Lastly, only *a paracentral temporal island of vision* persists, central vision being abolished.
- Ultimately, all the nerve fibers are eventually destroyed with *no perception of light.*

Investigations

- *Diurnal variation* of IOP.
- *Gonioscopy:* By definition, the anterior chamber angle is open, and grossly normal in eyes with POAG.
- *Tonography:* To estimate the facility of aqueous outflow, which is reduced in POAG. The POC ratio (more than 100) is thought to be more sensitive parameter in this situation.
- *Water drinking provocative test:* Fasting base line applanation tonometric reading is taken in the morning. The patient is instructed to drink 1 liter of water, following which applanation tonometry is performed every 15 minutes for 1 hour.

    Schiotz tonometry is unsatisfactory in this test, as water drinking reduces the ocular rigidity.

    A rise of 8 mm Hg is said to be significant. Performing tonography after water drinking test has an additional diagnostic value. The mechanism of IOP rise is due to increased aqueous secretion due to reduced serum osmolality.

> Other provocative tests, e.g. jugular vein compression, bulbar pressure test, priscol test, caffeine test, etc. are not used nowadays.

- *Slit-lamp examination* of the anterior segment is to rule out other (secondary) causes of open-angle glaucoma.
- *Perimetry and scotometry.*
- *To detect glaucoma in pre-perimetric stage:* Newer devices like—nerve fiber layer analyzer, optical coherence tomography (OCT), GDx VCC, etc. are important (*see* Chapter 28).

Treatment

The aim of the treatment is to prevent the field loss which results from too high an IOP. Optic nerve heads vary in susceptibility to pressure

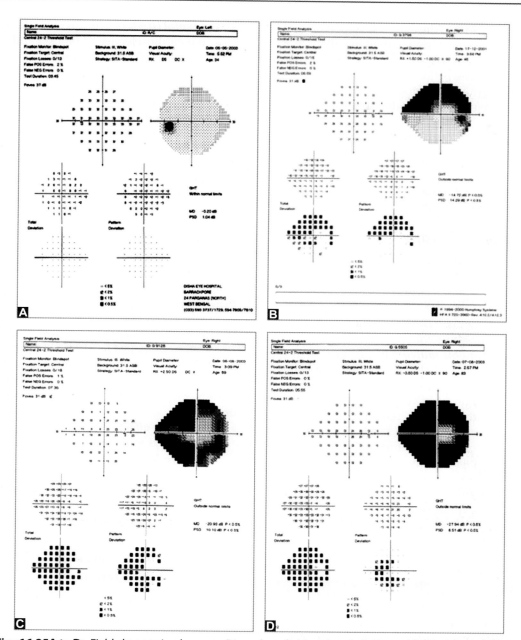

Figs 16.35A to D: Field changes in glaucoma (Humphrey field analyzer). **A.** Normal field; **B.** Upper arcuate field defect with nasal step; **C.** Double arcuate or ring scotoma with nasal step; **D.** Advanced field defect with only paracentral island of vision

damage, so that the danger level of IOP (target pressure) varies from patient to patient.

Treatment requires continued supervision, and it involves periodic tonometry, assessment of cupping (fundus photography is more valuable), and careful mapping of the visual fields.

Modes of Treatment

- Medical therapy
- Laser therapy
- Surgical therapy
- Combination therapy.

Medical Therapy

The treatment of POAG is in the first place, always medical, with operation as a last resort.

Topical therapy

1. **β-blockers:** Timolol maleate, betaxolol and levobunolol.

   1.a: Timolol maleate (0.25% or 0.50%) eye drops, at 12 hourly interval (twice daily).
   - **Mechanism of action:** It is a nonselective β-blocker. It lowers the IOP by reducing the aqueous secretion, as a result of direct action on the secretory epithelium of the ciliary body.
   - It has been seen that IOP responsiveness to timolol decreases with continued use in some patients, and timolol alone may not sufficient to control IOP after 3 months to 1 year after starting the treatment.

Side effects of timolol

- **Systemic:** Bradycardia, hypotension and arrhythmias due to β1 blocking effect; bronchospasm (due to β2 blocking effect); mental depression, sexual impotence, etc. It should not be used in heart block and asthmatic patients.
- **Ocular:** Superficial punctate keratitis, corneal anesthesia (due to membrane stabilizing effect) and reduced tear production.

1.b: Betaxolol (0.5%) eye drops twice daily.
- It is cardioselective β1 blocker and is almost as effective as timolol.
- It has little effects on cardiopulmonary system, and may be used safely in bronchial asthma.

1.c: Levobunolol (0.5%) eye drops twice daily. It is as effective as timolol with lesser ocular side effects.

Advantages of β-blockers
- It is equally effective as other antiglaucoma drugs.
- Convenient dose (twice daily).
- Does not alter the pupillary size or accommodation status.
- It can be safely used in hypertensive.
- Assessment of visual field is better as the pupillary size remains unaltered.

2. **Prostaglandin analogs (PGAs)**

   Prostaglandin analogs (PGAs) act by increasing the uveoscleral outflow by over 100% of physiological levels. It lowers IOP by 25–35% from baseline. The once daily dosing and minimal ocular side effects are advantageous. But there are expensive drugs.
   - **Ocular side effects:**
     - Increased growth and pigmentation of eye lashes (more with bimatoprost).
     - Hyperpigmentation of iris and periocular skin.
     - Conjunctival congestion.

   The common PGAs are:

   Latanoprost (0.005%) eye drop

   Travoprost (0.004%) eye drop

   Bimatoprost (0.03% or 0.01%) eye drop: It is a prostamide, a synthetic prostaglandin analog.

   Tafluprost (0.0015%) eye drop.

3. **Alpha agonists**

   3.a: **Brimonidine tartarate (0.1%, 0.15% or 0.2%) eye drop:**

   It is a selective α-2 adrenergic agonist. It has a peak ocular hypotensive effect occurring at two hours after instillation. Other medicines in this group are clonidine and aproclonidine.

Recommended dose is *two times daily*.

Brimonidine has a *dual mechanism of action*—(i) by reducing aqueous production and (ii) increasing uveo-scleral aqueous outflow.

It has minimal or no effect on cardiovascular or pulmonary functions. But, it *may cause fatigue and/or drowsiness* in some patients.

It is also thought to have some neuroprotective action.

3.b: *Epinephrine* (0.5%, 1% or 2%) eye drops twice daily, and is useful in young patients. It is a nonspecific adrenergic agonist

Mechanisms of action

– It reduces aqueous production due to vasoconstriction (α-adrenergic effect).

– It increases the aqueous outflow by stimulation of β-receptors in the outflow system (β-adrenergic effect).

■ Side effects of epinephrine

– *Systemic:* Increased BP, tachycardia, arrhythmias, tremor, etc. It should not be used in hypertensives.

– *Ocular:* Irritation, reactive hyperemia, conjunctival pigmentation and 'black cornea' (due to deposition of melanin), mydriasis, epinephrine maculopathy (a form of cystoid macular edema seen in aphakic individuals), discoloration of soft lenses, and may reduce the optic nerve head perfusion.

Dipivefrin or dipivalyl epinephrine (0.1%), a prodrug which is converted into epinephrine, after absorption into the eye. It penetrates the cornea better (17 times), and has fewer systemic side effects and does not discolor soft lens.

4. *Topical carbonic anhydrase inhibitors (CAIs)*

Dorzolamide (2%) and brinzolamide (1%) ophthalmic solution, 3 times daily. They lower IOP by reducing aqueous production. Most significant side effect is on corneal endothelium.

5. *Miotics*

Pilocarpine nitrate (1%, 2%, or 4%) eye drop 3–4 times daily. 2% solution is commonly used.

■ *Mechanism in lowering IOP in POAG:* Pilocarpine causes contraction of the longitudinal muscle of ciliary body → pull on the scleral spur → opens up the trabecular meshwork or Schlemm's canal, or both → increased facility of aqueous outflow → lowering of IOP.

■ Miotic effect of pilocarpine is useful in the management of angle-closure glaucoma.

■ Pilocarpine may be administered as ocusert, gel preparation, or with soaked soft contact lens.

Side effects of pilocarpine

■ *Systemic:* Increased perspiration, spasms of smooth muscles causing abdominal cramps or bronchospasm, increased glandular secretion, etc.

■ *Ocular:* Ciliary muscles spasm, leading to brow-ache and induced myopia (more in young patients); miosis may reduce the visual acuity and alter the visual fields, and retinal detachment (by exerting vitreoretinal traction).

Long-acting miotics (like ecothiophate, demecarium bromide, eserine, etc.) are not used nowadays.

Combination of topical therapy: There are multiple fixed-dose-combinations of glaucoma medications and are indicated when IOP control is not satisfactory with any one drug. Combination therapy has advantage of compliance and affordability than using the two same drugs separately.

Commonly used antiglaucoma combinations are: Timolol-Brimonidine; Timolol-PG analog; Timolol-CAI; Brimonidine-Brinzolamide, etc.

Drug group	Mechanism of action	Percentage IOP lowering effect	Examples
β-blocker	Decreased aqueous secretion	20–25%	Timolol, Betaxolol
Prostaglandin analogs	Increased aqueous outflow (uveoscleral)	25–30%	Latanoprost, Travoprost
α-adrenergic agonist	Decreased secretion and increased uveoscleral outflow	15–20%	Brimonidine
Carbonic anhydrase inhibitor	Decreased aqueous secretion	15–20%	Dorzolamide, Brinzolamide
Miotics	Increased aqueous outflow (trabecular)	15–20%	Pilocarpine

Systemic therapy

- **Carbonic anhydrase inhibitors (CAIs)** are used orally to control IOP. They are acetazolamide (250 mg), dichlorphenamide (50 mg), methazolamide (50 mg) and ethoxzolamide (125 mg). Among these, acetazolamide (250 mg), 1–2 tab 4 times daily is used most popularly.
  - **Mechanism of action:** It lowers the IOP by a 50–60% reduction of aqueous production. It acts on secretory epithelium of the ciliary body by creating a local acid environment, as well as by developing metabolic acidosis (**diuretic effect is not a factor in the reduction of IOP**).

Pressure lowering effect is additive when it is used along with topical pilocarpine or β-blockers.

Side effects of carbonic anhydrase inhibitors

- **Systemic:** Metabolic acidosis, hypokalemia (so a potassium supplement is necessary), gastrointestinal upset, renal calculi, paresthesia (tingling sensation) of finger and toes, and blood dyscrasias.
- **Ocular:** Transient acute myopia and rarely dry eye (due to Stevens-Johnson syndrome, an effect of sulfur drug).

Laser Therapy

Argon laser trabeculoplasty (ALT) is indicated when POAG is not well controlled with medical therapy.

- **Mechanism:** Burns in the trabecular meshwork for 360° by argon laser → shrinkage and fibrosis of collagen opening up of intertrabecular spaces → increase in aqueous outflow. It works better in whites than among blacks.

It is safe, noninvasive OPD procedure. The average drop in IOP is 8–10 mm Hg.

Surgical Therapy

The indications for surgical therapy are:

- POAG cannot be controlled with maximal medical therapy.
- The patient cannot tolerate medical treatment, due to toxicity.
- The compliance of the patient is poor, or when the follow-up is unreliable.
- Some surgeons prefer early surgical intervention.

Types of surgery

- **Free-filtering (full-thickness fistula) surgery,** e.g. Scheie's thermosclerostomy, Elliot's sclerocorneal trephining operation, iridencleisis operation, etc. They are no longer practised nowadays.

- **Guarded-filtering (partial-thickness fistula) surgery,** e.g. trabeculectomy, which is routinely practised nowadays (*see* Chapter 25).
- **Newer modifications**
  - Trabeculectomy with antimetabolites, e.g. with Mitomycin-C (MMC) or 5-fluorouracil (5-FU). Here, these drugs act as wound modulators because of their anti-fibroblastic activities. So the chance of fibrosis and postoperative bleb failure is less.
  - **Glaucoma drainage devices (shunt/valve):** Examples are Molteno, Kurpin-Denver, Baerveldt implant, Ahmed glaucoma valve, or Aurolab aqueous drainage implant (AADI) are designed to divert aqueous humor from anterior chamber to an external reservoir, where a fibrous capsule forms about 4–6 weeks after surgery and regulates flow.

    This is done in recalcitrant cases, like previously failed *trabeculectomy* and complicated glaucoma, such as uveitic glaucoma, neovascular glaucoma, iridocorneal endothelial (ICE) syndrome, pediatric glaucoma and also in conjunction with keratoprosthesis.

    The tube is usually placed in the anterior chamber (rarely through pars plana route). In valved variety, when IOP rises, the valve opens and aqueous drains into the subconjunctival space; but as soon as the IOP decreases, the valve automatically closes.

Combination Therapy

A combination of therapy may be required in some cases of POAG, e.g. trabeculectomy and medical therapy, or argon laser trabeculoplasty and medical therapy, etc.

Treatment of ocular hypertension

- The patients with ocular hypertension should be regarded as **glaucoma suspect**.

- They must be kept under observation for periodic analysis of the IOP, cup/disc ratio, and field of vision.
- But, when the IOP is more than 30 mm Hg, the patients are to be treated medically with topical timolol or PGA (latanoprost).

Treatment of low-tension glaucoma

- In this form of POAG, there is no firm evidence that treating the IOP, improves the visual prognosis.
- The most important aspect of the management is the treatment of any cardiovascular abnormality to ensure maximum perfusion of the optic nerve head.
- Nevertheless, most ophthalmologists try to keep the IOP as low as possible with topical antiglaucoma medication.
- Surgery does not help much, if required; trabeculectomy with MMC is the method of choice.

▌SECONDARY GLAUCOMA

It means glaucoma secondary to some preexisting or simultaneous ocular pathology.

While the open-angle and angle-closure aspects are useful in classifying the primary glaucoma, but they are of less value with regard to the secondary glaucoma, since many of these may involve more than one mechanism of outflow obstruction, depending upon the stage of the disease.

Common Types

Associated with Lens Disorders

Pseudoexfoliative glaucoma

Secondary glaucoma with pseudoexfoliation syndrome (Figs 16.36A and B).
- It is due to deposition of fibrillar basement membrane like material, and pigment granules in the trabecular meshwork.
- Characteristic white exfoliative material is seen on the anterior lens capsule in three distinct concentric zone.
- Treatment is same as POAG.

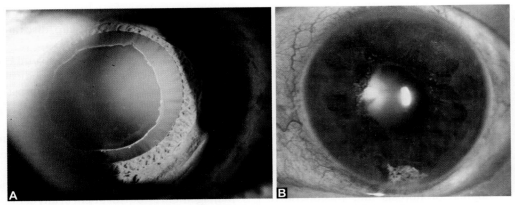

Figs 16.36A and B: A. Pseudo-exfoliation of lens capsule; **B.** Pseudo-exfoliative glaucoma

Phacomorphic glaucoma (Figs 16.37A and B)

- A swollen intumescent cataract (immature or hyper-mature) may cause secondary angle-closure glaucoma.
- Initial treatment is to reduce acute rise in IOP medically, followed by extraction of cataract with or without IOL implantation.

Phacolytic glaucoma (Fig. 16.38)

- A secondary open-angle glaucoma due to microleak of lens capsule in a hyper mature or rarely in a mature cataract.

- IOP-rise is due to obstruction of trabecular meshwork by macrophages which ingest the lens protein.
- Treatment is initially by medical means, followed by cataract extraction.

Lens particle glaucoma

- It occurs typically following extracapsular cataract extraction, or after penetrating injury of the lens.
- It is due to obstruction of the trabecular meshwork by the lens particles, with associated inflammation.
- Residual lens material should be removed surgically either by irrigation or by

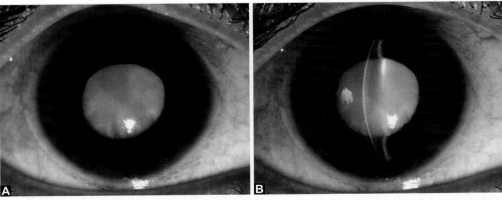

Figs 16.37A and B: A. Phacomorphic glaucoma—with corneal edema; **B.** Phacomorphic glaucoma—note the shallow anterior chamber

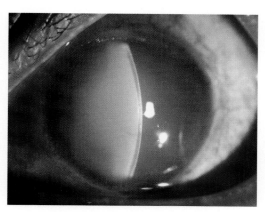

Fig. 16.38: Phacolytic glaucoma—deep anterior chamber with milky cortex

vitrectomy (if associated with rupture of the posterior capsule).

Phacoanaphylactic glaucoma

- Always associated with a latent period, and during that period sensitization to lens protein occurs.
- The typical finding is a chronic 'granulomatous' uveitis.
- Corticosteroids therapy along with antiglaucoma medication is required. When medical treatment fails, the retained lens material should be surgically removed.

Associated with ectopia lentis

- Secondary glaucoma may develop in congenital ectopia lentis, traumatic or spontaneous lens subluxation and dislocation.
- *The mechanisms are* pupillary block, phacolytic glaucoma or angle anomaly with peripheral anterior synechiae.
- Treatment by iridectomy (in pupillary block), or lens extraction (in phacolytic type and when the lens is cataractous).

Pigmentary Glaucoma (Figs 16.39A and B)

- Secondary open-angle glaucoma, occurs in a young, myopic male.
- Pigment dispersion occurs throughout the anterior segment, with loss of pigment from the iris pigment epithelium.
- Deposition of pigment on the corneal endothelium in a vertical line called *Krukenberg's spindle.*
- The glaucoma is due to pigmentary obstruction and subsequent damage to the trabecular meshwork.
- Gonioscopy shows, accumulation of pigment along the Schwalbe's line,

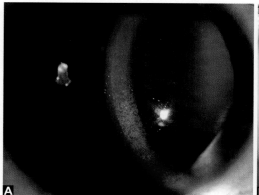
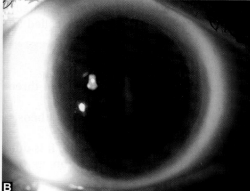

Figs 16.39A and B: Pigmentary glaucoma—Krukenberg's spindle

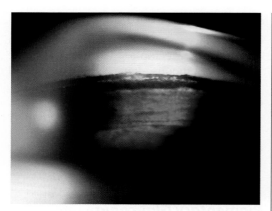

Fig. 16.40: Pigmentary glaucoma—Sampaolesi's line

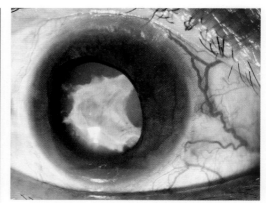

Fig. 16.41: Neovascular glaucoma—rubeosis iridis

especially inferiorly, as a dark line—***Sampaolesi's line*** (Fig. 16.40).

- Iris transillumination shows a characteristic radial spoke like pattern.
- Management is same as POAG and the prognosis is good if detected early.

Neovascular Glaucoma

- Secondary glaucoma is associated with neovascularization of the iris (rubeosis iridis) (Fig. 16.41) and angle of the anterior chamber.
- It is classically seen in:
  - Diabetic retinopathy
  - Central retinal venous occlusion (CRVO) (as the glaucoma usually develops after 3 months, it is called 90 days glaucoma)
  - Sickle cell retinopathy
  - Caroticocavernous fistula.
- Neovascular glaucoma occurs in three stages:
  1. ***Pre-glaucomatous stage*** (rubeosis iridis).
  2. ***Open-angle glaucoma stage:*** It is due to intense neovascularization at the angle.
  3. ***Angle-closure glaucoma stage:*** It is due to contracture of fibrovascular

membrane at the angle leading to goniosynechiae.

- Recurrent hyphema may occur due to hemorrhage from these new vessels.
- Treatment is very difficult
  - ***Prophylactic*** panretinal photocoagulation, panretinal cryocoagulation, or gonio-photocoagulation is helpful in the pre-glaucomatous stage.
  - ***After establishment*** of glaucoma the treatment:
    - Maximal medical therapy
    - Cyclocryotherapy
    - Filtering surgery with antimetabolites or valve implant may be helpful
    - Ultimately, a painful blind eye may require enucleation.

Inflammatory Secondary Glaucoma

The form of ocular inflammation, which most frequently produces secondary glaucoma is iridocyclitis. Other forms of ocular inflammations are keratitis or corneal ulcer, choroiditis, or scleritis.

Associated with iridocyclitis

- It occurs in all forms of iridocyclitis.

- In acute phase, it is due to plasmoid aqueous; and also due to associated trabeculitis (trabecular edema).
- In healed phase, or in chronic iridocyclitis → it is due to posterior synechiae → iris bombe → goniosynechiae and peripheral anterior synechiae.
- Treatment is usually medical. But sometimes, it requires surgical intervention, like iridectomy or synechiolysis, or even filtering surgery.

Glaucomatocyclitic crisis (Hypertensive uveitis)

- It is known as ***Posner Schlossmann's (PS) syndrome (Fig. 16.42).***
- It is an unilateral disease, of middle-aged patients, which is characterized by recurrent attacks of mild acute iridocyclitis with marked elevation of IOP.
- Patient may experience ***slight ocular discomfort with colored halos.***
- Slit-lamp examination (for cells and KPs), and gonioscopy (open-angle) confirm the diagnosis.
- ***Treatment*** is as acute iridocyclitis, in addition, topical timolol, and tablet acetazolamide (***but not pilocarpine***).

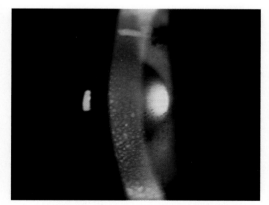

Fig. 16.42: Glaucoma with iridocyclitis—Posner Schlossmann's syndrome

Following perforated corneal ulcer

- If a greater part of iris is adherent with the scar, a secondary glaucoma is developed.
- This is due to shallow anterior chamber with angle-closure in the affected quadrant.
- ***Treatment*** is synechiolysis, and if necessary, trabeculectomy operation.

Glaucoma in keratitis, scleritis or choroiditis

It is usually due to associated secondary iridocyclitis which consequently causes posterior synechiae and rise in IOP.

Traumatic Glaucoma

Blunt injury

- A blunt injury to the eye may cause secondary glaucoma by several mechanisms. In many cases, more than one mechanism is involved. They are:
  - Traumatic iridocyclitis,
  - Hyphema,
  - Massive intraocular hemorrhage,
  - Subluxation or dislocation of the lens,
  - Trabecular damage, and
  - ***Angle-recession (Figs 16.43A and B):*** A late secondary glaucoma occurs with angle-recession. It is due to tear between longitudinal and circular muscles of the ciliary body, and later, by the formation of scar tissue (Descemet's-like membrane) at this area.
- ***Treatment*** is medical. Sometimes, surgical intervention is necessary in case of hyphema, trabecular damage, or in angle recession.

Penetrating injury

- The secondary rise in IOP is due to gross disruption of the ocular tissue (e.g. synechiae, hyphema, dislocation or rupture of the lens, inflammations, etc.).

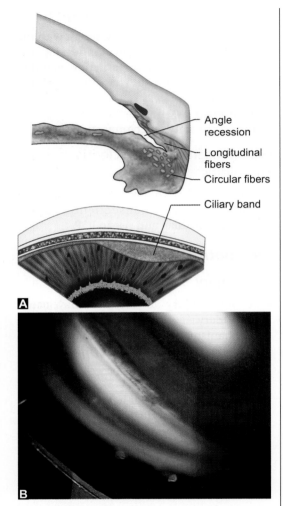

or subnormal pressure; then a slow and sustained rise in IOP occurs, associated with release of prostaglandins.

- **Treatment** is by antiglaucoma medication. Miotics are usually avoided as there is associated anterior uveitis.

Glaucoma with Intraocular Tumors

All intraocular tumor (retinoblastoma, malignant melanoma, metastatic carcinoma, diktyoma, etc.) may cause a secondary glaucoma.

Mechanisms (not by increased volume alone).
- Obstruction of the angle by seeding of neoplastic tissue.
- Angle-closure glaucoma due to forward displacement of lens iris diaphragm by ciliary body tumor.
- Neovascularization of the angle in eyes with retinoblastoma or melanoma.
- Direct extension of the tumor in the angle.
- *Melanomalytic glaucoma:* Due to blockage of trabecular meshwork by melanin containing macrophages (ingestion of necrotic tumor cells by macrophage).

The emphasis of treatment should shift from prevention of blindness to preservation of life.

Steroid-induced Glaucoma

- It is caused by topical, and sometimes, by systemic administration of corticosteroids.
- It occurs more commonly in individuals who have POAG, or a family history of POAG.
- It may occur in chronic (more common) or acute form.
- *Mechanism:* It is an open-angle type of secondary glaucoma, due to reduction in facility of aqueous outflow which is:
  - Due to accumulation of polymerized mucopolysaccharides in the trabecular meshwork, and

Figs 16.43A and B: A. Angle recession with irregular widening of the ciliary band; **B.** Angle recession in gonioscope

- *Siderosis bulbi,* results from intraocular retention of ferrous metal may also cause secondary glaucoma.

Chemical injury

- Both alkali and acid burns produce a rapid rise in IOP, due to shrinkage of the outer collagenous layer of the eye.
- This is followed by a return of normal

Angle recession
Longitudinal fibers
Circular fibers
Ciliary band

- Due to suppressed phagocytic activity of trabecular endothelial cells.
- In general, the anti-inflammatory potency of a topical steroid is proportional to its pressure-inducing effect, and β methasone is most dangerous.
- It is most serious with sub-Tenon or intravitreal injection of triamcinolone; and also with intravitreal injection of depot dexamethasone (Ozurdex).
- Weak steroids, like medrysone and fluorometholone have least pressure-inducing effect.
- Loteprednol (etabonate), a weak corticosteroid has the least pressure-inducing effect. Enzymatic degradation of loteprednol occurs quickly because of its ester based formulation (Other corticosteroids have ketone-based formulations which stay prolonged within tissues with good therapeutic effect).
- *Treatment:* (i) IOP normalizes with steroid withdrawal and antiglaucoma medication, within 1–4 weeks. (ii) trabeculectomy may be rarely needed.
- *Prevention* is by use of weak or dilute steroid (1:10), or nonsteroidal anti-inflammatory drops in susceptible individuals.

Glaucoma Following Ocular Surgery

Secondary glaucoma may be a complication of any intraocular surgical procedure. The important ones are:

Steroid-induced glaucoma

Most common cause after any extraocular or intraocular surgery where steroid drops are given to reduce inflammation.

Malignant (Ciliary block) glaucoma (Fig. 16.44)

- It includes the following features:
  - Shallowing of both the central and peripheral anterior chamber,

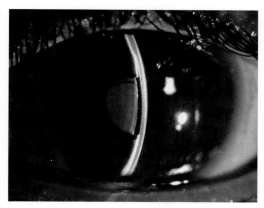

Fig. 16.44: Malignant glaucoma—very shallow (flat) AC following trabeculectomy

- Elevated IOP, and
- Poor response to conventional medical therapy.
- It occurs following peripheral iridectomy or filtering surgery (classical malignant glaucoma), and following aphakia or pseudophakia.
- *Mechanisms:* It is due to posterior pooling of the aqueous as a result of cyclorotation [ciliolenticular or ciliovitreal block (Figs 16.45A and B)] and anterior hyaloid face obstruction. The aqueous accumulates in the vitreous cavity (vitreous pockets), and further pushes lens iris diaphragm forward.
- It must be differentiated from pupillary-block glaucoma, where there is moderate depth at the central anterior chamber with peripheral bowing of iris.
- *Treatment*
  - Mydriatic (phenylephrine) and cycloplegic (atropine) therapy.
  - USG-localization of vitreous pockets and then pars plana vitrectomy and air injection into the anterior chamber.
  - Lens extraction in phakic cases.
  - YAG laser anterior hyaloidotomy.
  - Vitrectomy in aphakic cases.

Glaucoma in aphakia

There are many mechanisms by which cataract surgery can lead to glaucoma.

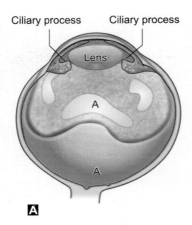 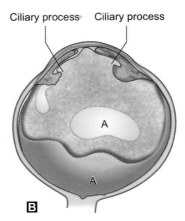

Figs 16.45A and B: A. Concept of ciliolenticular block as the mechanism of malignant glaucoma. Apposition of ciliary processes to the lens equator causes a posterior diversion of aqueous (A) which pools in and behind the vitreous, with a forward shift of the lens-iris diaphragm; **B.** Concept of ciliovitreal block as the mechanism of malignant glaucoma in aphakia. Apposition of ciliary processes against the anterior hyaloid leads to posterior diversion of aqueous (A) which causes a forward shift of the vitreous

- ***In early postoperative period***
  - By distortion of the anterior chamber angle, induced by tight suturing.
  - Delayed reformation of the anterior chamber, and subsequent development of peripheral anterior synechiae.
  - Pupillary-block by air or vitreous, leading to secondary angle-closure glaucoma.
  - Angle is blocked by vitreous or viscoelastic substance itself, leading to secondary acute open-angle glaucoma.
  - Hyphema and iridocyclitis.
  - ***Enzyme glaucoma:*** By use of α chymotrypsin for zonulysis during ICCE, (not used nowadays).
- ***In late postoperative period***
  - Epithelial downgrowth
  - Fibrous ingrowth
  - Peripheral anterior synechiae, presumably due to a flat anterior chamber, or iridocyclitis in early post-operative period.

Treatment
- In early period with antiglaucoma medic-ation, cycloplegics, or laser peripheral iridotomy.

- In late stages, antiglaucoma drugs or conventional trabeculectomy does not help much. Cyclocryotherapy is the treatment of choice in most cases. One may also try for trabeculectomy with antimetabolites.

Glaucoma in pseudophakia

The specific forms of secondary glaucoma in pseudophakic eyes are due to:
- ***Use of viscoelastic materials (like, hydroxy propyl methyl cellulose (HPMC), or Na hyaluronate):*** It causes a marked elevation of IOP during first few post-operative days.
- ***UGH (uveitis glaucoma hyphema) syndrome:*** It means uveitis, glaucoma and hyphema syndrome, and is associated with anterior chamber IOL implantation and sulcus fixation of single-piece hydrophobic IOL implantation.
- ***Pupillary-block glaucoma:*** It occurs more with anterior chamber or iris-supported lens.
- ***Fibrinous iridocyclitis:*** It is particularly in children.
- ***Prolonged use of corticosteroids (steroid-induced):*** It may be an important cause.

Following penetrating keratoplasty, pars plana vitrectomy and retinal detachment surgery

- In PK the additional mechanisms are steroid-induced glaucoma, trabecular collapse due to 360° suturing, and flat anterior chamber.
- In detachment surgery, due to tight buckling, congestion and shallowing of the anterior chamber.
- In vitrectomy, the main mechanism is excessive use of intraocular gas, or silicone oil.
- After intravitreal injection of triamcinolone or Ozurdex (dexamethasone implant).

Due to Elevated Episcleral Venous Pressure

- The features are—(i) dilatation and tortuosity of episcleral and bulbar conjunctival vessels, (ii) moderate rise of IOP and (iii) open-angle with blood reflux into the Schlemm's canal.
- The causes are—(i) thyroid ophthalmopathy, (ii) superior vena cava syndrome, (iii) caroticocavernous fistula, (iv) orbital varices and rarely, (v) idiopathic.
- *Treatment:* Anti-glaucoma medications with treatment of the cause.

Associated with Intraocular Hemorrhage

With fresh hemorrhage in the anterior chamber (traumatic hyphema)

- The pressure elevation is due to obstruction of the trabecular meshwork by fresh blood, and more with clotted blood.
- If the tension is not relieved, blood-staining of the cornea may result within a few days.
- Paracentesis, or opening of the anterior chamber to remove the clots may be necessary to prevent corneal blood-staining and permanent optic nerve damage.

With long-standing hemorrhage (in vitreous hemorrhage)

- *Ghost cell glaucoma:* The degenerated RBCs (less-pliable, spherical, ghost cells) from vitreous cavity enter the anterior chamber where they obstruct the outflow.
- It is a temporary process, and is usually responded by antiglaucoma medication.
- *Hemolytic glaucoma:* Here, the macrophages ingest the contents of RBC in intraocular hemorrhage, and block the trabecular meshwork. It is self-limiting and should be managed medically.
- *Hemosiderotic glaucoma:* Iron in the hemoglobin causes siderosis (in massive intraocular hemorrhage) which produces tissue alterations in trabecular meshwork, and cause obstruction to aqueous outflow.

Epidemic Dropsy Glaucoma

- It rarely occurs in an epidemic form, due to consumption of adulterated mustard oil by *Argemone mexicana.* The poisonous alkaloid is called *sanguinarin*.
- It is associated with massive generalized edema, cardiomegaly, widespread capillary dilatation, and rarely peripheral neuritis.
- *Mechanism:* Increased capillary permeability of the ciliary epithelium, leads to increased formation of aqueous (*hypersecretion glaucoma*).
- The IOP-rise is bilateral, acute and very high (above 50 mm Hg), and the patient presents with colored halos, eye ache and dimness of vision in both eyes.
- The eyes are non-congested, with normal anterior chamber depth and the angles are open.
- *Treatment:* Tablet acetazolamide and topical timolol are very effective in reducing IOP. With general treatment, the IOP usually comes down to normal.

CHAPTER 17

Diseases of the Vitreous

VITREOUS HUMOR

The vitreous humor is an inert biologic gel, which serves only optical function. It has a volume of about 4.5 mL. It comprises two-thirds of the volume of the eyeball and three-fourths of the weight. Although, its viscosity is derived from hyaluronic acid, 99% part of the vitreous humor is water. It possesses no blood vessels in postnatal life and is incapable of becoming inflamed.

Composition of Vitreous Humor

The vitreous humor (80% of the volume of the eyeball) is a delicate, optically clear gel composed of a highly-hydrated double network of protein fibrils and charged polysaccharide chains. By weight, vitreous is composed of ~99% water and 0.9% salts. Protein and polysaccharide components constitute remaining 0.1%.

The composition of vitreous humor:
- Water (~99%)
- Inorganic salts
- Sugar
- Ascorbic acid
- Large molecules of hyaluronic acid
- Peripheral cells (hyalocytes)
- A network of collagen fibrils (type II fibers with glycosaminoglycan).

   Vitreous humor has a viscosity 2–4 times that of water, giving it a gelatinous consistency and a refractive index of 1.336.

   Metabolic exchange between systemic circulation and vitreous humor is very slow. That is the reason why vitreous humor is sometimes the fluid of choice for postmortem analysis of glucose levels or other substances.

Symptoms and Signs of the Diseases of the Vitreous

- *Three main symptoms*
  1. Decreased vision due to opacities, hemorrhage or membranes.
  2. Floaters (visualization of materials floating in the vitreous).
  3. Flashes of light on ocular movement (photopsia).
- *Examination of the vitreous*
  - Gross vitreous opacities can be seen with a direct ophthalmoscope.
  - With indirect ophthalmoscopy, opacities are visible against red background of the fundus.
  - Slit-lamp microscope with –40D or 50D contact lens equipped with inclined mirror (three-mirror gonioscope).
- *Ultrasonography A-scan or B-scan* to find out the exact anatomical location of the vitreous pathology in presence of hazy media.

Degenerations

Syneresis

- The vitreous humor becomes partially or completely fluid, creating an appearance of strands or membranes floating freely in the vitreous.

- It occurs in aging, myopia, and following injury or inflammation of the eyes.
- They are easily visible with the ophthalmoscope or slit-lamp.
- No treatment is available to restore the integrity of the vitreous.

Normal attachment of the vitreous

It is firmly attached in the following regions:
- *At the vitreous base:* It is a 3–4 mm wide zone at the ora serrata, where the cortical vitreous is firmly attached to the peripheral retina and pars plana.
- *At the optic disc margin:* It is firmly attached.
- *Around the fovea:* It is rather a weak attachment. In other areas, the cortical vitreous is attached loosely to the internal limiting membrane of the sensory retina.

VITREOUS DETACHMENT

Vitreous detachment occurs in three forms— (1) posterior, (2) anterior and (3) basal.

Posterior vitreous detachment (Fig. 17.1)
- It is a senile phenomenon and more common in diabetics.

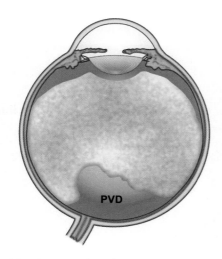

Fig. 17.1: Vitreous detachment
PVD—Posterior vitreous detachment

- It appears spontaneously, and produces sudden onset of floaters and photopsia.
- The photopsia are more common on the temporal field, and are due to vitreoretinal traction.
- On examination, floaters are seen in front of an optically empty space, adjacent to the posterior retina.
- The condition is benign, unless it is associated with other pathology like retinoschisis, a retinal break or diabetic retinopathy.
- At the onset, the patient must be examined carefully, especially the peripheral retina with an indirect ophthalmoscope.

Anterior and basal vitreous detachment: They occur secondary to blunt trauma, and are accompanied by vitreous hemorrhage.

VITREOUS OPACITIES

Many foreign substances may be suspended in the vitreous humor—(i) exogenous material, e.g. parasites or foreign bodies, or (ii) endogenous materials, e.g. leukocytes, red blood cells (RBCs), tumor cells, pigments, cholesterol crystals or calcium salts. All opacities cause the symptoms of floaters and some of them may cause severe impairment of vision.

Muscae Volitantes

- These physiologic opacities represent the residues of primitive hyaloid vascular system.
- The patient sees them as fine dots and filaments, often drift in and out of the visual field, against a bright illumination or background (e.g. blue sky).
- The opacities may cause disturbances to sensitive individuals, especially among myopes.
- Correction of ametropia (if required), with reassurance is the only treatment.
- Laser vitreolysis may be a treatment option in sensitive individual.

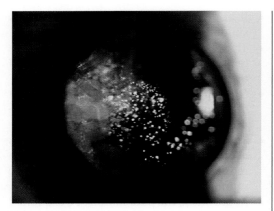

Fig. 17.2: Asteroid hyalosis

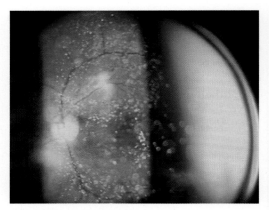

Fig. 17.3: Synchysis scintillans

Asteroid Hyalosis (Fig. 17.2)

- This is an involutional, mainly binocular phenomenon that affects the aged male patients.
- They appear as white, round or discoid bodies suspended throughout, or in a portion of the solid vitreous.
- The opacities exhibit slight oscillations in normal vitreous with ocular movements.
- They consist of various calcium containing lipids, and apparently result from the degeneration of vitreous fibrils.
- They do not cause symptoms, or do not require treatment (although they may obscure the view of the fundus).
- Pars plana vitrectomy may be required if it is very dense.

Synchysis Scintillans (Fig. 17.3)

- It affects the damaged eyes which have suffered trauma or inflammation in the past.
- It is due to deposition of the cholesterol crystals in the liquid vitreous.
- The crystals appear as multicolored glittering particles which settle at the bottom of the vitreous cavity, and can be thrown up by ocular movements to form a golden shower.

- If the lens is removed intracapsular cataract extraction (ICCE), the crystals may be observed both in the anterior chamber and in the vitreous cavity.
- Associated diseased condition may be responsible for poor vision in these eyes.
- No effective treatment is known.

Persistent Hyperplastic Primary Vitreous (Fig. 17.4)

- The hyaloid vascular system is atrophied by the 8th month of gestation, and sometimes, leaving only minute remnants which are visible as muscae volitantes.

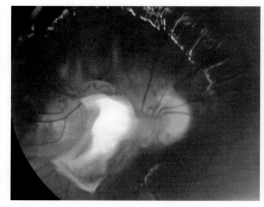

Fig. 17.4: Persistent hyperplastic primary vitreous—posterior type

- Failure of the hyaloid artery to regress, combined with the hyperplasia of the posterior portion of vascular meshwork, produces persistent hyperplastic primary vitreous (PHPV).
- It is a unilateral condition and the eye is smaller than the fellow eye due to faulty development. Bilateral cases of PHPV may be associated with Patau's syndrome (Trisomy 13) or Norrie's disease.
- A white pupillary reflex is noticed in the full-term infant shortly after birth.
- Associated abnormalities are microphthalmos, cataract, glaucoma, long and extended ciliary processes, and intraocular hemorrhage.
- The anterior chamber is shallow and the retrolental tissue contracts to pull the ciliary processes inward.
- The cause of cataract is rupture of the posterior lens capsule.
- It must be distinguished from other causes of white pupillary reflex, e.g. congenital cataract, retinopathy of prematurity, retinoblastoma, endophthalmitis and retinal dysplasia.
- Lens removal (preferably by pars plana lensectomy with vitrectomy) should be done as early as possible (1 day to 4 weeks of age) to preserve some vision.
- Visual prognosis is often poor due to development of amblyopia.

▌VITREOUS HEMORRHAGE

Vitreous hemorrhage may occur as a preretinal phenomenon, or an intravitreal phenomenon or a combination of both.

Etiology

- *Retinal break:* Due to *trauma* or by *vitreous traction* causing retinal tear, and subsequent rupture of the retinal blood vessels.
- *Rupture of newly formed blood vessels* originating from the optic disc and retinal capillaries. The causes are:

  ▪ *Eales' disease:* It is the retinal periphlebitis (probably due to hypersensitivity of vessels to tuberculoprotein) and subsequent development of neovascularization. Rupture of these new vessels lead to recurrent vitreous hemorrhage. It occurs in young male patients.
  ▪ *Retinal venous occlusion:* Usually after 3 months of occlusion, capillary microaneurysm and new vessels formation occur, and vitreous hemorrhage may arise from these delicate new vessels.
  ▪ *Proliferative diabetic retinopathy:* It may be due to rupture of fine new vessel arising from the disc (NVD) or from elsewhere (NVE) (Fig. 17.5).
  ▪ *Sickle-cell retinopathy:* Sea-fan neovascularization occurs, particularly at the superior temporal peripheral areas of the retina.
  ▪ Retinopathy of prematurity (ROP).
- *Operative:* Following retinocryopexy, retinal detachment surgery or vitrectomy (rebleeding).
- *Terson's syndrome:* Rupture of a subhyaloid hemorrhage secondary to subarachnoid hemorrhage.

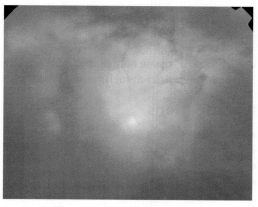

Fig. 17.5: Vitreous hemorrhage from neovascularization at the disc (NVD)

Symptoms

- Sudden onset of floaters to significant loss of vision.
- Blurring of vision with a red haze.

Signs

- In mild cases, there may not be any sign ophthalmoscopically.
- In moderate to severe cases, the fundus cannot be visualized with an ophthalmoscope. Indirect ophthalmoscopy may be helpful in moderate vitreous hemorrhage.
- No fundal glow is visible by distant direct retinoscopy with a plain mirror.
- With slit-lamp, a reddish mass may be visible in the anterior vitreous.

Fate of Vitreous Hemorrhage

- The blood (small or massive) may be evenly distributed throughout the vitreous humor, localized or distributed in sheets.
- Absorption of blood usually takes place without organization and the vitreous becomes clear within 4–8 weeks. In a young person resorption may be rapid.
- Organization of hemorrhage does occur in persistent or recurrent bleeding, and is followed by formation of yellow or white debris and fibrous membrane in the vitreous (Fig. 17.6).
- Ultimately, retinitis proliferans develops, which is more common near the optic disc from which the fibrous strands stretch forward.
- This fibrous tissue contracts, and leads to a tractional retinal detachment.

Investigations

- Blood pressure
- Routine hemogram
- Estimation of blood sugar
- Tests for tuberculosis

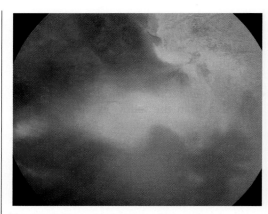

Fig. 17.6: Organized vitreous hemorrhage

- ***Ultrasonography:*** B-scan is helpful to establish the diagnosis, as well as to rule out any associated retinal pathology (e.g. retinal detachment)
- ***Macular function tests*** before surgery.

Treatment

Medical

- Bed rest with head elevation and eyes are padded, so as to minimize the dispersion of blood.
- Patient is periodically followed up and indirect ophthalmoscopy is done whenever possible.

Surgical: If the hemorrhage remains unabsorbed even after 6 months, a closed pars plana vitrectomy with laser photocoagulation (endolaser) should be considered.

Fellow eye: The fellow eye should be examined thoroughly and treated actively.

Prevention: Whenever a neovascularization is diagnosed, as in proliferative diabetic retinopathy, retinal venous occlusion or sickle cell retinopathy, laser photocoagulation should be done so that the new vessels are regressed.

PROLAPSE (LOSS) OF THE VITREOUS (FIG. 17.7)

- After removal of the intact lens (ICCE), or rupture of the posterior lens capsule [in extracapsular cataract extraction (ECCE)], the anterior vitreous may herniate into the anterior chamber to fill it completely.
- The consequences that result from operative loss of vitreous, are not at all related to the loss of vitreous bulk itself, but to the morphologic changes those occur in the vitreous body.

The complications of vitreous prolapse (loss) are related to one of the following mechanisms:
- Direct contact of the vitreous with other structures (such as the cornea or the angle structures).
- Incarceration of the vitreous into the operative wound.
- Fibroplasia of the residual vitreous.
- Inflammation.

The list of consequences is as follows:
- Excessive degree of astigmatism
- Bullous keratopathy due to damage of the corneal endothelium
- Epithelial and fibrous ingrowth
- Secondary glaucoma

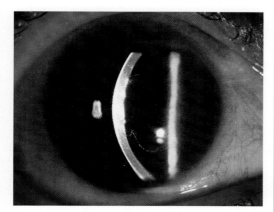

Fig. 17.7: Vitreous prolapse in anterior chamber after posterior capsular rent—vitreocorneal touch

- Updrawn or hammock pupil
- Wound infection and endophthalmitis (Vitreous Wick Syndrome)
- Vitreous opacities and formation of tractional bands
- Cystoid macular edema
- Tractional retinal detachment
- Chronic ocular irritability
- In case of posterior chamber intraocular lens (PCIOL) implantation the lens cannot be placed properly and the implantation is abandoned, due to fear of further problems.

Treatment

Therapeutic

- Vitreous loss at the time of surgery is treated by means of an anterior (open-sky) vitrectomy to ensure that no vitreous is between the wound edges and no traction upon the vitreous base.
- A sector iridectomy is usually done, and this may be combined with inferior sphincterotomy.

Preventive

- Readjustment of the preoperative medication and choice of anesthesia.
- Surgery on a soft eye which is achieved by hyperosmotic agents (e.g. injection mannitol) and bulbar massage after giving peribulbar block.
- Satisfactory anesthesia and akinesia.
- Reduction of external pressure on the globe.
- Use Flieringa's ring to prevent scleral collapse in selected cornea grafting cases.
- Microscopic visualization and proper instrumentation are necessary in ECCE.

VITRECTOMY

Removal (excision) and replacement of the vitreous is known as ***vitrectomy***.

Indications for vitrectomy

- **Persistent vitreous opacities**
  - Hemorrhage
  - Preretinal membranes
  - Vitreous membrane and strands.
- **Complications of cataract extraction**
  - Vitreous touch with bullous keratopathy
  - Malignant glaucoma
  - Loss of vitreous (posterior capsular tear)
  - Incarceration of vitreous in wound with traction
  - Removal of dropped nucleus or intraocular lens from the vitreous cavity.
- **Endophthalmitis with vitreous abscess**
- **Trauma**
  - Removal of intraocular foreign body
  - Removal of subluxated or dislocated lens.
- **Complicated retinal detachment**
  - Giant retinal tear
  - Retinal dialysis
  - Massive vitreous traction.
- **Congenital cataract and ectopia lentis**
- **Persistent hyperplastic primary vitreous.**

Types

There are two types of vitrectomy—(1) open-sky vitrectomy and (2) pars plana (closed) vitrectomy.

Open-sky Vitrectomy

It is performed through a large corneal or limbal section. It is necessary to remove the lens first. It is especially indicated in:

- Vitreous loss occurred during cataract extraction
- Aphakic keratoplasty
- Removal of dislocated or subluxated lens
- Anterior chamber reconstruction after trauma.

Pars Plana (Closed) Vitrectomy

It is employed to restore the optical pathway of the eye. If the opacities are confined to the vitreous cavity the prognosis is good.

Vitrectomy is done through a 1–3 mm incision via the pars plana route, called pars plana vitrectomy (PPV). As the vitreous is removed from the eyeball by cutting and suction, physiologic solution is infused into the eye to balance the suction.

An operative microscope with coaxial illumination and fine sophisticated instruments are necessary for vitrectomy.

Now-a-days, 23G pars plana vitrectomy is commonly used by the vitreoretinal surgeons. It does not require conjunctiva and Tenon's dissection and sclerotomy wound suturing. Modern 25G or 27G PPV is also transconjunctival sutureless procedure.

TA-assisted Vitrectomy

In both types of vitrectomy, triamcinolone acetonide (TA) injection is given routinely to stain the vitreous for better visualization.

Vitreous Substitutes

The vitreous replacement is necessary for:

- Restoration of intraocular pressure, and
- Repositioning the retina in different vitreoretinal surgeries.

Vitreous substitutes

- **Air:** As an internal tamponade.
- **Physiological solutions,** e.g. Ringer's lactate and balanced salt solution (BSS).
- **Gases:** They are better than air and give longer period of internal tamponade, e.g. sulfur hexafluoride (SF_6) and octafluoropropane (C_3F_8). They are used as a 40% mixture with air.
- **Silicone oil**
- **Sodium hyaluronate**
- **Perfluorocarbon liquid (PFCL):** It is heavy and mainly used to assist removal of dislocated lens nucleus or IOL from the vitreous cavity.

Diseases of the Retina

SYMPTOMS AND SIGNS

- Diminution of vision without pain.
- *Night blindness:* In diseases those predominantly affect the function of rods.
- *Peripheral constriction of the visual field* or *scotoma* may be present corresponding with the areas, especially affected.
- *Metamorphopsia (distorted images) micropsia (small images), or macropsia (large images):* It may be present in macular lesions.
- *Photopsia* (sparks or lightning flashes) occurs due to traction upon the retina.
- *Frequently*, the patient is unaware of symptoms, and the abnormality is only detected during routine ophthalmoscopic examination.

OPHTHALMOSCOPIC FINDINGS

- *Disturbances of the blood vessels:* Examples are vascular pulsation, venous dilatation, arteriovenous ratio and arteriovenous crossing changes, any abnormal vascular reflex, neovascularization of the disc (NVD, and/or elsewhere—NVE), hemorrhages (superficial or deep), and microaneurysms.
- *Opacities in the sensory retina*: Examples are soft exudates (cotton-wool patches), hard exudates, hemorrhages, edema residues and glial tissue proliferation.
- *Disturbances in the attachment of the sensory retina:* Examples are rhegmatogenous retinal detachment (with a retinal break) and non-rhegmatogenous retinal detachment (without a retinal break).
- *Disturbances in the retinal pigment epithelium (RPE):* Examples are decreased or increased pigmentation (dark areas).
- *Abnormalities of Bruch's membrane:* Examples are breaks in Bruch's membrane with replacement by fibrous tissue, as in angioid streak and drusen. Both of these conditions favor the formation of subretinal neovascular membrane.
- *Peripheral retinal lesions*, are best seen with an indirect ophthalmoscope, or Goldmann's three mirror gonioscope by a slit-lamp.
- Appearance of the normal fundus as seen with the direct ophthalmoscope (Fig. 18.1).

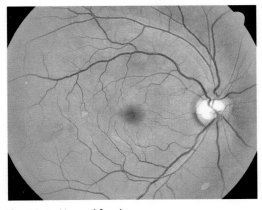

Fig. 18.1: Normal fundus

EXAMINATION OF THE FUNDUS

- *Examination with a retinoscopic plane mirror from 1 m distance:* To know the fundal glow and refractive status of the patient's eye.
- *Examination by an ophthalmoscope or a plane mirror at 22 cm distance (distant direct ophthalmoscopy):* Opacities in the anterior segment can be readily visualized.
- *Direct ophthalmoscopy:* The details of central retina are examined under higher magnification (15 times). The image is direct and erect, seen uniocularly.
- *Indirect ophthalmoscopy:* With this up to the peripheral portion of retina is visualized. Magnification is 3–5 times. But the image is real and inverted. Depth of lesion is better judged as it is binocular.
- *Slit-lamp* and special lenses:
  - Hruby lens
  - Fundus contact lens
  - Three-mirror contact lens
  - +90 D or +78D lens.

Fundus examination includes:
- *Fundal glow:* Good, poor or absent.
- *Optic disc:* Margin, color, size, shape, cup-to-disc ratio, neural rim, venous pulsation, any abnormal vessels or lesions.
- *Retinal blood vessels:* Vascular reflexes, A-V ratio, A-V crossing, any abnormal or new vessels.
- *Macula and foveal reflex:* Any abnormality, i.e. cyst, hole, hemorrhages, edema, scar, etc.
- *General fundus:* Any abnormality, e.g. exudates, hemorrhage, pigmentation, scar, new vessels, detached area, coloboma, folds, etc.
- *Peripheral fundus:* It is (best seen by an indirect ophthalmoscope) for retinal break (hole/tear), degenerated area, pigmentation, exudation, etc.

- *Choroidal blood vessels:* Normally not visible, but in case of sclerosis they are visible as ribbons.

METHODS OF OPHTHALMOSCOPY

There are two forms of ophthalmoscopy—(1) *Direct* and (2) *indirect*.

Direct Ophthalmoscopy

The hand-held direct ophthalmoscope is designed to provide a direct magnified (×15) view of the fundus. The source of illumination is projected by means of a mirror or prism coinciding with the observer's line of vision through the aperture.

- The ophthalmoscope is held close to the observer's eye and approximately 15 cm from the patient's eye.
- It is held in the right hand to examine patient's right eye and in the left hand to examine patient's left eye.
- The observer uses his/her right eye to examine patient's right eye and left eye for patient's left eye.
- The patient should fix on a distant target with the eye as steady as possible.
- The observer have to adjust ophthalmoscope power setting to accommodate for the patient's refractive error and/or his/her own.
- If both patient and observer are emmetropic, the lens is set at zero. A red reflex will be seen and is considered normal.
- Moving the ophthalmoscope as close to the patient's eye as possible and using the plus or minus lens, the observer will able to see central retina in detail up to the equator.
- Lens setting at more plus power will focus the ophthalmoscope in the vitreous or more anterior.

Indirect Ophthalmoscopy

This technique is generally used by retina specialist and involves the use of a head mounted, prism directed light source coupled with use of a high condensing lens (+14, +20 or +30D) to see the retinal image. A +20D condensing lens is more commonly used.

The retinal image formed by indirect ophthalmoscopy is inverted, real and capable of being seen at the focal plane of the lens.

The image is brilliantly illuminated, binocular stereoscopic one that covers approximately 10 times of the area compare to direct ophthalmoscope. The image is, however, smaller (×3 times). It is essential to see retinal periphery to locate different types of lesions. Because of its stronger illumination, it allows light to pass through moderate opacities in the media which are obstructive to direct ophthalmoscope.

CONGENITAL AND DEVELOPMENTAL ABNORMALITIES

Myelinated Optic Nerve Fibers (Fig. 18.2)

- The myelin sheaths of the optic nerve fibers cease normally at the lamina cribrosa.

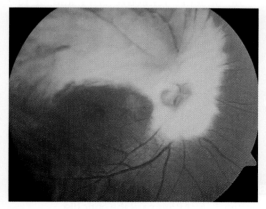

Fig. 18.2: Myelinated optic nerve

- Sometimes, this myelination extends a short distance over the retinal surface adjacent to the disc.
- **Ophthalmoscopically**, they appear as white patches with radial striations at peripheral edges. Usually the patches are continuous with the disc, but occasionally they are isolated. The retinal vessels are covered at places by the opaque fibers.
- When present, the blind spot is often enlarged, or a scotoma corresponds with the position of the patch.
- They must be differentiated from soft exudates, as seen in hypertensive retinopathy, and from papilledema.
- The myelin sheaths disappear in optic atrophy (due to any cause) and no trace of abnormality remains.
- No treatment is required.

Phakomatosis

This is a group of conditions (hamartomas) in which there are congenital, disseminated, usually benign tumors of the blood vessels or neural tissues. They are often ocular, cutaneous, and intracranial in location.

The variety of conditions are:
- Neurofibromatosis **(von Recklinghausen)**
- Tuberous sclerosis **(Bourneville)**
- Angiomatosis retinae with cerebellar hemangioblastoma **(von Hippel-Lindau)**
- Encephalotrigeminal angiomatosis **(Sturge-Weber)**
- Ataxia telangiectasia **(Louis-Bar)**
- Encephalo-retino-facial angiomatosis **(Wyburn Mason).**

Neurofibromatosis (von Recklinghausen's Disease)

- It is the most common type, with typical subcutaneous nodules and *cafe-au-lait spots*.
  Ocular manifestations: Plexiform tumors of lids with ptosis, thickened corneal nerves, Leish's spot (Fig. 18.3) on the iris

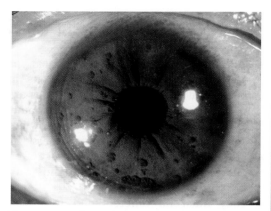

Fig. 18.3: Leish's nodules in neurofibromatosis

pulsating proptosis (due to transmitted cerebral pulsations through the defects in the orbital walls), glioma of the optic nerve, and congenital glaucoma.

- Operative measures are seldom satisfactory.

Tuberous Sclerosis (Figs 18.4A and B) (Bourneville's Disease)

- The diagnostic triad are epilepsy, mental retardation and adenoma sebaceum (angiofibroma). It is also called *epiloia-epi* (epilepsy)-*loi* (low IQ)-*a* (adenoma sebaceum).
- *Ocular lesion:* Multiple nodular tumors are seen springing from the optic disc, like white mulberries (astrocytoma).

- Glial hamartomas of the cerebrum result in seizures, and acoustic nerve is most frequently involved.

Angiomatosis Retinae (Fig. 18.5) (von Hippel-Lindau's Disease)

- It is classically seen in the retina and in the cerebellum.
- *Ophthalmoscopically:* It is a reddish, slightly elevated tumor is seen in the retina, which is nourished by dilated large retinal artery and vein. The retina becomes spattered with hemorrhages and exudates, ultimately leading to vitreous hemorrhage, retinal detachment and secondary glaucoma.
- When localized, the secondary complications can be prevented by photocoagulation.

Encephalotrigeminal Angiomatosis (Sturge-Weber's Syndrome) (Fig. 18.6)

- There is *nevus flammeus* (Port-Wine stain) along the distribution of the trigeminal nerve of the affected side.
- There is an associated *choroidal hemangioma* which may result in a congenital or childhood glaucoma.

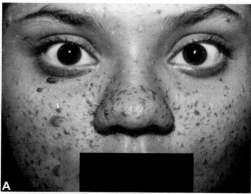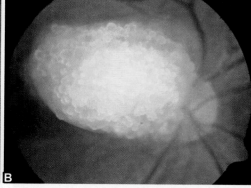

Figs 18.4A and B: Tuberous sclerosis. **A.** Adenoma sebaceum; **B.** Astrocytoma of the optic disc

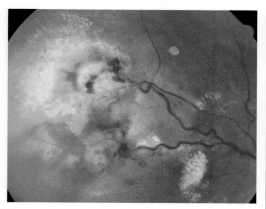

Fig. 18.5: Angiomatosis retinae

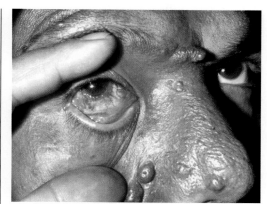

Fig. 18.6: Sturge-Weber's syndrome

- Focal seizures and mental retardation are also common.
- A characteristic X-ray finding is cortical calcifications which appear as double densities (***train-tract*** or ***rail-road*** sign).

Coats' Disease (Figs 18.7A and B)

- This is a chronic, progressive, vascular abnormality in which telangiectatic retinal vessels leak fluid, which results in an exudative bullous retinal detachment.
- It usually affects boys between 18 months and 18 years of age.
- It is usually unilateral, but both eyes may also be affected.

- The main symptoms are decreased visual acuity and a ***white pupillary reflex***.
- ***Ophthalmoscopically,*** yellowish-white exudative patches are seen behind the retinal blood vessels. The blood vessels may have a tortuous course with aneurysms, fusiform dilatations, and loop formations. Hemorrhage in the vitreous may occur subsequently. Eventually, there may be detachment of retina with iritis, cataract and glaucoma.
- Treatment is frequently ineffective in established cases, but early photocoagulation or cryotherapy is helpful.

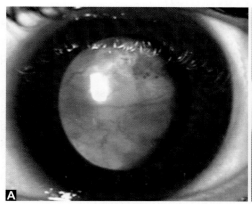

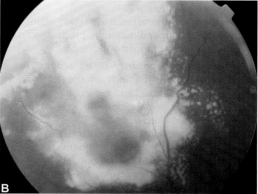

Figs 18.7A and B: Coats' disease. **A.** White pupillary reflex; **B.** Fundus picture

RETINOPATHY OF PREMATURITY (FIG. 18.8)

- It is a bilateral abnormality with retinal neovascularization.
- It occurs some weeks after birth, in premature infants (less than 1,500 g birth weight), who have been given high concentration of oxygen during the first 10 days of life.
- The earliest signs are dilatation of the retinal veins, and the appearance of hazy white patches in the peripheral retina.
- This is due to neovascularization in the retina itself which hubs into the vitreous.
- This is followed by the development of fibrous tissue which eventually proliferates to form a continuous mass behind the lens, appearing as a type of pseudoretinoblastoma (pseudoglioma).
- In many cases the retina gets detached, and of course, the vision is lost.

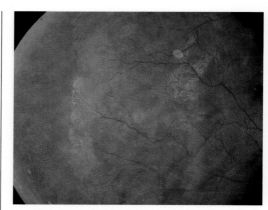

Fig. 18.8: Retinopathy of prematurity

Pathogenesis

- Retinal vascularization is only completed by the end of full-term gestation, and the retina anterior to the equator (especially that of the upper temporal quadrant) being the last to develop its vessels.
- In prematures, these immature vessels may be occluded by high oxygen concentration. On return to normal atmospheric air, there is intense new vessels formation at the border of these ischemic areas.
- Milder forms of disorder result in tractional bands in the upper temporal quadrant, producing an ectopic macula or dragged optic disc.

Retinopathy of prematurity (ROP) stages: To describe the fundus findings at the junction between the vascularized and avascular retina.
- Stage 1 = a faint demarcation line
- Stage 2 = an elevated ridge
- Stage 3 = extraretinal fibrovascular tissue
- Stage 4 = subtotal retinal detachment
- Stage 5 = total retinal detachment
- In addition, ***plus disease*** may be present at any stage. It describes a significant level of vascular dilation and tortuosity observed at the posterior retinal vessels.

Treatment

- In 80% of infants, the retinopathy of prematurity will regress spontaneously.
- Treatment is required, only when the definite progressive lesion are noted in the vitreous:
  - Photocoagulation or cryotherapy to ablate the avascular immature retina.
  - Scleral buckling for retinal detachment.
  - *Vitamin E* (100 mg/kg/day) may protect the susceptible infants.

Prevention

- Monitor arterial (umbilical) PaO_2 levels during treatment of asphyxia neonatorum, and it should be preferably between 50–100 mm Hg.
- Premature infants (less than 32 weeks) or weighing less than 1,500 g, who have received oxygen therapy, should be screened for retinopathy of prematurity (ROP).
- Once the signs of retinopathy develop, the child should be reexamined every 3 to 4 months up to the age of 4 years, to learn the progress of the disease.

RETINAL VASCULAR DISORDERS

Retinal Artery Occlusion

The occlusion may affect the central retinal artery occlusion (CRAO) (Fig. 18.9) itself, when the entire retina is involved, or a peripheral branch (arteriole), when the effect is localized.

Etiology

- Emboli from the carotid artery, e.g. atherosclerotic plaques in older patient
- Emboli from valvular heart disease in young patient
- Thrombus from arteriolosclerosis
- Hypertension
- Arteritis.

Symptoms

- Painless, unilateral sudden loss of vision.
- *Amaurosis fugax* (transient sudden loss of vision lasting for few minutes, due to occlusion by minute emboli) may be a premonitory symptom.

Signs

Ophthalmoscopically, the fundus shows a typical picture:

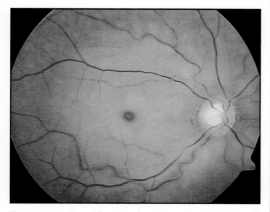

Fig. 18.9: Central retinal artery occlusion with cherry-red spot

- Larger arteries are thread-like, and the smaller arterioles are invisible.
- Veins are almost normal.
- Within a few hours, the retina loses its transparency, and becoming opaque and milky-white, especially around the posterior pole.
- A day or two later, a *cherry-red spot* appears at the fovea, since the vascular choroid is visible underneath. It is beautifully seen against strong contrast of the cloudy-white background.

A *cherry-red spot* is also seen in:
- Blunt injury (Berlin's edema of the macula),
- Tay-Sach's disease,
- Niemann-Pick disease,
- Sandhoff's disease, and
- Quinine amblyopia.

- When the obstruction is incomplete, the blood flow is partially restored. In that case, gentle pressure upon the globe may break up the column of venous blood into red-beads which move in a jerky fashion—the *cattle-track* appearance.
- After a week or so, the retina resumes its normal ophthalmoscopic appearance, but the optic nerve becomes atrophic and appears white.
- The vision is no perception of light (PL), and there is no direct pupillary reaction.
- *In obstruction of a branch of the retinal artery,* the occlusion is usually at a bifurcation, and invariably due to embolism. An atheromatous embolus may be visible as a pale refractile body within the artery (*Hollenhorst plaque*), and the distal area of the retina that the vessel supplies, becomes edematous. A sectorial scotoma corresponding to the affected area is detected in visual field charting.

Diagnosis

It depends on the history, since the patient is very rarely seen during an acute attack. All the patient of *amaurosis fugax* should be thoroughly investigated for *cardiovascular problems*.

Treatment

It is only effective, if given within the first few hours of such an occlusion.

- Immediate intermittent digital message to the globe.
- Intravenous acetazolamide, if available.
- Inhalation of 5% CO_2 and 95% O_2 mixture for 10 min may be helpful.
- Paracentesis of the anterior chamber.
- Retrobulbar injection of acetylcholine may produce vasodilatation.
- Anticoagulants, as intravenous heparin.

Prognosis

- As the patient usually presents after few hours, the most frequent result of an occlusion of central retinal artery, however, is blindness.
- No return of macular vision is anticipated if the obstruction has lasted over 6 hours.
- Where a cilioretinal artery is present (about 25% of cases), blood from the choroid will reach the posterior pole, preserving a useful island of vision which often includes the macular vision.

RETINAL VEIN OCCLUSION

Retinal vein occlusion may involve the central retinal vein which causes immediate severe loss of vision, or a branch retinal vein which results in partial loss of vision, depending on the affected region drained by the vein.

Predisposing Factors

- *Age:* Sixth and seventh decades.
- *Systemic hypertension:* The vein is compressed by a thickened artery where the two shares a common adventitia (at the arteriovenous crossing).

- *Raised intraocular pressure:* Patients with primary open-angle glaucoma (POAG) or ocular hypertension are at increased risk of central retinal vein occlusion (CRVO), but no correlation with branch retinal vein occlusion (BRVO).
- *Diabetes:* Increased risk of CRVO/BRVO.
- *Hyperviscosity syndrome:* As in chronic leukemia and polycythemia vera (hypercellularity of blood): In macroglobulinemia and cryoglobulinemia (change in plasma proteins) or obstructive pulmonary diseases (COPD).
- *Periphlebitis* as in sarcoidosis and Behcet's disease.

> Three basic mechanisms involved both in CRVO and BRVO are:
> 1. External compression on the vein,
> 2. Venous stasis, and
> 3. Degenerative diseases of the venous endothelium.

CENTRAL RETINAL VENOUS OCCLUSION (FIG. 18.10)

Types

There are two main types of CRVO:
1. *Nonischemic CRVO (Fig. 18.11):* It is also referred as venous stasis retinopathy

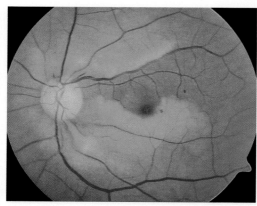

Fig. 18.10: Central retinal artery occlusion—macular sparing due to patent cilioretinal artery

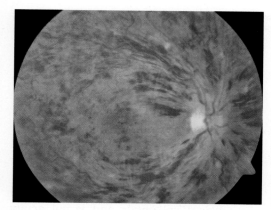

Fig. 18.11: Non-ischemic central retinal venous occlusion

or partial CRVO. This accounts for 75% of cases.

2. *Ischemic CRVO (Fig. 18.12):* It is also called complete CRVO, this accounts for the remaining 25% of cases.

Nonischemic Central Retinal Venous Occlusion

- *Clinical features*
  - Visual acuity is slightly or moderately reduced.
  - Relative afferent pupillary defect (Marcus-Gunn pupil) is usually mild, indicating mild retinal ischemia.

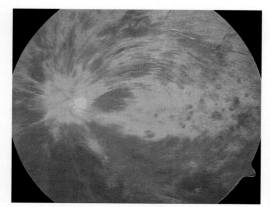

Fig. 18.12: Ischemic central retinal venous occlusion

- *Ophthalmoscopically*
  - Mild tortuosity and dilatation of all branches of the central retinal vein.
  - *Dot/blot and flame-shaped hemorrhages,* are seen throughout all four quadrants and most numerous in the periphery.
  - Cotton-wool exudates are usually absent.
  - Mild to moderate swelling of the optic disc.
  - Macular edema may or may not be present.
- *Fluorescein angiography:* It shows, venous stasis but with good retinal capillary perfusion.
- *Prognosis:* In 50% of cases, the retinopathy resolves, and visual acuity returns to normal or near normal. The permanent impairment of vision is due to chronic macular edema.
- *Treatment:* No specific treatment is required except to treat the predisposing factor, if any.

Ischemic Central Retinal Venous Occlusion

- *Clinical features*
  - Marked reduction in visual acuity.
  - Relative afferent pupillary defect marked.
- *Ophthalmoscopically*
  - Marked tortuosity and engorgement of the retinal veins.
  - Massive superficial and deep hemorrhages throughout the fundus.
  - Cotton-wool exudates are common.
  - Optic disc is swollen and hyperemic.
  - Macular edema and hemorrhages.

  This appearance is sometimes called *blood and thunder* fundus.
- *Fluorescein angiography* in early stage is not useful because of hemorrhages, but in less severe cases or in late stage, there are extensive areas of capillary non-perfusion.

- ***Course and prognosis:*** About 50% of eyes develop rubeosis iridis and neovascular glaucoma within 3 months of the initial occlusion ***(90-days glaucoma)***. A small percentage of eyes develop pre-retinal or vitreous hemorrhage, secondary to NVD and/or NVE.
- ***Treatment***
  - Patient should be followed-up closely for rubeosis iridis, as prompt treatment in early cases, by panretinal photocoagulation (PRP) (or cryoapplication if the media is hazy), prevents the subsequent development of neovascular glaucoma.
  - The management of established neovascular glaucoma is discussed in Chapter 16.

BRANCH RETINAL VENOUS OCCLUSION

It (Fig. 18.13) may occur near the optic disc and involves a major quadrant of the retina, or it may occur at a peripheral crossing with an artery. Blockage of the superior temporal vein frequently involves the macula.

- ***Symptoms:*** These depend on the location of the occlusion. Visual loss is marked, if the superior temporal branch is occluded.

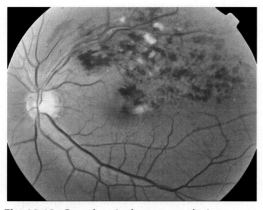

Fig. 18.13: Branch retinal venous occlusion

Ophthalmoscopically the affected part of the retina, drained by the obstructed vein shows:
- Dilated and tortuous veins
- Flame-shaped, and dot and blot hemorrhage in the affected quadrant
- Retinal edema and cotton-wool spots.

- ***Course and prognosis:*** Following a major branch retinal vein occlusion, visual acuity is initially reduced due to macular hemorrhage and edema.
  - Within 6 months, 50% of eyes develop efficient collaterals and visual acuity returns to 6/12, or better. However, complications may arise from vascular leakage and capillary nonperfusion.
  - Two most important vision-threatening complications are:
    1. Macular edema
    2. Vitreous hemorrhage due to neovascularization.
  - Secondary neovascular glaucoma occurs very rarely.
- ***Treatment***
  - Fundus fluorescein angiography to know the macular non-perfusion, or macular edema with good perfusion, and also to identify the ***collateral vessels*** (because they must not be treated by laser).
  - For macular edema, grid photocoagulation with argon laser or double-frequency yttrium aluminium garnet (YAG) (532) laser may be helpful.
  - ***Role of anti-VEGF:*** They are available to treat macular edema due to BRVO including ranibizumab (Lucentis, bevacizumab (Avastin), and aflibercept (Eylea).
  - For neovascularization following BRVO, the eye should be treated by scatter argon laser photocoagulation, in order to prevent vitreous hemorrhage.

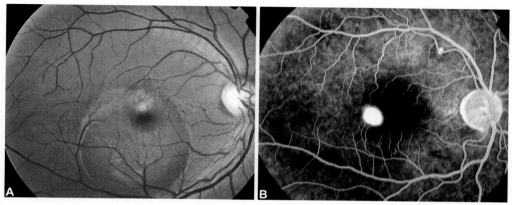

Figs 18.14A and B: A. Central serous retinopathy; **B.** Ink-blot pattern on fundus fluorescein angiography

CENTRAL SEROUS RETINOPATHY

Central serous retinopathy (CSR) (Figs 18.14A and B) is characterized by sudden edema of the macular area, which typically affects the young adult males due to unknown cause. It is basically a localized retinal detachment, and caused by exudation from the parafoveal or choroidal capillaries.

Symptoms

- Sudden onset of blurring of vision in one eye.
- Black fixed spot (a positive scotoma) at the center of the visual field.
- Metamorphopsia.

Signs

- Visual acuity reduced to 6/9 to 6/18, and often correctable to 6/6 with weak plus lens. This is due to elevation of neuro-sensory retina which gives rise to an acquired hypermetropia.
- **Ophthalmoscopically,** macula appears as an oval or circular dark swelling, larger than the size of the optic disc, which is surrounded by a glistening **ring-reflex.**

FUNDUS FLUORESCEIN ANGIOGRAPHY

Fundus fluorescein angiography (FFA) is helpful for a definitive diagnosis of CSR. Two patterns are seen on FFA:

1. **Ink-blot pattern:** Small hyperfluorescent spot, gradually increases in size.
2. **Smoke-stack pattern (Figs 18.15A to C):** A small hyperfluorescent spot, ascends vertically like a smoke-stack, and gradually

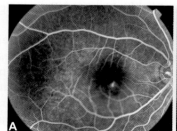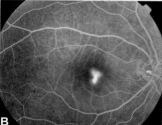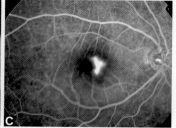

Figs 18.15A to C: Central serous retinopathy—smoke-stack pattern on fundus fluorescein angiography

spreads laterally taking on a mushroom or umbrella configuration.

Prognosis

- Eighty to ninety percent cases of CSR undergo spontaneous resolution, and the visual acuity returns to normal or near normal, within 4–12 weeks.
- Mild metamorphopsia or micropsia may persist for a longer period.
- Fourty percent of patients develop recurrent attacks.

Treatment

- In majority of the cases, no treatment is required except reassurance.
- Argon laser or double-frequency YAG (532) laser photocoagulation to the site of leakage may be considered in some cases:
    - Recurrent CSR with visual loss.
    - If the vision in fellow eye is permanently reduced due to previous attacks of CSR.
    - If the duration is more than 4 months.
    - In presence of turbid subretinal fluid.

CYSTOID MACULAR EDEMA (FIG. 18.16)

Cystoid macular edema (CME) is an accumulation of fluid in the outer plexiform (Henle's) layer and inner nuclear layer of the retina, in the macular region.

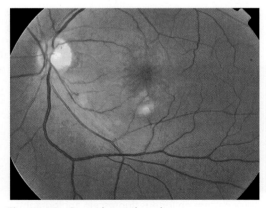

Fig. 18.16: Cystoid macular edema

Etiology

Cystoid macular edema is a very common macular disorder that has many diverse causes:

- *Irvine-Gass syndrome:* Probably, it is the most common cause of CME, which occurs as a common complication of cataract extraction, especially when associated with vitreous prolapse. The majority of the cases are transient and have little clinical significance.
- *Background diabetic retinopathy:* CME is an important cause of visual impairment among diabetics.
- *Retinal vein occlusion:* Chronic CME may occur following CRVO or BRVO.
- Pars planitis and acute iridocyclitis.
- *Retinitis pigmentosa:* Typical CME may be present up to 70% of eyes with retinitis pigmentosa.
- *Epinephrine:* CME may develop in aphakic eyes treated with epinephrine for open-angle glaucoma (epinephrine maculopathy).

Clinical Features

- Visual acuity is often reduced to 6/60.
- *Ophthalmoscopy* shows an irregularity and blurring of the foveal reflex.
- The macula is wrinkled, edematous, and may show multiple small cystic changes.
- In long-standing cases, there is formation of lamellar holes at the fovea with irreversible damage to central vision (Fig. 18.17).

Fluorescein angiography demonstrates leakage of the dye from the perifoveal capillaries, and accumulation within the macular region. The accumulation of dye in the outer plexiform layer, with its radial arrangement of fibers (Henle's layer) is responsible for the typical *flower-petal* (Fig. 18.18) or *spoke-pattern* of CME on FFA.

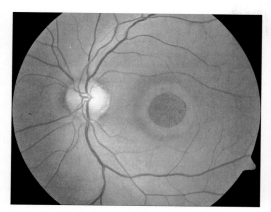

Fig. 18.17: Macular hole formation

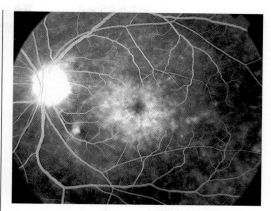

Fig. 18.18: Cystoid macular edema—flower-petal pattern on fundus fluorescein angiography

Treatment

- The edema is usually self-limited and improvement is spontaneous.
- Systemic steroids are often used in vascular or inflammatory conditions.
- Systemic steroids, sub-Tenon long-acting steroid, and nonsteroidal antiinflammatory agents (systemic or local) are helpful in postoperative cases.

AGE-RELATED MACULAR DEGENERATION

Age-related macular degeneration (ARMD) or senile macular degeneration (SMD) is a bilateral disease, characterized by formation of subretinal neovascular membranes (SRNVMs) or choroidal neovascular membranes (CNVMs) at the macula. It is one of the leading causes of blindness in the Western world.

Histopathologically drusen, retinal pigment epithelial degeneration and/or atrophy, SRNVMs, retinal pigment epithelium (RPE) and sensory retinal detachment due to subretinal hemorrhage, and disciform scars at the macula, are the different manifestations of the disease in different stages.

Drusen

Drusens or colloid bodies are the most frequent clinical manifestation of aging, and are present in about 70% of people after the age of 50 years.

Clinical Features

They appear as small, discrete, yellow-white, slightly elevated spots at the posterior poles of both fundi. With advancing age, they increase in size and number.

Secondary calcification in long-standing lesions gives them a glistening-white appearance.

Classification

- **Hard drusen (nodular) (Fig. 18.19):** It appear as small, discrete yellowish-white nodules.
- **Soft drusen (Fig. 18.20):** It have indistinct edges, are larger than hard drusens, and frequently become confluent.
- **Diffuse drusen** (confluent): It represent a widespread abnormality of RPE.
- **Calcified drusen:** It have glistening-white appearance with conspicuous margin.

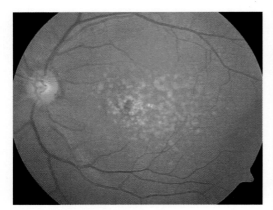

Fig. 18.19: Central hard drusen

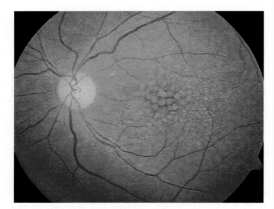

Fig. 18.20: Central soft drusen

Histopathology

Drusens consist of focal aggregation of hyaline material located between the basal lamina of the RPE and inner collagenous layer of the Bruch's membrane.

- Localized thickening and thinning of the Bruch's membrane.
- Variable degrees of RPE atrophy and depigmentation.
- Degenerative changes of the retinal receptors.

Fluorescein Angiography

- *Retinal pigment epithelium window defects* appear as multiple hyperfluorescent spots.

- *Staining of the drusens* by the dye, which may persist for a long time.

Drusen and ARMD
• The exact role of drusen in the pathogenesis of ARMD is still not clear. • But a significant number of elderly patients with drusens may develop impairment of vision due to ARMD. • Increased risk of subsequent visual loss in patient with confluent drusens, particularly if one eye has already developed visual loss from ARMD.

Types of Age-related Macular Degeneration

They are of two main types:
1. Non-exudative (dry) ARMD
2. Exudative (wet) ARMD.

Non-exudative (Dry) Age-related Macular Degeneration

- It is the most common type, and is due to a slow and progressive atrophy of RPE and photoreceptors.
- Progressive loss of vision for several months to years.
- *Clinically,* it appears as sharp circumscribed areas of RPE atrophy with varying degrees of loss of choriocapillaries. In late stage, the larger choroidal vessels become visible within the atrophic areas.

Treatment
- There are no definite medical treatments for dry AMD at this time.
- *Lifestyle changes:* It can slow down the process or contribute to the development and progress of AMD.
- Antioxidant medication that included vitamin C, vitamin E, beta carotene (or vitamin A), and zinc can slow the progression of the disease by 25%.
- Changing the diet which includes more fruits and vegetable, choosing healthy unsaturated fats, such as olive oil, refined

grains and adding fish with high omega-3 fatty acids.

- *Low vision rehabilitation:* The use of magnifying devices, e.g. binoculars or telescopes can often improve vision in macular degeneration to allow for reading or watching of television.
- Use of tablet devices or large smart phone—as reading device or to watch video.
- Miniature implantable telescope may help to improve the central vision. It involves surgical removal of crystalline lens and replace it with a miniature telescope. This is followed by an extensive training program.

Exudative (Wet) Age-related Macular Degeneration

- It is also sometimes referred to as *neovascular* or wet ARMD, and is less common than non-exudative type (Fig. 18.21).
- This is a more serious form, and the patient may lose all central vision within a few weeks. *Amslers grid test* (Figs 18.22A to C) is convenient and accurate way to detect ARMD in early stage.
- Two important features of exudative ARMD are *detachment* of the RPE and *choroidal neovascularization*.

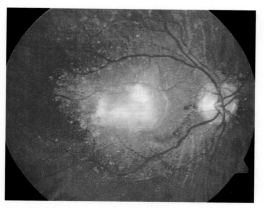

Fig. 18.21: Age-related macular degeneration—exudative type

- *RPE detachment* appears as sharply circumscribed dome-shaped elevation with ophthalmoscope.
- Subretinal neovascular membranes (SRNVMs), consisting of proliferations of fibrovascular tissue, begin to grow from the choriocapillaries → through the defects of the Bruch's membrane → into the sub-RPE space → and later into the subretinal space.
- *Clinically,* SRNVMs are undetectable in early stage. But later, they appear as gray-green elevated lesions in the macular region.
- *Fluorescein angiography* plays an important role in the detection and localization of SRNVMs in relation to foveal avascular zone (FAZ).

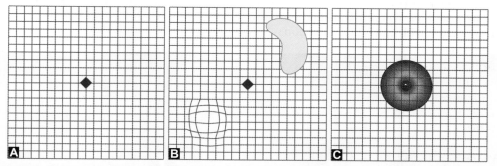

Figs 18.22A to C: Amsler grid test in ARMD, total number of square—20 × 20 in the chart. One square denotes 10 from the central part of fovea. Central diamond-shaped black spot represents foveola; **A.** Normal grid pattern; **B.** Distorted or missing pattern and **C.** Dark central spot

- *Sequelae of exudative—ARMD*
  - Hemorrhagic detachment of the RPE and neurosensory retina
  - Vitreous hemorrhage
  - Disciform scarring of the macula
  - Exudative retinal detachment.

Treatment

Wet macular degeneration cannot be cured. If diagnosed early, treatment may help slow progress of wet macular degeneration and reduce the amount of vision lost.

There are three main treatment options for wet AMD:

1. Anti-VEGF (vascular endothelial growth factor) medication to prevent the growth of new blood vessels in the eye.
2. Photodynamic therapy (PDT) to treat foveal abnormal vessels.
3. Laser surgery to destroy abnormal blood vessels in the eye.

- *Anti-VEGF* intravitreal injection are considered the first-line treatment for all stages of wet macular degeneration. They include (*see* anti-VEGF in Chapter 5):
  - Bevacizumab (Avastin)
  - Ranibizumab (Lucentis)
  - Pegaptanib (Macugen)
  - Aflibercept (Eylea).
- *Photodynamic therapy:* Using cold laser light to activate an injected medication called, verteporfin to prevent progression of SRNVMs. PDT is still used to treat some cases of Wet AMD sometimes in conjunction with anti-VEGF injection.

- *Photocoagulation:* Using an Argon (blue-green) laser to destroy abnormal extrafoveal SRNVMs outside the area of FAZ. Only a small number of patients are eligible for this procedure, as most patients have growth in the area of the fovea, which cannot be treated by laser.
- Counseling of the patients reading continued therapy.

RETINITIS PIGMENTOSA (FIGS 18.23A TO C)

Retinitis pigmentosa (RP) is a group of hereditary diseases, characterized by progressive night blindness and constricted visual fields.

Typical Retinitis Pigmentosa

Typical RP is a bilateral symmetrical diffuse pigmentary retinal dystrophy, predominantly affecting the rods.

Inheritance

- *Autosomal recessive:* Most common.
- *Autosomal dominant:* Benign nature.

Pathogenesis

- Degeneration of the rods and cones.
- Migration of pigments into the retina.
- Degenerated ganglion cells and their axons are replaced by neuroglial tissue.
- Attenuation of the blood vessels.
- Atrophy of the optic disc.

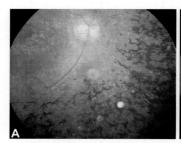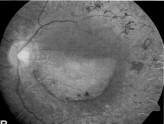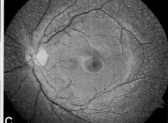

Figs 18.23A to C: **A.** Retinitis pigmentosa; **B.** Retinitis pigmentosa with cystoid macular edema; **C.** Retinitis punctate albicans

Clinical Features

- **Symptoms:** Include night blindness and progressive visual field defect.
- **Signs:** The classical triad of RP are:
  - Bony-spicule pigmentation
  - Arteriolar attenuation
  - Waxy-pallor of the optic disc.
- Pigmentary changes are typically perivascular, and have a bone-spicule appearance, which are observed mostly at the equatorial region of the retina.
- In late stages of the disease, the unmasking of the larger choroidal vessels (due to pigment migration), gives the fundus a tessellated appearance.
- **Macular lesions**
  - **Cystoid macular edema** may be present up to 70% of the patients with RP
  - Cellophane maculopathy
  - Atrophic maculopathy.

Investigations

They are helpful in early stages:
- **Electroretinography (ERG):** Markedly sub-normal in amplitude.
- **Electrooculography (EOG):** Absence of light peak.
- **Visual field:** Initially shows annular or ring-like scotoma. But ultimately, the progressive constriction of the visual field leaves only a tiny island of central vision, which may be lost eventually.

Atypical Retinitis Pigmentosa

- **Retinitis punctata albescens:** This is characterized by multiple scattered white dots, mostly between the posterior pole and the equator. Other findings are similar to typical RP.
- **Retinitis pigmentosa sine pigmento:** The typical pigmentary changes appear very late, while the presence of arteriolar attenuation and waxy-pallor of the disc with subnormal ERG, confirm the diagnosis.

- **Sectorial retinitis pigmentosa:** Involvement of only one quadrant (usually nasal), or one half (usually inferior) of the fundus.
- **Pericentric retinitis pigmentosa:** It is similar to typical RP, except that the pigmentary changes are confined to pericentral area, sparing the periphery (Fig. 18.24).

Systemic Associations of Retinitis Pigmentosa

- **Laurence-Moon-Biedl syndrome (Bardet Biedl) (Fig. 18.25):** Autosomal recessive; RP, mental retardation, polydactyly, obesity and hypogonadism.
- **Bassen-Kornzweig syndrome (abeta-lipoproteinaemia):** Autosomal recessive; RP, ataxia, acanthocytosis and fat malabsorption. Jejunal biopsy is diagnostic.
- **Refsum's syndrome:** Autosomal recessive; RP, peripheral neuropathy, cerebellar ataxia, elevated cerebrospinal fluid-proteins (CSF-proteins), deafness and ichthyosis. It is due to defective metabolism of **phytanic acid** which accumulates in the body.

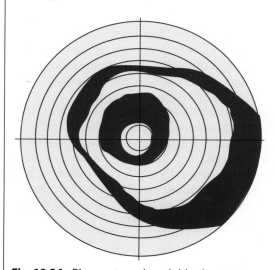

Fig. 18.24: Ring scotoma in retinitis pigmentosa

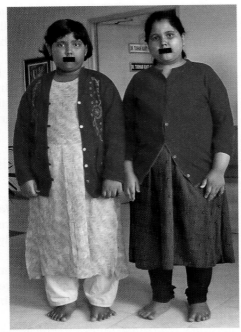

Fig. 18.25: Laurence-Moon-Biedl syndrome

- **Usher's syndrome:** Autosomal recessive; RP and sensorineural deafness.
- **Cockayne's syndrome:** Autosomal recessive; RP, dwarfism, 'bird-like' facies, flexion contracture of the limbs, mental retardation, ataxia and premature aging.
- **Kearns-Sayre syndrome:** The classical **triad** of RP, chronic progressive external ophthalmoplegia (ocular myopathy) and heart block; a rare mitochondrial DNA (mtDNA) deletion syndrome.
- **Friedreich's ataxia:** Autosomal recessive; RP, posterior column disease, cerebellar ataxia, nystagmus and subaortic stenosis.
- **Neuropathy, ataxia, and retinitis pigmentosa (NARP) syndrome:** It is a rare hereditary condition. It is related to changes in mitochondrial DNA (mutations in the MT-ATP6 gene).

Treatment

- No definite treatment is available for RP patients.

- However, there are therapies available to maximize their vision with refraction and low-visual aids (LVA).
- They should be examined annually for visual field testing and ERG evaluations. Often after this, the patients may be reassured that the changes are slow. Additionally, regular examinations can ensure appropriate time to seek community and legal assistance.
- **Medications**
  - Antioxidants and omega-3 fatty acid; or vitamin A (15,000 IU/day) may be useful in long-term to slow the progression.
  - **Acetazolamide:** It may be useful in macular edema in the later stages of RP.
  - Some medications have potential adverse effects in RP like, isotretinoin, vitamin E (400 IU) and sildenafil (viagra).
  - It may worsen night vision and ERG response.
- **Cataract extraction:** Often beneficial in RP with posterior subcapsular opacity with an improvement by 2 lines on Snellen chart.
- **Miscellaneous:** Dietary plan as in Refsum disease, audiology in Usher's syndrome, etc.
- Stem cells transplantation and retinal prosthesis (photoconducting chip on retinal surface) are being used in clinical trials in patients with RP, AMD and Stargardt disease.
- **Gene therapy:** It is also under investigation.
- **Counseling:** Genetic testing and counseling to know the mode of inheritance. Counseling can also help the patients for their future plans, such as pregnancy, job choices, medical treatments and psychological boost up.

RETINAL DETACHMENT

- **Retinal detachment (RD):** It is the separation of the sensory retina from the retinal pigmentary epithelium (which represent the two layers of the primary optic vesicle) by subretinal fluid (SRF).

- *Retinoschisis:* It is the splitting of the sensory retina into two layers.
- *Retinal break:* It is the full-thickness defect in the sensory retina.
  - *Hole:* It is a small retinal break (usually circular) without any vitreous traction.
  - *Tear:* It is a retinal break (usually horse-shoe-shaped) with the tractional element. A tear is more dangerous than a hole.
- *Syneresis:* It is the contraction of vitreous gel which separates its liquid from solid components.
- *Synchisis:* It is the liquefaction of the vitreous gel.
- *Choroidal detachment*: It is an effusion of fluid into the suprachoroidal space.

Classification

- Rhegmatogenous (primary) (Greek word *rhegma* means a break).
- Non-rhegmatogenous (secondary)
  - Tractional
  - Exudative.

Rhegmatogenous

Subretinal fluid, derived from the fluid vitreous gains access into the subretinal space through a retinal break. Rhegmatogenous RD may be traumatic or spontaneous.

Non-rhegmatogenous

- *Tractional:* The sensory retina is pulled away from the RPE by the vitreoretinal traction membranes. Two important causes of tractional RD are proliferative retinopathies, and penetrating ocular injury. The source of SRF is unknown.
- *Exudative:* SRF, derived from the choroid gains access to the subretinal space through the damaged RPE. Exudative RD may be due to choroidal tumors and inflammation.

RHEGMATOGENOUS RETINAL DETACHMENT (FIGS 18.26 AND 18.27)

Etiology

- *Incidence*: 1 in 10,000 population each year, and bilateral in 10% of the cases.
- *Trauma*: Most common in young adult males.
- *Myopia:* Over 40% of all RDs occur in myopic subjects. This is due to higher incidence of lattice degeneration, liquefaction of the vitreous, and posterior vitreous detachment.
- *Peripheral retinal degeneration:* Lattice is the most important degeneration directly related to RD, and is found more commonly in myopes over—3.0D.

Peripheral retinal degeneration

About 60% of all retinal breaks develop in the peripheral retina that shows specific changes. These lesions may be associated with a spontaneous hole formation, or they may predispose to retinal tear formation. The important predisposing degenerations are:
- *Lattice degeneration:* It is present in about 8% of general population, and 40% of eyes with RD. It is characterized by white arborizing lines, arranged in a lattice pattern occurring in the upper peripheral fundus between the equator and posterior border of the vitreous base, with long axis parallel to the ora seratta.
- *Snail-track degeneration:* It consists of sharply, demarcated bands of tightly packed snowflakes with a white frost-like appearance.
- *White-with-pressure:* It is a grayish-white appearance of the retina, induced by indenting the sclera (in case of normal fundus, scleral indentation induces a reddish elevation).
- *White-without-pressure:* It is an exaggeration of the above phenomenon, and is present without scleral indentation.
- *Focal pigment clumps:* It may be found with a retinal tear.

Contd...

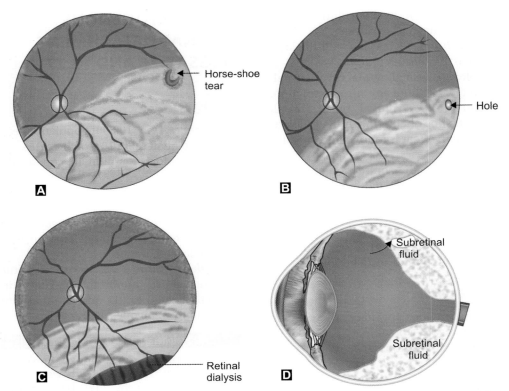

Figs 18.26A to D: Rhegmatogenous retinal detachment. **A.** Horse-shoe tear; **B.** Hole; **C.** Retinal dialysis; **D.** Accumulation of subretinal fluid

Contd...

> **Other benign degeneration are:**
> - *Peripheral (micro) cystoid degeneration:* It may be a constant finding in old age with increasing severity. This is not itself causally related to RD.
> - *Paving-stone degeneration:* It consists of yellowish-white areas of chorioretinal atrophy (present in 25% of normal eyes).
> - *Snowflakes:* They are minute, yellowish-white dots which are scattered diffusely in the periphery.

- *Cataract surgery:* It is more common with intracapsular cataract extraction, particularly if there had been vitreous loss. The incidence following extracapsular cataract extraction (ECCE) is less, possibly because the intact posterior capsule acts as a support to the vitreous, lessening its pull on the retina. It is also common after repeated needling in congenital cataract or after YAG-laser capsulotomy.

> ### Pathogenesis of rhegmatogenous
> - The breaks responsible for RD, are caused by interplay between vitreoretinal traction, and an underlying weakness of the peripheral retina.
> - 30% of horse-shoe tears proceed to RD within 6 weeks, and often within a few hours.
> - If the retinal operculum becomes completely detached from the tear to lie separated from the retina, the risk of RD is reduced.
> - Once the fluid (from liquefied vitreous) accumulates between the sensory retina and RPE, the retina becomes detached.
> - As the subretinal fluid (SRF) accumulates, it tends to gravitate downward.
> - The final shape of the RD is being determined by the position of the break, and the anatomical limits of the disc and ora serrata.

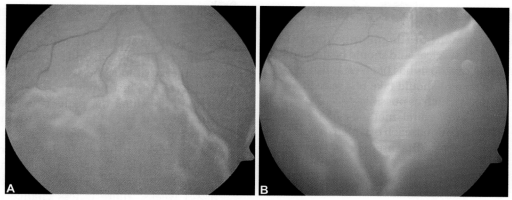

Figs 18.27A and B: Rhegmatogenous retinal detachment

Symptoms

- The classical premonitory symptoms reported in 60% patients with RD, are:
  - *Photopsia:* It is a flash of light and this is due to vitreoretinal traction.
  - *Floaters:* Which may appear as large ring, small black spots or cobwebs.
- *Visual field defect:* It is due to the spread of SRF posterior to the equator, and is perceived by the patient as a black curtain.
- *Loss of central vision:* It is due to involvement of the fovea.

Signs

In fresh RD:
- Relative afferent pupillary defect (Marcus-Gunn pupil) in eyes with extensive RD.
- Intraocular pressure is low.
- Mild anterior uveitis.
- *Posterior segment:* Indirect ophthalmoscopy is more important.
  - Detached retina is slightly opaque, convex and corrugated in appearance (due to intraretinal edema), with loss of underlying choroidal pattern.
  - Detached retina undulates freely with ocular movements.
  - There is no shifting of fluid.
  - Breaks appear as red areas (holes or tears) of discontinuities mainly in the peripheral retina.

- Vitreous shows *tobacco dust* in the anterior vitreous, with posterior vitreous detachment.

In long-standing RD:
- Retinal thinning.
- Subretinal demarcation lines.
- Secondary intraretinal cysts.
- Multiple opaque strands of subretinal fibrosis.
- Subsequently, proliferative vitreoretinopathy (PVR) develops.
- If untreated, the vast majority of RDs become total, and eventually give rise to complicated cataract, chronic uveitis, hypotony and eventually phthisis bulbi.

Investigations

- *Indirect ophthalmoscopy* is most important, and both eyes should be examined. Scleral indentation is necessary to enhance visualization of the extreme peripheral retina.
- Fundus drawing with appropriate color codes on a fundus chart.
- *Slit-lamp examination* with three-mirror gonioscope:
  - To detect breaks
  - To evaluate vitreous condition.
- *Ultrasonography (USG):* Both A-scan and B-scan are helpful when the media is hazy.

Treatment (Figs 18.28A to C)

The treatment of rhegmatogenous RD is essentially surgical, and should be immediate, once the diagnosis has been established.

The patient should take rest in recumbent position as much as possible.

- There are several methods of treating a detached retina, each of which depends on retinal breaks. The three general principles are:
  1. To find out the retinal breaks
  2. To seal the breaks
  3. To relieve present (and future) vitreo-retinal traction.

- **Sealing the retinal breaks:** It is required in any form of rhegmatogenous RD surgery—retinal breaks are closed by producing an area of chorioretinitis in the region of the defect, so that, the adhesions between the edge of the break and the RPE will seal the opening.

  The chorioretinal reaction may be produced by cryosurgery (cryoretinopexy) at –70°C, or diathermy to the sclera, or by laser photocoagulation.

Three types of retinal detachment surgery are practiced:

1. **Vitrectomy:** Pars plana vitrectomy (PPV) is the most commonly performed operation treatment for retinal detachment. It works by removing the vitreous from the eye and replacing it with either a gas (SF6 or C3F8) or silicone oil. This helps in reattaching retina.

   Small dissolving sutures are used to close the wound. It is also possible to perform such surgery without the use of stitches, using 23G or 25G instruments.

   After the procedure, the patient requires positioning of the head for a while, so the bubble settles in the correct position.

   - **Advantages** of using gas in this surgery is that there is no myopic shift after the operation and gas is absorbed within a 2–3 weeks. There is less chance of future vitreoretinal traction. Silicone oil is more commonly used in cases associated with PVR changes. Silicone oil, if filled needs to be removed 2–6 months after surgery depending on surgeon's preference.

   - **Disadvantage:** Vitrectomy always leads to more rapid progression of a cataract in the operated eye. Emulsified silicone oil may sometime seep into the anterior chamber, causing keratopathy and inverse hypopyon.

2. **Scleral buckling:** It is a surgical procedure to create an inward indentation of the sclera and the choroid. Scleral buckling is achieved by inserting a plomb (exoplant), which is usually a solid silicone band or a silicone sponge, and sutured firmly to the sclera.

   - **Radially-oriented** plombage is most effective in sealing an isolated

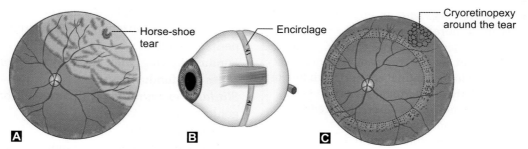

Figs 18.28A to C: Treatment of rhegmatogenous retinal detachment. A. Preoperative appearance; B. Encirclage (360°); **C.** Postoperative appearance

horse-shoe tear, and *circumferential* plombage (encirclage) is indicated when multiple holes are present parallel to the equator.

- *Subretinal fluid drainage:* It is customary to drain SRF by inserting a fine needle through the sclera and choroid, into the subretinal space, and allowing SRF to drain away.

3. *Pneumatic retinopexy:* If the retinal detachment is relatively small and uncomplicated, a procedure called pneumatic retinopexy may be used. This involves injecting a small bubble of gas (SF6 or C3F8 gas) into the eye, and may be followed by laser photocoagulation or cryoretinopexy to create scar tissue around the break. The patient's head is then positioned so that the bubble rests against the retinal hole. Patients may have to keep their heads tilted for several days to keep the gas bubble in contact with the retinal hole. The bubble is slowly absorbed into the eye over the following weeks.

This strict positioning requirement makes the treatment of the retinal holes and detachments that occurs in the lower part of the eyeball impractical.

Pneumatic retinopexy has significantly lower success rates compared to scleral buckle surgery and vitrectomy.

When an expansile gas is used with vitrectomy or for pneumoretinopexy, there is restriction of another surgery under GA or on flying.

- *Prognosis*: About 80–90% of RDs can be reattached, often with excellent visual results with immediate surgery, particularly, when macula is not involved. As, a detachment in the other eye occurs later in a high proportion of cases, a thorough retinal examination (indirect ophthalmoscopy), and prophylactic cryoretinopexy or laser photocoagulation is done, if there is any retinal break.

TRACTIONAL RETINAL DETACHMENT (FIGS 18.29 AND 18.30)

Symptoms

- Photopsia and floaters are usually absent, because the vitreoretinal traction develops slowly.
- Slow and progressive loss of visual field.

Signs

- Retinal breaks are usually absent.
- Rhegmatogenous configuration is concave. The highest elevation of retina occurs at the site of vitreoretinal traction.

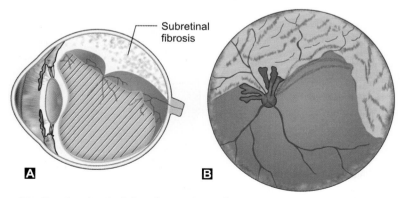

Subretinal fibrosis

A **B**

Figs 18.29A and B: Tractional retinal detachment (note the concave appearance of the detached retina)

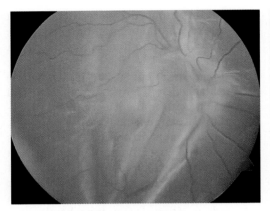

Fig. 18.30: Tractional retinal detachment

- Mobility of the detached area is severely reduced.
- Subretinal demarcation lines are absent.

EXUDATIVE RETINAL DETACHMENT (FIGS 18.31 AND 18.32)

Symptoms

- Floaters are present occasionally.
- Photopsia is absent, as there is no vitreoretinal traction.
- Sudden and rapid loss of visual field.

Signs

- Retinal breaks are absent.
- Rhegmatogenous configuration is convex. The detached retina is smooth, noncorrugated and bullous, and it may even touch the back of the lens.
- Shifting of fluid is **the hallmark of exudative RD**. The SRF responds to the force of gravity, and detaches the area under which it accumulates.
- Other associated ocular features (e.g. choroidal tumors), or systemic features (e.g. rheumatoid arthritis, Harada's disease, toxemia of pregnancy, etc.) may be present.

HYPERTENSIVE RETINOPATHY

- In systemic hypertension, it is important to consider two aspects separately—the severity and the duration.
- The **severity of hypertension** is reflected by the degree of hypertensive vascular changes and retinopathy.
- The **duration of hypertension** is reflected by the degree of arteriolosclerotic changes and retinopathy.
- The **primary response** of the retinal arterioles to systemic hypertension is

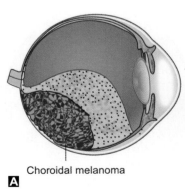

Choroidal melanoma

A

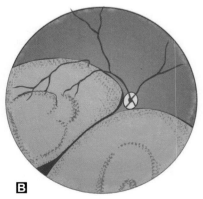

B

Figs 18.31A and B: Exudative retinal detachment (note the bullous appearance of the detached retina)

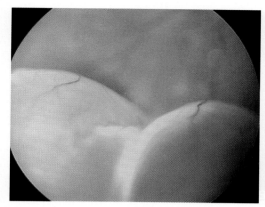

Fig. 18.32: Exudative retinal detachment—bullous detachment

narrowing, and it occurs only in young individual in its pure form.
- But, the degree of response in aged patient, also depends on the amount of preexisting involutional sclerosis.
- So, the grading of retinal changes in hypertension has caused confusion, because of the replacement fibrosis of arterial hypertension, and that of aging are identical.

Pathogenesis

- Systemic chronic hypertension → narrowing of retinal arterioles → retinal ischemia → hypoxia → increased capillary permeability → focal retinal edema, retinal hemorrhage and hard exudates.
- Hard exudates deposit around the fovea in the Henle's layer, and lead to their radial distribution, in the form of *macular star*.
- In severe or acute hypertension → obstruction of the precapillary arterioles → fibrinoid necrosis of the axons of nerve-fiber layer → interruption of axoplasmic flow → build-up of transported material within the nerve axons → *cotton-wool spots*.

Classification

Keith-Wagner-Barkan

This is traditional and widely cited. It relates only systemic hypertension and arteriolar sclerosis (not for involutional sclerosis).

- *Grade-1:* Mild generalized arteriolar narrowing.
- *Grade-2:* More narrowing of the arterioles and also focal arteriolar attenuation. Arteriovenous crossing changes (e.g. nicking) present.
- *Grade-3:* Grade II changes with hemorrhage, cotton-wool spot and exudates.
- *Grade-4:* All the changes of grade III with papilledema including the neuroretinal edema.

Scheie's Classification

Here, the retinal changes of hypertension and arteriolar sclerosis are graded separately.

Hypertensive features

- *Normal:* No ophthalmoscopic retinal changes.
- *Grade-1:* Narrowing of smaller retinal arterioles.
- *Grade-2:* Severe narrowing with localized irregular constriction of the arterioles.
- *Grade-3:* Narrowing and irregularities of the arterioles, with retinal hemorrhage and exudates.
- *Grade-4:* All changes in grade-3 along with neuroretinal edema, and/or papilledema (Figs 18.33A and B).

Arteriolosclerotic features

These changes develop if the hypertension is present over a period of many years, and are mainly seen in aged individual.
- *Normal:* No sclerotic changes.
- *Grade-1:* Widening of arteriolar light reflex with simple venous concealment.
- *Grade-2:* Grade-1 changes with deflection of veins at the arteriovenous crossing (Salus' sign).
- *Grade-3:* Grade-2 changes with copper wire arterioles, and marked arteriovenous crossing changes.
- *Grade-4:* All changes of grade-3 with silver wire arterioles and marked arteriovenous crossing changes. It may be associated with branch vein occlusion.

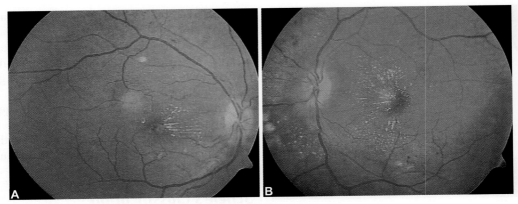

Figs 18.33A and B: Hypertensive retinopathy (Grade IV) with macular star

Arteriovenous crossing changes may be (Figs 18.34A to D):
- Banking of the vein where it appears dilated, distal to the crossing *(Bonnet's sign)*.
- Tapering of the vein on either side of the crossing *(Gunn's sign)*.
- Right-angled deflection of the vein, which gives the vein as S-shaped bend.

Associated choroidal changes:
- Severe hypertension may cause fibrinoid necrosis of the choroidal vessels which leads to atrophy of the RPE.

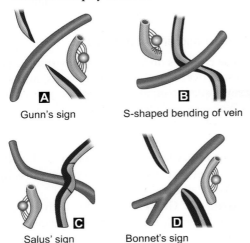

A Gunn's sign **B** S-shaped bending of vein

C Salus' sign **D** Bonnet's sign

Figs 18.34A to D: Arteriovenous crossing changes in hypertensive retinopathy

- Pigment deposition along the course of occluded choroidal vessels, is called *Seigrist's line*.
- Irregular scattered bright-yellow spots are also seen, called *Elschnig's spots*.
- Exudative bullous retinal detachment may occur in severe cases.

Renal retinopathy

The term describes the retinal changes seen in chronic renal failure. These may mimic a hypertensive retinopathy of Grade-III or IV, but the tendency to exudate formation is marked, particularly at the macula.

The severe hypertension in eclampsia may precipitate a florid retinopathy of Grade-IV, often with exudative retinal detachment. This detachment clears rapidly with the termination of pregnancy when the hypertension is under control.

Treatment

The treatment of hypertensive retinopathies is, necessarily, control of hypertension and that of underlying disease.

▌DIABETIC RETINOPATHY

- The prevalence of diabetic retinopathy (DR) is about 4–28%, and about 2% of diabetic population is blind as a result of retinopathy.

- The **best predictor** of diabetic retinopathy is the duration of diabetes. There is no clinically apparent diabetic retinopathy for 5 years after initial diagnosis.
- The severity of the diabetic retinopathy, generally parallels the duration of the disease and the adequacy of its control, and not the severity of the diabetes.
- The incidence of diabetic retinopathy is more with insulin dependent diabetes mellitus (IDDM) than with non-insulin dependent diabetes mellitus (NIDDM), but the severity of maculopathy is more with NIDDM.
- The course and severity of DR are affected by the presence of nephropathy, systemic hypertension, pregnancy, and positive family history of DR.

Pathogenesis

- The exact pathogenesis of DR is still not clearly understood.
- Diabetic retinopathy is essentially a *microangiopathy* which affects the retinal precapillary arterioles, capillaries and venules.
- This microangiopathy causes microvascular occlusion and leakage.
- Microvascular occlusion → retinal ischemia → retinal hypoxia.
  Two main effects of retinal hypoxia are neovascularization and arteriovenous shunts formation.
- *Microvascular weakness* is due to loss of pericytes and damage to the endothelial cells → saccular pouch formation → microaneurysm, which may leak.
- *Microvascular leakage* → increased vascular permeability → hemorrhage and retinal edema.
- *Chronic localized retinal edema* leads to the deposition of hard exudates at the junction of healthy and edematous retina. The hard exudates are composed of lipoprotein and lipid laden macrophages,

and they are typically arranged in a circinate pattern.

Classification

- Background diabetic retinopathy
- Diabetic maculopathy
  - Focal
  - Diffuse
  - Ischemic
- Pre-proliferative diabetic retinopathy
- Proliferative diabetic retinopathy (Fig. 18.35)
- Advanced diabetic eye diseases (PDR)
  - Vitreous hemorrhage
  - Tractional retinal detachment
  - Preretinal membrane
  - Neovascular glaucoma.

Background diabetic retinopathy or non-proliferative diabetic retinopathy (NPDR) (Fig. 18.36).

Clinical Features

- *Microaneurysms:* They are the most characteristic ocular lesions in diabetics. *They also occur in:*
  - Retinal venous occlusion
  - Coat's disease
  - Arterial hypertension

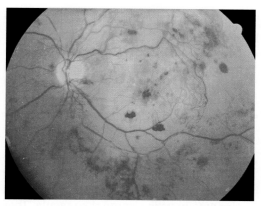

Fig. 18.35: Proliferative diabetic retinopathy—neovascularization elsewhere (NVE)

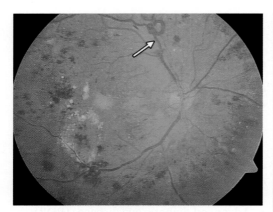

Fig. 18.36: Non-proliferative diabetic retinopathy—loop (arrow), dot and blot hemorrhage

- Anemia
- Dysproteinemia, etc.

Microaneurysms associated with diseases other than diabetes, are located on the arterial side of the capillary, rather than on the venous side at the posterior pole.

Microaneurysms consist of minute, round or ovoid distensions ranging from 20–200 μ in size, located on the venous side of capillary network at the inner nuclear layer.

> The resolving power of the direct ophthalmoscope is about 70–80 μ. Thus, majority of microaneurysms are not seen with the direct ophthalmoscope. They are visible with FFA.

They may be indistinguishable from 'dot' hemorrhages.

- **Dot and blot hemorrhages:** They originate from the venous end of the capillaries, and are situated in the inner nuclear layer of the retina.
- **Flame-shaped hemorrhages:** They are located superficially in the nerve-fiber layer.
- **Hard exudates** have a yellow-waxy appearance with a distinct margin, and become confluent, and may form a circinate pattern around the macula. They are located between the inner plexiform and inner nuclear layer of the retina.

Diabetic Maculopathy

Diabetic maculopathy is the most common cause of visual impairment in patients with diabetic retinopathy, and is more frequent in NIDDM. Maculopathy is of three types— focal, diffuse and ischemic.

Focal

- Background diabetic retinopathy
- Macular edema
- Hard exudates, may be ring-shaped
- Microaneurysms [absent within foveal avascular zone (FAZ)]
- Visual acuity is severely impaired
- It is caused by leakage from microaneurysms and dilated capillaries
- FFA shows—focal area of leakage, but adequate macular capillary perfusion.

Diffuse

- Microaneurysms and hemorrhages
- Focal retinal thickening around the macula
- Few hard exudates
- Cystoid macular edema in long-standing cases
- Lamellar hole may result
- FFA shows diffuse leakage at the posterior pole with typical flower-petal pattern (as in CME).

Ischemic

- Clinically, it may be similar to those seen in diffuse maculopathy.
- Fluorescein angiography is necessary to differentiate it from the diffuse type. FFA shows areas of capillary non-perfusion in the macular and paramacular regions.

Pre-proliferative Diabetic Retinopathy

It develops in some eyes, those initially show only simple background retinopathy. The lesions are caused by retinal ischemia (Fig. 18.36).

- *Cotton-wool patches (soft exudates)* are due to capillary occlusion of the nerve fiber layers.
- *Intraretinal microvascular abnormalities (IRMA):* They are seen adjacent to the areas of capillary closure. IRMA may resemble focal areas of flat retinal neovascularization. The main features of IRMA are intraretinal location, absence of profuse leakage on FFA, and failure to crossover the main retinal vessels.
- Venous changes consist of dilatation, beading, looping, and sausage-like segmentation.
- *Arteriolar* narrowing resembling branch retinal arteriolar occlusion.
- Large dark blot hemorrhages due to hemorrhagic retinal infarcts.

Recent classification of diabetic retinopathy

- Non-proliferative diabetic retinopathy (NPDR)
- Proliferative diabetic retinopathy (PDR)

NPDR: The lesions include microaneurysms, small dot and blot hemorrhages, IRMA and cotton wool spots. NPDR is further classified as mild, moderate, severe and very severe NPDR.

- *Mild NPDR:* At least one microaneurysms, and also dot and blot or flame-shaped hemorrhages in all four quadrants.
- *Moderate NPDR:* The findings are more severe than mild NPDR. Cotton-wool spots venous beading and IRMA are present but mild.
- *Severe NPDR:* At least one of the following should be present: (a) Severe hemorrhages and microaneurysms in all four quadrants, (b) Severe venous beading in two quadrants, and (c) IRMA-more severe in one quadrant.
- *Very severe NPDR:* Two or more of above criteria, but without any proliferative changes.

Diabetic maculopathy: Clinically significant macular edema (CSME) (Fig. 18.37) is described as:
- Retinal thickening at or within 500 μm at the center of macula.
- Hard exudates at or within 500 μm of the center of macula.
- An area of retinal thickening greater than 1 dd area in size, at least a part of which is within 1 dd of the center of the macula.

PDR: Neovascularization is the hallmark of PDR.

Advanced PDR: Same as advanced diabetic eye diseases.

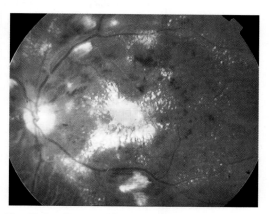

Fig. 18.37: Non-proliferative diabetic retinopathy—clinically significant macular edema (CSME)

Proliferative Diabetic Retinopathy

It affects about 5% of the diabetic population, and more with insulin-dependent diabetes mellitus (IDDM).

Clinical Features

- *Neovascularization* is the hallmark of PDR.

  It may be on the optic nerve head [NVD—*new vessels at the disc (Fig. 18.38)*], or along the course of major blood vessels (NVE—new vessels elsewhere). Over one-fourth of the retina has to be ischemic (non-perfused),

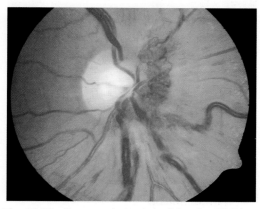

Fig. 18.38: Neovascularization of the disc (NVD)

before NVD appear. The new vessels start as endothelial proliferations, arising from the veins. The vessels are enveloped by mesenchymal fibroblasts forming a fibrovascular epiretinal membrane. NVD are more dangerous than NVE, as they have a greater propensity to bleed.

FFA shows hyperfluorescent areas with leakage from the new vessels.

- *Posterior vitreous detachment* is extremely important in the progression of PDR.
- *Hemorrhage* may occur in the form of intraretinal, preretinal and vitreous hemorrhage.

Apreretinal [subhyaloid (Fig.18.39)] hemorrhage has a crescentic or boat-shaped configuration, which demarcates the level of posterior vitreous detachment.

Advanced Diabetic Eye Diseases

The end results of uncontrolled PDR are:
- Recurrent vitreous hemorrhages.
- Tractional retinal detachment.
- *Burn-tout proliferative diabetic retinopathy:* In persistent PDR, after a variable period of time, the fibrous component of the fibrovascular proliferation becomes more evident, and the vascular component decreases. Then, the blood vessels become nonperfused, and no further proliferation occurs. This is called *burnt-out PDR*.

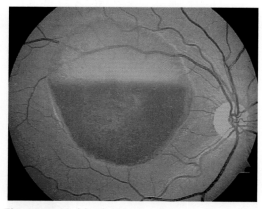

Fig. 18.39: Subhyaloid hemorrhage

- *Neovascular glaucoma:* Rubeosis iridis is a fairly common finding in eyes with PDR, and may lead to the development of neovascular glaucoma. It is more in patients following unsuccessful pars plana vitrectomy.

Management of Diabetic Retinopathy

General

- *Metabolic control:* Careful control of diabetes during first 5 years of the disease may reduce the severity, or delay the onset of DR. But, it apparently has little, or no effect on the established condition.
- *Control of hypertension:* Strict control of systemic hypertension is important.
- *Anemia:* Should be treated promptly.
- *Aspirin and dipyridamole:* It may have beneficial effect as they decrease platelet adhesiveness.
- *Clofibrate:* It is used to decrease lipid concentration.

Specific Treatment

- *Background DR:* No treatment is required for BDR with normal visual acuity except, periodic annual examination.
- *Diabetic maculopathy*
  - *Focal maculopathy:* Focal argon-laser photocoagulation is required, around the microaneurysms or leaking vessels.
  - *Diffuse maculopathy:* Macular grid (Fig. 18.40) photocoagulation is required, but avoiding the fovea (the burns should not be closer than 500 μ from the foveola). The results are much less favorable than for focal maculopathy.
  - *Ischemic maculopathy:* Photocoagulation will not improve vision. Follow-up is essential, as about 30% will develop PDR within 2 years.

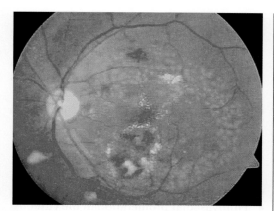

Fig. 18.40: Macular grid in diabetic maculopathy

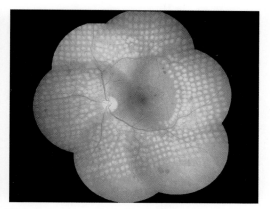

Fig. 18.41: Panretinal photocoagulation

- *Pre-proliferative DR:* The patients should be watched very closely. Treatment by photocoagulation is usually unnecessary, unless FFA shows extensive areas of capillary non-perfusion. Gentle argon laser photocoagulation is done to the areas of capillary non-perfusion, or in a panretinal fashion.
- *Proliferative DR:* Photocoagulation is the most important modality for the treatment of PDR. Double frequency YAG (532) laser, argon laser or diode laser is used for photocoagulation. Xenon arc photocoagulation is no longer used. Pituitary ablation, to treat PDR, is abandoned.

  Argon laser or double frequency YAG (532) laser photocoagulation: The treatment of choice in PDR, is panretinal photocoagulation (PRP) (Fig. 18.41) with a slit-lamp delivery system.

  The aim of the treatment is to convert the hypoxic area into anoxic area, and thereby, to induce involution of new vessels, and to prevent recurrent vitreous hemorrhage.

  PRP is performed in two or more sessions, as, if done in one session, it causes more serious complications. The new vessels usually take 4–8 weeks' time to regress after adequate PRP.

- *Advanced diabetic eye diseases*
  - *Vitreous hemorrhage:* Pars plana vitrectomy with panretinal photocoagulation (endolaser).
- *Tractional RD:* Pars plana vitrectomy is only to be undertaken when detachment has progressed to involve the macula.
- *Neovascular glaucoma:* As described in Chapter 16.

OTHER OCULAR SIGNS IN DIABETES MELLITUS

Visual defects
- Transient variations in refraction:
  - Hyperglycemia → increased refractive index of the lens → myopic shift
  - Hypoglycemia → decreased refractive power of the lens → hypermetropic shift
- Photopsia and diplopia in cerebral hypoglycemia
- Decreased accommodation
- Diplopia in ophthalmoplegia caused by neuropathy
- Decreased vision in cataract, maculopathy and vitreous hemorrhage
- Complete blindness from tractional RD, massive vitreous proliferation and neovascular glaucoma.

Ocular movements
- Neuropathy with muscle paralysis (pupillary sparing in third nerve palsy)
- Painful ophthalmoplegia.

Lids
- Increased incidence of stye or internal hordeolum
- Xanthelasma (due to associated hyperlipidemia).

Conjunctiva
- Tortuous and constricted blood vessels
- Sludging of the blood.

Cornea
- Delayed epithelial healing due to abnormality in epithelial basement membrane
- Punctate keratopathy
- Increased incidence of infective keratitis with delayed healing
- Wrinkling of the Descemet's membrane
- Decreased corneal sensation (due to trigeminal neuropathy)
- Increased prevalence of dry eye.

Iris
- Hydrops of the pigment epithelium (due to transient glycogen storage) release of pigment into the anterior chamber during surgery, or simply, even after dilatation of the pupil.
- Rubeosis iridis.

Lens
- Variation in refractive power [during hyperglycemia increased glucose content (sorbitol) of the lens cortex → imbibition of water → increased thickness of the lens → increased refractive power].
- Typical snowflake (sugar) cataract in IDDM
- Posterior cortical cataract
- Early onset of senile cataract.

Vitreous
- Vitreous hemorrhage
- Fibrovascular proliferation in the vitreous.

Retina
- Diabetic retinopathy (as already discussed)
- Lipemia retinalis (due to associated triglyceridemia, in ketoacidosis)
- Central retinal venous occlusion
- Diabetic retinopathy with superimposed changes of severe vascular hypertension—as seen in IDDM with renal failure.

Intraocular pressure
- Decreased in diabetic ketoacidosis (due to increased plasma bicarbonate level)
- Increased in neovascular glaucoma
- Increased incidence of POAG.

RETINOBLASTOMA

Discussed in Chapter 20.

Diseases of the Optic Nerve

OPTIC NERVE

Optic nerve is divided into four parts:
1. *Intraocular:* 1 mm
2. *Intraorbital:* 24 mm
3. *Intracanalicular:* 9 mm
4. *Intracranial:* 16 mm

Total length: 5.0 cm

- Its diameter increases from about 1.6 mm within the eye (intraocular) to 3.5 mm in the orbit to 4.5 mm within the cranial space (intracranial).
- The non-myelinated intraocular portion contained within the scleral canal may be divided into three parts—(1) *inner* retinal, (2) *middle* choroidal and (3) *outer* scleral.
- The retinal portion is seen ophthalmoscopically as the disc, or optic papilla (*papilla is a misnomer* because the disc is at the same level or slightly deeper than retinal nerve-fiber layer).
- A central depression, the *physiological cup* with its edges concentric to those of the disc, is lined with glial tissue, which may be sparse, so that the perforations of the lamina cribrosa are often visible.
- Human optic nerve contains between 7.7 lakh and 17 lakh nerve fibers, which are axons of the retinal ganglion cells of the retina. They synapse either in the lateral geniculate body (visual pathway), or in the pretectal region (papillary pathway).
- Optic nerve has the structures and shares the diseases of a neuron of second order of the central nervous system (CNS) rather than a peripheral nerve.
- The nerve fibers have myelin sheaths normally proximal to the lamina cribrosa. These sheaths are separated by glial tissue, and *neurilemma is absent.* For this reason, they do not regenerate after damage, as the tracts in the CNS.

OPTIC NERVE DISEASES

Symptoms

- *Loss of vision:* The main symptom.
- *Scotoma:* Loss of central vision.
- Disturbances in color vision.
- Pain is conspicuously absent, except it may be a prominent symptom in retrobulbar neuritis.

Signs

- Conduction defects in the optic nerve usually cause ill-sustained pupillary reaction, and *relative afferent pupillary defect* (RAPD) or Marcus-Gunn pupil.
- *Ophthalmoscopy* plays an important role in the diagnosis of optic nerve diseases. Attention is directed specially, to the margins of the disc, the surface of the disc and its color, pulsation of the central retinal vein, and the size and shape of the physiological cup.
- The variety of diseases affecting the optic nerve is large, and accurate diagnosis

requires a complete history, search for systemic diseases, and awareness of variety of diseases that may cause similar findings.

DEVELOPMENTAL ABNORMALITIES

Persistent Hyaloid Artery

- The hyaloids artery nurtures the lens during the first 10 weeks of embryonic life. After the fetal fissure closes, the hyaloids artery enters the eye at the optic cup and then obliterates.
- Occasionally, a short stub of this vessel projects into the vitreous cavity from the center of the optic disc and is surrounded by a small mass of glial tissue called *Bergmeister's papilla (Fig. 19.1)*. It is usually of no clinical significance, although it may rarely cause a recurrent vitreous hemorrhage.
- Failure of hyaloids artery to regress cause *persistent primary vitreous* which may proliferate.
- Minute residual fragments of the hyaloids system, may be seen as faint thread or small floaters *muscae volitantes*.

Drusen

Two kinds of drusen (*drusen* means stony nodule) occur in the intraocular portion of the optic nerve.

1. *Common drusens* are laminated, nodular, and may give the disc margins a blurred appearance (differentiated from papilledema by the absence of dilated retinal veins). Drusens often cause visual field defects but rarely affect visual acuity (Fig. 19.2).
2. The second type is *giant drusens,* which are astrocytic hamartomas that occur with *tuberous sclerosis*.

Conus

- In conus, or congenital crescent, the choroid and retinal pigment epithelium do not extend up to the optic disc.
- A large, white, semilunar area of sclera is seen adjacent to the disc, in the region of primitive retinal fissure (*inferonasal*).
- Defective vision, hypermetropic astigmatism and visual field defects are often present.
- A myopic crescent has a similar appearance, and is located at the temporal side of the disc.

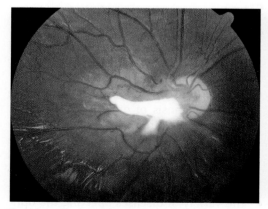

Fig. 19.1: Persistent hyperplastic primary vitreous— Bergmeister's papilla

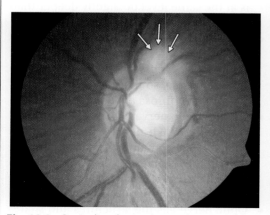

Fig. 19.2: Optic disc drusen (arrows)

- It is not present at birth and is associated with high myopia.

Coloboma of the Optic Disc

- In complete closure of the embryonic fissure causes optic nerve defects ranging from a deep physiological cup to a pit in the optic disc, or to a deeply excavated optic nerve.
- The condition is usually unilateral, but bilateral optic disc colobomas occur as an autosomal dominant hereditary defect.
- The disc looks large and the vessels have an abnormal distribution appearing only around the edges (morning glory syndrome) (Figs 19.3A and B). The apparent disc is really the sclera and the inner surface of the sheath, of the nerve. The nerve itself being spread out as a pink horizontal linear band at the upper part. The floor of the coloboma is white and measurably depressed, often quite ectatic. The eye usually has defective vision.
- *Pit in the optic disc* is probably an incomplete coloboma. It is usually single, and located in the inferotemporal region surrounding the fissure, and usually round or oval. A central scotoma is often present,

and in 30% of the cases, a central serous retinopathy (CSR) develops (Fig. 19.4).

Hypoplasia of the Optic Disc

- Failure of the axons of the ganglionic cells to develop or to reach the disc causes a small hypoplastic optic disc.
- It is bilateral in 60% of cases, and often associated with decreased size of the optic foramina.
- Typical appearance consists of a small gray optic disc surrounded by yellowish peripapillary halo of hypopigmentation due to concentric choroidal and retinal pigment epithelial abnormality often called *double-ring sign.*
- Despite the small optic disc the retinal vessels are of normal caliber. Sometimes, it may be associated with CNS anomalies, especially following the maternal ingestion of an anticonvulsant drug—*phenytoin sodium*.

Tilted Disc

This is due to an oblique entrance of the optic nerve into the globe and usually bilateral.
- The appearance of the disc is extremely oval, with the vertical axis directed obliquely, so

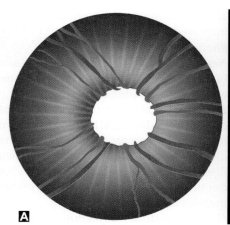
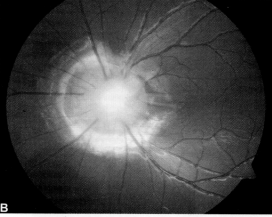

Figs 19.3A and B: Optic disc coloboma—morning glory syndrome. **A.** Schematic representation; **B.** Photograph

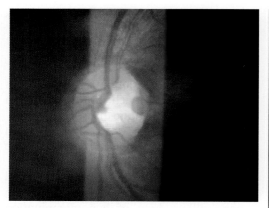

Fig. 19.4: Optic disc pit

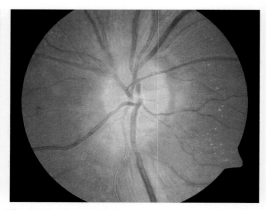

Fig. 19.6: Optic neuritis

that, its upper temporal portion lies anterior to the lower margin (Fig. 19.5).

- Eyes with tilted discs frequently have inferior crescent, myopia, a moderate degree of oblique astigmatism, and hypopigmentation of the inferonasal aspect of the retina.
- Tilted disc may be associated with upper temporal field defect which may be mistaken for chiasmal compression.

OPTIC NEURITIS (FIG. 19.6)

Optic neuritis is an inflammatory or demyelinating disorder of the optic nerve (from the optic disc to the lateral geniculate body).

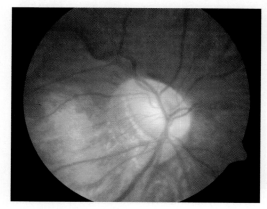

Fig. 19.5: Tilted optic disc

Classification

- Optic neuritis
- Retrobulbar neuritis—acute and chronic (toxic amblyopia)
- Neuroretinitis.

Etiology

- **Idiopathic**
- **Demyelination** or **multiple sclerosis (MS):** Optic neuritis is the presenting feature in about 25% of MS patient, and in 70% cases, it occurs in established disease. Recurrence in the same eye or opposite eye occurs in about 25% patient. The impairment of vision is more with increased body temperature (**Uhthoff's phenomenon**).
- **Neuromyelitis optica (of Devic):** An acute bilateral optic neuritis in young patient with paraplegia (due to myelitis).
- **Post-viral:** They are the most common causes in children, and frequently bilateral. It usually follows an episode of influenza-like symptom, then followed by acute disseminated encephalomyelitis. Less frequently, it is associated with mumps, measles or chickenpox.
- **Granulomatous inflammation:** Like sarcoidosis, tuberculosis or syphilis, and these are rare.

- *Infection of the adjacent structures:* Like uveitis, retinitis, meningitis, orbital cellulitis, sinusitis (sphenoidal or ethmoidal), etc.
- *Metabolic disturbance:* Like diabetes, anemia, pregnancy, vitamin deficiency, etc.

Clinical Features

Optic neuritis of the idiopathic type, or from demyelination, typically affects the patients between 20 years and 40 years of age, but post-viral type typically occurs in children.

Symptoms

- Uniocular sudden dimness of vision which may vary in severity (from a small scotoma to complete blindness).
- Visual loss progresses very rapidly, and usually maximum by the end of second week.
- A discomfort or pain behind the eyeball, especially when the eye is moved superiorly (due to involvement of the origin of superior rectus muscle).

Signs

- Visual acuity may be 6/60 or even less, although some patients have only mild loss of vision (6/12).
- Presence of local tenderness, especially near the site of attachment of superior rectus tendon.
- Pupillary reactions may be:
  - Sluggish and ill-sustained.
  - Relative afferent papillary defect (Marcus-Gunn's pupil).
- Impaired colored vision.
- A delayed dark adaptation.
- Field of vision—central, centrocecal or paracentral scotoma.

Ophthalmoscopic Features

- *Optic neuritis* is most common in children and is frequently post-viral.

Here, the intraocular portion of the optic nerve is involved and gives rise to engorgement and edema of the optic disc with obliteration of the physiological cup, small hemorrhages on the disc and inflammatory cells into the adjacent vitreous.

- *Retrobulbar neuritis* is the most common findings in adults. Here, the optic disc and retinal nerve-fiber layer are normal, as the site of involvement is behind the globe.
- *Neuroretinitis* is the least common type. It has all the signs of optic neuritis in addition to a macular star (Fig. 19.7). This form of optic neuritis is not usually associated with multiple sclerosis.

Differential Diagnosis

- *Papilledema:* Discussed in table (*see* page 369).
- *Pseudoneuritis (pseudopapillitis)* is seen in:
  - High hypermetropia
  - Congenital malformed disc
  - Myelinated nerve fibers
  - Optic nerve drusen or
  - Opacity in the media (nuclear sclerosis).

In these cases, the disc appears hyperemic with blurred margin, but is not significantly elevated, there are no vascular changes and the condition is stationary.

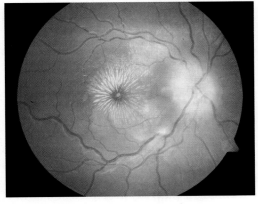

Fig. 19.7: Neuroretinitis with macular star

Investigations

Usually X-ray skull, CT scan (computed tomography scan) and MRI (magnetic resonance imaging) are unnecessary in a typical case. In some cases, these tests (especially the MRI scan) are required to establish demyelinating disorders. They should also be done in order to exclude papilledema due to intracranial lesions.

Course and Prognosis

- The rate of visual recovery is slower than that of the initial visual loss and usually takes 4–6 weeks of time.
- Almost 90% of the patients recover normal or near normal visual acuity, but minor defects in color vision may persist.
- There is no correlation between the initial visual loss and the final outcome.
- In 10% of cases, the patient may develop partial or total optic atrophy (secondary or post-neuritic optic atrophy).

Treatment

- Treatment must be directed to the cause.
- **Oral prednisolone** (1–1.5 mg/kg/day) is given to accelerate the speed of recovery of vision. Intravenous injection of **methylprednisolone** (10 mg/kg/day) for 3 consecutive days followed by oral prednisolone is advocated recently.
- Simultaneous posterior periocular injection of depot steroid may be tried.
- **Injection hydroxycobalamin** (in the form of B_1, B_6 and B_{12} injection) may be added.

TOXIC AMBLYOPIAS (TOXIC OPTIC NEUROPATHIES)

These include a number of conditions in which optic nerve fibers are damaged by exogenous toxins.

- Although, generally described as a form of chronic retrobulbar neuritis, the primary lesion is probably demyelination of the nerve-fiber layer.
- These toxic effects are of two types:
  1. In **the majority** initially affect the papillomacular bundle, presenting with **central** or **centrocecal** (between blind spot and fixation point) scotoma (Fig. 19.8).
  2. In **the minority,** there is simply a general depression of vision with contraction of the visual field.

Etiology

The common agents are tobacco, ethyl alcohol, methyl alcohol, lead, carbon disulfide, cannabis, or drug-induced, e.g. quinine, ethambutol, isoniazid or isonicotinylhydrazide (INH), etc.

Tobacco-alcohol Amblyopia

- A deficiency of protein and B vitamins (particularly thiamine) is an important association among heavy drinkers and pipe-smokers.
- The onset of visual impairment is gradual, progressive and bilateral.
- Visual field shows bilateral centrocecal scotomas, especially prominent with colored (red) targets.

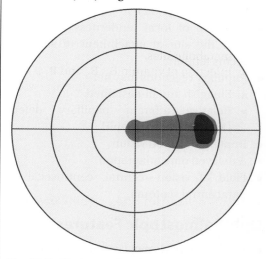

Fig. 19.8: Centrocecal scotoma

- **Treatment** is by means of weekly injection of 1,000 units of hydroxycobalamin for 3 months. Patient should abstain from drinking and smoking and also be advised to take a balanced diet.

Methyl-alcohol Amblyopia (Hooch Poisoning)

- Poisoning from wood-alcohol occurs sporadically, from drinking methylated spirit (mixed with country-liquor).
- Methyl alcohol is a severe neurotoxin which is lethal to the retina. It is oxidized into formic acid and formaldehyde, in the vitreous, causing destruction of the ganglion cells resulting total optic atrophy.
- It may occur in **acute** or **chronic** form.
  - **In acute form:** Vomiting, prostration, coma, and sometimes death, if more than one ounce (30 mL) has been consumed.
  - **If the patient survives:** Complete blindness is usually noticed within 1–2 days due to total optic atrophy.
  - **In chronic form:** Progressive loss of vision due to progressive optic atrophy.
- **Treatment**
  - Rapid correction of acidosis.
  - Correction of dehydration.
  - Administration of ethyl alcohol, which competes with methyl alcohol for metabolic sites.
  - Injection of vitamin B_1, B_6 and B_{12}.
- **Prognosis:** The vision may improve temporarily but usually relapses, again becoming gradually diminished to complete blindness.

Drug-induced Toxic Amblyopia

Ethambutol

- This is a standard oral chemotherapeutic agent, used in tuberculosis.
- It may produce optic neuritis, resulting in sudden impairment of vision, and color vision (especially for red-green).

- The optic disc is edematous and hyperemic with an eventual central scotoma.
- The optic neuritis is usually **dose dependent**. It does not occur if the dosage of not more than 15 mg/kg/day is administered (**upper limit of safety**).
- **Treatment:** The neuritis is reversible when the drug is discontinued, and the majority recovers their vision by 6–12 months. Injection hydroxycobalamin has an important role for the successful treatment.

Quinine

- Sudden, total loss of vision may follow even in small dosage (60 mg) in susceptible persons. 150 mg is the maximum amount of quinine sulfate which should be given within 24 hours.
- The pupil is dilated and non-reacting.
- **Ophthalmoscopically,** there are extreme narrowing of the arterioles, retinal edema with cherry-red spot and pallor of the optic disc.
- It may be associated with deafness and tinnitus.
- **Treatment:** Treated by vasodilator drugs and withdrawal of quinine.

ANTERIOR ISCHEMIC OPTIC NEUROPATHIES

Anterior ischemic optic neuropathy (AION) is a segmental or generalized infarction of the anterior part of the optic nerve caused by the occlusion of short posterior ciliary arteries. It causes a severe visual loss with an **altitudinal visual field defect** in the middle-aged, or elderly.

Causes

- **Atherosclerosis:** Non-arteritic AION
- **Giant cell arteritis:** Arteritic AION
- **Systemic collagen vascular disorders:** Like polyarteritis nodosa or systemic lupus erythematosus.

- ***Miscellaneous:*** Examples are emboli, malignant hypertension, anemia or migraine.

Non-arteritic Anterior Ischemic Optic Neuropathies

- Elderly patient with systemic hypertension.
- Visual loss is monocular, sudden, and painless, without any premonitory symptom.
- Moderate to severe loss of vision.
- Typical visual field defect is an altitudinal hemianopia, mainly involving the inferior half (Fig. 19.9).
- ***Ophthalmoscopy*** shows, sectorial (usually upper part) edema with hyperemic disc which may be surrounded by splinter hemorrhages (Fig. 19.10).
- No effective treatment is available.

Arteritic Anterior Ischemic Optic Neuropathies

- It occurs in 25% of patients with untreated giant cell arteritis, in elderly individuals.
- The visual loss is sudden, profound and usually permanent. Premonitory symptoms like periocular pain and transient blurring of vision are usually present.
- Visual acuity is reduced to hand movements or counting fingers.
- Visual field defect is profound.
- ***Ophthalmoscopy*** shows a swollen white or pale disc with splinter hemorrhages around. With time, the entire optic disc becomes pale.

Systemic associations include: Headache, scalp tenderness (with ischemic necrosis of the scalp in severe cases), jaw claudication, and pain and stiffness of the proximal muscles.

A ***high erythrocyte sedimentation rate (ESR)*** (more than 100 mm/hour), raised C-reactive protein and temporal artery biopsy confirm the diagnosis.

Treatment: Heavy doses of systemic steroids (intravenous hydrocortis one 250 mg along with prednisolone—80 mg orally), and then with gradual reduction of oral prednisolone over a period of 3 months. In many cases, treatment may be needed for 1–2 years with a small maintenance dose.

PAPILLEDEMA

Papilledema is the bilateral, noninflammatory passive swelling of the optic disc, produced by raised intracranial tension (ICT).

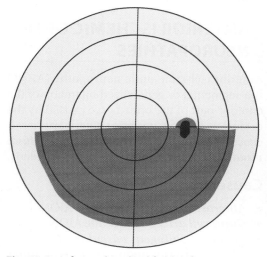

Fig. 19.9: Inferior altitudinal field defect

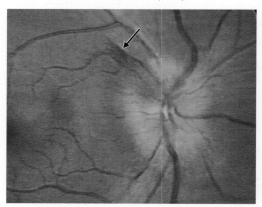

Fig. 19.10: Anterior ischemic optic neuropathy (arrow showing splinter hemorrhage)

- Papilledema (due to raised ICT) is one of the causes of disc edema, and they are not synonymous. The other causes of disc edema are mentioned in the next page.
- Generally, unilateral causes of disc edema should be considered to be due to a local inflammation, vascular disorders, or compressive lesions in the orbit.
- Unilateral papilledema with optic atrophy, on the other side, suggests a frontal lobe tumor or olfactory meningioma of the opposite side—the *Foster-Kennedy syndrome*.
- As a rule, papilledema does not develop if the optic nerve has already become atrophic.

Etiology

- *Raised intracranial tension* in papilledema may be due to:
  - *Congenital stenosis* of ventricular system.
  - *Blockage of the ventricular system* by space occupying lesions, e.g. tumors abscess, hemorrhage, etc.
  - *Obstruction of cerebrospinal fluid (CSF) absorption by the arachnoid villi*—e.g. direct blockage of villi by blood or protein, or due to cavernous sinus thrombosis.
  - *Hypersecretion of CSF by the choroidal plexus tumors.*

Any intracranial tumor in any position excepting of medulla oblongata may induce papilledema. It is most evident with tumors in the posterior fossa which obstruct the aqueduct of Sylvius, and least with pituitary tumors. The site of the tumor is, thus, more important than its nature, its size and rate of growth.

- *Idiopathic intracranial hypertension (IIH)* or *pseudo-tumor cerebri* causes gross papilledema without any striking neurological changes. It occurs mainly following intake of certain drugs, e.g. tetracycline, nalidixic acid, high doses of vitamin A, corticosteroids, oral contraceptive, etc. Presence of normal-size ventricles (as seen in CT scan of brain) and CSF study by lumbar puncture confirm the diagnosis.
- Malignant hypertension (Fig. 19.11).

Causes of disc edema
- Optic papillitis, neuroretinitis
- Ocular hypotony
- Anterior ischemic optic neuropathy
- Leber's optic neuropathy
- Optic nerve glioma or meningioma
- Central retinal venous occlusion
- Orbital cellulitis
- Metastasis on the optic nerve head
- Chronic anterior uveitis.

Symptoms

General Symptoms

- Headache (made worse by coughing or straining).
- Vomiting without nausea.
- Focal neurological deficit with changes in level of consciousness.

Ocular Symptoms

- *Visual acuity remains fairly normal* until the latest age of the disease.
- *Amaurosis fugax:* It is a transient black out of vision for a few seconds may be present in some patients.

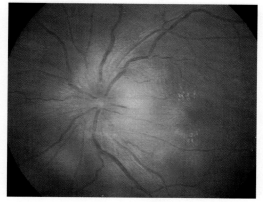

Fig. 19.11: Disc edema in malignant hypertension

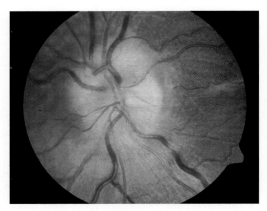

Fig. 19.12: Early papilledema

- Visual fields are usually normal, unless the lesion itself causes a hemianopia.

Signs

Pupillary reactions are normal until the secondary optic atrophy sets in.

Ophthalmoscopy: The features are different in the different stages of the disease:
- ***Early papilledema (Fig. 19.12)***
  - ***Earliest change*** is blurring of superior and inferior margins of the disc.
  - Disc hyperemia and dilated capillaries.
  - Spontaneous venous pulsation is absent.
  - Splinter hemorrhages at or just off the disc-margin.
  - Normal optic disc cup is preserved.

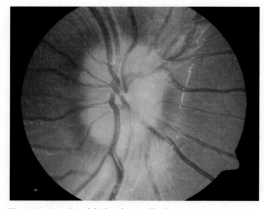

Fig. 19.13: Established papilledema

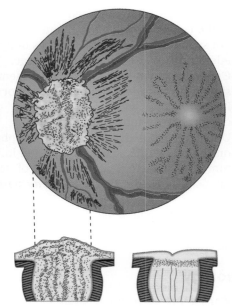

Fig. 19.14: Established papilledema with macular star (Note the disc elevation compared to normal disc).

- ***Established papilledema (Fig. 19.13)***
  - Disc margins become indistinct and central cup is obliterated.
  - Disc surface is elevated above the retinal plane [more than +3D (1mm) with direct ophthalmoscope].
  - Venous engorgement and peripapillary edema.
  - Flame-shaped hemorrhages and cotton wool spots.
  - Radiating folds around the macula, macular star (Fig. 19.14).
- ***Chronic papilledema (Fig. 19.15)***
  - Central cup remains obliterated.
  - The hemorrhagic and exudative components gradually resolve.
  - Optic disc appears as a champagne cork (Fig. 19.16).
- ***Atrophic papilledema***
  - Retinal vessels are attenuated with perivascular sheathing.
  - Dirty-white appearance of the optic disc due to reactive gliosis leading to secondary optic atrophy.

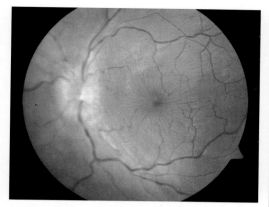

Fig. 19.15: Chronic papilledema—Patton's line

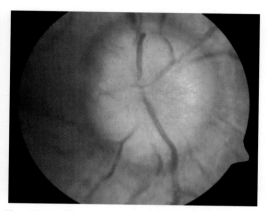

Fig. 19.16: Chronic papilledema—champagne cork appearance

Field Changes

- *In early stage* there is no field defect.
- *In established stage* there is enlargement of the blind spot.
- *In chronic stage* there is associated peripheral constriction of the visual field with appearance of nerve-fiber bundle defects.

- *Finally,* there is total loss of visual field.
- *In addition,* the lesion itself may cause hemianopic or quadrantic field defect.

Treatment

- Treatment must be directed to detect the cause, and then to treat it.

Difference between papilledema and optic neuritis		
Features	**Papilledema**	**Optic neuritis**
History	Headache and vomiting initially no visual symptom	Sudden loss of vision: History of fever or upper respiratory tract infection
Laterality placement	Usually bilateral	Usually unilateral
Visual acuity	Remains normal until late stage	Severely reduced (6/60 or less)
Pain or tenderness of the eyeball	Absent	May be present
Pupil	Normally reacting	Relative afferent pupillary defect (Marcus-Gunn's pupil)
Disc swelling	More than +3D (1 mm) elevation in the established case	Usually + 2D to +3D elevation
Hemorrhage and exudates	More in established case	Relatively less
Visual fields	Enlargement of blind-spot and later gradual constriction Colored field not much affected	Central or centrocaecal scotoma More with colored objects
CT scan or MRI	Intracranial space occupying lesion may be detected	Demyelinating disorder may be seen
Recovery of vision	May not be complete even after treatment	Usually complete with adequate treatment

Abbreviations: **CT**—Computed tomography; **MRI**—Magnetic resonance imaging

- Surgical decompression of the optic nerve may be indicated to preserve vision.

OPTIC ATROPHY

Optic atrophy is the degeneration of optic nerve fibers with loss of their myelin sheaths, and characterized by the pallor of the optic disc.

The pallor of the disc is not due to atrophy of the nerve fibers, but to loss of vascularity owing to obliteration of the disc capillaries.

Classification

Etiological

- **Primary optic atrophy:** It occurs without any local disturbance, but associated with CNS disease, or without any discoverable cause. The important causes are:
  - Tabes dorsalis (classical cause)
  - Multiple sclerosis (most common)
  - Leber's optic atrophy
  - Glaucomatous optic atrophy
  - Tumor compression of the optic nerve.
- **Secondary optic atrophy:** It is preceded by swelling of the optic disc, e.g.
  - Papilledema (Fig. 19.17)
  - Optic neuritis
  - Neuroretinitis.

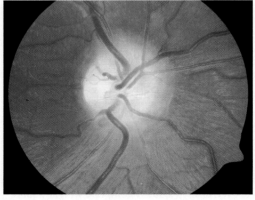

Fig. 19.17: Post-papilledemic optic atrophy

- **Consecutive optic atrophy:** Optic atrophy that follows extensive disease of the retina, causing extensive degeneration of the ganglion cells, as in:
  - Retinitis pigmentosa
  - Central retinal arterial occlusion
  - Extensive retinochoroiditis.

Anatomical

- **Ascending optic atrophy:** If the lesion is in the retina, an ascending optic atrophy occurs, which terminates at the lateral geniculate body, e.g. retinitis pigmentosa, central retinal arterial occlusion, etc.
- **Descending optic atrophy:** It follows diseases involving the optic nerve fibers anterior to the lateral geniculate body, and terminates at the optic disc, e.g. chiasmal compression, retrobulbar neuritis, etc.

Symptoms

- The chief symptom is loss of central or peripheral vision which may be sudden or gradual.
- Impairment of color vision (red-green).

Signs

- Visual acuity is impaired in proportion as the nerve fibers die.
- **Relative afferent pupillary defect:** In total optic atrophy the pupil is dilated and immobile.
- **Ophthalmoscopically**
  - **Primary optic atrophy (Fig. 19.18)**
    - Pallor of the disc, with gray or white color.
    - The margins of the disc are sharply defined, and peripapillary retina is normal looking.
    - There is slight atrophic cupping.
    - The blood vessels are only slightly constricted without any sheathing.
  - **Secondary optic atrophy (Fig. 19.19)**
    - Pallor of the disc (dirty-gray color) with blurred margins.

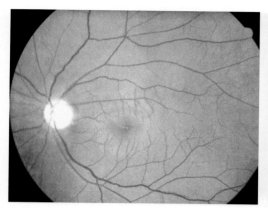

Fig. 19.18: Primary optic atrophy

- Physiological cup is full and lamina cribrosa is obscured.
- Narrowing of the blood vessels with sheathing.
- Gliosis over the disc surface extending towards the peripapillary retina.

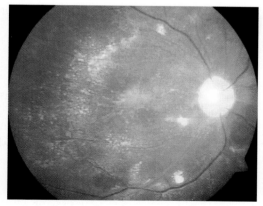

Fig. 19.19: Secondary optic atrophy—neuroretinitis

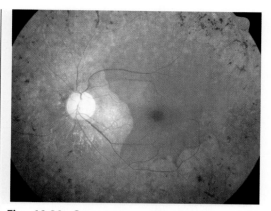

Fig. 19.20: Consecutive optic atrophy—retinitis pigmentosa

- **Consecutive optic atrophy (Fig. 19.20)**
  - Yellowish-waxy pallor of the disc.
  - Disc margins are less sharply defined.
  - Marked narrowing (even obliteration) of the retinal blood vessels.

Investigations

- *Field of vision:* In partial optic atrophy, the central vision is depressed with concentric contraction of the visual field, according to the cause.
- Fluorescein angiography of the optic nerve head.
- Visual evoke potential (VEP) is useful, especially in children.
- Total neurological evaluation by a neurophysician, and investigations, like, X-ray skull, CT scan and MRI of brain and optic nerve, etc.

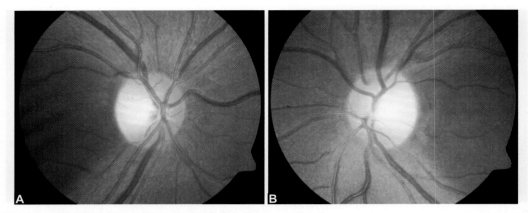

Figs 19.21A and B: Bilateral temporal pallor. **A.** Right eye; **B.** Left eye

Treatment

- Treatment of the cause.
- As the prognosis is usually poor, community based rehabilitation is important in bilateral cases.

Temporal pallor (Figs 19.21A and B)

Most forms of partial optic atrophy involve a loss of temporal fibers including the papillomacular bundles. This results in temporal pallor, which is an important sign of an evanescent neuritis as in multiple sclerosis. But, this should be confirmed by special investigations, since, temporal side is normally relatively pale, because the retinal vessels emerge from the nasal side and the temporal side is normally less vascular.

OPTIC NERVE TUMORS

Discussed in Chapter 21, page 398–399.

Intraocular Tumors

Tumors of the uvea and retina are rare. They are of great importance, since most of them are malignant and endanger the life of the patient.

IRIS TUMORS

Iris Nevus (Fig. 20.1)

- It consists of slightly elevated, localized, discrete, small pigmented mass and is composed of proliferated melanocytes.
- The nevi are not progressive, and do not distort the pupil.
- As a rule, this is benign, but occasionally it takes on malignant proliferation.

Such a development is suggested by an increase in size, vascularization and pigmentation, which sometimes distorts and everts the pupillary margin *(ectropion uveae)*.

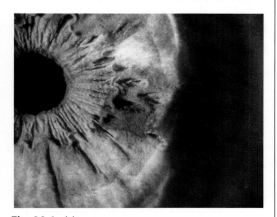

Fig. 20.1: Iris nevus

Malignant Melanoma (Figs 20.2A and B)

- It often arises from pre-existing nevus.
- It is usually symptomless, and the tumor is noticed by the relatives or friends as a brown mass on the iris surface.
- It has blood vessels growing in it and may be associated with seeding.
- Pupil is distorted and there may be glaucoma when it extends into the anterior chamber angle.
- The growth should be watched carefully and is best treated by broad iridectomy or iridocyclectomy if the angle is involved.

CILIARY BODY TUMORS

Medulloepithelioma (Diktyoma)

- Intraocular medulloepithelioma arises in the nonpigmented epithelium of the ciliary body and resembles embryonic tissue of the primitive retina and ciliary body.
- It is thought to be congenital, though it occurs between 4 years and 12 years of age.
- The chief symptoms are pain and poor vision.
- A white pupil (leukocoria), secondary cataract and secondary glaucoma are often present.
- Enucleation is often delayed due to failure to diagnose the condition.

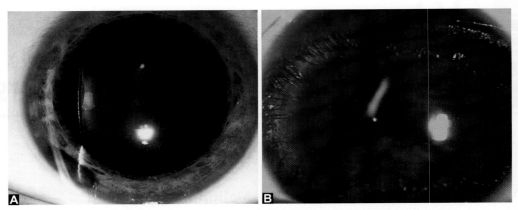

Figs 20.2A and B: A. Iris melanoma at anterior chamber angle; **B.** Malignant melanoma—iris

Malignant Melanoma

Ciliary body melanoma is more common than iris melanoma, but less common than the choroidal melanoma.

- It tends to involve either the choroid or the iris, or both.
- It cannot usually be visible unless the pupil is widely dilated.
- Clinically, it may present in a variety of ways:
  - As subluxation of the lens with secondary glaucoma.
  - As dilated episcleral blood vessels in the same quadrant as with the tumor *(sentinel vessels)*.
  - As retinal detachment.
  - As diffuse mass in a ring around the ciliary body (Fig. 20.3).
- Because of its location and minimal symptoms, the diagnosis may be often delayed.
- Indirect ophthalmoscopy, three-mirror gonioscopy, transillumination test and USG B-scan or ultrasonic biomicroscopy (UBM) are helpful for early diagnosis.
- Treatment is by enucleation (for large tumors), or by local resection (for small tumors).
- Since, ciliary body melanomas have a low degree of malignancy, the prognosis is usually good.

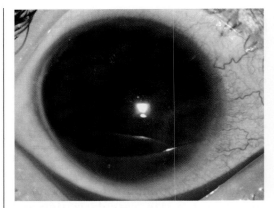

Fig. 20.3: Ciliary body melanoma

CHOROIDAL TUMORS

Benign Melanoma (Nevus) (Fig. 20.4)

- Typical benign melanomas of the choroid are flat or slightly elevated, oval or circular state-gray lesions.
- They are usually less than three disc diameters in size and occur most frequently at the posterior half of the fundus.
- They are usually present at birth and maximum growth occurs during puberty.
- Most of the benign melanomas are asymptomatic, although those near the macula may present with impairment of central vision.

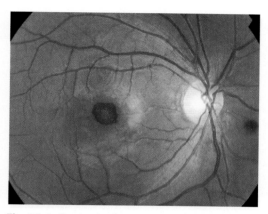

Fig. 20.4: Benign melanocytoma of the choroid

- Benign melanomas may become malignant. An increase in size, elevation of the mass, irregular pigmentation over the tumor and visual field loss suggest malignancy.
- Treatment is not indicated except the patient should be followed up regularly with serial fundus photographs.

MALIGNANT MELANOMA OF THE CHOROID

The most common primary intraocular tumor in adults is malignant melanoma of the choroid (Fig. 20.5).

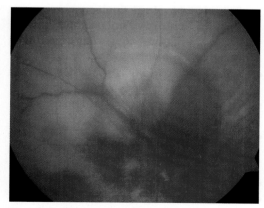

Fig. 20.5: Choroidal melanoma

- The average age of the patients with choroidal melanoma is 50 years.
- They are extremely rare among blacks, and slightly more common in males.
- Most malignant melanomas develop from pre-existing benign melanomas (nevi).
- They originate most frequently in the outer layers of the choroid, and may spread like a carpet between the sclera and the Bruch's membrane.
- Tumors may remain quiescent for many years, and then without apparent reason, suddenly begin to grow rapidly.
- Eventually, the Bruch's membrane perforates and the growth appears as mushroom or collar-button shaped mass.

Histological Classification (Callender's)

Uveal malignant melanomas can be divided into six types (Figs 20.6A to D) according to cellular features:

1. *Spindle-A cell type:* Tumors composed of this cell type have the best prognosis.
2. *Spindle-B cell type:* It is having the second best prognosis.
3. *Fascicular type:* The cells in a palisading arrangement are composed of either spindle-A or spindle-B cells and has the same prognosis as primary cell type.
4. *Epithelioid cell type:* This is the least common type and these cells carry the worst prognosis.
5. *Mixed-cell type:* This is composed of a combination of spindle and epithelioid cells with intermediate prognosis. This is the most common type of malignant melanoma.
6. *Necrotic type:* This is the tumor in which the specific cell type cannot be recognized. The necrotic process may initiate a severe inflammatory reaction which may be mistaken clinically, as endophthalmitis or uveitis.

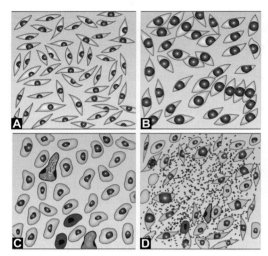

Figs 20.6A to D: Histological types of uveal melanoma. **A.** Spindle-A type; **B.** Spindle-B type; **C.** Epitheloid type; **D.** Mixed type

Clinically, malignant melanoma of the choroid is commonly divided into four stages:
1. Quiescent stage
2. Glaucomatous stage
3. Stage of extraocular extension
4. Stage of metastasis.

The chief symptoms result from the exudative retinal detachment and secondary glaucoma caused by increase in the choroidal volume. The patient may present with decreased visual acuity, or a defect in the visual field, and ocular pain accordingly.

In some of the cases, the patient is *asymptomatic,* and the tumor is detected by a routine ophthalmoscopic examination.

Ophthalmoscopically
- The tumor is invariably unilateral and solitary.
- A typical melanoma appears as a pigmented and elevated oval mass.
- The color of the mass is frequently brown, although it may be mottled with black or dark-brown pigment or it may be amelanotic (Fig. 20.7).
- As the tumor grows a brown exudative detachment results owing to break in the Bruch's membrane.

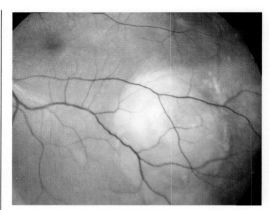

Fig. 20.7: Choroidal amelanotic melanoma

- An accumulation of orange pigment *(lipofuscin)* in the retinal pigment epithelium is commonly seen over the detached area but is not diagnostic.
- *Other ocular features include* choroidal folds, subretinal hemorrhage, vitreous hemorrhage, secondary glaucoma cataract and posterior uveitis.
- The lymph nodes are not affected, but distant metastasis in the liver and elsewhere are the common cause of death.

Investigations

- *Medical evaluation:* It is to exclude the possibility of a metastatic tumor of the choroid and to check for distant metastasis from the primary ocular growth. Liver function tests and X-ray chest are most valuable.
- *Indirect ophthalmoscopy* for better depth assessment.
- Three-mirror and contact lens examinations of the fundus.
- *Transillumination* test is useful in differentiating a pigmented tumor from a non-pigmented lesion.
- Fundus photography.
- *Fluorescein angiography:* In general, most melanomas show a mottled fluorescence during the arteriovenous phase of the angiogram with a progressive staining

of the lesion and prolonged retention of the dye.

- **Ultrasonography:** It is especially useful in detecting the presence of a tumor in an eye with hazy media. Both A-scan and B-scan are helpful to detect the solid nature of the mass. It shows a solid mass with homogenous appearance arising from the choroid with collar-button appearance, acoustic hollow and choroidal excavation.
- **P32-uptake:** Malignant melanoma has an increased rate of phosphate uptake and retains **P32-isotope** longer than other nonmalignant lesions.
- **Visual field examination:** It is of limited value.
- **CT scan and MRI:** They are valuable in detecting the extraocular extension.
- **USG-guided tissue biopsy:** It is to obtain cellular aspirates for analysis.

Differential Diagnosis

Rhegmatogenous retinal detachment (RD), metastatic tumor of the choroid, choroidal hemangioma, large choroidal nevus, and choroidal detachment.

Management

The correct management at present is controversial as the traditional treatment of enucleation has been questioned by many ophthalmologists, especially for small tumors.

- **Observation:** It is indicated for small tumors, where the diagnosis is not certain; patients over the age of 65 years; patients with liver metastasis; and with a slow growing tumor with normal vision.
- **Enucleation:** It is indicated for very large melanomas, especially, if all useful vision has been irreversibly lost. The overall 5 years survival rate is 75% after enucleation for all types of melanoma.
- **Radioactive scleral plaques (Cobalt-60 or Iodine-125):** They are suitable for small to medium size tumors.

- **Heavy-charged particle irradiation (protons or helium):** It is a new approach to radiotherapy and may be better than enucleation in eyes with large tumors. It is not available widely.
- **Photocoagulation:** Xenon arc photocoagulation is better than argon laser and indicated for small tumors away from the fovea.
- **Choroidectomy (local resection):** This difficult and complicated operation may be useful for the selected peripheral tumors.
- **Palliative therapy:** Chemotherapy and immunotherapy may be useful in cases with distant metastases.

METASTATIC CARCINOMA OF THE CHOROID (FIG. 20.8)

Metastatic choroidal tumors are probably the most common type of intraocular malignancy (which are often undetected).

- The most frequent primary sites are the bronchus (bronchogenic carcinoma) in males and breast (breast carcinoma) in females (Fig. 20.9).
- Other primary sites are kidney, testis and gastrointestinal tract. The prostate is an extremely rare primary site.

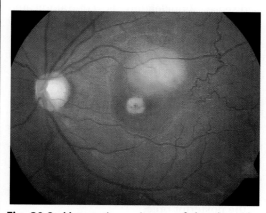

Fig. 20.8: Metastatic carcinoma of the choroid—from bronchogenic carcinoma

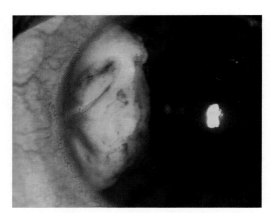

Fig. 20.9: Metastatic carcinoma of the iris from breast carcinoma

- Choroidal metastases have a definite predilection for the posterior pole of the fundus, with early loss of central vision.
- Typically, they appear as solitary or multiple, creamy-white, placoid or oval lesions which infiltrate laterally.
- They rarely become significantly elevated and have ill-defined borders.
- A careful examination of the opposite eye is important as bilateral metastases are common.
- *Diagnosis* depends mainly on accurate history and careful general physical examination.
- *Treatment* must be directed to the primary disease. Enucleation is contraindicated unless the eye is painful and blind. Palliative treatment is carried out with chemotherapy in conjunction with external-beam irradiation.

CHOROIDAL HEMANGIOMA

This is rare and is associated in about half of the patients with skin angioma (as in ***Sturge-Weber syndrome***).
- Typically, it appears as a dome-shaped or diffuse, reddish-orange lesion mostly at the posterior pole.
- Frequently, secondary changes, like exudative retinal detachment, pigment mottling and cystoid degeneration may occur.
- A useful clinical sign is the blanching of the lesion with pressure on the globe.
- P32-uptake test, ultrasonography (USG) and fluorescein angiography are helpful to differentiate it from other lesions (e.g. metastatic tumors and amelanotic melanoma).
- *Treatment:* Asymptomatic tumors do not require treatment. If the vision is threatened, extensive photocoagulation should be applied around the tumor.

RETINOBLASTOMA

It is the malignant intraocular tumor originating in the outer nuclear layer of the retina and strongly resembles fetal retina.

Etiology

- ***Incidence:*** 1 in 20,000 live births.
- ***Laterality:*** 25–30% of cases are bilateral.
- ***Age:*** The neoplasm is probably congenital, but the average age of diagnosis is 18 months. The vast majority of cases become clinically apparent before the age of 3 years. It is exceptional after the age of 7 years.
- ***Inheritance:*** A positive family history is present only in 6% of cases (mostly in bilateral cases). Mode of inheritance is autosomal dominant. Remaining 94% of cases are sporadic.
- ***Chromosomal abnormalities:*** In 5% of cases, it is associated with deletion of the long arm of chromosome-13 and with trisomy-21.

Other Facts

- Orbital sarcoma may occur in the irradiated field in children with enucleated retinoblastoma.
- Osteogenic sarcoma of femur and skull bones are more common in patients who have survived from bilateral retinoblastoma.

- Very rarely pinealoblastoma may be associated with some cases of bilateral retinoblastoma and then it is called *trilateral retinoblastoma*.

Clinical Features

Clinical Presentation

- *Leukocoria or amaurotic cat's eye reflex:* The most common mode of presentation (60% of cases) and is due to reflection of light from the yellowish-white mass in the retrolental area (Fig. 20.10).
- *Squinting of the eye:* The second most common mode of presentation (20%).
- *Secondary glaucoma* which may be associated with buphthalmos.
- *Proptosis* (due to orbital involvement) (Fig. 20.11).
- *Endophthalmitis or anterior uveitis* may also be a presenting feature.
- *Visual difficulties:* Noticed by the parents.
- Nystagmus in bilateral cases if it occurs within 6 months.

Signs

- Unilateral dilated pupil
- White pupillary reflex
- Strabismus
- Intraocular tension is higher

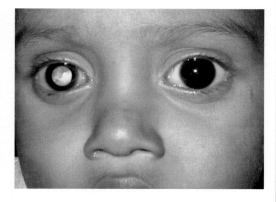

Fig. 20.10: Right-sided retinoblastoma—amaurotic cat's eye reflex

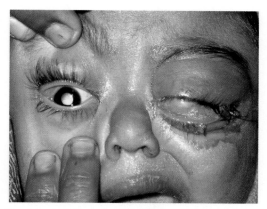

Fig. 20.11: Bilateral retinoblastoma with proptosis of the left eye due to orbital involvement

- *Heterochromia of the iris:* It is due to rubeosis irides owing to massive posterior segment ischemia.

Stages of Retinoblastoma

Stage 1: The quiescent stage (6–12 months).
Stage 2: The glaucomatous stage.
Stage 3: The stage of extraocular extension.
Stage 4: The stage of metastasis.

Spread of Retinoblastoma

- *Direct spread*
  - Into the intraocular tissues.
  - Into the extraocular tissues:
    - Extension into the central nervous system (CNS) via optic nerve.
    - Extension into the orbit as a fungating mass (Fig. 20.12).
- *Lymphatic spread:* Along the orbital lymphatics into the preauricular and cervical lymph nodes.
- *Spread by blood stream:* Choroidal invasion is the main route of escape. Most common sites are the bones and liver, and lung is the least common site.

Diagnosis

Indirect Ophthalmoscopy

Indirect ophthalmoscopy with scleral indentation, following full dilatation of pupil

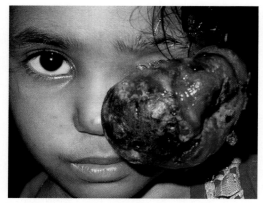

Fig. 20.12: Retinoblastoma—extensive direct extension into the orbit

should be performed in both eyes under general anesthesia. Tumors arising anterior to the equator are missed with direct ophthalmoscope. The appearance of the tumor may be:

Endophytic type (glioma endophytum) (Fig. 20.13)

- This projects from the retina into the vitreous cavity.
- White or pearly-pink colored mass with sharply demarcated margin.
- Presence of calcium deposits in most cases gives the appearance of **cottage-cheese**.
- Multiple seeding of the tumor cells may be seen in the vitreous cavity.

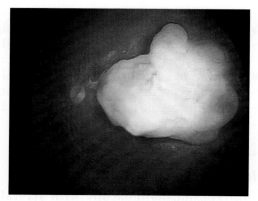

Fig. 20.13: Large endophytic retinoblastoma

Exophytic type (glioma exophytum)

- This grows in the subretinal space and gives rise to a total exudative retinal detachment.
- The tumor itself is difficult to visualize.

Plane type (glioma planum): It is difficult to visualize the tumor.

Special Investigations

- **X-ray of the orbit:** It is for the presence of calcification and erosion of the optic foramen.
- **Ultrasonography:** USG B-scan shows presence of tumor with calcification.
- **CT scan of the orbit and brain** to demonstrate calcification and CNS spread.
- **Aqueous humor paracentesis**: It is for cytology and lactate dehydrogenase (LDH) enzyme assay. An aqueous to serum LDH ratio of greater than 1.0 is suggestive of retinoblastoma.
- **Carcinoembryonic antigen (CEA)** may be found in retinoblastoma patient.
- **Enzyme-linked immunosorbent assay (ELISA)** test to differentiate it from Toxocara endophthalmitis.
- **Lumbar puncture** and bone marrow aspiration for the evidence of metastases.
- **Fine needle aspiration cytology (FNAC)** when other diagnostic tests are inconclusive.
- **Fluorescein angiography:** It is not done routinely.

Histopathology

- **Gross examination:** A chalky-white, friable tumor with dense foci of calcification.
- **Microscopic:** Retinoblastoma consists of small, round, densely packed cells with large basophilic nuclei. It may be well differentiated or poorly differentiated. Well-differentiated retinoblastoma is characterized by presence of **rosettes** and **fleurettes** (Figs 20.14A to D).
  - **Flexner–Wintersteiner rosette:** Cells arrange in a single layer around a central clear lumen. This is true rosette and highly characteristic.

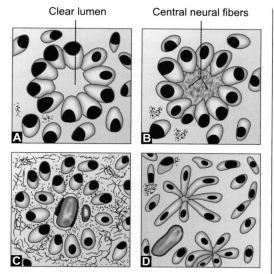

Clear lumen Central neural fibers

Figs 20.14A to D: Microscopic appearance of retinoblastoma. **A.** Flexner–Wintersteiner rosette area of necrosis; **B.** Homer–Wright rosette; **C.** Pseudorosette; **D.** Fleurettes

- **Homer–Wright rosette:** It is a radial arrangement of cells around a central triangle of neural fibers (rather than clear lumen) and is mainly found in neuroblastoma or medulloblastoma.
- **Pseudorosette:** In necrotic retinoblastoma, several layers of cells may be seen around a blood vessel, within the areas of extensive necrosis with the formation of pseudorosette.
- **Flurette:** It is composed of group of tumor cells and contains pear-shaped eosinophilic processes which project through a fenestrated membrane.
- **Histology of metastatic lesions** outside the retina shows a change of character of the cells. They resemble sarcomatous cells and rosettes are in rarity.

Treatment

- **Enucleation:** Excision of the eye with a long optic nerve stump is the treatment of choice for most tumors affecting the first eye. The treatment of the second eye depends on the size and location of the tumor.
- **Exenteration:** Exenteration of the orbit is indicated in case of orbital involvement of the tumor.
- **Radiotherapy:** It is done by external irradiation or by a Cobalt-60 scleral plaque. Cataract, radiation retinopathy and scleral necrosis may occur. It is indicated in small to medium size tumors and for recurrent or residual tumor of the orbit.
- **Photocoagulation:** Xenon arc photocoagulation is useful for certain small retinoblastomas not involving the optic nerve or the macula.
- **Cryotherapy:** It is useful for small peripheral tumors. The tumor should be frozen by triple-freeze and thawing technique.
- **Chemotherapy:** It is indicated following enucleation in advanced cases and in presence of distant metastases. Cyclophosphamide and vincristine are used every 3 weeks for 12–15 months.
- **Combination of therapy:** To achieve best results.

Genetic counseling: This is important in bilateral cases and if two or more cases of retinoblastoma occur in a family.

- Normal parents with one affected child in sporadic case—the chance of transfer to next sibling is 1.3–6%.
- When an affected person survives to maturity and procreates—chance of having retinoblastoma in offspring is about 25–30% in unilateral case, and the risk is more in bilateral cases.

Prognosis: The overall mortalities from retinoblastoma are between 15 and 20%. Mortality rate is higher with optic nerve involvement, large size tumor, poorly differentiated tumor and when there is choroidal invasion.

Follow-up

Follow-up is extremely important in case of treated retinoblastoma.

In general, the rule is every 4 months until 3 years of age, every 6 months until 4 years of age and yearly for next 3 years.

Examination under anesthesia (EUA) is done in each visit. The examination includes:
- Inspection and palpation of the socket after removing the prosthesis.
- Indirect ophthalmoscopy of the fellow eye.
- USG B-scan of the fellow eye to know the status of the tumor (if treated with other methods).

DIFFERENTIAL DIAGNOSIS OF LEUKOCORIA IN CHILDREN

The common causes of leukocoria or white pupillary (Figs 20.15 and 20.16) (*amaurotic cat's eye*) reflex in children are:
- Retinoblastoma
- Pseudoretinoblastoma (pseudoglioma)
- Congenital cataract
- Retinopathy of prematurity
- Toxocara endophthalmitis
- Persistent hyperplastic primary vitreous
- Retinal dysplasia
- Coat's disease
- Choroidal coloboma.

Retinoblastoma
- Usually unilateral (Figs 20.10 and 20.15)
- Usual age at diagnosis is 18 months
- No inflammatory sign in anterior segment
- Ophthalmoscopy shows, a pearly-white mass with presence of secondary calcification
- Lens is usually transparent
- Intraocular pressure is high
- The lesion is progressive
- X-ray orbit, USG and enzyme assay of the aqueous confirm the diagnosis.

Congenital cataract (Fig. 20.16)
- Unilateral or bilateral
- Opacity in the lens clearly indicates the presence of cataract
- It does not cause diagnostic problem, but a cataract does not exclude other causes of leukocoria especially persistent hyperplastic primary vitreous (PHPV).

Retinopathy of prematurity
- History of prematurity and low birth weight are present.
- History of prolonged exposure to oxygen.
- Bilateral in 100% of cases.
- First noted in neonatal period.
- Presence of tractional retinal detachment.
- Intraocular pressure is normal.

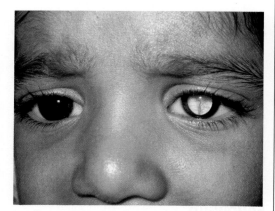

Fig. 20.15: White pupillary reflex—retinoblastoma in left eye

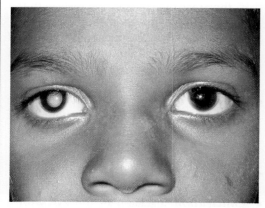

Fig. 20.16: White pupillary reflex—congenital cataract

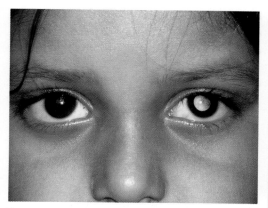

Fig. 20.17: White pupillary reflex—toxocariasis

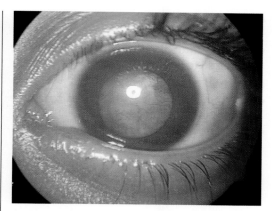

Fig. 20.19: White pupillary reflex—Coats' disease

Toxocara endophthalmitis (Fig. 20.17)
- Usual presentation is between 2 years and 9 years of age.
- History of contact with pet cat or dog.
- Usually unilateral.
- Signs of inflammation in anterior segment and vitreous are present.
- Intraocular pressure is low and eventually the eye may be phthisical.
- ELISA test is very diagnostic.

Persistent hyperplastic primary vitreous (Fig. 20.18)
- Developmental disorder of the vitreous.
- Usually unilateral, and first noted in the neonatal period.

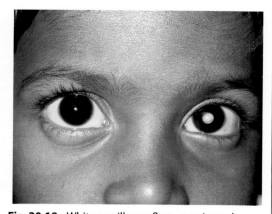

Fig. 20.18: White pupillary reflex—persistent hyperplastic primary vitreous

- Associated with microphthalmos.
- Lens may be cataractous.
- Elongated ciliary processes are visible through the dilated pupil.
- Intraocular pressure may be high.
- USG B-scan confirms the diagnosis in presence of cataract.

Retinal dysplasia
- Unilateral or bilateral usually present at birth.
- Pink or white retrolental mass.
- The eye is microphthalmic with shallow anterior chamber and elongated ciliary processes.
- It is due to failure of the retina to develop normally.
- Usually associated with severe systemic abnormalities.
- USG B-scan helps to differentiate it from PHPV in unilateral cases.

Coats' disease (Fig. 20.19)
- It is almost always unilateral.
- It occurs primarily in older boys (although, it may occur at an early age).
- Large areas of retinal or subretinal exudates with cholesterol crystals.
- Dilated and tortuous retinal blood vessels at the posterior pole.
- Exudative detachment as a retrolental mass occurs over a period of years.

- It is a severe form of retinal vascular telangi-ectasia.
- Fundus fluorescein angiography may be required to confirm the diagnosis.

Choroidal coloboma

- Leukocoria is only with a large complete choroidal coloboma.
- Usual presentation is at birth.

- Unilateral or bilateral.
- They are always located inferonasally.
- The eye is usually microphthalmic in case of large coloboma.
- Ophthalmoscopy shows the defect is at the embryonic position of choroidal fissure with shiny-white sclera.

Diseases of the Orbit

Symptoms of orbital diseases	
Symptoms	**Causes**
Forward displacement of the globe (proptosis) • Unilateral • Bilateral • Rapidly progressive • Slowly progressive • Periodic exacerbation and remission with upper respiratory tract infection (URTI)	• Space-occupying lesion within the orbit • Thyroid ophthalmopathy • Orbital cellulitis • Rhabdomyosarcoma • Pseudotumor • Benign neoplasm • Lymphangioma
Backward displacement of the globe (enophthalmos)	• Microphthalmos • Horner's syndrome • Blow-out fracture of the orbital floor
Ocular pain	• Orbital cellulitis • Rhabdomyosarcoma • Pseudotumor
Diplopia	• Space-occupying lesion outside the muscle cone
Visual loss	• Optic nerve compression by the neoplasm • Posterior scleral indentation by the tumors
Congestion of the conjunctiva	• Inflammatory orbital diseases • Thyroid ophthalmology

Signs of orbital diseases	
Signs	**Causes**
Reduced visual acuity	• Optic nerve compression • Exposure keratopathy • Induced hypermetropia • Choroidal folds
Relative afferent pupillary defect (Marcus-Gunn)	• Optic nerve compression • Optic neuritis
Lid lag and retraction	• Thyroid ophthalmopathy

Contd...

Contd...

Signs	Causes
Increased resistance to orbital compression	• Neoplasms • Thyroid ophthalmopathy
Ocular movement abnormality	• Neurological lesions • Thyroid myopathy • Blow-out fracture • Optic nerve-sheath meningioma
Optic disc • Optic atrophy • Disc edema • Opticociliary shunt vessels	• Optic nerve compression • Raised intraorbital pressure • Optic nerve-sheath meningioma
Pulsatile proptosis	• Carotid-cavernous fistula • Orbital roof defect
Presence of bruit	• Carotid-cavernous fistula
Change of proptosis by head posture	• Capillary hemangioma • Orbital varices
Positive forced duction test (FDT)	• Blow-out fracture • Contracture of muscle

DEVELOPMENTAL ANOMALIES

The orbit and its contents may be affected by a number of developmental anomalies involving the bones of the skull or face.

They are commonly hereditary (autosomal dominant) in nature.

Frequently, there is a characteristic shape of the head or facial appearance, associated with proptosis, papilledema, optic atrophy and strabismus.

Common Abnormalities

Craniosynostosis

It follows premature closure of one or more cranial sutures. This closure causes a complete arrest of bone growth perpendicular to the closed suture and the compensatory growth of the cranium in other diameters, which causes the typical shape of the skull.

Types:

- *Scaphocephaly (boat-shaped skull):* Premature closure of sagittal suture.
- *Oxycephaly (tower-shaped skull):* Premature closure of coronal suture.
- *Trigonocephaly (egg-shaped skull):* Premature closure of frontal suture.
- *Brachycephaly (clover-leaf skull):* Premature closure of all sutures.

The common clinical features are:

- Bilateral proptosis due to shallow orbit.
- Esotropia or exotropia.
- Papilledema, due to increased intracranial pressure.
- Optic atrophy, primarily due to traction on the optic nerve, or secondary to papilledema.

Treatment by craniotomy or orbital decompression to reduce cerebrospinal fluid (CSF) pressure and papilledema.

Craniofacial Dysostosis (Crouzon) (Figs 21.1A and B)

- Brachycephaly is combined with hypoplasia of the maxilla.
- *Ophthalmic features*
  - Widely separated eyeballs (hypertelorism)
  - Shallow orbits with bilateral proptosis
  - Corneal problems due to exposure
  - Divergent squint
  - Optic atrophy.
- *Non-ophthalmic features*
  - High-arched palate
  - Irregular dentition
  - Hooked (parrot-beak) nose
  - Mental retardation.

Mandibulofacial Dysostosis (Treacher Collins)

- Hypoplasia of the zygoma and mandible.
- *Ophthalmic features*
  - Indistinct inferior orbital margin
  - Coloboma (notching) of the lower lid
  - Anti-mongoloid slanting.
- *Non-ophthalmic features*
  - Bird-like face
  - Macrostomia with high-arched palate
  - External ear deformity.

Median Facial-Cleft Syndrome

- Hypertelorism with telecanthus
- Cleft nose, lip and palate
- V-shaped frontal hair line (widow's peak)
- Divergent squint.

Oxycephaly-Syndactyly (Apert)

- Tower skull with flat occiput
- Mental retardation
- Ventricular septal defect
- High-arched palate
- Hypertelorism, shallow orbits and proptosis
- Anti-mongoloid slanting with ptosis and exotropia
- Syndactyly of the fingers and toes.

Hypertelorism (Figs 21.2A and B)

- Increased separation of the eyes.
- Widely separated orbits, and broad nasal bridge.
- The interpupillary distance (IPD) may be 85 mm or more.
- Divergent squint, telecanthus and anti-mongoloid slanting.
- There may be optic atrophy due to associated narrowing of the optic canals.

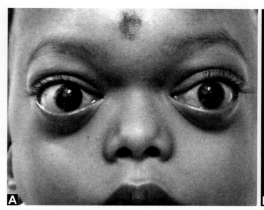 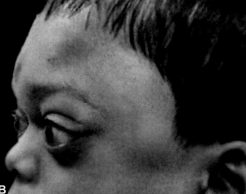

Figs 21.1A and B: Cruozon syndrome. **A.** Front view; **B.** Lateral view

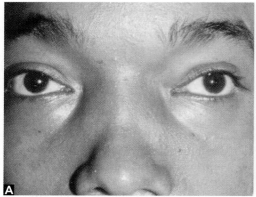 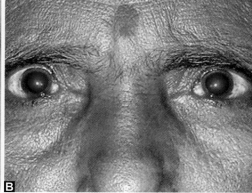

Figs 21.2A and B: A. Hypertelorism; **B.** Telecanthus

- *Hypertelorism also occurs in:*
  - Median facial-cleft syndrome,
  - Apert's syndrome,
  - Crouzon's syndrome, etc.

PROPTOSIS AND ITS INVESTIGATIONS

Forward protrusion of the eyeball beyond the orbital margin is called *proptosis* or *exophthalmos*.

In general, proptosis and exophthalmos are loosely synonymous. But in strict sense:

- *Exophthalmos means* an active or dynamic protrusion of the eyeball (usually bilateral). Classically seen in thyroid ophthalmopathy.
- *Proptosis means* a passive protrusion of the eyeball, classically seen in space occupying lesion in the orbit and hence, usually unilateral. Proptosis may be:
  - Unilateral
  - Bilateral
  - Rapidly-growing (acute)
  - Slowly-growing (chronic)
  - Intermittent
  - Pulsating.

Unilateral Proptosis (Fig. 21.3)

Inflammatory

- *Acute:* Orbital cellulitis, panophthalmitis.
- *Chronic:* Periostitis, pseudotumor.

Neoplastic

- *Benign:* Hemangioma, osteoma, fibroma, neurofibroma, dermoid, lymphangioma, glioma of the optic nerve, xanthomatosis, mixed tumor of the lacrimal gland, etc.

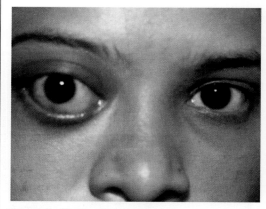

Fig. 21.3: Right-sided proptosis

- *Malignant:* Lymphosarcoma, rhabdomyo-sarcoma, meningioma (optic nerve-sheath or sphenoidal-ridge); retinoblastoma and malignant melanoma extending into the orbit, maxillary antral carcinoma, metastatic deposit into the orbit (from CA-breast or CA-lung), etc.

Vascular

- Retrobulbar hemorrhage (RBH)
- Orbital varices
- Aneurysm of the blood vessels.

Parasitic

- Cysticercosis
- Hydatid cyst.

Systemic Diseases

- Leukemic deposits in acute myeloid and lymphoid leukemia (*chloroma*)
- Thyroid ophthalmopathy.

Bilateral Proptosis (Exophthalmos) (Fig. 21.4)

- *Congenital:* Craniosynostosis, uveal colo-bomatous cyst
- *Endocrine:* Thyroid ophthalmopathy
- Cavernous sinus thrombosis
- Xanthomatosis of orbit
- *Metastatic:* Leukemia, neuroblastoma.

Rapidly-growing (Acute) Proptosis

- *Orbital emphysema* due to fracture of the medial wall of the orbit.
- *Orbital hemorrhage (RBH)*
- Orbital cellulitis
- Rhabdomyosarcoma.

Slowly-growing (Chronic) Proptosis

Proptosis that grows over months or years.
- Optic nerve glioma
- Optic nerve meningioma
- Orbital hemangioma
- Thyroid ophthalmopathy
- Benign neoplasm of the orbit.

Intermittent Proptosis

- Orbital varices (most common)
- Lymphangioma (Fig. 21.5) (periodic enlargement with upper respiratory tract infection)
- Recurrent orbital hemorrhage
- Recurrent orbital emphysema.

Pulsating Proptosis

- *Transmitted vascular pulsation*
  - Caroticocavernous fistula

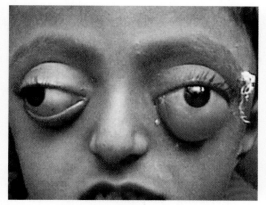

Fig. 21.4: Bilateral proptosis—Crouzon's syndrome

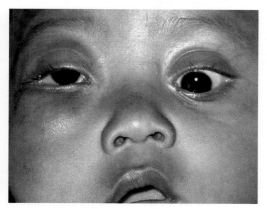

Fig. 21.5: Lymphangioma

- Saccular aneurysm of the ophthalmic artery
- Highly vascular tumor in the orbit.
- *Transmitted CSF pulsation*
  - Congenital absence of the orbital roof, as in meningocele and encephalocele.
  - Erosion of the orbital roof, as in neurofibromatosis and dermoid cyst.

Investigations

Careful history and clinical examination should precede radiological and laboratory investigations.

History

- Benign lesions tend to have a longer history than malignant lesions.
- Acute onset with pain suggests an inflammatory lesion (orbital cellulitis or pseudotumor); and also in rhabdomyosarcoma.
- In the past history, enquire about thyroid dysfunction, malignancies, orbital trauma, and sinus diseases.

Clinical Examination

- *Measurement of the degree of protrusion* is most readily assessed clinically by standing behind the patient and viewing the eyes from above.
  First rule out the possibilities of the pseudoproptosis and enophthalmos of the opposite eye.
  - *Pseudoproptosis:* The important causes are:
    - Enlargement of the same eye from high axial myopia and buphthalmos.
    - Retraction of the eyelids on the same side.
    - Shallow orbits as in craniosynostosis.
    - Enophthalmos of the opposite eye.
  - *Enophthalmos:* About 50% of patients with enophthalmos are initially misdiagnosed as having contralateral proptosis, or ipsilateral ptosis.

The important causes are:
- Microphthalmos
- Phthisis bulbi
- Horner's syndrome
- Absence of greater wing of the sphenoid as in neurofibromatosis
- Blow-out fracture of the orbital floor.

- *Measurement of proptosis (exophthalmometry):*
  - It measures the distance between corneal apex to the deepest portion of the lateral orbital margin.
  - It is measured by simple plastic ruler, and by *Hertel's exophthalmometer* (in both eyes simultaneously).
    - Normal value less than 20 mm (average 16 mm).
    - In *proptosis* a reading of 21 mm or more; or a difference of more than 2 mm between the two eyes.
- *Exophthalmometry may be:*
  - *Absolute:* As compared to normal value (i.e. more than 20 mm).
  - *Comparative:* As compared, from time to time in the same eye.
  - *Relative:* As compared between the two eyes.
- *Detailed ocular examination:* Already discussed in table under *signs of orbital diseases* (*see* page 385–386).
- *Palpation of the orbital rim:* It may reveal a mass, bony erosion or bony thickening. The character of the mass (surface, consistency, thrill, tenderness, etc.) is noted carefully.
- *Dynamic properties of proptosis:*
  - *Try to precipitate proptosis:* By dependent head posture, a Valsalva maneuver or by jugular venous compression. A proptosis may be induced or exacerbated, in orbital varices or in capillary hemangioma.
  - *Look for pulsation:* A mild pulsation is better judged with a slit-lamp. A pulsating exophthalmos is seen in defect in the orbital roof (transmitted

CSF pulsation), or in arteriovenous communication.

- *A bruit on auscultation:* It may be heard in carotid-cavernous fistula or a highly vascular tumor. CSF pulsation is not associated with a bruit.
- *Transillumination:* It is often valuable in evaluation of anterior orbital lesions, either solid or cystic.
- *Systemic examination:*
  - Thyroid evaluation.
  - Examination particularly for paranasal sinuses and nasopharynx.
  - To search for primary neoplasm elsewhere in the body, whenever a metastatic deposit are suspected in the orbit.
  - The important primary sites are breast, lungs, stomach, prostate, kidney and adrenals. Liver and spleen must be examined in leukemic patients.

Special Investigations

- *Laboratory tests*
  - *Hematologic study:* Total leukocyte count (TLC) and differential leukocyte count (DLC) for inflammatory lesions, or blood dyscrasias, e.g. leukemia.
  - *Thyroid function tests:* Examples are serum T3, T4 and thyroid stimulating hormone (TSH) levels.
  - *Casoni's test:* For hydatid cyst.
  - *Urine analysis:* Bence-Jones protein in multiple myeloma.
- *Plain X-rays of the orbit*
  - *The standard frontal anterior posterior (AP) view:* For a composite view of the bones of the orbits, and to compare between the two orbits.
  - *Caldwell view:* To demonstrate the superior orbital fissure.
  - *Water's view:* To detect orbital floor fractures.
  - *Rhese view:* To visualize the optic foramina.
  - *Lateral view:* To study the nasopharynx.

X-ray signs in proptosis
Enlargement of the orbit • *Symmetrical:* In intraconal lesions (optic nerve glioma, hemangioma, etc.) • *Asymmetrical:* In extraconal lesions (rhabdomyosarcoma, dermoid cyst, etc.)
Change in bone density • *Increased:* In meningioma, Paget's disease, fibrous dysplasia and osteoblastic metastasis. • *Decreased or destruction:* In malignant-tumors.
Intraorbital calcification: Seen in orbital varix (Figs 21.6A and B), optic nerve-sheath meningioma, retinoblastoma, etc.
Superior orbital fissure enlargement: Seen in infraclinoid carotid aneurysm, intracavernous aneurysm, intracranial extension of orbital tumors, etc.
Optic canal enlargement: In optic nerve glioma.
Dehiscence of orbital bones: In neurofibromatosis, mucocele, aneurysm, etc.

- *Orbital venography:* Presently, orbital venography is only indicated in patients who are clinically suspected to have *orbital varices.*
- *Computed tomography (CT) scan*
  - CT scan is the most valuable noninvasive method of diagnosis for orbital lesions.
  - It is capable of visualizing the eyeball, extraocular muscles and the optic nerve.
  - It is extremely useful in determining the location and size of the orbital lesion.
- *Ultrasonography (USG) B scan*
  - USG B scan gives an anatomical display which is easier to interpret than A scan.
  - USG is superior to CT scan in specific tissue diagnosis, and can usually differentiate a vascular lesion from a solid tumor, or an inflammatory pseudotumor from thyroid ophthalmopathy.
- *Magnetic resonance imaging (MRI)*
  - MRI is major recent advance in imaging method, and superior to CT scan.
  - It distinguishes between the lesions based on their location, tissue structures and metabolic profile.

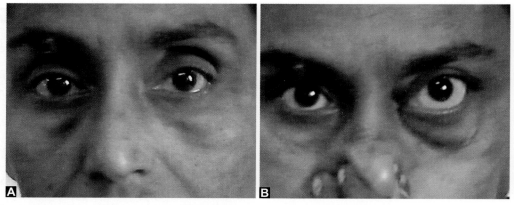

Figs 21.6A and B: Orbital varix with proptosis in left eye on Valsalva maneuver

- ▪ The imaging is not hampered by the bony shadow.
- • *Fine needle aspiration cytology (FNAC)*
  - ▪ The aspirate is obtained under CT scan or ultrasound guidance using a 23-gauge needle.
  - ▪ It is especially valuable in suspected cases of orbital metastasis or secondary neoplasm, from the adjacent structures.
  - ▪ Diagnostic accuracy may be up to 95%.
- • *Incisional biopsy*
  - ▪ It may have a deleterious effect on the course of the tumor.
  - ▪ Incisional biopsy along with frozen section tissue study is a better alternative.
- • *Excisional biopsy*
  - ▪ It should always be preferred to incisional biopsy, for orbital tumors which are well encapsulated or circumscribed.
  - ▪ Exact diagnosis in many orbital lesions can only be made by histopathological studies of the orbital mass.

Principles of Treatment in Proptosis

- • *Medical:* For orbital cellulitis, pseudo-tumor, thyroid ophthalmopathy, leukemic deposits in the orbit, etc.

- • *Radiotherapy:* For secondary deposits and rapidly-growing malignant tumors.
- • *Surgical*
  - ▪ *Tarsorrhaphy:* To protect the exposed cornea.
  - ▪ *Orbitotomy:* For benign lesions, e.g. hemangioma, glioma, lacrimal gland tumor, dermoid cyst, etc.
    - – *Anterior orbitotomy:* For a mass in the anterior part of the orbit.
    - – *Lateral orbitotomy (Kronlein's):* For a mass in the posterior (retrobulbar) part or at the apex of the orbit.
    - – *Transcranial approach:* For tumors extending into the cranial cavity.
    - – *Transconjunctival approach:* For the lesions which are anterior or inferior.
    - – *Transnasal or transantral approach:* These are endoscopic approach—used more frequently to gain access to orbital lesions.
  - ▪ *Exenteration of the orbit:* Total excision of the orbital contents and eyelids, followed by immediate grafting of the orbit. This is performed for secondary malignancy of the orbit from contagious ocular structures (e.g. advancing malignant melanoma of lid or tarsal conjunctiva) or radio resistance orbital malignancy.

ORBITAL INFLAMMATIONS

Orbital Cellulitis

Etiology

- *Age:* Usually child or young adult.
- *Sinus infections:* From the frontal, maxillary or ethmoidal sinusitis (sphenoidal sinusitis is very rare). This is the most common cause.
- *Penetrating orbital injury:* It may be with retained intraorbital foreign body.
- *Thrombophlebitis:* From a focus in the adjacent skin.
- *Postoperative:* Following enucleation of the globe.
- Dental or nasopharyngeal infection.
- *Causative organisms: Streptococcus pneumoniae, Staphylococcus aureus, Streptococcus pyogenes* and *Haemophilus influenzae* in children under 5 years of age.

Types

The **orbital septum**, the dense fascia (which separates the anterior structures from the orbit), divides the cellulitis into two types: (1) Pre-septal and (2) Orbital.

1. *Pre-septal cellulitis (Fig. 21.7)*
   - Acute periorbital swelling and redness.
   - Increased warmth and tenderness of the eyelids.
   - Conjunctival chemosis.
   - Sometimes, fever with leukocytosis.
   - A fluctuating mass signifies abscess formation.
   - *Treatment:* Hot compress oral antibiotics and analgesics, and topical antibiotics.

2. *Orbital cellulitis (Fig. 21.8A)*
   Symptoms
   - A sudden onset of unilateral severe pain and swelling of the lids.
   - Diplopia due to limitation of movements.
   - Lacrimation and photophobia.
   - Impairment of vision lately.
   - Frequently associated with fever.

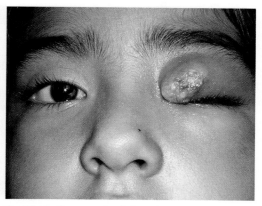

Fig. 21.7: Pre-septal cellulitis

Signs
- Lid marked edema and tenderness.
- Conjunctiva chemosis and congestion.
- Proptosis commonly the eyeball is displaced laterally and downwards.
- Limitation of ocular movements.
- Ophthalmoscopy may show features of optic neuritis in severe cases.

Course and Complications

- Subsides completely with prompt treatment.
- *Orbital abscess* (Fig. 21.8B) formation, which may point and burst on the skin near the orbital margin.
- Meningitis, brain abscess, and cavernous sinus thrombosis, which may be fatal.
- Central retinal arterial occlusion, optic neuritis and optic atrophy may lead to blindness.

Management

- Patient should be admitted immediately.
- *Intravenous (IV) broad-spectrum antibiotics* should be started immediately and the choice of antibiotics can be changed based on cultures.
  - *In children under 5 years of age:* The antibiotics should cover *H. influenzae.* Choice of IV antibiotics are ampicillin-

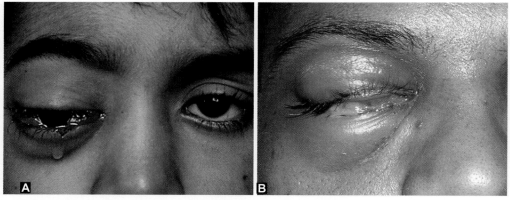

Figs 21.8A and B: A. Orbital cellulitis; **B.** Orbital abscess—severe chemosis

sulbactam; ceftriaxone, cefotaxime, ceftazidime.

- ■ ***In adult or older children:*** Cefuroxime or piperacillin-tazobactam is given every 4 hourly.
- If methicillin-resistant *Staphylococcus aureus* (MRSA) is suspected, add vancomycin (15 mg/kg) twice daily to the above regimen.
- IV metronidazole may be required along with antibiotics.
- Once the improvement is documented within 48–72 hours of IV antibiotics use, switch to oral antibiotics.
- ***Oral options:*** Amoxicillin-clavulnate (20–40 mg/kg/day); cefpodoxime (5 mg/kg/day) or cefdinir 14 mg/kg/day for 2–3 weeks.
- A ***multidisciplinary approach*** is usually required for patients with orbital cellulitis under the care of pediatrician, ENT surgeon, ophthalmologist and general physician.
- Hot compress and analgesics to relieve pain.
- Simultaneously, the patient should be ***investigated*** for etiological factors:
  - ■ Nasal and conjunctival swab culture.
  - ■ X-ray of the paranasal sinuses (PNS).
  - ■ Complete hemogram [may have normal erythrocyte sedimentation rate (ESR) and white blood cell (WBC) count].
  - ■ Ultrasonography B scans to detect an orbital abscess.
  - ■ Cerebrospinal fluid study and CT scan of the brain, if intracranial spread is suspected.
- ***Surgery***
  - ■ Drainage of the orbital abscess.
  - ■ Incision and drainage of the lid abscess.
  - ■ In most cases, it is necessary to drain the infected sinuses as well.

Inflammatory Orbital Disease (Pseudotumor) (Fig. 21.9)

Inflammatory orbital disease (IOD) is a term for idiopathic, non-neoplastic, non-microbial

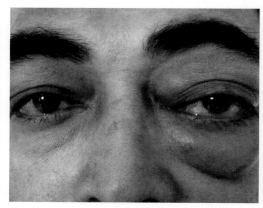

Fig. 21.9: Inflammatory orbital disease (left eye)

space-occupying periocular lesion, which may simulate an orbital neoplasm (pseudotumor).

Clinical Features

- Typically affects the middle-aged males.
- Most cases are unilateral.
- The onset is sudden with:
  - Periocular pain,
  - Edema of the lids and conjunctiva,
  - Conjunctival congestion,
  - Limitation of ocular movements, and
  - Proptosis.
- Depending on the site of involvement, a palpable mass may be present.

Investigations

- **Ultrasonography B scan:** It shows a sonolucent area (edema) posterior to the globe with thickening of the extraocular muscles.
- **CT scan:** Shows muscle enlargement and scleral thickening.

Differential Diagnosis

- **Thyroid ophthalmopathy:** More gradual onset, bilateral, presence of lid signs, and altered thyroid function tests.
- **Orbital cellulitis:** Usually affects the children and with more severe picture.

Clinical Course

- Spontaneous remission after a few weeks.
- Intermittent course and eventual remission.
- Severe prolonged inflammation → progressive fibrosis of orbital tissues → frozen orbit with visual impairment.

Treatment

- **Observation:** Mild cases require no specific treatment, except close observation.
- **Systemic corticosteroids:** Oral prednisolone, 60–80 mg/day for 2 weeks. The

dose is gradually tapered according to the response. 50–75% of patients show a favorable response.
- **Radiotherapy:** In patients who are steroid-resistant. A biopsy or fine needle aspiration cytology should be performed to rule out true neoplasm, prior to the initiation of orbital irradiation.
- **Cytotoxic agents:** In few cases who are resistant to both steroids and radiotherapy, cyclophosphamide 200 mg/day may be the choice.

THYROID OPHTHALMOPATHY (FIGS 21.10A AND B)

The ophthalmopathy may be present in hyperthyroid, hypothyroid or euthyroid state.
- **Grave's disease** is the most common variety of hyperthyroid state with an auto-immune basis.
  It typically affects the women between 20–45 years of age, and is characterized by goiter, infiltrative ophthalmopathy, thyroid acropathy (clubbing) and pretibial myxedema.
- **Ophthalmic Grave's disease (OGD)** is a variant of Grave's disease where usual clinical and laboratory findings of hyperthyroidism are absent.
- Smokers have more severe thyroid ophthalmopathy than non-smokers. Smoking delays or worsens the outcome of treatment.

Pathogenesis

- Neither LATS (long-acting thyroid stimulator), nor EPS (exophthalmos producing substance) is responsible for ophthalmopathy.
- It has been proposed recently that circulating thyroglobulin (Tg) and anti-Tg immune-complex may bind to the eye muscle and orbital tissue to produce thyroid ophthalmopathy.

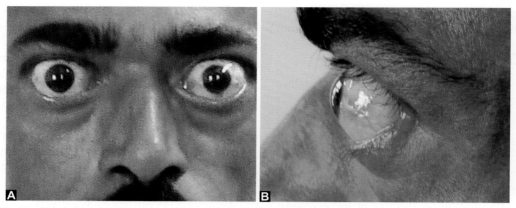

Figs 21.10A and B: Thyroid ophthalmopathy. **A.** Front view; **B.** Lateral view

Pathology

Ophthalmopathy is due to:
- Hydrophilic mucopolysaccharide deposition and inflammatory cells infiltration (plasma cells and lymphocytes) in the orbital tissues including the muscles.
- Proliferation of retrobulbar fat and connective tissues.

Clinical Features

They consist of one or more following signs.
- Retraction of the eyelid, due to:
  - Muller's muscle overaction due to sympathetic stimulation.
  - Overaction of levator-superior rectus muscle complex.
  - Contraction of the levator muscle due to infiltration.
- Lid lag
- Exophthalmos (unilateral or bilateral)
- Extraocular muscle involvement
- Conjunctival chemosis and hyperemia
- Optic neuropathy.

Warner's NO SPECS classification:

Class	Ocular changes	Grading
0	**N**o physical signs or symptoms	
I	**O**nly signs (lid retraction or lag)	

Contd...

II	**S**oft tissue involvement **Symptoms**— photophobia, watering, foreign body sensation, **signs**—hyperemia and chemosis of conjunctiva, retrobulbar resistance, palpable lacrimal gland	0 = absent a = minimal b = moderate c = marked
III	**P**roptosis (3 mm or more)	0 = absent a = 3–4 mm b = 5–7 mm c = 8 mm or more
IV	**E**xtraocular muscle involvement (most common: inferior rectus, then—medial rectus; least common: lateral rectus)	0 = absent a = limitation of movement at extreme gazes b = evident restriction of movement c = fixation of globe or globes
V	**C**orneal involvement (due to lagophthalmos or exposure keratitis)	0 = absent a = punctate keratitis b = ulceration c = clouding, melting and perforation

Contd...

Contd...

VI	Sight loss (due to optic nerve involvement)	0 = absent a = disc or field changes; vision: 6/6–6/18 b = same, but vision: <6/18– 6/60 c = blindness, vision less than 6/60

VISA classification by the International Thyroid Eye Disease Society is popularly used in North America. It consists of **4 parameters** which are scored of total 20 points. The parameters are: **V**ision; **I**nflammation/congestion; **S**trabismus/ motility restriction and **A**ppearance/exposure.

The European Group of Grave's Orbitopathy (EUGOGO) follows the modified Clinical Activity Score (CAS) which consists of 10 parameters. **Seven points** are assessed initially and all 10 points during follow-up visits—each parameter is scored 0 or 1. The disease severity is then graded as mild, moderate, severe and sight-threatening based on the CAS and the impact of the disease on the eye. The advantage of VISA and EUGOGO is that the grading and severity is used to guide the level and mode of therapy in thyroid eye diseases.

Key lid and other signs with their eponyms

	Ocular signs	Eponyms
1.	Lid retraction	Dalrymple
2.	Upper lid-lag on downgaze	von Graefe
3.	Staring and frightened appearance	Kocher
4.	Infrequent blinking	Stellwag
5.	Tremor of the closed lid	Rosenbach
6.	Poor forehead wrinkling on up gaze	Joffroy
7.	Upper lid resistance to downward traction	Grove
8.	Lower-lid lags behind the globe on, upward gaze	Griffith

Contd...

Contd...

9.	Globe lags behind upper lid on up gaze	Means
10.	Increased pigmentation of the lid-skin	Jellinek
11.	Prevent eversion of upper lid	Gifford
12.	Fullness of the eyelids	Enroth
13.	Weakness of convergence	Mobius

Investigations

- *Thyroid function tests:* Serum T3, T4 and thyroid-stimulating hormone (TSH); thyrotropin-releasing hormone (TRH) test; T3 suppression test and tests for thyroid antibodies.
- *Ultrasonography:* Both A scan and B scan show enlargement of extraocular muscle. It can also demonstrate orbital involvement, and optic nerve involvement in some cases.
- *CT scan:* Enlargement of the extraocular muscles is a common finding. Optic nerve compression can be well demonstrated by CT scan.
- *Forced duction test (FDT):* To rule out contracture of the muscles.

Treatment

- *Urgent cessation of smoking: An important* independent *risk factor which can alter the outcomes of therapy.*
- *Medical treatment for thyrotoxicosis*
  - *Antithyroid drugs:* Carbimazole (neomercazole) or propyl thiouracil, and beta-blockers (propranolol).
  - Radioactive iodine therapy.
- *Ocular treatment*
  - Topical therapy
    - Decongestant eye drop and lubricants, in the form of artificial tears for symptomatic relief.
    - Guanethidine (5%) eye drop for lid retraction.

- **Systemic therapy**
  - **Corticosteroids:** They are indicated for optic neuropathy and rapidly progressive exophthalmos. A high dose of 80–100 mg/day, oral prednisolone is started initially, and then tapered gradually. Alternately, single dose of intravenous injection of methyl prednisolone—10–15 mg/kg body weight is given to reduce the acute proptosis more rapidly.
  - **Cytotoxic agents:** Azathioprine or cyclophosphamide may be tried in steroid-resistant cases.
- **Radiotherapy:** It is reserved for those patients who are unresponsive to steroid therapy, or have contraindication to steroids. Complications of radiotherapy include keratitis, cataract, radiation retinopathy, and localized erythema.
- **Surgical therapy**
  - **Lateral tarsorrhaphy** to prevent exposure keratitis.
  - **Recession of levator and Muller's muscle** to correct lid retraction.
  - **Extraocular muscle surgery** to correct diplopia and squint.
  - **Blepharoplasty** to remove excess fat and redundant skin from around the eyelids.
  - **Orbital decompression** should only be considered when systemic steroids and/or radiotherapy are ineffective. The indications are:
    - Severe exposure keratitis
    - Compressive optic neuropathy
    - Cosmetically unacceptable exophthalmos.

Orbital decompression may be one-wall, two-wall, and three-wall or four-wall decompression—depending upon the severity of proptosis.

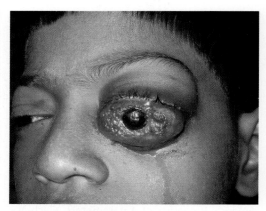

Fig. 21.11: Rhabdomyosarcoma

RHABDOMYOSARCOMA (FIG. 21.11)

- It is the most common primary malignant orbital tumor in children.
- It occurs at about 7 years of age.
- Tumor arises from voluntary muscles and presents as a rapidly-growing proptosis.
- Typically, a mass is palpable in the **superonasal quadrant**.
- Diagnosis is confirmed by biopsy where **cross-striations of tumor cells** are seen.
- Three different histological types of rhabdomyosarcoma are **embryonal, alveolar** (most malignant variety), and **pleomorphic** (best prognosis).
- Ultrasonography and CT scan show, that the tumor appears to arise from the extraocular muscles.
- **Treatment:** Combination of radiotherapy and chemotherapy. The survival rate is 90% when the tumor is confined to the orbit. In **unresponsive cases**, exenteration of the orbit may be required.

OPTIC NERVE TUMORS

These may be divided into two groups:
1. Ectodermal tumor of nerve—glioma.
2. Mesodermal tumor of the optic nerve-sheath—meningioma.

Glioma of the Optic Nerve (Fig. 21.12)

- Most prevalent in childhood (4–8 years of age).
- Presents as unilateral proptosis with visual impairment.
- Proptosis is slow-growing and axial (Fig. 21.13).
- Marcus-Gunn pupil and optic atrophy.
- About 50% of cases, it is associated with neurofibromatosis.
- Plain X-ray of the orbit (Rhese view) shows, a uniform enlargement of the optic foramen in 90% of the cases.
- Ultrasonography B scan and CT scan show fusiform or irregular enlargement of the optic nerve. Intracranial extension may be demonstrated by CT scan.
- *Treatment:* Local resection of tumor with preservation of the globe, by lateral orbitotomy. Radiation is helpful for tumors beyond surgical excision. Prognosis for life is excellent.

Meningioma

Meningiomas are invasive tumors which occur predominantly in middle aged women. The ocular features are related to primary site of involvement by the tumor.

- *Tuberculum sellae meningioma:* It may compress the chiasma or optic nerve. The patient is having a junctional scotoma (an ipsilateral central scotoma and a contralateral upper temporal field defect).
- *Sphenoidal-ridge meningioma (Fig. 21.14):* It typically causes fullness in the temporal fossa, and a slowly-growing

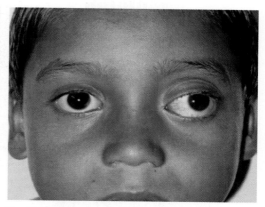

Fig. 21.13: Axial proptosis in glioma of the optic nerve

proptosis due to hyperostosis of the roof and lateral wall of the orbit, as well as invasion into the orbit itself.

- *Optic nerve-sheath meningioma (Fig. 21.15):* The patient presents with a progressive impairment of vision in one eye, or a slowly-growing unilateral axial proptosis (Fig. 21.16). The triad of long-standing visual impairment, a pale swollen optic disc, and opticociliary shunt vessels are virtually pathognomonic of optic nerve-sheath meningioma.

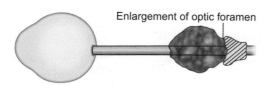

Fig. 21.12: Glioma of the optic nerve

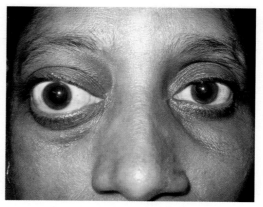

Fig. 21.14: Sphenoidal-ridge meningioma.
Note: Temporal fossa fullness on the right side

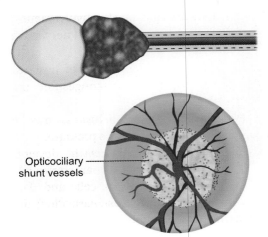

Opticociliary shunt vessels

Fig. 21.15: Optic nerve-sheath meningioma—with opticociliary shunt vessels

Investigations

- ***Plain X-rays show:*** Hyperostosis of the roof and lateral wall of the orbit in sphenoidal ridge meningioma.
- Computed tomography scan shows a segmental or diffuse enlargement of the optic nerve in optic nerve-sheath meningioma.

Treatment

- Surgical excision of the tumor by lateral orbitotomy. Prognosis for vision is extremely poor, but for life is good.

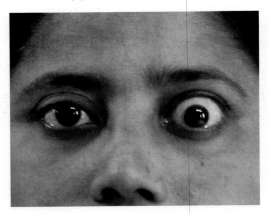

Fig. 21.16: Optic nerve-sheath meningioma—axial proptosis

- Radiotherapy may be encouraging to treat the tumor, with improved visual prognosis.

CAVERNOUS SINUS THROMBOSIS

This is an acute thrombophlebitis that originates from a purulent infection of the face, peripheral nervous system (PNS), ear or orbit that drains through the veins into the cavernous sinus.

Clinical Features

- The onset in usually violent with severe pain along the ophthalmic division of the fifth nerve, fever and prostration.
- These are rapidly followed by proptosis, with congestion and edema of the lids and conjunctiva.
- Ophthalmoplegia occurs, and the lateral rectus is the first muscle to be affected.
- Edema of the mastoid region (a pathognomonic sign) indicating back-pressure in the mastoid emissary vein.
- There may be papilledema and visual loss.
- The other eye becomes similarly affected within a few hours, due to intercavernous communication.
- Death may occur from meningitis or pulmonary infarction.

Investigations

Imaging-contrast-enhanced CT scan and MRI of the orbit and/or nasal sinuses; complete hemogram, ESR blood cultures, and sinus cultures help establish and identify an infectious primary source. Lumbar puncture is necessary to rule out meningitis.

Treatment

Intensive intravenous antibiotic is necessary to control infection, and anticoagulant to prevent extension of the clot.

CAROTID CAVERNOUS FISTULA (FIGS 21. 17A AND B)

It results from an abnormal communication between the cavernous sinus and the internal carotid artery, giving the classical picture of a pulsating exophthalmos.

Etiology

- **Trauma:** As in fracture of the base of the skull.
- **Spontaneous:** Due to rupture of an intracavernous aneurysm or an atherosclerotic internal carotid artery in a hypertensive individual.

Clinical Features

- The onset is usually unilateral, sudden and dramatic.
- A marked proptosis, which is typically pulsatile, and is associated with a thrill and bruit. The pulsation can be abolished by compression of the ipsilateral carotid artery at the neck.
- **Chemosis, redness** and **dilatation** of the episcleral blood vessels [**caput medusae**—appearance (Fig. 21.17B)].

- **Ophthalmoplegia** due to involvement of the 3rd, 4th and 6th nerve (6th nerve most common).
- **Reduced visual acuity** due to posterior segment involvement (congestion and disc edema).
- **Raised intraocular pressure**, due to elevated episcleral venous pressure.
- **Anterior segment ischemia** develops in some patients. It is characterized by corneal edema, aqueous cells and flare; iris atrophy and neovascularization; and cataract formation.

Treatment

- In 5% of the cases, the fistula closes spontaneously.
- **Surgical treatments include:** Ligation of the common carotid or internal carotid artery, direct intracavernous surgery, and balloon catheter embolization.

FRACTURES OF THE ORBIT

Discussed in Chapter 24.

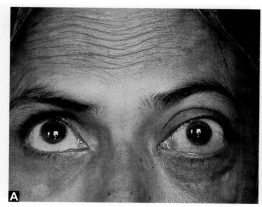 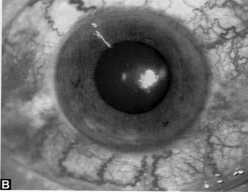

Figs 21.17A and B: A. Carotid cavernous fistula (left eye); **B.** Caput medusae of the same patient

Diseases of the Lacrimal Apparatus

SYMPTOMS AND SIGNS

The diseases of the lacrimal apparatus are divided into two groups: Abnormalities of the lacrimal glands; defects in the drainage system.

1. *Abnormalities of the lacrimal glands*
   - *Excessive tear secretion:* Reflex stimulation of the main lacrimal gland.
   - *Deficient tear formation:* Atrophy of the lacrimal gland and conjunctival scarring leading to occlusion of the main and accessory lacrimal glands.
   - *Characteristic swelling with S-shaped upper lid:* Neoplasms or inflammatory diseases of the lacrimal gland.

2. *Defects in lacrimal drainage system*
   - Cause watering from the eye.
   - Obstructed lacrimal sac may be chronically or acutely inflamed.
     - *Acute inflammation* causes cellulitis of the sac and surrounding structures, and lacrimal abscess formation.
     - *Chronic inflammation* causes painless swelling in the sac region, with regurgitation of pus through the puncta, when pressure is applied to the sacarea.
   - *Excessive tear formation* or poor drainage is a nuisance, since the vision is blurred by tears and discomfort caused by overflow of tears onto the cheek.
   - *Deficient tear formation* may cause loss of the eye and is associated with ocular surface diseases (OSD), i.e. keratinization of the cornea and conjunctiva.

DISEASES OF THE LACRIMAL GLAND

Acute Dacryoadenitis (Fig. 22.1)

- It usually accompanies a systemic disease like mumps, influenza or glandular fever.
- It is characterized by acute local pain, swelling and tenderness, and drooping of the outer part of upper lid with a characteristic S-shaped curve.
- *Treatment:* The infection is usually self-limiting. Antibiotics with local hot compress may be required in some cases.

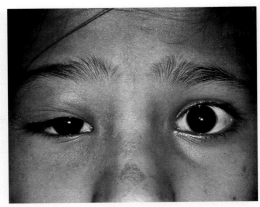

Fig. 22.1: Acute dacryoadenitis right side—S-shaped right upper eyelid

Chronic Dacryoadenitis

A proliferative inflammation of the lacrimal gland may occur as a part of generalized granulomatous disorders (e.g. syphilis, tuberculosis or sarcoidosis). It presents as a painless, firm, mobile swelling of the lacrimal gland.

Mikulicz Syndrome

It is characterized by a symmetrical swelling of the lacrimal and salivary glands, and may occur as a part of sarcoidosis, Hodgkin's disease or one of the lukemias.

Dacryops (Fig. 22.2)

It is a cystic swelling in the upper fornix due to retention of secretion owing to blockage of one of the lacrimal ducts.

Treatment is surgical excision or marsupialization of the retention cyst via the conjunctival route.

Lacrimal Gland Tumors

- They are relatively rare, and show a marked resemblance to the parotid gland tumors.
- They present in middle-aged, progress slowly, until they become palpable as hard, nodular and slightly mobile lumps.

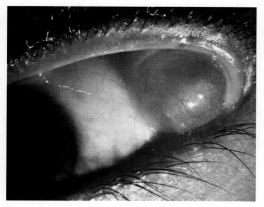

Fig. 22.2: Dacryops of the lacrimal gland

- *Proptosis* occurs in downwards and medially, along with limitation of movements and diplopia.
- *Benign mixed tumors* form the majority, and have an excellent prognosis if they are excised completely with their capsule.
- *Carcinomas* have a more rapid onset, often with pain and lymph node involvement. Local hyperostosis of the orbital bone is often evident on X-ray.

Treatment

A biopsy may be needed to confirm the diagnosis. If malignant, a radical surgical removal, or a full exenteration of the orbit is often advisable.

▌DRY EYE SYNDROME

A dry eye syndrome is said to exist when the quantity or the quality of the precorneal tear-film is insufficient to ensure the well-being of ocular epithelial surface.

Dry Eye

Dry eye is a multifactorial disease of the tears and ocular surface that results in discomfort, visual disturbance and tears film instability with potential damage to the ocular surface. It is accompanied by increased tear osmolarity and inflammation of the ocular surface [definition given by dry eye workshop (DEWS) in 2007].

> **DEWS II report redefines dry eye in 2017**
>
> "Dry eye is a multifactorial disease of the ocular surface characterized by a loss of homeostasis of the tear film, and accompanied by ocular symptoms, in which tear film instability and hyperosmolarity, ocular surface inflammation and damage, and neurosensory abnormalities play etiological roles."

In most of the situations, it results from a localized immune-mediated inflammatory response affecting both the lacrimal gland and the ocular surface.

Other commonly used terms:
- *Tear-film dysfunction:* It is a disturbance in the tear-film function owing to change in lipid, water or mucin component of the tears.
- *Ocular surface disorders*
- *Keratoconjunctivitis sicca (KCS):* It is a deficiency of aqueous component of the tear-film.
  - *Primary KCS:* Involvement of the lacrimal gland alone.
  - *Secondary KCS:* When there are additional features of connective tissue disorders.
- *Sjögren syndrome (primary):* It is an autoimmune disease, characterized by a dry eye (xerophthalmia) and a dry mouth (xerostomia), due to involvement of both lacrimal and salivary glands.
  - *Secondary Sjogren syndrome:* When they are associated with a connective tissue disorders, such as seropositive rheumatoid arthritis, systemic lupus erythematosus (SLE), systemic sclerosis, polymyositis, etc.
- *Xerosis:* It is a dryness of the conjunctiva, and presents as wrinkling, thickening, pigmentation and dryness of the conjunctiva.
- *Xerophthalmia:* When the same xerotic process spreads over the cornea, mainly caused by vitamin A deficiency.
- *Keratomalacia:* It is the softening and aseptic necrosis of the cornea, usually due to vitamin A deficiency along with malnutrition.

Symptoms

The symptoms are typically worse during night-time, or awakening from sleep (as sleep decreases the tear production) and they include:
- Foreign body (sandy/gritty) sensation
- Transient blurring of vision
- Excessive stringy mucus
- Burning sensation
- Photophobia
- Intolerance to drafts and winds
- Constant awareness about the eye itself.

Causes

Categories	Causes
Aqueous tear deficiency	<ul><li>Keratoconjunctivitis sicca</li><li>Sjögren syndrome</li><li>Riley-Day syndrome</li><li>Trauma to lacrimal gland</li><li>Surgical removal of lacrimal gland</li><li>Infiltrations by— sarcoidosis, lymphoma, amyloidosis, etc.</li></ul>
	<ul><li>Drug-induced, like antihist-aminics, antimuscarinics, thiabendazole, etc.</li><li>Neuroparalytic hyposecretion</li></ul>
Mucin-deficiency	<ul><li>Goblet cell dysfunctions, as in hypovitaminosis A</li><li>Goblet cell destruction, in alkali burn, trachoma, phemphigoid, Stevens-Johnson syndrome</li><li>Drug-induced: Beta-blockers (practolol), ecothiophate iodide</li></ul>
Lipid abnormalities	<ul><li>Anhydrotic ectodermal dysplasia (congenital absence of Meibomian glands)</li><li>Various types of blepharitis including Meibomianitis</li></ul>
Lid surfacing abnormalities	<ul><li>Lagophthalmos</li><li>Exposure keratitis</li><li>Entropion, ectropion</li><li>Lid-notching</li><li>Coloboma of the lid</li></ul>
Epitheliopathies	<ul><li>Recurrent erosions</li><li>Limbal lesions</li><li>Hard contact lens</li><li>Topical anesthesia</li></ul>

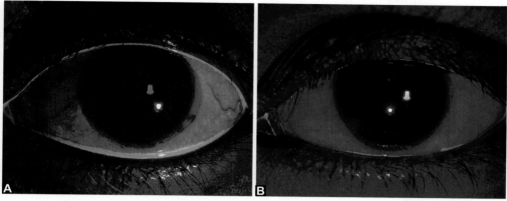

Figs 22.3A and B: A. Normal tear-meniscus height after fluorescein staining. Normal lower tear-meniscus height = 0.3 mm; **B**. Diminished lower tear-meniscus height after fluorescein staining in keratoconjunctivitis sicca

Signs

- *Precorneal tear-film:* Increased amounts of mucus strands and debris in the upper and lower tear-menisci (meniscus floaters).
- *Marginal tear-strip (tear-meniscus):* Marginal tear-strip is reduced and it contains mucus and debris (normal lower tear meniscus height is about 1 mm) (Figs. 3A and B).
- *Conjunctiva*
  - Hyperemia of the conjunctiva.

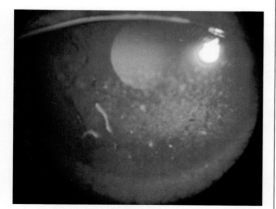

Fig. 22.4: Punctated keratopathies and corneal filaments after fluorescein stain in keratoconjunctivitis sicca

  - Appearance of folds on the temporal side, especially on abduction.
  - Papillary conjunctivitis (a nonspecific reaction).
- *Cornea*
  - *Superficial punctuate keratitis (Fig. 22.4)* involving the inferior cornea, which is stained by fluorescein and Rose-Bengal.
  - *Filaments (Fig. 22.5)* are short tails that hang from the corneal surface. They are composed of central mucus core encased by epithelial cells and stained with the Rose-Bengal and fluorescein.
  - Mucus plaques are attached loosely to the corneal surface and are also stained by Rose-Bengal dye.

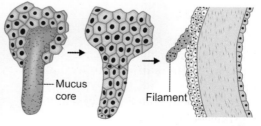

Fig. 22.5: Pathogenesis of filamentary keratopathy

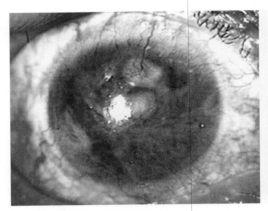

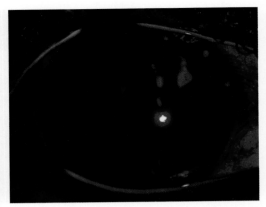

Fig. 22.6: Dellen and superficial vascularization in severe dry eye

Fig. 22.7: Fluorescein stain—filamentary keratopathy and corneal staining

- ■ *Dellen (Fig. 22.6)*, but not associated with limbal lesions.
- ■ *Thinning* occurs in severe dry eye and sometimes with perforation.

Special Clinical Tests

Vital Dye Staining

- • *Fluorescein (2%) staining (Fig. 22.7):* It stains precorneal tear-film and intercellular tissue. It does not stain the mucus and devitalized epithelial cells.
- • *Rose-Bengal (1%) staining (Figs 22.8A and B):* It has an affinity for devitalized

epithelial cells, mucus and filaments. It is very useful to detect mild cases of dry eye by staining the interpalpebral conjunctiva in the form of two triangles with their bases towards the limbus. Topical anesthesia should not be used prior to Rose-Bengal staining, as it may induce false-positive result.

- • *Alcian blue staining:* It is used to stain the mucus more selectively (not commonly used).
  - ■ *Lissamine green (Fig. 22.9):* It is also used to stain the surface similar to Rose-Bengal stain.

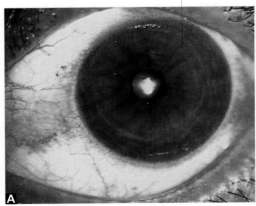

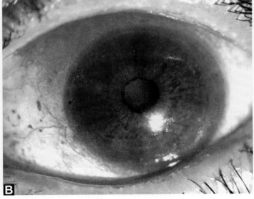

Figs 22.8A and B: Keratoconjunctivitis sicca typical Rose-Bengal staining. **A.** Conjunctiva; **B.** Cornea

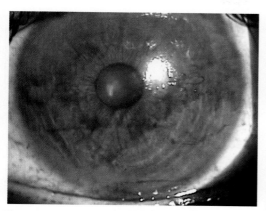

Fig. 22.9: Lissamine green staining in dry eye

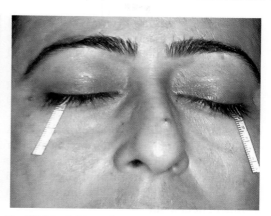

Fig. 22.10: Schirmer's test

Tear-Film Break-up Time

It is a simple test to assess the stability of the precorneal tear-film.

- A drop of fluorescein is instilled and the patient is asked to blink 2–3 times to distribute the dye.
- The patient is then asked not to blink while the cornea is studied by the cobalt blue filter with the slit lamp.
- The tear-film break-up time (TBUT) is the time in seconds between the last blink and the appearance of dry (black) spots on the cornea.
- A normal TBUT is more than 10 seconds (11–35 seconds), and a TBUT value less than 10 seconds is abnormal.

Schirmer's Test (Fig. 22.10)

- A 5 mm wide and 35 mm long special filter paper (Whatman no. 41) is placed in the lower fornix at the junction of the middle and outer-third of the eyelid after folding it at 5 mm. After 5 minutes, the amount of wetting from the fold is measured. Patient may blink or close the eyes as necessary during the test.
- This is **Schirmer's test I** and done without anesthesia. It measures the total secretion (i.e. basic plus reflex).

- ▪ *Values of Schirmer's test I*
  Normal value: 11–25 mm
  Borderline: 5–10 mm
  Impaired secretion: Less than 5 mm
- ▪ Schirmer's test I may be done after topical anesthesia, which measures only the **basic secretion**.
- *Schirmer's test II* measures the **reflex secretion** only. The procedure is same except, instillation of topical anesthesia, in the eye and irritation of ipsilateral nasal mucosa with a camel hair brush or cotton swab during the test.
  The reading is taken after 2 minutes and a measurement of less than 15 mm indicates failure of reflex secretion. This test is seldom used.

Laboratory Tests

- *Tear lysozyme assay:* It is estimated by placing a tear-wetted filter strip in an agar plate containing the bacteria **Micrococcus lysodeikticus,** and zone of lysis is measured after incubation at +37°C for 24 hours. In KCS there is reduction in tear lysozyme.
- *Tear osmolarity:* Its normal range is 290–311 mOsm/L, and it increases in KCS. Tear osmolarity value above 316 mOsmol/L is diagnostic of dry eye disease.

- *Fluorescein dilution test:* One drop of fluorescein is instilled in the eye and the dilution over a period of time is measured photometrically to calculate the tear volume.
- *Tear mucin measurement:* By measuring the hexosamine content (one of the principal moieties of mucus) of tears.
- *Goblet-cell count of the conjunctiva:* A biopsy specimen is taken from the inferior nasal conjunctival fornix for this. Average goblet-cell count in normal eyes is 8–15 cells/sqmm. The number is diminished in mucin deficiency states.
- *Conjunctival impression cytology (CIC):* The impression is taken with a cellulose acetate filter paper strip from the bulbar conjunctiva, and then stained by Papanicolaou's technique. The specimen is then analyzed for normal and abnormal cells, goblet cells and distribution of different cells. It is important in mucin deficiency states as well as in KCS.
- *Hematological tests:* They are important to detect etiological factors responsible for dry eye, as in collagen vascular disorders [rheumatoid factor, antinuclear factor (ANF), erythrocyte sedimentation rate (ESR), etc.].

Levels of Severity of Dry Eye (DEWS Classification)*

Levels	Previous term	Clinical features
Level 1	Mild dry eye	Mild conjunctival signs; normal Schirmer; slightly lower TBUT; no other problems
Level 2	Moderate dry eye	Mild corneal signs, abnormal TBUT, abnormal Schirmer's value
Level 3	Severe dry eye	Marked conjunctival and corneal sign; abnormal TBUT and Schirmer; symptomatic

Contd...

Contd...

Level 4	Extremely severe dry eye	More visual symptoms; severe corneal erosions; constant features

* International Dry Eye Workshop (DEWS) 2007.
Abbreviation: TBUT—Tear-film break-uptime

Treatment

There is no permanent cure for the dry eye, but there are some options available to relieve symptoms.

- *Preservation of the existing tears*
  - Reduction of the room temperature.
  - *Humidifiers:* Examples are swimmer's goggles, moist-chamber goggles, etc.
  - Plenty of intakes of drinking water.
  - Lid taping and tarsorrhaphy to prevent exposure keratitis.
  - *Punctal occlusion:* It is to preserve the natural or artificial tears in contact with the ocular surface for a longer time.
    - *Temporary:* By solid gelatin rods, collagen plugs, cyanoacrylate glue, '2-0' catgut pieces, or heat cautery.
    - *Permanent:* For severe cases of KCS when the Schirmer's value is less than 2 mm. This is done by silicone plugs, thermodynamic acrylic plugs, electrocautery or by small patch graft over the puncta.
- *Supplementation of tears:* Essentially four types of tear substitutes are currently available in the market. The compositions of tear substitutes are cellulose (methyl cellulose, hydroxypropyl methyl cellulose, hypermellose), polyvinyl alcohol, povidone and sodium hyaluronate. They are used either alone or in combination.

A preservative-free eye drop is more preferable for long-term use, as some of the preservatives may cause dryness, e.g. benzalkonium chloride (BAK). Nobel preservatives, like Purite and perborate containing tears substitute are more important when the frequency of instillation is more than six times per day for a prolonged period.

- **Drops:** Frequency of instillation may vary with the severity of dry eye 4 times/daily to half-hourly interval.
- **Ointments:** Petroleum mineral oil or jelly is used at bed time as an ointment.
- **Slow-releasing inserts (ocusert):** Lacrisert, formerly known as SRAT (slow releasing artificial tear), is a small 5 mg pellet of hydroxypropyl cellulose in a cylinder form. It is placed in the lower fornix once daily. It dissolves slowly, and releases its polymer into the tear-film. In advertent loss of insert and blurred vision are the common problems.
- **Gel-tears:** The gel is a clear synthetic polymer of acrylic acid which dissolves very slowly. It persists in the conjunctival sac for several hours after instillation. Temporary blurring of vision may be a problem.

- **Stimulation of tears production: Bromhexine and eledosin** are sometimes used for stimulation of the lacrimal gland to produce more tears. **Oral pilocarpine or pilocarpine-like drug (Cevelamine)** may also be used to stimulate tears production. But, they have systemic muscarinic like toxicity.
- **Mucolytic agent:** Acetylcysteine (5% or 10%) drops 4 times daily, when there is excessive production of mucus strands. It has an unpleasant sulfurous odor.
- **Bandage soft contact lenses:** High hydrated bandage contact lenses occupy a unique place in the treatment of dry eye. They are most valuable in filamentary keratopathy, recurrent epithelial erosions and exposure keratitis.

- **Systemic and topical corticosteroids:** They are useful for underlying systemic diseases, in patients with secondary KCS.
  Topicals of steroids (like loteprednol) may be used 4–6 times daily for a short period of time (pulse therapy) to reduce ocular surface inflammation in selective cases.
- **Cyclosporine:** Topical cyclosporine (0.05%) is now currently recommended in patient with moderate to severe dry eye due to primary or secondary KCS.
  Cyclosporine, an immune modulator inhibits activation of T lymphocytes and prevents T cells in releasing cytokines. It is given twice daily for at least 6 months.
- **Major surgical procedures**
  - **Parotid duct transplantation:** It is rarely performed nowadays.
  - **Tarsorrhaphy or botulinum toxin:** It is to reduce the exposed ocular surface area.
  - Limbal cell transplantation (autograft or allograft).
  - **Corneal transplantation and kerato-prosthesis:** They are more heroic measures used to treat severe form of dry eye. But, they are often unsuccessful in preserving vision in severe dry eye.
- **Treatment of associated problems:** These include treatment of blepharitis, meibomianitis, conjunctivitis, corneal ulcer, entropion, symblepharon, etc.
- **Change in working environment:** This is also important especially who works in air-conditioned environment and spend along time with the computer.
- **Psychotherapy:** This includes explaining to the patient about the disease and its future course. Because of its chronic nature, most patients go through periods of despondency and depression. Ophthalmologists must actively encourage these patients to continue to pursue their normal activities.

Management outline of dry eye diseases (DEWS recommendation)

Level 1

(i) Counseling, (ii) dietary modification, (iii) tears substitute (any type) 4 times/day, (iv) environmental management, (v) systemic medication review, (vi) control ocular allergy and (vii) address contact lens problems.

Level 2

(i) Steps from level one, (ii) tears supplement–preservative-free (6–8 times), (iii) oral tetracycline analogs, (iv) topical anti-inflammatory agents, (v) topical cyclosporine (0.05%): twice daily, (vi) reversible lacrimal occlusion and (vii) lid hygiene/nutritional support (omega-3 fatty acid).

Level 3

(i) Steps from level one and two, (ii) tears substitute (preservative-free) 1 hourly, (iii) autologous serum eye drop (20–50%), (iv) bandage contact lens and (v) permanent punctal occlusion.

Level 4

(i) Steps from level one, two and three, (ii) tears supplement (P/F)—1/2 hourly to 1 hourly, (iii) oral anti-inflammatory medications, (iii) oral cyclosporine, (iv) acetyl cysteine 20% eye drop, (v) tarsorrhaphy or botulinum toxin and (vi) limbal cell transplantation (auto/allograft).

▌WATERING FROM THE EYE

Watering is associated with blurring of vision and continuous discomfort caused by tears running down the cheek.

In all instances, it is necessary to find out, whether there is excessive production of the tears (lacrimation), or its defective drainage (epiphora).

Lacrimation: Excessive secretion of tears, due to reflex stimulation of lacrimal gland.

Causes
- Psychic stimulation, as in weeping or laughing.
- Irritation of the cornea or conjunctiva, by dust, fumes, chemicals, foreign body, inflammation, etc.
- In yawning, coughing, sneezing or vomiting.
- Exposure to bright lights.

Epiphora: Defective drainage of tears due to fault in the lacrimal passage.

Causes: Mechanical obstruction in the drainage system, due to:
- Congenital absence or occlusion of the puncta
- Canaliculitis, canalicular obstruction
- Congenital dacryocystitis
- Chronic or acute dacryocystitis
- Neoplasms of the lacrimal sac
- Nasal pathology, like polyps, tumors in the inferior meatus of the nose.
  - *Lacrimal pump failure due to:*
    - Lower lid laxity.
    - Weakness of the orbicularis oculi, as in Bell's palsy.
    - Ectropion due to other causes.

Special Investigations

Special investigations of watering from the eye have been described in Table 22.1. Evaluation of Watering from the Eye

History

- Watering due to epiphora is usually unilateral and is not associated with irritation. On the other hand, watering due to lacrimation is usually bilateral and associated with irritation, itching orphotophobia.
- Past history of Bell's palsy is important, and it suggests lacrimal pump failure rather than a mechanical obstruction.
- History of medications like topical idoxuridine (IDU), latonoprost, mitomycin-C and systemic 5-FU (fluorouracil) may cause *punctual stenosis.*

Examinations

Inspection
- *Eyelids:* For trichiasis, ectropion, lower lid laxity, blocked puncta, etc.
- *Medial canthal (sac) area:* For swelling (e.g. mucocele, acute dacryocystitis), fistula, etc.

TABLE 22.1: Special investigations of watering from the eyes

Types of test	Procedure
Saccharine, or **quinine test** *(alternately chloramphenicol)*	Sweet or bitter taste after instillation of solution in conjunctival sac. One eye is to be tested at a time.
Patency test (syringing)	Irrigation of lacrimal passage is done with distilled water by lacrimal cannula. Presence of water in the nasopharynx indicates a patent nasolacrimal passage.
Dye disappearence test	Fluorescein dye disappearance from the cul-de-sac (normal 2 minutes). A prolonged retention of dye indicates inadequate lacrimal drainage.
Jones I (primary) test	Appearance of fluorescein in the nose (5 minutes), after its conjunctival instillation. If no dye is recovered the test is called negative.
Jones II (secondary) test	Appearance of fluorescein in the nose after its lacrimal sac irrigation and indicates partial obstruction of nasolacrimal duct (NLD). If no dye is recovered the test is called negative, and probably due to canalicular block.
Probing test (Figs 22.11A and B)	After insertion of a probe or cannula, an attempt is made to touch the medial wall of the lacrimal sac and the lacrimal bone. The interpretation may be a hard stop or a soft stop. • **Hard stop:** A firm to hard feeling caused by the probe–touching the medial wall of the sac against the lacrimal bone. It indicates that the lacrimal passage is patent up to the lacrimal sac and also indicates that the obstruction is below, i.e. at the NLD. • **Soft stop:** A spongy (soft) feeling as the probe presses the common canaliculus (CC) against the medial wall of the sac. It indicates either stenosis or obstruction of the canalicular system. However, an iatrogenic kinking of canalicular system during probing may also result in soft stop.
Intubation dacryocystography (DCG)	X-rays (anteroposterior and lateral view) after injection of radio-opaque dye into the lacrimal sac. It demonstrates the location of obstruction, fistula, diverticula and tumors.
Dacryoscintigraphy	Gamma camera tracing of technetium (99 mmTC) after instillation into cul-de-sac and its progress through the drainage system.

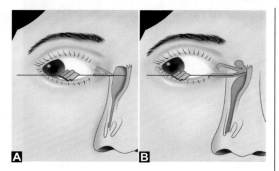

A **B**

Figs 22.11A and B: Probing test. **A.** Hard stop; **B.** Soft stop

• **Orbicularis functions:** By forcible closure of the eyelids.

Palpation

• **Pressure over the sac area**—regurgitation of mucus or mucopurulent material in nasolacrimal duct (NLD) block (e.g. chronic dacryocystitis).

• **Tenderness** on palpation—in acute dacryocystitis.

Slit-lamp examination

• **Puncta:** Look for stenosis, foreign body, malposition, etc.

- *Pressure over the canaliculi* with glass rod and look for pus coming out through the puncta.
- *Marginal tear-film strip* for a high lower marginal tear-strip.
- Look for any corneal or conjunctival pathology.

Nasal examination

- To detect deviated nasal septum (DNS), polyps or tumor.
- To detect hypertrophy of the inferior turbinate.
- To detect the position of anterior end of the middle turbinate when dacryocystorhinostomy (DCR) is contemplated.
- To know the condition of the nasal mucosa (*atrophic rhinitis* is a contraindication for DCR).

Patency (syringing) test (Figs 22.12A and B):
A drop of 4% lignocaine is instilled into the conjunctival sac. The lower punctum is dilated with a punctum dilator. A lacrimal cannula, on a 5 mL distilled water-filled syringe is inserted into the lower canaliculus. The piston is then pushed to irrigate the lacrimal passage. The result may be:
- Water is going freely into the nasopharynx— lacrimal passage is patent.

Contd...

Contd...

- Water is regurgitating through the upper, and partly through the lower puncta:
  - *Fast regurgitation:* The fluid is clear and the regurgitation is rapid. It is due to common canalicular (CC) block.
  - *Slow regurgitation:* The fluid is turbid (as mixed with mucopus), and the regurgitation speed is slow. It is due to NLD block.
- Sometimes, fluid is going partially into the throat (and partly coming out through the puncta). It is due to partial NLD block.

Investigations for Surgery

- Blood for Hb%, total leukocyte count (TLC), differential leukocyte count (DLC) and erythrocyte sedimentation rate (ESR) is done.
- Bleeding time and clotting time to be checked.
- Blood sugar and blood pressure to be checked.
- General anesthesia fitness, if necessary.

DISEASES OF THE LACRIMAL PASSAGE

Canaliculitis

- *Acute canaliculitis* is usually due to herpes simplex infection and self-limiting.

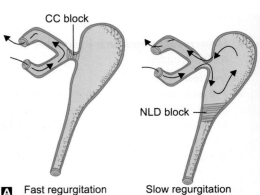
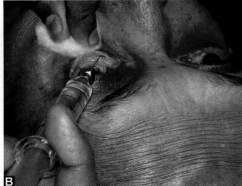

Figs 22.12A and B: A. Patency (syringing) test; **B.** Syringing of the lacrimal passage
CC—Common canalicular; **NLD**—Nasolacrimal duct

- *Chronic canaliculitis* is most commonly caused by *Actinomyces israelii* (streptothrix)
  - *Chronic infection causes:* Discharge, a pouting punctum and concretions within the canaliculi.
  - It also causes stone formation (dacryolith) in the lacrimal sac.
  - A gritty foreign body sensation during probing establishes the diagnosis.
  - *Treatment* of dacryolith is by a linear incision into the conjunctival side of the canaliculus (canaliculotomy).

Occlusion of the puncta and canaliculus
- *Causes*
  - Congenital closure or mal development.
  - Foreign body, e.g. eyelash (Figs 22.13A and B) (most common) and concretion due to actinomycosis.
  - *Scarring:* It is due to burns, cosmetics, trauma or infections (trachoma and herpes simplex).
  - *Medications:* The examples are IDU or phospholine iodide drop, systemic 5-FU.
- Slit-lamp examination is essential to establish the diagnosis.
- *Treatment* is by removal of foreign body, or by dilating the canaliculus, and slitting it with a canaliculus knife. In case of CC block, conjunctivo-dacryocystorhinostomy (C-DCR) with a bypass tube is helpful.

Dacryocystitis

Dacryocystitis is an acute (Fig. 22.14) or chronic inflammation of the lacrimal sac. It is the sequel to obstruction of the NLD, or the sac itself, followed by bacterial infection.

Etiology

- It is commonly seen among newborn infants (congenital type) and middle-aged women (7 times more common than men).
- Left side is more commonly affected (left:right = 9:1).
- More common in lower socioeconomic status.
- *Causes*
  - *Lacrimal passage proper:* NLD block due to narrowness or chronic inflammation of the sac.
  - *Nasal factors:* DNS, hypertrophied inferior turbinate, nasal polyps, etc.
- Following a primary conjunctivitis.
- Infection spreading from the nasopharynx.
- *Organisms responsible: Pneumococcus* (most common), *Streptococcus, Staphylococcus, Mycobacterium, Chlamydia*, etc.

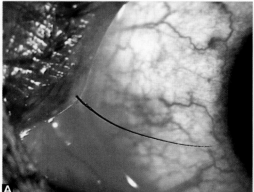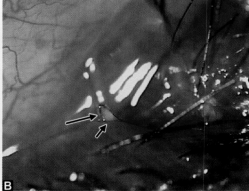

Figs 22.13A and B: Eyelash. **A.** In upper punctum; **B.** In lower punctum (arrows)

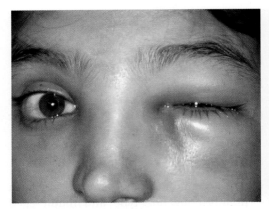

Fig. 22.14: Acute dacryocystitis

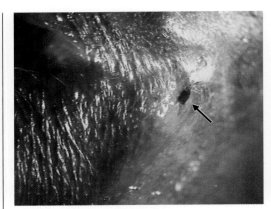

Fig. 22.16: Lacrimal fistula (arrow)

Types

- Acute dacryocystitis
- Chronic dacryocystitis
  - Congenital type
  - Adult type.

Acute dacryocystitis (Fig. 22.15)

- It is a suppurative inflammation of the lacrimal sac with an associated cellulitis of the overlying tissues.
- The onset is acute, and there is a painful swelling below the inner canthus, often combined with widespread cellulitis.

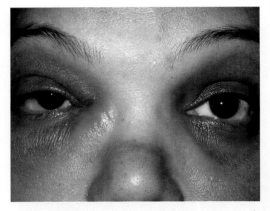

Fig. 22.15: Resolving acute dacryocystitis—right side

- The swelling is exquisitely tender with enlargement of the submandibular lymph node.
- Constitutional symptoms like fever, malaise, etc. are present.
- An abscess may often form, with perforation of the skin just below the medial palpebral ligament leading to formation of *lacrimal fistula (Fig. 22.16)*.

Treatment

- Local hot compresses 3–4 times daily
- Broad-spectrum systemic antibiotics
- Topical antibiotics 4–6 times daily
- Systemic analgesics with antacids
- In case of *lacrimal abscess* (Fig. 22.17) it is best drained by ask in incision.
  - In case of *lacrimal fistula* (whether formed naturally or artificially by drainage). It usually closes when the patency has been restored by DCR operation. Otherwise, the tract is excised along with dacryocystectomy (DCT) operation.
  - When everything is resolved a DCR or DCT operation has to be done as an elective procedure.

Chronic Dacryocystitis (Figs 22.18 and 22.19)

- This is seen most frequently in newborns, infants and middle-aged women.

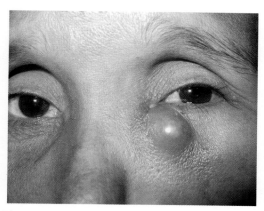

Fig. 22.17: Lacrimal abscess

- The chief symptoms are watering and a chronic mucopurulent discharge at the inner-angle of the eye.
- There is regurgitation of pus or mucopus through the puncta, on pressure over the sac area.

Congenital Chronic Dacryocystitis (Fig. 22.18)

- It occurs in infants because of failure of the NLD to open into the inferior meatus of the nose, which normally occurs about third week of life.
- The initial symptom is constant watering of one eye and it is followed by the regurgitation of pus through the puncta.

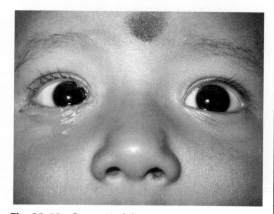

Fig. 22.18: Congenital dacryocystitis (right eye)

- Congenital acute dacryocystitis is exceptional.
- *Differential diagnosis*
  - *Neonatal conjunctivitis (ophthalmia neonatorum:* Usually bilateral, stickiness of the eyelids, no regurgitation of pus and quick response with antibiotic drops.
  - *Congenital glaucoma (buphthalmos):* There are associated blepharospasm and photophobia; cloudy cornea and raised intraocular tension.
- *Management*
  - *Hydrostatic sac massage and antibiotic drops:* By giving downward strokes, with index or little finger (10 strokes in each time) four times daily.
    This should be followed by antibiotic or sulphacetamide (10%) drops four times a day. This treatment is to be continued until the age of 6 months (some surgeons prefer till the age of 12 months). With this conservative treatment, canalization occurs in about 95% of cases.
  - *Probing:* It is usually done 10–12 months of age, under general anesthesia. The success rate decreases significantly after the age of 4 years. If there is no improvement after 4 weeks the probing should be repeated.
  - *Intubation:* It may be done with silicone tube. If two probings fail to cure the obstruction, the tube should be kept *in situ* for 6 months.
  - *Dacryocystorhinostomy:* It is required only in exceptional circumstances, and wisely delayed until the child is 4 years of age.

Adult Chronic Dacryocystitis (Fig. 22.19)

- It typically occurs in postmenopausal women and either occurs spontaneously, or follows a lacrimal sac infection.
- There may be spontaneous atresia of NLD, or weakness of the orbicularis, and it is often associated with nasal pathology.

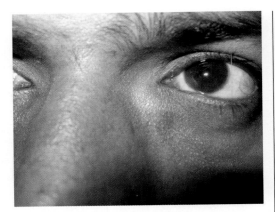

Fig. 22.19: Chronic dacryocystitis (left eye)

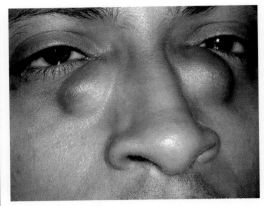

Fig. 22.20: Bilateral mucocele of the lacrimal sac

- In long-standing cases, there is extra-ordinary dilatation and thinning of the lacrimal sac called **mucocele** or **hydrops** of the lacrimal sac (Fig. 22.20).
- *Complications*
  - Chronic conjunctivitis
  - Recurrent attacks of acute conjunctivitis
  - *Acute-on-chronic* dacryocystitis
  - From acute dacryocystitis, there may be chance of:
    - Lacrimal abscess pyogenic granuloma (Fig. 22.21A)
    - Lacrimal fistula
    - Orbital and facial cellulitis

    - Cavernous sinus thrombosis
    - Lacrimal osteomyelitis, etc.
  - *Hypopyon corneal ulcer:* Chronic dacryocystitis (Fig. 22.21B) is in fact a constant menace to the ophthalmologist or to the patient, as mild corneal abrasion due to any cause may be turned into a hypopyon corneal ulcer, which is mostly due to *Pneumococci.*

Treatment
- *Symptomatic relief* is often obtained by antibiotic (e.g. ciprofloxacin) and a stringent (e.g. zinc sulfate) eye drops.

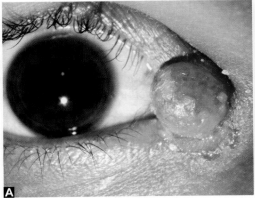
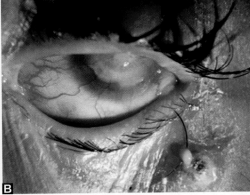

Figs 22.21A and B: A. Lacrimal abscess with pyogenic granuloma at the puncta; **B.** Chronic dacryocystitis with corneal ulcer

- ***Dacryocystorhinostomy:*** The surgical procedure of choice is DCR operation, in which a communication is established between the lacrimal sac and the middle meatus of the nose.
- ***Dacryocystectomy:*** It means simple removal of the lacrimal sac. The main idea is to eliminate the reservoir of infection and regurgitation of pus into the conjunctival sac. But watering will continue throughout the life.
  - In extreme old age.
  - When the sac is shrunken and fibrotic.
  - In presence of growth of the sac.
  - In obvious nasal pathology, like atrophic rhinitis.

(For operative details *see* Chapter 25).

TUMORS OF THE LACRIMAL SAC (FIG. 22.22)

- Tumors of the lacrimal sac are extremely rare and represent a potentially life-threatening condition.
- Most neoplasms are squamous cell carcinomas, transitional cell carcinomas and adenocarcinomas.

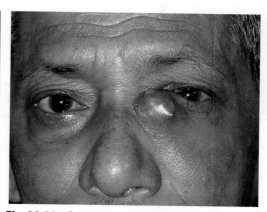

Fig. 22.22: Carcinoma of the lacrimal sac

- The triad of malignancy are:
  - A mass below the medial palpebral ligament (Fig. 22.22)
  - A chronic dacryocystitis that irrigates freely and
  - Regurgitation of bloody mucopus.
- Dacryocystography shows a filling defect.
- ***Treatment*** is by complete excision of the sac followed by irradiation.

CHAPTER

23

Ocular Motility: Squint

OCULAR MOVEMENTS

The ocular movements are of four types—*ductions, version, vergences, supranuclear movements.*

Ductions (Fig. 23.1)

Ductions refer to the movement of one eye, and consist of adduction, abduction, supraduction (elevation), infraduction (depression), incycloduction (intorsion) and excycloduction (extorsion).

- **Agonist:** It is the primary muscle, moving the eye in any given direction.
- **Synergist:** It is a muscle which acts together with the agonist to produce a given movement.
- **Antagonist:** It is the muscle which acts in the opposite direction to the agonist.

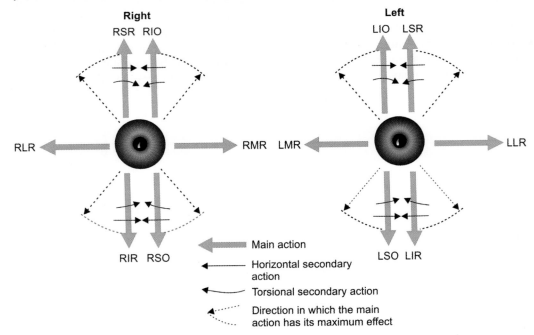

Fig. 23.1: Actions of extraocular muscles
RSR—Right superior rectus; **RIO**—Right inferior oblique; **RMR**—Right medial rectus; **RSO**—Right superior oblique; **RIR**—Right inferior rectus; **RLR**—Right lateral rectus; **LIO**—Left inferior oblique; **LSR**—Left superior rectus; **LLR**—Left lateral rectus; **LIR**—Left inferior rectus; **LSO**—Left superior oblique; **LMR**—Left medial rectus

- When a person is looking toward his right side, right lateral rectus is the agonist, left medial rectus is the synergist, and right medial rectus and left lateral rectus are the antagonists.
- **Sherrington's law of reciprocal innervation:** Implies that increased contraction of a muscle is automatically associated with a reciprocal decrease in contraction (relaxation) of its antagonists.

Versions

Versions are binocular movements, in which the two eyes move synchronously and symmetrically in the **same direction**.

The movements are:
- Dextroversion (right gaze), levoversion (left gaze), supraversion (up gaze), and infraversion (down gaze). These are secondary positions of gaze.
- Dextroelevation (gaze up and right), dextrodepression (gaze down and right), levoelevation (gaze up and left) and levodepression (gaze down and left). These oblique movements are tertiary positions of gaze.

- Dextrocycloversion (rotation of upper limbus of both eyes to the right) and levocycloversion (rotation to the left).

Six cardinal positions of the gaze (Fig. 23.2) are dextroversion and levoversion, dextroelevation and levoelevation, dextrodepression and levodepression.

Yoke muscles (Fig. 23.3): A muscle of one eye is paired with a muscle of the opposite eye, while moving the eyes into each of the six cardinal positions of gaze.

For example: In **dextroversion**, two yoke muscles are right lateral rectus and left medial rectus. In **dextroelevation**, the yoke muscles are right superior rectus and left inferior oblique.

For oblique movements, the **mnemonics**— the muscles responsible for particular gaze are **same named rectus muscle** (in right superior area, i.e. in dextroelevation, right superior rectus) and **cross named oblique muscle** (i.e. in right superior area, the left inferior oblique muscle).

Hering's law of equal innervation: States that during any conjugate eye movement, equal and simultaneous innervation flows to the yoke muscles. Hence, a paresis of one muscle is always accompanied by an apparent

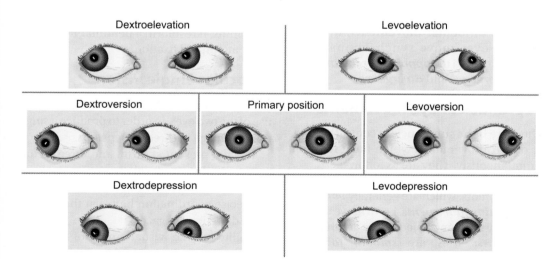

Fig. 23.2: Six cardinal positions of version

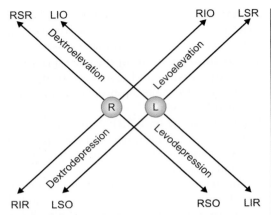

Fig. 23.3: Yoke muscles in diagonal movements
RSR—Right superior rectus; **LIO**—Left inferior oblique; **RIO**—Right inferior oblique; **LSR**—Left superior rectus; **LIR**—Left inferior rectus; **RSO**—Right inferior oblique; **LSO**—Left superior oblique; **RIR**—Right inferior rectus

overaction of yoke muscle or its contralateral synergist (left inferior oblique is contralateral synergist of right superior rectus), which receives the same amount of stimulation as its lagging fellow. This is responsible for more *secondary angle of deviation* in paralytic squint.

Vergences

They are binocular movements, in which the two eyes move synchronously and symmetrically in the *opposite directions*. They are *convergence* and *divergence.*

Supranuclear Eye Movements

There are basic supranuclear control systems of ocular movements, which must function simultaneously. They are as follows:

- *Saccades:* They are the rapid eye movements, which are generally *voluntary refixation movements*, i.e. to move the eyes quickly from one object to the another.
- *Pursuits:* They are *smooth following movements* which maintain the visual axes on any slow moving object.

- *Vestibuloocular movements:* They are the coordinated eye movements with respect to gravity and head positions, e.g. vestibular nystagmus (as in *caloric test*), Doll's eye maneuver, etc.

VISUAL DEVELOPMENT

- *At birth*, the eyes appear to move randomly, and there is no central fixation. The fovea is not fully developed, and the visual acuity is roughly 6/60 (as estimated by other means).
- *At 6 weeks of age,* the fixation reflex first becomes apparent, and the eyes can follow a bright light for a short distance.
- *At 4–6 months of age,* the refixation reflex develops firmly.
- *At 6 years of age,* the fovea develops completely with the full visual acuity of 6/6.
- If the visual developmental process is interrupted during this process, by any means (e.g. congenital cataract, high anisometropia, or squint), it results in a degree of amblyopia which becomes irreversible after few years.
- If the *stimulus deprivation* occurs bilaterally and severely (e.g. in bilateral congenital cataract) by the age of 6 months, it results in a pendular nystagmus on attempted fixation.

Binocular Single Vision

Binocular single vision (BSV) is the coordinated use of the two eyes, in order to produce a single unified image in three dimensions.

It is not present at birth, and three factors are required for its development:

1. Reasonably clear vision in both eyes.
2. Precise coordination between the eyes for all directions of gaze.
3. Ability of the visual areas of brain to promote fusion of the two slightly dissimilar objects.

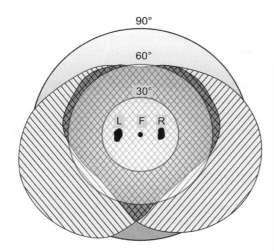

Fig. 23.4: Binocular field of vision
F—Fixation point; **R**—Blind-spot of the right eye;
L—Blind-spot of the left eye

The three advantages of BSV:
1. An enlarged field of vision (Fig. 23.4) with compensation of each blind spot.
2. An ability to appreciate depth with stereoscopic vision.
3. A combined binocular visual acuity is better than the uniocular visual acuity.

Three components (grades) of BSV are; simultaneous macular perception (SMP), fusion and stereopsis (Fig. 23.5).

Grade-1 (SMP): This means the ability to see two dissimilar (but not mutually antagonistic) images simultaneously, and to superimpose them.

Grade-2 (Fusion): This is the ability to see the slightly dissimilar images formed in each eye and blend them into one.

The normal range of fusion is about 30° of convergence to 5° of divergence, and 2° deviation in vertical meridian.

Grade-3 (Stereopsis): This is the appreciation of the third dimension, allowing the perception of depth. For stereopsis to occur, disparate points must be stimulated.

Monocular Perception of Depth (Fig. 23.6)

The perception of a single eye, is in fact, two dimensional, but an "one-eyed" person achieves a considerable power of depth perception by a number of indirect methods:
- ***Overlapping of contours:*** They readily indicate their relative distances from the observer.

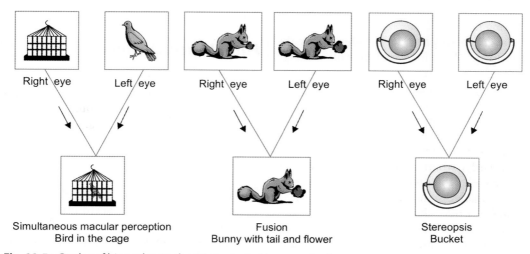

Fig. 23.5: Grades of binocular single vision—tested by synoptophore

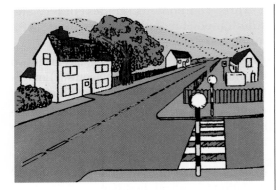

Fig. 23.6: Methods of monocular perception of depth.

Note: The above features are apparent: overlapping of contours, relative size of houses, 'aerial perspective' evidenced in the blurring of the horizon, perspective convergence of parallel lines, shading of circular objects to give the impression of a sphere

- *Relative size of the objects:* Objects whose size is familiar, will produce a retinal image of a size, which is inversely proportional to their distance from the observer. This distance can then be judged by the distance relative to that of another object whose size is also known. In addition, the definition of the object will be proportionately reduced. These two factors together are traditionally employed by the military in assessing their firing range.
- *Aerial perspective:* It is evidenced by the blurring of outlines, and the color change of the horizon, caused by intervening atmospheric scatter. It can estimate the intervening distance by the contrast of different objects.
- *Perspective convergence of parallel lines:* They are receding away from the observer. Similarly, when circular objects are seen obliquely, they will appear as oval, with one smaller than the other.
- *Light and shades:* A simple two-dimensional circle, can be made into a sphere by adding the contrast of light and shades on its surface.

- *Parallax:* Movement of the head from side to side will cause nearer objects to move in the opposite direction, in relation to more distant objects.
- *Accommodation:* Within a limited range of distance, the amount of accommodative effort required to focus on an object, clearly gives an indication of the proximity of that near object.

DIPLOPIA

Diplopia (double vision) means that an object appears double.

Classification

- Physiological
- Pathological
  - Uniocular
  - Binocular
    » Homonymous or uncrossed (Fig. 23.7A)
    » Heteronymous or crossed (Fig. 23.7B).

Physiological Diplopia

It is a normal phenomenon, in which objects not within the area of fixation, are seen double. It is easily demonstrated by looking at a near object with attention directed toward a distant object. Usually, it does not impinge on the consciousness.

Pathological Diplopia

Uniocular diplopia

An object appears double even when only one eye remains open. It occurs when two images of the same objects forms on the two different parts of the retina. More commonly, there is uniocular polyopia (multiple vision) due to multiple images.

Causes

- Immature cortical cataract (due to multiple water clefts within the lens).
- Subluxated clear lens (pupillary area is partly phakic and partly aphakic).

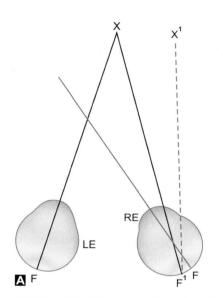 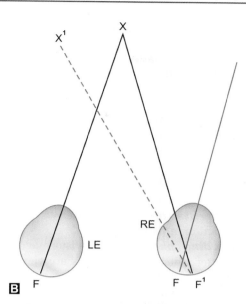

Figs 23.7A and B: Pathological diplopia. **A.** Homonymous diplopia in convergent squint; **B.** Heteronymous diplopia in divergent squint (**LE**—Left eye; **RE**—Right eye)

- Large peripheral iridectomy, iridodialysis or polycoria (multiple pupil).
- Retinal detachment due to dialysis when the retina becomes inverted.

Binocular diplopia

An object appears double with both eyes remain open. This occurs when the image of an object does not fall on the corresponding points of the retina of the both eyes. Image of an object fall on the fovea of one eye, and on the extrafoveal area of the opposite eye.

Causes
- Paralysis or paresis of the extraocular muscles (most common).
- Displacement of the eyeball, by a space-occupying lesion in the orbit, by fracture of orbital wall or by pressure of fingers.
- Mechanical restriction of the movements of the globe, e.g. pterygium, symblepharon, thyroid ophthalmopathy, etc.
- Deviation of rays of light in one eye, as in decentered spectacles.
- Disparity of image size between two eyes, as in acquired high anisometropia (e.g.

aphakia with spectacle correction in one eye, and the other eye being normal). Congenital high anisometropia causes amblyopia of the more ametropic eye rather than diploid.

In diplopia, one image is distinct (*true image*), and the other is indistinct (*false image*). Binocular diplopia disappears when one eye is closed. Depending on the position of the false image in relation to midline, binocular diplopia may be *uncrossed (homonymous)*, or *crossed (heteronymous)*.

In a convergent squint, the diplopia is uncrossed *(homonymous)*—that means, the false image is on the same side of the deviation.

In a divergent squint, the diplopia is crossed *(heteronymous)*—that means, the false image is thrown across the midline.

Treatment

- Investigation to find out the cause and treat accordingly.
- For relief of symptom:
  - Occlusion of the worse eye.

- Prism correction if the deviation is small in paralytic squint.

AMBLYOPIA

Amblyopia denotes a unilateral or bilateral reduction in form vision, without any detectable organic ocular lesion.

The most sensitive period of developing amblyopia is in the first 6 months of life; and after about the age of 6 years, amblyopia does not usually develop.

Characteristics of an amblyopic eye:
- Reduction in visual acuity.
- *Crowding phenomenon:* Visual acuity is better when the test letters are viewed singly (optotype), rather than in a series (Snellen's chart).
- *Neutral density filter test:* Amblyopic eye shows no change in visual acuity with a neutral density filter. But a normal eye shows a drop in acuity of about one or two lines, whereas an eye with macular lesion may have a large drop in visual acuity.
- *Color vision is unaffected.*
- *Eccentric (extrafoveal) fixation* is common, and the degree of amblyopia is proportionate to the distance of the eccentric point from the fovea.

Types

- *Stimulus deprivation amblyopia (amblyopia ex anopsia):* Results from the nonuse of one eye in infancy or early childhood and is caused by opacity in the media (cataract or leukoma), ptosis, or by occlusion (occlusion amblyopia).
- *Strabismic amblyopia:* Develops in a squinting eye, as a result of continued suppression, and it persists even when the deviated eye is forced to fixate.
- *Anisometropic amblyopia:* Occurs in the more ametropic eye, as a result of constantly blurred image of an object falling onto its fovea. This is more with

high anisohypermetropia and anisoastigmatism than with anisomyopia.
- *Ametropic amblyopia:* It is bilateral, and associated with almost equally high refractive error of both eyes. It is also more with bilateral high hypermetropia.

Treatment

Principles of Treatment

- Removal of opacity in the media
- Full correction of refractive errors
- Occlusion therapy.

The treatment should be started as early as possible. The younger the patient is, the more rapid improvements in visual acuity will be, and the better will be the ultimate prognosis.

Occlusion therapy: The aim is to occlude the sound eye, and to force to use the amblyopic eye.

This is *conventional occlusion*.
- It may be total (to occlude both form and light senses), or partial (to occlude only the form sense).
- If the vision in the amblyopic eye is worse than 6/18, occlusion must be total (with the help of a direct patching of the eye).
- If the vision is better than 6/18, the occlusion may be partial (with the help of cellotape or nail polish over the spectacles lens).
- Occlusion must be given in ratio (e.g. 3:1, i.e. 3 days in sound eye and 1 day in amblyopic eye) in younger children to prevent occlusion amblyopia of the sound eye.
- Occlusion therapy is to be carried out until the visual acuity develops fully, or there is no further improvement of vision after 3 months of continuous occlusion.
- *Inverse occlusion:* This is done when amblyopia is combined with eccentric fixation. The initial step is to return the normal foveal fixation by patching the amblyopic eye, with simultaneous stimulation of the fovea.

After the development of central fixation in the amblyopic eye, patching of the sound eye is to be continued until maximum visual acuity is attained.

Other modes of therapy:
- ***Atropine penalization:*** An alternative to occlusion, atropine is used to blur the sound eye only (and may be with pilocarpine to the amblyopic eye).
- ***Pleoptics:*** They are the methods of reestablishment of foveal fixation and may be helpful in older children.
- ***CAM stimulator therapy:*** This consists of the viewing of rotating high contrast stripes of different sizes with the amblyopic eye.

▌SQUINT (STRABISMUS)

It is a condition in which only one of the visual axes is directed toward the fixation object, the other being deviated away from this point.

Normally, the visual axes of the two eyes are essentially parallel in all directions of ocular movement, except in convergence and in divergence.

Orthophoria is that ideal condition, in which the eyes are parallel without the effort of fusion faculty for distant fixation and have the proper convergence for near vision. This in normal ocular-muscle balance. Only a few people are orthophoric, and some degree of heterophoria is almost universal.

Position of rest is usually a mild divergence as in sleep, deep anesthesia, or after death.

Apparent Squint (Pseudostrabismus) (Fig. 23.8A)

Here, the visual axes are in fact parallel, but the eyes seem to have squint.

Causes

- Prominent epicanthic folds (Fig. 23. 8B) in infants—may simulate the appearance of a convergent squint.
- Hypertelorism—an apparent divergent squint.
- Hypermetropia—an apparent divergent squint due to large angle "kappa".
- Myopia—an apparent convergent squint due to smaller, or even negative angle "kappa". Squint in these conditions is easily excluded by checking the relative position of corneal light reflections, and also by other means.

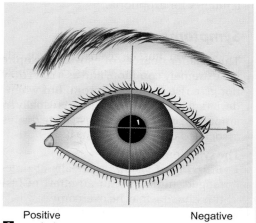
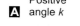

Positive angle *k*   Negative angle *k*

A

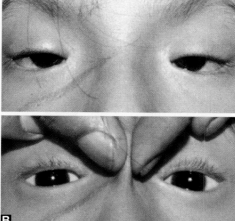

B

Figs 23.8A and B: A. Pseudostrabismus (schematic representation); **B.** Pseudoconvergent squint in telecanthus and epicanthic folds (photographs)

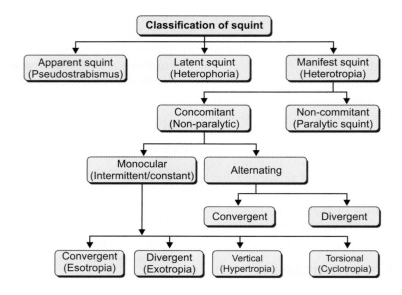

Latent Squint (Heterophoria) (Fig. 23.9)

This is a tendency for the eyes to deviate, but that is prevented by the fusion mechanism for the interest of BSV.

But, under condition of stress, or when the fusion is interrupted the deviation readily becomes manifest.

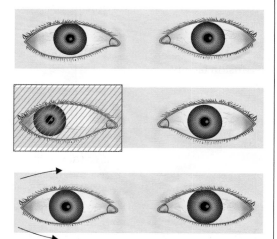

Fig. 23.9: Latent divergent squint (exophoria). Note the eye deviates under the cover

Types

- **Esophoria:** Tends to deviate inward.
- **Exophoria:** Tends to deviate outward.
- **Hyperphoria:** Tends to deviate upward.
- **Cyclophoria:** Torsional deviation.

  In general, esophoria is common among hypermetropes, and exophoria in myopes. In presbyopia, as the near point recedes, the convergence becomes weaker and there is a tendency for exophoria.

Symptoms

The smaller degrees of eso- and exophoria are extremely common, and as a rule, they do not give rise to any symptom. But when the deviation is more than 5°, there is usually some amount of distress. The most acute distress is associated with cyclophoria.

The symptoms are:

- **Blurring of vision**, especially at times of fatigue. Initially, with an effort of fusion, this blurring may be overcome.
- **Headache** and **eyeache** (strains) are extremely common.
- **Intermittent diplopia** due to exhaustion of fusional reserve intermittently.

Diagnosis

- **Cover test:** One eye is covered and the other eye is made to fix on an object. In presence of heterophoria, the eye under cover, deviates. When the cover is removed, the covered eye corrects the deviation, and regains its normal position quickly. Cover test should be done both for near and distant objects with or without spectacles.
- **Maddox rod:** It consists of a series of parallel high-power, plus cylinders, that convert a point light as a red straight line, at right angle to the axis of rod. When Maddox rod is held in front of one eye, the images of the point source of light in two eyes become dissimilar, and fusion becomes dissociated (dissimilar image test). This test is performed at a distance of 6 meters and at 33 cm.
  In heterophoria, the red line of light becomes separated from the point source of light.
- **Maddox wing:** It is a device to find out the amount of heterophoria for near vision (at 33 cm).
- **Prism vergence tests:** The strength of the involved muscles are to be tested by forcing them to a maximum effort against the prism.
- **Synoptophore evaluation:** To know the range of fusion.

Treatment

- Smaller degrees of heterophoria which give rise to no symptom—require no treatment.
- **Errors of refraction must be corrected** fully by spectacles, which should be worn constantly.
- **Orthoptic exercises:** With the help of a synoptophore, to increase the fusional range and muscle power.
- **Exercises with prism (adverse prism)** are practiced against prisms with their bases turned toward the direction of deviation.
- **Relief of symptoms with the prisms (relieving prism):** Prisms are incorporated with the spectacles to correct the defect optically. The base of the prism is placed in the opposite side of the direction of deviation, and the power is equally divided between the two eyes.
- **Operative treatment:** It is rarely indicated, especially in a large deviation, and then the heterophoria is to be treated as heterotropia.

▍CONCOMITANT SQUINT

It is the dissociation of the eyes, wherein the angle of deviation remains the same in all directions of gaze, irrespective of eyes of fixation.

Etiological Factors

- **Poor vision in one eye,** e.g. uncorrected refractive errors, opacities in the media, diseases of the retina or optic nerve, etc.
- **Disturbances of ocular muscle-balance,** e.g. congenital malinsertion or maldevelopment of the extraocular muscles.
- **Dissociation between accommodation convergence relationship,** e.g. in case of hypermetropia → more accommodation is exerted to correct the error → more convergence → chance of convergent squint. Conversely, in myopia→ minimum or no effort of accommodation to correct the error → weakness of convergence → tendency for divergent squint.
- **Decompensated heterophoria** → manifest heterotropia.
- **Central cause:** As in cerebral palsy or mental retardation, due to deficient development of fusion faculty.

Types

Monocular Squint

Squint is normally monocular (about 85% of cases), in the sense, that one eye habitually takes up fixation, and the other eye, therefore, becomes the squinting eye. It may be convergent, divergent, or vertical.

- **Convergent concomitant squint (Figs 23.10A and B):** One eye always deviated inward, and it typically develops in early

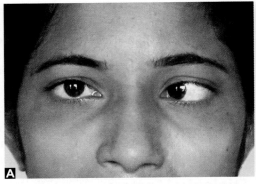
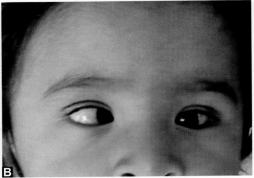

Figs 23.10A and B: A. Left convergent squint; **B.** Cross-fixation in convergent squint

childhood before the binocular reflexes are firmly established. Amblyopia is a frequent association.

Causes

- *Hypermetropia* with excessive use of accommodation is the common cause, and frequently becomes obvious after a debilitating illness.
- *Congenital myopia:* Due to excessive use of convergence for near vision.
- *Uncompensated esophoria.*
- *Anatomical factors*, e.g. orbital asymmetry, enophthalmos, etc.
- *Divergent concomitant squint (Fig. 23.11):* One eye always deviates outward. It is characteristically seen in older children and adults, and less frequently associated with amblyopia.

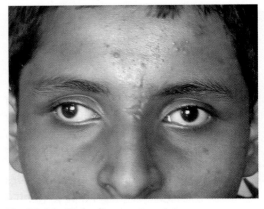

Fig. 23.11: Right divergent squint

Causes

- *Inherent neuromuscular incoordination:* It is the cause of primary divergent squint in a child. It is initially intermittent, and later on, becomes constant. The angle of deviation is usually greater for distant fixation than for the near.
- *Uncorrected myopia.*
- *Complete loss of vision in one eye:* As in unilateral cataract, after injury, etc. (blind eye takes the position of anatomical rest—*secondary divergent squint*).
- *Consecutive divergent squint:* Due to overcorrection of a convergent squint by operation.
- *Craniofacial anomalies:* As in hypertelorism and Crouzon syndrome, due to widely separated orbits.
- *Decompensated exophoria.*
- *Vertical concomitant squint (Figs 23.12A and B):* It is rare. Most of the cases are those of hyperphoria which become manifest.

Alternating Squint (Figs 23.13 to 23.15)

Alternating squint means when one eye fixes, the other eye deviates, and either of the eyes can adopt fixation alternately and freely. It may be convergent or divergent.

In an alternate squint, the visual acuity remains normal (or near normal) in each eye.

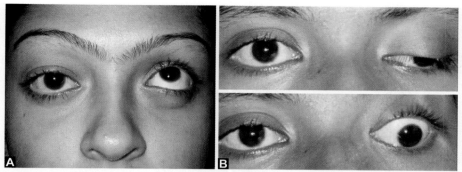

Figs 23.12A and B: A. Vertical squint left hypertropia; **B.** Vertical squint left hypotropia (right eye fixing)

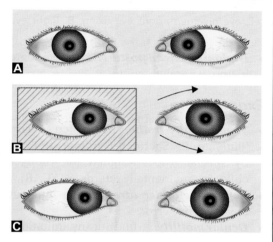

Figs 23.13A to C: Alternate convergent squint. **A.** Left eye convergent; right eye fixing; **B.** On cover test—left eye taking fixation and right eye converging; **C.** On uncover—right eye convergent; left eye fixing

There is no diplopia, as the image formed in the deviating eye is completely suppressed by the brain.

Alternating squint may be either, due to congenital weakness of either of lateral or medial rectus of each eye, or due to refractive errors.

Clinical Features (in General)

Usually, there is no symptom. The squinting of the eye is noticed by the parents or relatives.

There is no diplopia, as the suppression develops easily in the young age.

- In case of uniocular squint, visual acuity in usually poor (strabismic amblyopia). This is maximum with convergent squint.
- There is no limitation of eye movements.

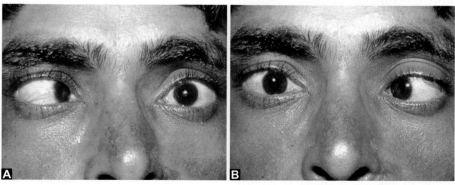

Figs 23.14A and B: Alternate convergent squint. **A.** Right eye convergent; left eye fixing; **B.** Left eye convergent; right eye fixing

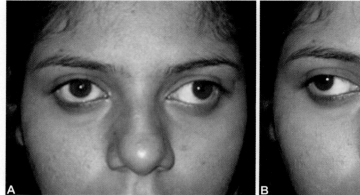
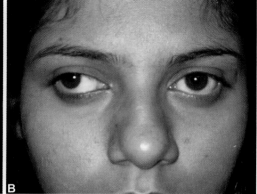

Figs 23.15A and B: Alternate divergent squint. **A.** Left eye divergent; right eye fixing; **B.** Right eye divergent; left eye fixing

- Primary angle of deviation is equal to the secondary angle of deviation the primary deviation means, the angle of deviation of the squinting eye, when the other eye fixes an object, secondary deviation means, the angle of deviation of the normal eye under cover, when the squinting eye is made to fix an object by covering the normal eye.

Evaluation of Concomitant Squint

History

- *Age of onset:* The older the age of onset and shorter the squinting period, the better is the prognosis.
- *History of an acute illness or debility* at the time of onset.
- *Family history* may often be positive.
- *Intermittent or constant:* The prognosis is better in the intermittent cases than in constant type, as it is likely, that some form of binocularity is still present in intermittent type.
- *Unilateral or alternating:* In constant unilateral squint, the presence of amblyopia should be suspected.

- *Diplopia or head posture:* To differentiate it, from a paralytic squint.

Examination

- *Visual acuity testing:* By Snellen's chart, 'illiterate E', Sheridan-Gardiner test, or by special tests, designed for younger children and mentally retards (STYCAR).
- *Refraction under atropine:* To find out any refractive error.
- *Ocular motility:* To find out any limitations of ocular movement.
- *Cover test:* To find out the squint is uniocular or alternating.
- *Fixation behavior:* To find out foveal (centric) fixation or eccentric fixation.
- *Anterior segment and fundus:* To rule out any organic lesion which may be the cause of squint.
- Measurement of the angle of squint
  - *Corneal reflection test (Hirschberg) (Fig. 23.16):* A reasonable assessment of the angle is made by holding a fixation light at 30 cm distance from the patient, and estimating the distance of the corneal light reflex (Purkinje's first image) from the pupillary center. One mm decentration of reflex corresponds to about 7° of ocular

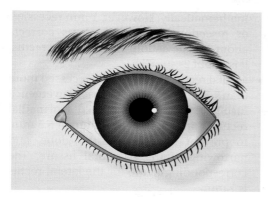

Fig. 23.16: Hirschberg's corneal reflection test

deviation. For example, if the reflex is situated at the pupillary margin, the angle is about 15°, and if it is at the limbus, the angle of squint is about 45°. This test is also useful to differentiate it from pseudostrabismus.

- **Prism reflex test (Krimsky):** Prisms are placed in front of the deviating eye until the corneal light reflexes become symmetrical.
- **Prism-bar-cover test (PBCT):** The prism power required to negate the ocular movements, equals to the angle of deviation, and it is measured in prism diopter (Δ). Roughly, 1° of ocular deviation equals to 2 prism diopter (2Δ) deviation. It is the most accurate method of measuring the angle of deviation.
- **Perimeter or tangent screen:** It is rarely used nowadays.
- **Synoptophore (major amblyoscope):** This is one of the accurate methods of estimation of the angle of squint.
- **Worth's 'four-dot' test:** To diagnose the presence of suppression and abnormal retinal correspondence in a manifest squint.
- **State of binocular vision:** All three grades of binocular vision (SMP, fusion and stereopsis) are determined by synoptophore. The alternating squint does not possess any grade of binocular vision. In intermittent squints, binocular vision is being maintained for the part of the time.

Treatment of Concomitant Squint

The aim of the treatment is to make the eyes straight, and to ensure BSV.

The treatment should be started as early as possible, so that the restoration of BSV is not delayed.

The prognosis decreases significantly after the age of 6 years and in adults the correction is purely for cosmetic reason.

Remember 4 'O's during treatment:
- *Optical correction of refractive errors:* By suitable spectacle. Some squints (particularly fully accommodative convergent squint) are completely controlled by spectacle correction.
- *Occlusion therapy:* To treat the amblyopia as already discussed.
- *Orthoptic exercises:* They are given with a synoptophore or prism-bar to overcome suppression, to improve the range of fusion, and to ensure easy stereopsis.
  These are initial steps to restore BSV, earlier before the surgical intervention. Fusional exercises are to be continued when the eyes become straight after the operation.
- *Operative measures:* Surgical intervention should be undertaken after initial occlusion therapy, when there is no further improvement of vision in the squinting eye.

Types of Squint Operation

Weakening Procedures (Figs 23.17A and B)

- *Recession:* It can be performed on any extraocular muscle. Here, the muscle insertion site is moved posteriorly toward the equator of the globe.
- *Marginal myotomy:* It is done by cutting partially through the muscle margin.
- *Myotomy (tenotomy):* It is commonly performed on an overacting inferior

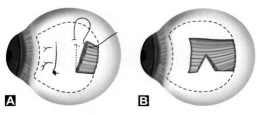

Figs 23.17A and B: Weakening procedure. **A.** Recession; **B.** Marginal myotomy

oblique muscle, by cutting across the muscle near its insertion (tenotomy for superior oblique muscle).

- **Disinsertion:** It is almost a similar procedure, done in case of contracted rectus muscle as in thyroid ophthalmopathy.
- **Faden procedure** (Faden means suture) (posterior-fixation suture): It is the suturing of the muscle belly to the globe at about 12 mm behind its insertion. This will weaken its effective action.

Strengthening Procedures (Figs 23.18A and B)

- **Resection:** Effective pull of the muscle is enhanced by making it shorter, and is suitable only for rectus muscles.
- **Advancement:** The muscle is first disinserted, and then reinserted nearer to the limbus.
- **Tucking (plication):** This effectively shortens the muscle, and is usually reserve for superior oblique muscle in 4th nerve palsy.

General principles of squint surgery:
- The degree of resection or recession, that is required, cannot be determined

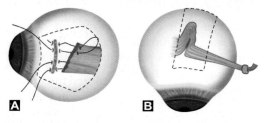

Figs 23.18A and B: Strengthening procedure. **A.** Resection; **B.** Tucking of superior oblique muscle

mathematically. However, 1 mm recession or resection of medical rectus corrects about 3° of deviation; and for lateral rectus, it is about 2°.

- Medial rectus should not be recessed more than 5.5 mm, as this may cause convergence insufficiency. Similarly, resection of medial rectus is limited to a maximum of 5.5 mm, to prevent retraction of the globe, and narrowing of the palpebral fissure. The corresponding figure for the lateral rectus is 7 mm.
- It is wise to aim toward under correction especially in children, as a residual 5–10° may well disappear, once the stereoscopic vision is established.
- It is preferable to operate on elevators, rather than on depressors which are important in reading and walking. A 3 mm muscle recession corrects about 10° of vertical squint.

Choice of Surgery

- *In convergent squint*
  - Medial rectus recession and lateral rectus resection of the squinting eye.
  - Medial rectus recession of the both eyes (bimedial recession).
- *In divergent squint (Figs 23.19A and B)*
  - Lateral rectus recession and medial rectus resection of the squinting eye.
  - Recession of lateral rectus of the both eyes (bilateral recession).
- *In alternating squint:* Treatment is only for cosmetic purpose, as fusional faculty does not develop in this type of squint. Both eyes are to be tackled to correct the deviation (e.g. bimedial recession or bilateral recession).

  Depending upon the amount of deviation, 'two', 'three' or 'four' muscles of two eyes are to be tackled.

  As there is good visual acuity in each eye, the patient must be warned that diplopia may follow the operation, and may persist for months.

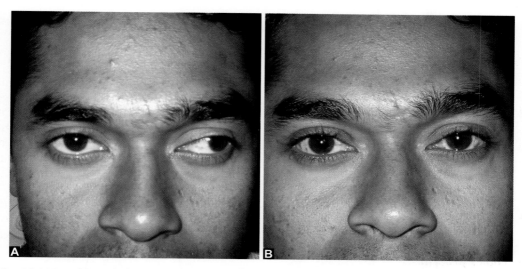

Figs 23.19A and B: Left divergent squint. **A.** Before correction; **B.** After surgical correction

PARALYTIC SQUINT

It is the misalignment of the visual axes as a result of paresis, or paralysis of one or more extraocular muscles. It is characterized by impaired movement in the field of action of the muscle(s), and thus the angle of deviation varies in different directions of gaze and with fixation of eyes.

Etiology

- *Lesions affecting the cranial nerve supplying the muscle:*
  - *Nuclear lesions*—cerebrovascular accidents, infection, neoplasm, aneurysm, toxin (diphtheric), etc.
  - *Lesions of the nerve*—head injury, meningitis, cavernous sinus thrombosis, fracture of the base of the skull, pressure from a neoplasm or aneurysm.
- *Lesions in the muscle:*
  - *Congenital maldevelopment* of a muscle.
  - *Direct injury* to the muscle.
  - *Diseases of the muscles*—as in ocular myopathy, thyroid myopathy, myasthenia gravis, etc.

Clinical Features

- *Diplopia:* Paralytic squint in an adult with previously single binocular vision, causes diplopia. It is the chief symptom, and most marked when the eye is rotated into the field of action of the paralyzed muscle. Diplopia may be crossed, uncrossed, or may be with tilting.
- *False orientation of the object:* Object is projected too far in the direction of paralyzed muscle, due to increase in secondary deviation.
- *Vertigo and nausea:* They are partly due to diplopia, and partly due to false orientation.
- *Secondary angle of deviation is more than* the primary deviation (Fig. 23.20). This is because of excessive innervation is required to move and maintain the eye in primary position when the patient fixates with the paralytic eye (Hering's law of equal innervation).
- *Restriction of ocular movements* in the direction of action of paralyzed muscle.
- *Compensatory head posture:* In paralytic squint, to neutralize diplopia the chin may be elevated or depressed, the face is turned

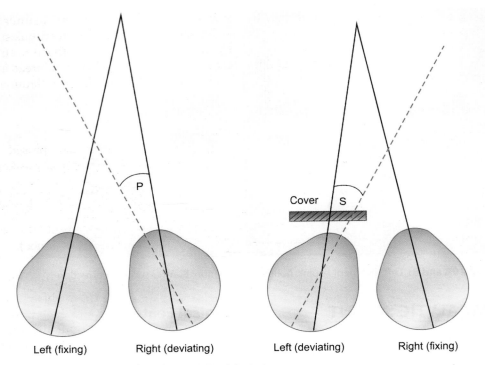

Fig. 23.20: Primary angle and secondary angle of deviation

In *concomitant squint* (right eye), the primary deviation (P) is equal to the secondary deviation (S), obtained when the non-squinting eye is occluded. In *paralytic squint*, the secondary deviation is greater than the primary

Difference between concomitant and paralytic squint	
Concomitant squint	**Paralytic squint**
Mostly developmental, usually not associated with trauma/disease	Mostly acquired, usually associated with trauma/disease
Occurs in infants and children	Usually in adults
Diplopia absent	Diplopia present
No abnormal head posture	Abnormal head posture to avoid diplopia
Absence of false projection (i.e. false localization of object)	False projection is present
Angle of squint is usually constant in all directions of gaze	Angle of squint is variable in different directions of gaze
Ocular movements are normal and there is no restriction	Ocular movement is restricted in the direction of action of paralyzed muscle
Secondary angle of deviation is always equal to primary deviation	Secondary deviation is greater than primary deviation
Amblyopia is present	No amblyopia
Surgical result is usually good	Surgical result is not satisfactory, and at times, surgery may be contraindicated

to right or left side, and the head may be tilted to the right or left shoulder (ocular torticollis). This head posture, is to neutralize the angle of deviation, or to separate the images maximally, so as to avoid diplopia.

In *paralysis of horizontal rectus* muscle, the face is turned to field of action of the paralyzed muscle, but the head is not tilted. As, in right lateral rectus palsy, the patient keeps his face turned to the right. In case of *cyclovertical muscle palsy*, it is more complicated, and less valuable diagnostically. Face turn and chin position are toward the main action of the paralyzed muscle, and the head tilt is toward the hypotropic eye. As in *superior oblique palsy*, the head is tilted on the side of the normal eye, the face is turned to normal side, and the chin is depressed.

- *Visual acuity is normal* in both eyes, and there is no amblyopia.

Different Types of Ocular Paralysis

Total ophthalmoplegia (Fig. 23.21): It means involvement of both extrinsic and intrinsic muscles of the eyeball. In unilateral cases, the lesion is in the cavernous sinus, or in the superior orbital fissure, and in bilateral cases, the lesion is widespread in the brainstem due to vascular or inflammatory cause.

Clinical signs
- Ptosis.
- The eyeball is slightly proptosed and divergent (due to anatomical position of rest).
- No movement of the eyeball in any direction.
- Fixed dilated pupil (no reaction to light, accommodation and convergence).
- Total loss of accommodation.

External ophthalmoplegia: It is due to paralysis of extrinsic muscles which includes six extraocular muscles and the levator. It is due to nuclear lesion without affecting the Edinger-Westphal nucleus, which supplies the intrinsic muscles.

Signs are same as total ophthalmoplegia except, that the pupillary reactions and accommodation are normal.

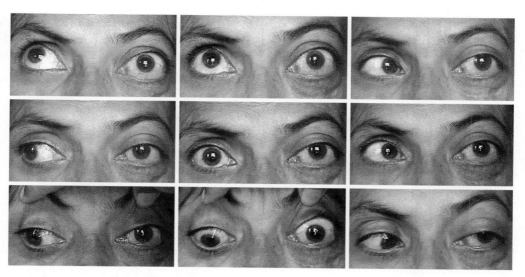

Fig. 23.21: Total ophthalmoplegia

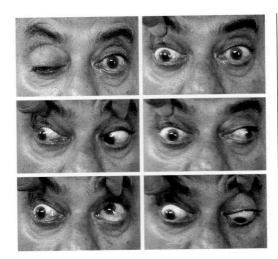

Fig. 23.22: Right third nerve palsy

Third (Oculomotor) Nerve Palsy (Fig. 23.22)

- Ptosis due to weakness of levator.
- Eyeball rotates outward (divergent) and slightly downward due to unopposed action of the lateral rectus (N VI) and superior oblique (N IV) muscles.
- Intorsion of the eyeball on attempted down gaze, due to action of superior oblique muscle.
- Ocular movements are restricted in all direction, except outward (due to lateral rectus).

- Pupil is dilated, and does not constrict to light or convergence.

Fourth (Trochlear) Nerve Palsy

Trauma is the most common cause of isolated fourth nerve palsy, which may be bilateral. It causes paralysis of the superior oblique muscle. The clinical features are as follows:

- *Abnormal head posture:* Chin depression, head tilt and slight face turn to the opposite (normal) side.
- Diplopia is most troublesome, as it is more in downgaze.
- Eyeball deviated upward and inward (ipsilateral hypertropia).
- Extorsion of the globe (excyclotropia).
- Restriction of the ocular movements on downward and inward.
- Bielschowsky's 'three-step' test is useful to diagnose a fourth nerve (superior oblique) palsy (Figs 23.23A and B).

When a healthy individual tilts their head, the superior oblique (SO) and superior rectus of the eye closest to the shoulder keep the eye level. The inferior oblique and inferior rectus keep the other eye level.

In patients with SO palsy: The SR muscle's action is not counteracted by the SO. This leads to vertical deviation of the affected eye when the head is tilted toward the effected eye.

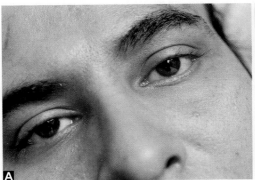
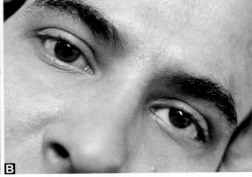

Figs 23.23A and B: Bielschowsky's head tilt test in left superior oblique palsy

However, there is no deviation when the head is tilted toward the unaffected eye because the SO muscle is not stimulated in the effected eye, but rather it is stimulated in the unaffected eye.

Sixth (Abducens) Nerve Palsy

This is the most common type, and commonly occurs in raised intracranial tension.

The long intracranial course, and its angulation over the petrous-tip of the sphenoid bone, make it vulnerable in raised intracranial tension. In this situation, the sixth nerve palsy is a false localizing sign.

Signs: They are due to paralysis of lateral rectus (Fig. 23.24).
- The eyeball is rotated inward (convergent squint).

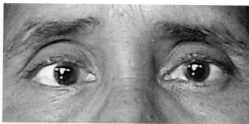
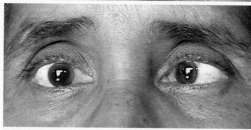
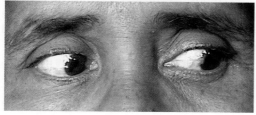

Fig. 23.24: Right sixth nerve (lateral rectus) palsy. **Note**—absence of abduction in right eye

- Defective abduction of the eye, partially or completely.
- Face turn toward the field of action of paralyzed muscle (e.g. a patient with right sixth nerve palsy will turn his face to the right).

Investigations

- ***Diplopia charting (Fig. 23.25):*** It is done in a dark room, with red glass placed in front of right eye and green glass in front of left, to dissociate the images. A streak light is moved in different areas of binocular vision, with the head being held stationary. Position of two images are recorded on a chart with nine squares (representing nine diagnostic positions of gaze) marked on it.
  Now, note
  - The direction of gaze, where the separation of images are maximum.
  - The farther displaced image (outer image) belongs to which eye. This can be done by covering one eye of the patient, and asking him which one of the two images

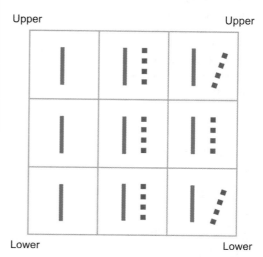

Fig. 23.25: Diplopia chart showing the position of the images in right lateral rectus palsy
The dotted lines show the positions of the false image in different parts of the field of diplopia

has disappeared. The farther displaced image belongs to the affected eye.

- **Hess screen (chart) (Fig. 23.26):** The eyes are dissociated similarly with red and green goggles, and note the patient's response to the dissimilar images formed by each eye while viewing a different targets (dot and line) on Hess screen.
  - The results of the test is interpreted by comparing the grids, charted for each eye, and they depend on **Herring's law of equal innervation**.
  - In paralytic squint, the greatest restriction occurs in the direction of paretic muscle, with corresponding overaction of the contralateral synergistic muscle. (Shorter chart is of paralytic eye and the larger chart is due to overacting contralateral synergists). It also provides the accurate measurement of commitance.
- **Worth's four-dot test:** Patients eyes are dissociated with red glass placed in front of right eye and green glass in front of left. He then views at a box with four lights (dots); one red, two green and one white (Fig. 23.27).
- **Forced duction test (FDT):** This test is used to differentiate defective ocular movements due to physical restriction, from a muscle paralysis.
  After topical anesthesia, the insertion of the affected muscle is grasped with

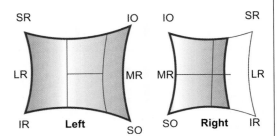

Fig. 23.26: Hess chart in right lateral rectus palsy
SR—Superior rectus; **IO**—Inferior oblique; **LR**—Lateral rectus; **MR**—Medial rectus; **IR**—Inferior rectus; **SO**—Superior oblique

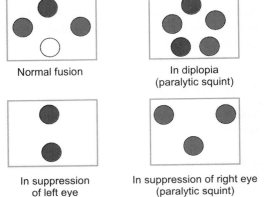

Normal fusion	In diplopia (paralytic squint)
In suppression of left eye	In suppression of right eye (paralytic squint)

Fig. 23.27: Worth's four-dot test

fixation forceps, and gently attempted to rotate the eyeball in the field of action of weak muscle.

The interpretations of Worth's four-dot test are as follows:

If the patient sees	Presence of
All four lights	Normal fusion
All four lights, even in presence of a concomitant manifest squint	Abnormal retinal correspondence (ARC)
Two red and three green lights	Diplopia (paralytic squint)
Two red lights	Suppression of left eye
Three green lights	Suppression of right eye
Two red or three green lights alternately	Alternate suppression

FDT 'positive' means, it is difficult to move the globe with the forceps (e.g. contracture of muscle as in thyroid myopathy, trapped muscle in orbital floor fracture, etc.).

FDT is 'negative' in case of muscle paralysis.

- **Investigations of find out the cause,** e.g. neurological consultation, X-ray skull, CT scan of brain and orbit, MRI scan, blood sugar, thyroid function tests, 'Tensilon test' for myasthenia gravis, etc.

Sequelae of extraocular muscle palsy:
- Overaction of contralateral synergist (Herring's law of equal innervation).
- Contracture of ipsilateral antagonist.
- Inhibitional (secondary) palsy of the contralateral antagonist (Sherrington's law of reciprocal innervation).

For example
- ***In right lateral rectus palsy***
  - Overaction of left medial rectus
  - Contracture of right medial rectus
  - Inhibitional palsy of left lateral rectus.

- ***In right superior oblique palsy***
  - Overaction of left inferior rectus
  - Contracture of right inferior oblique
  - Inhibitional palsy of left superior rectus.

Treatment

- Treatment must be directed toward the cause of paralysis.
- For the relief of diplopia:
  - Occlusion of affected eye temporarily.
  - Suitable prism correction for minor diplopia.
- Observation for at least 6 months, so that maximum amount of spontaneous recovery could take place.
- Recession of contralateral synergist may be done for the nerve palsy. Alternately, various type of muscle transposition operations may be undertaken.
- Botulinum toxin injection may be tried in some cases—to prevent contracture of the antagonist muscle.

DUANE'S RETRACTION SYNDROME (FIG. 23.28)

This type of non-commitant squint, occurs because of aberrant innervation which causes contraction of lateral rectus muscle instead of relaxation, when the medial rectus muscle contracts (i.e. co-contraction of medial and lateral rectus muscles during adduction).

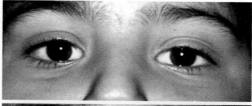
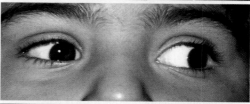
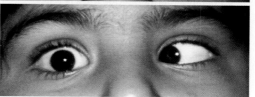

Fig. 23.28: Duane's retraction syndrome

Clinical Features

- Marked restriction, or absence of abduction.
- Slight restriction of adduction.
- Retraction of the globe on attempted adduction.
- Narrowing of the palpebral aperture on adduction, and widening on attempted abduction.
- Deficiency of convergence of the affected eye.
- 'Up-shoot' or 'down-shoot' of the eye on adduction.

  This is Type I (most common type), and the other types are:

  Type II: Limitation of adduction with relatively normal adbuction.

  Type III: Limitation of the both abduction and adduction.

  Girls are more commonly affected than boys. The left eye is affected more commonly than the right eye, and in few cases, it may be bilateral.

Treatment is only indicated, when there is ocular deviation in primary position. But, no method can restore a full and normal range of ocular movement.

Superior oblique tendon-sheath syndrome (Brown's syndrome)

It is usually congenital, but acquired Brown's syndrome may occur following trauma, tenosynovitis of the superior oblique tendon-trochlea apparatus.

Clinical features
- Limitation of elevation of the eye on adduction, simulating inferior oblique muscle palsy.
- Normal elevation on abduction.
- The eyes are straight on primary position, and there is no overaction of superior oblique muscle.
  - *Diagnosis* is confirmed by FDT, which is 'positive' in attempting to elevate the eye from adducted position.
  - *Surgical intervention* (superior oblique tenotomy) should only be considered in extreme cases.

NYSTAGMUS (FIGS 23.29A AND B)

This is an involuntary, rhythmic, to-and-fro oscillation of the eyeballs.

It is usually detected by simple observation of the eyes. But when minimal, it may be observed during slit-lamp examination or ophthalmoscopy, under magnification.

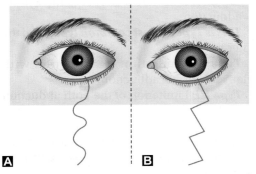

Figs 23.29A and B: Nystagmus. **A.** Pendular; **B.** Jerky

On the basis of rhythm, nystagmus may be classified as:
- *Pendular nystagmus (Fig. 23.29A):* To-and-fro oscillation of the eyes are equal in velocity and amplitude in each direction. The movements may be horizontal, vertical, oblique or rotatory.
- *Jerky nystagmus (Fig. 23.29B):* It has a slow component in one direction, and a fast component in the opposite direction. The direction of nystagmus is defined by the direction of the fast component, although the slow movement reflects the basic disability.
- *Mixed:* Pendular nystagmus in primary position, and jerky in lateral gaze.

Clinical Types

Physiological Nystagmus

- *End-gaze nystagmus:* Fine jerky nystagmus in extreme gaze positions. It is common after administration of barbiturates and other tranquillizers.
- *Optokinetic nystagmus (OKN):* It is a jerky nystagmus induced by moving repetitive visual patterns across the visual field. It has a slow phase in the direction of moving pattern, followed by a fast phase in the opposite direction, to refixate the eye on the next target. It is also called *rail-road nystagmus*.
  - *Clinical applications:* For testing visual acuity in infants or young children (Catford drum test), and for detecting malingering.
- *Vestibular nystagmus:* It is a jerky nystagmus, caused by altered input from the vestibular nuclei to the horizontal gaze centers. Clinically, caloric test is done to induced vestibular nystagmus in suspected gaze paralysis.
  - If hot water is irrigated into right ear—the patient will develop right jerky nystagmus; and if cold water into right ear—the patient will develop left jerky nystagmus (mnemonic 'C-O-W-S', cold-opposite and warm-same).

TABLE 23.1: Types of nystagmus.

Types	Characteristics	Causes
Congenital nystagmus	Jerky type and horizontal, absent during sleep, and persists throughout life	Usually hereditary
Latent nystagmus	Bilateral jerky, horizontal nystagmus, elicited by covering one eye. Fast component is towards the uncovered eye. With both eyes open, patient has normal vision, but when one eye is covered, visual acuity of the open eye may be 6/60 or less	Unknown, but convergent squint is a common association
Spasmus nutans	Pendular nystagmus, abnormal head posture, and head nodding. Occurs between 4 months to 2 years of age. Spontaneously cured by 3 years of age	Unknown
Ataxic (gaze-paretic) nystagmus	Nystagmus of abducted eye	Internuclear ophthalmoplegia
Down-beat nystagmus	Jerky nystagmus, with fast phase downwards	Lesion at the cervicomedullary junction at the foramen magnum
Up-beat nystagmus	Fast phase in upward direction	Phenytoin sodium intoxication, or posterior fossa lesions
See-saw nystagmus	One eye rising and intorting, while the other eye falls and extorts	Chiasmal lesion (with bitemporal hemianopia)
Periodic alternate nystagmus (PAN)	Jerky nystagmus, with rhythmic changes in amplitude and direction	Demyelinating brainstem disease of the brainstem
Nystagmus retractorius	Jerky nystagmus, with convergent movement of two eyes, and retraction of the globe. May be associated with vertical gaze palsy, lid retraction. Light-near dissociation of pupils, and accommodative spasm (**Parinaud's syndrome**)	Lesions in the pretectal area, e.g. vascular lesions or pinealoma
Miner's nystagmus	Rotatory rapid nystagmus, defective vision at night with dancing of lights and movements of objects	Fixation difficulties in dim illuminations in coal mines
Nystagmus blockade syndrome	Occurs in some cases of congenital nystagmus in which a 'purposive esotropia' dampens the horizontal nystagmus	Compensatory phenomenon

- If both ear are stimulated—for cold water the patient develops up-beat jerky nystagmus and for warm water, down-beat jerky nystagmus (mnemonic—'C-U-W-D,' cold-up and warm-down).
- In pathological vestibular nystagmus, the fast phase of jerky nystagmus is directed to the opposite side, and is associated with deafness, vertigo and tinnitus, e.g. in Meniere's disease, or labyrinthitis.

Types of nystagmus are described in Table 23.1.

Ocular (Sensory-Deprivation) Nystagmus

This is typically provoked by lowered central vision in the first few months of life, before the fixation reflexes have matured.

- Nystagmus occurs, if the lesion occurs before the age of 6 months. In later life, there is nystagmoid excursions, but after the 6 years this type of nystagmus does not occur.
- Ocular nystagmus is typically pendular and horizontal, but on looking to either side, it may break down into a jerky nystagmus.
- *Common causes* are—bilateral congenital cataract, albinism, aniridia, congenital high myopia, macular hypoplasia, Leber's optic atrophy, etc.

Motor Imbalance Nystagmus

This is due to primary defect in the efferent mechanism and acquired in nature.

Treatment

Basic aim of the treatment is, *to transfer the 'neutral point'* (where the nystagmus is least apparent) *from an eccentric point to a straight ahead position*. So, there is elimination of the compensatory head posture, and improvement of vision in primary gaze. This is done by:

- Prismotherapy
- Surgical treatment:
  - *Kestenbaum's operation:* The aim of the surgery is to shift the null (neutral) point to the primary position.
  - *Faden* or posterior-fixation suture operation may be better in this situation.

Ocular Injuries

CLASSIFICATION OF MECHANICAL INJURIES

Classification of mechanical injuries

- **Closed globe injury**
  - Contusion
  - Lamellar laceration
  - Superficial foreign body
  - Mixed

  Zone I: Conjunctiva, cornea and sclera involved

  Zone II: Anterior chamber and lens is involved

  Zone III: Posterior part is involved.
- **Open globe injury**
  - Rupture
  - Penetrating
  - Intraocular foreign bodies
  - Perforating
  - Mixed

  Zone I: Only cornea is involved

  Zone II: Cornea and sclera up to 5 mm

  Zone III: Wound extends >5 mm of the sclera.

CONTUSIONS (BLUNT INJURY)

- Ocular injuries by blunt instruments vary in severity, from simple subconjunctival hemorrhage to rupture of the globe.
- Every part of the globe may be so injured by contusion, that may seriously cause diminished vision. Moreover, in some cases the effects are progressive or delayed. So, in all cases of contusions, a guarded prognosis should be given.

- The *mechanisms* of ocular tissue damage are:
  - *Direct effect* of injury,
  - *Indirect effect* against bony orbit, and
  - *Contrecoup effect* due to propagation of wave of thrust, to-and-fro within the globe.

The various ocular effects resulting from contusions are briefly enumerated below.

Eyelids

- Lid lacerations
- Swelling and ecchymosis (black eye) (Fig. 24.1)
- *Emphysema* of the eyelids [crepitation on palpation, due to orbital fracture with involvement of paranasal sinuses (PNS) (Fig. 24.2)].

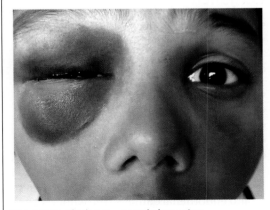

Fig. 24.1: Black eye—panda bear sign

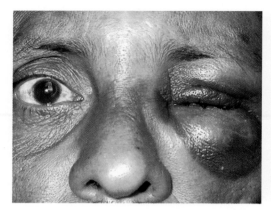

Fig. 24.2: Ecchymosis with emphysema of the lids

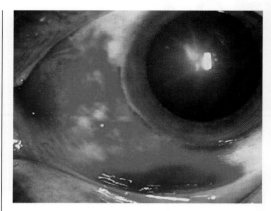

Fig. 24.3: Subconjunctival hemorrhage

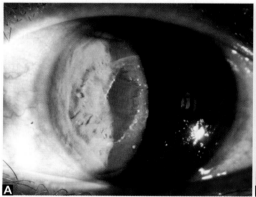
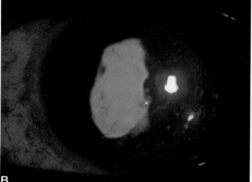

Figs 24.4A and B: Corneal abrasion and with fluorescein staining

Conjunctiva

- Conjunctival lacerations and chemosis
- Subconjunctival hemorrhage (Fig. 24.3).

Cornea

- Simple abrasions (Figs 24.4A and B)
- Recurrent corneal erosion syndrome
- Rupture of the Descemet's membrane
- Corneal stromal edema
- *Blood-staining of the cornea (Figs 24.5A and B):* Usually it occurs after a traumatic hyphema with raised intraocular pressure and endothelial damage. The whole cornea is stained (reddish-brown or greenish). Cornea gradually and very slowly clears up from the periphery towards the center, for a period of 2 years or more. Usually, some amount of permanent visual impairment results. Penetrating keratoplasty may be necessary in future.
- *Corneal rupture* may also occur.

Sclera

Scleral rupture (rupture of the globe) (Fig. 24.6): The force usually comes from the direction of down and out, as there the globe is least protected by the orbital rim. The sclera gives way at its *weakest part,* near the canal of Schlemm and the wound runs concentrically with the limbus. The conjunctiva is often intact. There may be associated uveal prolapse,

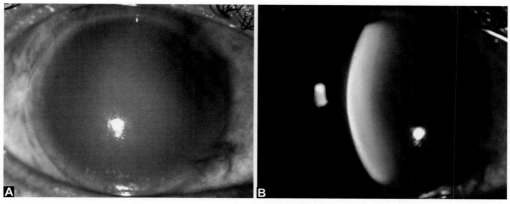

Figs 24.5A and B: Blood staining of the cornea (slit-section on right)

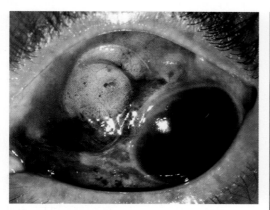

Fig. 24.6: Scleral rupture with subconjunctival dislocation of intraocular lens

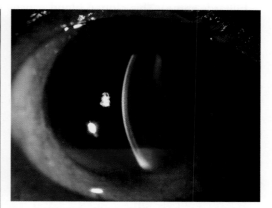

Fig. 24.7: Blood in anterior chamber—traumatic hyphema partially settled

subconjunctival dislocation of lens, vitreous prolapse and intraocular bleeding. Prognosis is often very poor as the eye usually shrinks with total loss of vision.

Anterior Chamber

Hyphema (Blood in the Anterior Chamber) (Fig. 24.7)

Sources of Bleeding

- Small branches of the major arterial circle due to tear between longitudinal and circular fibers of the ciliary muscle.
- Capillaries of the minor arterial circle, when there is sphincteric tear.
- Radial vessels at the iris root, associated with iridodialysis.

Other causes of hyphema

- Intraoperative and postoperative
- Herpetic iridocyclitis
- Rubeosis iridis (as in diabetes)
- Blood dyscrasia
- Intraocular malignancies
- Idiopathic
- Juvenile xanthogranuloma (recurrent spontaneous hyphema in a young child).

Clinical features

- The blood usually does not get clotted and settles at the most dependent portion of the anterior chamber, and a fluid meniscus is formed.
- Frequently, original minor hyphema is followed by a more severe bleeding within 24–48 hours of injury.
- Sometimes, the blood may be clotted, especially in presence of sphincteric tear or iridodialysis.
- *'8' ball (or blackball) hyphema:* When the blood gets clotted, the hyphema appears as small blackball (like no. '8' ball in billiards game). This clotted blood causes secondary glaucoma more frequently (Fig. 24.8).

Complications

- Secondary glaucoma—due to blockage of angle by red blood cells, or breakdown products of the blood.
- Secondary optic atrophy due to chronic glaucoma.
- Blood staining of the cornea.

Treatment

- Complete bed rest with propped up position.
- Sedation.

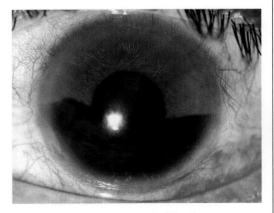

Fig. 24.8: Blunt trauma—'8' ball hyphema

- Patching of the eyes (binocular is better).
- Corticosteroid eye drops to minimize traumatic uveitis.
  Mild hyphema without secondary glaucoma usually responds with above therapy. Aspirin should not be used, as it increases the risk of secondary hemorrhage.
- Secondary glaucoma is treated with:
  - Tablet acetazolamide (250 mg), half to one tablet—4 times daily.
  - Timolol (0.5%) eye drops, twice daily.
- *Indications of paracentesis:*
  - Blood does not get absorbed quickly by 5–7 days.
  - Persistent high intraocular pressure (IOP) for 3–7 days depending upon the height of intraocular pressure.
  - Early signs of blood staining of cornea.
- Limbal incision and removal of the clots may be urgently required in blackball hyphema.

Iris

- *Iridodialysis:* Iris is partially torn away from its ciliary attachment. A black biconvex area is seen at the periphery, and pupillary margin bulges slightly inward, causing a D-shaped pupil (Figs 24.9 and 24.10). A fundal glow is obtained through the peripheral gap. There may be uniocular diplopia.
- *Antiflexion of the iris:* In extensive iridodialysis, the detached portion of the iris may be rotated completely, so that

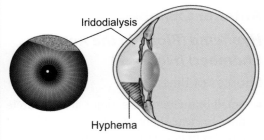

Fig. 24.9: Iridodialysis and hyphema. Note the D-shaped pupil in iridodialysis

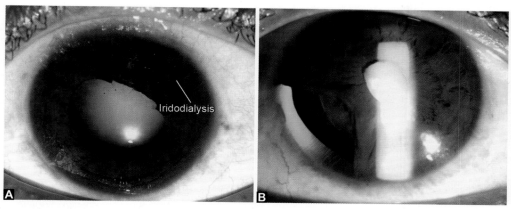

Figs 24.10A and B: A. Traumatic iridodialysis—D-shaped pupil; **B.** Iridodialysis—note the gap at the iris root

pigmented back surface of the iris faces forward. Torn peripheral edge of the iris may be sutured just behind the limbus.

- **Traumatic aniridia (irideremia):** The iris is completely torn away (360°) from its ciliary attachment, contracts into a small ball, and sinks at the bottom of the anterior chamber.
- **Retroflexon (total inversion) of the iris:** The whole iris may be doubled back into the ciliary region. When partial, it may appear as coloboma of the iris.
- **Iridoschisis:** Partial thickness tearing of the iris.
- **Traumatic iridocyclitis:** Usually mild.

Pupil

- Traumatic miosis
- Traumatic mydriasis
- D-shaped pupil (due to iridodialysis)
- Irregular pupil (due to sphincteric tear).

Ciliary Body

- Spasm of accommodation
- **Angle recession (Fig. 24.11):** There is longitudinal tear in the face of the ciliary body which splits the circular fibers from the longitudinal fibers of the ciliary muscle. There is deepening of the anterior chamber, widening of the ciliary band on

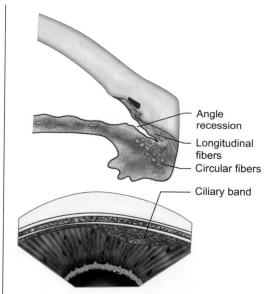

Fig. 24.11: Angle recession with irregular widening of the ciliary band

gonioscopy (Fig. 24.12), and tendency to develop glaucoma in future.

Crystalline Lens

- **Vossius's ring:** A circular pigmented imprint of the miosed pupil on the anterior surface of the lens.
- **Concussion cataract:** This is largely due to imbibition of aqueous through the

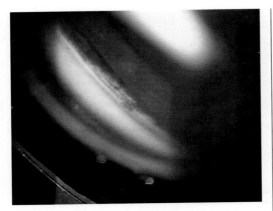

Fig. 24.12: Gonioscopic view of angle recession

damaged capsule, and partly due to direct mechanical effect on the lens fibers. The capsular tear commonly occurs at the posterior pole of the lens.

- *Types of concussion cataract*
  - Minute discrete subcapsular opacities.
  - Localized cataract, often behind the iris, which may remain stationary.
  - Total cataract (in large capsular tear).
  - ***Typical rosette-shaped cataract (Figs 24.13 to 24.15):*** It is a star-shaped cataract, usually in the posterior cortex. Accumulation of fluid marks out the architectural pattern of the lens. Star-shaped cortical sutures are delineated

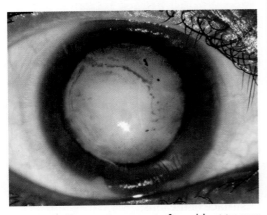

Fig. 24.13: Traumatic cataract after a blunt trauma

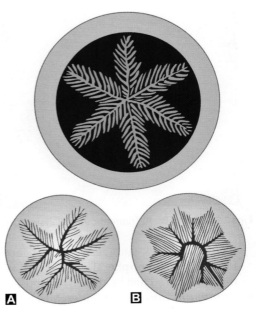

Figs 24.14A and B: Rosette-shaped cataract. **A.** In *early rosette*, leaves of the feathery opacities are formed by the suture acting as a backbone from which the opacities radiate outwards; **B.** In *late rosette*, feathery opacities stream outward from which lie in the angle between neighboring leaves

and radiating feathery line of opacities outlines the lens fibers. Sometimes, it remains stationary, and sometimes, it may progress into a total cataract.

  - ***Late rosette-shaped cataract:*** It usually develops in the posterior cortex, 1–2 years after a concussion. It is smaller and more compact than early type, and its sutural extensions are short.
- ***Subluxation of the lens.***
- ***Dislocation of the lens:*** In the anterior chamber or in the vitreous cavity.

Vitreous

- Disorganization and liquefaction of the vitreous.
- Anterior and/or posterior vitreous detachment.

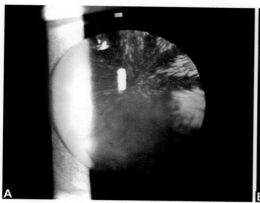 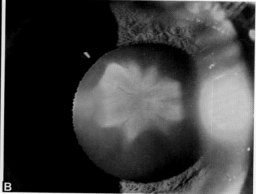

Figs 24.15A and B: Rosette cataract. **A.** Early; **B.** Late

- Fine pigmentary opacities.
- *Vitreous hemorrhage* with its sequelae.

Choroid

- *Choroidal rupture (Fig. 24.16):* Immediately after the injury, choroidal rupture is not visible due to extravasation of blood. After the blood gets absorbed, the rupture is seen as two curved white lines, concentric with the disc margin and on its temporal side. These lines become rapidly pigmented along its edge.

  Simple rupture without macular involvement, causes little visual impairment.

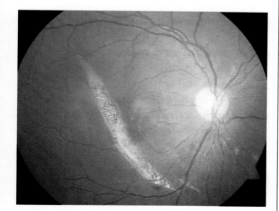

Fig. 24.16: Choroidal rupture

Treatment is by bed rest (with upright head) and atropine ointment.

- *Choroidal hemorrhage:* It appears as a red-dark patch underneath the retinal vessels.

Retina

- *Commotio retinae (Berlin's edema):* It is the milky-white cloudiness at the macular area due to edema. Since the fovea is very thin the edema is not visible, it appears more reddish (cherry-red) in the white surroundings.
- Central vision may be permanently impaired due to pigmentary deposits at the macula.
- *Traumatic macular degeneration* with the formation of a *macular cyst* and subsequently, a *macular hole.*
- *Retinal hemorrhage,* due to rupture of the retinal vessels.
- *Retinal tears:* Particularly at the retinal periphery, if the eye is already myopic or having peripheral degeneration.
- *Retinal detachment* following a tear in the retina.
- *Traumatic proliferative vitreoretinopathy (Fig. 24.17)* is usually secondary to vitreous hemorrhage, leading to fibrovascular tractional bands.

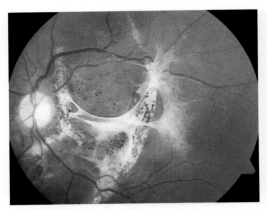

Fig. 24.17: Traumatic proliferative vitreoretinopathy

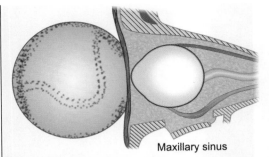

Fig. 24.18: Blow-out fracture of the orbital floor

Optic Nerve

- Optic nerve sheath hemorrhage.
- *Avulsion of the optic nerve* leading to optic atrophy, which may be partial or total.

Intraocular Tension

- *Hypotony* due to vasomotor reaction.
- *Secondary glaucoma due to*
  - Vasomotor reaction
  - Trabecular edema
  - Hyphema
  - Subluxation or dislocation of the lens
  - Ghost cell glaucoma
  - Angle recession glaucoma.

Lacrimal Apparatus

- Traumatic subluxation of lacrimal gland
- Injury to the lacrimal canaliculus.

Orbit

- Proptosis and displacement of the globe.
- Orbital (retrobulbar) hemorrhage.
- Orbital emphysema following orbital bone fracture involving PNS.
- *Fracture of the orbital bones:* It most commonly affects the margin of the orbit. Fractures near the orbital margin are easy to diagnose from unevenness of the margin, and tenderness on pressure.

Fracture of the superior rim of the orbit may dislocate the trochlea of superior oblique tendon, causing paresis of superior oblique muscle with diplopia.

- *Blow-out fracture:* Pure blow-out fracture is typically caused by a sudden rise in intraorbital pressure by a striking object which is greater than 5 cm in diameter, such as a tennis-ball or a fist. The fracture usually involves the floor of the orbit, along the thin bone covering the infraorbital canal (Figs 24.18 and 24.19).

Clinical Features

- *Diplopia*—typically occurs in both upgaze and downgaze *(double diplopia), due to entrapment of the inferior rectus and inferior oblique muscles.*
- *Periocular ecchymosis and edema.*
- *Enophthalmos with pseudoptosis* usually appears after 10–14 days.
- *Infraorbital nerve anesthesia* involving the lower eyelid, side of the nose, cheek, upper lip and teeth.
- *Nasal bleeding* from maxillary sinus.
- *Subconjunctival hemorrhage is common, but other ocular damage is very rare*, due to natural protection by the type of injury.

Investigations

- *Plain X-ray (Water's view) of orbit:* The classic finding is the presence of a polypoid mass *(the tear-drop sign)* protruding

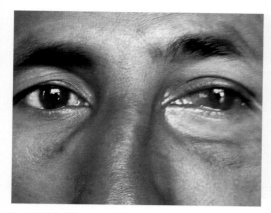

Fig. 24.19: Blow-out fracture on the left side

from the floor of the orbit into the maxillary antrum. The tear-drop represents the herniated orbital contents, periorbital fat and inferior rectus muscle.

- *CT scan* demonstrates the soft tissue involvement in more details.
- *Forced duction test (FDT)* is positive if the muscle is entrapped.

Treatment

- Small cracks or minor fracture without herniation of the orbital content does not require any treatment.
- A blow-out fracture needs to be repaired only if:
  - There is permanent diplopia with restriction of ocular movement, and
  - There is significant enophthalmos.
- Larger fracture with herniation, should be repaired *within 2 weeks*, to prevent secondary contracture of the muscles.
- The fracture opening is bridged with bone graft or silicone rubber sheet.

Blow-in fracture of the orbital floor is just opposite and may be rarely caused by a sudden rise in pressure in the maxillary antrum as a result of trauma to the face with subsequent elevation of bone fragments into the orbit.

PENETRATING (PERFORATING) INJURY

They are caused by sharp objects or foreign bodies. Perforating injuries are potentially serious, and the patient should be urgently admitted and treated promptly.

Penetrating injuries by definition penetrate into the eye but not through and through; there is no exit wound. *Perforating injuries* have both entry and exit wounds (a through and through injury).

The seriousness arises from—the immediate effects of trauma, the introduction of infection, sympathetic ophthalmitis.

The Immediate Effects of Trauma

Two important signs of perforation are— wound of entry and a low intraocular tension.

- *Wounds of the lid and conjunctiva:* They are common and should be stitched meticulously in three layers.
  A lid-notching is common following repair of the lids.
- *Wounds of the cornea:* These may be linear or lacerated. The margins soon swell-up after the injury, and become cloudy, due to imbibition of fluid. Adhesion of the iris or its prolapse is almost certain (Figs 24.20A and B).
  Treatment
  - Antibiotics and atropine eye drop are applied immediately, and then a pad and bandage.
  - *The prolapsed iris must be abscised (Fig. 24.21).*
  - The wound is repaired with 10-0 nylon under operative microscope (preferably, under general anesthesia).
- *Wounds of the sclera:* It is recognized by the uveal prolapse. In deep injury, vitreous may come out through the wound.
- *Wounds of the lens*
  - If the wound is very small (e.g. with a needle), there is localized lens opacity,

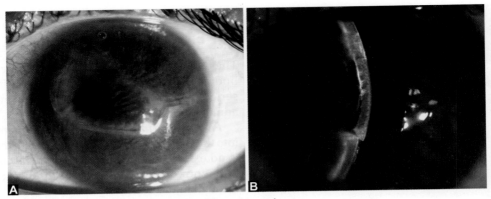

Figs 24.20A and B: Large corneal rupture without iris prolapse

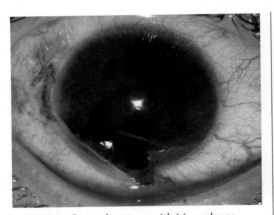

Fig. 24.21: Corneal rupture with iris prolapse

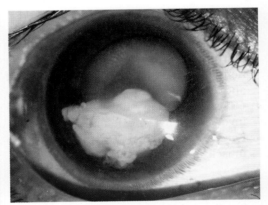

Fig. 24.22: Penetrating injury with lens capsular tear and lens matter in anterior chamber

or after sometimes, there may be formation of rosette-shaped cataract.

- In case of large capsular wound— the flocculent white cortical matters protrude through the capsular opening, and sometimes, the whole anterior chamber is full of white flocculi (Fig. 24.22).

- *Treatment*
  - *For mild injury* of the lens, cataract is better managed as a secondary procedure.
  - *For severe injury*—the aim of the surgery is to remove the cataract with or without posterior chamber intraocular lens implantation, to

perform an anterior vitrectomy if necessary, and repair of the wound of entry at the earliest.

Signs of globe perforation

Any one or combination of the following suggests possible perforation of the globe.
- Decreased visual acuity
- Hypotony (marked decrease in IOP)
- Shallow or flat anterior chamber
- Alteration of pupillary size, shape and location
- Focal iris tear or hole
- Injury tract in the cornea, lens or vitreous
- Marked conjunctival chemosis
- Wound leak (a positive Seidel's test) (Figs 24.23A and B).

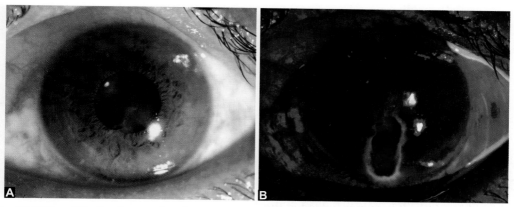

Figs 24.23A and B: Small corneal perforation and Seidel's test positive

Introduction of Infection

The organisms are introduced into the eye, by a dirty sharp object. The pyogenic organisms may lead to:

- Purulent keratitis
- Purulent iridocyclitis with hypopyon
- Endophthalmitis (Fig. 24.24) and panophthalmitis.

Sympathetic Ophthalmitis

One of the most dreadful complications of penetrating injury has already discussed (*see* Chapter 14).

▌FOREIGN BODIES

- *Extraocular foreign bodies (EOFB)*—corneal or conjunctival.
- *Intraocular foreign bodies (IOFB)*—with a perforating injury of the eyeball.

Extraocular Foreign Bodies

Small foreign body, e.g. coal, dust, sand, iron particles, eyelash, wood-piece, husks of seeds, wings of insect, etc. may pitch upon the conjunctiva or the cornea.

A history of injury, and the probable character of the foreign body help in its detection and removal.

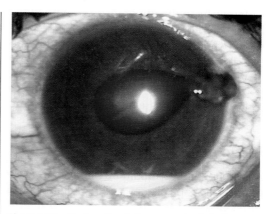

Fig. 24.24: Perforating injury—endophthalmitis

The symptoms vary from mild or no discomfort to severe pain, and watering. There may be associated photophobia and redness.

Corneal

- Patient cannot localize a foreign body on the cornea, as there is no kinesthetic sensation in the cornea. Instead, it is very often referred to the tarsal conjunctiva of the upper lid against which the foreign body rubs.
- The particle is usually embedded in the epithelium or in the anterior stroma.
- Foreign body is best localized by careful inspection of the cornea, aided by magnification with a loupe or slit-lamp.
- A fluorescein stain is also very helpful.

- Ciliary congestion may be present.
- When the removal is delayed, there may be surrounding infiltration, or even frank ulceration of the cornea.
- In all cases of corneal foreign bodies, *two clinical procedures* are important:
  1. *Eversion of the upper lid* to check the subtarsal sulcus.
  2. *Pressure over the sac area* to exclude the presence of chronic dacryocystitis.

Conjunctival

- Most frequently, it becomes lodged at the middle of the *upper subtarsal sulcus*.
- It may be in the upper fornix or embedded in the bulbar conjunctiva.
- Upper eyelid must be everted (sometimes double eversion is necessary), otherwise the foreign body may be overlooked.
- The foreign body in the subtarsal sulcus (Fig. 24.25) rubs against the cornea and causes linear (vertical) corneal abrasions.

Removal of Extraocular

All foreign bodies should be removed as early as possible. Topical anesthesia (4% lignocaine) must be used to prevent pain and eyelid closure during removal.

- *Corneal: Steps of removal*
  - First, an attempt should be made to remove the foreign body by means of

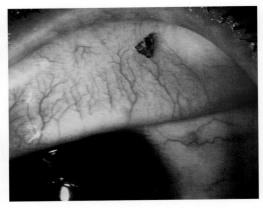

Fig. 24.25: Foreign body (subtarsal sulcus)

irrigation with sterile saline solution by a syringe.
- If it is not possible to remove by irrigation, it can be removed by a sterile cotton-tipped swab, or by a triangular piece of sterile blotting paper.
- If not possible, the foreign body is lifted gently out of the corneal substance by means of a sterile (disposable) hypodermic 23 or 24 G needle. *Do not scratch the cornea, and do not cross the pupillary zone of the cornea*.
  It is always wise to use some magnification during removal of corneal foreign body (Fig. 24.26A).
- If a ferrous metal is embedded for several days, a rust-ring (Fig. 24.26B)

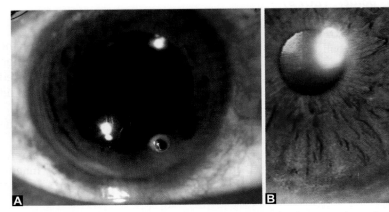

Figs 24.26A and B: A. Foreign body cornea; **B.** Foreign body cornea (rust-ring)

may remain after removal of the main portion of foreign body. That is to be removed in the same manner as the foreign body.

- If the foreign body is impacted into the deeper stroma, it is to be removed under operative microscope with a sharp needle.
- After removal, antibiotic ointment and if necessary, cycloplegic (in presence of ciliary congestion, or for large foreign body) are applied. Pad and bandage is given for 24 hours.
- Since, a foreign body may introduce microorganisms into the cornea—the eye should be examined daily until the area no longer stains with fluorescein.
- *Conjunctival*
  - Foreign bodies of the conjunctiva can easily be removed with *irrigation, a sterile cotton-swab, or with needle or a spud*.
  - The ophthalmologist must be prepared to remove the foreign body while he everts the upper lid, because the foreign body may be dislodged and difficult to locate again, if the eyelid is released.
- *Prophylactic measures:* Foreign bodies in the eye are extremely common among industrial workers. Such accidents could be almost entirely prevented by the use of protective goggles.

Intraocular Foreign Bodies

The common foreign bodies which penetrate the eyes and retain, are minute chips of iron or steel (most common), stones, glass, lead pellets, copper, spicules of wood, etc.

While chipping the stone, with an iron chisel and a hammer, it is a chip of the chisel (from cutting edge, or from its mushroomed head) which enters the eyes, but not the chip of the stone.

The entry of the foreign body into the eye may cause ocular damage in three ways:

1. By mechanical effects.
2. By introduction of infection.
3. By specific reaction, caused by the particular type of foreign body.

Mechanical Effects

The mechanical effects largely depend upon the size and velocity of the foreign body.

They are usually small and travel at a high velocity. The effects are:
- After penetrating the cornea or sclera, it may:
  - Retain in the *anterior chamber (Fig. 24.27)*.
  - *Pass into, or through the lens*, either by way of the iris or pupil, and causing a *traumatic cataract*. Thus, a hole in the iris is of great diagnostic value (Fig. 24.28).
  - Retain in the *vitreous*, causing its liquefaction.
  - Rest onto the *retina*; and if the media is clear, the foreign body may be seen ophthalmoscopically in the vitreous, or on the retina.
  - Rarely, pierce the coat of the eyeball and comes to rest within the orbital tissue *(double perforation)*.

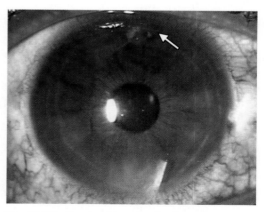

Fig. 24.27: Retained intraocular foreign bodies—angle of the anterior chamber. Arrow shows wound of entry

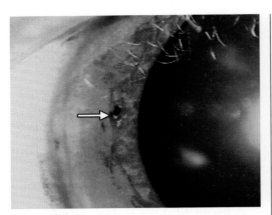

Fig. 24.28: Retained intraocular foreign bodies—iris hole (arrow)

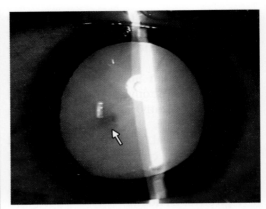

Fig. 24.29: Retained intraocular foreign bodies within the crystalline lens with cataract and siderosis (arrow)

- The lodgement of the foreign body in the posterior segment often leads to degenerative changes (apart from the changes which occur due to chemical reaction).
- The vitreous usually turns fluid, fibrous bands from along the path of foreign body, hemorrhage may be extensive, and subsequently, retinal detachment may occur.
- A particle greater than 2 mm in size usually leads to destruction of the eye.

Infection

- Small flying metallic objects are usually sterile, owing to the heat generated partly on their emission, and partly by their high velocity.
- But pieces of wood or stone, usually cause a notorious intraocular infection, leading to severe endophthalmitis or panophthalmitis.
- Despite treatment, the visual prognosis is seldom good.

Specific Reaction by a Foreign Body

It varies with the chemical nature of the foreign body, which may be **non-organized** or **organized material**.

Non-organized materials cause:

- **Minimal or no reaction**—by inert materials e.g. glass, plastics, porcelain, gold, silver, platinum or tantalum.
- **A local irritation and often with encapsulation,** e.g. lead, aluminium.
- **A suppurative reaction**, e.g. zinc, mercury, nickel or pure copper.
- **Specific degenerative changes**, e.g. iron and copper undergo chemical dissociation, and are widely deposited throughout the ocular tissues, causing **siderosis** (Fig. 24.29) and **chalcosis** respectively.

Siderosis bulbi (Figs 24.30A to C)

- It is the chronic **irreversible** degenerative changes of the ocular tissues, caused by retained intraocular iron (and also steel, in proportion of its ferrous content) foreign body.
- Epithelial structures are preferentially affected.
- **Characteristic signs**
  - **Rusty deposition on the anterior lens surface** (earliest clinical sign): Oval patches of rusty deposit are arranged radially in a ring, corresponding to the edge of the dilated pupil. This is due to deposition of iron in the anterior cubical

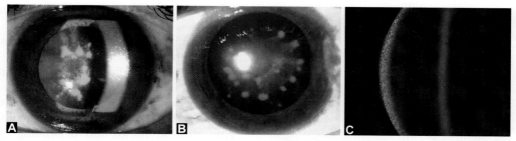

Figs 24.30A to C: Siderosis bulbi. **A.** Rusty deposits on the lens surface; **B.** Rusty deposits on anterior lens capsule with cataract; **C.** Rusty discoloration of the cornea

cells of the lens, and ***pathognomonic*** (Figs 24.30A and B).

- ***Heterochromia of the iris:*** The iris is first greenish, and later reddish-brown.
- ***Retinal pigmentary degeneration:*** It is associated with great attenuation of the blood vessels.
- ***Rusty discoloration of the cornea*** may also occur (Fig. 24.30C).
- Secondary ***open angle glaucoma*** is a common late complication.
- Ultimately, most of these eyes go blind.
- ***Electroretinography response*** of the eye is ***reduced*** even before the appearance of clinical signs.
- ***Histochemically***, the deposition of iron is revealed by the Prussian blue reaction with Pearl's microchemical stain.

Chalcosis bulbi

- It is the tissue reaction caused by intra-ocular retention of copper foreign body (in the form of an alloy). ***Unlike siderosis, it is reversible, if the particle is removed***.
- With ***pure copper***, a violent suppurative reaction ensues, which eventually results in shrinkage (phthisis) of the globe.
- ***Chalcosis, a milder reaction***, occurs when the metal is heavily alloyed, e.g. brass (as from percussion caps), or bronze.
- ***Clinical features***
  - ***Kayser-Fleischer's ring (KF ring):*** A golden-brown ring at the level of Descemet's membrane of the cornea.

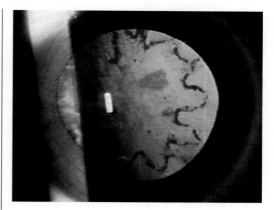

Fig. 24.31: Chalcosis bulbi—sunflower cataract

- ***Sunflower cataract:*** A brilliant golden-green sheen in the form of petals of sunflower (with good prognosis) (Fig. 24.31).
- ***Retinal changes:*** Lustrous golden plaques which reflect the light at posterior pole.
- As the degenerative changes do not appear, vision may remain good indefinitely.

Organized materials
- ***Wood and vegetable materials***—produce a proliferative reaction with giant cell formation.
- ***Eyelashes***—cause proliferation of the hair root epithelium leading to the formation of intraocular cysts (Fig. 24.32).
- ***Caterpillar hairs***—excite a severe irido-cyclitis with granulomatous nodules ***(ophthalmia nodosa).***

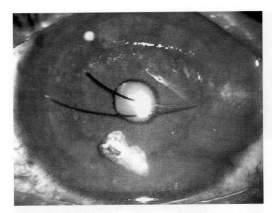

Fig. 24.32: Penetrating injury with intraocular foreign body with eyelashes

Diagnosis and Localization of Intraocular Foreign Body

- Careful history regarding the nature of injury.
- *Slit-lamp microscopy and gonioscopy.* A hole in the iris, or an opaque-track through the lens is pathognomonic.
- If the media is clear, the entire fundus is searched under full mydriasis, with the help of direct and indirect ophthalmoscope, and if necessary, with a Goldmann's three-mirror lens.
- *Plain X-rays* of the orbit (anterior posterior and lateral) for radiopaque materials.
- *Limbal-ring X-rays* of the orbit, for localization of the foreign body.
- *Ultrasonography B-scan and CT-scan* are important for radiolucent foreign bodies.
- Metal locator *(Berman or Roper-Hall)* to detect metallic foreign body, and to differentiate between magnetic from a nonmagnetic foreign body.

Removal of an Intraocular Foreign Body

- An intraocular foreign body should be removed unless:
    - It is inert and probably sterile.

- A little damage has been done to vision, and
- The process of removal will almost inevitably destroy vision.

Minute foreign bodies on the retina are typical examples to fulfil above criteria.

- In other cases, early removal is essential, because the foreign body may become enmeshed in fibrin, and depending on the site of location of the foreign body, its removal will vary.

In the anterior chamber or iris (Fig. 24.33):
- *If it is magnetic*—removal by a point magnet or by forceps.
- *If nonmagnetic*—removal by forceps.
- *Iridectomy* is necessary, if it is embedded in the iris tissue.

In the lens: Removal along with extraction of the lens with or without an IOL implantation.

In the vitreous or retina:
- *For a magnetic foreign body*—the particle is removed directly through the posterior route by an electromagnet, and it is by the shortest possible route.

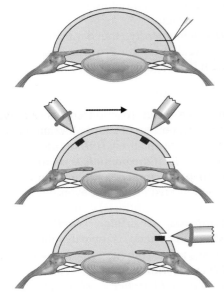

Fig. 24.33: Removal of a magnetic foreign body from the anterior chamber with hand magnet

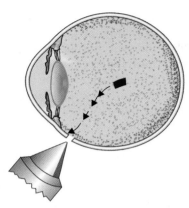

Fig. 24.34: Removal of a magnetic foreign body from the vitreous cavity via pars plana route using a giant magnet

- *For a nonmagnetic foreign body*—via pars plana route (Fig. 24.34), by vitrectomy, and with the help of special forceps and other instruments.
- Now, because of advancement in vitreoretinal surgery, any IOFB (either magnetic or nonmagnetic) is removed by forceps via pars plana route after doing good vitrectomy. Additional surgery of retina is performed in the same sitting if required.

CHEMICAL INJURIES (BURNS)

In most cases, chemical injuries (e.g. with household detergents, and cleaning agents) of the eye are relatively minor and are easily treated. But occasionally, *alkaline and acidic substances may cause severe ocular damage and permanent loss of vision*.

Alkali burns are much more dangerous than acid burns because:

- Alkalies produce a high pH (by hydroxide ion) in the tissue-water, which saponifies the fatty component of the cell membrane, leading to cell disruption.
- Alkali's cations bind to the proteins, to form gel-like soluble alkaline-protinates (unlike acids which cause instant coagulation of proteins).
- Alkali makes the collagen more susceptible to enzymatic degradation.

All these changes lead to increased penetration of alkalies deep into the tissue. Along with it, there are accelerated proteolytic effects (by collagenase enzyme) and defective collagen synthesis, make the damage more serious.

Whereas in acid burn, there is instant coagulation and precipitation of proteins, which are insoluble. These *acid-protein complexes have a buffering effect*, on the further action of the acid, and so there is no penetration of the acid in the deeper tissues. Thus, most acid burns are limited and localized. But, accelerated proteolytic enzymatic activity and defective collagen synthesis may also occur in severe acid burns.

Common alkalies responsible, are lime (chuna), liquid ammonia, caustic soda, caustic potash, etc. among which liquid ammonia is the most dangerous, and lime is the least.

Common acids are sulfuric acid (used in battery), hydrochloric acid, nitric acid, muriatic acid, acetic acid and commercial toilet cleaners; among which sulfuric acid is the most dangerous.

All alkalies and acids produce their effects not only by their chemical effects, but also by release of heat during the process of chemical reactions within the tissue.

Clinical Features

Severity of the injury depends on the type of chemical and its quantity, pH of the solution, duration of exposure, and the time of presentation following chemical burns. As already discussed, alkali burns cause more serious damage than acid burns. The effects are:

- *Acute phase (up to 1 week) (Figs 24.35 and 24.36A)*
  - Conjunctival chemosis, congestion and discharge

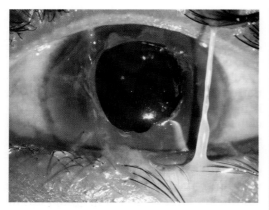

Fig. 24.35: Acid burn in acute phase

- ■ Perilimbal ischemia (Fig. 24.36B)
- ■ Corneal epithelial defects and stromal clouding
- ■ Increased intraocular pressure.
- • *Early reparative phase (1–3 weeks)*
  - ■ Conjunctival and corneal epithelia begin to regenerate
  - ■ Corneal opacity of various degree with vascularization
  - ■ Iridocyclitis.
- • *Late reparative phase (3 weeks to several months)*
  - ■ Irregular scarring of the cornea.
  - ■ Descemetocele formation or even perforation.

- ■ Dry eye, due to scarring of the ducts of lacrimal glands and goblet cells.
- ■ Posterior synechia and cyclitic membrane formation.
- ■ Cataractous changes of the lens.
- ■ Hypotony due to atrophy of the ciliary body, followed by phthisis bulbi.
- ■ Development of entropion, trichiasis and symblepharon.

Acid burns produce less severe injury than alkali burns. Deeper intraocular tissue damage usually does not occur, except in burns with *sulfuric acid* which penetrates well inside the eye and causes as much damage as alkali.

Treatment

- • *First and immediate treatment*
  - ■ *A thorough irrigation* of the ocular surface with plain water, normal saline or distilled water, whichever is available.
  - ■ *No time must be spent in searching for neutralizing substances* (e.g. 3% sodium bicarbonate solution for acids, or boric acid for alkalies), as their efficacy is doubtful.
  - ■ *Removal of particles*, carefully with the help of a sterile swab or forceps.
  - ■ Excision of necrotic conjunctival tags.

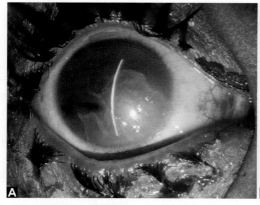
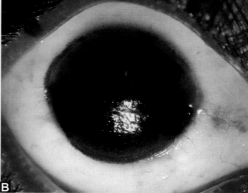

Figs 24.36A and B: A. Alkali burn in acute phase; **B.** Alkali burn with 360° limbal ischemia

- A careful assessment of the grade of chemical burn with the help of a slit-lamp.
- *Treatment in acute phase*
  - For grade I and II, the patient is treated at outpatient department (OPD), and for Grade III and IV, the patient must be admitted (Tables 24.1 and 24.2).
  - Antibiotic drops, cycloplegic, topical corticosteroids and antiglaucoma therapy are important.
  - A collagenase inhibitor (10–20% acetyl cysteine drop) is very effective.
  - Amniotic membrane transplantation (AMT) in acute phase is giving much better results, especially in alkali burn.

- *Intermediate treatment*
  - Therapeutic bandage contact lens for persistent epithelial defect (Fig. 24.37).
  - A conjunctival flap may be helpful in stromal ulceration.
  - Prevention of symblepharon formation by sweeping a glass rod twice daily.
- *Surgical rehabilitation*
  - When the eye is totally healed, the potential for useful vision in the eye, is assessed.
  - Conjunctival limbal autograft (CLAU) from the other eye if only one eye is affected with limbal stem cell deficiency. CLAU is the best type of limbal stem cell transplantation (Fig. 24.38).

TABLE 24.1: Roper-Hall (modified Hughes) Classification for ocular surface burn

Grade	Prognosis	Corneal findings	Limbal ischemia
I	Good	Corneal epithelial damage	No limbal ischemia
II	Fair	Corneal haze; Iris details visible	<1/3 limbal ischaemia
III	Guarded	Total epithelial loss, stromal haze; Iris details obscured	1/3 to 1/2 limbal ischemia
IV	Poor	Cornea opaque; Iris and pupil obscured	>1/2 limbal ischemia

It is based on the degree of corneal involvement and limbal ischemia. Dua's classification is found to be superior to the Roper-Hall in predicting outcome in severe ocular surface burns

TABLE 24.2: New classification of ocular surface burn (Dua's classification)

Grade	Prognosis	Clinical findings	Conjunctival involvement	Analog scale*
I	Very good	0 clock hour limbal ischemia	0%	0/0%
II	Good	≤3 clock hour limbal ischemia	≤30%	0.1–3/1–29.9%
III	Good	>3–6 o'clock hour limbal ischemia	>30–50%	3.1–6/31–50%
IV	Good to guarded	>6–9 o'clock hour limbal ischemia	>50–75%	6.1–9/51–75%
V	Guarded to poor	>9–<12 o'clock hour limbal ischemia	>75–<100%	9.1–11.9/75.1–99.9%
VI	Very poor	Total limbus – 12 o'clock hours limbal ischemia	Total conjunctiva (100%) involved	12/100%

*The analog scale records accurately the limbal involvement in clock hours of affected limbus/percentage of conjunctival involvement. While calculating the percentage of conjunctival involvement, only involvement of bulbar conjunctiva, up to and including conjunctival fornices is considered.

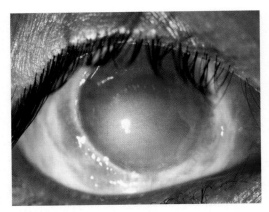

Fig. 24.37: Chemical burn in intermediate phase—persistent epithelial defect

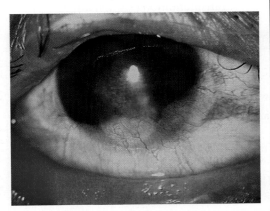

Fig. 24.38: Chemical burn—late phase corneal opacity with limbal stem cell deficiency

- Penetrating keratoplasty—success rate is not encouraging.
- Keratoprosthesis in drastic cases.
- *Cultivated limbal epithelial transplantation (CLET):* It is ex vivo expansion of limbal cells (a small limbal tissue is taken from the healthy eye) on an amniotic membrane—requires sophisticated laboratory. It is expensive and a staged procedure.
- *Simple limbal epithelial transplantation (SLET):* It is a more recent single stage procedure. Here, 2 × 2 mm or 3 × 2 mm limbal tissue is harvested from the healthy donor eye; cut into multiple pieces and finally placed on amniotic

membrane which is fixed with the diseased ocular surface by fibrin glue. It is least expensive and does not require sophisticated laboratory support.

THERMAL BURNS

- Thermal burns of the eyelids (Fig. 24.39) usually do not involve the eyeball proper, since blinking reflex provides the natural protection.
- In addition, tightly closed eyelids usually prevent involvement of eyelid margins themselves.
- Thermal burns of the eyelids require ***prompt care to prevent ectropion formation***. Early skin grafting in severe burns may speed up the recovery and prevent late complications.
- Severe body burns are often associated with carbon monoxide poisoning and asphyxia. The ocular changes then resemble those seen in ***altitudinal hypoxemia***. There are retinal hemorrhages, arterial and venous congestion, and hyperemia of the optic disc.

RADIATIONAL INJURIES

The ocular media should ideally allow maximum transmission of light, with minimum absorption and reflection.

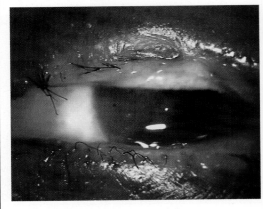

Fig. 24.39: Thermal burn—eyelids

Only energy that is absorbed, causes a reaction and injury to the ocular tissue. The effects are with:

- **Ultraviolet (UV) rays:** The cornea transmits the longer UV rays (300–400 nm), but its epithelium absorbs the UV rays with wavelengths below 300 nm. This results photokeratitis (UV keratitis) or snow blindness or photophthalmia.
- **Visible spectrum (400–700 nm):** It is perceived as lightw The lens is normally transparent to all the wavelengths of visible spectrum but becomes progressively more impervious with advancing age with nuclear sclerosis and restricts the violet end of the spectrum in old age.
- **Infrared rays (above 700 nm):** They are absorbed by the iris, and the resultant heat is transmitted to the lens, which becomes cataractous **glass-blower's cataract** (Fig. 24.40). Observation of a solar eclipse with the naked eye causes **solar retinopathy**. As the pupil is dilated due to low light intensity, the infrared (heat) rays are focused on the fovea centralis, causing a focal macular burn **(eclipse burn or eclipse blindness) (Fig. 24.41)**.
- **Electromagnetic energy of short-wave lengths** (X-rays, gamma-rays): They may damage any part of the eye, e.g. blepharo-conjunctivitis, keratitis, radiation cataract (Fig. 24.42) and retinopathy.

Adequate prophylactic measures are to be taken to prevent radiational injuries.

Different types of protective glasses are available, which can prevent lesions caused by UV and infrared rays.

Adequate and necessary protection is also to be taken during watching a solar eclipse.

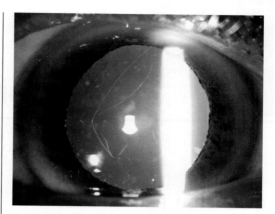

Fig. 24.40: Glass-blower's cataract—true exfoliation

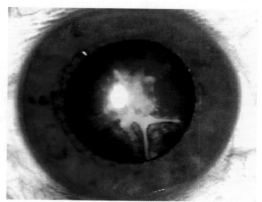

Fig. 24.41: Radiation cataract

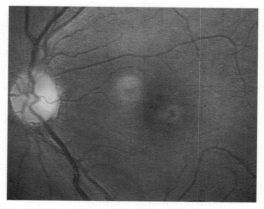

Fig. 24.42: Solar retinopathy (eclipse burn)

CHAPTER 25

Common Eye Surgeries

GENERAL PRINCIPLES

- For eye operations which are not urgent, it is essential to have the patient in a good state of health as possible.
- There must be no septic lesions (e.g. infected teeth, or otitis media).
- Culture swab is taken from the conjunctival sac, and a broad-spectrum antibiotic drop (e.g. gatifloxacin or moxifloxacin) is started 3–4 times daily for 3 days prior to surgery.
- Lacrimal passages are irrigated, and any evidence of infection is noted, the presence of which will necessitate dacryocystorhinostomy (DCR) or dacryo-cystectomy (DCT) operation before intraocular surgical procedures.
- Diabetes and hypertension must be controlled.
- Cardiovascular, respiratory and renal diseases must receive medical attention.
- Hemorrhagic tendency must be investigated routinely.
- The patient should not smoke for one week before operation and about one month after it.
- The psychological state of the patient is reviewed, and every effort is made to encourage a state of optimism.
- Fitness for general anesthesia is required for children, very nervous patients and for extensive operations.

PREOPERATIVE PREPARATION

Day of Admission (1-day Before Surgery)
- Informed written consent for operation.
- Antibiotic drops are instilled frequently.
- Mild tranquillizer at bed time.
- Tab acetazolamide; 1–2 tablet at night (for cataract or glaucoma surgery).
- Lashes of upper and lower lids are cut short (many surgeons now prefer to leave the lashes uncut, relying on the speculum and drape to isolate them from the operative field).
- Mild purgative if necessary.

Day of Operation
- Light breakfast in the morning.
- Shaving for male patients.
- The face is washed thoroughly with soap and water.
- Diabetic patient must omit the morning dose of medicine.
- Blood pressure is checked, and if necessary, antihypertensive drugs are to be administered.
- Appropriate premedication for general anesthesia.
- Mild sedative if required.
- Tablet acetazolamide—2 tablets, may be given 1–2 hours before surgery, if necessary.
- Injection mannitol (20%) 200–300 mL, is given intravenously at least 30 minutes

before surgery (for young and selective patients with high intraocular pressure (IOP).

- Start dilating the pupil (when necessary) with phenylephrine and tropicamide (or phenylephrine and homatropine) along with flurbiprofen or nepafenac eye drop 3–4 times 1 hour before surgery.
- Flurbiprofen or nepafenac eye drops prevent intraoperative miosis, and also decreases postoperative pain and inflammation.

Day Care Eye Surgery

In recent years, there has been a major switch from inpatient care to day care for ophthalmic surgeries, provided to the patients who do not require overnight hospital stay. Rate of day care cataract surgery is as high as 100% in Denmark and as low as 0% in Austria. In India, about 50% cataract surgery is performed as day care basis.

This change has been accepted by the patients and treating surgeon. This has been greatly facilitated by the advent of small incision cataract surgery (Phaco or SICS); newer microsurgical procedures in retina, glaucoma or oculoplasty.

Advantages of Day Care Surgery

- Less requirement of hospital beds
- Cost saving for the patients and caregivers
- Less nosocomial infections
- Early recovery in home environment with the family
- Insurance/Medicare prefers day care surgery.

Day care surgery demands the highest standards of professional skills and management. Patient selection is the key of success of day care surgery. Sometimes, concept of day care surgery may not be acceptable to the patient and relatives.

Disadvantages of Day Care Surgery

- For far away patients
- Physically unfit patients
- Children and mentally unstable patients
- If close monitoring is required after surgery
- In some eye surgeries, like retina or cornea surgeries, head positioning is important.

In adults above 40 years, in addition to complete blood count (CBC), electrocardiography (ECG) and serum glucose are advised. The detailed preoperative assessment by the anesthetist is similar to inpatients surgery.

After the surgery, the vital signs are monitored till the patient is discharged. The first follow-up is usually recommended for the next day.

POSTOPERATIVE CARE AND TREATMENT

- Avoid unnecessary jerky movements of the head and the body.
- Avoid sudden strain, e.g. sneezing, coughing, weight lifting, etc.
- While the patient is in bed, he should be made comfortable. It is preferable to place the patient at night, either supine or onto the unoperated side.
- As the wound security is excellent, prolonged bed rest is unnecessary, on the other hand, early mobility is encouraged for the elderly patients.
- Postoperative pain, which comes on half to one hour after the operation, must be treated with analgesics.
- A mild sedative is useful to promote sleep for some patients.
- Some disturbance of bowel rhythm is expected for a few days following major surgery. This should not cause concern unless the patient is suffering from discomfort. This can be easily tackled by mild laxatives.
- A normal, easily digestible balanced diet is reintroduced from the next day.

- A postoperative dressing is important to protect a healing wound from injury and exogenous infection to afford support and to soak up the discharge for first 24 hours.
- An eye pad is better replaced by a protective dark glasses, or a shield, after 4 to 24 hours. It may be better to use the dark glasses during night to avoid accidental trauma by finger or by a corner of a pillowcase.
- The patient is instructed to clean the ocular discharge daily in the morning with sterile cotton (in boiling water).
- Instillation of eye drop and application of ointment at bed time as directed by the treating surgeon.
- *Removal of sutures*
  - *Conjunctival sutures* are usually removed after 5 to 7 days.
  - *Corneal sutures*
    - 8-0 virgin silk, is usually removed 4–6 weeks after the surgery.
    - 10-0 nylon sutures, when continuous or interrupted with buried knots, it is not necessary to remove them. But for exposed knots, they should be removed carefully. A bent disposable 26-gauge needle is often sharp enough for this purpose *[Katzin's method (Fig. 25.1)]*.

Corneal sutures are removed either because of irritation, or as a mean of adjusting corneal astigmatism. It is to be done under magnifica-

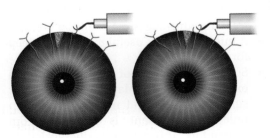

Fig. 25.1: Katzin's technique of suture removal using a bent 26-gauge disposable needle

tion with full aseptic measure in the operation theatre.

Prescription of glasses: As most of the cataract surgery are sutureless, the glasses are prescribed for 1 to 3 weeks depending upon the type of surgery.

ANESTHESIA AND AKINESIA

A good anesthesia, either local anesthesia (LA) or general anesthesia (GA), is essential for smoother surgery to save sight and indeed a bad anesthesia may be disastrous.

Local Anesthesia

Most eye surgeons still prefer to perform cataract and other operations under local anesthesia.

Advantages

- It is easy to administer, and there is no need of trained anesthetist (though an anesthetist is required in the operation theatre as a protocol to handle any systemic emergency).
- Patient can cooperate during surgery.
- It does not require any special and costly investigations.
- There is no major complication of GA, e.g. cardiorespiratory problems, coughing, vomiting, etc. Immediate postoperative recovery is uneventful.
- It is less expensive.

Disadvantages

- It is difficult and sometimes, hazardous for the nervous and noncooperative patients.
- Head movements and straining may cause serious complications.
- Cardiac shock may also occur in susceptible individual.
- Rarely, there may be globe perforation, which is sight-threatening.

General Anesthesia

The chief advantage of GA is that, control is where it should be, entirely with the surgeon and the anesthetist.

Indications of General Anesthesia in Ophthalmic Practice

In children
- Examination under anesthesia (EUA)
- Surgeries like:
  - Probing of nasolacrimal duct (NLD)
  - Cataract operations
  - Glaucoma operations
  - Enucleation as in retinoblastoma
  - Injury repair
  - Squint and DCR operation.

In adults
- Repair of perforating injury
- Mentally retarded and noncooperative patients
- The patient is too nervous and apprehensive
- Enucleation, evisceration or exenteration operations
- Major cornea and oculoplastic surgeries
- Major posterior segment surgeries
- Surgeon's preference for GA.

Types of Local Anesthesia

- **Surface (topical) anesthesia:** This is either by instillation of 4% lignocaine, 0.5–1% amethocaine or 0.5% proparacaine thrice at an interval of 5 min. It is most commonly required for the removal of corneal foreign body, syringing, tonometry or gonioscopy. Many cataract surgeons prefer to perform phacoemulsification or other minor surface procedures under topical anesthesia.
- **Infiltration (regional) anesthesia:** There is no need to say more than a few words of encouragement and assurance, and to give a preliminary warning about the prick of the needle which injects the anesthetic solution.

The agents commonly used are:
Anesthetic agents
- **Injection lignocaine (2%)**
  - **Onset of action:** 5–10 min
  - **Duration of action:** 45 minutes to 2 hours.
- **Injection bupivacaine (0.50–0.75%)**
  - Onset of action: 15–20 minutes
  - Duration of action: 5–8 hours.

Adjuvants
- **Injection adrenaline (1 in 100,000):** It decreases the systemic absorption of the anesthetic agent by local vasoconstriction. It also reduces the chance of bleeding and prolongs the duration of action. It is contraindicated in hypertension and heart diseases.
- **Injection hyaluronidase:** It enhances the diffusion of anesthetic agents through the tissues. It is used 75–150 units/10 mL of anesthetic solution.

  Infiltration anesthesia is best achieved by a *mixture* containing 50% of injection lignocaine with adrenaline (for rapid onset) + 50% of injection bupivacaine (for longer duration of action) + injection hyaluronidase.

Types of Infiltration Anesthesia

Facial Block (Fig. 25.2)

It is to block the facial nerve or its zygomatic branch to paralyze the orbicularis oculi muscle. The aim is to prevent closure and squeezing of the eyelids during operation.
- O'Brien's technique: About 4–5 mL of anesthetic solution is infiltrated at the neck of the mandible just in front of the tragus.
- Van-Lint's method: The needle is introduced about 1 cm below and behind the lateral canthus. About 4 mL of solution is infiltrated along the superolateral and inferolateral orbital margins in a V-shaped manner.

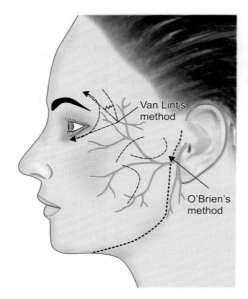

Fig. 25.2: Facial block

Retrobulbar (Ciliary) Block (Fig. 25.3)

The patient is asked to look up and opposite side. A long needle (35 mm) is introduced at the junction of middle third and lateral third along the inferior orbital margin, and then directed backwards and medially, towards the apex of the orbit. 1–2 mL of anesthetic solution is injected. Onset of action is indicated by mydriasis.

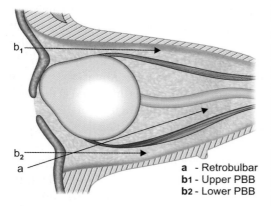

a - Retrobulbar
b1 - Upper PBB
b2 - Lower PBB

Fig. 25.3: Retrobulbar and peribulbar block (PBB)

The aim is to block the ciliary ganglion, and to paralyze the extraocular muscles.

Effects

- Anesthesia of the deeper intraocular structures (e.g. iris)
- Akinesia of all extraocular muscles (except superior oblique)
- Mydriasis
- Hypotony is due to loss of tone of extraocular muscle and bulbar massage
- Proptosis, which is desirable in deep-seated and sunken eyes
- Decreased oculocardiac reflex.

Complications

- Retrobulbar hemorrhage (RBH): Immediate proptosis, subconjunctival hemorrhage and ecchymosis, operation is to be postponed for 2–3 weeks. *Treatment* is by tight pressure bandage (lateral canthotomy if required), tab acetazolamide and reassurance.
- Perforation of the globe (especially in myopic eyes).
- Central retinal artery occlusion.
- Injection of anesthetic solution into the subarachnoid space may cause brainstem anesthesia leading to convulsion and respiratory arrest.
- Optic nerve damage and atrophy.

Peribulbar Block

Most surgeons have abandoned the retrobulbar block in favor of peribulbar injections (Figs 25.4 and 25.5) at inferior and superior parts of peripheral space of the orbit, with a 23- or 24-gauge needle.

The *inferior injection* is given at the junction of middle and outer-third of the lower orbital margin. With the patient looking up, the needle is directed towards the floor of the orbit.

An additional *superior injection* may be given superonasally beneath the superior orbital notch, with the needle directed towards the orbit roof.

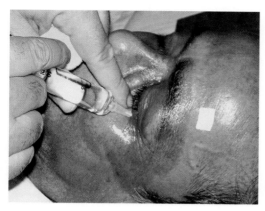

Fig. 25.4: Peribulbar injection—lower

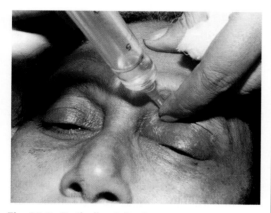

Fig. 25.5: Peribulbar injection—upper

- An intermittent pressure is given against the closed eyelids for 10 min with the help of fingers, ***super pinky*** or Honan's balloon. This is to achieve lowering of IOP, and reduction in orbital volume of the fluid injected.
- It has all the effects of facial, retrobulbar and surface anesthesia.

Advantages

- Least chance of RBH, globe perforation or optic nerve damage.
- Less painful procedure.
- No need of additional facial block and surface anesthesia.

Disadvantages

- In takes little longer time to achieve anesthesia, akinesia and hypotony.
- Chemosis of lid and conjunctiva, and subconjunctival hemorrhage are common. Injection hyaluronidase is essential for spreading the anesthetic solution.
- Rarely, additional facial or retrobulbar block is necessary.

Sub-Tenon Block (Anesthesia)

The use of sharp needles for the peribulbar or retrobulbar block may cause possible serious and even life-threatening complications—like, globe perforation, retrobulbar hemorrhage, optic nerve damage and subarachnoid diffusion. Sub-Tenon block is a relative new and safest technique that can avoid all these serious complications.

The sub-Tenon's space is a virtual space between the Tenon's capsule and the sclera. The injection of local anesthetic agents into this space produces analgesia and akinesia by diffusing posteriorly into the retrobulbar space to block the traversing sensory and motor nerves.

Technique: First the conjunctiva is anesthetized with topical agent. An eyelid speculum is inserted to improve access and prevent blinking. Then, it is cleaned by few drops of povidone iodine. Ask the patient to look up and out to expose the inferonasal quadrant. A small tent of conjunctiva with Tenon's capsule is raised with a forceps approximately 6–8 mm from the inferonasal to limbus then a small incision is made using a tenotomy scissors, exposing the sclera below. The special sub-Tenon's cannula is then inserted, with the syringe filled with anesthetic agent, and passed posteriorly, following the curvature of the globe, until its tip is perceived to crossed the equator. 3–5 ml anesthetic solution is then injected slowly.

On injection of the local anesthetic, little resistance is usually encountered and most of the solution should disappear behind the eyeball resulting in slight proptosis. The onset of analgesia is usually rapid, whereas maximal akinesia develops by 5-6 minutes.

This technique is very safe. The main complications are chemosis and subconjunctival hemorrhage, both of which will usually resolve with gentle pressure.

Regional Blocks (at Other Sites)

The sites are different, for different extraocular operations, e.g. for DCT or DCR operation, for lid tumors, for ptosis, chalazion, etc.

Preparatory steps just before operation:

- Periocular skin is cleaned painted with rectified spirit and povidone iodine (10%) solution.
- Conjunctival sac is washed with sterile normal saline or weak (5%) povidone iodine solution.
- Two or three drops of antibiotics are to be instilled.
- Sterile towels are draped around the head, neck and chest. The face is covered with a mask or 'Steri Drape' in which an aperture has been made to get access to the eye.

CONVENTIONAL ECCE WITH PCIOL IMPLANTATION

Surgical steps: Pupil should be widely dilated preoperatively and an operative microscope (Fig. 25.6) is essential.

- *Separation of the eyelids:* Either by lid stitches or wire eye speculum.
- *Superior rectus stitch (Bridle suture):* It helps to keep the globe rotated downwards and to retract a fornix-based conjunctival flap. It also aids in lifting a deep-seated globe from the orbit.
- *Conjunctival flap preparation (Figs 25.7A and B):* There are two types of conjunctival flap: fornix-based and limbal-based. The former provides better visualization of the upper limbus and is

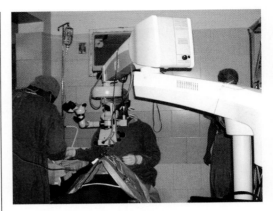

Fig. 25.6: Operative microscope

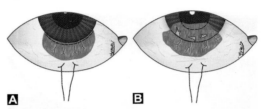

Figs 25.7A and B: Conjunctival flaps; **A.** Fornix-based flap; **B.** Limbal-based flap

preferred by most surgeons. Here, the conjunctiva is dissected at the upper limbus and retracted towards the fornix. Whereas, in limbal-based flap, the conjunctiva is incised 4–5 mm away from the limbus and reflected over the cornea.

- *Hemostasis of bleeding points:* It is most satisfactorily done with a wet-field coagulator. Alternately, it may be done with a thermocautery, which causes more tissue charring.
- *Limbal-grooved incision:* A partial thickness limbal-groove is made along the entire length of the intended section, with a knife (no. 11 or no. 15 blade), or with a razor blade-fragment in a blade-breaker.
- *Anterior chamber (Fig. 25.8) is entered* with a bent-tipped 26-gauge needle (capsulotome), fitted with balanced salt solution (BSS) or Ringer's lactate filled 2 mL syringe. (Alternately, anterior chamber may be entered with the tip of the

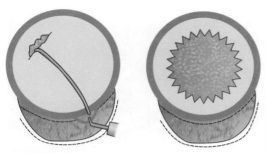

Fig. 25.8: Anterior capsulotomy with a bent tipped 26-gauge disposable needle

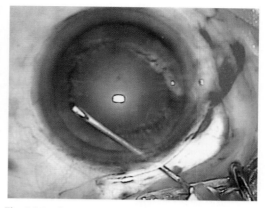

Fig. 25.9: Can-opener capsulotomy with 26 G needle cystotome

knife, and then anterior chamber is filled with viscoelastic solution).

- *A can-opener anterior capsulotomy (Fig. 25.9)* is performed with the tip of the 26-gauge needle. Alternately, a *continuous curvilinear capsulorhexis* (CCC) is preferable for smooth edge of the anterior capsular opening which increases the strength of the capsular bag. Or, an envelope technique may be done.
- *Limbal section is enlarged* with corneal scissors for 10–12 mm (110°–120°), at the upper limbus.
- Anterior capsule is removed.
- *Lens nucleus is delivered (Figs 25.10A and B)* by scleral depression with the help of a lens hook and lens spatula, or vectis.
- *Simultaneous irrigation and aspiration* (I/A) with a two-way cannula (Fig. 25.11),

to clear all the cortical matter of the lens. The cannula is fitted with an infusion system of Ringer's lactate, or BSS. The posterior capsule may be polished with special polisher to remove/small residual cortical plaque.

- Viscoelastic substance is injected into the capsular bag and anterior chamber, to facilitate subsequent insertion of intraocular lens (IOL).
- *Intraocular lens insertion:* A posterior chamber IOL is grasped by the optic with MacPherson forceps. The anterior surface of the lens is coated with viscoelastic material. The implant is introduced into the

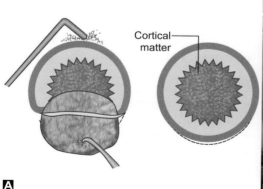

Cortical matter

A

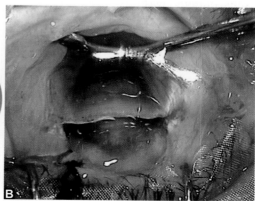

B

Figs 25.10A and B: A. Delivery of the lens nucleus; **B.** Nucleus delivery by sliding technique

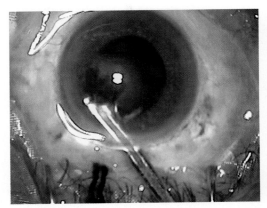

Fig. 25.11: Cortical cleaning by Simcoe irrigation and aspiration cannula

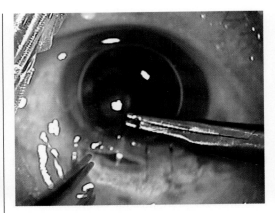

Fig. 25.12: Corneoscleral suturing by 10–0 nylon.

eye without retracting or lifting the cornea. The leading loop is placed in the inferior portion of the capsular bag or ciliary sulcus. The trailing loop is flexed towards the optic, and with slight pronation of the wrist, the loop is engaged slightly posterior to the capsular bag or in the ciliary sulcus.

- *The implant is then dialed* into horizontal position by engaging into the dialing holes with an IOL–dialer and checked for correct centration of the IOL.
- *Removal of viscoelastic substance* by irrigation and aspiration.
- *Constriction of the pupil* with injection pilocarpine (0.125%) into the anterior chamber may be required and subsequently wash is given to remove pilocarpine.
- *A peripheral iridectomy* is not mandatory in routine cases of extracapsular cataract extraction (ECCE). It is required in complicated cataract (e.g. uveitic cataract), when combined with trabeculectomy, if posterior capsular rent occurs during surgery or in case of anterior chamber intraocular pressure (ACIOL) if required.
- *Closure of the wound* with four to five interrupted 10-0 nylon sutures (Fig. 25.12) with buried knots.
- *Reformation of the anterior chamber* with BSS or Ringer's lactate solution.

- Subconjunctival injection of gentamicin and dexamethasone may be given.
- Topical antibiotic and steroid ointment.
- Pad and bandage.

MANUAL SMALL INCISION CATARACT SURGERY

Small incision cataract surgery (SICS) (Figs 25.13A to L) is now the method of choice of cataract surgery all over the world. Manual or non-phaco techniques are becoming popular in the developing countries. Phacoemulsification (phaco) technique is the excellent procedure of doing SICS. But, it has got its own limitations like, lack of training facilities, cost and maintenance of the machine, and the serious complications by the beginners. Manual SICS provides the best of both worlds—the simplicity of ECCE and the excellent results of phacoemulsification procedure.

Aims

- Early ambulation and rehabilitation of the patient
- Least complication
- To achieve low astigmatism.

Principles

- Self-sealing sclerocorneal tunnel incision
- Working under high IOP in close chamber

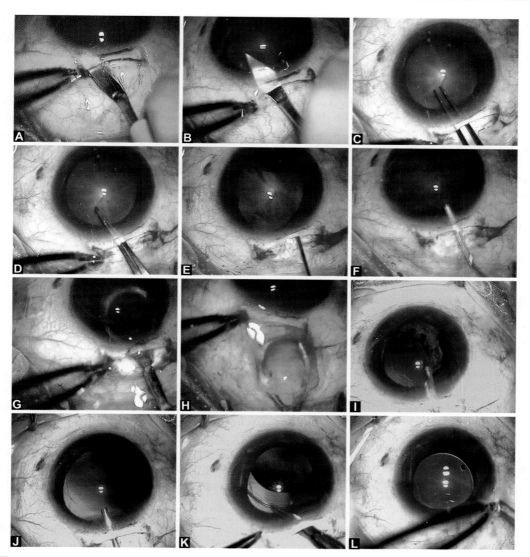

Figs 25.13A to L: Manual small incision cataract surgery (SICS). **A.** External scleral incision with tunneling; **B.** Corneal internal incision; **C.** Initiation of capsulorhexis; **D.** Completion of capsulorhexis; **E.** Hydrodissection—note the fluid wave; **F.** Nulear rotation and its prolapse into the anterior chamber; **G.** Irrigating vectis behind the nucleus; **H.** Nucleus delivery by the same vectis; **I.** Cortical cleaning with Simcoe irrigation and aspiration cannula; **J.** Viscoelastic in the anterior chamber and capsular bag; **K.** Posterior chamber intraocular lens implantation in-the-bag; **L.** Wound closure after completion of surgery

- Working in deep anterior chamber
- Protection of corneal endothelial layer with good viscoelastics HPMC (hydroxypropyl methylcellulose) or sodium hyaluronate throughout the procedure.

Technical Steps

- 5.5–6.5 mm sclerocorneal tunnel incision.
- Routine capsulorhexis or may be can-opener capsulotomy.

- Hydrodissection of the lens nucleus from its capsule.
- Nuclear prolapse into anterior chamber.
- Nucleus delivery by irrigating Vectis or phacosandwich or fish hook technique.
- Cortical cleaning by Simcoe I/A cannula.
- Viscoelastic agent to fill the bag and anterior chamber.
- Intraocular lens placement in-the-bag or may be in ciliary sulcus.
- Anterior chamber wash and reformation.
- Closure of the conjunctiva.

Some surgeons use anterior chamber maintainer (ACM) during manual SICS.

Irrigating Vectis and phacosandwich techniques are the most popular methods for nucleus delivery in manual SICS.

Advantages

- Low cost, no expensive instruments
- Learning curve smooth and easy
- Same results as phacoemulsification
- Within reach of every cataract surgeon
- Can be performed in any type of cataract (hard, black or hypermature)
- Lesser complications than phacoemulsification by the beginners.

PHACOEMULSIFICATION (FIGS 25.14 AND 25.15)

Phacoemulsification is now the standard form of extracapsular cataract extraction. The machine is known as phacoemulsifier which has three functions:

1. *Irrigation:* It is a gravity flow system, and the fluid BSS is allowed to flow to the phaco handpiece (Figs 25.16A and B) being used, through foot switching.
2. *Aspiration:* It occurs through a peristaltic or venturi pump, and the aspiration force is also controlled by surgeon's foot, by foot switching.
3. *Fragmentation and Emulsification:* It occurs through a piezoelectric ultrasonic

mechanism which activate a hollow 0.9 mm titanium needle, vibrating at 40,000/ sec. The amplitude of vibration is also controlled by same foot switch.

Steps of Surgical Procedure (in brief)

- Selection of the patient (difficulty in eyes with supra hard nucleus) with dilated pupil.
- Most of the surgeons prefer under topical anesthesia.
- A 2.2 mm to 2.8 mm clear corneal incision on temporal side. This is for foldable IOL. It is preferable to create two-step or three-step incision (for phaco with rigid lens a 5.5 mm posterior-limbal tunnel or sclerocorneal tunnel is required; internal incision in that case will be 2.8 mm for entry of phacotip).
- Viscoelastic agent is injected into the anterior chamber.
- Continuous curvilinear capsulorhexis is performed using a bent-tipped 26-gauge needle or rhexis (utarata) forceps.
- Hydrodissection and hydrodelamination to separate lens nucleus and cortex from the capsular bag.
- Sculpting the lens nucleus from the anterior surface.
- A phaco chopper is passed into the anterior chamber through a separate stab incision.
- The chopper keeps the nucleus away from the corneal endothelium, simultaneously fragments the nucleus and feeds smaller pieces of nucleus into the ultrasonic tip, until the whole nucleus is fragmented and aspirated. The different techniques used are; chip and flip technique for soft nucleus, four quadrant divide and conquer technique, stop and chop technique or direct chop technique for nucleus fragmentation and emulsification.
- Epinucleus removal by phaco hand piece.
- Lens cortex is aspirated completely from the peripheral part, using bimanual irrigation and aspiration probes.
- Polishing of the posterior capsule, if necessary.

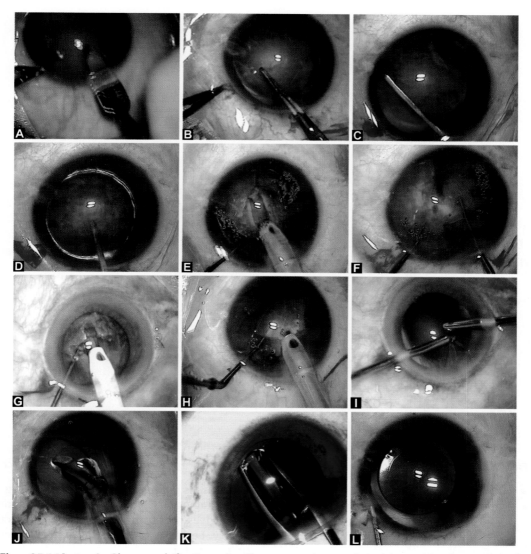

Figs 25.14A to L: Phacoemulsification. **A.** Clear corneal tunnel incision with diamond knife; **B.** Continuous curvilinear capsulorhexis with rhexis forceps; **C.** Hydrodissection—note the fluid wave; **D.** Hydrodelamination—appearance of "golden ring"; **E.** Deep sculpting in stop and chop method; **F.** Bimanual nuclear division (halving); **G.** Deep sculpting in divide and conquer technique; **H.** Nucleus piece emulsification and removal; **I.** Cortical cleaning by automated I/A probes; **J.** Foldable intraocular lens in-the-bag by an injector; **K.** Foldable intraocular lens in-the-bag by folder-holder; **L.** Intraocular lens in-the-bag and hydration of the wound

- Viscoelastic is injected to inflate the capsular bag.
- A foldable IOL is implanted within capsular bag using IOL injector system [incision is enlarged to 5.5 mm for insertion of a rigid polymethyl methacrylate (PMMA) PCIOL in-the-bag].
- Viscoelastic material is washed thoroughly.

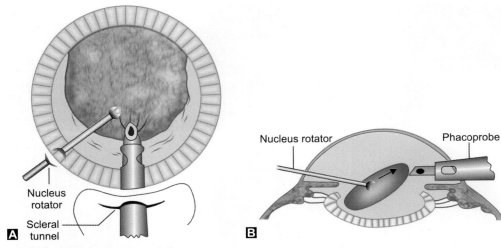

Figs 25.15A and B: Phacoemulsification

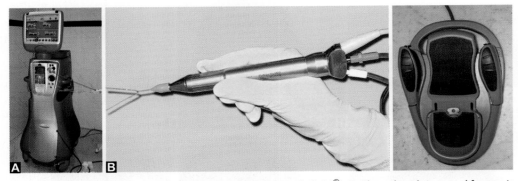

Figs 25.16A and B: **A.** Phacoemulsification machine (Alcon–Infiniti®); **B.** Phaco handpiece and foot switch

- Hydration of the side port(s).
- No suture (sutureless surgery) is required for foldable IOL with 2.2 to 3.0 mm incision (one suture may be required if the incision is 5.5 mm).
- Repose the conjunctival flap if required.
- Subconjunctival injection of gentamicin and dexamethasone may be given.
- No pad and bandage if under topical anesthesia.

FEMTOSECOND LASER CATARACT SURGERY

It is the latest development in cataract surgery. A femtosecond-assisted cataract procedure is guided by in built anterior segment imaging (OCT or Scheimpflug) system which gives maximum precision in cataract surgery. Femtosecond laser used in cataract surgery are for:

- A perfect centered anterior capsulorhexis.
- Phacofragmentation (by microphotolysis of the lens nucleus in multiple small fragments).
- The creation of single and multiplane incisions in the cornea.
- Astigmatic relaxing incisions when required.

Nevertheless, the need for ultrasound phaco is still there, further to emulsify the nuclear fragments and to aspirate them.

Although the cost of the procedure is at present much higher compared to phacoemulsification, femtosecond laser cataract surgery is likely to become the gold standard in the near future.

INTRACAPSULAR CATARACT EXTRACTION (FIGS 25.17A AND B)

Very rarely done nowadays as in anterior dislocation of the lens, grossly subluxated lens (*ectopia lemtis*) or along with keratoprosthesis procedure, etc.

Surgical Steps

1–5. Same as conventional ECCE.
6. Anterior chamber is entered with the tip of the blade, with slow release of the aqueous.

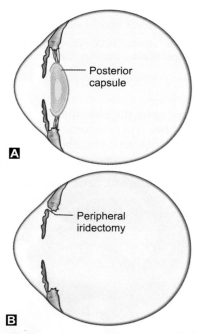

A

Posterior capsule

B

Peripheral iridectomy

Figs 25.17A and B: Postoperative appearance. **A.** After extracapsular cataract extraction; **B.** After intracapsular cataract extraction

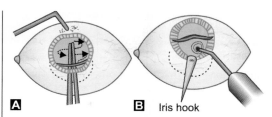

A   **B**   Iris hook

Figs 25.18A and B: Methods of intracapsular cataract extraction. **A.** By intracapsular forceps; **B.** By cryoprobe

7. Limbal section is enlarged with corneal scissors about 150–180° (i.e. from 3 o'clock to 9 o'clock position).
8. A peripheral iridectomy is done at 11 o'clock to 10 o'clock position. This is a must for intracapsular cataract extraction (ICCE).
9. Lens (with its capsule) is extracted by either a cryoprobe (Figs 25.18A and B), or by intracapsular forceps, or, by tumbling method.
10. Iris is reposited back.
11. Limbal section is closed with 10–0 nylon by five interrupted stitches.
12. Anterior chamber is reformed by air or BSS.
13. Subconjunctival injection of gentamicin and dexamethasone.
14. Pad and bandage are given after applying antibiotic ointment or the incision may be like SICS and the lens delivery via wire Vectis.

A very good anterior vitrectomy (triamcinolone assisted) is required in ICCE before implantation an IOL either ACIOL or scleral fixation IOL.

INTRAOCULAR LENS IMPLANTATION

Nowadays, IOL implantation has become the standard surgical procedure in the management of cataract. The main aim is to replace the function of the natural crystalline lens, and to restore the vision approximating to pre-cataractous stage.

Differences between intracapsular cataract extraction (ICCE) and extracapsular cataract extraction (ECCE)		
Features	**ICCE**	**ECCE**
Indications	• In camps or other places, where the facilities for ECCE are not available. • Subluxated or dislocated lens.	• All types of cataract except mentioned in ICCE.
Technique	• Relatively easy	• Relatively difficult
Intraoperative complications	• Vitreous loss is more common. • Hyphema is more frequent. • Accidental capsule rupture causes problem for cortical cleaning.	• Vitreous loss is very rare. • Hyphema is less frequent. • No such problem.
Postoperative complications	• Iridocyclitis is less common. • No question of after-cataract formation PCO, and so no need for second operation. • Incidence of retinal detachment is more. • Incidence of CME is more. • Chance of pupillary block glaucoma is more.	• Iridocyclitis is more common. • Chances of after-cataract formation, and consequent need for second operation, like needling or yttrium aluminium garnet (YAG) laser capsulotomy. • Incidence of retinal detachment is less. • Incidence of CME is less. • Chance of pupillary block glaucoma is much less.
Provision for IOL	• ACIOL may be implanted, which is not popular due to its complications.	• PCIOL is usually implanted, which is an ideal IOL.
Cost	• Less costly due to less costly instrumentation.	• More costlier due to more investment for operative microscope and instruments.

(*Abbreviations:* **ACIOL**—Anterior chamber IOL; **CME**—Cystoid macular edema; **ECCE**—Extracapsular cataract extraction; **ICCE**—Intracapsular cataract extraction; **IOL**—Intraocular lens; **PCIOL**—Posterior chamber IOL; **PCO**—Posterior capsular opacification)

Intraocular lens implantation is usually performed along with extraction of cataract at the same sitting (as a primary procedure), and it is called ***primary implantation*** (Fig. 25.19). But, an implantation can also be done in selected cases any time after primary cataract surgery, it is then called ***secondary implantation***.

Intraocular lens implantation was first performed by Dr Harold Ridley, on 29th November 1949 at St. Thomas Hospital, London. It was a posterior chamber IOL.

Indications

Any type of cataract for primary implantation, except in congenital cataract, before 2 years of age. A secondary IOL implantation may be considered after 3 years of age.

Types

Depending upon the placement of the optic, they are of two types—anterior chamber IOL (ACIOL) and posterior chamber IOL (PCIOL).

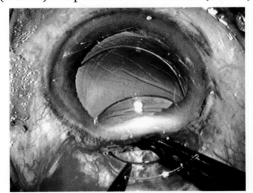

Fig. 25.19: Intraocular lens implantation in the posterior chamber

1. ***Anterior chamber IOL (ACIOL) (Figs 25.20A to C):*** They are placed in the anterior chamber, usually following ICCE. Here, the optic of the lens lies in front of the pupil, and the haptics are either placed at the chamber-angle (angle-supported, e.g. Kelman Multiflex lens) or are fixed with the iris (iris-supported, e.g. Worst-Singh's iris claw lens).

ACIOL implantation is practically discarded now, by all surgeons as a primary procedure owing to its own complications, like:

- Corneal decompensation leading to pseudophakic bullous keratopathy.
- Uveitis glaucoma hyphema (UGH) syndrome (a triad of uveitis, glaucoma and hyphema).
- Iris tuck and pupillary capture, which may cause chronic irritable eye.
- Iris fixation lens has more complications.

It is now popularly used for secondary implantation with encouraging results, the other eye is being treated primarily with ECCE with PCIOL (Phaco or SICS).

2. ***Posterior chamber IOL (PCIOL):*** They are placed in the posterior chamber following ECCE.

The implants are intended for placement either in the ***capsular bag*** or on the ***ciliary sulcus*** (a potential space between the posterior iris-root and ciliary processes). It is more physiological to place the IOL in-the-bag.

A scleral fixation or iris retrofixation PCIOL may be more useful after ICCE or after complicated ECCE where the posterior capsular support is absent.

Types of PCIOLs

- ***Single-piece*** (both optic and haptics are in one-piece) or multipiece or three-piece (optic and two pieces of haptic) (Fig. 25.21).
- ***Uniplaner*** (no angulation between the optic and haptics) or angular (angulation between the haptics and the plane of optic approximately 50–100).
- With or without dialing holes.
- J-looped, C-looped, modified J-looped, cap-C haptic, plate haptic, etc.
- Rigid (conventional), disc IOL (without haptics) or foldable IOL (made of soft materials).

Though technically difficult, PCIOL implantation gives the best visual results with relatively a fewer complications, like.

- Decentration of the lens.
- Sunset syndrome, windshield wiper syndrome
- Posterior dislocation of the IOL.
- Corneal decompensation or edema, or pseudophakic bullous keratopathy (relatively less).
- Posterior capsular opacification (PCO) or after cataract, etc.

Parts (Fig. 25.22)

An IOL has two parts—optic and haptics.

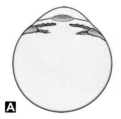 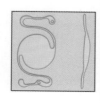 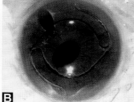 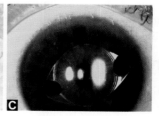

Figs 25.20A to C: Anterior chamber intraocular lens. **A and B.** Kelman multiflex—angle supported type; **C.** Worst-Singh iris-claw lens

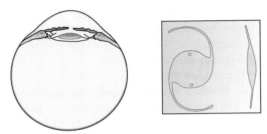

Fig. 25.21: Posterior chamber IOL (single-piece)

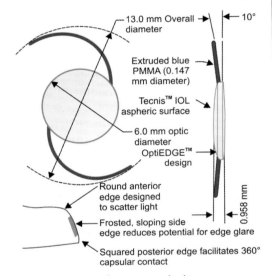

- 13.0 mm Overall diameter
- 10°
- Extruded blue PMMA (0.147 mm diameter)
- Tecnis™ IOL aspheric surface
- 6.0 mm optic diameter
- OptiEDGE™ design
- Round anterior edge designed to scatter light
- Frosted, sloping side edge reduces potential for edge glare
- 0.958 mm
- Squared posterior edge facilitates 360° capsular contact

Fig. 25.22: Parts of an intraocular lens

Optic

It is made of PMMA, silicone, or acrylic materials and it is about 5.5 to 6.5 mm in diameter. Optic may be planoconvex or biconvex. There may be 2–4 min holes at the periphery of the optic, called **dialing holes** (some optics do not have holes). Power of the optic varies from –5.0 to +40D.

Types of IOL

- **Optic materials**
  - **Rigid IOL–PMMA** material: This is time-tested over 70 years. Refractive index –1.49.

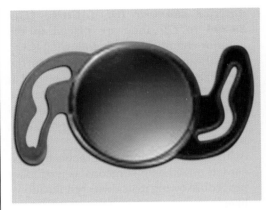

Fig. 25.23: Hydrophilic foldable intraocular lens

- **Foldable IOL**
  - Acrylic material
    i. Hydrophobic acrylic refractive index –1.55
    ii. Hydrophilic acrylic refractive index –1.46 (Fig. 25.23).
  - Silicone material refractive index –1.43.
  - Hydrogel (poly HEMA) material refractive index –1.47.
- **Spherical or aspherical:** Aspheric IOL has better contrast acuity.
- **Monofocal or multifocals (Fig. 25.24):** Multifocal IOLs may be refractive or diffractive types—provide for simultaneous viewing of both distance, intermediate and near vision.

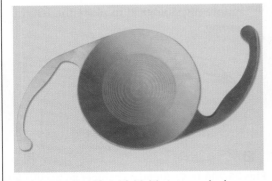

Fig. 25.24: Multifocal foldable intraocular lens

- *Accommodative IOLs:* They allow for both distance vision and midrange near vision.
- *UV-filtering; violet shielding and blue-blockers IOLs:* Specific for light protection like human crystalline lens.
- *Toric IOLs:* To correct preexisting corneal astigmatism.
- *Toric multifocal IOLs:* To correct preexisting astigmatism and to provide distance and near vision simultaneously.
- *Square edge IOL:* A square edge IOL is always preferable than round edge optic because of low incidence of PCO formation.
- *Phakic IOLs:* Mainly used to correct very high myopia in presence of crystalline lens:
    - *Anterior chamber type:* Either angle-fixated or iris-fixated.
    - *Posterior chamber type:* In the ciliary sulcus just in front of natural crystalline lens.

Haptics

They are made of PMMA, prolene or polypropylene or same material as IOL optic. They may be transparent (colorless) or blue in color (for better identification). The shape of the haptic varies, e.g. J-looped, modified J-looped, C-looped or S-shaped-loop (Kelman Multiflex ACIOL), etc. In multi-piece type, the haptics are fixed with optic by biological glue (Figs 25.25A to D).

The main function of the haptics is to anchor the IOL in position.

Other Specifications of Intraocular Lens

- The overall diameter = 12.0–13.5 mm
- Average weight = 20 mg in air and 3.0–3.2 mg in aqueous.
- Thickness of the optic = 1.2–2.0 mm.
- Sterilization = Presterilized by ethylene oxide. A thorough wash with BSS or Ringer's lactate is necessary before insertion of IOL into the eye.

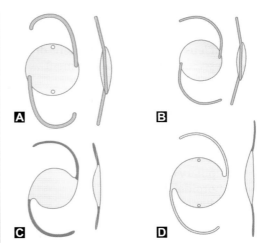

Figs 25.25A to D: Different types of posterior chamber intraocular lens (PCIOL). **A.** Multi-piece, biconvex, modified 'J' loop, **B.** Multi- piece, biconvex, short 'C' loop (without hole); **C.** Single-piece, biconvex, small optic (phaco lens); **D.** Single-piece, biconvex, 'C' loop

- 'A' constant = is fixed for a particular type of IOL, like, 118.0, 118.4, 118.7, etc. for PCIOL and 115.0 for ACIOL.

Overall Complications of Cataract Surgery

Intraoperative
- *Anesthesia-related*
    - Retrobulbar hemorrhage (RBH)
    - Injury to the optic nerve
    - Globe perforation
    - Lignocaine shock, acute anaphylaxis, and convulsion following injection into the optic nerve or its sheaths.
- *Surgery-related (on table)*
    - Subconjunctival hemorrhage
    - Poor wound construction
    - Run away rhexis
    - Iridodialysis
    - Hyphema
    - Positive vitreous pressure (upthrust)
    - Zonular dialysis
    - Subluxation or posterior dislocation of the lens

- Posterior capsular tear (rent)
- Vitreous prolapse (loss)
- Nucleus drop, or part of the lens drop
- Descemet's tear and detachment
- Corneal endothelial damage
- Expulsive hemorrhage.

Early postoperative (within 1 week)
- Striate keratopathy (SK).
- Shallow anterior chamber due to:
  - Wound leak
  - Pupillary block
  - Choroidal detachment
  - Malignant glaucoma.
  - Hyphema
  - Iris prolapse
  - Postoperative uveitis
  - Retained lens matter (cortex or nuclear fragment)
  - Postoperative secondary glaucoma
  - Hypotony
  - Bacterial endophthalmitis
  - Toxic anterior segment syndrome (TASS).

Late postoperative (weeks to months)
- Posterior capsular opacification or after cataract
- Cystoid macular edema or Irvine-Gass syndrome
- Epithelial downgrowth
- Fibrous ingrowth
- Filtering bleb formation (cystoid cicatrix)
- Unpredictable astigmatism
- Persistent chronic uveitis
- Intraocular lens related complications
- Retinal detachment
- Corneal edema
- Bullous keratopathy (pseudophakic or aphakic).
- Late postoperative endophthalmitis.

Complications of Cataract Surgery: Specific to Type of Surgery

Conventional ECCE/PCIOL
- Complications of peribulbar or retrobulbar block (PBB/RBB)

- Positive vitreous upthrust
- Expulsive hemorrhage
- Suture-related problems
- High astigmatism
- Improper cortical cleaning.

Manual SICS
- Complications of PBB/RBB
- With sclerocorneal tunnel preparation:
  - Buttonholing
  - Premature entry
  - Bleeding within the tunnel.
- Zonular dialysis during prolapsing the nucleus into AC
- Inferior iridodialysis during nucleus delivery
- Hyphema.

Phacoemulsification
- Posterior capsule blowout during forcible hydrodissection in case of smaller rhexis
- Wound burn especially with hard cataract
- Runaway rhexis
- Iris chafing/iridodialysis
- Intermittent floppy iris syndrome (IFIS) with its problem. It specially happens with patient taking oral alpha-1 adrenergic receptor antagonists (e.g. tamsulosin) for prostate-related urinary problem
- Zonular dehiscence
- More chances of corneal endothelial damage especially in hard cataract and with shallow AC.

Vitreous loss (prolapse): It may occur during ICCE and following accidental posterior capsular tear or zonular dehiscence during phaco or manual SICS. It is a serious complication because, it is associated with the following unpleasant sequela:
- Updrawn pupil (hammock-shaped)
- High astigmatism
- Iris irregularities
- Uveitis
- Cystoid macular edema
- Retinal detachment
- Vitreous touch syndrome which may lead to corneal decompensation

- Vitreous wick syndrome which may lead to delayed endophthalmitis
- Increased risk of postoperative endophthalmitis.

Intraoperative signs of imminent vitreous loss are—creasing of the cornea along the chord of the wound, gaping of the incision, bulging of the iris diaphragm and deepening of the anterior chamber as vitreous passes into it.

Prevention: Good akinesia of the globe, bulbar massage, release of superior rectus stitch after limbal section, preoperative intravenous mannitol to shrink the vitreous, careful nucleus delivery/fragmentation and cortical cleaning during surgery.

Management: By sponge vitrectomy or by triamcinolone–assisted automated anterior vitrectomy. If the capsulorhexis margin is well preserved a sulcus-fixated PCIOL is given; otherwise a Kelman type ACIOL is implanted. A peripheral iridectomy (PI) is mandatory in case of ACIOL. Sometimes, a secondary scleral fixation IOL may be implanted later on when the eye is quiet.

▮ GLAUCOMA OPERATIONS

Trabeculectomy

It is a ***partial thickness*** filtering operation, where the fistula is guarded by a superficial scleral flap (Fig. 25.26).

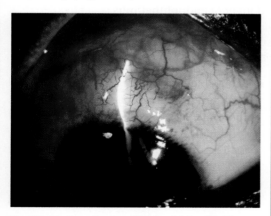

Fig. 25.26: Functioning filtering bleb with PI

Indications

- Primary open-angle glaucoma, not controlled medically
- Chronic angle-closure glaucoma
- Secondary glaucoma's
- Developmental or congenital glaucoma.

Possible Mechanisms of Action

- Filtration around the margins of the scleral flap.
- Filtration through the connective tissue substance of the scleral flap.
- Filtration through outlet channels of the scleral flap.
- Cyclodialysis, if the tissue is dissected posterior to the scleral spur, leading to increased uveoscleral outflow.
- Aqueous flow through the cut ends of the Schlemm's canal (rare).

Operative Steps (Figs 25.27A to D)

- A limbal-based conjunctival flap is made by giving an incision 10 mm posterior to the limbus.
- An area, triangular (5 mm × 5 mm × 5 mm), or square (4 mm × 4 mm), based at limbus, is outlined on the sclera with a wet field cautery.
- A partial thickness (half to two-thirds) superficial scleral flap is dissected, along the cautery mark, and hinged at the limbus.
- A deep rectangular block of sclera (1.5 mm × 3 mm) is excised anterior to the scleral spur, along with trabecular tissue.
- A peripheral iridectomy is performed.
- The superficial scleral flap is repositioned and sutured with 10-0 nylon.
- The conjunctival flap is reposed and sutured meticulously.

Scheie's Thermosclerostomy

It is a free filtering operation, where the fistula is made through the entire thickness of the sclera.

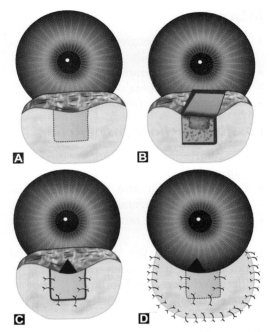

Figs 25.27A to D: Steps of trabeculectomy. **A.** Limbal-based conjunctival flap with marking on sclera; **B.** Scleral-flap dissection with removal of deeper sclera along with trabecular tissue; **C.** Peripheral iridectomy with suturing of scleral flap; **D.** Suturing the conjunctival flap

Indications: Same as trabeculectomy operation except, in developmental or congenital glaucoma.

Operative Steps

- A limbal-based conjunctival flap is made.
- A partial thickness groove, about 4 mm long, is created behind the corneo-limbal junction.
- The posterior lip of the groove is cauterized.
- The incision is extended into the anterior chamber, and cautery is applied to the depth of the wound, while a dry field is maintained with a sponge.
- A peripheral iridectomy is performed.
- The conjunctiva is sutured.

Iridencleisis: A wedge of the iris is incarcerated into the limbal incision with an effort to maintain a patent channel for aqueous outflow. Endothelial cells of the iris proliferate and line the wound, and the iris stroma atrophies to act like a filtering wick. This was once a popular procedure, but is obsolete now, due to the associated higher incidence of sympathetic ophthalmitis.

Complications of Glaucoma Surgery

Early Complications

- Changes in refraction
- A shallow or flat anterior chamber
- Hyphema
- Endophthalmitis
- Total loss of visual field
- Malignant glaucoma.

Late Complications

- Nonfunctioning filtering bleb.
- Bleb infection (blebitis) which may lead to endophthalmitis.
- Cataract formation.

Full-thickness filtering procedure is more complicated, by excessive aqueous filtration leading to a flat anterior chamber associated with corneal decompensation and synechia formation. In addition, the filtering blebs often become very thin and may rupture creating the danger of endophthalmitis.

Minimally Invasive Glaucoma Surgery

- Trabeculectomy is regarded as the gold standard in glaucoma surgery; however, there are less invasive procedures called minimally invasive glaucoma surgery (MIGS) have gained popularity in recent years among patients and surgeons.
- *MIGS:* The new procedures and devices are relatively safe and can easily be combined with cataract surgery.

- *Main advantage:* They are non-penetrating and/or bleb-independent procedures with shorter surgery time. Major complications of fistulating surgery related to blebs and hypotony are also minimum.
- MIGS procedures do not preclude the possibility of future, more traditional conventional surgeries, like, trabeculectomy or tube/shunt surgery.
- *Main disadvantage:* They are expensive and may not be suitable in lowering IOP for moderate to severe glaucoma.

MIGS may be of ab interno and ab externo types:

Surgical approach

- *Ab interno:* Done under gonioscopic view usually through a small side port. By removing tissue or by implanting a shunt device.
- *Ab externo:* By using external approach to reach surgical side, like suprachoroidal space, either to remove/modify tissue or to implant device.

Internal filtration

- Trabeculotomy (excimer laser)
- Trabecular microbypass
- Suprachoroidal stent
- Intracanalicular scaffold
- Canaloplasty (canal expander)
- Suprachoroidal gold micro shunt.

External filtration: Subconjunctival implant.

CYCLOCRYOTHERAPY (FIG. 25.28)

This is most commonly practiced cyclodestructive procedure, which involves freezing of the ciliary body, to reduce the rate of aqueous production.

Indications

- Painful absolute glaucoma
- Aphakic glaucoma

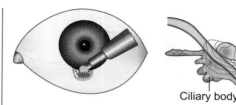

Fig. 25.28: Cyclocryotherapy

- Post-keratoplasty secondary glaucoma
- Neovascular glaucoma (may be needed along with panretinal photocoagulation).

Mechanism

Cyclocryotherapy destroys the ability of the ciliary body to produce aqueous humor.

This is by destruction of the ciliary epithelial cells, due to intracellular ice crystal formation and ischemic necrosis.

In addition, it provides relief of pain by destruction of the corneal nerves.

Steps

- Surface and retrobulbar anesthesia.
- The nearest edge of the cryoprobe (glaucoma probe) is placed 2.5 mm from the limbus.
- Cryoprobe is applied for 60 sec, at a temperature of –60° to –80°C. A rapid freeze, and slow unassisted thaw is desirable, as it produces maximum cell death.
- In each treatment session, six cryo-applications are recommended over 180° of the globe.
- Subconjunctival injection of dexamethasone and atropine are preferably given.
- Two or more sessions may be required for a few patients.

Intense postoperative pain (for first 24 hours), is treated with strong analgesics. In addition, topical corticosteroids and cycloplegics are to be used from the day of surgery.

Complications: Excessive treatment may cause uveitis, hyphema, vitreous opacities, iris atrophy, pupillary distortion and hypotony (phthisis bulbi).

CYCLOPHOTOCOAGULATION

Cyclophotocoagulation (CPC) is also another way to perform cyclodestruction. It can be performed using different laser wavelengths. Previously, neodymium-doped yttrium aluminum garnet (Nd:YAG) laser was used for CPC.

But, presently, diode laser (810 nm wavelength) is preferred to perform CPC over other wavelengths since the melanin in the ciliary epithelium better absorbs this wavelength than others and therefore causes more targeted destruction with less inflammation.

Two main types of CPC: Transscleral CPC (TS-CPC) or endocyclophotocoagulation (ECP). TS-CPC requires LA (retrobulbar or peribulbar) and can often be performed in outpatient department (OPD) setting. ECP requires local (topical with intracameral, retrobulbar/peribulbar block) or general anesthesia and is performed in operation theatre setting.

Both are performed for similar glaucoma conditions. In general, TS-CPC and ECP are indicated for refractory glaucoma, or eyes with poor visual acuity and/or visual potential.

Indications for TS-CPC or ECP:
- Elevated IOP with poor vision and/or visual potential.
- Pain relief due to very high IOP in a painful blind eye.
- Poor candidates for glaucoma filtration surgery or glaucoma drainage devices.
- Pseudophakic/aphakic glaucoma.
- Intractable pseudoexfoliation glaucoma.
- Glaucoma after penetrating keratoplasty or other corneal transplant surgery.
- Neovascular glaucoma.
- Refractory cases of pediatric glaucoma.
- Uveitic glaucoma or silicone oil induced glaucoma.
- Uncontrolled glaucoma in the presence of conjunctival scarring from previous surgery.
- Patient's medical condition preclude going to operating room.

Complications: Conjunctival burn in TS-CPC; chronic hypotony in both procedures; retreatment is required in some cases.

OPERATIONS UPON THE IRIS

Iridectomy

It consists of abscission of a portion of the iris, usually done in the upper part where it is covered by the upper eyelid.

There will be diplopia (in case of peripheral iridectomy) or dazzling of light (in case of complete iridectomy), if the iridectomy is done in the lower part, as the lower part of the iris is not covered by the lower lid.

Types of iridectomy with indications (Figs 25.29A to C):
- Peripheral buttonhole iridectomy: It is usually done at 11 o'clock to 1 o'clock meridian.

Indications
- Angle-closure glaucoma.
- As a part of trabeculectomy operation.
- In intracapsular cataract extraction.
- In some cases of extracapsular cataract extraction.
- In penetrating keratoplasty operation.
- Inferior peripheral iridectomy at 6 o'clock—in vitreoretinal surgery and also in endothelial keratoplasty [like descemet's stripping endothelial keratoplasty (DSEK) or descemet's membrane endothelial keratoplasty (DMEK)].

A peripheral iridectomy is done to prevent postoperative pupillary block glaucoma. As the aqueous can flow freely

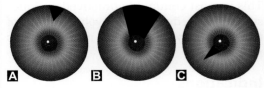

Figs 25.29A to C: Different types of iridectomy. **A.** Peripheral button–hole; **B.** Sector (complete); **C.** Optical

into the anterior chamber via this bypass channel. An equilibrium is thus maintained between the anterior and posterior chamber, following operations.

Steps

- Eyeball is rotated downwards with superior rectus stitch.
- A small conjunctival flap is made from 11 o 'clock to 1 o'clock meridian.
- A small ab externo incision is given to open the anterior chamber.
- Slight pressure is given on the posterior lip of the wound, which causes prolapse of a knuckle of iris.
- A portion of the iris near its base is abscised, leaving the sphincter intact. Care should be taken to retain the anterior chamber during this maneuver.
- A stitch may be required to close the wound, and then conjunctiva is repositioned.

- *Board (complete) iridectomy:* To facilitate the extraction of the lens when the pupil is small and rigid, or there is extensive synechia (combined extraction of cataract). A sector of iris is abscised from the pupillary margin to the base of the iris.
- *Optical iridectomy:* It is rarely done nowadays.

Indications

- In case of small central corneal opacity where keratoplasty is not possible.
- In case of axial congenital cataract, if the child is mentally retarded.

It is done in the lower pupillary margin of the iris, as in the upper part of new opening will become covered by the upper lid. The best site for optical iridectomy is judged by stenopaeic slit test, and it should correspond to the clear zone at the lower half of the cornea.

- *Iridectomy for prolapsed iris:* After successful abscission of the prolapsed iris, the stumps of iris retract into the anterior chamber, and should be free from the wound.

- *Iridectomy to remove foreign bodies or small cysts or tumors of the iris.*

Iridotomy

It consists of section of the iris without abscising any portion of it.

Indications

- *To create an artificial pupil,* when the normal pupil is closed or severely updrawn.
- *Laser iridotomy* for primary angle closure glaucoma or postoperative pupillary block glaucoma. It may be carried out with an argon laser or a Nd:YAG laser.
- *Four-point iridotomy (quadri-puncture):* It is done to treat secondary glaucoma in *iris bombe.* A von Graefe's cataract knife is useful for this purpose.
- *Division of anterior synechiae,* is also a form of iridotomy.

OPERATIONS OF THE CORNEA

Paracentesis

Paracentesis means opening the anterior chamber for the purpose of aspiration of its contents, partially or completely.

Indications

Diagnostic: Aqueous humor study for:
- Intraocular malignancy
  - Cytology
  - Lactate dehydrogenase enzyme assay.
- Intraocular parasite infestation
- Polymerase chain reaction (PCR) diagnosis in infective uveitis or viral endotheliitis.

Therapeutic
- Massive hyphema to control secondary glaucoma, and to prevent blood staining of the cornea.
- Corneal ulcer with massive hypopyon to improve corneal nutrition.
- Impending corneal perforation.
- Central retinal artery occlusion.

Steps

- Eyeball is steadily fixed with forceps.
- An incision is made at the temporal limbus within 2 mm, with the help of a keratome, MVR blade, a paracentesis needle or a sideport knife or a 26-gauge needle.
- The knife or needle is inserted at the iris plane. Then posterior lip is slightly depressed so that the aqueous is drained out slowly with a minimum of disturbance.

Keratoplasty

It means surgical replacement of a scarred or diseased cornea with a viable donor cornea.

Classifications

Morphological

- Full thickness or penetrating keratoplasty (PK)
- Partial thickness or lamellar keratoplasty (LK) (Fig. 25.30)
  - Anterior lamellar keratoplasty (ALK) (Figs 25.31A and B)
  - Deep anterior lamellar keratoplasty (DALK) (Figs 25.32A to E)
  - Posterior lamellar keratoplasty (PLK)
    - Deep lamellar endothelial keratoplasty (DLEK)
    - Descemet stripping (automated) endothelial keratoplasty (DSEK/DSAEK)
    - Descemet membrane endothelial keratoplasty (DMEK).

According to purpose (Table 25.1)

- *Optical:* Primary purpose is being the improvement of vision (e.g. leucoma, keratoconus, etc.).
- *Tectonic:* Restoration of altered corneal structure (e.g. thinning, perforation, etc.).
- *Therapeutic:* Tissue substitution for refractive corneal diseases (e.g. nonhealing corneal ulcer, pterygium, etc.).
- *Cosmetic:* Replacement, without the hope for visual improvement.

Frequently, several purposes are addressed when a keratoplasty is performed.

According to donor material Employed

- *Homograft (allokeratoplasty):* Donor material from the same species (human to human).

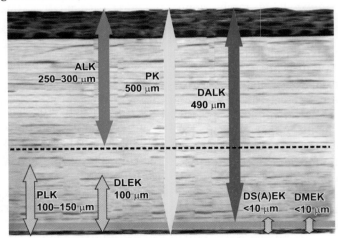

Fig. 25.30: Level of dissection in recipient's eye in different types of keratoplasty

ALK—Anterior lamellar keratoplasty; **DALK**—Deep anterior lamellar keratoplasty; **DLEK**—Deep lamellar endothelial keratoplasty; **DMEK**—Descemet membrane endothelial keratoplasty; **DS(A)EK**—Descemet stripping (automated) endothelial keratoplasty; **PK**—Penetrating keratoplasty; **PLK**—Posterior lamellar keratoplasty

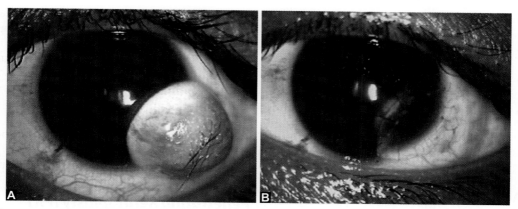

Figs 25.31A and B: Anterior lamellar keratoplasty in dermoid. **A.** Before operation; **B.** After operation

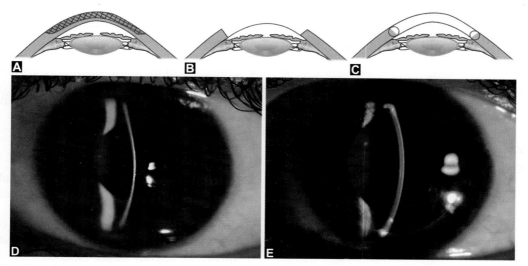

Figs 25.32A to E: Deep anterior lamellar keratoplasty (DALK). **A.** With anterior corneal disease; **B.** Removal of diseased part and only descemet membrane (DM) and endothelium remained; **C.** Replacement of donor cornea without DM and endothelium; **D.** In keratoconus (before surgery); **E.** In keratoconus (after surgery)—that shape and thickness like normal cornea

TABLE 25.1: Indications of keratoplasty		
Indications	**India (%)**	**USA (%)**
Corneal scar (ulcer related)	28.1	7.9
Therapeutic penetrating keratoplasty	12.2	2.9
Pseudophakic corneal edema/bullous keratopathy	10.6	27.2
Non-Fuchs' dystrophy	7.2	9.3
Keratoconus	6.0	15.4
Fuchs' dystrophy	1.2	15.2
Failed graft	17.1	10.9
Others	17.7	2.7

- **Autograft (autokeratoplasty):** Donor material from the same individual.
- **Isograft:** Transplants between homozygous twin.
- **Heterograft (xenograft):** Graft obtained from another species.
- **Keratoprosthesis:** The grafted material is an optical cylinder made of PMMA and the carrier may be a donor cornea [Boston Keratoprosthesis (Kpro)] or a canine tooth [osteo-odonto-keratoprosthesis (OOKP)].

According to type of surgery

- **Simple keratoplasty:** Keratoplasty is performed alone.
- **Combined keratoplasty:** When combined with:
  - Cataract extraction (ICCE/ECCE)
  - ECCE with PCIOL implantation (**triple procedure**)
  - Trabeculectomy
  - Vitrectomy.

Indications for Lamellar Keratoplasty

Indications
- **Anterior lamellar keratoplasty**
  - **Tectonic:** For marginal thinning, e.g. Mooren's ulcer, Terrien's degeneration, etc.
  - **Therapeutic:** With pterygium surgery, limbal dermoids, etc.
- **Deep anterior lamellar keratoplasty (DALK) (for optical purpose):** Any anterior corneal disease/scar without involvement of descemet membrane and endothelium.
  - Reis-Buckler's dystrophy
  - Granular dystrophy
  - Lattice dystrophy
  - Keratoconus (most common)
  - Anterior corneal scar after an ulcer
  - Macular dystrophy (in some cases, endothelium is also involved and in that case, PK is indicated).
- **Posterior lamellar keratoplasty (DSEK/DSAEK, DMEK):** Any disease affecting the

descemet and endothelium (endothelial dysfunctions) without any stromal scar (Figs 25.33A to E).
  - Pseudophakic corneal edema/bullous keratopathy (most common)
  - Fuchs' dystrophy
  - Posterior polymorphous dystrophy
  - Post PK failed graft
  - Iridocorneal endothelial syndrome (Chandler's syndrome)
  - In some cases of congenital hereditary endothelial dystrophy.

Penetrating Keratoplasty (PK) (Figs 25.34 to 25.36)

Surgical technique

This technique aims:
- Minimal manipulation of the donor tissue.
- Protection of the intraocular structures of the recipient.
- Attaining a water-tight host-graft junction at the end.

Steps
- Preoperative miosis and hypotony
- Anesthesia and akinesia
- Exposure, globe fixation and scleral support (flieringa ring is used to prevent scleral collapse).
- **Trephination of the donor cornea:** It is better from the endothelial side and should be slightly larger (0.25–0.50 mm) than the recipient corneal hole.
- **Trephination of the recipient button:** It is usually 7.0 to 7.5 mm diameter in size. Cutting of the recipient button is completed with fine scissors.
- Management of the iris, lens, vitreous, and IOL implantation in selected cases.
- Graft placement and maintenance of anterior chamber by viscoelastic agent.
- **Suturing the corneal button:** The first four sutures, placed at 12, 6, 3 and 9 o'clock meridians, are known as cardinal sutures. Subsequent sutures are given with 10-0 nylon (at 75–90% of depth) by continuous or interrupted fashion.

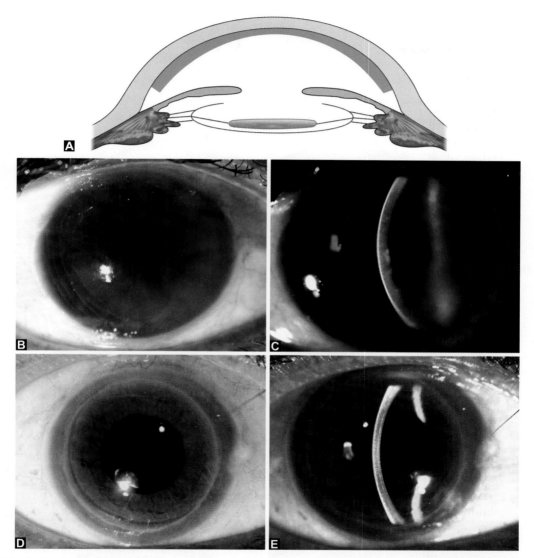

Figs 25.33A to E: A. Descemet stripping endothelial keratoplasty (DSEK). Here, recipient's diseased "DM and endothelium complex" is replaced with healthy donor tissue (endothelium, DM and thin layer of posterior stroma); **B.** Pseudophakic bullous keratopathy; **C.** Pseudophakic bullous keratopathy—severe corneal edema; **D and E.** Same eye after DSEK surgery in diffuse illumination and slit section

- Wound margin is checked for fluid leak and iris adherence.
- Anterior chamber is reformed.
- Subconjunctival injection of dexamethasone and gentamicin.
- Pad and bandage.

Complications of Penetrating Keratoplasty

Early complications
- Primary graft failure
- Wound leak and iris prolapse

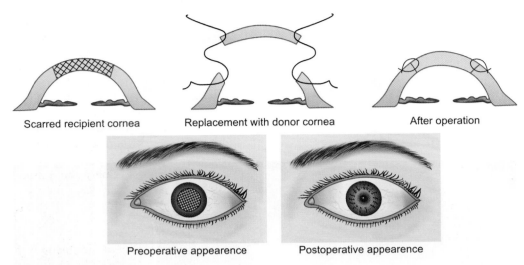

Scarred recipient cornea   Replacement with donor cornea   After operation

Preoperative appearence   Postoperative appearence

Fig. 25.34: Penetrating keratoplasty

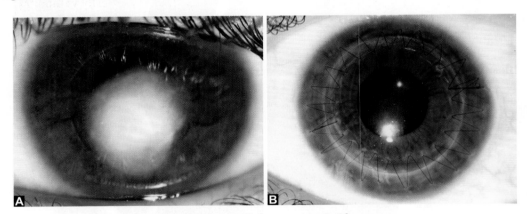

Figs 25.35A and B: Penetrating keratoplasty. **A.** Before surgery; **B.** After surgery

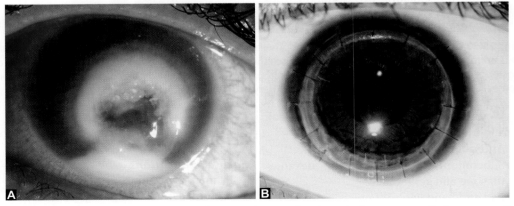

Figs 25.36A and B: A. Corneal ulcer with impending perforation—before surgery; **B.** Same eye after therapeutic penetrating keratoplasty

- Postoperative glaucoma
- Iridocyclitis
- Hyphema
- Wound infections
- Persistent epithelial defect.

Intermediate complications
- Graft rejection (immunological)
- Epithelial
- Subepithelial
- Stromal
- Endothelial (Khodadoust line)
- Graft infections
- Wound dehiscence.

Late complications
- Recurrence of host disease (e.g. herpes simplex keratitis, lattice dystrophy, Reis-Buckler's dystrophy, etc.)
- Retrocorneal membrane (RCM) formation
- Late graft failure
- Cataract formation
- Transmission of donor disease to the host
- Post-keratoplasty astigmatism.

EYE BANK AND DONOR CORNEA

Objectives of an Eye Bank

- Collection of donor eyes.
- Process and storage of donor cornea.
- Distribution and utilization of the highest quality of donor tissue for transplantation.
- Provide for soliciting eye donation from potential donors.
- Provide and process eye tissue for teaching or research, as needed.
- To promote public education relation system.
- To promote hospital cornea retrieval program (HCRP) to improve collection of donor eyes from hospital deaths.

Collection

Person pledges before death to donate his eyes (no living person can donate his one eye, because the law does not permit it. Similarly, eye tissue cannot be sold or purchased). After getting information of death, and proper written consent from the next of kin, eye bank personnel collects the eyes. The eyeballs should be collected with 4–6 hours of death (traditional postmortem time).

It is important to know the *age of the donor, time of death* and *cause of death* before enucleation of the donor globe. Most eye banks accept eyes from donors between 6 months and 80 years of age.

Methods

There are two methods of procuring donor tissue for the eye banks:
1. Voluntary donation (mostly without prior pledge).
2. Hospital cornea retrieval program.

Voluntary Donation

It is the result of realization of one's social responsibility towards people with corneal blindness. However, in the moment of grief, this realization may not materialize to actual donation, because the near relatives may not be in a position to make such noble decisions. Currently, the total donor cornea collection all over India is between 60,000 to 70,000 per year. Maximum collections occur from Gujarat, Maharashtra, Tamil Nadu and Andhra Pradesh. Among these, 75–80% of eye donation is from voluntary aged donors who die in their homes, hospitals, or nursing homes. Only 40–45% of the eyes from voluntary donation are utilized for transplantation.

The reasons are:
- Age of the donor
- Longer death-to-enucleation time
- Nonavailability of donor's complete medical history.

It is to address the nonavailability of *quality* corneal tissue. The Eye Bank Association of India (EBAI) along with Government of India has come up with this new cornea collection strategy called HCRP. This program was initiated by Ramayamma International Eye Bank at LVP Eye Institute, Hyderabad in 1990.

Hospital Cornea Retrieval Program

Here, an *eye donation counselor* (EDC, or previously called *grief counselor*) makes a timely and sensitive request to the near relatives of the bereaved in a hospital set up to make an eye donation. With several leaflets and close intimate education, he or she wins the heart of the relatives of the deceased.

If the consent is given, he organizes quick collection of donor tissue (whole eyeball or in situ corneoscleral rim) so that the family is not inconvenienced.

The overall conversion (request by EDC vs. actual donation) is between 5% and 35% in different hospitals. The donor cornea collection through HCRP is around 20–25% of total collection in last 2 years (i.e. approximately 15,000 cornea per year).

Advantages of HCRP
- Access to younger and healthier tissues.
- Availability of donor medical history.
- Reduce death–to–enucleation time.
- Higher tissue utilization rate (65% or more).
- More scope of training and future research.
- Cost-effective.

Choice of hospitals
- Large multispeciality hospitals with 500 beds or more.
- Death rate = 3–4 per day or greater than 10 per week.
- Should be close vicinity (within 5–15 Km) to the linked eye bank.
- Should have signed memorandum of understanding (MoU) between both.
- Help and active support is required from all level of the staff of the hospital.

Pledged eyes cannot be retrieved without the consent of the family members (next of kin). The near relatives of those who have not pledged their eye can also decide, at the time of death, to donate the eyes of the deceased on his or her behalf. However, at the time of death of near and dear one, in the midst of grief and confusion, even the best of intention may not lead to actual eye donation. HCRP (with the help of trained counselor) plays a key role in this situation.

Contraindications for donor eye collection:
- *Medical:* Acquired immunodeficiency syndrome (AIDS) or human immuno-deficiency virus (HIV), seropositivity, rabies, active hepatitis B, hepatitis C, septicemia, death from unknown cause, Creutzfeldt-Jakob disease, leukemia, syphilis, etc.
- *Ophthalmic:* Previous intraocular surgery, corneal pathology, retinoblastoma and malignant melanoma, iridocyclitis, endoph-thalmitis, etc.

Storage (preservation) of the donor eye:
- Short-term preservation (up to 96 hours)
  - *Moist chamber method:* Whole globe is preserved in a moist chamber at +4°C in a refrigerator for 24 hr.
  - *McCarey-Kaufman (M-K) medium (Fig. 25.37A):* Composition: Tissue culture (TC)–199: 5%: Dextran-40; 4-(2-hydroxyethyl)-1-piperazi-neethanesulfonic acid (HEPES) buffer to adjust pH at 7.4; gentamicin 0–1 mg/mL; color-pink.
  - *Corneoscleral button (Fig. 25.37B)* is preserved in M-K medium at +4°C for up to 96 hours. It is superior than conventional moist chamber method and practised widely.
- *Intermediate-term preservation (up to 2 weeks):* Optisol-GS, Cornisol, Eusol-C and Life4C media.
- *Long-term preservation (months to years).*
  - *Viable:* Organ culture method, cryopreservation.
  - *Non-viable:* Glycerine preservation.

Evaluation of the donor tissue:
- *Gross examination* with torch and loupe.

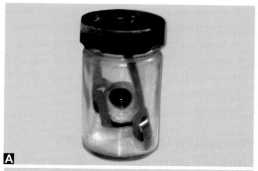

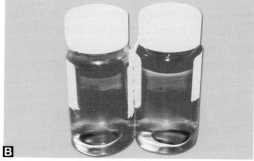

Figs 25.37A and B: A. Corneal preservation—moist chamber method (whole globe); **B.** Sclerocorneal button preservation in McCarey-Kaufman medium

- *Slit-lamp* examination.
- Specular microscopy (for endothelial cell count and morphology).
- Vital staining (trypan blue dye).
- Microbial evaluation by culture.
- Serological screening (for HIV, hepatitis B, hepatitis C and syphilis).
- Human leukocyte antigen typing of the donor not done.

TARSORRHAPHY

Aims of the Surgery

- To reduce the length of the palpebral aperture, when this is abnormal.
- To close the eye temporarily, to protect the cornea.

Types and Indications

- Permanent (lateral) (Figs 25.38A and B)
  - Residual Bell's palsy

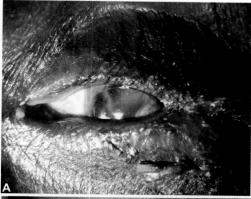

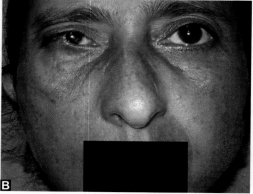

Figs 25.38A and B: A. Temporary lateral tarsorrhaphy in perforated corneal ulcer; **B.** Permanent tarsorrhaphy in operated cerebellopontine angle tumor

  - Abnormal length of the palpebral fissure
  - Mild degree of exophthalmos.
- Temporary (paramedian or lateral)
  - Neuroparalytic keratitis
  - Moderate to severe exophthalmos
  - To assist healing of skin grafting
  - During reconstruction of a contracted socket
  - Small perforation of corneal ulcer
  - Impending perforation of corneal ulcer
  - In severe dry eye.

Steps: Apart from placement of sutures both the operations almost follow the same technique.

- Dissection of the mucous membrane from the margin of lower lid just posterior to the grey line in rectangular (5–6 mm long) fashion.

- The edge of the upper lid is similarly dissected at the corresponding position.
- A horizontal mattress suture is passed through the rubber beads and the skin, so that they come out at the posterior edge of the bare surface of both lids. Suture is then tied firmly.
- The lids will be firmly adherent within a few days (7–10 days) when the suture and rubber beads are removed.

PTERYGIUM OPERATION

Anesthesia

- Surface anesthesia with 4% lignocaine.
- Infiltration anesthesia with 2% lignocaine with adrenaline into the body of the pterygium.
- Peribulbar anesthesia as cataract surgery. May be performed under topical anesthesia.

Indications of Surgery

- Pterygium approaches towards the pupillary area.
- Chronic irritation due to fleshy pterygium.
- Causing much astigmatism.
- Purely cosmetic—in rare situation.

Bare Sclera (D'Ombrian's) Technique

- Eye speculum is inserted.
- The neck is held with a fixation forceps, and the head (apex) of the pterygium is shaved from the cornea with a 15 number blade.
- Two diverging incisions are given along the upper and lower borders of the pterygium.
- The pterygium is lifted with a hook and rotated nasally, while the dissection is carried out subconjunctivally.
- The subepithelial thick triangular pathological tissue is removed in one piece.

- The conjunctiva over the head, neck and 2 mm of the body of the pterygium is excised to leave an area of exposed (bare) sclera.
- Conjunctiva is repositioned and sutured, the bleeding vessels of the bare area is cauterized.
- Pad and bandage.

Pterygium Operation with Limbal Conjunctival Autograft

Here, the pterygium is resected (Fig. 25.39A) first as bare sclera technique. Then the steps are as follows:

- A rectangular piece of limbal conjunctiva is dissected from upper temporal area and taken out as graft tissue. This is usually from the same eye, but sometimes from the other eye (Fig. 25.39B).
  - The tissue is placed over the bare area to cover it. Limbal side is matched carefully.
  - Grafted tissue is sutured by 10-0 vicryl or 10-0 nylon. Donor site is also closed by the same suture.
- Nowadays, graft fixation is preferably done with biological tissue (fibrin) glue. It is faster and easier. The postoperative reaction is minimal with quicker rehabilitation. The recurrence rate is also much lower.
- If required, the sutures may be removed after 3 weeks.

CHALAZION OPERATION

Most chalazion requires incision and curettage, for very rarely does spontaneous resolution occur (Fig. 25.40).

Anesthesia

- Surface anesthesia by 4% lignocaine.
- Infiltration by 2% lignocaine with adrenaline into the skin around the chalazion.

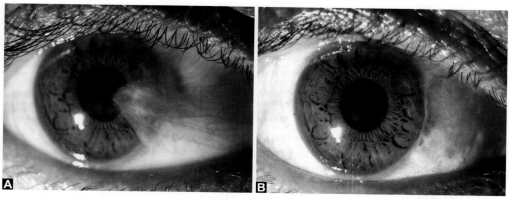

Figs 25.39A and B: A. Pterygium before surgery; **B.** Pterygium resection with conjunctival autograft with fibrin glue

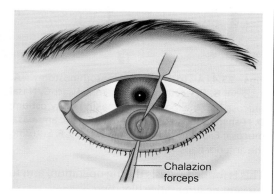

Fig. 25.40: Chalazion operation (vertical incision)

Operative Steps

- Chalazion is fixed with chalazion clamp or forceps, the plate of which is passed over the skin and the ring is placed on the palpebral conjunctiva with the chalazion in its center.
- Chalazion clamp is closed by tightening the screw, and the lid is everted.
- A vertical incision is made through the tarsal conjunctiva with a sharp knife.
- Cheesy granulomatous tissue is thoroughly scooped out with the help of a chalazion scoop.
- The walls of the cavity is scraped carefully with the same scoop.

- Fibrous tissue wall may be excised entirely, if it is thick.
- Clamp is removed, and pressure is applied for 2–3 minutes to secure hemostasis.
- Pad and bandage for 4–6 hours.

DACRYOCYSTECTOMY

Anesthesia (Local)

- Two drops of 4% lignocaine into the conjunctival sac.
- Infiltration: Anesthetic agents are injected at the following sites:
  - At the junction of the inferior orbital margin with the beginning of the anterior lacrimal crest—0.5 mL solution is injected, and then along the line incision to a point 3 mm above the medial palpebral ligament.
  - Second injection is made at the above point and needle is directed posteriorly for about 8 mm, and the tissues around the fundus are injected with about 0.5 mL. The needle is then carried out further downwards to the upper half of posterior lacrimal crest and injected with 0.5 mL solution.
- Nasal mucosa of the inferior and middle meatus is anesthetized with 4% lignocaine and adrenaline (with spray or nasal pack).

Operative Steps

- A slightly curved incision with its concavity towards the inner canthus is made (care is taken not to injure the angular vein). The incision is about 2.0 cm, and one-third of its lies above the medial palpebral ligament.
- Separation of skin and orbicularis oculi along the line of incision with lacrimal dissector, and then retracted with Muller's retractor.
- Medial palpebral ligament is then exposed, and disinserted form the anterior lacrimal crest by a rougine.
- Lacrimal sac is dissected from the floor, at the fundus, and from its connection with the canaliculi.
- After the sac is well dissected, it is grasped with a straight artery forceps up to its lower end and twisted until it is torn off from nasolacrimal duct.
- The torn end of nasolacrimal duct is curetted and then cauterized with iodine solution.
- Skin is closed by interrupted or continuous, 5–0 or 6–0 silk.
- Pad and pressure bandage are applied for 24–48 hours. Stitches are removed after 6–7 days.

DACRYOCYSTORHINOSTOMY (FIGS 25.41A TO F)

Anesthesia

- ·In adult: Same as dacryocystectomy. It is better with anesthetic mixture.
- ·In children: General anesthesia.

Operative Steps

Nasal pack: In dacryocystorhinostomy (DCR), before starting the operation a nasal pack is given on the same side with a roller gauze, soaked with 4% lignocaine, adrenaline and hemostatic agent.

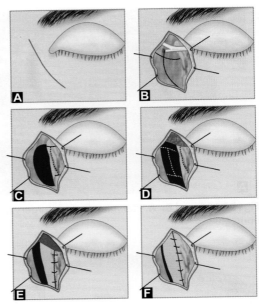

Figs 25.41A to F: Dacryocystorhinostomy. **A.** Incision; **B.** Dissection of the lacrimal sac; **C.** Nasal mucosa being exposed after making bony ostium; **D.** H-shaped incisions on the lacrimal sac and nasal mucosa; **E.** Suturing the posterior flaps; **F.** Suturing the anterior flaps

This is for hemostasis during operation, and to prevent postoperative bleeding.

1–3. Same as dacryocystectomy.

4. Lacrimal sac is separated from the medical wall and floor only. Lacrimal fossa is now exposed.

5. A 10 mm bony ostium is made by cutting the lacrimal bone, part of the adjacent nasal bone, and frontal process of the maxilla. Nasal mucous membrane of the middle meatus is thus exposed.

6. Two horizontal H-shaped incisions are given on the nasal mucosa, and the medial wall of the lacrimal sac; and thereby, two anterior flaps and two posterior flaps are created.

7. First posterior, and then the anterior flaps are sutured with 6-0 or 8-0 chromic catgut or vicryl. Sometimes, it is difficult to suture both the flaps. In that case, only two anterior flaps are sutured together, while the posterior flaps are excised.

8. Skin is sutured by 5-0 or 6-0 silk.
9. Nasal pack is removed after 48–72 hours.

EVISCERATION (FIG. 25.42)

It is a destructive surgical procedure, in which intraocular contents are removed along with inner two coats, retaining the sclera and optic nerve.

Indications

- Panophthalmitis
- Very rarely expulsive hemorrhage to assist in removing the contents, if the process is incomplete.

Special consent: An informed written consent has to be taken prior to surgery.

Anesthesia

- General anesthesia is preferable, as the procedure is painful and psychologically traumatic.
- Local anesthesia when GA is contraindicated
  - Surface by 4% lignocaine.
  - Infiltration by 2% lignocaine with adrenaline at 4 quadrants in retrobulbar space.

Steps of Operation

- Universal eye speculum is applied.

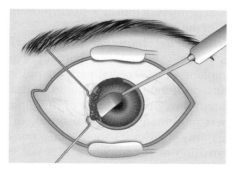

Fig. 25.42: Evisceration. Note the introduction of evisceration scoop between the sclera and uveal tract

- Conjunctiva is dissected 360° around the limbus.
- Whole cornea is removed with a knife and scissors.
- After fixing the sclera, the evisceration scoop is introduced between the sclera and the uveal tract and swept circumferentially 360° to separate the uveal tissues from the sclera and optic nerve.
- Intraocular contents are scooped out thoroughly, precaution being taken to remove all the uveal tissues, especially around the vortex veins and optic nerve.
- Bleeding is stopped by applying pressure with warm saline-soaked gauze.
- Double pad and pressure bandage is applied for 48 hours.

Variations of Evisceration

- ***Frill excision:*** If the entire sclera is left out, there is considerable reaction, and delayed wound healing. These disadvantages may be avoided, by cutting the insertion of the recti muscles and excising a greater part of the sclera, leaving only a small collar of sclera around the optic nerve, so as to leave the nerve sheath unopened.
- ***Insertion of an acrylic ball implant***
  - A small acrylic or silicone ball (about 14–16 mm in diameter) is placed within the scleral cup (pocket) after proper hemostasis.
  - Sclera is sutured over the implant.
  - Tenon's capsule and the conjunctiva are sutured separately.
  - Artificial eye (cosmetic shell) is given after 4–6 weeks.
  - Cosmetic result after this implant is very satisfactory.

ENUCLEATION

Enucleation is the surgical removal of the eyeball with a portion of the optic nerve from the orbit.

Indications

- **Absolute indications:** When there is risk of life or risk to the other eye of the patient
  - Retinoblastoma in children
  - Malignant melanoma in adults
  - Severely traumatized eye with no perception of light (PL) to prevent sympathetic ophthalmitis of contraindication.
  - Enucleation of whole eye ball—from donor, as a part of collection procedure in eye banking.
- **Contraindication:** Panophthalmitis, because the infection can spread via the cut ends of optic nerve sheath, causing meningitis.Special consent: An informed written consent has to be taken prior to surgery.
- Anesthesia: Same as evisceration.

Steps of Operation

- Universal eye speculum is applied.
- Conjunctiva is dissected all around the limbus, and Tenon's capsule is separated from the sclera up to the insertion of the extraocular muscles.
- Each rectus muscle is hooked with a squint hook and cut with scissors, in the order of superior, lateral, inferior and medial rectus muscle (SLIM). For insertion of the implant, transfix each muscle with 5-0 chromic catgut suture.
- Speculum is depressed, and the eyeball is made to be luxated out.
- Enucleation scissors are introduced with closed-tip along the lateral side of the globe. Scissors are opened, and optic nerve is severed.
- Oblique muscles are severed lastly with the same scissors.
- Bleeding is stopped by applying pressure within the socket.

In case of malignant intraocular tumor, it is essential to **cut the optic nerve at least 10 mm** behind the globe, near the optic foramen.

To do this, the eyeball is rotated laterally by a traction suture in the medial rectus tendon, and the optic nerve is tensioned. Enucleation spoon with optic nerve guide is introduced from the lateral side and optic nerve is then transected with one bold cut with a pair of **straight enucleation scissors** from the medial side of the globe.

- Tenon's capsule and conjunctiva are sutured separately.
- Pressure bandage is applied for 48 hours.

Enucleation with Implants

Implants are inserted within the Tenon's capsule, and the aim is:
- To provide a mobile base for the prosthesis to pivot upon.
- To prevent bony deformity of the orbital wall (i.e. contracted socket) in children.
- To maintain orbital socket in adults.

Types of Implants

- **Buried implants**
  - **Non-integrated:** It is an acrylic sphere, which is inserted within the Tenon's capsule to maintain shape of the eyeball. The recti muscles are tied in a cruciate manner over the implant.
  - **Semi-integrated:** It has holes or tunnels in which the four recti muscles are tied separately. It moves with the movement of the opposite eye.
- **Semi-buried implants (integrated):** It is partially buried and partially expose implant. In its exposed part, the posterior surface of the prosthesis could be exactly fitted. Though it is capable of affording the best movement of the prosthesis, in the majority of the cases, there is infection and extrusion of the implants. It is not used nowadays.

- *Hydroxyapatite implant:* It is from natural source coral. It is a costly type of integrated implant in which an artificial eye is pegged. It gives the best cosmetic appearance with excellent movements of an artificial eye.

A *prosthesis (or an artificial eye)* may be fitted in the 3rd or 4th week after the operation. The person who is responsible for making and fitting of an artificial eye, or prosthesis is called an *ocularist*.

AMNIOTIC MEMBRANE TRANSPLANTATION

Human amniotic membrane transplantation (AMT) is used for a variety of ocular surface surgeries.

Source

Innermost layer of human placenta from cesarean section deliveries. Necessary serology tests are done before using it. The amnion is cut into square pieces and stored in special storage medium (Dulbecco's modified Eagle's medium) at 80°C.

Mechanism

The amniotic membrane transplantation works in two ways.

1. Provides physical protection to damaged surface and forms a scaffold for newer epithelial regeneration.
2. Secretes several growth factor and tissue factors which promote proliferation and differentiation of the epithelial cells and fibroblasts.

Indications of Use

- Chemical injury
- Pterygium excision
- Simple limbal epithelial transplantation (SLET)
- Persistent corneal epithelial defects
- Shield ulcer in vernal keratoconjunctivitis
- Some corneal ulcers
- Conjunctival mass excision
- Glaucoma filtering bleb repair
- Socket or fornix reconstruction.

26

CHAPTER

Blindness and its Prevention

BLINDNESS

"Too blind to perform work for which eyesight is essential." —*Parsons.*

The term *blindness* means inability to perceive light. There are at least 65 definitions of blindness throughout the world and they differ widely.

Uniform Definition of Blindness (WHO)

"Visual acuity in the better eye is less than 3/60 (Snellen's) or its equivalent" or in the absence of visual acuity chart-"inability to count fingers in daylight at a distance of 3 meters" (to indicate less than 3/60 or its equivalent).

Categories of Visual Impairment (WHO) (Tables 26.1 and 26.2)

Levels of visual impairment, recommended by World Health Organization (WHO), has been incorporated in International Classification of Diseases (ICD).

Definition of Blindness (National Program for Control of Blindness)

The definition of Blindness under NPCB is modified in line with 'WHO definition': "Presenting distance visually acuity less than 3/60 (20/400) in the better eye and/or limitation of field of vision to be less than 10 degrees from center of fixation". (Previously it was 6/60 and/or <20 degrees visual field).

Few More Definitions

- *Legal blindness:* Visual acuity in the better eye is less than 3/60, and/or, visual field constricted to less than 10° (in India).
- *Economical blindness:* Visual acuity in the better eye is less than 6/60, and/or, visual field constricted to less than 20° (in India).
- *Visually handicapped:* Visual acuity in the better eye is less than 6/18 (in India).

TABLE 26.1: Categories of visual impairment (World Health Organization)		
Categories of visual impairment	**Visual acuity with best correction (better eye)**	
	Maximum vision (less than)	**Minimum vision (equal to or more than)**
Low vision	• 6/18 • 6/60	6/60 3/60
Blindness	• 3/60 (finger counting at 3 m) or, visual field constricted to <10° • 1/60 (finger counting at 1 m) or visual field constricted to <5° • No perception of light (no PL)	1/60 (finger counting at 1 meter) PL (perception of light)

TABLE 26.2: Visual impairment disability categories based on its severity and proposed disability percentages **(Government of India)**

Categories	All with best corrections		Percentage impairment
	Better eye	**Worse eye**	
Category 0	6/9–6/18	6/24 to 6/36	20%
Category I	6/18–6/36	6/60 to no PL	40%
Category II	6/60–4/60 or Field of vision 10–20°	3/60 to no PL	75%
Category III	3/60 to 1/60 or Field of vision <10°	FC at 1 feet to no PL	100%
Category IV	FC at 1 feet to no PL or Field of vision less than 10°	FC at 1 feet to no PL or Field of vision less than 10°	100%
One-eyed person	6/6	FC at 1 feet to No PL	30%
Category I to IV = Visually handicapped (challenged)			

(**PL**—Perception of light; **FC**—Finger counting)

- *Avoidable blindness:* This includes both preventable blindness and curable blindness. 85% of the blindness is estimated to be avoidable.
  - *Preventable blindness:* The blindness which can be easily prevented by attacking the causative factors, e.g. corneal blindness (vitamin A deficiency, trachoma, infectious keratitis, etc.), industrial blindness (by improving occupational safety conditions), retinopathy of prematurity (ROP), diabetic retinopathy, etc.
  - *Curable blindness:* It is almost synonymous with cataract blindness. Others are glaucoma, inflammation of ocular tissues, etc.

In the World, 82% of people, 50 years and older are with visual impairment. The major causes of visual impairment are uncorrected refractive errors (43%) and cataract (33%); the first cause of blindness is cataract (51%) (Table 26.3 and Fig. 26.1).

TABLE 26.3: Causes of blindness in World and India

Causes	World (Vn <3/60)	India (Vn <6/60)
Cataract	51%	62%
Refractive errors	3%	20%
Glaucoma	8%	6%
Corneal opacity	4%	0.9%
Trachoma	3%	0
Posterior segment diseases	–	4.7%
• AMD	5%	–
• DR	1%	–
PCO		0.9%
Surgical complication		1.2%
Childhood blindness	4%	–
Miscellaneous/ undetermined	21%	4.5%

Vn—Vision; **AMD**—Age-related macular degeneration; **DR**—Diabetic retinopathy; **PCO**—Posterior capsular opacification

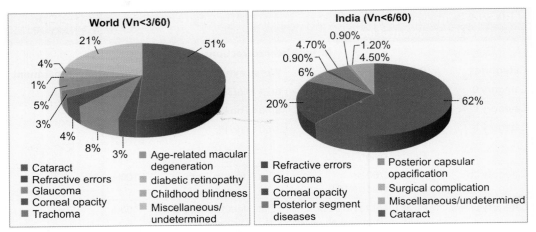

Fig. 26.1: Causes of blindness in World and India

Prevalence of blindness in India
Vision <6/60 in better eye
1986–1989   - 1.49%
2001-2004   - 1.10%
2007 (RAAB/NPCB)   - 1.05% and 0.62% (3/60)

Increase in prevalence is due to population explosion and more old-aged patient.

RAAB = Rapid Assessment of Avoidable Blindness
NPCB = National Program for Control of Blindness

Blindness Data of India

Prevalence of visual impairment and blindness in different age-group statistical data have been described in Tables 26.4 and 26.5.

NATIONAL PROGRAM FOR THE CONTROL OF BLINDNESS

One of the basic human rights is the right to see. We have to ensure that no citizen goes blind needlessly, or being blind does not remain so, if, by reasonable deployment of skill and resources, his sight can be prevented from deteriorating, or if already lost, can be restored.

—*National policy pronounced in 1975*

Overall Objectives of NPCB (1976)

- Provision of comprehensive eye care facilities for *primary, secondary, and tertiary levels* of eye-health care.
- Substantial reduction in the prevalence of eye diseases in general and *reduction in the prevalence of blindness from 1.40% to 0.3% by 2000 AD.*
- National Program for the Control of Blindness (NPCB) was launched by the Government of India, Ministry of Health and Family Welfare in the year 1976 and is a 100% rally sponsored scheme/program with the goal of reducing the prevalence of blindness.
- To reduce the backlog of blindness through identification of treatment of blind and visually handicapped.
  - To develop eye care facilities in every district.
  - To develop human resources for providing eye care services.
  - To improve the quality of service delivery.
  - To secure participation of voluntary organization in eye care.
  - To enhance community awareness of eye care.

TABLE 26.4: Prevalence of visual impairment (WHO-2010)

Blindness	(BCVA <3/60 in better eye)	Low vision (BCVA <6/18 in better eye)	Total visual impairment
World	39 million	246 million	285 million
India	8 million	54.5 million	62.5 million

(*Abbreviation:* **BCVA—Best corrected visual acuity**)

TABLE 26.5: Blindness in different age groups

Age-groups	Causes of blindness
Infants and preschool age	• Congenital cataract • Congenital glaucoma • Optic atrophy • Xerophthalmia • Rare congenital • Anomalies • Trauma • Retinoblastoma • ROP
School-age	• Congenital/developmental anomalies • Neurological (optic neuritis, papilledema) • Trauma
Adult life (20–50 years)	• Pathological myopia • Neurological diseases • Industrial injuries • Diabetes • Infectious diseases
Late adult life (51–70 years)	• Cataract • Glaucoma • Diabetes • Retinal vasculopathies • Trachoma
Elderly life (above 70 years)	• Cataract • Glaucoma • Age-related macular degeneration • Diabetes • Retinal vasculopathies • Trachoma

In 2017, *National Program for the Control of Blindness (NPCB) was changed to National Program for the Control of Blindness and Visual Impairment (NPCBVI).*

Best practices adopted under this new program:

- To reach every part of the country to provide eye care services, provision for setting up Multipurpose District Mobile Ophthalmic Units in the District Hospitals of States/ UTs as a new initiative under the program.
- Provision for distribution of free spectacles to old persons suffering from presbyopia as a new initiative under the program.
- Emphasis on the comprehensive eye care coverage by covering diseases other than

cataract like diabetic retinopathy, glaucoma, corneal transplantation, vitreoretinal surgery, treatment of childhood blindness including retinopathy of prematurity (ROP) etc.

- Strengthening of tertiary eye care centers by providing funds for purchase of sophisticated modern ophthalmic equipment.
- Ensure setting up of superspecialty clinics for all major eye diseases including diabetic retinopathy, glaucoma, retinopathy of prematurity, etc. in state level hospitals and medical colleges all over the country.
- Linkage of teleophthalmology centers at PHC/Vision centers with superspecialty eye hospitals to ensure delivery of best possible diagnosis and treatment for eye diseases, especially in hilly terrains and difficult areas.
- Development of a network of eye banks and eye donation centers linked with medical colleges and RIOs to promote collection and timely utilization of donated eyes in a transparent manner.

Current Infrastructure (2010–2011)

• Apex Institute	1
• Regional Institute of Ophthalmology	20
• Upgraded Medical College	150
• District Hospitals equipped	550
• District Blindness Control Society (DBCS)	575
• Central Mobile Ophthalmic Units	155
• District Mobile Ophthalmic Units	250
• Ophthalmic Assistant training center	100
• Vision Center in Primary Health Center	3,000
• Eye Bank and Eye Donation Centers	650

- ***Ophthalmologists:*** Approximately 20,000 (about one-third in government sector)
- ***Paramedical ophthalmic assistant (PMOA)*** approximately 25,000
- ***Need:*** One ophthalmologist and one ophthalmic assistant per 50,000 population
- Cataract operation performed in the year 2017–2018 = 6.32 million.
- Donor eye collection in the year 2017–2018 = 69,343.

Source: NPCB, Ministry of Health and Family Welfare, Government of India (http://npcb.nic.in)

Methods of Intervention (Fig. 26.2)

Peripheral (Primary) Sector

- Community health worker
- Ophthalmic assistant at primary health center (PHC), block primary health center (BPHC), and rural hospitals.

Service: Primary eye-health care

- Treatment of common eye ailments, e.g. acute conjunctivitis, trachoma, superficial foreign body, etc.
- Treatment of xerophthalmia
- Vitamin A prophylaxis
- Correction of refractive errors
- Screening for cataract
- Teleophthalmology services via vision center.

Intermediate (Secondary) Sector

- Sub-divisional hospitals
- District hospitals

Service: Secondary eye-healthcare (in addition to primary eye care).

- Treatment of common blinding conditions, e.g. cataract, glaucoma, trichiasis, entropion, ocular trauma, etc.
- Mobile ophthalmic units (MOU)
- Eye camp via outreach program.

Central (Tertiary) Sector

- Medical colleges
- State eye hospitals/institutes
- Regional institutes of ophthalmology (RIOs)
- National (Apex) eye institute

Service: Tertiary eye-healthcare (in addition to secondary eye care).

- Sophisticated eye care, e.g. retinal detachment, corneal grafting, and other complex surgeries
- To provide eye bank services
- To provide specialized training programs for all staffs

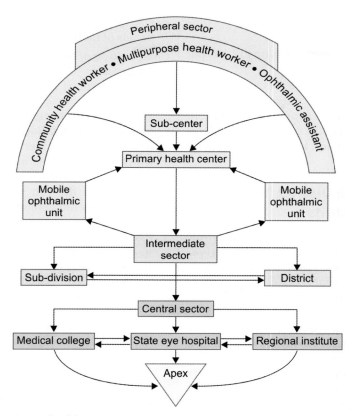

Fig. 26.2: Community eye health care

- To arrange continuing medical education program for the ophthalmologists
- To undertake and promote research activities in ophthalmology.

Apex center (National Eye Institute) is to function as a center of excellence to provide overall leadership, supervision, and guidance in technical matters in planning and implementation of the program.

Dr Rajendra Prasad Center for Ophthalmic Sciences, AIIMS, New Delhi, is identified for this purpose.

Guidelines for Presbyopia under the NPCBVI

This is a new program initiated by the NPCBVI to combat presbyopia-related visual impairment.

Objective of the scheme:
- To further extend eye care services by distributing free spectacles for near work to old persons suffering from presbyopia.
- To take care of elderly people in weaker section of the society.

Criterion for selection of beneficiary and distribution under the scheme:
- Elderly people—45 years and above: Suffering from presbyopia are eligible for free spectacles on the prescription of government eye specialist.
- These patients will be screened for the presbyopic correction in District Hospitals; Medical Colleges and RIOs; and any other Government Hospitals.

- Preference will be given to the persons below poverty line.
- The amount of assistance is up to ₹ 100 per presbyopic spectacles.

The procurement of the spectacles will be made by the respective State/District Health Society by following proper procurement procedures similar to the purchase procedures being followed for purchase of spectacles for school children.

Multipurpose District Mobile Ophthalmic Units

Multipurpose District Mobile Ophthalmic Units (MDMOU) are the new initiatives introduced under the 12th Five Year Plan with a view to further expand eye care coverage in remote and underserved areas. Earlier, it was known as mobile ophthalmic unit (MOU).

It has been approved to develop 400 MDMOU in District Hospitals in a phased manner in the States/UTs during the 12th Five Year Plan. Preference will be given to remote/hilly areas including NE States and underprivileged regions to expand eye care coverage.

The objectives of the scheme are:
- To operationalize MDMOU in district hospitals for improved access to eye care services.
- To further expand eye care coverage.
- To make eye care services available in remote and underprivileged areas of the country.

The activities to be undertaken by MDMOU:
- Screening via eye camps
- School eye health screening
- Transporting patients from screening centers to the nearest district hospital/referral centre for further management
- On the spot refraction and provision for glasses
- Diagnosis of diseases like diabetic retinopathy, glaucoma, etc.

- Display of IEC messages on the outer panels of mobile van.

Composition of the MDMOU:
1. *Manpower:*
   a. Paramedical ophthalmic assistant (PMOA)
   b. Driver and cleaner/helper
2. *Mobile van with following specifications:* It will be a 10-seater passenger carrier which includes driver and helper, a PMOA and six eye patients/school children. The back of the van will be utilized for placing lens box, emergency tray and as store for spare essential material/items.
3. *Essential equipment in mobile van:*
   a. Battery operated torch (2)
   b. Illuminated vision testing drum
   c. Illuminated handheld near vision testing drum
   d. Snellen and near vision charts
   e. Trial lens set with trial frames (2)
   f. Streak retinoscope
   g. Stationary (Glass prescription, OPD slips)
   h. Direct ophthalmoscopes
   i. Tonometers (Schiotz)
   j. Binocular loupe
   k. Epilation forceps
   l. Lignocaine eye drops (4%)
   m. Ishihara color vision chart
   n. Mini storage cabinet with lock facility.

Administrative board of MDMOU:
- District Programme Manager (DPM) will be the officer-in-charge at district level
- The medical officer in the PHC of the area will facilitate the eye camps
- PHC or sub-centre staffs and members of the village health committee
- The post of driver and helper shall be filled up on contractual basis.

Specific National Programs

- *Trachoma control program:* Early diagnosis and treatment can cure trachoma. This program launched in 1963, and has merged with NPCB in 1976.

- *Vitamin A prophylaxis:* 200,000 IU of vitamin A as oil are given orally at 6 months interval between the age of 1 year and 5 years.
- *School eye-health services:* It is estimated that 5–7% of children aged 5–14 years have problems with their eye-sight affecting their participation and learning at the school. This can be easily corrected by a pair of spectacles.

  Other diseases, like, vitamin A deficiency, squint, amblyopia, congenital anomalies, etc. can be detected earlier for further and better management.

The school eye screening program seeks to:
- Screen all children in the age group of 5–14 years for refractive errors (difficulty in clearly seeing distant or near objects).
- Train teachers, preferably with science background, female teachers and those wearing spectacles for identifying children with eye problems.
- Refer children with suspected refractive errors, to the Ophthalmic Assistant at the PHC for refraction.
- Prescription of spectacles.
- Provide children from poor families with free glasses.
- Screening should be on an annual basis. In 2017–2018, more than 7.7 lakh free spectacles have been distributed among school children.
- *Occupational eye-health services:* This is to prevent and treat eye hazards in industries. Education on the prevention of occupational eye hazards and use of protective devices in some occupations are important.

District Blindness Control Society (DBCS)

Features
- Autonomous society to implement NPCB
- Representation consists of government, non-governmental organization, and private sectors

- Decentralized planning, management, and monitoring
- Direct funding from Government of India
- Empowered to utilize and raise funds
- Forum for community participation.

Composition of DBCS

Chairman	District Magistrate/ District Collector/ Deputy Commissioner
Vice-Chairman	Chief Medical Officer (CMO)
Technical Advisor	Head, Department of Ophthalmology of Medical College/District Ophthalmic Surgeon
Member Secretary	Deputy CMO or any Government Officer of equal rank or higher
Members	Representative of non-governmental organization (NGO), private sector and media.

Functions of DBCS
- *Planning:* Preparation of the district micro-plan based on magnitude and distribution of blind persons and resources available for eye care.
- *Implementation of program* through utilization of government facilities, involvement of NGOs, and community participation.
- *Monitoring of program* activities and quality control.
- *Financial and material management.*
- *Social mobilization and public awareness.*
- *Orientation of various functionaries of health* and other sectors, formal and non-formal leaders.
- *Procurement* of good quality refraction sets, drugs, consumable, cataract sets, etc. and maintenance of the equipment.
- *Arrangement* for screening camps, intraocular lens (IOL), spectacles, generator sets, etc.
- *Monitoring and financial assistance* to eye banks and eye donation centers.

Manpower Development

Technical manpower development is an important priority for effective implementation of its services and time-bound targets achievement.

The priority training programs are:
- Training of ophthalmic assistants
- Training of mid-level ophthalmic personnels (MLOPs)
- Orientation training to the medical officers of PHC, BPHC, and rural hospitals about the need of the NPCB
- Refresher training course to the district ophthalmologists and ophthalmic assistants
- Fellowship training to ophthalmologists and teachers of medical colleges under the prevention of blindness program.

Information, Education, and Communication

- Information, education, and communication (IEC) is an important component of the program to increase community awareness on eye health.
- National Program for the Control of Blindness utilizes the print, electronic, and social media to propagate IEC messages in public.
- Information, education, and communication strategy is developed in various states and subsequently followed at district level.
- Local IEC activities include identification, motivation of potential beneficiaries, information through media, educating voluntary groups, teachers and other community-based volunteers including Accredited Social Health Activists (ASHA) identified under National Rural Health Mission (NRHM).
- Interpersonal communication is the most effective method for motivation of target population.

- Select group may be given one day orientation on blind registry, motivation and assistance for providing services for the affected population.
- The orientation program is organized at PHC/CHC.
- National Program for the Control of Blindness coordinates with other national programs like RBSK (Rashtriya Bal Swasthya Karyakram) and Ministry of Social Welfare and Empowerment.
- People suffering from incurable blindness are provided rehabilitation from Ministry of Social Welfare and Empowerment for physical, vocational, and social therapy.

National Program for the Control of Blindness at the district level carries out screening in blind schools where children and adolescents are treated and referred for rehabilitation.

Voluntary organizations

Voluntary organizations or NGOs have played a vital role in the control of blindness in India. They are active in the field of educative, preventive, rehabilitative, and surgical services to control blindness for many years.

Some of the active organizations:
- Vision-2020 India with its members across the country
- The Royal Commonwealth Society for the Blind (sight savers)
- Lions International (sight first)
- Rotary International and its branches
- International Agency for Prevention of Blindness (IAPB)
- Helen Keller International
- ORBIS International and its branches
- Helpage India, etc.
- SightLife International

Other assistances
- WHO assistance
- Danish assistance
- Indo-UK collaboration
- World Bank assistance.

NUTRITIONAL BLINDNESS VITAMIN A DEFICIENCY

Vitamin A deficiency (VAD) along with protein–energy malnutrition (PEM) causes severe blinding corneal destruction.

Most of the time, VAD is precipitated by PEM and other diseases which precipitate malnutrition (e.g. measles, diarrhea, malaria or other acute illness in children).

Again malnutrition is caused by VAD. Together, this blindness is termed as *nutritional blindness*, though the main factor is *VAD*.

Vitamin A deficiency is a systemic disease that affects cells and organs throughout the body.

The resultant changes in epithelial architecture are termed as *keratinizing metaplasia*.

The characteristic ocular manifestations of VAD ranging *from night blindness to corneal melting* are termed as *xerophthalmia (Figs 26.3 and 26.4).*

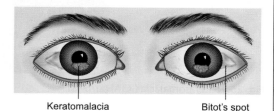

| Keratomalacia | Bitot's spot |

Fig. 26.3: Xerophthalmia

Approximately, one-fifth of preschool-age population of the world is estimated to be vitamin A deficient, with just less than 1% being night blind at any given time.

Vitamin A deficiency is largely limited to the first 4–6 years of life and is especially frequent among those 6 months to 3 years.

In India, about 15,000–20,000 preschool children suffer from VAD at any point of time.

Major Signs and Symptoms of Xerophthalmia (WHO Classification)

```
XN  =  Night blindness
X1A =  Conjunctival xerosis
X1B =  Bitot's spot
X2  =  Corneal xerosis
X3A =  Corneal ulceration/keratomalacia
       (<1/3 corneal surface)
X3B =  Corneal ulceration/keratomalacia
       (>1/3 corneal surface)
XS  =  Corneal scar
XF  =  Xerophthalmic fundus
```

- *XN (night blindness):* It is usually the *earliest manifestation* of VAD; sometimes termed as *chicken eyes* (chicken lack rods and are thus night blind).

Night blindness responds rapidly (within 24–48 hours) to vitamin A therapy.

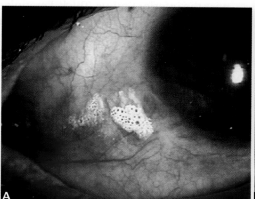
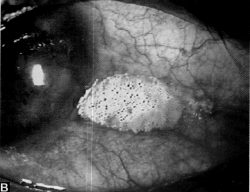

Figs 26.4A and B: Bilateral conjunctival xerosis and Bitot's spot (X1A and 1B)

- **X1A and X1B (conjunctival xerosis and Bitot's spot):** The conjunctival epithelium in VAD, is transformed from normal columnar to stratified squamous with a resultant loss of goblet cells, formation of agranular cell layer and keratinization of the surface.

Conjunctival xerosis (Fig. 26.4A) first appears at the temporal side as an isolated oval or triangular patch, adjacent to the limbus in the interpalpebral fissure. It is almost always present in both eyes.

In some cases, keratin and saprophytic bacilli accumulate on the xerotic surface, giving it a foamy or cheesy appearance. These lesions are known as *Bitot's spots (Fig. 26.4B).*

Isolated, usually temporal, patches of conjunctival xerosis or Bitot's spots are sometimes encountered in absence of active VAD (Fig. 26.5).

In most instances, these patches represent persistent areas of squamous metaplasia induced during an earlier episode of VAD. The only certain means to distinguish an active lesion from an inactive lesion is to observe its response to vitamin A therapy. Active conjunctival xerosis and Bitot's spot begin to resolve within 2–5 days and mostly disappear by 2 weeks.

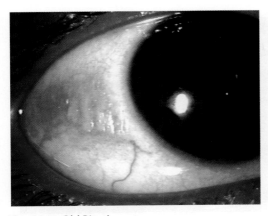

Fig. 26.5: Old Bitot's spot

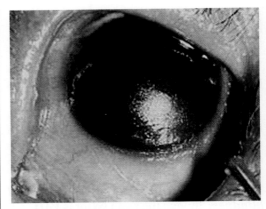

Fig. 26.6: Corneal xerosis (X2)

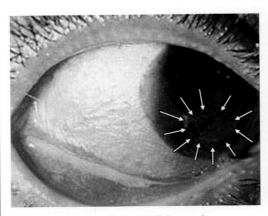

Fig. 26.7: Keratomalacia (X3A) (arrows)

- **X2 (corneal xerosis):** A hazy, lusterless dry appearance of the cornea, is first seen near the inferior limbus. Thick, keratinized plaques may form on the corneal surface and often more dense in the interpalpebral zone (Fig. 26.6).
- Corneal xerosis responds within 2–5 days to vitamin A therapy and it returns to normal appearance by 1–2 weeks.
- **X3A and X3B (corneal ulceration/ keratomalacia) (Fig. 26.7):** They indicate permanent destruction of a part, or all the corneal stroma, resulting in permanent structural alteration.

These ulcers are classically oval or round punched out defects. The surrounding

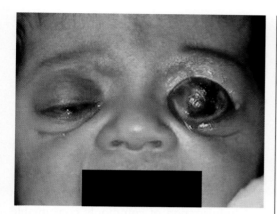

Fig. 26.8: Keratomalacia (right eye) (X3B) and anterior staphyloma (left eye) (Xs)

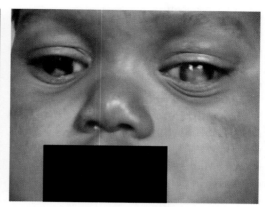

Fig. 26.9: Bilateral xerophthalmic scar (XS)

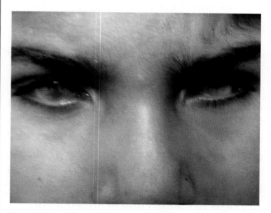

Fig. 26.10: Bilateral old xerophthalmia—phthisis bulbi

cornea is usually xerotic. The ulcer usually starts from slightly inferior and nasal aspects.

Perforation if occurs, becomes plugged with iris, thereby preserving the anterior chamber.

With therapy, superficial ulcers often heal with surprisingly little scarring, but deeper ulcers with perforation form adherent leukoma. Sometimes, a bigger perforation results with extrusion of intraocular contents leading to phthisis bulbi or pseudo-cornea formation leading to anterior staphyloma (Fig. 26.8).

An emergency vitamin A therapy may still save the child's eye to some extent.

- **XS (xerophthalmic scar):** They are usually bilateral and indicate healed sequelae of prior corneal disease related to VAD (Fig. 26.9).

  They include **nebula, macula, leukoma, adherent leukoma, anterior staphyloma or phthisis bulbi (Fig. 26.10).**

- **XF [xerophthalmic (Uyemura's) fundus]:** Small white lesions on the retina, seen in some cases of VAD, are only of academic interest. They may be associated with constriction of the visual fields.

Treatment

Xerophthalmia is a medical emergency as it carries a high risk of corneal destruction and blindness and/or sepsis and death.

Effective therapy is immediate administration of massive doses of vitamin A with concomitant treatment of underlying systemic illness and PEM, and prevention of any recurrence.

Treatment Schedule for Xerophthalmia

Vitamin A (WHO recommendation):
- Immediately upon diagnosis: 200,000 IU vitamin A orally

- Next day: 200,000 IU vitamin A orally
- Within 1–4 weeks: 200,000 IU orally
- Children between 6 months and 11 months old, or less than 8 kg—half the above dose
- Children less than 6 months old: One-quarter of the above dose.

Intramuscular injection of vitamin A (water-soluble) 100,000 IU is usually given, when:
- The children cannot swallow
- In case of persistent vomiting
- In severe malabsorption
- Where the compliance is poor.

Oral liquid, oil-based preparation of retinyl palmitate or retinyl acetate is preferred. It is safe, cheap, and highly effective even in presence of mild diarrhea (as it is also helpful for the intestinal epithelium).

Medical status and diet: Proper treatment includes rehydration, frequent feeding with easily digestible and protein-rich food, and general supportive care. Concurrent illness, e.g. respiratory infection, diarrhea, worm infestation, etc. should also be treated.

Eye care: In case of corneal involvement:
- Board-spectrum antibiotic ointment, e.g. chloramphenicol or ciprofloxacin: 4 times daily
- Atropine eye ointment: 2 times daily
- If secondary infection is present—second antibiotic is added. Subconjunctival injection of gentamicin and atropine may also be given.
- Artificial tears (PVA or povidone iodine or both) eyedrop—4 to 8 times daily.

Preventing recurrence: This is for the vulnerable children.

By inexpensive, readily available vitamin A rich diet.

Periodic administration of a large dose of vitamin A at an interval of 4–6 months to ensure adequate vitamin A store in children (*see* later).

Vitamin A Prophylaxis

Three main intervention strategies are as:
1. Increasing the dietary intake of foods rich in vitamin A and pro-vitamin A
2. Periodic administration of large doses of oral vitamin A
3. Administration of commonly consumable fortified food items (vitamin A fortification).

Increased Intake of Dietary Vitamin A

Dark-green leafy vegetables are usually the least expensive and most widely available source of vitamin A.

> The daily requirement of vitamin A is obtained from a handful of fresh spinach (65 g) as from a small portion of liver (65 g), 4 medium-sized hen's eggs, 1.7 L of whole cow's milk or 6 kg of mutton. The dark-green leafy vegetables should be boiled, shredded (mashed or sieved for the infants), and should be combined with a small amount of edible oil to improve vitamin A absorption.

Sources of vitamin A
- *Vegetable sources:* Dark-green leafy vegetables, spinach, carrot, tomato, pumpkin, etc.
- *Animal sources:* Liver, meat, cod-liver oil, shark-liver oil, egg-yolk, etc.
- *Fortified food items:* Vitamin A enriched commercially available food items.

Daily requirements
- *School children, adolescent and adults:* 2,250 IU (750 µg).

- ***Children (0–4 years):*** 1,000–2,000 IU (300–400 µg).
- ***Pregnancy and lactation:*** 3,000–3,500 IU (750 µg + 300 µg).

Periodic Supplementation

Target group:
- Infants 6–11 months of age (including HIV+): 100,000 IU vitamin A once.
- Children 12–59 months of age (including HIV+): 200,000 IU vitamin A every 4–6 months

Target group is determined by: Where vitamin A deficiency is a public health problem—prevalence of night blindness is 1% or higher in children 24–59 months of age or where the prevalence of vitamin A deficiency (serum retinol 0.70 µmol/L or lower) is 20% or higher in infants and children 6–59 months of age.

This prophylaxis may be for entire neighborhood ***(mass prophylaxis)***, or for high-risk group ***(selective prophylaxis)***.

The high-risk conditions are as follows:
- Children with severe PEM
- Children with measles
- Children with diarrhea, lower respiratory tract infection, or other acute infection (e.g. malaria, chickenpox, etc.).

They should receive a dose of 200,000 IU vitamin A orally at the time of diagnosis by the pediatrician.

Children below 1 year should receive half dose.

Fortification of Dietary Items

Fortification, the addition of selected nutrients to common dietary items, is a successful means of protecting nutritional status of the children.

Dalda, milk, sugar, tea, cereal grains, bread, butter, margarine, etc. may be fortified with vitamin A.

The fortified foods should be inexpensive, stable and virtually undetectable in food vehicle selected, and they should be acceptable to the community.

Ocular Findings in Other Vitamin Deficiencies

Vitamins	Ocular manifestations
Vitamin B₁ (Thiamine)	• Retrobulbar neuritis • Corneal hypoesthesia • Corneal and conjunctival degenerative changes
Vitamin B₂ (Riboflavin)	• Corneal vascularization Punctate epithelial keratitis • Blepharoconjunctivitis
Vitamin B₁₂	• Retrobulbar neuritis
Vitamin C	• Delayed wound healing • Hemorrhage in the conjunctiva, retina or orbit • Keratoconjunctivitis
Vitamin D	• Zonular cataract • Papilledema
Vitamin K	• Hemorrhages in different ocular tissues

VISION 2020: THE RIGHT TO SIGHT

VISION 2020: The Right to Sight is the global initiative for the elimination of avoidable blindness, a joint program of the World Health Organization (WHO) and the International Agency for the Prevention of Blindness (IAPB).

It was launched in 1999.

Aim

To intensify and accelerate present prevention of blindness activities so as to achieve the goal of eliminating avoidable blindness by the year 2020.

"World Sight Day is an annual day of awareness held on the second Thursday of October every year".

Present Position

- Up to 80% of global blindness is avoidable
- 180 million people worldwide are visually disabled
- 40–45 million people are totally blind
- Sixty percent of blind population resides in sub-Saharan Africa, China, and India.

Blindness will continue to increase by 2 million cases/year—unless more aggressive intervention is taken.

Action needed

- Disease control and eye care
- Human resource development
- Provision of appropriate technology and infrastructures.

VISION 2020 will be implemented through 4 five-year plans. The first three have already expired in the year 2015. This last phase will be completed by the year 2020.

Five conditions have identified as immediate priorities within the framework of VISION 2020 program.

1. Cataract
2. Trachoma
3. Onchocerciasis
4. Childhood blindness
5. Refractive errors and low vision.

In India, as there is no onchocerciasis, and trachoma is declining, *two* more diseases have been included recently in VISION-2020 India program.

These are *diabetic retinopathy* and *glaucoma*. They need special attention by all levels of eye healthcare personnel.

Cataract

Problem

- 20 million cataract backlog
- 8 million cataract operation/year globally
- Worldwide problem.

Action

- To eliminate backlog by 2020
- To provide good qualities of surgery:
  - Accessible and affordable to all people
  - High success rate with IOL for all.
- Global cataract operation *target:*
  - 2000 AD—12 million
  - 2010 AD—20 million
  - 2020 AD—32 million.

Trachoma

Problem

- 146 million with active disease
- 10 million trichiasis
- 6 million blind
- Mostly in Africa, South-East Asia, Western Pacific, and Eastern Mediterranean.

Action

- Implementation of SAFE in all endemic countries
- 5 million trichiasis surgery (by 2010)
- Treatment of 60 million people (by 2010).
- Total elimination by 2020.

SAFE strategy for trachoma:

- **S**urgery for trichiasis—the immediate precursor to corneal blindness
- **A**ntibiotics—to treat active diseases—oral azithromycin or 1% tetracycline ointment
- **F**acial cleanliness—to reduce person to person transmission
- **E**nvironmental improvement—to affect the determinants of vulnerability.

Onchocerciasis

Problem

- 17 million people infected
- 0.3–0.6 million blind
- Mainly in African countries.

Action

- Implementation of control program in endemic countries
- Community-directive distribution of *ivermectin*
- Surveillance

- Elimination by 2010 AD
- In 2015, Colombia, Ecuador, and Mexico were the three countries declared free of onchocerciasis.

Dr Satoshi Ōmurao and Dr William C Campbell have been awarded Nobel Prize in Medicine, 2015 for the development of "Ivermectin".

Childhood Blindness

Problem

- 1.5 million blind children in the world:
  - Asia—1 million
  - Africa—0.3 million
- 5 million visually disabled

Action

- Promotion of primary eye care by:
  - Elimination of vitamin A deficiency
  - Measles immunization
  - Prevention of newborn conjunctivitis.
- Development of pediatric eye care services:
  - Surgery for squint, congenital cataract, congenital glaucoma, and retinopathy of prematurity.
  - Low visual aids.

Refractive Errors and Low Vision

Problem

- *Refractive errors*
  - Magnitude not actually known
  - Varies from country to country.
- *Low vision*
  - 35 million in need of low visual aids
  - Will rapidly escalate because of aging and retinal problems.

Action

- Introduction of refractive services at the primary eyecare level
- Vision screening
- Low cost production of glasses and low visual optical devices.

Glaucoma

Glaucoma has been declared to be the second most common cause of blindness in adult population in India. Glaucoma accounts for 8–13% of the blind and 12 million have estimated to have glaucoma. Studies have estimated that this number will increase to 31.6 million by 2020.

Primary angle-closure glaucoma (PACG) is more common than primary open angle glaucoma (POAG) (2–4 times) in Indian population. The high rate of blindness in Indian population is due to high proportion of undiagnosed glaucoma. Glaucoma was undetected in more than 90% of individuals in the population studied.

Diabetes

India has the highest number of people with diabetes in the world with 31.7 million in 2000. This figure is estimated to rise to 79.4 million by 2030.

The prevalence of diabetic retinopathy in general population was 3.5%. The prevalence of diabetic retinopathy in the population with diabetes mellitus was 18.0%.

Human Resource Development

- Number of ophthalmologists per million population has to be increased especially in Africa and Asia.
- Equal distribution of eye care services for urban and rural population.
- *Training of eye care supporting staffs*
  - Ophthalmic medical assistants
  - Ophthalmic nurses
  - Refractionists.
- *Management training*
  - For ophthalmologist
  - For paramedical staffs.
- Ophthalmic technician training.

Mission of VISION 2020 Program

To eliminate the main cause of blindness in order to give all people in the world, particularly the millions of needlessly blind, the right to sight (Fig. 26.11).

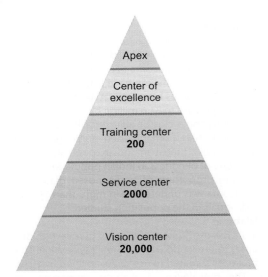

Fig. 26.11: The proposed structure for VISION 2020 program

National Apex Center 1

Centers of excellence 20:
- Profession leadership
- Strategy development

- Continued medical education (CME)
- Laying of standards and quality assurance
- Research.

Training Centers 200

- Tertiary eye care including retinal surgery, corneal transplantation, glaucoma surgery, etc.
- Training and CME.

Service Centers 2000

- Cataract surgery
- Other common eye surgeries
- Facilities for refraction
- Referral services.

VISION Centers 20,000

- Refraction and prescription of glasses
- Primary eye care
- School eye screening program
- Screening and referral services
- Teleophthalmology services with the training centers.

Surgical Instruments

EYE SPECULUMS

The types are—(1) Universal eye speculum, (2) guarded eye speculum, (3) wire speculum.

Universal Eye Speculum (Fig. 27.1A)

Identification: It has a spring and two limbs, and a screw to adjust the limbs. It is called universal because it can be used on either side.

Method: It is fixed to the eyelids in such a way that screw should face outward and forward.

Uses: It is used to separate both eyelids for good exposure of the eyeball mainly during extraocular operations, e.g.

- Pterygium excision
- Squint operation
- Evisceration and enucleation
- Debridement and cautery of corneal ulcer
- To give subconjunctival or sub-Tenon's injection
- Removal of corneal foreign body

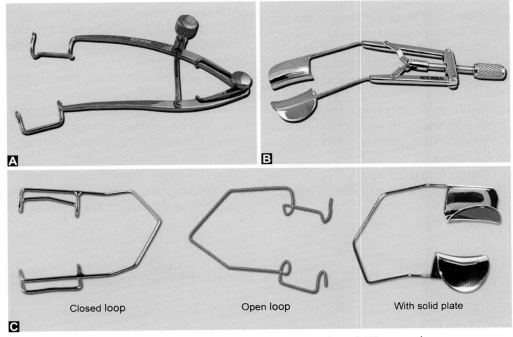

Figs 27.1A to C: A. Universal eye speculum; **B.** Guarded eye speculum; **C.** Wire speculum

- Removal of conjunctival cyst or mass
- During suture removal.

It is not used routinely in intraocular operations as it gives pressure over the globe. This causes rise in intraocular pressure (IOP) during operation. One can put a cotton pellet or assistant can lift the instrument during intraocular operation to avoid rise in IOP. Otherwise, stay sutures to the lids are commonly used for intraocular operation.

Disadvantages

- Since it has no guard, eyelashes of upper lid (larger) come in the field of operation.
- Not used in intraocular operation because of more vitreous up thrust and risk of vitreous loss by direct pressure on the globe.

The speculum should not be confused with Muller's retractor, which has got two or three right-angle sharp-pointed pins (teeth) underneath to engage the skin flap.

Guarded Eye Speculum (Fig. 27.1B)

Identification: The upper limb of the speculum is having a guard plate which keeps the eyelashes of the upper lid away from the field of operation. So, two instruments are required, one for the right eye and the other for the left eye.

Uses: Same as universal eye speculum. It is especially useful in squint operation in children and in pterygium operation.

Disadvantages

- Operating field is reduced
- It is heavier, hence gives more pressure on the globe.

Wire Speculum (Fig. 27.1C)

It is made up of a stainless steel wire and there is no screw. It is of universal type.

It is very light and hence gives little pressure on the eyeball. So, it can be used safely during intraocular operations as well as extraocular operation.

SILCOCK'S NEEDLE HOLDER (FIG. 27.2A)

Identification: This stout instrument has two limbs (one short and one long) and a catch. The short limb has a concave impression at its end for giving pressure with thumb. This is to hold the needle, and an upward stroke with thumb on short limb will automatically release the needle.

ARRUGA'S NEEDLE HOLDER (FIG. 27.2B)

Identification: This stout instrument also has two limbs and a catch similar to Silcock's type. But its long limb is having a broad platform, and thumb rest on short limb is wider without any impression on it.

Uses: It is used to hold the needle (larger needles).

- During suturing the skin and conjunctiva.
- To pass stay sutures through the skin and underneath the superior rectus muscle during intraocular operations.
- To pass stay sutures underneath the rectus muscles in detachment surgery. Needles of 6-0 suture, 8-0 suture or more

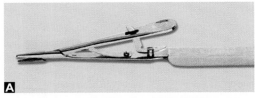
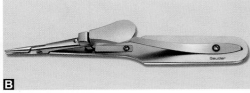

Figs 27.2A and B: A. Silcock's needle holder; **B.** Arruga's needle holder

fine sutures should not be held with these needle holders.

ARTERY FORCEPS (HEMOSTAT) (FIG. 27.3)

Identification: This is a medium-sized, fully serrated forceps with catch. It may be straight or curved. The curved forceps are used more frequently.

Uses

- To hold lid stitches and superior rectus stitch, and then to fix the suture ends with head towel.
- To crush lateral canthus in lateral canthotomy.
- For hemostasis during dacryocystorhinostomy (DCR) or dacryocystectomy (DCT), especially if the angular vein is damaged.
- Fasanella-Servat operation in ptosis (to clamp conjunctiva, tarsal plate, Muller's muscle, and levator muscle).
- To hold muscle stump during enucleation.
- To make irrigating cystitome from a 26-gauge needle.
- To hold whole lacrimal sac prior to excision in DCT.

FIXATION FORCEPS (EYEBALL FIXATION FORCEPS) (FIG. 27.4)

Identification: It is a medium size forceps with 2:3 teeth (maybe 3:4) at its tip.
Method: The conjunctiva and episcleral tissue are firmly held at 6 o'clock position within 3–4 mm of limbus with left hand. Because, the conjunctiva is firmly adhere to episcleral tissue and sclera around the limbus, and it is 4–5 layers thick. It may be used at other part around the limbus (e.g. 3 o'clock, 9 o'clock, etc.).
Uses

- To fix the eyeball during operative procedures, like:
    - Cataract surgery

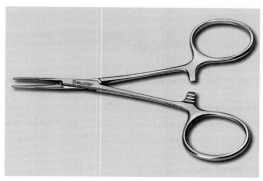

Fig. 27.3: Artery forceps (hemostat)

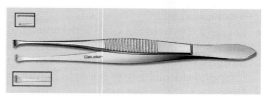

Fig. 27.4: Fixation forceps

- Paracentesis
- Pterygium surgery
- Needling, etc.
- To catch superior rectus muscle to pass bridle suture.
- To catch other tissues, e.g. skin, Tenon's capsule, etc.
- To lift bulbar conjunctiva during sub-conjunctival or sub-Tenon injection.
- Used in forced duction test (FDT) in case of squint to know any mechanical restriction is present or not.
- To hold the sponge piece, gauze piece or cotton ball for swabbing in depth.

VON GRAEFE'S CATARACT KNIFE (FIGS 27.5A AND B)

Identification: It has a thin straight blade with sharp-pointed tip and a cutting edge, the other edge is blunt. The blade may be thin or thick. It may have sliding case arrangement where the sharp blade end is kept in a cover to protect its tip when it is not in use.

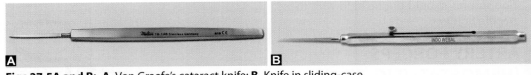

Figs 27.5A and B: A. Von Graefe's cataract knife; **B.** Knife in sliding-case

Method: It is used for **ab interno** corneoscleral section in cataract operation (**ab interno** means—the section is given from inside to outside).

Steps of knife section:
- Lid sutures and superior rectus suture.
- Fix the eyeball with fixation forceps at 6 o'clock position.
- For right eye, hold the knife with right hand and for left eye ideally with the left hand (otherwise surgeon has to move to the left temporal side, if he uses his right hand).
- Hold the knife as pen holding position.
- The tip is introduced into anterior chamber from the temporal limbus; then make the knife horizontal.
- Quickly cross over the iris, pupil, and opposite iris.
- When the tip reaches near the opposite limbus, counter-puncture the cornea just 1 mm inside the limbus (because of refraction of the tip of the blade in aqueous, the tip appears to be displaced).
- When the tip is pierced out the opposite limbus, knife is moved as see saw movement toward 12 o'clock position and the section is completed at upper half of cornea.
- It is preferable to make a triangular flap of conjunctiva along with section at its completion.

Nowadays this knife is not used for routine cataract surgery. It was mainly used in eye camps because:
- It is a quicker procedure.
- Bleeding is minimum.
- Uniform fine section.

Disadvantages
- This type of section is not "guarded", i.e. sudden release of aqueous—leads to sudden decompression of the globe which may cause uveal prolapse or effusion in subchoroidal space.
- Not "stepped", i.e. uniplanar section, so wound closure may not be well secured.

Complications may occur during knife section:
- Loss of anterior chamber and incomplete section. In that case, the section is completed with the help of corneal scissors.
- Involuntary iridectomy or iridotomy.
- Injury to the lens or its capsule.
- Scleral section which may lead to bleeding.
- Subluxation or dislocation of hypermature cataractous lens.
- Conjunctival tear by the fixation forceps.

Test of sharpness of the tip:
- **Drum test:** Touch a mini drum (commercially available previously) with the tip—it will break immediately.
- Sweep a cotton ball along the blade—if there is any catch in cotton fiber, knife tip is not that sharp.

Uses
- **Ab interno** section in case of cataract operation
- Optical iridectomy
- Paracentesis
- Glaucoma iridectomy
- Suture removal after cataract operation
- In pterygium operation to dissect the head, or in chalazion operation to give incision
- Four-point iridotomy in iris bombe (**quadripuncture**).

SCALPEL HANDLE (BARD-PARKER HANDLE) (FIG. 27.6)

Identification: It is a flat handle with a short grooved neck. Handle no. 3 is used in ophthalmic surgeries. The blades are fitted with the neck no. 11 or no. 15 (no. 11 is triangular blade and no. 15 has curved elliptical tip).

Method: In cataract operation.

- The knife is held in pen holding position. Eyeball is fixed with fixation forceps.
- A groove (partial thickness) is made at the limbus with the knife (preferable with no. 15 blade).
- A puncture is made at 11–12 o'clock position to enter into the anterior chamber (preferably with "no. 11" blade).
- Posterior or scleral lip is depressed to drain aqueous very slowly.
- Then the section is enlarged with the corneal scissors.

Uses

- *Ab externo* corneoscleral section for cataract surgery.
- Trabeculectomy operation.
- Skin incision as in DCR, ptosis or other lid surgeries.
- To dissect the pterygium head from the cornea.
- To give incision in chalazion operation.
- For suture removal after cataract operation or keratoplasty.

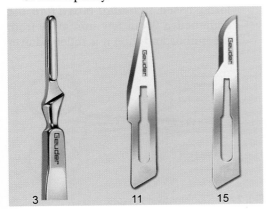

3   11   15

Fig. 27.6: Scalpel handle and blades

Advantages in cataract operation

- It is a "guarded" section. As there is slow release of aqueous, the chance of quick decompression of the globe is almost nil.
- It is "stepped", i.e. biplanar or triplanar incision—so wound security is better.
- Easier for the beginners.

Disadvantages

- Conjunctival flap is usually necessary before giving section.
- It is time-consuming.

BLADE BREAKER

Identification: It is an instrument to break the razor blade (must be a carbon-steel blade, e.g. "Bharat" blade). It is of medium size, with two jaw-like plates at its tip to catch the razor blade firmly. The other end of the instrument is having catch for better grip of the blade. At least eight blade fragments can be made from a single razor blade (Figs 27.7A to C).

Advantages

- It is cheaper than any other knife-blade.
- It is sharper than no. "11"or no. "15" blade.

Disadvantages: As only the breakable carbon-steel razor blade is used—rust formation is a problem.

Uses: Blade breaker with razor blade fragments is having the same uses as Bard-Parker handle with knife.

Instruments used for corneoscleral or clear corneal incision are: (a) Cataract knife, (b) Bard-Parker knife, (c) Blade breaker with razor blade, (d) Disposable super-blades, (e) Keratome, (f) Diamond knife, (g) Laser (femtosecond).

THERMOCAUTERY (HEAT CAUTERY) (FIG. 27.8)

Identification: It is a metallic ball with pointed tip, attached to the end of a handle. The ball is made up of steel or brass (*brass retains heat for a longer time*).

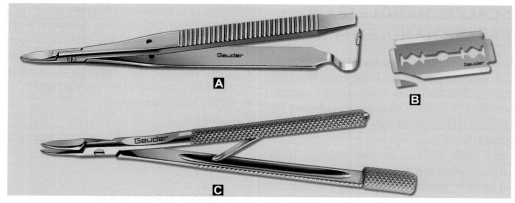

Figs 27.7A to C: A and B. Carbon-steel blade; **C.** Blade breaker

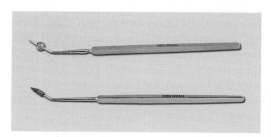

Fig. 27.8: Thermocautery

Method: The metallic ball is heated over the flame of a spirit lamp before cauterization. When it is sufficiently hot, the pointed tip is applied to the bleeding points for hemostasis.

Uses
- To cauterize any superficial bleeding points during operation on the eyeball (e.g. in cataract operation and glaucoma operation after making the conjunctival flap).
- To cauterize the bare scleral area in pterygium surgery.
- To cauterize the margin of a progressive corneal ulcer.
- To cauterize small iris prolapse.
- Temporary punctal occlusion.

Advantages: It is cheap and easily available.

Disadvantages
- As the application of heat is not uniform— there may be more tissue charring at the beginning of cautery.

- More tissue charring may excite more tissue reaction.
  The best method of hemostasis is by diathermy or wet field cautery (*hemostatic eraser*), where the hemostasis is uniform and tissue reaction is minimal.

CONJUNCTIVAL SCISSORS (FIG. 27.9)

Identification: It is a straight fine scissors with pointed tips. It may be curved.

Uses
- It is used to dissect the bulbar conjunctiva in some operations:
  - Conjunctival flap in cataract operation. Here the flap may be limbal-based or fornix-based. In *limbal-based flap*, the conjunctiva is cut few mm away from the limbus and then it is reflected over

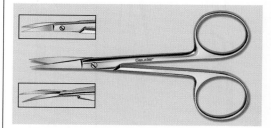

Fig. 27.9: Conjunctival scissors

the cornea from its attached base at the limbus.

In *fornix-based flap*, conjunctiva is cut at the limbus and retracted toward fornix. Fornix-based flap may be better than limbal-based flap in some operations.

- Conjunctival flap in trabeculectomy operation.
- Squint, retinal detachment, enucleation operation, etc.
- It may be used to cut the suture ends.
- It is used to cut other tissues, e.g. Tenon's capsule, pterygium, skin edges, etc.

PLAIN DISSECTING FORCEPS (FIG. 27.10)

Identification: It is an ordinary straight forceps without any teeth at its tips. The ends are little blunt, and on their inner surface, there are fine serrations for better grip.

Uses

- To hold the bulbar conjunctiva during its dissection.
- To hold episcleral tissue during its dissection.
- It is also used during suturing of conjunctiva.
- To hold conjunctiva during subconjunctival injection.
- It may be used to hold small sponge swabs.

CORNEAL SPRING SCISSORS (UNIVERSAL) (FIG. 27.11A)

Identification: It is a small curved spring scissors with sharp small blade. It is called universal, as it is used to cut both right and left half of the section (right half means temporal half of right cornea and nasal half left cornea, left half means temporal half of left cornea and nasal half right cornea).

Note: Right sided corneal scissors means to cut right half of the section and left sided corneal scissors for left half of the section (Fig. 27.11B). In case of universal scissors to cut the right half of the section, surgeon must use his left hand and to cut the left half, use right hand, to avoid any inconvenience. But those who are not proficient with the left hand—they use right and left corneal scissors, and both are operated by right hand.

Method: In case of cataract surgery, after making corneoscleral groove and entering into anterior chamber, one blade of the scissors is introduced into the anterior chamber, the other blade is being outside. Scissors are held

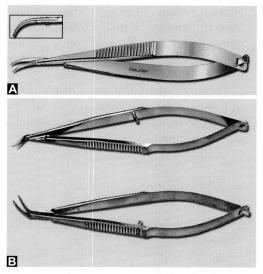

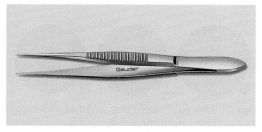

Fig. 27.10: Plain dissecting forceps

Fig. 27.11A and B: A. Corneal spring scissors (universal); **B.** Corneal scissors—right and left sided

in pen holding position, and with small snips, the section is enlarged both on temporal and nasal side up to 120°–160° in upper half. Left hand is used for making right half of the section.

Uses

- To extend **ab externo** section in cataract operation.
- To cut the corneal button from the donor and recipient eyes in case of keratoplasty.
- It may be used to cut the 8-0 suture ends.
- It may be used to cut the iris for iridectomy.
- To make conjunctival flap in cataract or trabeculectomy operation.

IRIS FORCEPS (FIG. 27.12)

Identification: It is a small light-weight forceps with 1:2 teeth on the inner side of its tips. If the limbs are closed, teeth cannot be seen or felt. The shape of the forceps may be straight, curved or angular.

Method of iridectomy

- Hold the instrument in such a way that its tips face toward 12 o'clock position and angle toward 6 o'clock position.
- Now enter into the anterior chamber with close tips and touch the peripheral iris.
- Open the forceps a little to catch a pinch of iris tissue and take out as a triangular fold of iris outside the section.
- Cut a small triangular piece of iris tissue radially with de-Wecker's scissors. Always check the severed iris tissue by rubbing it over face mask.

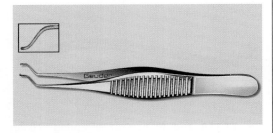

Fig. 27.12: Iris forceps

This is to see the pigmented layer has cut or not, i.e. if there is release of pigment—it means iridectomy has done in full thickness.

Uses: To grasp the iris tissue in various types of iridectomies.

Iridectomy: It is usually done in upper part as it is covered by the upper lid. There will be diplopia (in case of peripheral iridectomy) or dazzling (in case of complete iridectomy) of light, if the iridectomy is done in the lower part, as the lower part of iris is not covered by the lower lid.

There is usually *no bleeding during iridectomy* as iris vessels are highly contractile. Iridectomy is avoided in case of diabetic cataract and rubeosis iridis as there may be chance of bleeding.

Types of iridectomy with indications (Figs 27.13A to C)

- *Peripheral button-hole iridectomy:* (At 11 and/or 1o'clock position) one full thickness iridectomy is equally effective as two iridectomies. The indications are:
  - In intracapsular cataract extraction
  - Angle-closure glaucoma
  - As a part of trabeculectomy operation
  - Sometimes, in penetrating keratoplasty operation.
  - When an ACIOL is implanted
  - In endothelial keratoplasty procedures (DSEK/DMEK)
  - In vitreoretinal surgeries.

  It is not mandatory in extracapsular cataract extraction. Peripheral iridectomy is done to prevent papillary block glaucoma and consequent iris prolapse in case of intracapsular

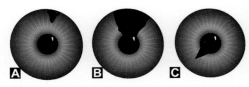

Figs 27.13A to C: Different types of iridectomy. **A.** Peripheral button-hole; **B.** Sector (complete); **C.** Optical

cataract extraction (ICCE). As the aqueous can flow into the anterior chamber via this bypass channel, equilibrium between the anterior chamber and posterior chamber is maintained after ICCE.

- **Optical iridectomy:** In case of central corneal opacity where facilities for keratoplasty are not available and rarely in polar cataracts.

  It is done in the lower part of the iris, as in upper part, the new opening will be covered by upper lid. The best site for optical iridectomy is judged by stenopeic slit test, and it must be at the clearest zone. Customarily, it is said that the site of election will be down and in for the literates, and down and out for illiterates.

- **Broad or complete iridectomy:** To facilitate the extraction of lens (combined extraction of cataract) when pupil is small and rigid, or if there is extensive synechiae, and if there is vitreous loss after cataract extraction.

- **Iridectomy for prolapsed iris.**
- **Iridectomy to remove foreign body on the iris.**
- **Iridectomy to remove tumor or cyst of the iris.**
- **Inferior iridectomy** in cases of vitreo-retinal surgery with silicon oil injection.
- **Yttrium aluminum garnet (YAG) laser peripheral iridectomy** is better in acute attack of angle closure glaucoma as it is a noninvasive (so no chance of infection) outpatient department (OPD) procedure. It is also less expensive for the patient.

Iridotomy: Puncture of the iris without abscission of any portion.

- To create an artificial pupil when the true pupil is closed or severely updrawn.
- **Four point iridotomy** is done by a von Graefe's cataract knife to treat secondary glaucoma in iris bombe.

DE-WECKER'S IRIS SCISSORS (FIG. 27.14)

Identification: It is a butterfly-shaped spring scissors with the cutting blades bent at an angle of 60° with the handle. On the handle, there are two wings for index finger and thumb. Its one blade has pointed tip and the other blade has rounded tip.

Method: Scissors is held in such a way that the plane of blade lies at the same plane as of iris, whereas the handle is almost vertical.

De-Wecker's can be replaced by angular Vannus' scissors for the same uses.

Uses

- It is used to cut a piece of iris tissue in iridectomy.
- It is used for anterior or open-sky vitrectomy, if there is any vitreous loss during cataract extraction.
- It is used to cut the trabecular tissue with a part of sclera in trabeculectomy operation.
- It may be used to cut the suture ends (8-0 or 10-0 sutures) during corneascleral suturing.

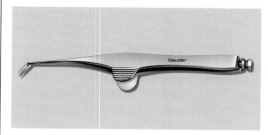

Fig. 27.14: De-Wecker's iris scissors

INTRACAPSULAR FORCEPS

Identification: There are two types of intracapsular forceps.

1. **Elschnig's:** It has no tooth, and is double curved with blunt tips (Fig. 27.15A).
2. **Arruga's:** It has also no tooth, and is single curved. Its tips are more blunt (knob-like) and have cups on their inner surfaces (Fig. 27.15B).

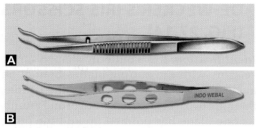

Figs 27.15A and B: Intracapsular forceps
A. Elschnig's; **B.** Arruga's

Methods

- *Lower pole delivery (Arruga's method)*
  - Here mid-peripheral lens capsule is grasped at 6 o'clock position by intracapsular forceps carefully, without catching the iris.
  - Side-to-side movement is made and simultaneous pressure over the zonules is given by the lens expressor (taken in the left hand) from outside to tear them.
  - Cataractous lens is taken out by tumbling (i.e. lower pole is delivered first).
- *Upper pole delivery (Kirbi's methods)*
  - Here mid-peripheral lens capsule is grasped at 12 o'clock position after retracting the iris (sometimes, a complete iridectomy is done to facilitate upper pole delivery).
  - (Same as above) Pressure from outside at limbus is given by lens expressor to break the zonules.
  - Lens is delivered by sliding (i.e. upper pole is delivered first).

Lower pole delivery (i.e. tumbling) is better as tumbling itself gives support to the anterior vitreous face, so there is less chance of vitreous loss.

Uses

- Intracapsular cataract extraction
- To remove capsular tags in extracapsular cataract extraction (ECCE)
- As a suture tier
- To hold suture ends during suture removal
- To remove clots from the anterior chamber as in clotted hyphema
- To remove caterpillar hair.

Advantages of intracapsular forceps in cataract extraction:

- No assistant is required
- It is cheap and quick procedure—useful for camp surgery.

Disadvantages

- It is not preferred in intumescent or hypermature morgagnian cataract, where the capsule may be torn.
- It is a difficult procedure for the beginners.

Complications of Intracapsular Forceps Extraction

- Iris may be caught—leading to iridodialysis and hyphema.
- Capsule may be torn—leading to accidental ECCE.
- Lens may get dislocated into the vitreous due to excessive pressure.
- Corneal endothelial damage by the tip of the forceps.
- Capsular grasp may open up in the midway of the procedure.

Cryoextraction of Cataract (Fig. 27.16)

It is a very safe procedure and useful for the beginners. The gases used for the formation of iceball are: (i) Nitrous oxide and (ii) Freon.

Temperature at cryoprobe tip is about –40°C to –60°C.

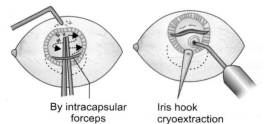

By intracapsular forceps   Iris hook cryoextraction

Fig. 27.16: Methods of intracapsular cataract extraction

Here a pencil-tipped insulated cryoprobe is applied over the anterior surface of the lens while retracting the iris. The assistant lifts the cornea during the whole procedure. When the iceball forms (i.e. when the adhesion of cryoprobe with the lens capsule and cortex is good) little side-to-side movement is made to tear the zonules. Thereby cataractous lens is extracted by sliding.

Advantages
- It is useful in all types of cataract, e.g. immature, mature, and hypermature.
- Safe technique—for the beginners.

Disadvantages
- Accidental cryotouch to the cornea or iris may cause damage.
- Mechanical failure of the instrument.
- More costly and sometimes not portable.

LENS EXPRESSOR (LENS HOOK) (FIG. 27.17)

Identification: It has a flat corrugated handle with a curved, olive-pointed blunt tip. The plane of the flatness of the handle is perpendicular to the plane of curvature of the limb.

Uses
- During intracapsular extraction of the lens, either by intracapsular forceps or by Smith-Indian technique.
  Pressure is applied from outside at the limbus and adjacent part of the cornea at 6 o'clock position. This is to facilitate zonular tear. Then a gradual support is given at the lower pole of the lens.

- In case of extracapsular cataract operation—to deliver the nucleus.
- Milking out the cortical materials with the knee or bend of the instrument in ECCE.
- It may be used to hook the extraocular muscles.
- It may also be used as a fine tissue retractor, particularly in DCR operation to retract the sac during punching or breaking the bone.

McNAMARA'S SPOON (LENS SPATULA)

Identification: It is a straight long instrument with two flat spoons or spatula at the two ends. One of the spoons may be perforated at its center (Fig. 27.18).

Uses
In intracapsular cataract extraction: Along with lens hook, the lens is delivered by pressure and counter-pressure (Smith-Indian technique). Spoon is in the left hand outside the section and lens expressor is in the right hand at the lower limbus. By giving pressure and counter-pressure, lens is delivered out by tumbling or by sliding.

Advantages
- No instrument is introduced into the anterior chamber, so endothelial damage is less.
- Useful in camp surgery—as this method works best in hypermature cataract (in camp number of hypermature cataract is more).
- No assistant is needed.

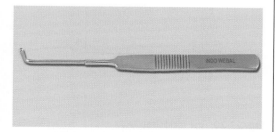

Fig. 27.17: Lens expressor (hook)

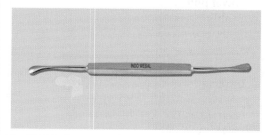

Fig. 27.18: Lens spatula

Disadvantages

- Not a very good method for immature cataract.
- Chance of vitreous loss is more.
- A difficult technique.
  - To deliver the nucleus in extracapsular cataract operation.
  - The perforated spoon end may be used as a vectis to deliver the subluxated or dislocated lens.

Erysiphake extraction of ICCE: It is an instrument that uses vacuum or negative pressure to grasp the lens (anterior lens capsule and cortex) in intracapsular cataract extraction.

It is not used nowadays. It was used previously to deliver the immature cataractous lens where intracapsular forceps could not be used.

VECTIS (WIRE VECTIS) (FIG. 27.19)

Identification: It is a ring of wire (round or oval) at the end of an arrow limb, attached to a handle (like a large platinum loop). It may be little curved like a spoon.

Method: Pupil must be fully dilated. Never pass it blindly. The lens edge should be visible. Carefully pass the vectis behind the lens. Lift the lens and then take the lens out. Vitreous loss is inevitable in vectis delivery. Sometimes, a sector iridectomy is needed instead of peripheral iridectomy. Open-sky vitrectomy is done after lens delivery.

Uses

- To remove a subluxated or dislocated lens.
- To deliver the nucleus in ECCE with irrigating vectis.

  If the vectis is not available, the instruments may be used as vectis:
  - Perforated end of McNamara's spoon.
  - Intracapsular forceps—here apply forceps with closed tips, carefully pass it behind the lens and then open the tips little bit so that lens sit well on it. Now, lift the lens and remove it.

IRIS REPOSITOR (FIG. 27.20)

Identification: It is an elongated "S" or "Z"-shaped instrument with a stout handle and two long narrow flattened extremities. Both the edges and tips are blunt. Its one end may be curved and other end may be angulated.

Method: A few strokes over the peripheral iris on its upper part are required to reposit the iris. When the iris is properly repositioned the pupil becomes perfectly circular and central.

Uses

- To reposit the iris after the delivery of lens in ICCE or after nucleus delivery in ECCE. In fact, the assistant must be ready with this instrument when the surgeon is delivering the lens or nucleus.
- To reposit the iris after iridectomy.
- To retract the iris during cryoprobe application over the anterior surface of the lens in ICCE.

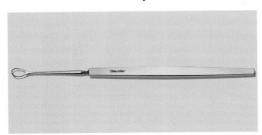

Fig. 27.19: Wire vectis

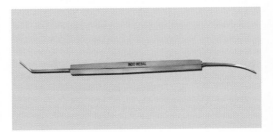

Fig. 27.20: Iris repositor

- To bring air from posterior chamber to anterior chamber during intracapsular cataract surgery.
- To break the adhesions in synechiae (synechiolysis).
- To bring back the folded conjunctiva to cover the wound.
- Lamellar dissection of the cornea in lamellar keratoplasty.

Precaution: Iridectomy site should be avoided during repositioning of the iris. If reposition is not done properly there may be:
- Iris incarceration at the wound
- Prolapse of the iris
- Chance of infection
- Gaping of the wound
- Non-reformation of the anterior chamber.

NEEDLE HOLDER (BARRAQUER'S AND CASTREVEIJO'S) (FIGS 27.21A AND B)

Identification: It is a medium-sized spring needle holder with two narrow and fine curved jaws. It may be available with or without a catch.
Uses: It is used to hold the fine needles (of 6-0, 8-0 and 10-0 sutures) for:
- Corneoscleral suturing after cataract operation.
- Scleral suturing in squint, detachment, and trabeculectomy operations.
- Corneal suturing in penetrating injury or keratoplasty.

- Suturing the mucosal flaps in DCR operation.
- Sometimes in conjunctival suturing.

Castroveijo's needle holder is mainly required to hold slightly large needles (of 4-0 to 6-0 sutures) for conjunctival suturing as in squint, glaucoma, pterygium or retinal detachment.

COLIBRI FORCEPS (FIG. 27.22A)

Identification: It is a curved or angular forceps with fine limbs, having 1:2 teeth at its tip. It is thicker and stout.

ST. MARTIN'S FORCEPS (FIG. 27.22B)

Identification: It is a straight small but stout forceps with 1:2 teeth at its fine tip.
Uses: Both instruments have similar uses:
- To hold the cornea and sclera lips during corneoscleral suturing after cataract surgery, and corneal lips in repair of penetrating injury or wound closure in keratoplasty.
- It is also used to hold the scleral lip for dissection and sclera suturing (as in trabeculectomy operation).
- It is used to hold the corneal lip in cataract operation to extend the section with corneal scissors.
- To lift the cornea upward during application of the cryoprobe.

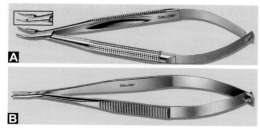

Figs 27.21A and B: Needle holder. **A.** Barraquer's; **B.** Castreveijo's

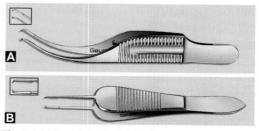

Fig. 27.22A and B: **A.** Colibri forceps; **B.** St. Martin's forceps

- It may be used to catch the iris for iridectomy.

SUPERIOR RECTUS HOLDING FORCEPS

Identification: It is a stout forceps with double curvature (S-shaped) at its ends. It has 1:2 teeth at its tip. Its curvature at the tip is to fit with the curvature of the globe (Fig. 27.23).

Uses: It is used to catch the superior rectus muscle belly for passing stay (bridle) sutures, so that the eyeball can be rotated and fixed downward in cataract, glaucoma or other surgery. It is also used to catch the inferior rectus muscle as in keratoplasty.

There is always a chance of superior rectus muscle injury while passing SR bridle suture. Many surgeons prefer to give limbal corneal stay suture during glaucoma surgery.

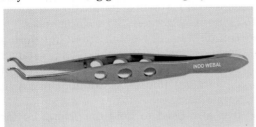

Fig. 27.23: Superior rectus holding forceps

SUTURE TIER FORCEPS (FIG. 27.24)

Identification: It is a small straight or curved forceps with long fine limbs. It does not have any tooth at its tip. The tips are made stout by extra thick platform.

Uses
- To hold the suture ends during tying the sutures after proper tightening.
- To hold the cut ends of the suture during its removal.
- May be used to catch the margin of incised conjunctiva during suturing.
- To remove caterpillar hair.

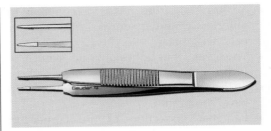

Fig. 27.24: Suture tier forceps

BOWMAN'S DISCISSION NEEDLE (FIG. 27.25)

Identification: It is a straight fine needle, attached to a handle. Its tip is very sharp, pointed and diamond-shaped. There may be a guard at the middle of the needle to prevent deeper penetration into the eye.

Uses
- Discission or needling of congenital and childhood traumatic cataract.
- Needling of "after-cataract" to create an aperture in the papillary area.

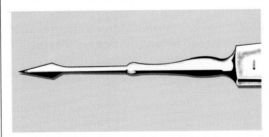

Fig. 27.25: Bowman's discission needle

ZEIGLER'S KNIFE (FIG. 27.26)

Identification: It is a tiny curved or sickle-shaped, sharp-pointed knife blade at the end of narrow limb, attached to a handle.

Uses
- Discission of "after-cataract" to create a gap in the papillary area.
- In discission or needling of congenital or traumatic cataract.

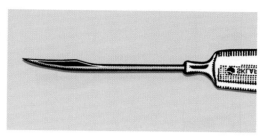

Fig. 27.26: Zeigler's knife

- To incise the iris, in up-drawn pupil complicated by cataract surgery.
- To cut and separate the iris in adherent leukoma.

Surgery in congenital, developmental or childhood-traumatic cataract: Operation should be done as early as possible to prevent amblyopia (may be within 6 weeks after birth).
- *Needling and aspiration*
  - *Single stage:* As in total cataract.
  - *Two stages:* As in partial cataract. Not used nowadays because repeated surgeries are needed due to quick posterior capsule opacification (PCO) or after-cataract formation in almost all cases.
- *Planned extracapsular cataract extraction (ECCE):* As in adult ECCE. Posterior chamber intraocular lens (PCIOL) implantation may be considered along with ECCE if the child is more than 3 years.
- Extracapsular cataract extraction with PCIOL with primary posterior curvilinear capsulorhexis.
- Pars plana lensectomy with anterior vitrectomy is also an alternative choice.

LASER TREATMENT FOR POSTERIOR CAPSULE OPACIFICATION

This is especially useful in PCO following ECCE with PCIOL implantation. It is known as *YAG laser capsulotomy*. It is done with Nd-YAG laser beam by a slit-lamp delivery system (Nd means *neodymium*; YAG means *yttrium aluminum garnet*).

This laser acts by photodisruption of the tissues.

Advantages
- It is a noninvasive procedure, chance of infection is nil.
- It is an OPD procedure.
- It is safe and painless.

Disadvantages
- Not widely available in district or sub-divisional level as it is costly.
- Retina check-up is essential after the procedure.
- It is very difficult in children and non-cooperative patient.

CAPSULOTOMY FORCEPS

Identification: It is a small curved forceps having 3:4 teeth hanging downward from the end of the curved limbs (Fig. 27.27A).
Uses: To tear the anterior capsule in extra-capsular cataract operation.

It is not used nowadays as the capsular opening is not perfect and there may be damage to the corneal endothelium. It was done by open method, i.e. after limbal section.

Nowadays a bent tipped 26 gauge needle is used as a capsulotome or cystitome (Fig. 27.27B) which is fitted with a 2 mL syringe. Here, the capsulotomy is done by a close method after making limbal groove. The syringe is filled with balanced salt solution (BSS) or Ringer's lactate to keep the anterior chamber well formed during needle manipulation. The

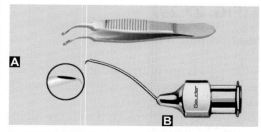

Figs 27.27A and B: A. Capsulotomy forceps; **B.** Cystitome

capsule is cut with the bent tip of the needle in a continuous circular fashion capsulorhexis, or by interrupted multiple puncture by can-opener technique or stamp-hole technique. After withdrawing the needle, the limbal section is extended and loose circular anterior capsule is removed.

CAPSULORHEXIS FORCEPS (UTRATA FORCEPS) (FIG. 27.28)

Identification: It is a fine long forceps with curved sharp tip without any tooth.

Uses: To perform continuous curvilinear capsulorhexis (CCC) in case of manual SICS or in phacoemulsification.

The initiation of rhexis is started with a 26 gauge needle, and then completed with the rhexis forceps, or it may be with the rhexis forceps alone.

It may be used to remove small capsular tag.

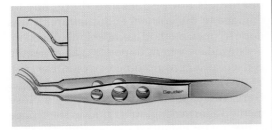

Fig. 27.28: Capsulorhexis forceps (Utrata)

IRRIGATING VECTIS (FIG. 27.29)

Identification: It is a hollow vectis fitted with a needle base. Its tip has 3–5 small openings for free passage of irrigating solution. The maximum horizontal diameter of the vectis is 5.0–5.5 mm.

Use: The vectis is connected with the tubing system of a Ringer's lactate or BSS bottle, or it may be fitted with a Ringer's lactate or BSS filled 2cc syringe during nucleus delivery.

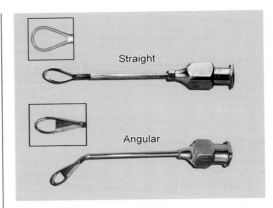

Fig. 27.29: Irrigating vectis

The irrigating fluid creates hydrostatic pressure and at the same time mechanical pull by the vectis is to deliver the nucleus out. Posterior scleral lip depression and simul-taneous counterbalancing force by superior rectus bridle suture are the important steps during nucleus delivery.

IRRIGATION-ASPIRATION TWO-WAY CANNULA (SIMCOE CANNULA)

Identification: It is a two-way cannula, one end of which is attached to a blunt needle via a silicone tube. Normally, this end is fitted with an irrigation or infusion system and the two-way cannula itself is fitted with a 2 mL or 5 mL syringe for aspiration (Fig. 27.30). *Method:* After delivery of the nucleus in ECCE, the cannula is introduced into the anterior chamber. The infusion is slowly started either from a hanging Ringer's lactate or BSS bottle (or, alternately assistant may irrigate via BSS filled 10 mL syringe). As the anterior chamber is formed, the surgeon starts aspirating cortical material slowly till the posterior capsule is cleaned (as appreciated by brilliant fundal glow under co-axial illumination of the operative microscope).

Uses
- For simultaneous irrigation and aspiration of cortical materials in case of ECCE or ECCE with PCIOL.

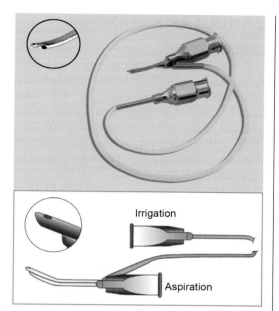

Fig. 27.30: Irrigation-aspiration two-way cannula (Simcoe cannula)

- To remove viscoelastic material after insertion of IOL.
- May be used to remove blood in hyphema.

McPHERSON'S FORCEPS (FIG. 27.31)

Identification: It is a fine medium-size toothless forceps with an angulation at about 7–8 mm from its tip.

Uses
- It is used to hold the intraocular lens during its placement in the posterior chamber.
- It is used to catch and remove the loose anterior capsule after completion of capsulotomy.
- It may be used as a suture tier during suturing with 10-0 nylon.

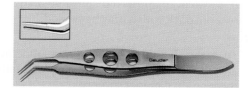

Fig. 27.31: McPherson's forceps

VANNAS' SCISSORS (FIG. 27.32)

Identification: It is much smaller scissors with spring action. It may be straight, curved or angular.

Uses
- To prepare conjunctival flap.
- To cut 10-0 sutures in cataract or keratoplasty operation.
- To cut trabecular flap in trabeculectomy.
- To cut anterior capsular tags in ECCE.
- To cut vitreous in open-sky vitrectomy, as in vitreous loss during ICCE or ECCE.
- To cut corneal button after trephination in corneal grafting.
- To cut iris in different types of iridectomy.

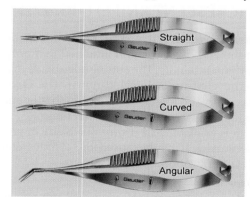

Fig. 27.32: Vannas' scissors

INTRAOCULAR LENS DIALLER (SINSKY'S HOOK) (FIG. 27.33)

Identification: It is an angular fine hook attached to a long round solid handle.

Methods and uses
- It is used to dial the IOL for the purpose of centration and bringing the IOL-haptics in horizontal position. The hook is positioned in the dialing holes of the optic of IOL, and then to rotate in clockwise manner.
- It may be used as a left hand instrument during phacoemulsification:
  - To rotate the lens nucleus.

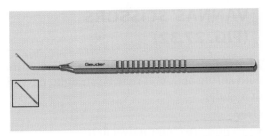

Fig. 27.33: Intraocular lens dialler (Sinsky's hook)

- To crack the lens nucleus after doing quadrant trenching.
- To chop the nucleus.
- It is used to break the posterior synechiae (synechiolysis) during ECCE.

SCLEROCORNEAL SPLITTER (CRESCENT KNIFE) (FIG. 27.34)

Identification: It has a thin crescentic blade, at the end of a neck and attached to a poly-carbonate handle. The cutting edge blade may be beveled-up or beveled-down. The blade has a forward angulation of 45° for better and parallel movement during dissection.

It is available as a disposable blade in pre-sterile pack. It may be reused for 3–4 times after ETO sterilization.

Uses
- Used to make sclerocorneal tunnel in manual SICS or phacoemulsification.
- Used for lamellar dissection of the cornea in lamellar keratoplasty.

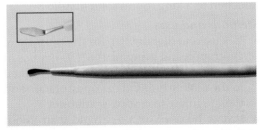

Fig. 27.34: Sclerocorneal splitter (Crescent blade)

ANGULAR KERATOME

Identification: It has a thin triangular blade, at the end of a neck and attached to a poly-carbonate handle. The cutting edge blade may be beveled-up or beveled-down. The blade has a forward angulation of 45° for better and parallel movement during dissection. The width of the blade may be 2.8–3 mm diameter (for phacoemulsification) or 4.5–5.5 mm for manual SICS (Fig. 27.35).

It is also available as a disposable blade in pre-sterile pack. It is advisable not to reuse these disposable blades.

Uses
- Used to enter into the anterior chamber after making sclerocorneal tunnel in manual SICS or phacoemulsification.
- It may be used directly for making corneal section in phacoemulsification.
- 4.5–5.5 mm diameter keratome is used to enlarge the tunnel.

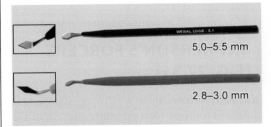

Fig. 27.35: Angular keratome

SIDE-PORT BLADE (FIG. 27.36)

Identification: It has a thin, long straight blade, at the end of a neck and attached to a polycarbonate handle. Sometimes, it has got 15° angulation. The maximum width of the blade is to pass a 20 G needle.

It is also available as a disposable blade in pre-sterile pack which may be reused.

Uses
- To make the side-port (to enter into the anterior chamber from the side of main incision) in cataract surgery.

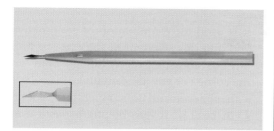

Fig. 27.36: Side-port blade (15 degree)

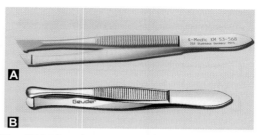

Figs 27.37A and B: A. Rhomboidal tip; **B.** Elliptical tip

Indication of side-port

- For paracentesis
- To inject viscoelastic substance
- To inject trypan blue dye
- To clean subincisional lens cortex by irrigation aspiration cannula
- To manipulate second instrument (like phaco-chopper, Sinsky hook, etc.) in case of phacoemulsification. Some-times, two side-ports are given on either side of main port for bimanual irrigation and aspiration
- To insert the anterior chamber main-tainer.
- It is also used for paracentesis to drain blood in hyphema.
- To remove small intracameral foreign body.

EPILATION FORCEPS (CILIA FORCEPS)

Identification: It is a small stout forceps with blunt flat ends. Near the tip, the inner surfaces are reinforced by extra-thick platform which may be rhomboidal or elliptical (Figs 27.37A and B).

Uses

- To remove the offending, misdirected eyelashes in trichiasis.
- To remove the involved eyelash in stye.

No anesthesia is required for epilation. It is not an ideal technique as it is not a permanent procedure. As the root is not destroyed, eyelash grows again within 6–8 weeks and causes same irritation.

Ideal method should be permanent where the hair-root is destroyed.
Ideal methods are:

- *Electrolysis:* Anesthesia is required. A fine needle (the negative pole) is introduced into the hair follicle and a current of 2 mA is passed. Endpoint is noted by:
  - Appearance of foam due to liberation of nascent hydrogen and saponification, at the root.
  - Eyelash can be easily lifted (no pulling against resistance).
- *Electrodiathermy:* A current of 30 mA is applied for 10 seconds.
- *Cryosurgery:* Pigmentation is a problem.
- If more than one-third lid margin is involved with trichiasis—partial entropion correction operation is better choice.

STRABISMUS HOOK (MUSCLE HOOK OR SQUINT HOOK) (FIG. 27.38)

Identification: It has a solid handle with a long narrow limb with 90° bent at its tip. The tip may be sharp or knobbed. The handle is not corrugated and the plane of curvature of the limb is same as the plane of handle.

Uses

- It is used to hook the extraocular muscles during:
  - Squint operation
  - Retinal detachment operation
  - Enucleation operation.
- Occasionally, it may be used as tissue retractor.

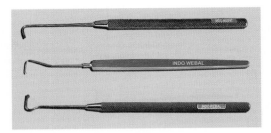

Fig. 27.38: Strabismus hooks

LID RETRACTOR (DESMARRE'S) (FIG. 27.39)

Identification: It is a saddle-shaped folded instrument at the end of a metallic handle. It is of varying size depending upon the size of the palpebral aperture. It is not self-retaining.

Method (for children)
- Patient is made to lie on the table and an assistant must fix his head.
- Lignocaine (4%) eye drop is instilled.
- Lid retractor is introduced in the eye from the temporal side sliding against the eyeball.
- Upper lid is retracted and the eye is examined.
- As the lower lid can be easily retracted by finger normally, lower lid retractor is not necessary. But in some cases of severe blepharospasm, two retractors are needed.

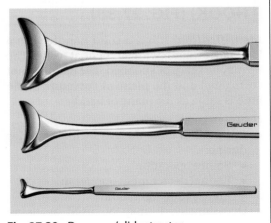

Fig. 27.39: Desmarre's lid retractor

Uses
- It is used for examination of conjunctiva and anterior segment of the eye—to find out any abrasion, ulcer, foreign body on the cornea or any abnormality:
  - In children and noncooperative patient.
  - In case of severe blepharospasm and photophobia.
  - In case of lid edema.
- For removal of corneoscleral stiches (better than eye speculum) after cataract surgery.
- To examine upper fornix by double eversion of the lid.
- It may be used as a tissue retractor (e.g. to retract conjunctiva and Tenon's capsule in squint and detachment operation).

FOREIGN BODY SPUD AND NEEDLE (FIGS 27.40A AND B)

Identification: The spud has a straight narrow limb with blunt tip with a handle. One surface of the limb is flat and the other is convex. The needle is tiny scoop with sharp pointed tip on a narrow limb with a handle. These two instruments may be available with one handle—one on either end.

Methods and uses
- The spud is used to remove the superficial corneal foreign body. With the convex smooth surface of the spud, foreign body is removed by gentle stroke.
- The needle is used to remove the embedded foreign body from the cornea.

In both the cases, the direction of the stroke is from the central part toward the periphery. Otherwise, the central part of the cornea may be damaged.

Both the instruments are not used now-a-days because of their broader tip which may cause more damage to the cornea.

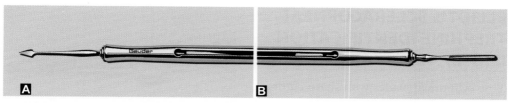

Figs 27.40A and B: A. Foreign body spud; **B.** Foreign body needle

Steps for removal of foreign body:

- Search for the foreign body with a good torchlight and if necessary with a loupe (a slit-lamp is much better).
- Evert the upper lid to find out any foreign body in the subtarsal sulcus. *This is the most common site of lodgement of a foreign body.* If it is there, remove it with a sterile cotton swab or pellet, even without anesthesia.
- If the foreign body is on the cornea, put 4% lignocaine or 1% proparacaine drop to anesthetize the ocular surface.
- If it is superficial, remove the foreign body with a sterile cotton swab or a sterile triangular blotting paper simply by touching it.
- If it is not possible to remove it, take a disposable sterile hypodermic needle of any size and remove the foreign body by lifting. It will cause only a point damage. Do not scratch and cross the pupillary zone of the cornea.
- If the foreign body is embedded into the deeper stroma of the cornea, take the patient to the operation theater and remove the foreign body with a needle under operative microscope.
- In all cases apply antibiotic ointment and if necessary cycloplegic drop. Put a pad and bandage for 24 hours. Examine the patient on the next day, and frequent antibiotic drops for the next few days.
- In case of old iron foreign body, there is formation of rust-ring around the foreign body. It is also to be removed carefully with a needle.
- In all cases of corneal foreign body, always examine the lacrimal sac by giving pressure over the sac region to rule out any chronic dacryocystitis.

If it is present, the puncta is temporarily occluded by thermocautery and antibiotic drops and ointment are to be applied frequently after removal of foreign body.

TOOKE'S KNIFE (SCLERACORNEAL SPLITTER) (FIG. 27.41)

Identification: It is a short, flat blade with semicircular cutting edge at its tip. It is beveled on both sides at its distal end. It is attached to a stout handle with short neck. Note: Rougine has a long neck, the blade is more flat and beveled on one side.

Uses

- For splitting the sclerocorneal junction during trephining operation in glaucoma.
- Used to clear the sclerocorneal junction or episcleral tissue in cataract or trabeculectomy.
- May be used for lamellar dissection of the sclera.

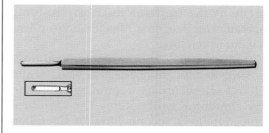

Fig. 27.41: Tooke's knife

ELLIOT'S SCLERACORNEAL TREPHINE IDENTIFICATION (FIG. 27.42)

- Fine cylindrical blades with sharp cutting edge
- A stout aluminum cylindrical handle.

These two portions can be detached. The diameter of the blade may be 1.0 mm, 1.5 mm, 1.75 mm or 2.0 mm.

Use: To cut the sclerocorneal disc in a circular fashion in trephining operation for glaucoma. *Trephine* means—circular blade. Larger diameters of trephine (6.0–10.0 mm) are widely used in keratoplasty operation to make corneal button both from the donor and the recipient.

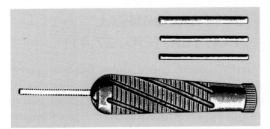

Fig. 27.42: Elliot's trephine with handle

DISC-HOLDING FORCEPS (FIG. 27.43)

Identification: It is a fine forceps with 1:2 teeth on the under surface at the tip the limbs. The blade of the forceps has large hexagonal hole for holding.

Use: It is used to hold the sclerocorneal disc, made by the trephine during trephining operation for glaucoma. After holding the disc, it is cut by scissors.

Tooke's knife, Elliot's trephine and disc-holding forceps are not used nowadays, and Elliot's sclerocorneal trephining operation for glaucoma is obsolete. The standard procedure for glaucoma filtration operation is trabeculectomy for the last 20 years.

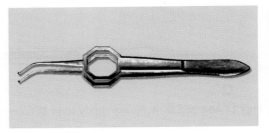

Fig. 27.43: Disc-holding forceps

CHALAZION FORCEPS (CLAMP) (FIG. 27.44)

Identification: It is a forceps with a large screw for fixing or tightening the limbs like a clamp. One limb has got a solid disc-shaped plate and the other limb has a ring at its end. It is hemostatic and self-retaining.

Method: The solid plate is applied on the skin surface of the lid and the ring side is applied on the tarsal conjunctiva, encircling the chalazion. The screw is tightened and the lid is everted and then chalazion is exposed for incision.

The functions of the screw are:
- Fixation of the lid
- Hemostasis by means of tightening.

Uses
- To fix the chalazion for surgery and also to ensure hemostasis.
- To give intralesional injection of steroids in chalazion after fixing it with forceps.
- Excision of a small granuloma or papilloma of the lid.

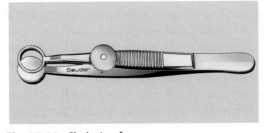

Fig. 27.44: Chalazion forceps

BEER'S KNIFE (FIG. 27.45)

Identification: It is a large triangular knife with a sharp pointing cutting edge.

Method and uses

- It is used to give incision on palpebral conjunctival side of the chalazion after fixing it with forceps. The Beer's knife is not used routinely. Nowadays the incision is given by a no. 11 blade attached to the Bard-Parker handle or by side-port blade.
- Beer's knife may be used to give incision over skin in any lid surgery.

The incision is vertical to avoid injury to the meibomian glands and ducts as they are arranged vertically.

Sometimes, when the pus is pointing toward the skin surface, the fixation plate and ring of the chalazion clamp is reversed. Then a horizontal incision is given on skin surface. This reverse type of incision is given because:

- Vascular arcades are running horizontally so less chance of bleeding.
- The scar mark will be along the natural crease of lid skin.

CHALAZION SCOOP (CURETTE) (FIG. 27.46)

Identification: It is a small scoop with sharp edge, attached to a handle. The size of the scoop may vary. Two different sized scoops may be attached to the two ends of same handle for convenience.

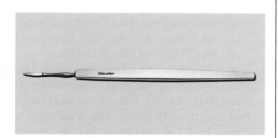

Fig. 27.45: Beer's knife

Uses: To scoop out the granulation tissue after giving incision on chalazion. Scooping of the chalazion must be complete, otherwise there may be chance of recurrence. After removal of the chalazion forceps, the bleeding is controlled by pressure over the lid, against the incised area. A pressure bandage is applied for few hours with antibiotic ointment.

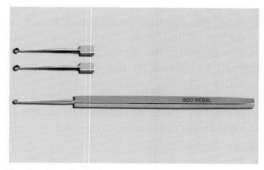

Fig. 27.46: Chalazion scoop

PUNCTUM DILATOR (NETTLESHIP'S) (FIG. 27.47)

Identification: It is a long narrow solid cylindrical instrument with a smooth conical pointed tip. Its body is corrugated for better gripping with thumb and index finger.

Method of syringing

- Anesthetize the eye with 4% lignocaine or 1% proparacaine drop.
- Pull the lower lid and identify the lower punctum in bright light.
- Hold the punctum dilator vertically by right index and thumb and place it on the punctal opening.
- Twist it with light pressure and introduce into the punctum.
- Then hold the punctum dilator horizontally and push it medially by rotatory movement—following the course of the canaliculus (first vertically then horizontally). Then withdraw it.

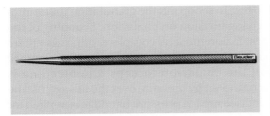

Fig. 27.47: Punctum dilator

- Take the lacrimal cannula, fitted in a syringe, filled with distilled water and introduce it in the same direction.
- Push the piston of the syringe to inject water into the canaliculus and ask the patient whether water has reached the throat or not. Alternatively, note the swallowing movement of the neck.

Uses
- To dilate the punctum and part of the canaliculus before introducing lacrimal cannula for syringing.
- To dilate the punctum for probing in case of congenital dacryocystitis.
- To dilate the punctum and then probing to identify lacrimal sac during DCR operation.
- For dilatation of the punctum in congenital or acquired punctal stenosis.
- Before dacryocystography (DCG).
- May be used as a marker (by dipping the pointed tip in gentian violet) in squint or retinal detachment operation.

LACRIMAL CANNULA (FIG. 27.48)

Identification: It is a small straight angulated or curved cannula with blunt tip. It can be fitted to any hypodermic syringe.
Method: Same as punctum dilator.

Uses
- Syringing or patency test of the lacrimal passage.
- For DCG.
- During probing and syringing in congenital dacryocystitis.

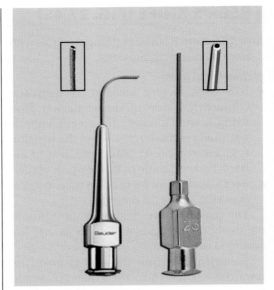

Fig. 27.48: Lacrimal cannula

- Postoperatively, it is used to check the patency after DCR operation.

In patency test or syringing, the interpretation may be:
- Water is going freely into the throat—lacrimal passage is patent.
- Water is not going into the throat, instead it is regurgitating through the upper punctum and partly through the same punctum.
  - *Fast regurgitation:* The fluid coming out through the upper puncta is clear and it is rapid. It is due to common canalicular block (CC block) (Fig.27.49A).
  - *Slow regurgitation:* It is turbid fluid (i.e. water is mixed up with pus, mucopus or mucoid material) and the regurgitation speed is slow. It is due to nasolacrimal duct (NLD) block (Fig. 27.49B).
- If little water is going into the throat after forced syringing (some part is coming out through punctum). It is partial NLD block. In case of NLD block—the treatment of choice is DCR operation. But in case of CC block, the treatment of choice is CDCR (canaliculo-DCR).

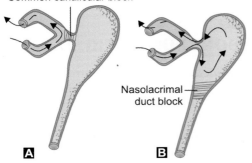

Common canalicular block

Nasolacrimal — duct block

A　　　　　**B**

Figs 27.49A and B: Patency test. **A.** Fast regurgitation; **B.** Slow regurgitation

LACRIMAL DISSECTOR WITH SCOOP (LANG'S) (FIG. 27.50)

Identification: It is a narrow long instrument with a stout pointed dissector at one end, and the other end is having an elongated scoop.

Uses
- ***Dissector end***
  - It is used for blunt dissection of lacrimal sac after giving skin incision (both in DCT and DCR operation).
  - It is used to clean the bone pieces from the punch, while punching or cutting the bone of DCR.
- ***Scoop end:*** To scoop out the tissue remnants by scraping from the upper end of bony NLD after excision of the lacrimal sac (only in DCT).

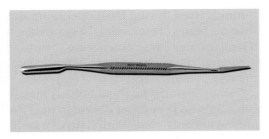

Fig. 27.50: Lacrimal dissector with scoop

ROUGINE (FIG. 27.51)

Identification: It is rectangular blade attached by a narrow neck to a corrugated handle. The blade is sharp at its distal end which is beveled on one surface, the other surface being plane. It is basically a small periosteal elevator.

Uses
- To dissect and disinsert the medial palpebral ligament to find out cleavage between lacrimal sac and the lacrimal fossa.
- Dissection of the lacrimal sac from the medial wall and the floor of the lacrimal fossa, by separating the periosteal tissue surrounding the sac.

It is used both in DCT and DCR operation.

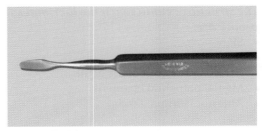

Fig. 27.51: Rougine

MULLER'S (SELF-RETAINING ADJUSTABLE HEMOSTATIC) RETRACTOR (FIG. 27.52)

Identification: It is made up of two limbs with a screw to fix the limbs in a retracted position. Each limb has got two or three right-angled curved pointed hooks (pins) for engaging

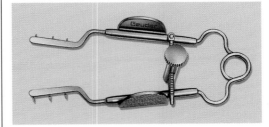

Fig. 27.52: Muller's retractor

the incised edges of the skin and deeper tissues.

Uses: To retract the incised edges of the skin and deeper tissues during dacryocystectomy and dacryocystorhinostomy operations.

Its hemostatic effect is due to angled hooks causing compression of the blood vessels by the spring action of the retractor.

This instrument has disadvantage of reducing field of operation. Instead, one can pass three deep stay sutures on each skin-edge of incision to achieve retraction and hemostasis.

The complications may occur during giving incision to the skin are:

- Injury to the angular vein
- Cutting the medial palpebral ligament
- Injury to the lacrimal sac inadvertently.

The structures cut to reach the lacrimal sac proper are:

- Skin
- Subcutaneous tissue
- Few fibers of orbicularis oculi
- Medial palpebral ligament
- Anterior lacrimal fascia.

CAT'S PAW RETRACTOR (FIG. 27.53)

Identification: This instrument is just like a small dinner fork. The ends of the fork are bend downward.

Uses

- It is used to retract the skin, subcutaneous tissues and ligament during lacrimal sac surgery.

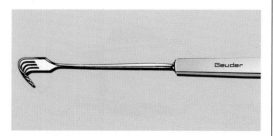

Fig. 27.53: Cat's paw retractor

- It may also be used in other plastic operations of the eyelid.

BONE PUNCH (FIG. 27.54)

Identification: It is a large instrument, which consists of a spring handle and two long blades. The upper blade has a hole with sharp cutting edge and the lower blade has a cup like depression with sharp edge.

Use: It is used to punch or break the bones (lacrimal bone, adjacent nasal bone, and frontal process of the maxilla) in DCR operation to create a bony ostium. Ideally, two different sized bone punches are required to make a round bony opening of about 10 mm diameter.

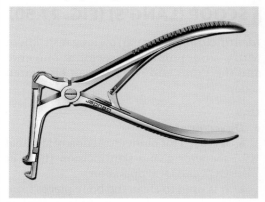

Fig. 27.54: Bone punch

HAMMER, CHIESEL AND BONE GOUGE (FIGS 27.55A TO C)

These stout and heavy instruments are not routinely used during DCR operation. But when the bones of the lacrimal fossa are seem to be hard, these instruments are then used for making a bony ostium (osteotomy) in DCR surgery.

Usually, first the lacrimal bone is broken with a lens hook or blunt dissector, then the bony window is made with help of a bone punch.

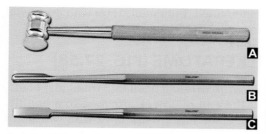

Figs 27.55A to C: A. Hammer; **B.** Bone gouge; **C:** Chisel

EVISCERATION SPOON OR SCOOP (FIG. 27.56)

Identification: It has a large rectangular or oval shallow spoon attached to a handle. Its shape is almost like a spade.

Uses: It is used to scoop out the intraocular contents during evisceration. Evisceration is the removal of the contents of the globe with inner two coats while leaving the sclera and the optic nerve intact.

The structures scooped out are:
- Lens
- Vitreous
- Whole uvea
- Whole retina.

Indications of evisceration:
- Panophthalmitis
- In case of expulsive hemorrhage—to assist auto-evisceration if the process is incomplete—rarely performed.

Method: Steps of operation (*see* Chapter 10). In case of painful blind eye or disfigured eye—evisceration is relatively contraindicated, as the remnant of healthy uveal tissue may excite sympathetic ophthalmia. In case of malignancy, evisceration may cause spread of the tumor cells via the bloodstream.

But in case of panophthalmitis as the uveal tissue is dead and necrotic, there is no antigenicity of the uveal tissue, so there is no chance of sympathetic ophthalmia.

ENUCLEATION

Scissors (Fig. 27.57A)

Identification: It is a broad, stout scissors having uniformly curved blades with blunt tips. The scissors is curved to fit the curvature of the globe.

Use: It is used to cut the optic nerve with its sheaths during enucleation operation. Enucleation is the surgical removal of the globe and a portion of the optic nerve from the orbit.

Spoon (Fig. 27.57B)

Use: After severing all the recti muscles, it is passed from the lateral side deep inside the orbit to get hold the optic nerve. Then, the scissors is used to cut the optic nerve.

Indications of enucleation
- *Absolute indications:* When there is risk of life, or risk to the other eye due to the disease.

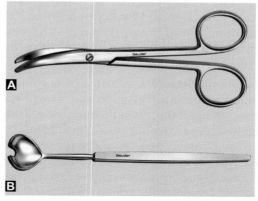

Figs 27.57A and B: Enucleation. **A.** Scissors; **B.** Spoon with optic nerve guard

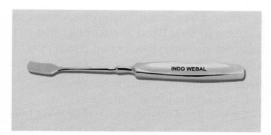

Fig. 27.56: Evisceration scoop

- Malignant melanoma in adult
- Retinoblastoma in children
- Nonrepairable severely injured eye to prevent sympathetic ophthalmia in the other eye.
- *Relative indications:* Enucleation may be done in case of:
  - Painful blind eye due to absolute glaucoma, chronic iridocyclitis, intraocular hemorrhage, etc.
  - Phthisis bulbi with calcification
  - Disfigured eye, e.g. anterior staphyloma, ciliary staphyloma, etc.
  - Sympathetic ophthalmia.
- *To collect donor eyes from the cadaver for eye bank for keratoplasty:* By and large, this is the most common indication of enucleation in ophthalmic practice.

Method: Steps of operation (*see* Chapter10). The structures cut by enucleation scissors are:
- Optic nerve with its meningeal sheaths
- Central retinal artery and vein
- Two long posterior ciliary arteries
- Two long ciliary veins
- Short posterior ciliary vessels and nerves
- Lastly, two oblique muscles.

In case of malignant tumors of the eyeball, at least more than 10 mm optic nerve stump is to be cut behind the globe. This is because the central retinal artery enters the optic nerve at this distance. So when the extraocular vascular spread occurs—it may be detected by histopathological examination of the optic nerve. Thereby subsequent treatment by radiation or exenteration may be considered.

In panophthalmitis, enucleation is contra-indicated because infection may spread via the meningeal sheaths or their spaces into the brain leading to meningitis or encephalitis.

The cosmetic appearance of the artificial eye is better with evisceration than with simple enucleation. Because the muscle attachments are still present to the scleral shell (later form a ball like structure) in case of evisceration, the movements of the artificial eye are well maintained. But enucleation with an orbital implant has a better cosmetic result.

KERATOME (FIG. 27.58)

Identification: It has a thin triangular blade, at the end of a neck attached to a handle. The blade has a sharp apex with two sharp cutting edges. Keratome may be angular or straight.

Uses
- It is used to make small limbal section for cataract surgery. Then the section is enlarged with a corneal scissors.
- To make small limbal section for glaucoma iridectomy or optical iridectomy.
- Newer disposable angular keratomes are widely used in phacoemulsification, for making sclerocorneal or corneal tunnel incisions.
- May be used for paracentesis.

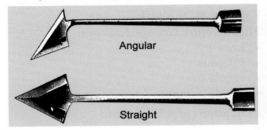

Fig. 27.58: Keratome

LACRIMAL PROBE (BOWMAN'S) (FIG. 27.59)

Identification: It is a thin, long probe with round lip. It is made up of stainless steel or silver. They are of different diameters (size 00 to 08). Each instrument has two different size probes attached centrally with a flat handle.

Uses: To probe nasolacrimal passage in:
- Congenital punctal stenosis.
- Congenital dacryocystitis—if probing fails to achieve the patency of nasolacrimal passage then one should go for DCR.

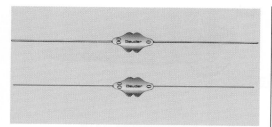

Fig. 27.59: Lacrimal probes (Bowman's) of different size

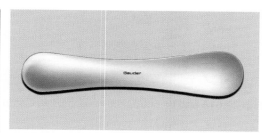

Fig. 27.60: Lid plate (spatula)

- During DCR to identify the exact position of lacrimal sac for giving incision on the sac wall.

Method (probing and syringing):
- Under general anesthesia.
- Probing is usually done through the upper punctum.
- Start with a smaller size probe and gradually increase the size.
- Always follow the direction of nasolacrimal passage during probing.
- Syringing is done 2–3 minutes after the probing.

Complications of probing:
- False passage
- Nasal bleeding
- Orbital cellulitis.

LID PLATE (SPATULA) (FIG. 27.60)

Identification: It is a flat solid instrument of about 10 cm long. Its both ends are round and convex. It is little curved or grooved at right angle to its long axis, near its end.

Method: Before its application, eyeball is smeared with antibiotic ointment to prevent corneal abrasion. It is introduced under the lid to provide a solid support during lid surgery. Three stay sutures are usually passed along the lid margins so that the assistant can hold the sutures together along with lid plate for better support during dissection.

Use: It is used in various lid surgeries, e.g. ptosis, entropion, etc. It gives more exposure of operative field than a clamp, but it does not help in hemostasis.

ENTROPION

Forceps (Fig. 27.61A)

Identification: It is just like chalazion forceps except its shape is horizontally oval, and it is bigger in size. It is used for both sides.

Clamp (Fig. 27.61B)

Identification: It is a stout clamp with two limbs, and one screw for fixation. One limb has got a solid semilunar plate and the other limb has U-shaped curved rim corresponding to the semilunar plate. Right and left-sided clamps are different.

Method: Same for both instruments. Eye is smeared adequately with antibiotic ointment before its application to prevent corneal abrasion. Its solid plate is applied on the tarsal conjunctival side and the fenestrated or rim-side is on the skin surface (in reverse order of chalazion forceps). The screw is tightened for fixation.

Use: Same for both. It is used to fix the lid during entropion operation. By tightening the screw, it helps in hemostasis during operation. But it reduces the area of operative field.

CALIPER (CASTROVEIJO'S) (FIG. 27.62)

Identification: It is a measuring caliper in which the measurement (in mm) is adjusted by spring action of a screw. The measuring ends are pointed like a compass, and the scale is fixed to the opposite end.

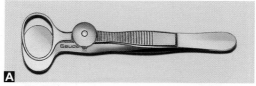 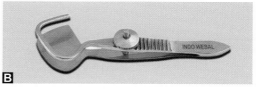

Figs 27.61A and B: Entropion. **A.** Forceps; **B.** Clamp

Methods: The exact measurement is taken by adjusting the spring action of the screw which is indicated by the pointed end on the scale.

Uses

- To measure the size of the cornea, as in buphthalmos, congenital hereditary endothelial dystrophy (CHED), megalocornea, microcornea, etc.
- *To use in various surgeries:*
  - Phacoemulsification or small incision cataract surgery—length of incision
  - Trabeculectomy—length of scleral flap
  - Squint operation—amount of resection or recession of the muscle
  - Keratoplasty—to determine the size of the donor and recipient corneal button.
  - Retinal detachment surgery—to measure the distance for passing encircling band or to make port at pars plana
  - Intraocular foreign body (IOFB) removal—to measure the site of incision for IOFB removal
  - Ptosis surgery—to measure the amount of lipopolysaccharide (LPS) to be resected.
  - To measure white-to-white diameter in phakic IOL or in case of ACIOL implantation.
  - To measure the length for any purpose.

CORNEAL TREPHINE (CASTROVEIJO'S)

Identification: It is a cylindrical instrument which has three parts (Fig. 27.63):
1. A circular blade
2. An adjustable inner core or "obturator"
3. A cover to protect the sharpness of the blade.

It is available in different diameters (like 6.0, 6.5, 7.0, 7.5...10, 10.5, etc. in mm). The obturator has a scale (marking 0, 2, 4, 6, etc. in 1/10th of mm) which helps the surgeon to select exact depth of the cornea to be cut. This is important in lamellar keratoplasty.

Uses: To cut the "donor" and "recipient" corneal button in penetrating and lamellar keratoplasty procedures.

Nowadays disposable corneal trephine is used.

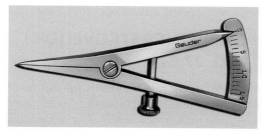

Fig. 27.62: Caliper

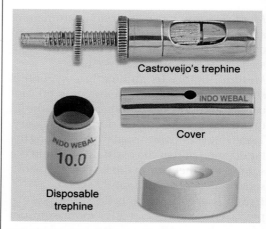

Fig. 27.63: Parts of corneal trephine

PIN-HOLE (FIG. 27.64)

Identification: It is a black disc with a small central hole, attached to a small handle.

Principle of pin-hole (PH): When it is held in front of eye, only a small pencil of rays get through, which passes through the axis of dioptric system of the eye, and is therefore, unaffected by it.

It follows that if the hole is small enough, all refraction would be eliminated and a clear image thus be formed in the same manner as seen in a pin-hole camera.

Method: Patient complaining of dimness of vision is asked to look at the Snellen's chart. Then a pin-hole is placed in front of his eye, the other eye is being closed. He is asked whether his vision is better or worse, or unchanged.

Uses

- To differentiate dimness of vision is due to refractive error or due to organic diseases of the media, or due to macular or neuro-ophthalmologic disease.
  - In case of refractive error or in minor opacity in the media, there will be a substantial improvement of vision.
  - In case of macular or neurological disease, and major opacity in the medial—there will be no improvement, rather some worsening may occur.

- During prescription of the glasses in refractive error, achieved by proper lenses or not.
- To assess potential visual acuity which may be achievable after surgical interventions— as after cataract surgery, keratoplasty, etc.

Note: Best visual acuity obtainable with a pin-hole is approximately 6/7.5 (20/25), not 6/6 (20/20); due to diffraction caused by pin-hole aperture.

STENOPEIC SLIT (FIG. 27.65)

Identification: It is black disc with a large slit-like opening at the center. It has small handle.

Method: Stenopeic slit is placed in front of the eye by means of a spectacles frame within the slot. It can be properly positioned by rotating it within the frame.

Uses

- Detection of the axis for prescribing cylindrical lens for astigmatic correction.
- Fincham's test to differentiate between glaucomatous halos from cataract halos.
- To find out the best meridian for optical iridectomy.
- As a low visual aid.
- Used as a part of Maddox wing.

The stenopeic slit is essentially an elongated pin-hole. When placed in front of the eye, it

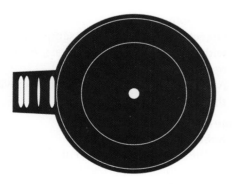

Fig. 27.64: Pin-hole

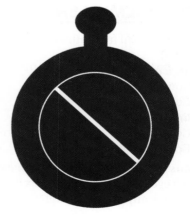

Fig. 27.65: Stenopeic slit

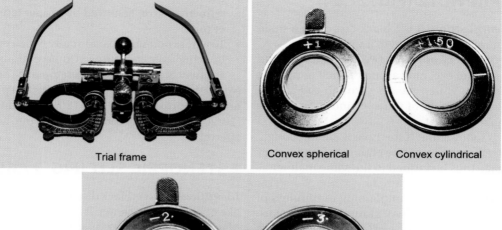

Fig. 27.66: Trial frame and ophthalmic lenses

allows only the rays of light in the particular meridian to enter into the eye. As for example, if the slit is placed horizontally, the vertical focal line passes through the pin-hole and reduced to almost point image.

OPHTHALMIC LENSES

Types of lens used in ophthalmic practice are (Fig. 27.66).
- *Spherical lenses:*
  - Convex and
  - Concave
- *Cylindrical lenses:*
  - Convex and
  - Concave

Methods of identification of a given lens: Close left eye. Hold the lens by index finger and thumb. Look any object through the lens with the right eye for magnification or minification.

Then hold the lens close to the right eye with thumb and index finger, left eye being closed. *Concentrate on a distant object* (some figure or a line) through the lens. Now move the lens in:
- Horizontal direction
- Vertical direction
- Rotatory fashion.

Note the following:
- Object is moving in the same direction with the movement of the lens, or in the opposite direction.
- Any distortion of the object while moving the lens in a rotatory fashion.

Now identification of the lens:
- *Spherical*
  - The object appears to move in both directions, i.e. horizontal and vertical,
  - No distortion of the image of the object in rotatory movement.

- **Cylindrical**
  - Object appears to move in one direction only,
  - There is distortion of the image when the lens is in rotatory movement.

Then identify whether the lens is convex or concave:
- **Convex lens (plus lens)**
  - Magnification of the image,
  - The object appears to move in the **opposite direction** as that of the lens.
- **Concave lens (minus lens)**
  - Minification of the image,
  - Object appears to move in the same direction as that of the lens.

So a given lens may be either:
- **Convex spherical**
  - Object appears to move in both meridians and in the **opposite direction.**
  - No distortion of the image.
  - Magnification of the image.
- **Concave spherical**
  - Object appears to move in both meridians and in the **same direction**.
  - No distortion of the image.
  - Minification of the image.
- **Convex cylindrical**
  - Object appears to move in one meridian and in the **opposite direction**.
  - Distortion of the image.
  - Magnification of the image.
- **Concave cylindrical**
  - Object appears to move in one meridian and in the **same direction**.
  - Distortion of the image.
  - Minification of the image.

Note: In a plane glass (plano): **Lens with "no" power**—no movement of the object, no distortion of the image, size remains same.

Some hints for identification of a given lens:
- **Spherical**
  - It has got a handle with the rim and
  - No axis marking on it.
- **Cylindrical**
  - Perfectly circular with no handle and

- Axis mark on the metallic or plastic rim in one side only.

Uses
- **Convex spherical**
  - **Correction of refractive status:**
    - Hypermetropia
    - Aphakia
    - Presbyopia
    - As a low visual aid (magnifier).
  - **Instrumental uses:**
    - Direct ophthalmoscope
    - Indirect ophthalmoscope
    - Microscope
    - Synoptophore
    - Corneal loupe or telescopic loupe.
  - **Diagnostic uses:**
    - Volk + 90D lens, or + 78D lens—to see the fundus
    - Placido's disc (+ 3.0D)
    - Malingering (with high plus lens)
    - Different condensing lenses for laser therapy.
- **Concave spherical**
  - **In refractive error:** Myopia.
  - **Instrumental use:**
    - Direct ophthalmoscope
    - Telescopic loupe (Galilean system).
  - **Diagnostic use:**
    - Hruby lens (–55D)
    - Fundus contact lens (–45D)
    - Central lens of gonioscope
    - Malingering test with high minus lens.
- **Convex cylinder:** Regular hypermetropic astigmatism.
- **Concave cylinder:** Regular myopic astigmatism.

In case of irregular astigmatism—one should use contact lens.

RED-GREEN GOGGLES (FIG. 27.67)

Identification: It is like a toy goggles with an elastic band. At one side, it is red and on other side, it is green.

Procedure: Conventionally, the red side of the goggles has to be placed in front of right eye (red for right, i.e. R for R).
Use: It is used to dissociate binocular single vision in various tests:
- Worth's four dot test
- Hess screen test
- Diplopia charting.

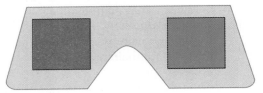

Fig. 27.67: Red-green goggles

PLACIDO'S DISC (FIG. 27.68)

Identification: It is a medium-size circular disc with a central hole and attached to a handle. On one surface of the disc, there are alternate black and white circle like Bull's eye.
Procedure: Placido's disc is held in front of the patient's eye while examiner looks through the hole in center of the disc. The examiner then observes the corneal image of the disc as reflected from the light behind the patient.

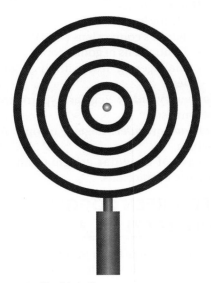

Fig. 27.68: Placido's disc

Use: It is used to assess the corneal anterior surface and anterior corneal curvature (astigmatism):
- A loss in sharpness of image denotes a loss of normal smoothness of the anterior corneal surface, e.g. corneal abrasion, dry eye, etc.
- Elliptical image is seen in regular astigmatism.
- Irregular image is seen in keratoconus.
- Small hand held surgical keratoscope is also used in penetrating keratoplasty or DALK to adjust sutures at the end of surgery.
- Many modern corneal topography instruments are based on Placido's disc principle.

PRISM (FIGS 27.69A AND B)

Identification: It is wedge-shaped refracting material (glass or plastic) with thin edge at one side and thick edge on opposite side. It is triangular in cross-section having an apex and a base.
Refraction through a prism: There is total deviation of light toward the base of the prism. The image is displaced toward the apex of the prism.

Positions

- **Frontal position:** Plastic prism—parallel to infraorbital margin.
- **Prentice position:** Glass prism—posterior face of the prism is perpendicular to the line of sight.

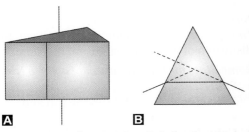

Figs 27.69A and B: **A.** Prism; **B.** Refraction through a prism

One prism diopter power produces a linear apparent displacement of 1 cm of an object situated at 1 meter.

Uses of Prisms in Ophthalmology

Diagnostic

Assessment of squint and heterophoria:
- Objective measurement of angle by prism cover test, prism reflex test of Krimsky.
- Subjective measurement of angle by Maddox rod.
- Assess likelihood of diplopia after squint surgery in adults.
- Measurement of fusional reserve.
- Diopter base out test for microtropia.
- To detect malingering.

Therapeutic

- Convergence insufficiency—synoptophore.
- To relieve diplopia—decompensated heterophorias, small vertical squints and some paralytic squints due to some surgical contraindications.

Forms of therapeutic prisms:
- **Temporary wear:** Clip on spectacle prisms (Fresnel prisms).
- **Permanent wear:** Incorporation into the spectacles by decentering the spherical lenses.

Instruments

- Goldmann applanation tonometer
- Indirect ophthalmoscope
- Slit-lamp microscope
- Keratometer
- Operating microscope
- Synoptophore
- Haidinger's brush
- Koeppe's goniolens.

Forms of instrumental prisms
- Right angle prism—angle of deviation 90°.
- Porro prism—angle of deviation is 180°, image is inverted but not transposed.

- Dove prism—no deviation, image is inverted but not transposed.

Miscellaneous

- Recumbent spectacles
- Hemianopic spectacles—8 diopter prism with base toward blind side
- Low visual aid (LVA)—base in prisms incorporated into binocular magnifier.

▌RETINOSCOPE (FIG. 27.70)

Identification: This is a circular plain mirror with a central aperture in a plastic frame with handle. Sometimes, a concave mirror of 2.0D may be attached with other end in a dumble-shaped frame.

Uses
- It is used for determination of refraction.
- It may be used for distant direct ophthalmoscopy (at 22 cm). This is:
  - To know any opacity in the media
  - To discover the edge of a subluxated or dislocated lens
  - To recognize a retinal detachment or tumor.
  - To confirm the results found by external examination.

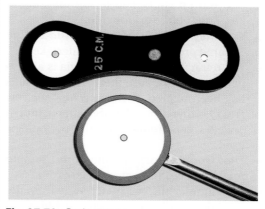

Fig. 27.70: Retinoscope

Optics of Retinoscopy

It entails a study of the movements of the retinal image produced by a beam of light that sweeps across the pupil.

The observer then watches this illuminated retinal image by looking down the path of incident light, through a hole in the center of a mirror (retinoscope).

- *If the eye is emmetropic:* Parallel rays of light come to a point focus on retina, so they are emerging in the same pathway.
- *If the eye is hypermetropic:* Parallel rays converge behind the retina and hence, the emerging rays are divergent.
- *If the eye is myopic:* Parallel rays converge in front of the retina and hence, the emerging rays are convergent.

The principle of retinoscopy is to make every observing eye emmetropic, so that the emerging rays should form a parallel beam.

Procedure

- *Cycloplegia:* It is only required in children and young patients. In adults and old patients, it is usually not necessary.
  - *If the patient is less than 5 years:* Atropine eye ointment (1%) is to be applied three times daily for 3 days.
  - *If the patient is between 5 and 15 years:* 1% cyclopentolate, or 2% homatropine eye drop is instilled for 3 times, about 1 hour before examination.
  - *If the patient is between 15 and 20:* The same procedure may be undertaken.

  The refraction under cycloplegia is always pathological because the shape of the lens has been altered. A *post-cycloplegic test (PCT)* is therefore advisable after 3 days to 3 weeks depending upon the cycloplegic used.
- *Dark-room test:* Retinoscopy should preferably be conducted in dark room.
  - Examiner sits at 1 meter away from the patient (point of reversal is at 1.0D). It is even more convenient to sit at arm's length, i.e. two-thirds meter away, so that the trial lenses can be held in the other hand while the light beam is passed. The point of reversal then be 1.5D.
  - The patient is normally seated and looking toward the far end of the room (relaxed eye).
  - Source of light is from behind the patient.
  - The surgeon looks through a *plane mirror* with central perforation, and light is reflected into the patient's eye.
  - The mirror is slowly moved from side to side in different meridians, and movement of the shadow is noted.
  - In hypermetropia, emmetropia and myopia less than 1.0D the reflex moves in the same direction.

    In myopia of −1.0D = there is no movement of shadow.

    In myopia of more than 1.0D = the shadow moves in the opposite direction.
  - Increasing convex (if the movement is on same side) or concave (if opposite side) lenses are placed before the eye until the *point of reversal* is reached. *At this point there will be no movement of the shadow, and pupil will be brightly illuminated.*
  - The procedure is done in each meridian separately.
    - In simple spherical refractive error— the movement and the point of reversal will be same in both meridians.
    - In astigmatism, they are different. If the axes are oblique, the shadow themselves will seem to move obliquely and the mirror is then tilted accordingly.
- *Calculation:* Refraction of patient's eye— lens required to reach end point = −1D (myopia). Since the surgeon is sitting at 1 meter distance, and if he is at 2/3 meter, it will be − 1.5D (myopic). So the refraction of the eye = −1.0D + lens.

Examples:
- *If the end point is with +4.0D lens: Refraction* = −1.0D + 4.0D = + 3.0D.

- *Similarly if, with –4.0D lens:*
  Refraction = –1.0D–4.0D = –5.0D.
- *If the end point is with +1.0D lens:*
  Refraction = –1.0D = 0, i.e. the patient
  is emmetropic.
- In case of astigmatism, each meridian is
  to be calculated separately.

Streak retinoscopy: Instead of circular light as
obtained by a plain mirror, a self-illuminated
streak of light is used. Here, the appearances
of the shadow are more dramatic. Axis of the
astigmatism is easily determined. It has certain
other advantages:

- Can be done in any position of the
  patient.
- Can be done in difficult patients, e.g. in
  children or non-cooperative patient.
- Can be used per-operatively.

MAGNIFYING LOUPE

Identification: It is a strong biconvex lens,
fitted in a metal-case (uniocular); or in a plastic
frame (binocular) with forehead band (Figs
27.71A and B).

Uses: It is used for examination of the anterior
segment of the eye with oblique illumination.
It is useful to search minute corneal foreign
bodies, keratic precipitates (KPs), superficial
punctate keratitis (SPK), caterpillar's hairs, etc.

Magnification
- Uniocular loupe—10 times
- Binocular loupe—3–4 times

Dioptric power of the loupe
- Uniocular = +40D
- Binocular = +12–16D.

Magnification = power in diopter/4

JACKSON'S CROSS CYLINDER (FIG. 27.72)

Identification: It is a sphero-cylindrical
combination of lens in which the spherical
component is half the power but of the
opposite sign of the cylindrical component.

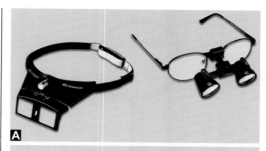
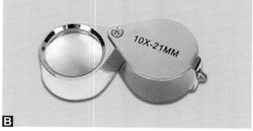

Figs 27.71A and B: Magnifying loupe. **A.** Binocular;
B. Uniocular

The most convenient form is a combination
of a –0.25D spherical with + 0.50D cylinder.
Method: The cylindrical axis of the cross-
cylinder is first placed in the same direction as
the axis of the cylinder in the trial frame and
then perpendicular to it. In the first position,
the cylindrical correction is enhanced by 0.5D,
and in the second, it is diminished by the same
amount. If the visual acuity is not improved in
either of these positions, the cylinder in the
trial frame is correct.

If the visual acuity is improved, a corresponding change should be made in the
correction, and the new combination is
verified by running through the cycle again.
Use: It is used to check the power and axis of
the cylinder in refractive correction.

MADDOX ROD (FIG. 27.73)

Identification: It consists of a series of parallel
high-power, plus cylinders (rods) of red glass
placed side by side in a supporting disc. It can
convert a point light into a red streak light at
right angle to the axis of rods.

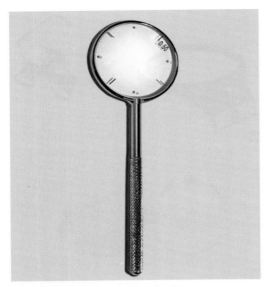

Fig. 27.72: Jackson's cross cylinder

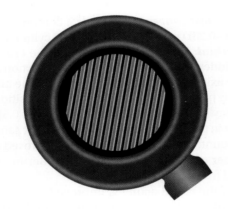

Fig. 27.73: Maddox rod

Methods: When a Maddox rod is held in a front of one eye, the image of a point source of light becomes dissimilar between the two eyes, and fusion becomes dissociated (dissimilar image test). This test is performed at 6 meters and at 33 cm from a bright spotlight in a dark room.

Uses
- To test the latent squint for distance.
- For orthoptic exercise in cyclophoria.
- To test macular function, in presence of opaque media.

METHODS OF STERILIZATION

The methods of sterilization commonly practiced in ophthalmic surgery are: (1) Autoclave, (2) Boiling, (3) Dry heat, (4) Chemicals, (5) Gamma-rays, and (6) Ultraviolet (UV) rays.

Autoclave

Steam under pressure is biocidal. A temperature of 134°C (321 lbs/sq. inch pressure) for 3 minutes, or 121°C (15 lbs/sq. inch pressure) for 15 minutes is used. It is used to sterilize towels, gowns, masks, sutures, dressings, irrigating solutions and blunt instruments. Sharp instruments should not be autoclaved.

Boiling

A traditional method of sterilization is still used routinely, not only in eye camps, but also in many hospitals. Boiling for 30 minutes usually kills most bacteria, but some spores may withstand boiling for this period. It is preferable to use distilled water to prevent salt deposition. Sharp instruments are better not to be sterilized by boiling.

Dry Heat

Dry heat kills bacteria by oxidative destruction of their protoplasm. In dry heat, a temperature of 150°C is used for 90 minutes in the hot air oven. It is better not to sterilize sharp instruments by dry heat.

Chemicals

- *Ethylene oxide:* The vapor of ethylene oxide can destroy all microorganisms, including spores. As undiluted ethylene oxide is highly explosive, it is diluted with an inert gas like carbon dioxide or Freon (12% ethylene oxide and 88% freon). Sharp instruments, plastic cryoprobes, IOLs, indirect ophthalmoscopy lens, diathermy wires, etc. can be sterilized by this method.

- *Glutaraldehyde solution (cidex):* 2% glutaraldehyde kills all microorganisms including spores. Its full potency persists for 2 weeks, then it is to be discarded. Cidex does not reduce the sharpness of the cutting instruments. In 10 minutes all microorganisms are killed and in 3 hours all spores are destroyed. The instruments, after removed from cidex, are thoroughly rinsed with sterile water and hollow instruments are to be flushed. All metallic instruments including the sharp-cutting instruments may be sterilized by this method.

- *Alcohol (rectified spirit):* Sharp cutting instruments and sutures may be dipped in 90% alcohol for 30 minutes for sterilization. It is not an excellent method.

- *Isopropyl alcohol (70%):* This is also used for sterilization of all kinds of metallic instruments. Dip the instruments for 15 minutes and then wash it with sterile water or saline before use.

- *Formalin vapor:* Keep the instruments in formalin vapor in a chamber (vapor released from formalin tablets) for overnight. Rinse thoroughly before use. *It is carcinogenic and now banned in many countries.*

Plasma Sterilization

Hydrogen peroxide plasma is a type of low temperature sterilization that is used widely today to sterilize such devices, such as endoscopes and other hollow instruments. It kills microorganisms including spores by a process called oxidation, which essentially deactivates their cellular components. It is safe for the environment and it has short cycle time.

Gamma Irradiation

Gamma rays from cobalt-60. This type of sterilization is used commercially, for disposable needles, disposable syringes, infusion sets, etc.

Ultraviolet Rays

Ultraviolet (UV) radiation is used in the disinfection of drinking water, operating room air and contact lenses. Bacteria and viruses are more easily killed by UV light than the bacterial spores.

LASER IN OPHTHALMOLOGY

Laser is the acronym of light amplification by stimulated emission of radiation.

Physics

Certain substances have the property to "lase", to absorb energy in one form, and to emit a new form of light. On pumping, these "lasing" substances are able to transfer electrons from a lower orbit to the higher metastable orbit *(Bohr's theory)*. The excited atoms in turn decay back to their original orbit to lower energy, thus emitting a new form of photons. This decaying can be spontaneous, or induced *(stimulate demission)*. These photons are then passed through a close system of mirrors, which leads to *light amplification*, and delivered as *laser*.

Common Types of Laser

Common types of laser used in ophthalmology have been described in Table 28.1.

Properties of Laser

- It is always *monochromatic* (has got one wavelength of light).
- It is *collimated* (all photons run parallel).
- It is *coherent* (always in the same phase).
- It is *polarized* at high energy level.

TABLE 28.1: Common types of laser

Types of laser	Wavelengths
Ruby laser (first laser)	550 nm
Argon laser • Blue-green • Puregreen	 488 nm 518 nm
Krypton laser	647 nm
Nd-YAG laser (Neodymium: Yttrium-Aluminum Garnet) • Single frequency • Double frequency (pulsed)	 1064 nm 532 nm
Diode laser Produced from semiconductor crystals Lasing substance: Gallium-aluminum-arsenate	810 nm
Excimer (excited dimer) laser Lasing substance: Argon fluoride	193 nm
Femtosecond laser Nd: Glass	1053 nm

Laser Effects on Ocular Tissues

- *Photocoagulation (controlled burn):* Argon laser, diode laser, krypton laser.
- *Photovaporization:* Argon laser, diode laser.
- *Photodisruption (optical breakdown to disrupt tissues by the formation of plasma):* NdYAG laser, femtosecond laser.

- *Photoablation (ablation of corneal tissue without thermal damage):* Excimer laser.

Indications of Laser (in General)

Common Indications

- Iridotomy for angle-closure glaucoma
- Pupilloplasty
- Argonlaser trabeculoplasty (ALT) in primary open-angle glaucoma
- Yttrium aluminum garnet (YAG) capsulotomy for posterior capsular opacification following extracapsular cataract extraction (ECCE)
- To create chorioretinal adhesions around the retinal breaks
- Panretinal photocoagulation (PRP) for proliferative retinal diseases and rubeosis iridis, e.g. diabetes, central retinal vein occlusion (CRVO)
- Central serous retinopathy (CSR)
- Direct photocoagulation to treat the vascular abnormalities
- "Macular-grid" photocoagulation to treat macular lesions
- Intraocular tumors and malignancy
- Photorefractive keratoplasty (PRK) in refractive errors, by excimer laser
- Laser assisted *in situ* keratomileusis or LASIK for the treatment of refractive errors (mainly myopia)
- Phototherapeutic keratoplasty (PTK) with excimer laser for superficial corneal scars
- Creation of LASIK flaps and trephination of donor and recipient button in penetrating and lamellar keratoplasty
- Femtosecond laser cataract surgery.

Miscellaneous

- Trichiasis (laser cilia-ablation)
- Suture removal (laser suturolysis)
- Pterygium (to treat the bare area)
- Cyclophotocoagulation in glaucoma.

- *Diagnostic:* Laser-interferometry with helium-neon (He-Ne) laser to test the potential visual acuity in presence of opacity in the media.

Femtosecond Laser in Ophthalmology

Femtosecond laser (FS) is an infrared laser (wavelength = 1,053 nm) with ultrashort pulse duration (10–15 sec). This laser has the ability to deliver laser energy with minimal collateral damage to the adjacent tissue. Thermal damage to neighboring tissue in the cornea has been measured to be around 1 μm.

- Femtosecond laser works by photodisruption like Nd-YAG laser, a process in which small volumes of tissue are vaporized resulting in the formation of cavitation gas (CO_2 and water) bubbles.
- Furthermore, the unique FS laser can be focused anywhere within or behind the cornea and is capable of passing through optically hazy media, such as an edematous cornea or cataractous lens. It may be applied in multiple geometric patterns including vertical, horizontal, spiral or zig-zag cuts.
- There are multiple commercially available femtosecond laser models in the market.

Femtosecond Laser in Refractive Surgery

- *Flap creation in LASIK:* Corneal flap creation in LASIK is the most common use of FS laser. It has many advantages over mechanical microkeratome flap, like— fewer flaprelated complications, thinner flap, improved thickness predictability and less induced higher order aberrations.
- *Femtosecond lenticule extraction (FLEx):* It is a new procedure to correct myopia and myopic astigmatism. This procedure

involves making two cuts (anterior and posterior) that intersect in the periphery, creating a lenticule which is ultimately removed.

- **Small incision lenticule extraction (SMILE):** A procedure in which the corneal flap is eliminated and instead a small incision is created in the mid-periphery of the cornea and the lenticule is removed through this self-sealing incision. SMILE has less tendency to induce post-refractive surgery dry eye, ectasia, and least flap complications.

Intracorneal Ring Segments (INTACS)

- Intracorneal ring segments are arcuate, polymethyl methacrylate (PMMA) implants for intrastromal insertion in mid-peripheral cornea for correction of milder cases of keratoconus with up to –3.50D of myopia and without central scarring.
- Femtosecond laser creates arcuate tunnels at 70% corneal depth. This method is easier and safer than manual dissection.

Femtosecond Laser for Presbyopia Correction

Femtosecond laser can be used to create intrastromal pockets for the implantation of INTRACOR or the Kamra small aperture corneal inlay which help to correct presbyopia.

Femtosecond Laser in Corneal Transplantation

- **Penetrating keratoplasty (PK):** Femtosecond laser creates complex pattern trephination cuts for enhanced wound integrity of the graft-host junction. Theoretically it may decrease suture-induced astigmatism and allow for faster visual recovery. The cuts include tophat (larger diameter cut posteriorly), mushroom (larger diameter ante-

riorly), zigzag and christmas tree pattern. Mushroom cut may be advantageous in keratoconus by providing a larger anterior refractive surface while the tophat may be useful in endothelial disorders by replacing more endothelial cells.

- **Anterior lamellar keratoplasty (ALK):** Femtosecond-assisted sutureless anterior lamellar keratoplasty can be used to treat anterior corneal pathologies with less irregular astigmatism and faster visual rehabilitation. Femtosecond-assisted DALK (deep anterior lamellar keratoplasty) is also a promising development.
- **DSAEK (Descemet's stripping automated endothelial keratoplasty):** Femtosecond laser can be used to create the lenticule for insertion in DSAEK procedure. The results are equal to or better than microkeratome assisted DSAEK.
- **DMEK (Descemet's membrane endothelial keratoplasty):** Femtosecond laser can be used in the donor preparation in DMEK and also for the creation of smooth stromal interface.

Femtosecond Laser and Astigmatic Keratotomy and Arcuate Wedge Resection

Femtosecond laser may be used in astigmatic keratotomy (AK) and/or arcuate wedge resection for the correction of high astigmatism following penetrating keratoplasty (PK) or cataract surgery. This laser procedure is easier, more precise and carries less risk of perforation than diamond blade method.

Femtosecond Laser-assisted Cataract Surgery (FLACS)

- Femtosecond laser are now used routinely in cataract surgery to create capsulotomy, clear corneal incision, limbal relaxing incisions, and lens fragmentation.

- Incisions (main incision and paracentesis) created by the laser are more precise, stable and with faster wound healing.
- The capsulorhexis created by the laser is more precisely centered and measured leading to better outcomes in premium intraocular lenses (IOLs) like multifocal and toric IOLs.
- Lens fragmentation with the laser leads to lesser phacoenergy being used and thus lesser endothelial damage.
- Visual recovery is also faster.
- Cystoid macular edema may be less in FS laser as compared to conventional phacoemulsification.

CRYOTHERAPY IN OPHTHALMOLOGY

Cryotherapy is a technique to injure, or to adhere tissues by the application of intense cold.

- This is achieved by a *cryoprobe,* a pencil-like instrument held by the surgeon, and it is cooled at a temperature of –40°C to –100°C by a freezergas under pressure. The gasflow to the cryoprobe is controlled by a foot-switch.
- The *gases used* are nitrous oxide (liquid nitrogen), freon or solid carbon dioxide.

Principle

Joule-Thomson effect—when a gas (cryogen) is released under high pressure through a micro-orifice, the gas expands to reach at its boiling point to reduce the temperature (e.g. liquid nitrogen boils at –195.6°C, and is an excellent cryogen).

Mechanism

When the freezing source is applied to a tissue, there is formation of hemispherical iceball which has different temperature zones.

- The temperature at any point within the iceball depends upon:
  - The distance from the cryogen.
  - The rate and duration of freezing.
- *Two basic mechanisms* involved in cryotherapy are:
  i. *Cryoadhesion* (as in ICCE or retinal breaks).
  ii. *Cryoinjury (in vivo* cell death), which has two phases:
    a. *Initial phase:* (i) Extracellular ice-crystal formation → dehydration → cell death. (ii) Intracellular icecrystal formation cell death.
    b. *Late phase:* Damage to the microcirculation of the cells → ischemic necrosis.

Maximum cell death is best achieved with a "rapid freeze" and a "slow thaw".
The three different probes are:
1. *Cataract probe:* –40°C to –50°C
2. *Retinal probe:* –50°C to –70°C
3. *Glaucoma probe:* –60°C to –80°C

Use of Cryo in Ophthalmology

- *Eyelids:* Papilloma, molluscum contagiosum, trichiasis, basal cell carcinoma, xanthelasma, etc.
- *Conjunctiva:* Cystoid cicatrix, giant papillae in vernal conjunctivitis and ocular surface squamous neoplasia (OSSN)
- *Cornea:* Herpes simplex keratitis (epithelial or stromal), epithelial downgrowth, carcinoma in situ
- *Iris and ciliary body:* Prolapsed iris, cyclocryopexy
- *Lens:* Intracapsular cataract extraction
- *Retina*
  - To seal the peripheral retinal breaks (cryoretinopexy).
  - To flatten retinoschisis.
  - To treat retinal neovascularization (when the media is opaque).

- To destroy retinal neoplasm, either simple (angioma), or malignant (retinoblastoma).

FLUORESCEIN DYE IN OPHTHALMOLOGY

Sodium fluorescein is a nontoxic, stable highly fluorescent dye. It does not penetrate the cell membrane, but remains on its surface.

When administered parenterally, the dye binds with albumin in the bloodstream, and circulates into the ocular tissues and intraocular fluids.

The dye absorbs light in the *blue* range of visible spectrum, with an *absorption peak* at 465 to 490 nm, and after excitation it emits light (fluoresce) in the *green* range of visible spectrum, with an *emission peak* at 520 to 530 nm. This color change can be detected even at a dilution of 1 in 1,000,000 by using ultraviolet light.

After intravenous (IV) injection, fluorescein dye is eliminated from the body through the kidneys and liver within 24–36 hours.

Dosages

- *For topical uses*—2% solution—1 drop.
- *Fluorescein paper strip* (available in sterile pouch) convenient to stain cornea and to assess tear film dysfunction.
- *For fundus fluorescein angiography:* 5 mL of 10% solution (most commonly), 10 mL of 5% solution, or 3 mL of 20% solution—as intravenous (IV) bolus injection.

Adverse Effects of Intravenous Fluorescein Dye

- Nausea and vomiting
- Vasovagal (syncopal) attack
- Painful local extravasation and phlebitis
- Pruritus and urticaria
  Anaphylaxis and bronchospasm (acute emergency) which may be fatal.

Uses of Fluorescein Dye

Topical uses
- Staining corneal abrasions or ulcer
- Hard contact lens fitting
- Tearfilm breakuptime (TBUT)
- To detect wound leak (Siedel's test)
- Applanation tonometry
- Patency of the lacrimal passage:
  - Dye disappearance test (DDT)
  - Jones test (I and II).
- To mark the radial cuts in radial keratotomy, etc.

Intravenous uses
- Fundus fluorescein angiography.
- Fluorescein fluorophotometry to study aqueous outflow or corneal endothelial cell function.
- Fluorescein iridography to study iris vascular pattern (e.g. in rubeosis iridis or angioma).
- As an antidote for aniline dye poisoning.

Fundus Fluorescein Angiography

It is a procedure of recording serial photographs (black and white) of retinal and choroidal circulation, and their integrity, after IV injection of fluorescein dye.

Normal Angiogram

The dye first appears at the choroid, then the retina, and finally it is drained via the central retinal vein. Normal *"arm-to-retina"* circulation is about 8–12 seconds (*average—10 seconds*). In the choroid, the dye appears about 1 second before the retina.

Fundus fluorescein angiography can be divided into following phases:
- *Choroidal (pre-arterial) phase:* When the dye enters into choroidal circulation, a bright glow is seen, known as *choroidal flush*. If a *cilioretinal artery* is present, it fills during this phase.

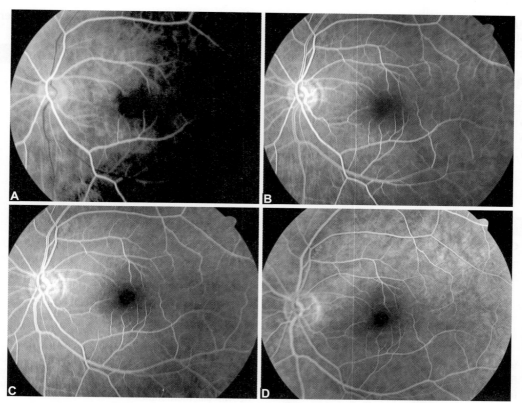

Figs 28.1A to D: Phases of fundus fluorescein angiography. **A.** Arterial; **B.** Early venous; **C.** Late venous; **D.** Recirculation phase

- *Arterial phase (Fig. 28.1A):* The dye appears in the retina through the central retinal artery. The superior and inferior branches fill quickly, and then the whole retinal arterialtree becomes brightly displayed.
- *Arteriovenous (capillary) phase:* The dye is seen both in the retinal artery and vein. The visualization of capillaries is at its best, during the venous phase.
- *Early venous phase (Fig. 28.1B):* This phase is marked by *laminar flow* which is due to presence of dye on the lateral wall of vein.
- *Late venous phase (Fig. 28.1C):* Soon the laminar flow reverses, and the entire blood column in the vein is mixed with the dye.

- *Recirculation phase (Fig. 28.1D):* This phase is marked by the *eventual fade of the dye.* If the blood-retinal barrier has been broken, the dye leaks out and stains the abnormal vessels, or pools into the tissue.
- *Normal macula:* It appears as a small hypofluorescent area. The perifoveal capillary arcade is seen during venous phase.
  Dark appearance of macula is due to:
  - Macular-RPE (retinal pigment epithelium) cells are taller and more pigmented
  - Presence of xanthophyll pigment
  - Foveal avascular zone (FAZ)
- *Optic disc:* The capillary fluorescence is seen at different stages, and valuable in differentiating pseudopapilledema, from papilledema and papillitis.

After 10 minutes, the fundus resembles that of pre-angiographic state, and any deviation from this is abnormal.

Abnormal Angiogram

It is based on two important features:
- The bloodretinal barrier
- The barrier between choroid and RPE.
1. *Hypofluorescence (Figs 28.2A and B):* It means a reduction or absence of normal fluorescence. It appears as dark area on the positive print of an angiogram.

Two possible causes of hypofluorescence	
Causes	**Example of lesions**
Blocked fluorescence	• *Pigments*—melanin, hemoglobin, xanthophyll • *Exudates*—hard, soft • *Hemorrhages*—subhyaloid retinal • Abnormal tissue materials—foreign body scar tissue
Vascular filling defects (dropout areas)	• Retinal artery, vein and capillaries, e.g. vascular occlusion • Choriocapillaris, e.g. sclerosis

2. *Hyperfluorescence (Figs 28.3 and 28.4):* It constitutes the appearance of an area that is more fluorescent than the surrounding area, or that stays fluorescent for a longer period of time.

Three possible causes of hyperfluorescence	
Causes	**Example of lesions**
Increased transmission	• *Atrophic:* RPE—drusen, RPE-window defect
Leak	• *Pooling* (in spaces) – *Retinal:* CME – *Subretinal:* CSR, RD • *Staining* (of tissues) – *Retinal*—soft exudates – *Subretinal*—drusen, scar
Abnormal vessels	• *Retinal*—neovascularization, aneurysms, shunts, collaterals, telangiectasis • *Subretinal*—SRNVMs, vessels in scar • *Tumors* – *Retinal*—retinoblastoma – *Subretinal*—malignant melanoma, choroidal hemangioma

RPE—Retinal pigmented epithelium; CME—Cystoid macular edema; CSR—Central serous retinopathy; RD—Retinal detachment; SRNVMs— Subretinal neovascular membranes

Fundus fluorescein angiography (FFA) is useful as an important diagnostic tool for certain clinical conditions. It is also important

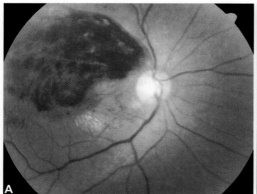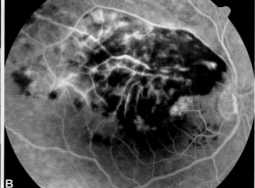

Figs 28.2A and B: A. Branch retinal vein occlusion—at the disc margin; **B.** Fundus fluoresce in angiography—same eye showing hypofluorescence

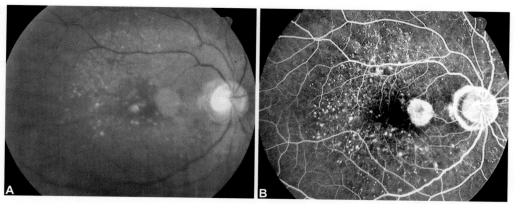

Figs 28.3A and B: A. Hard and calcified drusen; **B.** Fundus fluorescein angiography—same eye showing hyperfluorescence

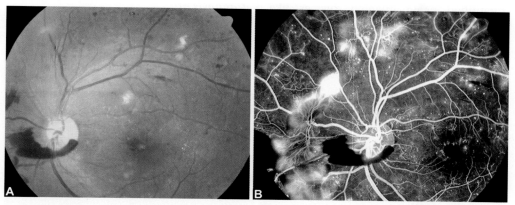

Figs 28.4A and B: A. Proliferative diabetic retinopathy; **B.** Fundus fluorescein angiography—both same eye showing hypo- and hyperfluorescence area, or that stays fluorescent for a longer period of time

to monitor laser photocoagulation treatment, in certain retina and choroidal diseases.

The common indications are:
- Diabetic retinopathy
- Retinal venous occlusions (CRVO or BRVO)
- Eales' disease
- Central serous retinopathy (CSR)
- Age-related macular degeneration
- Tumors of the retina and choroid
- Vascular anomalies of the retina and choroid
- Papilledema

Fundus Autofluorescence

- Fundus autofluorescence (FAF) is the emission of fluorescent light from ocular structures in the absence of sodium fluorescein. Pseudofluorescence occurs when the blue exciter and green barrier filters overlap.
- Retinal pigmented epithelium (RPE) is a monolayer which plays a critical role in phagocytosis and lysosomal breakdown of pigmented outer segments of photoreceptors. With aging, incomplete or partial

breakdown of these segments in the post-mitotic RPE cells causes the accumulation of lipofuscin. Excessive lipofuscin deposition is considered pathologic and is associated with visual loss.

- Because of its diverse composition, lipofuscin has a broad-spectrum of excitation (300–600 nm) and emission (480–800 nm). Thus, it can be excited by many wavelengths of visible light in the blue and green portion of spectrum. Autofluorescence uses the fluorescent properties of lipofuscin to generate images.
- The unique autofluorescent properties of RPE lipofuscin can be detected and quantified using imaging devices like, confocal scanning laser ophthalmoscope (cSLO) and FAF camera systems.
- Fundus autofluorescence imaging has potential role to provide useful information in conditions where the health of the RPE plays a key role (Figs 28.5A to D).

Reduced fundus autofluorescence:
- Retinal pigmented epithelium loss or atrophy
- Intraretinal fluid
- Reduction in RPE lipofuscin density
- Fibrosis
- Presence of luteal pigment.

Increased fundus autofluorescence:
- Drusen
- Excessive RPE lipofuscin accumulation
- Agerelated macular degeneration.

Fundus autofluorescence is useful in the diagnosis of:
- Agerelated macular degeneration
- Retinitis pigmentosa
- White dot syndromes
- Central serous chorioretinopathy

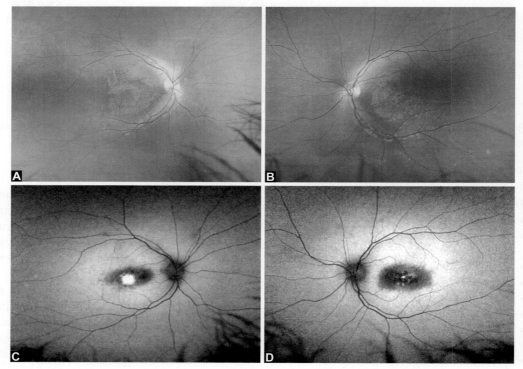

Figs 28.5A to D: Fundus autofluorescence showing heredo-macular dystrophy. **A and B.** Fundus as seen in normal digital fundus photography; **C and D.** Same eyes with FAF camera system

- Macular dystrophies like—Stargardt disease, cone dystrophies, and Best's disease
- Chloroquine maculopathy.

Indocyanine Green Angiography

Indocyanine green angiography (ICGA) is a diagnostic technique that uses ICG dye's infrared fluorescence to provide details about the choroidal circulation and its disorders (Figs 28.6A to D).

- Indocyanine green angiography is an amphophilic tricarbocyanine dye and the lyophilized powder is dissolved in water for injection. It is 98% bound to proteins and remains longer in large blood vessels with a lesser tendency to diffuse in the interstitial space. Hence, it is ideal for diseases affecting the choroidal tissues.
- Plasma halflife of ICG is 2–4 minutes. Maximal peak of absorption is at 790–805 nm and a peak emission of 835 nm.
- There are two types of ICG systems—modified fundus cameras and SLO -based systems. Dosage of dye varies from 20 mg to 50 mg dissolved in 2–4 mL of aqueous solvent. Preferred technique is to inject 25 mg dye in 5 mL of water slowly.
- Some iodine is present in the dye and cross over allergy can occur. Contraindications

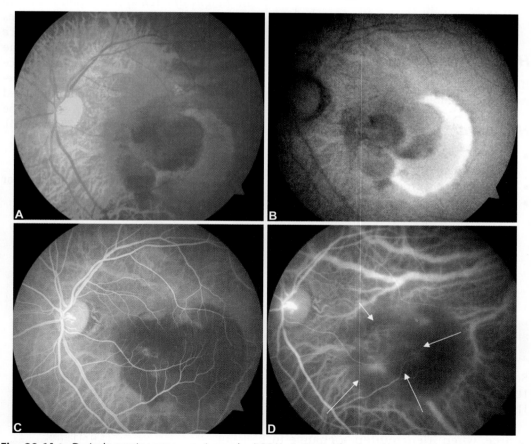

Figs 28.6A to D: Indocyanine green angiography (ICGA). **A.** Digital fundus photograph of a case of occult choroidal neovascular membrane (CNVM); **B.** Same lesion as visible under autofluorescence; **C.** Same lesion as seen in fundus fluorescence angiography; **D.** Same lesion best visible in ICGA (white arrows)

are prior anaphylactic reactions to iodine-based preparations, hepatic insufficiency, uremia and pregnancy.

Phases

- **Early phase:** It occurs 2 seconds after injection of ICG, choroidal arteries and choriocapillaris fills up, 3–5 seconds after injection, larger choroidal veins begin to fill.
- **Middle phase:** It occurs at 3–15 minutes after injection and marked by continuous fading of choroidal and retinal vessels.
- **Late phase:** It occurs at 15–60 minutes after injection.

Abnormal areas can be described as hypocyanescence or hypercyanescence.

Hypocyanescence

Blockage—blood/serous fluid/pigment/exudates/impaired choroidal perfusion.

Hypercyanescence

- Lack of overlying tissue—RPE dropout/lacquer cracks
- Leakage from surrounding vessels
- Leakage from abnormal blood vessels
  - Hot spots and plaques are used to define areas of intense hyperfluorescence during the middle and late phases.
  - Hot spots are defined as <1 DD (disc diameter) in size. Plaques are >1 DD in size and reveal less obvious leakage.

ULTRASONOGRAPHY IN OPHTHALMOLOGY

Sound frequencies between 16 Hz and 20,000 Hz are audible, and frequencies above 20,000 Hz are called ultrasound.

The ultrasound is reflected toward its source, when it encounters a change in elasticity or density of the medium through which it is passing. This reflecd vibration *(echo)* is converted into an electric potential by a *piezoelectrical crystal,* and displayed on an oscilloscope.

Ultrasonic frequencies in the range of 10 MHz are used in ophthalmic ultrasonography (USG). *Two types of USG are used: A-scan and B-scan.*

Ultrasonography A-scan (Fig. 28.7)

A transducer is positioned so that the ultrasonic beam passes through a chosen ocular meridian. The tracing records a series of spikes, at sites of change in intraocular impedance. The *height of each spike* depends on the acoustic density of the tissue, which varies with cellular composition. *The distance* between the spikes gives a measure of the distance from the transducer, as well as distance between intraocular structures. Ascan is *one-dimensional*, and hence, amplitude modulated display provides the information. A-scan may be axial or nonaxial *(di-scleral)* (Figs 28.8A and B).

Uses of A-scan

- Axial length measurement for intraocular lens power calculation.

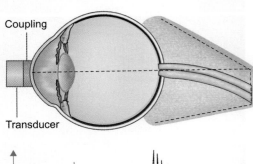

Coupling

Transducer

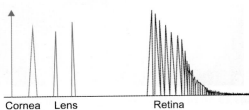

Cornea   Lens   Retina

Fig. 28.7: A-scan ultrasonography

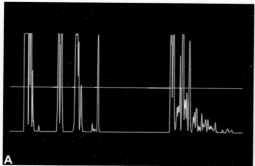
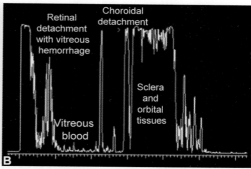

Figs 28.8A and B: Ultrasonography A-scan. **A.** Normal spikes in normal eye; **B.** Abnormal spikes in vitreous chamber indicating vitreous hemorrhage with retino-choroidal detachment

- Measurement of anterior chamber depth, lens thickness, or depth of a lesion.
- To detect pathological lesions preoperatively, in presence of opacities in the ocular media.
- To differentiate a preretinal membrane from a retinal detachment (***quantitative echography***).
- To differentiate between benign and malignant intraocular lesions.
- To measure corneal thickness (***ultrasonic pachymetry***) before radial keratotomy operation, or PRK or LASIK.

Ultrasonography B-scan (Fig. 28.9)

The testing transducer is moved in a linear fashion across the eye, to build up a ***two-dimensional*** picture of the intraocular structures, and the orbit.

Echoes are plotted as ***dots*** instead of spikes, and the brightness of the dot indicates the size of the received echoes. The resulting B-scan picture is comparable to a histological cross-section through the eye and the orbit. B-scan may be taken on the sagittal, horizontal or oblique planes of the eye.

Uses of B-scan (Figs 28.10A and B)

- To differentiate the space-occupying lesions within the eye and the orbit.

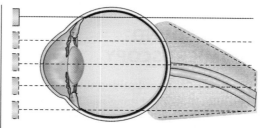

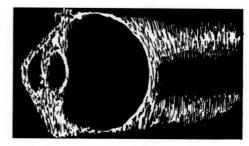

Fig. 28.9: B-scan ultrasonography

- To determine the vitreoretinal pathology (e.g. retinal detachment, or vitreous hemorrhage) in presence of opacity in the ocular media.
- To localize the intraocular foreign body, especially, if it is not radioopaque.
- To study the muscle thickness, e.g. in thyroid ophthalmopathy or orbital pseudotumor.
- To study the vitreous hemorrhage and its complications (e.g. vitreous bands) prior to vitreous surgery.
- To differentiate the types of retinal detachment (e.g. rhegmatogenous, exudative or tractional).

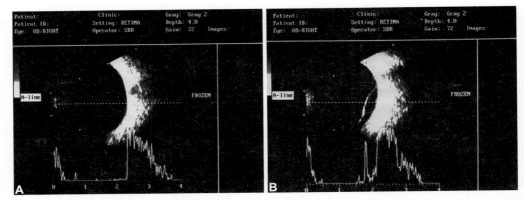

Figs 28.10A and B: A. Normal USG-B scan; **B.** Abnormal membrane (spikes) in front of lower retina indicating inferior retinal detachment

ULTRASOUND BIOMICROSCOPY

It is a new ultrasoundguided diagnostic tool which allows detailed imaging of the anterior segment of the eye *(like slit-lamp biomicroscopy)*.

High-frequency, high-resolution ultrasound biomicroscopy (UBM) is similar in principle to conventional USG B-scan.

In general, the resolution and depth of penetration of ultrasound waves are affected by transducer frequency.

The ocular USG B-scan uses a 10 MHz transducer, with approximately 150 μm resolution.

Whereas, an UBM is performed with a *high frequency (50 MHz)* transducer with a tissue resolution of 50 μm. But this is at the expense of decreasing tissue penetration depth of 4–5 mm which is sufficient to image the anterior segment (Figs 28.11A and B).

Ultrasound scanning of the cornea is possible with a 100 MHz transducer that increases the tissue resolution to less than 20 μm.

Uses

- High frequency UBM allows detailed imaging of the:
    - Anterior segment of the eye
    - Angle of the anterior chamber (Figs 28.11A and B)

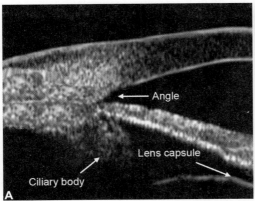
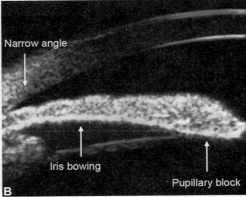

Figs 28.11A and B: A. Normal human eye; **B.** Pupillary block

- Ciliary body (e.g. tumor, etc.)
- Pars plana and peripheral vitreous (e.g. pars planitis).
- It also helps to identify position of intra-ocular lens and its haptics.

Advantage of UBM: To assess the above structures in patients with media opacity—like, edematous or scarred corneal tissue.

RADIOLOGY IN OPHTHALMOLOGY

Each orbit is a four-sided pyramidal cavity with apex aimed posteromedially and the base toward the face. It is made up of *parts of seven bones* and divided into the roof, medial wall, lateral wall and the floor. Radiological examination of the eye and orbit is useful for evaluating trauma, foreign body, and tumors.

X-ray

X-ray studies of the orbits are difficult because of superimposition of the other bones of the skull. The patient is placed on the radiographic table, usually in the prone position.

Several techniques are used to localize lesions at a particular depth and side:

- *Caldwell's view* is a PA projection of the orbit. This is important for orbital rim, roof, and superior orbital fissure.
- *Water's view* is useful for orbital floor.
- *Rheese view* is useful for optic canal.
- *Oblique view* is especially useful for orbital rim fracture.
- *Lateral view* is useful for localization of foreign bodies.
- *X-ray orbit with limbal marker* to localize intraocular metallic foreign body more precisely in relation to the limbus.
- *Dacryocystography* is an X-ray evaluation of the drainage system of lacrimal apparatus in an attempt to localize the precise site of obstruction.
- *Orbital venography* is an X-ray evaluation of the orbital veins with a contrast dye to diagnose orbital varix in case of proptosis.

CT Scan

The CT scan is the study of choice for soft tissue and bony abnormalities. The main diagnosis possible with CT scan is the orbital tumors. The other diagnosis possible with CT scan includes:

- Ruptured globe
- Intraocular or intraorbital foreign body
- Ocular tumors
- Fracture of any wall including, blowout fracture
- Secondary sinus involvement
- Neuroophthalmological diseases.

Magnetic Resonance Imaging

Magnetic resonance imaging (MRI) is the procedure of choice for soft tissue anatomy and pathology of vascularized lesions of ocular, orbital and neuro-ophthalmic structures from the orbit to the brain. MRI is also useful in early diagnosis of multiple sclerosis.

Magnetic Resonance Angiography

It is a noninvasive method for imaging the carotid and major cerebral arteries, helpful for neuro-ophthalmologic diagnosis, like carotid artery occlusion/stenosis, any aneurysm, arteriovenous malformation, vascular mass, etc.

OCULAR EMERGENCIES

Ocular emergencies are those situations that require immediate attention and management. The following situations need emergency care of the patients:

- *Chemical burns:* Alkali, acid or organic solvents in the eye.
- *Sudden painless total loss of vision:* This problem suggests an acute vascular occlusion and could cause permanent loss of vision if not treated immediately, especially in central retinal arterial occlusion (CRAO).

Above two conditions need real emergency management without any delay.

Others are:
- **Open globe** injury of the eyeball.
- **Severe blunt trauma** such as a forceful blow to the eyeball with a fist or by a cricket or tennis ball.
- **A foreign body** in the eye.
- **Corneal abrasion** caused by a foreign body or by trauma.
- **Sudden painless severe dimness of vision**— as in optic neuritis or retinal detachment.
- **Acute painful red eye with loss of vision**, e.g. acute attack of angle closure glaucoma, lensinduced glaucoma, etc.
- **Any emergency referral** from other physician or ophthalmologist.

Ocular Urgent Situations

The urgent situation requires the patient should be seen within 24–48 hours. The patients with urgent conditions may report with a variety of symptoms, some of which may suggest an emergency situation, while the others, although not serious, but may deserve prompt attention. Sometimes, it is difficult to distinguish an urgent situation from an emergency.

The following situations are generally considered to be urgent:
- Subacute or gradual loss of vision over a few days to a week
- Sudden onset of diplopia
- Recent onset of flashes and floaters especially in myopes
- Acute red eye with or without discharge and loss of vision
- Acute and progressively increasing ocular pain
- Sudden onset of photophobia
- Loss or breakage of glasses or contact lenses needed for work, driving or studies (though not all physicians consider losing or breaking glasses as urgent).

SUBCONJUNCTIVAL INJECTION

Subconjunctival injections are most useful for attaining effective concentration of drugs in the aqueous. Though, in most cases they can be replaced by frequent topical application of drugs.

Routes of absorption of drugs after subconjunctival injection:
- Part of the effects of a subconjunctival injection is due to gradual reflux of the drug along with the needle track, with subsequent transcorneal absorption.
- Partly, via the sclera adjacent to the injection site.

Disadvantages
- These injections may be painful, especially in case of inflamed eyes.
- Conjunctiva tends to become scarred.
- Accidental globe perforation may occur which is dangerous.

Indications
- Severe ocular infections, e.g. in bacterial corneal ulcers (mainly antibiotic and atropine).
- Severe intraocular inflammation, e.g. iridocyclitis (steroids and atropine) or endophthalmitis (antibiotics and atropine).
- At the end of any intraocular surgery, e.g. after cataract operation or penetrating keratoplasty (gentamicin and dexamethasone).
- To give subconjunctival anesthesia in certain operations, e.g. pterygium resection, or to remove a conjunctival cystor mass.

Procedure
i. Topical anesthesia by 4% lignocaine or 0.5% proparacaine. A small cotton palette soaked in anesthetic agent is held on the area for 2 minutes—very effective.
ii. Patient is lying on a bed.
iii. Care has to taken to minimize patient's apprehension.
iv. Wire speculum is applied.
v. Patient is asked to look upward or opposite side away from the site of injection.

vi. 0.5–1 mL of drug is taken in a 1 mL or 2 mL syringe with 26 gauge needle or (in an insulin syringe).

vii. Gently hold a fold of conjunctiva in a tent fashion, 3 mm away from the limbus with a plain forceps, avoiding the blood vessels.

viii. The needle tip with beveled up, is slid underneath the bulbar conjunctiva. The plunger of the syringe is withdrawn to ensure against any intravascular penetration.

ix. Inject about 0.5 mL solution at a time.

x. Gently withdraw the needle.

xi. Cover the eye with a pad for 1 hour.

SUB-TENON INJECTION

Here, the main route of absorption is via the trans-scleral route near the injection site. Posterior sub-Tenon injection is mostly preferred.

This is the most effective method of continuous drug delivery, especially in inflamed eyes. The most popular drug used for sub-Tenon injection is depot steroids, e.g. triamcinolone or methylprednisolone with or without atropine and antibiotic.

Indication: Chronic uveitis (pars planitis and posterior uveitis) and cystoid macular edema (CME).

Best site of injection: Upper temporal quadrant. Alternately, the inferotemporal quadrant may be selected for injection.

Procedure

Step (i) to (v) same as subconjunctival injection.

- Patient is instructed to look down and in, toward his nose.
- With the beveled side toward the globe, the needle is introduced into the superior bulbar conjunctival area avoiding the conjunctival blood vessels and moved from side to side and injected deep into the posterior sub-Tenon's space.

Disadvantages

- It is technically difficult.
- Chance of globe perforation is more than subconjunctival injection.
- Steroid-induced glaucoma which is difficult to manage. May have to dissect sub-Tenon space and remove the depot steroids.

INTRAVITREAL INJECTIONS

Injecting drugs directly into the vitreous cavity is indicated in various posterior segment pathologies. This route delivers the drugs at the target site and bypasses all absorption barriers. The gel-like vitreous also acts as a reservoir for the drug which acts slowly over time. Some patients may require multiple injections.

Indications of intravitreal injections:
- Various drug delivery
- Vitreous biopsy/tap for microbiology (smear, culture or PCR).

The various drugs given intravitreally are:

Drug group	Indications	Drugs
Antibiotics	Endophthalmitis	Vancomycin, Ceftazidime, Amikacin
Antifungals	Endophthalmitis	Amphotericin B, Voriconazole
Antivirals	Viral retinal necrosis or retinopathy	Ganciclovir, Foscarnet
Anti-VEGFs	Diabetic retinopathy, Wet ARMD, ROP	Ranibizumab, Bevacizumab, Aflibercept
Steroid*	CME in BRVO or chronic uveitis	Triamcinolone acetonide

*Steroids are sometimes administered as slow release implants for prolonged duration of action. The commonly used implants are: Dexamethasone implant—Ozurdex; and Fluocinolone implant—Retisert and Iluvien.

Procedure:
- Done usually under topical anesthesia (paracaine or lignocaine)

- Instil drop of povidone iodine 5% in conjunctival sac
- Insert eye speculum for exposure
- *Needle used:* 30 G; volume injected 0.05 to 0.1 mL
- *Injection location:* Commonly in infero-temporal region for ease of access (sometimes superotemporal)
- *Measure injection site location from limbus with callipers:* 3 mm in aphakia; 3.5 mm in pseudophakia, and 4 mm in phakic eyes
- Needle direction is toward center of globe. Nowadays usually a straight needle path is followed.
- A sterile cotton swab is placed at injection site immediately after withdrawing needle to prevent reflux.
- Post-procedure topical antibiotics are given for 5–7 days.

Complications: Transient rise in IOP; acute rise in IOP causing central retinal artery occlusion (CRAO); retinal or vitreous hemorrhage; retinal detachment, and endophthalmitis.

LABORATORY DIAGNOSIS OF OCULAR INFECTIONS

Conjunctival Swab

Laboratory diagnosis in bacterial conjunctivitis is not a routine. However, the *indications* of conjunctival scraping for microscopic examination are:

- Neonatal conjunctivitis
- Hyperacute purulent conjunctivitis
- Chronic recalcitrant conjunctivitis. Conjunctival swab is a routine procedure before any intraocular operation (e.g. cataract operation, glaucoma operation) in some places. But it is not a mandatory.

Methods

- Conjunctival scrapings should be taken prior to the use of topical anesthetics, as these agents and their preservatives may mask the recovery of certain bacteriae.
- Cultures are taken by moistering asterile alginate (not cotton) swab with saline and wiping the inner lid margin or conjunctival cul-de-sac.
- They are then inoculated in solid or liquid culture media (blood agar and/or chocolate agar).
- Simultaneous smear may be prepared for staining with Gram or Giemsa stain. This is to identify the organisms and inflammatory cell types. The cytologic features of each type of conjunctivitis are different and helpful in diagnosis.

Corneal Scraping

This is the most important step in early diagnosis of a corneal ulcer, for prompt and rigorous initiation of therapy.

- The scraping is performed after instillation of topical preservative-free anesthetic agents (e.g. proparacaine 0.5% or lignocaine 2–4%).
- The procedure should obtain as much material as feasible, particularly from the deeper areas (floor) and the margins of the ulcer.
- Scraping material is usually taken with a No. 15 blade or a Kimura's spatula.
- Smear is prepared for microscopic examination with KOH mount, Gram or Giemsa stain. In 30–40% cases in results may be negative for bacteria even if infection is present.
- Culture should be done on blood agar plate (at room temperature) and Sabouraud's media (for fungus) and into Page's medium (for acanthamoeba), if suspected.

Aqueous or Vitreous Tap

In suspected cases of infective endophthalmitis—to find out the causative agent.

CORNEAL TOPOGRAPHY (FIGS 28.12A AND B)

It is a method of qualitative and quantitative evaluation of the corneal surface by the reflected light.

- In 1619, Father Scheiner first found that corneal surface can be studied from reflection of a window on it *(window reflex)*.
- In 1880, Placido introduced a disc *(Placido's disc)* with alternate white and dark concentric circles with central aperture for viewing. These circles were reflected on the cornea. A qualitative assessment was made.

The invention of videography has been incorporated into the Placido image system. The image thus captured on a CCD camera and analyzed by computer software on the basis of relative distances between the rings. "Shorter the distance, steeper is the cornea" and vice versa. Normal cornea is a prolate surface, i.e. steeper in the center and flatter in the periphery.

The computer adds chosen color to the image and produces a color-coded map of the whole cornea. By standardization the:

- *Warm (hot) colors* such as red, yellow represent high corneal power *(steeper)*.
- *Cool colors* like violet, blue represent low corneal power *(flatter)*.
- *Yellow-green spectrum* represents the most normal corneas.

A scale is given alongside the colorcoded map which gives the numerical values in diopters to the specific colors.

Uses

- The curvature of the whole cornea can be studied.
- Early diagnosis of corneal ectatic disorders such as keratoconus, pellucid degeneration or secondary corneal ectasia, etc.
- Study of changes in corneal astigmatism following surgical procedures like keratoplasty, cataract surgery, refractive surgeries, etc.
- *Corneal tomography.*

SPECULAR MICROSCOPY

The ophthalmologist can visualize the corneal endothelium directly by performing specular reflection method of slit-lamp microscope. But, this is not enough to get sufficient information about cell density and morphology of the corneal endothelium.

Specular microscope is a useful instrument to visualize the corneal endothelium (at 500 x) to the ophthalmologists, especially the corneal surgeons.

It yields information that guides the physician in decision-making of certain corneal disorders and anterior segment surgeries. It also captures the pictures that are

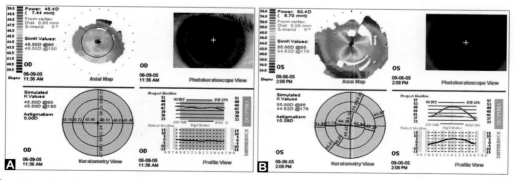

Figs 28.12A and B: A. Normal corneal topography; **B.** Corneal topography in keratoconus

useful for documentation and monitoring a patient over a period of time.

The corneal endothelium is a hexagonal monolayer that does not divide in human being.

The cell count of an infant is around 4,500–5,000 cells/sq.mm. With age, the cell count declines. The adults typically have 2,000–3,000 cell/sq.mm. of endothelium. The cell morphology is also changed with ages. In young adult, the percentage of hexagonal cells is more (>60%).

The critical *endothelial cell* count is around 500 cell/sq.mm. If the cell count is less than 500 cells/sq. mm, there may be chance of corneal decompensation and corneal edema (Figs 28.13A and B).

Specular Microscopy Analysis

- *Cell density (CD):* Number of endothelial cells/sq.mm.
- *Hexagonality:* Percentage of hexagonal cells among total endothelial cells.
- *Cell size and shape:* Percentage of cells that show polymegathism (different cell sizes) and pleomorphism (different cell shapes).
- *Coefficient of variation of cell size:* An automatic statistical index of polymegathism.

- *Corneal thickness (CT):* It gives the measurement of corneal thickness in µm in a noncontact way.

The additional software algorithm can analyze in depth the morphological changes of the corneal endothelium and can compare the results with other values.

Both contact and noncontact specular microscope are available. But practically, noncontact specular is more safe and popular.
Two types of specular microscopes:
1. *Clinical specular:* To study the endothelium in a clinical set-up.
2. *Eye bank specular:* To study the sclerocorneal donor button for keratoplasty purpose.

Uses

- To study the corneal endothelial diseases.
- To take decision about corneal surgery.
- Before cataract operation when there is any suspicion during slit-lamp examination (*see* Chapter 15).
- To study the safety of certain surgical procedures.
- To study the safety of certain drugs used intracamerally during surgery.
- During follow-up of keratoplasty and refractive surgery patients.

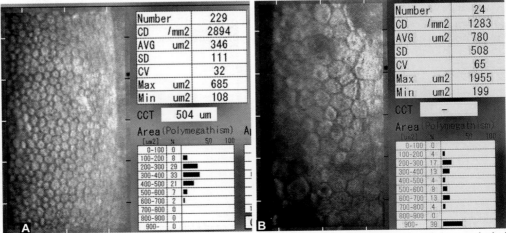

Figs 28.13A and B: A. Normal specular microscopic photograph; **B.** Corneal guttata with low endothelial cell count in early Fuchs' dystrophy

SCANNING LASER POLARIMETRY (GDxVCC) (FIGS 28.14A AND B)

Glaucoma detection with variable corneal compensation (GDxVCC) is a scanning laser polarimeter which helps to assess the thickness of the retinal nerve fiber layer (RNFL) without dilatation.

Patients with early glaucoma having normal optic nerves and visual fields may have RNFL defects and thus, GDx VCC helps in diagnosing glaucoma in *preperimetric stage*.

Principle: When polarized light passes through the RNFL, the birefringent properties of the axons cause polarized light to undergo a phase shift. The amount of phase shift or retardation is measured, and is proportional to the thickness of RNFL. This technique is known as *scanning laser polarimetry*.

Using a near infrared *diode laser* (780 nm) RNFL thickness is measured in a 15° × 15° grid centered on the optic nerve head.

The readings obtained are compared to a normative database.

The colored printout includes images and various parameters along with the probability of deviation of such values in compare to the normal database. RNFL thickness is represented using a color scale, with *dark blue being the thinnest* and the *red being thickest*.

Uses

- It is a noninvasive quick technique for diagnosis and monitoring of early glaucoma.
- It may also be used as a screening tool for the "*glaucoma-suspect*" patients.

OPTICAL COHERENCE TOMOGRAPHY (FIGS 28.15A TO D)

It is a new diagnostic tool mainly for the posterior segment disorders. It rapidly provides a quantifiable two (or three) dimensional crosssection (tomography) of the retina.

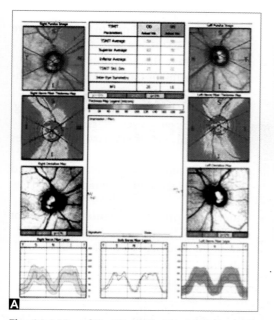
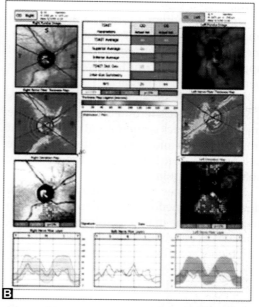

Figs 28.14A and B: GDx VCC pictures. **A.** Normal appearance of RNFL with normal thickness; **B.** Thinning of RNFL—more in right eye with advanced glaucoma and inferior part in left eye with early glaucoma

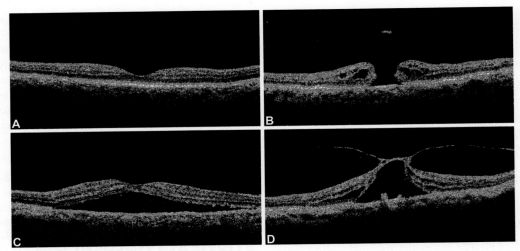

Figs 28.15A to D: A. Normal optical coherence tomography; **B.** Macular hole with detached; **C.** Central serous retinopathy; **D.** Vitreomacular traction

Ultrasonography B-scan mechanism has a similarity with optical coherence tomography (OCT). But instead of dynamic echoes of sound used in USG, OCT relies on differential reflections of light. Spatial resolution of OCT is approximately 5 µm, whereas that of USG Bscan is approximately 150 µm.

Optical coherence tomography is based on the principle of low coherence interferometry. It uses an infrared incident beam of approximately 830 nm in wavelengths. The beam is focused on retina by a +78D lens.

Optical coherence tomography unit employs a Michaelson interferometer to compare the magnitude of back scattered and reflected light from the retina and demonstrates it as a false colorcoded image in two/three dimensions by software manipulations.

Different types of OCT imaging have been developed: Timedomain and Fourierdomain techniques. The main advantages of Fourier-domain OCT are higher signal acquisition rates and higher sensitivity than timedomain OCT.

Uses of Optical Coherence Tomography

- *Macular imaging:* In today's clinical ophthalmology, OCT is used mainly for imaging in macular diseases, like:
  - Diabetic macular edema
  - Macular edema related to vaso-occlusive diseases
  - Cystoid macular edema
  - Epiretinal membrane (ERM), with or without vitreomacular traction (Fig. 28.15D)
  - Macular hole or pseudohole (Fig. 28.15B)
  - Choroidal neovascular membranes (CNVMs)
  - Central serous chorioretinopathy and pigment epithelial detachment (Fig. 28.15C).
- Anterior segment evaluation by anterior segment OCT.
- Quantification of peripapillary RNFL analysis.

Anterior Segment Optical Coherence Tomography

Optical coherence tomography is a noncontact optical device that provides cross-sectional images and quantitative analysis of the ocular tissues in the anterior and posterior segment.

Anterior segment OCT systems are categorized by the wavelength of the light sources.

- Dedicated systems using 1,310 nm, e.g. Zeiss Visante, Heidelberg SL-OCT, Tomey CASIA.
- Systems converted from a retinal scanner using 830 nm, e.g. Optovue, Zeiss Cirrus, Heidelberg Spectralis.

A shorter wavelength (830 nm, near infrared) provides a higher axial resolution, but its imaging depth is limited. A longer wavelength (1,310 nm) provides deeper penetration.

Uses

- *Refractive surgery and ectatic disorders:* Used in visualization of flap thickness, flap interface, and flap displacement post-LASIK.
- *Assessment of Descemet membrane:* ASOCT can help in prognosis, e.g. planar/nonplanar, local/extensive detachment, and rupture of DM. Also useful in knowing the status of DM post PK, DMEK, DSAEK, e.g. lenticule detachment, fluid in the interface and status after rebubbling.
- *Deep anterior lamellar keratoplasty (DALK), descemet stripping endothelial keratoplasty (DSEK), Descemet's membrane endothelial keratoplasty (DMEK):* Live intraoperative OCT is useful while performing DALK, DSEK and DMEK, e.g. dissection depth, insertion depth of cannula for Big bubble technique, lenticule insertion in DMEK and its attachment and interface quality.

- *Corneal deposits:* Useful in diagnosis of corneal dystrophies. Useful in the planning of PTK for superficial opacities, as in granular dystrophy.
- *Keratitis:* Useful in knowing the depth of the infiltrate and can help in the planning of therapeutic PK vs. therapeutic DALK.
- *Tumors and OSSN:* It has a supplementary role in some nonpigmented tumors.
- *Dry eye:* Useful in tear meniscus measurement viz. tear meniscus height (TMH), tear meniscus depth (TMD) and tear meniscus area (TMA).
- *Cataract surgery:* Useful in femtosecond assisted cataract surgery where a live image of the cornea and lens is available for detailed planning of mainport, sideports, relaxing incisions, and capsulorhexis.

Optical Coherence Tomography in Glaucoma

- *Angle assessment:* Anterior segment OCT can provide important parameters about the anterior chamber, like the anterior chamber angle (ACA), angle opening distance (AOD 500 and 750 μm) and trabecular iris space area (TISA).

  These parameters help in—angle assessment especially in angle closure screening, structural cause of angle closure, evaluation of efficacy of a laser iridotomy procedure and analysis of iris configuration.
- *Filtering bleb and tube:* ASOCT can reveal morphology of filtering blebs, the recently developed 3D ASOCT technique allows for a detailed evaluation of internal morphology of blebs. It can help determining which blebs are suitable for needling and for visualizing tube erosion in glaucoma drainage devices.
- *Glaucoma diagnosis and progression:* ASOCT allows for *in vivo* cross-sectional

imaging of the optic nerve head (ONH) and retina.

Spectral domain optical coherence tomography (SDOCT) with 3D images helps in glaucoma diagnosis by studying the RNFL thickness, rim area, and total macular thickness.

Ganglion cell layer with inner plexiform layer (GCIPL) is the most sensitive parameter for the diagnosis of glaucoma.

SDOCT is useful in detecting RNFL changes in glaucoma progression. SDOCT glaucoma progression algorithms measure changes based on either eventbased or trendbased analysis.

Retinal Nerve Fibers Layer (RNFL) OCT

- Optical coherence tomography technology can be used to quantitatively measure the thickness of the RNFL to assess glaucoma induced retinal nerve fiber damage.
- The newer OCT machines allow highly precise measurements. And since anatomical changes precedes field loss, RNFL OCT is a pre-perimetric test which allows detection of glaucomatous damage even before the patient is aware of any field loss. This makes it a valuable glaucoma screening test.
- RNFL is measured in microns in the peripapillary region with circular scan of 3.4 mm diameter centered around the optic nerve head.
- These measurements are arranged in **TSNIT** order (**T**emporal – **S**uperior – **N**asal – **I**nferior – **T**emporal) and are compared with age-gender matched normative data.
- The test result shows the RNFL thickness in a graphical pattern and are color coded as green (normal), yellow (suspicious) and red (abnormal) (Fig. 28.16A and B).

Subsequent tests can also pick up subtle thinning in each quadrant and is used to assess glaucoma progression.

HEADACHE IN OPHTHALMOLOGY

- *"Headache"* is defined by the dictionary, as continuous or prolonged dull pain in the region of the head.

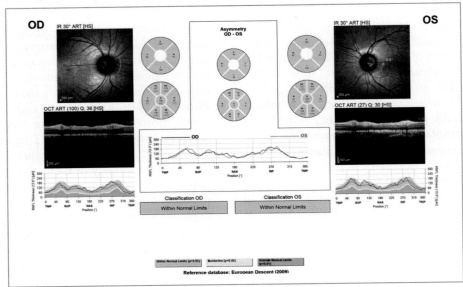

Fig. 28.16A: Normal image of RNFL OCT

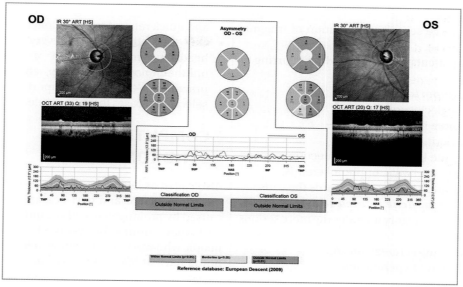

Fig. 28.16B: Image of RNFL OCT in glaucoma

- It is the ***most frequent and most ill-under-stood clinical symptom***, which depends to a great deal on the emotional background and pain threshold of the subject.
- Headache is usually mild, vague, brief lasting, and often innocuous, ***but some-times***, it is severe, persistent, or frequent, and could be a symptom of more serious conditions, in an apparently healthy individual.
- So, a patient presenting with headache as a primary symptom to an ophthalmologist, often presents a diagnostic challenge.

Causes of Ocular Headache

- Associated with refractive errors and ocular muscle imbalance.
- Secondary to organic diseases of the eye.
- Due to systemic disorders, but have prominent ocular symptoms.

Headache associated with refractive errors and ocular-muscle imbalance:
- Majority of the patients with ocular headache belong to this category, and the pain is dull, boring and often associated with eye-strain.
- Headaches are usually experienced towards the afternoon, and typically, experienced on undertaking tasks which entail binocular vision, e.g. reading, writing, knitting, etc.
- ***Conditions responsible***
    - ***Astigmatism and hypermetropia:*** Low grades of error cause more headache, because the ciliary muscle tries to overcome the defect by spasm. But this element is lacking in higher errors, which present as visual deficit than headache.
    - ***Presbyopia*** (mainly on near work)
    - ***Heterophoria (latent squint)***
    - ***Convergence insufficiency***
- These headaches are relieved by proper glasses and orthoptic exercises.

Headache secondary to organic eye-diseases:
- These headaches are usually unilateral, acute, continuous and located in and around the eyeball, and often aggravated by light.

- The pain is characteristically radiated along the sensory distribution of trigeminal nerve.
- The patients often have sudden blurring of vision.
- *The important causes:*
  - Angleclosure glaucoma
  - Acute iridocyclitis
  - Scleritis
  - Acute keratitis due to infection, contact lens overwear, or photokeratitis.
- Treatment is directed towards the cause.

Ocular headache related to systemic diseases: This category includes the more serious diseases:
- Raised intracranial tension
- Malignant hypertension
- Migraine
- Temporal arteritis
- Psychogenic (e.g. anxiety neurosis).

Ophthalmic Evaluation of Headache

- *Refraction under cycloplegia*
- Ocular movements
- *Orthoptic check-up*
- Slitlamp examination—to detect abrasion, ciliary congestion, KPs, etc.
- Ophthalmoscopy to check *papilledema*
- Cranial nerve examinations
- Intraocular pressure measurement
- Gonioscopy to know the anglestatus
- Palpation of the temporal artery for tenderness
- Automated perimetry for visual field.

Ophthalmologist's Approach

- The ophthalmologists are responsible for the management of headache due to refractive errors and ocular muscle imbalance, and those secondary to organic eye diseases.
- But, for the headaches related to systemic disease, his basic responsibility in early diagnosis (may be of an intracranial neoplasm by detecting the papilledema) and quick referral to other colleagues.
- On the other hand, every case of headache must undergo a thorough ophthalmological check-up, and general practitioner can play an important role to select such cases for proper referral.

COMPUTER VISION SYNDROME (CVS)

Also called as Digital eye strain, is a complex of various ocular and peri-ocular symptoms caused by prolonged use of computer, tablets and smartphones. Between 50% to 90% of people who work at a computer screen for 6–9 hours have at least some symptoms. This is also common in children who stare at tablets, smartphone or gaming devices can have the same problems. CVS symptoms are more with small screen smartphones devices than large screen tablets/computers.

The common symptoms are:
- Redness,
- Dry eyes (evaporative type),
- Blurred vision and double vision,
- Eye strain,
- Headache and brow-ache, and
- Stiffness of neck and shoulders.

The reasons for these symptoms are: Decreased blink rate while staring at the screen, constant accommodation for long duration, blue light, glare from screen, poor lighting, improper viewing distance and sitting posture.

Treatment: It consists primarily of ergonomic and lifestyle modifications. dry-eye component is treated with lubricants.
- Correct sitting position and viewing distance
- Anti-glare eye glasses; reduce screen brightness etc.
- Frequent blinking and making conscious effort to blink (15-20 times/min)
- *20-20-20 rule:* Every 20 minutes interval look at 20 feet distant object for 20 seconds. This relieves constant accommodation

- Lubricants/artificial tears drops in between work (every two hourly during long session of computer works)
- Cut down on excessive screen use in any form.

MIGRAINE (TABLE 28.2)

It is a familial disorder characterized by:
- Recurrent attacks of headache, widely varied in intensity, frequency and duration.
- Attacks are commonly unilateral, and usually associated with anorexia, nausea or vomiting.
- In some cases, they are preceded by, or associated with neurological and mood disturbances.

- *Incidence:* About 5–10%.
- *Age and sex:* It usually begins in childhood or early adult life, and is more common in women.
- *Pathophysiology:* Migraine represents a disorder of cerebrovascular regulation. In a typical migraine, there is cerebral vasoconstriction decrease in O_2 supply brain cell hypoxia biochemical and vascular changes reactive extracranial vasodilatation leading to typical headache.

Vasoconstriction initiates the prodromal symptoms including the neurological manifestations, and is due to:
- Release of serotonin and thromboxane A_2 from platelets (*vascular theory*).

TABLE 28.2: Features of different types of migraine	
Types	**Characteristic features**
Classical migraine	• Severe hemicranial throbbing pain • Preceded by an aura for 15 to 20 minutes • Visual symptoms are common, e.g. scintillating scotoma. In the dark field, zig-zag rays of various color are often seen, called 'fortification spectra' *(teichopsia)* • Sensory symptoms include paresthesia and numbness
Common migraine	• More common • Severe headache lasts for hours to 1–2 days • Associated with nausea, vomiting, and anorexia • No prodrome, no aura
Basilar migraine	• Bilateral visual symptoms with headache • Associated features of vertebrobasilar insufficiency (e.g. tinnitus, ataxia, vertigo) • More common in adolescent girls
Ophthalmoplegic migraine	• Common in children below 10 years of age • Ocular cranial nerve palsy (3rd most common) • Spontaneous recovery is common
Complicated migraine	• Associated with neurological deficit lasting for more than 24 hours after the headache
Hemiplegic migraine	• Associated with hemiplegia which outlasts headache
Retinal migraine	• Headache associated with transient unilateral visual loss
Migraine equivalent	• Auras occurring in isolation without headache • May be associated with abdominal pain • A variant of migraine
Cluster headache	• Severe unilateral headache in clusters, several times daily for several days or weeks • It is worse at night, and aggravated by alcohol ingestion

- Substance P, a neurotransmitter (*neurogenic theory*).
- *Trigger factors:* Migraine is often precipitated by some extrinsic or intrinsic factors, e.g. alcohol, cheese, chocolate, dairy products, change in weather, oral contraceptive pill, menstruation, change in sleep habit, stress, fatigue, depression, etc.

Treatment of Migraine

- *Treatment for an acute attack:* It may include analgesics, antiemetics, sedatives, ergotderivatives and sometimes systemic steroids. Ergots should be used cautiously. New drug, Sumatriptan, a 5-HT-receptor agonist is highly effective for the treatment of an acute attack, with fewer side effects.
- *Prophylactic therapy:* Prevention of future attacks is only considered with the frequency of attacks is more than two per months.
  The agents are beta-blockers (e.g. propranolol), cyproheptadine, anti-depressants, calcium-channel blockers (e.g. flunarizine), methysergide, etc.
- *Reduction of migraine trigger-factors:* Try to avoid all the "triggerfactors" which may precipitate a migraine attack.

SMOKING AND EYE DISEASES

It is well known that smoking is a risk factor for heart disease and lung cancer; however, smoking can also lead to different eye diseases. Avoiding smoking, or taking steps to quit lowers the risk of vision impairment and vision loss.

Smokers are at higher risk for:

- *Age-Related Macular Degeneration (AMD):* Smokers are 3–4 times more likely to develop AMD than non-smokers.
- *Cataract:* Heavy smokers (15 cigarettes/day or more) have 3 times the risk of cataract as non-smokers.
- *Dry Eye Syndrome:* is twice more common among smokers than non-smokers. Smokers who wear contact lenses have four times the increased risk of infection.
- *Grave's Disease (Thyroid ophthalmopathy):* is an autoimmune disease of thyroid gland and smoking is a major significant risk factor.
- *Diabetic Retinopathy:* Complications of diabetes made worse by smoking which include diabetic retinopathy and maculopathy.
- *Glaucoma:* Older smokers have a higher risk of developing increased eye pressure (intraocular pressure) as compared to non-smokers.
- *Uveitis:* Uveitis is more common in smokers than non-smokers.
- *Transient Ischemic Attack (TIA):* The most common cause of temporary vision loss is known as a transient ischemic attack. It is more commonly known as a TIA, or a "mini-stroke".
- *Pregnancy and Smoking:* Smoking during pregnancy is associated with premature births (thus more retinopathy of premeturity), and higher rates of strabismus, refractive errors, retinal and optic nerve problems.

OCULAR CHANGES IN PREGNANCY

The possible pregnancy-associated eye changes are broad. Many of these changes resolve during the postpartum period. Management thus involves watching simple findings, referring the patient who may require medical or surgical treatment.

Ocular changes pregnancy may be of 3 categories:

1. Physiological changes,
2. Pregnancy-specific eye diseases, and
3. Changes in pre-existing eye diseases.

Physiological changes
- *Corneal change:* Changes in both thickness and curvature—making change in refractive status—causing contact lens intolerance; and a contraindication for refractive surgery.
- Decrease in intraocular pressure (IOP)
- Temporary ptosis—which may be bilateral.

Pregnancy-specific eye diseases
- Hypertensive retinopathy secondary to pregnancy induced hypertension or pre-eclampsia. Exudative retinal detachment (usually bilateral) occurs in <1% of patients with preeclampsia and in 10% with eclampsia. Cortical blindness may also occur in pre-eclamptic and eclamptic women.
- Retinal vascular occlusive disorders – due to hypercoagulable state of pregnancy or amniotic fluid embolism to retinal vessels.
- Central serous retinopathy (CSR) – in women, it has a strong association with late pregnancy.

- Pituitary apoplexy – field changes due to optic nerve compression.

Changes in pre-existing eye diseases
- *Diabetic retinopathy (DR) progression:* Pregnancy is an independent risk factor for worsening of DR. No risk of retinopathy with gestational diabetes. Women with diabetes who plan to become pregnant should have a pre-pregnancy dilated fundus examination. During pregnancy, fundus examination to be performed in each trimester.
- *For chronic non-infectious uveitis:* Pregnancy may have a beneficial effect, possibly due to hormonal and immunomodulatory mechanisms.
- Latent ocular toxoplasmosis may reactivate during pregnancy, with a negligible risk to the fetus of acquiring congenital toxoplasmosis. Spiramycin is preferred over pyrimethamine as a safer alternative in pregnant women.

Index

Page numbers followed by *f* refer to figure, and *t* refer to table

Anterior uveitis 226, 235, 236, 379
  complications of 230
Antibiotic 50, 244
  drops 415
  intraocular injections of 50
  intravenous broad-
    spectrum 393
  subconjunctival 50
  systemic 50, 185
  therapy 244
  topical 50, 194
Antibody
  antinuclear 230f
  derivative 60
  monoclonal 59
Anticholinesterase 51
Anticonvulsant drug 361
Antifungal 51
  drugs 188
Antihistamines 49
Antihistaminic, topical 163
Antithyroid drugs 397
Anti-toxoplasmic drugs,
  systemic 237
Anti-vascular endothelial
    growth factor agents 59
Antivirals 50
Aphakia 81, 117, 213, 273f
  correction of 83f
  etiology 81
  hypermetropia in 82f
  signs of 280
  treatment 83
Aphakic glasses, conventional 262
Applanation tonometer 119, 283
Aqueous
  cells 227, 228f
  flare 226, 228f
  humor 30
    circulation of 31
    formation 30
    paracentesis 380
    normal flow rate of 31
    outflow channels 282f
    production, reduction of 283
    tap 574
    tear deficiency 404
Arcuate scotomata 305f
Arcuate wedge resection 560
Arcus juvenilis 201, 201f
Arcus senilis 201, 201f
Argon laser
  cilia ablation 127
  trabeculoplasty 559
Aristotle's theory 38
Arlt's triangle 226, 227f
Arruga's method 528

Arruga's needle holder 520, 520f
Arteriosclerosis 171
Arteriovenous crossing 94
Arteritis, temporal 582
Artery 22
  anterior ciliary 10, 23
  central retinal 23
  cilioretinal 562
  forceps 521, 521f
  lacrimal 23
  occlusion, central retinal
    333, 333f, 334f, 571
  ophthalmic 21-23
  recurrent 23
Arthritis
  idiopathic rheumatoid 235f
  juvenile rheumatoid 234
A-scan
  ultrasonography 568f
  uses of 568
Aspiration 474
Aspirin 356
Asteroid hyalosis 322, 322f
Astigmatic fan 80, 81f, 93
Astigmatism 70, 78, 213, 581
  against rule 82
  compound hypermetropic 78
  curvature 78
  degree of 81
  irregular 79, 81
  simple hypermetropic 78
Atherosclerosis 365
Atrophic
  bulbi 230
  papilledema 368
  pterygium 166
  rhinitis 412
Atropine 47, 52, 283
  intoxication 61
  penalization 425
  sulfate 185
Attack
  acute 291, 292
    congestive 290
  recurrent 215
  transient ischemic 584
Aurolab aqueous drainage
    implant 311
Autograft 490
  conjunctival 167
  limbal 167
Autokeratoplasty 490
Autosomal dominant 260, 342
Autosomal recessive 342
Autoxidation 27
Avastin 60
Axial length 3
Azathioprine 57

B

Balanced salt solution 326
Bandage soft contact lenses 409
Bard-Parker handle 523
Bare sclera technique 496
Basal cell carcinoma 142, 142f
Basal vitreous detachment 321
Bassen-Kornzweig syndrome 343
Bayonetting sign 300f, 301f
Bean-pot cupping 300, 302f
Beer's knife 541, 541f
Behçet's disease 238
Bell's palsy 195f, 410
Bell's phenomenon 133
Benzalkonium chloride 63
Bergmeister's papilla 360, 360f
Berlin's edema 449
Beta-blockers 53
Beta-irradiation 167
Bevacizumab 60
Bicarbonate system 31
Bick's procedure 125, 125f
Bielschowsky's head tilt test 436f
Bifocal lenses 88f, 88
Binocular loupe 97
Binocular single vision 420
  grades of 421f
Binocular vision 85
  state of 431
Biologic response modifiers 57, 58
Biomicroscopy, ultrasonic 374
Biopsy
  excisional 392
  incisional 392
Birth trauma 288f
Bitot's spot 173f, 511f, 512
Bjerrum scotoma 305
Bjerrum screen 303
Black eye 443f
Blackball hyphema 446
Blade breaker 523, 524f
Bleeding
  points, hemostasis of 470
  sources of 445
Blepharitis 135
  sequelae of 136
  squamous 135, 136f, 137
  types of 135
  ulcerative 136, 136f, 137
Blepharochalasis 129, 129f
Blepharophimosis 120, 121
  syndrome 121f
Blepharoplasty 398
Blepharoptosis 130
Blepharospasm 134
  essential 134

YUMMY
Easy
QUICK

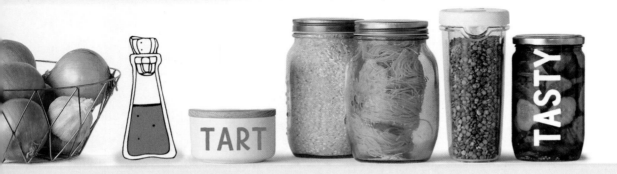

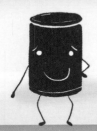
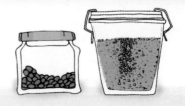

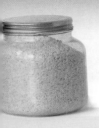

THIS BOOK IS DEDICATED TO JONATHAN, WILLIAM AND SADIE
because you make me proud, make me think, make me laugh,
and in the end make everything worth it.

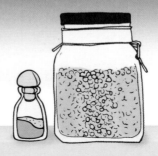

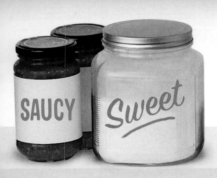
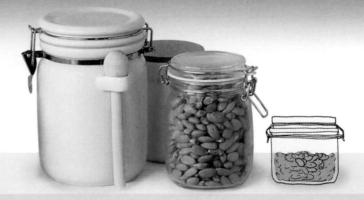

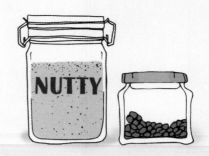

YUMMY
Easy
QUICK

127 DINNERS THAT TAKE 30 MINUTES OR LESS TO PREPARE

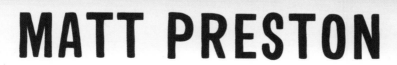

MATT PRESTON

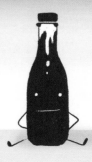

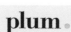plum.

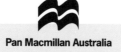Pan Macmillan Australia

CONT

ENTS

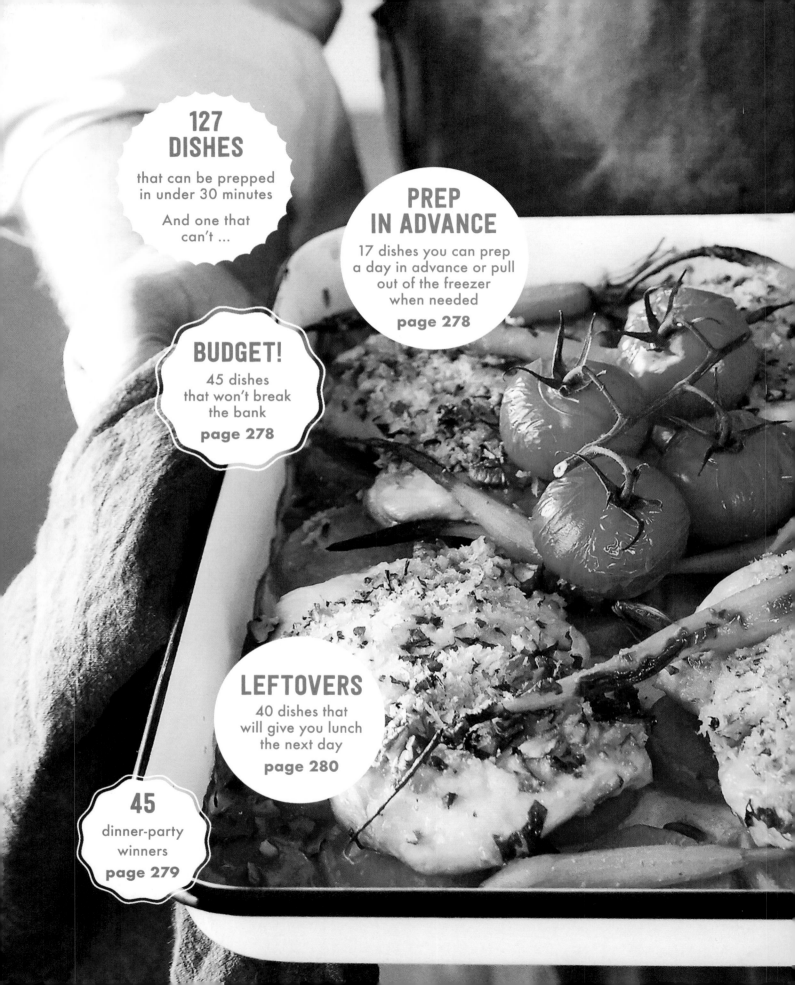

127 DISHES

that can be prepped in under 30 minutes

And one that can't ...

PREP IN ADVANCE

17 dishes you can prep a day in advance or pull out of the freezer when needed

page 278

BUDGET!

45 dishes that won't break the bank

page 278

LEFTOVERS

40 dishes that will give you lunch the next day

page 280

45

dinner-party winners

page 279

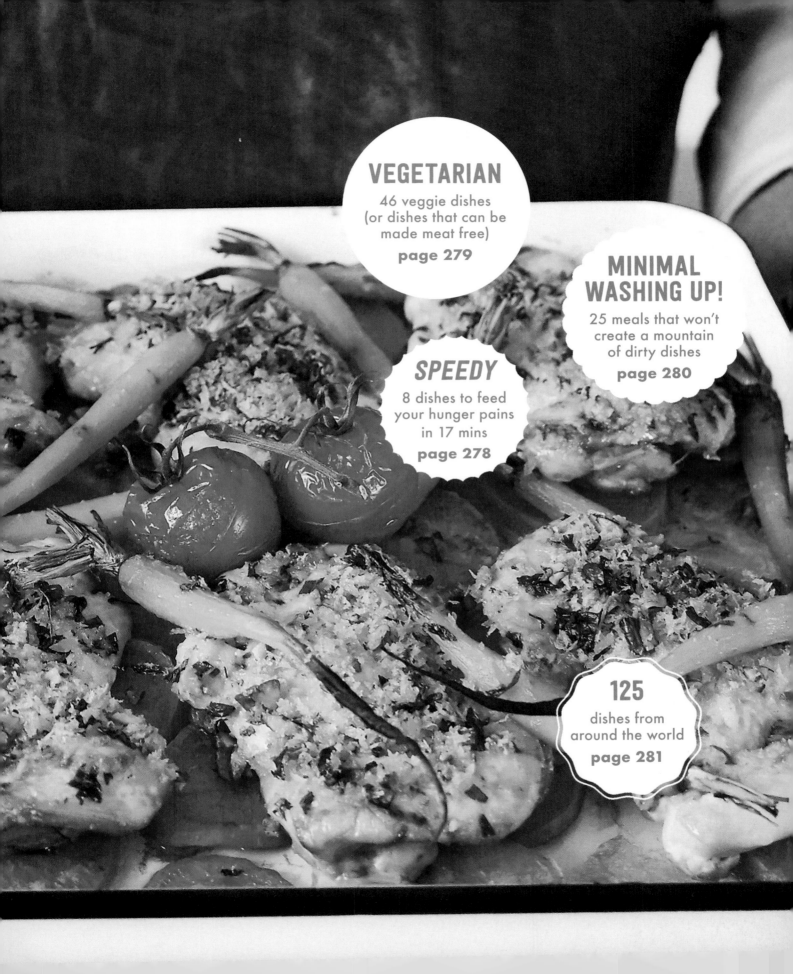

VEGETARIAN

46 veggie dishes
(or dishes that can be
made meat free)

page 279

**MINIMAL
WASHING UP!**

25 meals that won't
create a mountain
of dirty dishes

page 280

SPEEDY

8 dishes to feed
your hunger pains
in 17 mins

page 278

125

dishes from
around the world

page 281

WHAT'S FOR DINNER?

Answering this question is what this cookbook is all about.

We all have a selection of go-to dishes to cook for family and friends but, delicious though they are, even the best of us can get stuck in a rut, caught on a culinary hamster wheel, cooking from the same repertoire of nine or so recipes over and over again.

This book aims to break this cycle with dishes that are easy, delicious and nutritious … and that minimise the washing up along the way!

These dishes are my take on modern classics that will instantly become household favourites. Banging with flavour, they all use everyday fresh ingredients alongside fridge, freezer and pantry staples to make them easily achievable; whether you're whipping up a quick midweek meal, cooking a leisurely dinner for friends on the weekend, or wanting to get ahead and prepare next week's lunches.

In addition, we've packed this book to the gills with ideas for adapting dishes and suggestions that allow you to change some of the base recipes for ingredients you have to hand, ensuring that you will never be left wondering what to do with those neglected orphan vegetables at the back of the crisper drawer. Check out the Speedy Pasta Dishes on pages 262–263 for 19 suggestions for pasta sauces, or learn how to make fritters out of pretty much anything on pages 210–211. Feel all millennial with 44 ideas for bowl food, or rightfully return the baked spud to the dinner table with 43 toppings that will definitely leave your bank account intact.

Most Australians average just 32 minutes a night cooking dinner, so these recipes also champion a new approach to quick cooking in the kitchen by highlighting the amount of time required to prep each dish, instead of the time when the oven or stove is doing the work instead of you. All of the recipes can be prepared in 30 minutes or less (apart from one – answers on a postcard …), allowing you to spend your time on things that matter.

To make life even easier there are multiple indexes at the back of the book – a bog-standard one that lists recipes by their core ingredients, as well as numerous recipe collections that solve any number of dinner dilemmas: meals that you can prepare in advance, cheap mid-week feeds, meat-free meals for the vegetarians in your life and an around-the-world index that allows you to go culinary globetrotting whenever the urge takes you.

WHY YOU NEED THIS BOOK

YUMMY Whether it's the best bolognese or roast lamb you've ever tasted, modern takes on retro sweet 'n' sour, chow mein or rissoles, or fresh plates of vegetable tastiness that make you feel good to be alive, this cookbook is packed with modern classics you'll love cooking for your friends and family. And that they'll love eating.

EASY All the recipes rely on everyday ingredients; staples that you probably already have in your fridge, freezer or pantry. My recipe adaptations will give you inspiration after inspiration for how to take a basic recipe and turn it into a dozen different meals.

QUICK All of the dishes can be prepared in 30 minutes or less. Our new canny index system also allows you to immediately find recipes that suit your mood, budget and available time.

CLEVER This book will give you valuable advice on how best to stock your pantry and freezer so you've always got something delicious to eat, and always something interesting to help twist up dinner in new and exciting ways.

CLEAR Step-by-step instructions will help you create dishes without any added stress and encourage you to up your cooking game.

REAL This is a home cookbook written for home cooks by a home cook.

HELPFUL Our extended index will give you endless inspiration for different dinner dilemmas, so you're never stuck for what to cook.

WHAT I KNOW ABOUT GOING TO THE SUPERMARKET

Australians love supermarkets. We have more per capita than the USA and three times as many as the UK. And our 2000 or so supermarkets love us, because we give them well over $80 billion a year in cold hard cash. While much is made about freshness and price in supermarket advertising, only 11% of people rate these factors as the most important reasons for visiting a particular supermarket. Location, habit, familiarity and convenience are all between twice and over three times more important to us. In fact, in Australia, 76% of people shop 'All' or 'Most of the time' at the same supermarket.

Over the last decade or so we have also started going to the supermarket more often each week. The importance of the one-off weekly shop has waned, and the supermarket has taken on the role of 'community pantry'. On average, we visit the supermarket about 2½ times a week, more often than not buying only a few items instead of doing a huge shop. A University of South Australia study found that the average time we spend in a supermarket is 17 minutes a visit, and that almost 25% of all trips were under six minutes.

The upside of all these speedy visits is that we have developed our own strategies for getting the most out of each supermarket visit. Here are mine:

TROLLEY OR BASKET?

Greek philosopher Aristotle claimed that nature abhors a vacuum, but I can tell you from experience that groceries love one. Even if I go in to buy just a few items, if I use a trolley it will be half full in no time. So now every time I raid a supermarket for a couple of items to complete dinner, I avoid the trolleys and choose a basket instead.

THE LIST

I love the discipline of a list. It's a Virgo thing. I also love that working out what you need means that you don't get home and realise you've forgotten the mince that you needed for tonight's meatballs, which was the reason you went to the supermarket in the first place.

Eighty per cent of Australian grocery shoppers use a shopping list and about 88% of those then deviate from it. I am no different. Sometimes I deviate because apricots, cherries, plums, local strawberries or something equally delicious has come into season and is temptingly cheap. Other times it's because I just HAVE TO TRY that new ocelot-flavoured chocolate exploding breakfast cereal or strange pot of chemical dessert in the dairy section that has one of my favourite cartoon characters on it. Yes, I admit, I am a slave to marketing.

THE ANTI-LIST

There are two times when I don't take a list to the supermarket: when I'm lacking inspiration for what to cook for friends and when I am writing recipes. This always blows out the amount of time I spend in store, but by doing this I know that the ingredients I am using are readily available to readers across the country. This is a must for any recipe I write. Also, those shelves are filled with 40,000 jumping-off points for inspiration when it comes to working out what I'll cook for dinner. Maybe it's the fact that the ricotta looks particularly appealing and milkily fresh, or that there's a special on easy-carve lamb or some remaindered barbecued chooks going (forgive me) cheep, but once I have a starting point I find it much easier to angle down what I want to cook. Maybe I'll bake that ricotta to toss through a winter salad of bitter leaves, orange, fennel and sweet baked beets; or I might roast that lamb with crunchy potatoes, the Sicilian roast pumpkin on page 198 and a gravy cut with the bitter saltiness of olives; or make a chicken pie with some of that sweetcorn sitting at the back of my freezer, or whichever fresh vegetable is on special.

THINK ABOUT THE DEALS

There are two numbers that have had a huge impact on my supermarket shopping. The first is that an overwhelming majority of us (up to 96%) buy things we didn't realise we needed, and that each year Australians throw away well over $1000 of the food we buy! I've learnt to avoid the traps of buying perishable goods that seem like such a bargain in those 'two-for-one' deals unless I know I am going to use them in the next three days – in which case 'score'! I also try and buy the amount that I need for a recipe rather than ending up with those annoying almost-empty packets clogging up the pantry.

NEVER SHOP HUNGRY

It used to be that coffee 'n' cake was the reward after a successful shopping trip, but now I realise that I buy less if I am not hungry when I shop, so I start with a coffee or a bowl of porridge.

DON'T FORGET ...

Convenience is important, but there's a joy and connectivity with food that comes from building relationships with your butcher, baker, farmer (at the farmers' market), fishmonger and local international grocer.

THE SUPERMARKET MUST-BUYS

While I love shopping at excellent local bakers, fishmongers, butchers, specialist greengrocers, wholesalers and farmers' markets, much of what I eat is bought from the supermarket. It's just so convenient! Below is a list of the things that are always on my shopping list. As you will see, I am largely a perimeter shopper who only rarely ventures down those enclosed central aisles.

THE LISTS

There is a romantic notion that we should all be popping down the market and making our decisions of what to cook based on what looks best. I'm not sure that this is really sustainable. Far better is to have a core list of fresh ingredients you keep in your fridge and then cook these in different ways depending on what you feel like and what flavour enhancers you have in the pantry. That's the approach of this book – so here's a collection of ingredients to buy each week for a nice varied selection of dinners, drawn from the pages that follow.

CHOOSE FROM THESE FRESH STAPLES TO BUY EVERY WEEK

- **LOTS AND LOTS OF SEASONAL VEGETABLES THAT TAKE YOUR FANCY:** leeks, red or brown onions, garlic, potatoes, pumpkin, sweet potatoes, parsnips, broccoli, cauliflower, kale, cabbage, snow peas, carrots, beetroot, brussels sprouts, eggplant, capsicum, mushrooms, green beans and zucchini.
- **LOADS OF SALAD VEGETABLES:** cherry tomatoes, spring onions, cucumber, iceberg lettuce and chillies.
- **USEFUL FRUIT FOR SAVOURY DISHES:** lemons, limes and maybe mandarins, oranges, apples or pears depending on what proteins you are buying.
- **HERBS:** I pick herbs from my garden, but if you've yet to plant any you'll need some parsley, mint, coriander or dill depending on what you are cooking. It's far cheaper and lesss wasteful to grow your own.
- **DAIRY:** butter, Greek yoghurt, milk and eggs.
- **HARD CHEESE:** parmesan, cheddar, gruyere or manchego depending on what's run out.
- **SOFT CHEESE:** I usually buy feta and then some ricotta, goat's cheese or cream cheese.
- **FISH:** salmon (fresh fillets or smoked) or perhaps ocean trout, blue eye trevalla, ling or trevally for a change.
- **POULTRY:** chicken breasts, thighs or a whole chicken.
- **MEAT:** good bacon and some chorizo or ham every so often, minced beef, veal, chicken, turkey or pork, or red meat such as a leg of lamb or porterhouse steak.

PANTRY STAPLES TO MAKE YOUR FRESH INGREDIENTS SING

Also check out pages 254–255 on how to organise your pantry.

- **CANS:** chickpeas, lentils or cannellini beans, tomatoes, tuna, baked beans, tomato paste, chipotle chillies, anchovies, coconut milk and condensed milk.
- **BOTTLES AND JARS:** hoisin, char siu and oyster sauce, Kewpie mayonnaise, tamarind paste, three jars of hot pickles, capers, glucose syrup, liquid smoke and fish sauce.

- **DRIED GOODS:** flaked sea salt, pasta in myriad shapes and forms, various rices, such as jasmine, brown, risotto and short-grain, sugars, different flours including 00 flour, self-raising and plain, oats, barley, quinoa, pulses, crispy shallots, vac-packed fresh hokkien noodles, nori, rice paper, stock, wraps with a long use-by date, shredded coconut and various dried fruits.

- **NUTS AND SEEDS:** almonds, pistachios, walnuts, pumpkin seeds, sunflower seeds and sesame seeds (buy nuts in small bags as they can go rancid).

- **OILS:** grapeseed, vegetable, peanut, pumpkin seed and, importantly, good olive oil.

- **VINEGARS:** rice wine, cider, sherry and red wine vinegar.

- **ALCOHOL:** cooking sherry (medium), vermouth and any leftover wine. I also have a bottle of cooking gin but that tends to find itself into the cook rather than the cooking.

- **CONDIMENTS:** hot English and dijon mustards, horseradish, barbecue and tomato sauce.

- **SPICES:** all manner of, but especially cumin, coriander, curry powder, smoked paprika, fennel seed, cardamom and cinnamon.

I have far fewer spreads, jellies and jams than I used to, but mint jelly, redcurrant jelly and mango pickle all have a place.

There is also, I have to admit, a catering stack of two-minute noodles because sometimes that's all the time you've got. Don't judge me. Eighty-five per cent of what we eat is fresh, nutritious produce.

FLAVOUR BOMBS IN MY PANTRY FROM SPECIALIST FOOD STORES

Sometimes you need to make a little expedition to buy more interesting ingredients that put an immediate spin on what you're cooking. I have built these up over time.

- **ASIAN INGREDIENTS:** gochujang, miso, kombu, dried shiitake mushrooms, hondashi, XO sauce, black bean sauce, lap cheong sausage, kecap manis, Shaoxing rice wine and crispy laver seaweed snacks, mostly available from Asian grocers and food stores or fancy supermarkets.

- **MIDDLE EASTERN FLAVOURS:** pomegranate molasses, harissa, freekeh, good chilli powder and spices, purchased from specialist food stores and some supermarkets.

- **DELI GOODS:** good-quality anchovies, salted capers, big blocks of parmesan, cheap canned tomatoes, beans and pulses, porcini stock cubes and cheap pastas in unusual shapes, available from Italian delis and most supermarkets.

INGREDIENTS AND PRODUCE IDEAL FOR FREEZING

See the freezer as a hidden arsenal of produce that can be speedily deployed to enhance dinner. Check out the freezer chapter starting on page 228 for more freezer inspiration.

- **BREAD:** sliced, pita, tortillas, garlic, breadcrumbs and rolls.

- **SWEET STUFF:** ice cream, pastry for tarts, fruit, citrus juice and cookie dough.

- **LEFTOVERS:** stocks, casseroles, soups, sauces and herbs.

- **DAIRY:** butter and some cheese.

- **VEGGIES:** broad beans, sweetcorn, peas, broccoli florets, soy beans and spinach.

- **MEAT AND FISH:** bacon, chicken breasts and thighs, mince, sausages, prawns and smoked salmon.

- **ALCOHOL:** vodka.

CHIC

THI

KEN
GHS

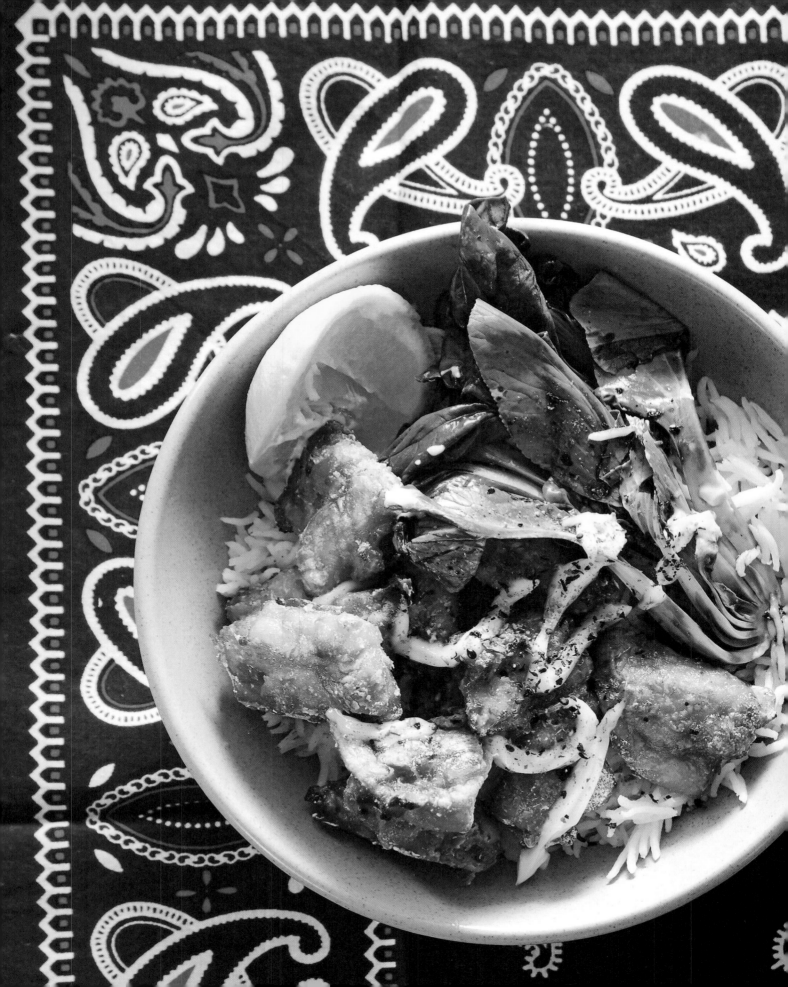

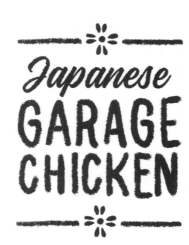

Japanese GARAGE CHICKEN

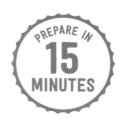

We call it 'Garage Chicken' in our house as the recipe is based on Tetsuya Wakuda's karaage chicken. This is ironic, as the first time I introduced Tets to a non-foodie mate late one night at a food festival in Noosa, she was sure I said his name was 'Tex'. She then spent the next 20 minutes quizzing the legendary chef about his cowboy leanings and how much time he'd spent in Texas – much to his bemusement.

This dish is far less confusing, but worth trying for the bok choy alone, which is cooked in the manner of *MasterChef* S9 contestant Sarah.

You can serve this baked not fried garage chicken with Kewpie mayo and shichimi togarashi (page 130), or sweet chilli sauce, or sriracha chilli sauce, or soy sauce, or teriyaki sauce, or with just about anything you blooming well like, including Texas barbecue sauce!!!

SERVES 4 PREP: 15 MINS (PLUS 1 HOUR MARINATING) COOKING: 20 MINS

2 tablespoons soy sauce, plus extra to serve
1 tablespoon cooking sake
4 cm knob of ginger, peeled and finely grated
1 teaspoon caster sugar
800 g chicken thigh fillets, cut into 3–4 cm pieces
100 g potato flour or cornflour

SOY-FRIED BOK CHOY
1 tablespoon vegetable oil
1 bunch baby bok choy, halved lengthways and rinsed
2 tablespoons soy sauce

TO SERVE
steamed rice
lemon cheeks
Kewpie mayonnaise
shichimi togarashi (page 130)

Combine the soy sauce, sake, ginger and sugar in a glass or ceramic dish. Add the chicken and toss to coat. Cover and place in the fridge for 1 hour to marinate.

Preheat the oven to 200°C/180°C fan-forced. Line two baking trays with baking paper.

Drain the chicken and toss it in the flour in small batches. Place in a single layer on the trays, not too squashed together. Bake, turning halfway through cooking, for 16 minutes, or until golden and tender.

Meanwhile, to make the soy-fried bok choy, heat the oil in a large frying pan over medium–high heat. Add the bok choy, cut-side down. Cover the pan and cook for 1–2 minutes, until just tender. Add the soy sauce and cook for a further 1–2 minutes without moving, so the bok choy gets sticky with the reduced soy and the cut side catches slightly. Remove from the heat and set aside for 2 minutes to absorb the flavours.

Divide the rice among serving bowls. Top with the bok choy and chicken. Serve with a lemon cheek, a squeeze of Kewpie mayo, a sprinkle of shichimi togarashi and a drizzle of extra soy sauce.

TIP

Combine the chicken and soy marinade mixture in a zip-lock bag. Seal and freeze for up to 3 months. Thaw overnight in the fridge; as it thaws it will marinate.

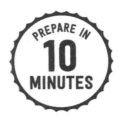

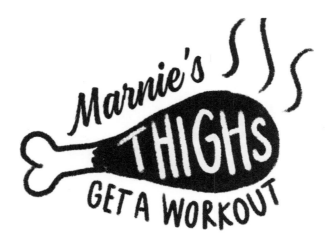

This recipe is the brilliant invention of my culinary muse, Ms Marnie. She is fierce. She is brilliant. She's not afraid of thumbing her nose at the culinary establishment. I'm a little scared of what she might do to me when she sees how her original recipe has evolved over the years in my kitchen. I am even more scared of what she'll do if she thinks that I think her thighs need a workout.

SERVES 4–6 **PREP:** 10 MINS (PLUS 30 MINS MARINATING) **COOKING:** 15 MINS

1 bunch coriander, roots and stems washed
125 ml (½ cup) sweet chilli sauce
2 tablespoons fish sauce
2 tablespoons peanut or rice bran oil
4 cm knob of ginger, peeled and finely grated
juice of 1 lime
8 chicken thigh fillets, excess fat trimmed
mint leaves (or Vietnamese mint if you've got it), to serve
Thai basil leaves, to serve

Remove the leaves from the coriander and set aside for another use. Finely chop the roots and stems and place in a bowl. Add the sweet chilli sauce, fish sauce, oil, ginger and lime juice. Mix to combine. Add the chicken and toss until well combined. Cover and leave to marinate in the fridge for 30 minutes, or up to 2 hours.

When you are ready to cook, preheat a barbecue grill or large chargrill pan over medium–high heat. Add the chicken and cook for 4 minutes on each side, or until cooked through with a few little charred bits on the edges. Transfer to a plate, cover loosely with foil and leave to rest for 5 minutes.

Divide the thighs among serving plates and scatter the herbs over the top for leafy goodness.

TIPS

Make extra for tomorrow's lunch boxes.

The thighs can also be baked in a 200°C/180°C fan-forced oven.

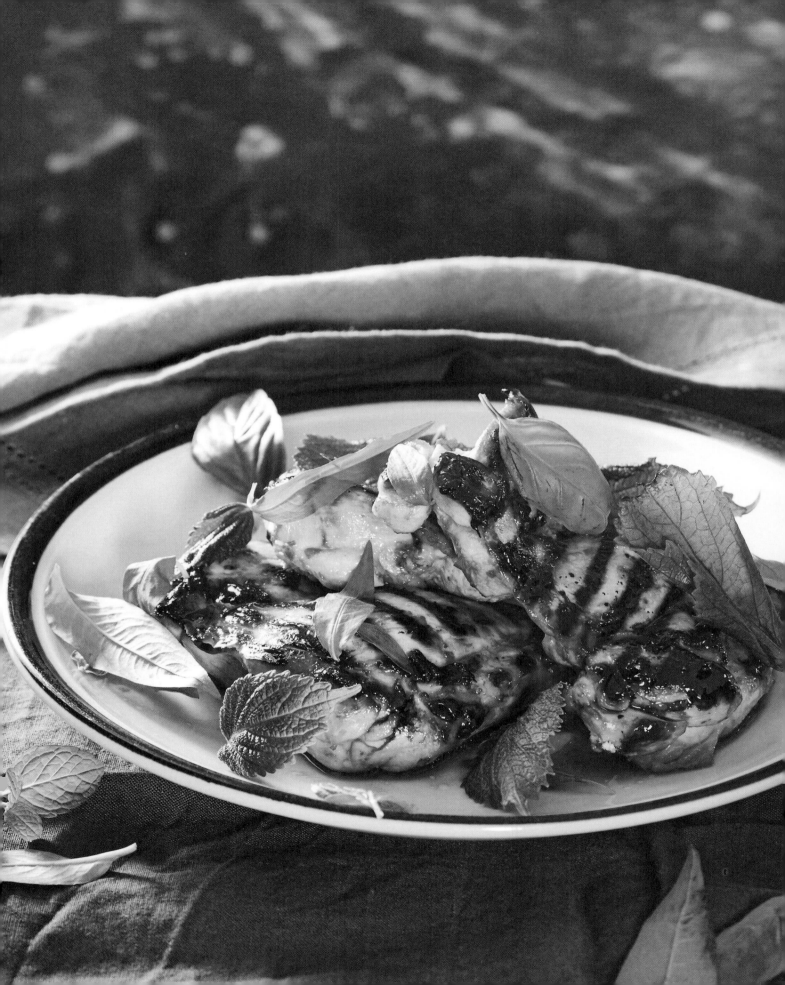

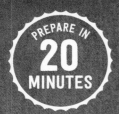

BAKED-NOT-FRIED CHICKEN NUGGET SAN CHOI WOW

Throughout 2017 I have been trying to make serving-things-in-leaves-rather-than-in-rolls-or-flatbread 'happen'. Sure, I know, it's as likely as a reality TV judge becoming the leader of the free world …

I started my campaign with this, the most obvious of propositions: basically mini schnitzels in a leaf with a funky mayo and something crisp. You and your family will love 'em.

First you've got to make the simple baked (but buttery-tasting) nuggets of schnitzel. Then serve them in iceberg lettuce cups or baby gem leaves with my Instant Miso-Bacon Mayo, Red Onion Rings and a squeeze of lemon. Or serve with my Maple-Candied Bacon, Red Onion Rings and Korean Mayo.

SERVES 4   PREP: 20 MINS   COOKING: 40 MINS

12 (about 1.5 kg) chicken
  thigh fillets
80 g butter, melted
120 g (2 cups) panko breadcrumbs
400 g thin sweet potatoes
sea salt
1 iceberg lettuce or 2 baby
  gem/baby cos lettuces,
  leaves separated

TO SERVE (SOME OR ALL OF THE FOLLOWING!)
Instant Miso–Bacon Mayo
  (see page 22)
Korean Mayonnaise (page 22)
Maple-Candied Bacon (page 23)
Red Onion Rings (page 23)

Preheat the oven to 180°C/160°C fan-forced. Line two baking trays with baking paper.

Flatten the chicken thigh fillets between baking paper using a mallet or rolling pin, until they are even in thickness. Cut into pieces about 3 cm square.

Toss the chicken, one piece at a time, in the warm melted butter, shaking off any excess. Then dunk into the panko breadcrumbs to coat.

Peel the sweet potatoes and use the peeler to cut them into thin ribbons. Spread out the sweet potato ribbons on a baking sheet in a single layer. Do NOT use any oil. Place in the oven until crisp and cooked. This will take about 15–20 minutes but watch them. When cooked, transfer to wire racks and leave in a warm place to dry out further. Season with salt.

Increase the oven temperature to 220°C/200°C fan-forced. Lay the chicken nuggets on the lined baking trays, leaving enough room between each nugget to allow crisping. DO NOT OVERCROWD THEM!

Bake, turning once halfway through the cooking time, for 15–20 minutes, until they are cooked and golden.

Pile the nuggets onto a serving board with the lettuce leaves and sweet potato chips. Serve with your favourite mayos, a sprinkle of maple-candied bacon and a few red onion rings.

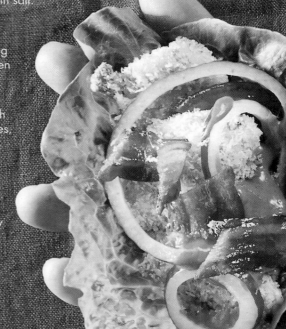

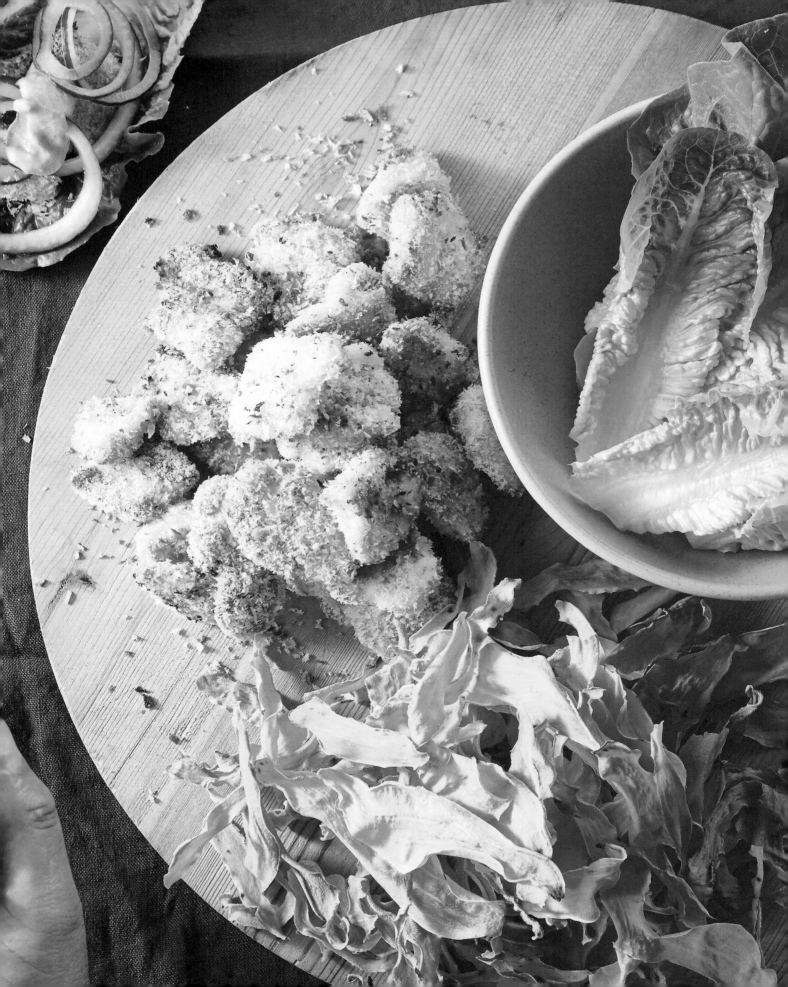

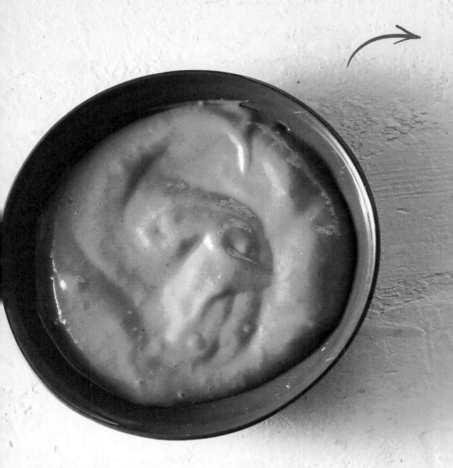

KOREAN MAYONNAISE

3 tablespoons gochujang chilli paste
2 tablespoons cider vinegar, rice wine
  vinegar or bog-standard white vinegar,
  plus extra if needed
1 generous teaspoon salt, plus extra
  if needed
1 egg, yolk and white
300 ml peanut oil
50 ml sesame oil

Place the gochujang chilli paste, vinegar and
salt in the beaker of a stick blender. Slip
the egg on top without breaking the yolk.
Combine the peanut oil and sesame oil and
add to the beaker. Place the stick blender in the
beaker so it covers and encloses the yolk of the
egg. Blend for 1–2 seconds to emulsify – you will
see ribbons trailing out from the blender head.
Continue to blend, pulling the blender up through
the oil, bouncing gently as you go, until a thick
mayonnaise forms. Keep the blender going the
whole time. Adjust the seasoning with more salt or
vinegar as required.

INSTANT MISO–
BACON MAYO

3 bacon rashers, coarsely chopped
1 generous tablespoon red miso paste,
  plus extra if needed
2 teaspoons mirin
2 teaspoons soy sauce
1 egg, yolk and white
350 ml peanut oil

Fry the bacon in a non-stick frying pan, or
microwave between paper towel until crisp and
golden, then drain briefly on paper towel.

Place the miso paste, mirin and soy sauce in
the beaker of a stick blender and briefly blend
to combine. Carefully crack in the egg without
breaking the yolk, then pour in the peanut oil.
Place the stick blender in the beaker and follow
the same technique as for the Korean mayo. Taste,
and blend in more miso if it needs it and then
blend in the warm chopped bacon.

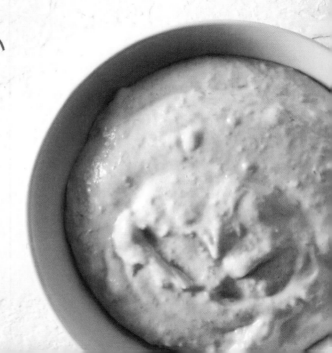

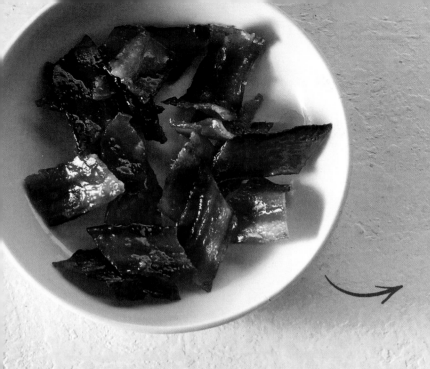

MAPLE-CANDIED BACON

6 smoked streaky bacon rashers
125 ml (½ cup) maple syrup

Fry the bacon rashers in a small non-stick frying pan until starting to crisp. Add the maple syrup and toss the bacon around. Leave on the heat for 3 minutes for the bacon to candy.

Set aside to cool, then chop into bite-sized pieces.

RED ONION RINGS

2 teaspoons caster sugar
½ teaspoon salt
1 red onion, cut into thin rounds
   and separated
splash of cider vinegar or white
   wine vinegar

Combine the sugar and salt in a zip-lock bag. Add the onion rings and mix well. Seal the bag and leave on the kitchen bench for 10 minutes. When the onion starts giving up its liquid, splash in the vinegar, reseal the bag and keep until required. Drain to serve.

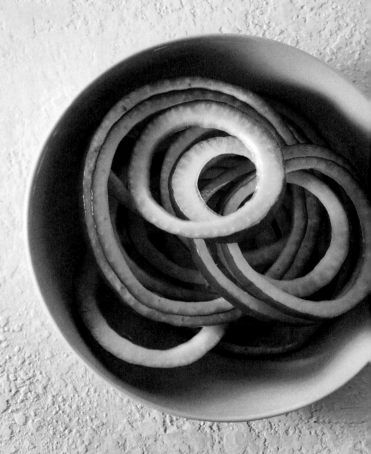

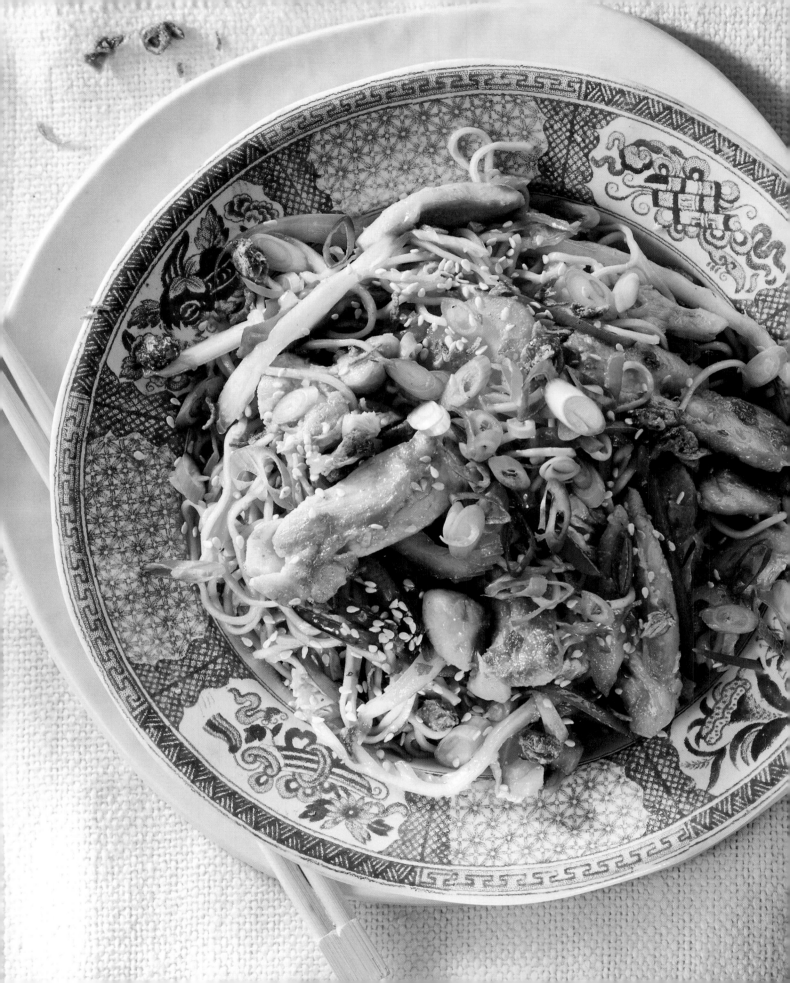

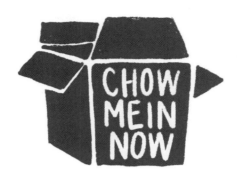

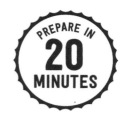

Let me stake my reputation – or at least the little bit of it that I have left – on this year being the year of the Chow Mein Resurgence. Your household will be clamouring for you to make this daggy 60s takeaway favourite, but they'll want more; they'll want something that justifies all the fuss. This recipe is it!

In essence, chow mein is chop suey with noodles, and this staple of the Chinese–American gold rush kitchen is based on a Guangdong dish called *tsap seui*, which translates rather prosaically as 'miscellaneous leftovers'. It's the perfect vehicle for those sad and lonely vegetable orphans, left abandoned at the bottom of the crisper drawer.

This version pays tribute to the Chinese miners who travelled from California to Victoria for our own gold rush, and it is interesting to note that many of the restaurateurs who built Melbourne's reputation for good (and bad) Chinese food came from Taishan – the area of Guangdong where *tsap seui* originated. What makes this recipe even more interesting is using the Chinese technique of 'velveting' the chicken to make it even silkier.

SERVES 4 PREP: 20 MINS (PLUS 30 MINS MARINATING) COOKING: 20 MINS

1 egg white
1 tablespoon cornflour
60 ml (¼ cup) Shaoxing rice wine or dry sherry
6 chicken thigh fillets, excess fat trimmed, thinly sliced
350 g packet fresh chow mein egg noodles
2 tablespoons soy sauce
2 tablespoons hoisin sauce
1 teaspoon sesame oil
¼ teaspoon Maggi seasoning liquid
60 ml (¼ cup) peanut oil
1 × 225 g can water chestnut slices
200 g snow peas, thinly sliced lengthways (or sugar snap peas or green beans)
3 celery stalks, thinly sliced diagonally
½ wombok or cabbage, finely shredded (use bean shoots or even julienned carrots instead, if you have them to hand)
2 garlic cloves, crushed

TO SERVE
sesame seeds, toasted
sliced spring onion
sesame oil (optional)
crispy shallots (optional)

Let's velvet! Whisk together the egg white, cornflour and 1 tablespoon of the rice wine in a bowl. Add the chicken and toss to coat. Cover and place in the fridge for 30 minutes to marinate.

In a heatproof bowl, cover the noodles with boiling water and set aside for 3 minutes. Drain and dry well on a tray lined with paper towel. Combine the soy, hoisin, sesame oil, Maggi seasoning and remaining rice wine in a jug.

Heat 1 tablespoon of peanut oil in a wok or large frying pan over high heat. Add the noodles and toss for 2–3 minutes to coat in the oil, then spread them out to cover the base and side of the wok. Cook for 2 minutes, or until the outside of the noodles are crisp. Transfer the noodles to a bowl.

Add another tablespoon of peanut oil to the wok. Add half the chicken and stir-fry for 3–4 minutes, or until a golden crust forms. Transfer to a bowl. Repeat with the remaining chicken.

Add the remaining peanut oil to the wok. Add the water chestnuts, snow peas and celery. Stir-fry, tossing continuously, for 2 minutes. Add the wombok, garlic, noodles and chicken, and toss until well combined. Add the reserved soy mixture and toss for 1 minute, or until well combined.

Sprinkle with sesame seeds and spring onion (and add a few drops of sesame oil and a pinch of crispy shallots, if you have them in the pantry) and serve.

TIP

If you find tossing the long noodles difficult, give them a little snip with scissors to make life easier.

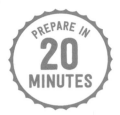

20 MINUTES

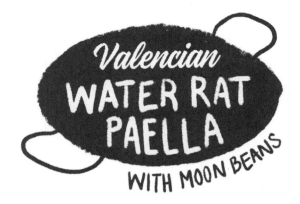

Valencian
WATER RAT PAELLA
WITH MOON BEANS

Actually this is a bog-standard paella that you can customise with whichever proteins you have in your fridge. That is if you decide you are bored of chicken thighs, or agree with the controversial claim that chorizo doesn't belong in a paella. Try chicken breast slices, prawns, calamari, fish, rabbit – anything you want, really. Of course, champions of the original paella would recommend the traditional water rats from the rice fields around Valencia, snails that have been purged on rosemary, and 'moon beans' (which sound suspiciously like butter beans). This might be a little too out there for most of us – those butter bean skins are just too ooky.

SERVES 4–6 PREP: 20 MINS COOKING: 50 MINS

875 ml (3½ cups) chicken stock
1 very large pinch of saffron threads
1 tablespoon olive oil
4 chicken thigh cutlets, skin on
2 chorizo sausages, sliced into rounds
2 red capsicums, deseeded and coarsely chopped
1 onion, finely chopped
1 tablespoon smoked paprika
440 g (2 cups) arborio rice – or use calasparra or bomba if you want to be a foodie purist
1 × 400 g can diced tomatoes
3 rosemary sprigs
300 g (2 cups) frozen broad beans, thawed and peeled

TO SERVE
chopped flat-leaf parsley, to serve (optional)
zest of 1 orange, to serve
sea salt, to serve

Combine the stock and saffron in a saucepan. Cover with a tight-fitting lid and bring to the boil over high heat. As soon as it boils, remove from the heat and set aside to infuse. Reserve 60 ml (¼ cup) of the stock mixture in a separate jug.

Heat the oil in a large deep frying pan or paella pan over medium–high heat. Add the chicken and cook on each side for 4 minutes, or until golden. Transfer to a plate. Wipe the pan of excess oil with paper towel.

Add the chorizo to the pan and cook for 2–3 minutes, until golden. Transfer to the chook plate.

Add the capsicum and onion to the pan. Cook, stirring, for 5 minutes, or until soft. Add the paprika and cook, stirring, for 30 seconds or until aromatic. Add the rice and cook, stirring, for 1 minute. Add the infused stock, tomatoes and rosemary and stir until well combined. Bring to the boil. From now on – no more stirring!!!

Add the chicken cutlets to the pan, skin-side up, nestling them into the rice. Reduce the heat to medium–low and simmer – without stirring, remember – for 20 minutes.

Add the chorizo and press it into the rice. Scatter over the broad beans and pour over the reserved jug of stock. Cover and cook for a further 5 minutes, or until the rice is just firm to the bite and the chicken is cooked through. Sprinkle over the parsley (if using), orange zest and a little sea salt to serve.

TIP

You don't want to stir the rice because you want the grains to remain separate and, most importantly, you don't want to disturb the crust that will form on the bottom of the pan – the treasured paella *socarrat*.

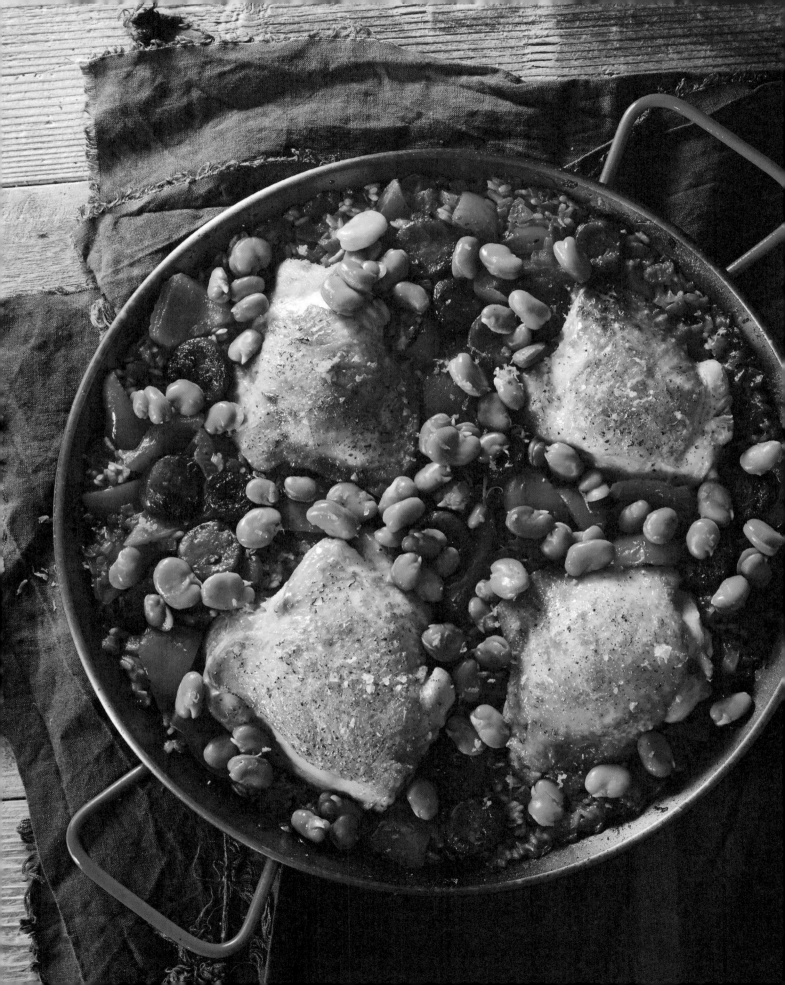

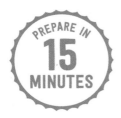

PREPARE IN
15
MINUTES

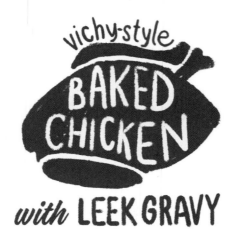

vichy-style
BAKED CHICKEN
with **LEEK GRAVY**

Your family will want to surrender after eating this simple tray bake that combines all the joy of chicken, leeks and potato with asparagus. Originally it was a one-pan bake but it's really worth dirtying another pan to get the potatoes nice and crispy – which is why we did it!

Seriously though, throughout this book it's always my aim to avoid creating extra washing up if I can absolutely help it. I suspect that, like me, you don't have an army of kitchen hands to clean up after you in your kitchen ... unlike some cookbook authors.

SERVES 4   **PREP:** 15 MINS   **COOKING:** 1 HOUR

8 chicken thigh cutlets, skin on
60 ml (¼ cup) olive oil
2 teaspoons thyme leaves
3 garlic cloves, crushed
sea salt and freshly ground
   black pepper
12 (about 850 g) baby red-skinned
   potatoes, halved (or use whatever
   potatoes you have, cut into
   small chunks)
3 leeks, cut into 2 cm thick slices
80 ml (⅓ cup) chicken stock
80 ml (⅓ cup) white wine
1 large bunch asparagus, trimmed
85 g (⅓ cup) crème fraîche or
   sour cream

Preheat the oven to 200°C/180°C fan-forced. Cut a few slashes into the skin of the chicken thighs.

Combine the oil, thyme and garlic in a bowl and season.

Place the potato, leek, stock and wine in a large roasting tin. Place the chicken thighs on top and drizzle with the thyme mixture. Bake for 20 minutes.

Add the asparagus to one end of the tin and bake for a further 25 minutes, or until the chicken is cooked through and golden.

Transfer the chicken and asparagus to a plate and cover with foil to keep warm.

Transfer the potatoes to a baking tray, leaving the liquid and leeks behind. Return the potato to the oven to crisp up while you prepare the leek gravy in the roasting tin. This will take about 15 minutes – both the crisping *and* the gravy, actually.

Place the roasting tin over medium heat for 10–12 minutes, until the sauce reduces and thickens. Don't forget to stir away happily, scraping any toastiness from the sides or base of the tin back into the sauce. Stir in the crème fraîche and warm through.

Strew the chook pieces and asparagus randomly back in the tin on top of the creamy leek gravy. Throw in the crispy potatoes. Serve!

TIP

For extra flavour place the chicken and thyme mixture in a zip-lock bag. Seal and place in the fridge until you are ready to make dinner. You can even freeze the raw chicken with the oil mixture for up to 3 months. Then as it thaws it will marinate.

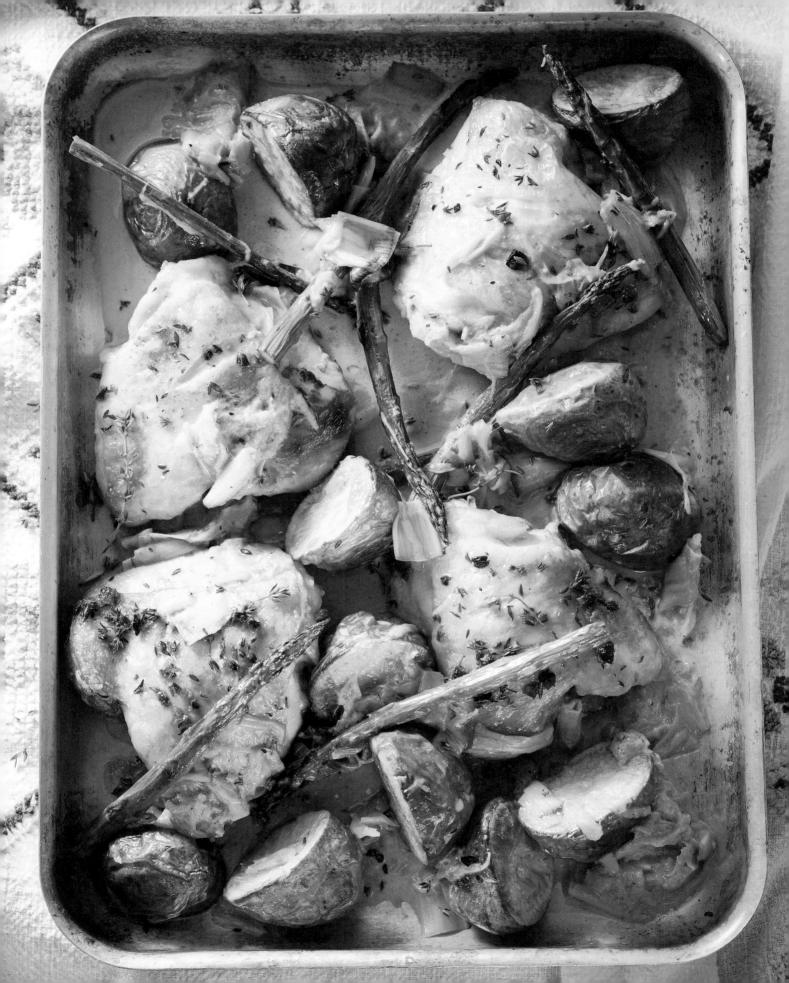

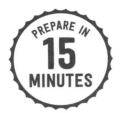

PREPARE IN
15
MINUTES

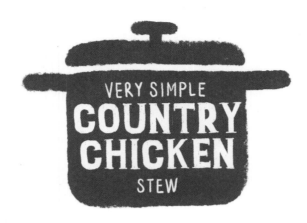

VERY SIMPLE
COUNTRY CHICKEN
STEW

This is a tasty crowd-pleaser that offends virtually no one. 'Nuff said. (Well, apart from the vegans and the vegetarians. But between you and me, you don't see many of their kind in the chicken-thigh section of any cookbook.)

SERVES 6–8 **PREP**: 15 MINS **COOKING**: 1 HOUR 20 MINS

1.5 kg (about 8) chicken thigh cutlets, skin on
2 tablespoons plain flour
2 tablespoons olive oil
4 bacon rashers, finely chopped
2 onions, coarsely chopped
3 garlic cloves, crushed
1 × 820 g can tomato soup
125 ml (½ cup) dry sherry
1 dried bay leaf or 2 fresh ones
1 bunch flat-leaf parsley, leaves picked and stems very finely chopped
145 g (1 cup) pitted olives of your choice (green are more elegant; black are more fruity and oomphy – which is a real word. I just checked and the internet wouldn't lie, would it?)
sea salt and freshly ground black pepper
buttered risoni or orzo pasta, to serve
steamed zucchini, to serve

Preheat the oven to 200°C/180°C fan-forced.

Sprinkle both sides of the chicken thighs with the flour. Heat the olive oil in a large frying pan over high heat. Cook the chicken thighs in batches, skin-side down, for 5–6 minutes, until a crisp golden crust forms. Turn the chicken pieces over and cook for a further 4 minutes, or until golden. Transfer to a casserole dish.

In the same frying pan, cook the bacon and onion for 5 minutes, or until soft. Wipe the pan with paper towel to remove excess oil, leaving about 1 tablespoon in the pan. Add the garlic and cook for 1 minute or so until it just starts to turn golden. Stir in the tomato soup, sherry, bay leaves, all the parsley stems and half the parsley leaves. Simmer for 5 minutes.

Tip the tomato sauce mixture over the chicken in the casserole dish and add the olives. Cover and bake for 45 minutes, or until the chicken is cooked through. Season.

Top the chicken with the remaining parsley leaves and serve with some buttered risoni or orzo pasta, and loads of steamed zucchini.

TIPS

If you have a flameproof casserole dish, use that for everything and dispense with the washing up of the frying pan!

This dish freezes well. Place in an airtight container and freeze for up to 3 months. Thaw overnight in the fridge and reheat in a large saucepan over low heat.

You can always leave out the olives if members of your household abhor them and just add them (warmed slightly in the microwave) to individual portions as you serve.

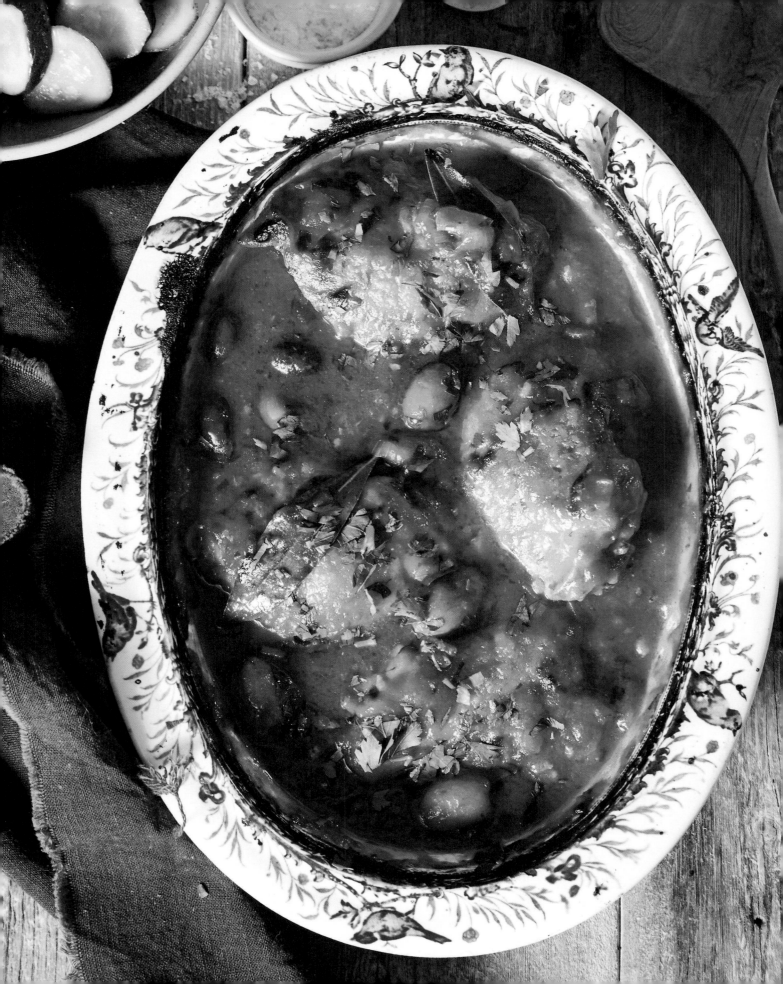

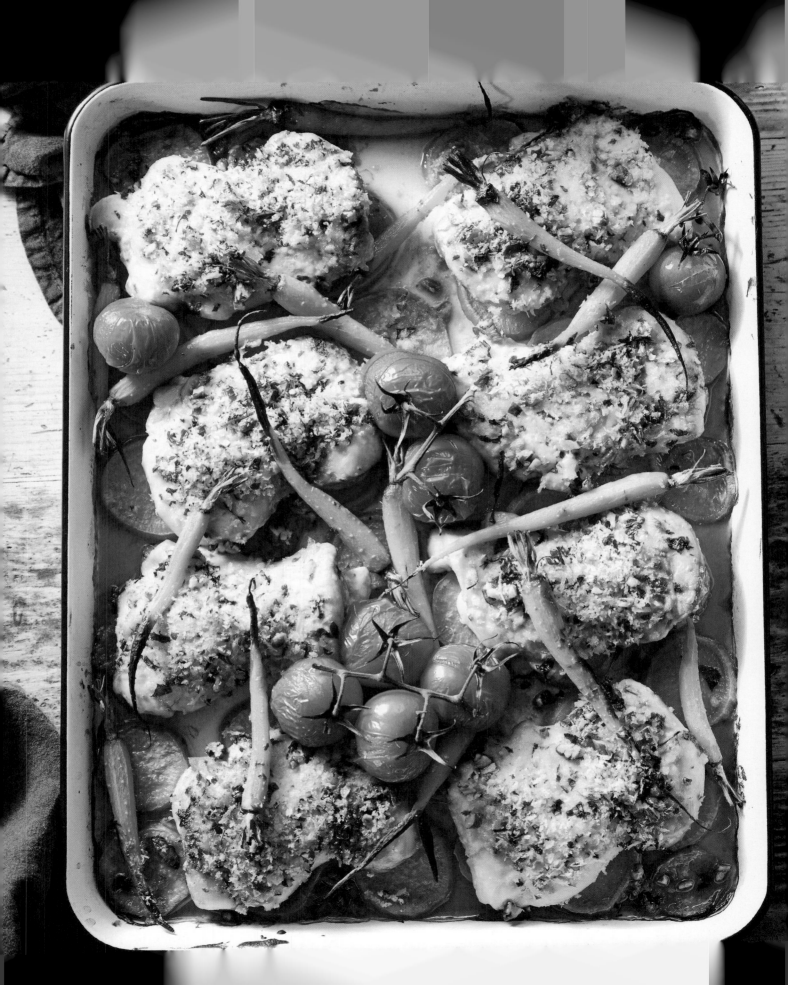

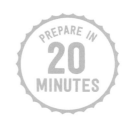

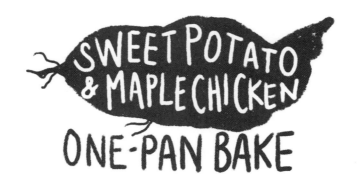

SWEET POTATO & MAPLE CHICKEN ONE-PAN BAKE

Read the title of this recipe. Do you really need to know any more? It should be immediately self-evident why you need to make this dish.

SERVES 4   **PREP:** 20 MINS   **COOKING:** 45 MINS

2 tablespoons maple syrup
1 tablespoon olive oil
zest and juice of 1 lemon
700 g sweet potatoes, peeled and thinly sliced
sea salt and freshly ground black pepper
35 g (½ cup) panko breadcrumbs
⅓ cup coarsely chopped flat-leaf parsley
45 g (⅓ cup) pecan pieces, coarsely chopped
40 g butter, melted
8 chicken thigh fillets, excess fat trimmed
2 tablespoons dijon mustard
1 bunch baby carrots, trimmed and peeled
260 g cherry truss tomatoes, trusses halved

Preheat the oven to 200°C/180°C fan-forced.

In a jug, whisk together the maple syrup, olive oil and 1 tablespoon of the lemon juice.

Place the sweet potato slices in a large shallow roasting tin. Drizzle with the syrup mixture and season. Bake for 15 minutes.

Meanwhile, combine the breadcrumbs, parsley, pecans, lemon zest and butter in a bowl. Mix until well combined.

Turn the sweet potato slices over, then place the chicken thighs on top. Spread the top of each chicken piece with mustard, then carefully and firmly press on the breadcrumb mixture to coat (don't worry if some falls onto the potato). Arrange the carrots around the chicken. Season. Bake for 20 minutes.

Add the tomatoes to the tin and bake for a further 10 minutes, or until the chicken is cooked through and the crumb topping is golden. Serve with the remaining lemon juice if you like.

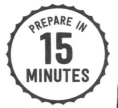

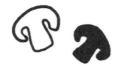

BAKED CHICKEN MUSHROOM RISOTTO *with* A CHEESY CRUST

Is it a risotto if you don't stir it? I'd love to know your views. Tell me via Insta, Facebook or whichever social media platform the young people are using these days. Twitter's totally dead, right???

SERVES 4–6 **PREP:** 15 MINS **COOKING:** 50 MINS

2 tablespoons olive oil
20 g butter
¼ cup sage leaves
200 g button mushrooms, halved
1 leek, thinly sliced
2 garlic cloves, crushed
sea salt and freshly ground
    black pepper
6 chicken thigh fillets, cut into
    4 cm pieces
330 g (1½ cups) arborio rice
1 litre chicken stock
60 g (¾ cup) shredded parmesan
    or pecorino
squeeze of lemon, to serve

Preheat the oven to 200°C/180°C fan-forced.

Melt the oil and butter in a flameproof casserole dish over medium–high heat until foaming. Add the sage leaves and fry for 2 minutes, or until crisp. Use tongs to transfer to a plate lined with paper towel. Set aside.

Add the mushroom, leek and garlic to the pan and cook, stirring, for 5 minutes, or until soft. Season.

Add the chicken and cook, tossing, for 2 minutes, or until the chicken changes colour.

Add the rice and stock and bring to the boil. Cover with a tight-fitting lid or foil and bake for 30 minutes.

Remove the lid and sprinkle over the parmesan. Bake for a further 5–10 minutes, until the cheese melts.

Sprinkle the surface of the risotto with the crisp-fried sage. Serve with a squeeze of lemon and salt.

TIP

Stocks and parmesans differ in saltiness, so don't add any extra salt until just before serving.

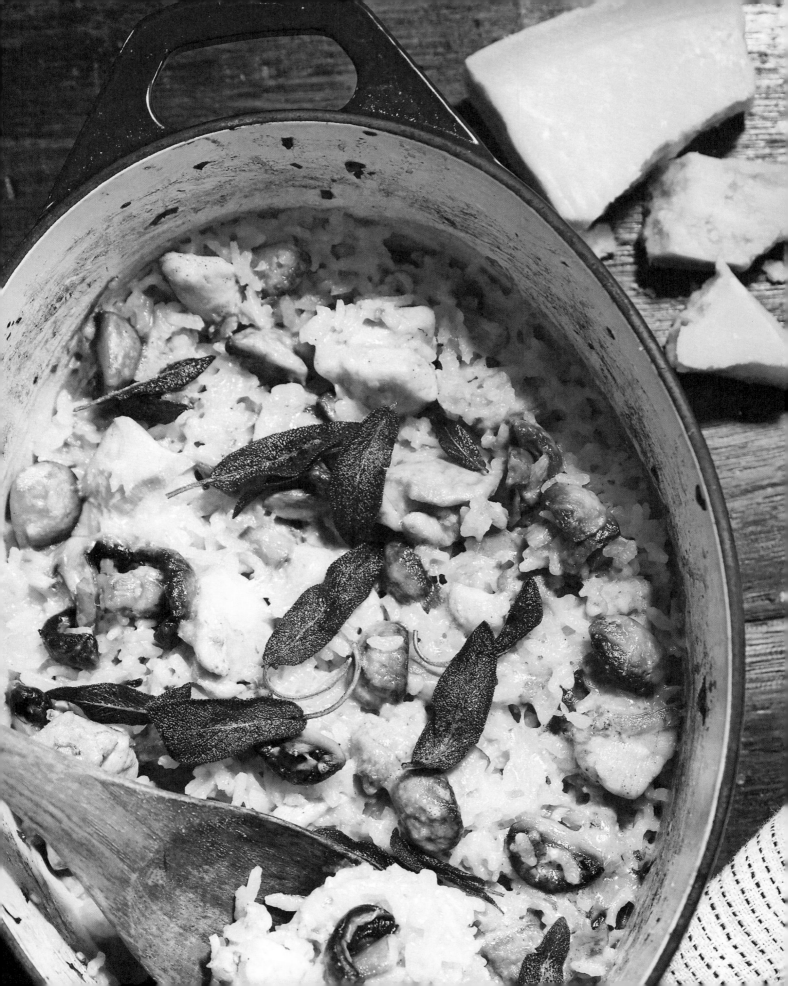

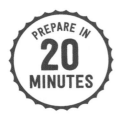

PREPARE IN
20
MINUTES

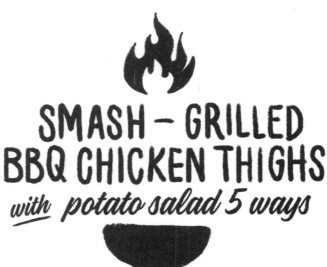

SMASH – GRILLED BBQ CHICKEN THIGHS
with potato salad 5 ways

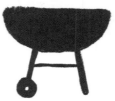

I am often accused of not being able to moderate a flame, however this method of cooking thighs requires you to turn the heat all the way up to get the grill REALLY hot before slapping on the chook, but then knocking the heat back to finish the cooking. It makes for thighs that are both crisply bar-marked and juicy, which is perfect in my book (which this is …).

This chook is terrific with potato salad so, in the interest of variety, what follows is a selection of marinades (inspired by some of my favourite restaurant kitchens) with potato salads to match.

SERVES 4 PREP: 20 MINS (PLUS 30 MINS MARINATING) **COOKING:** 20 MINS

8 chicken thigh cutlets, skin on
olive oil, to drizzle

GREEK MARINADE
70 g (¼ cup) tomato paste
3 garlic cloves, crushed
1 tablespoon dried oregano
zest and juice of 1 lemon

GREEK POTATO SALAD
1.2 kg red-skinned, waxy potatoes,
  skins on
60 ml (¼ cup) olive oil
60 ml (¼ cup) red wine vinegar
2 tablespoons coarsely chopped dill
2 tablespoons coarsely chopped
  oregano
sea salt and freshly ground
  black pepper
1 red onion, cut into thin wedges
145 g (1 cup) pitted Kalamata olives
100 g feta, crumbled

To make the marinade, combine the tomato paste, garlic, oregano, lemon zest and juice in a bowl. Add the chicken and rub well until completely coated. Cover and leave to marinate in the fridge for 30 minutes, or up to 2 hours.

While the chicken marinates, make the potato salad. Place the potatoes in a large saucepan of cold water and bring to the boil. Boil for 20 minutes, or until just tender (you know, so they slip off the blade of a small sharp knife when jabbed). Drain and set aside for 5 minutes to cool slightly.

Combine the oil, vinegar, dill and oregano in a bowl. Season.

While still warm, cut the potatoes into chunks and place in a large bowl. Add the onion, olives and dressing to the potato and toss gently until combined. Transfer to a serving bowl and sprinkle with the feta.

Preheat a barbecue grill or chargrill pan on high. Drizzle the chicken with oil. Place the chicken, skin-side down, on the grill. Turn the heat down to low and cook for 15 minutes on each side, or until cooked through and slightly charred. Transfer to a plate, cover loosely with foil and leave to rest for 5 minutes before serving with the Greek potato salad.

TIP

If you want to use skinless, boned thigh fillets, they will only take around 4 minutes on each side.

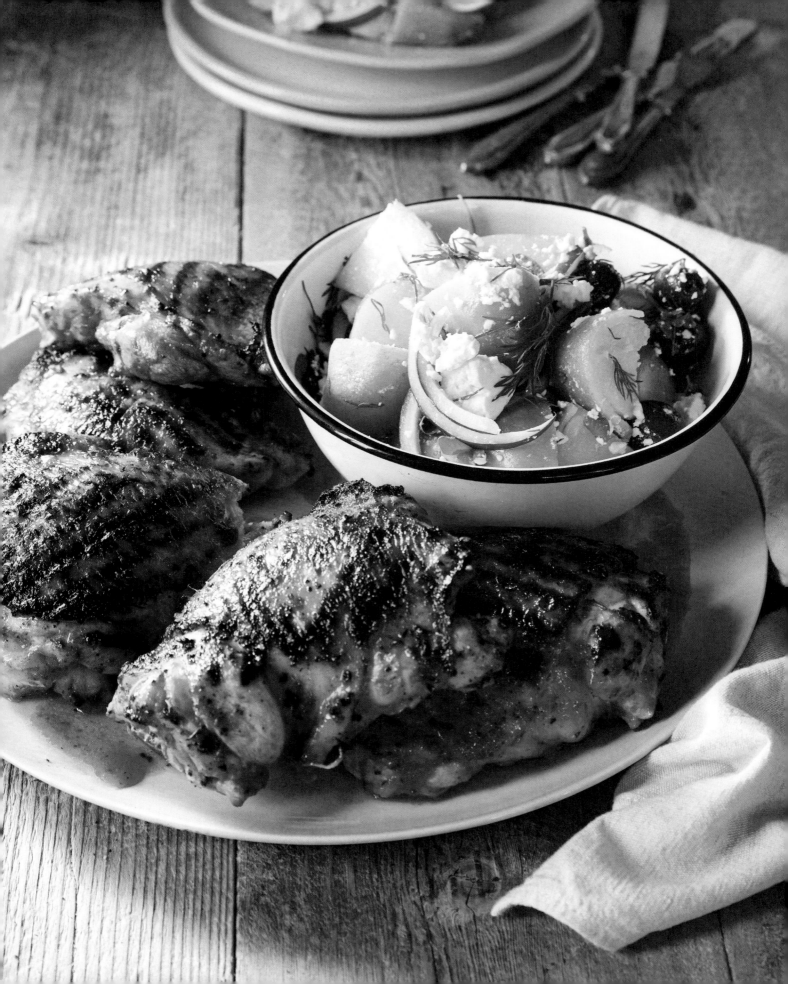

4 BRILLIANT WAYS TO CUSTOMISE YOUR BARBECUED THIGHS AND POTATO SALAD

1. THE PRINCE OF PERSIA'S THIGHS WITH AFGHAN POTATO SALAD

I love tenderising meat with onion juice. It's a Persian idea I picked up for the best lamb chops but it also works wonderfully as a marinade for chicken thighs. The matching potato salad takes it cue from an Afghani chatni.

FOR THE MARINADE

Toast a large pinch of saffron threads in a small frying pan, then crush with the back of a spoon and stir into 250 g (1 cup) of thick natural yoghurt. Add a finely grated onion with its juices (the secret ingredient to so many great Persian marinades) and the chicken thighs. Marinate in the fridge for at least 30 minutes, then barbecue following the instructions on the previous page until nicely charred and cooked through. Rest for 5 minutes before serving.

FOR THE POTATO SALAD

Boil whole unpeeled waxy potatoes, then drain, peel and chop into large chunks. Cook 150 g (1 cup) of frozen peas in 125 ml (½ cup) of stock. Strain the peas, reserving the stock, and add the peas to the potato. Reduce the stock by half, then toss through the potato and peas. Blitz a bunch of flat-leaf parsley with 4 chopped spring onions, 1 green chopped chilli, and the zest and juice of 1 lime. Pour the dressing over the potato and add finely diced green capsicum and finely chopped cornichons. Toss gently to combine. Top with chopped hard-boiled egg, shredded mint and chopped pistachios tossed in a little olive oil to make them shimmer.

2. TRAILER TRASH THIGHS WITH RED-EYE BACON POTATO SALAD

My recipe guru Michelle and I have a shared love affair with junky American diner food. We couldn't go past this potato salad! The red eye and classic Southern spice mix naturally came along for the ride like biscuits with gravy (which we'll have to do in the next book!).

FOR THE MARINADE

Combine 2 tablespoons of sweet paprika, 1 tablespoon each of onion powder, dried oregano leaves and ground cumin, and 1 teaspoon each of garlic powder, chilli powder and salt. Rub all over the chicken and marinate for at least 30 minutes. Barbecue following the instructions on the previous page until nicely charred and cooked through. Rest for 5 minutes before serving.

FOR THE POTATO SALAD

Boil small whole unpeeled sweet potatoes then drain, peel and chop into large chunks. Fry some frozen corn in a frying pan until lightly toasted, then add to the potato. Fry some large chopped pieces of bacon until golden, add a light sprinkle of instant coffee and 2 tablespoons of brown sugar and water, and cook until the sugar dissolves and the bacon is sticky. In a bowl, combine 125 g (½ cup) whole egg mayonnaise and a few good dessert spoons of sweet pickle relish, or sweetcorn relish and 1 teaspoon of mustard powder for kick. Toss the mayonnaise mixture through the potato with a small dessert spoon of poppy seeds. Sit 2 halved hard-boiled eggs on top, then sprinkle over finely chopped celery, blanched chopped onion, the bacon mixture and a sprinkling of paprika.

3. HARIYALI THIGHS WITH INDIAN-SPICED POTATO SALAD

There are so many ways to marinate meat in the Indian manner that it's hard to pick a favourite but my do I love the green herbaceousness of 'hariyali' kebabs. Of course it's not strictly a spice rub but then if I was following rules I could have just said rub them with curry powder but that wouldn't have been much of a recipe would it – or be as delicious!

FOR THE MARINADE

Blend 250 g (1 cup) thick natural yoghurt with 1 heaped tablespoon of grated ginger, 3 crushed garlic cloves, 1 long chopped green chilli, 1 tablespoon cream, 2 tablespoons chopped coriander, 1 tablespoon each of roasted cashews and almond meal, and 2 teaspoons lemon juice until smooth, adding more lemon juice and some salt and chilli if you like. Stir in 1 tablespoon melted butter so it marbles the mix. Massage this paste into the chicken thighs, then marinate in the fridge for 3 hours or overnight. Barbecue following the instructions on the previous page until nicely charred and cooked through. Rest for 5 minutes before serving.

FOR THE POTATO SALAD

Roast halved baby coliban potatoes in a preheated 200°C/180°C fan-forced oven for 30–40 minutes, until crisp (even better – use up your leftover roasties from yesterday's Sunday roast). Fry a few thinly sliced onions until very golden and crisp and blanch some peas. Combine 125 g (½ cup) yoghurt, a good spoonful of mango chutney (or apricot jam if that is easier), 1 teaspoon curry powder, a sprinkle of sea salt and the juice of ½ lemon. Toss through the potato and add the peas. Top with the fried onion, a few chopped coriander stems and leaves and toasted cashews.

4. RAS EL HANOUT THIGHS WITH NORTH AFRICAN POTATO SALAD

This is the worst sort of cultural appropriation. I'm sorry. Sure, it's very tasty misappropriation but I'm not sure that this helps.

FOR THE MARINADE/DRY RUB

Buy ready-made ras el hanout or make your own by dry-frying 4 cardamom pods, 2 teaspoons each of ground mace and coriander seeds, and 1 teaspoon each of cumin seeds, freshly ground black pepper and ground cinnamon in a small frying pan over low heat for 30 seconds, or until toasted. Transfer to a mortar and pestle and grind to a fine powder. Rub into the thighs and marinate for at least 30 minutes. Barbecue following the instructions on the previous page until nicely charred and cooked through. Rest for 5 minutes before serving.

FOR THE POTATO SALAD

Boil unpeeled baby coliban potatoes, then drain and halve while still warm. Combine a 1:3 ratio of white wine vinegar and olive oil with some crushed garlic and season well. Toss through the potato with finely chopped red onion, chopped coriander and mint, and toasted slivered almonds.

CHIC
BREA

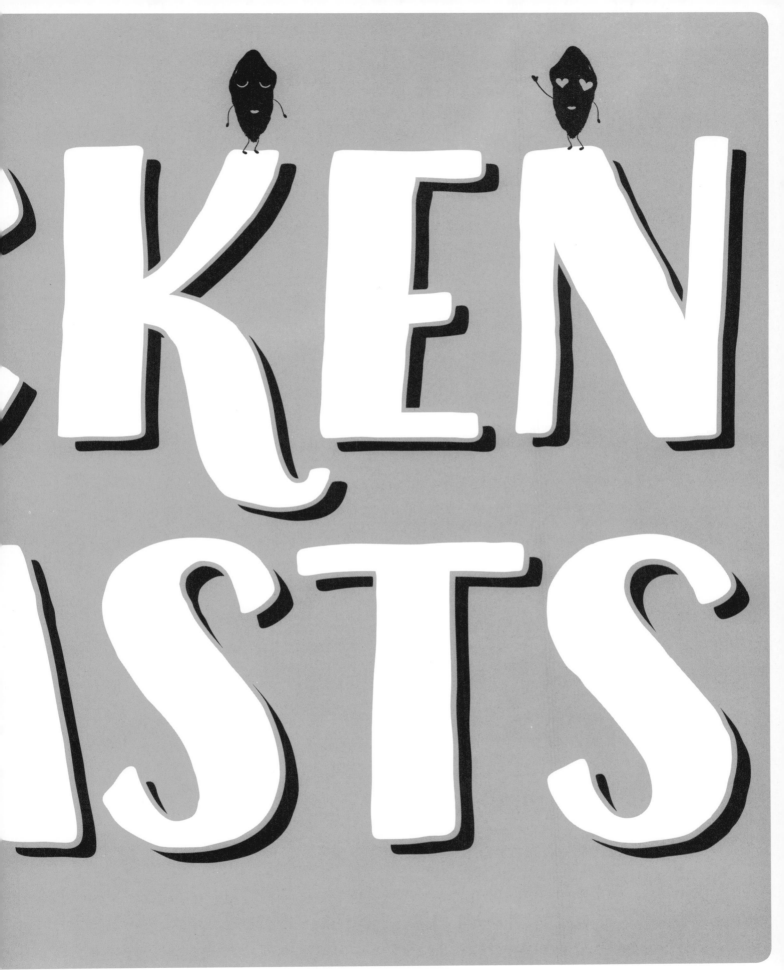

FLATTENED TENDERLOIN-STYLE US SPICE-RUBBED BBQ SKEWERS

Roger Miller's *King of the Road* was the second song I learned to play on the guitar when I was a kid. It's a romantic paen to being a railway hobo. I loved the free-wheelin' swagger of smoking 'old stogies' and the romance of the 'third boxcar, midnight train'. This is the sort of dish I imagine the hero dreaming of sitting down to after 'two hours pushin' broom'.

Ironically, the maple mustard is stolen, with much respect, from the guys at Joe Beef – Canadians who know as much about the pleasure of eating as they do about the pleasure of cooking, which is weirdly rare. Appropriately, their Montreal restaurant is on the site of the city's old railyards. What was that about 'every lock that ain't locked when no one's around ...'?

SERVES 6 PREP: 30 MINS COOKING: 1 HOUR 15 MINS

6 small sweet potatoes, unpeeled
1 kg chicken tenderloins
melted butter, to brush
sea salt and freshly ground
   black pepper
6 streaky bacon rashers,
   coarsely chopped
1 spring onion, thinly sliced
Simple Lettuce Salad (page 175),
   to serve

MAPLE MUSTARD
200 ml maple syrup
125 g (½ cup) dijon mustard
1½ tablespoons yellow
   mustard seeds
½ teaspoon freshly ground
   black pepper

SMOKY BBQ RUB
3 tablespoons dried oregano leaves
3 tablespoons smoked paprika
1½ tablespoons ground cumin
1½ tablespoons brown sugar
3 teaspoons smoked salt (or just
   use plain salt)

Preheat the oven to 220°C/200°C fan-forced. Place the sweet potatoes on a baking tray and cover the tray tightly with foil. Roast for 1 hour or until tender. While this is happening, make the mustard and prepare the chicken.

To make the maple mustard, heat the maple syrup in a small saucepan over medium heat for about 7 minutes, or until really big bubbles start to form. Set aside to cool slightly. Whisk in the mustard, mustard seeds and ground pepper. Pour into a bowl and refrigerate until serving.

Combine all the ingredients for the barbecue rub in a bowl and stir to combine. Place half the rub in a zip-lock bag. Add the chicken tenderloins and toss until well coated. Weave the chicken onto 18 soaked bamboo skewers.

Leave the cooked sweet potatoes on the tray and slit them down the centre without cutting all the way through. Use a fork to press open the potatoes slightly and roughly mash the flesh inside. Brush the outside of the skins with butter. Season. Bake for a further 10–15 minutes, until crisp. Cover with foil to keep warm.

Heat a large frying pan over medium–high heat. Add the bacon and cook, tossing, for 2–3 minutes, until super-crisp. Transfer to a plate. Add the chicken skewers to the pan and cook for 2–3 minutes on each side, or until cooked through and slightly charred. Alternatively, if you want to use the barbie, heat the barbecue grill and flat plate on medium. Cook the chicken on the grill and the bacon on the flat plate.

Transfer the chicken to a plate, cover loosely with foil and leave to rest.

Top the potatoes with a drizzle of maple mustard and scatter with bacon bits and spring onion. Serve with the chicken skewers and the simple lettuce salad.

TIP

You'll only need half the rub for these skewers, so store the rest in an airtight container or zip-lock bag in the cupboard for up to 1 month. It's a great all-purpose rub to have on hand for other meats, such as lamb, pork and beef when barbecuing. You can also try it on your Sunday roast chicken or lamb or on roast veggies.

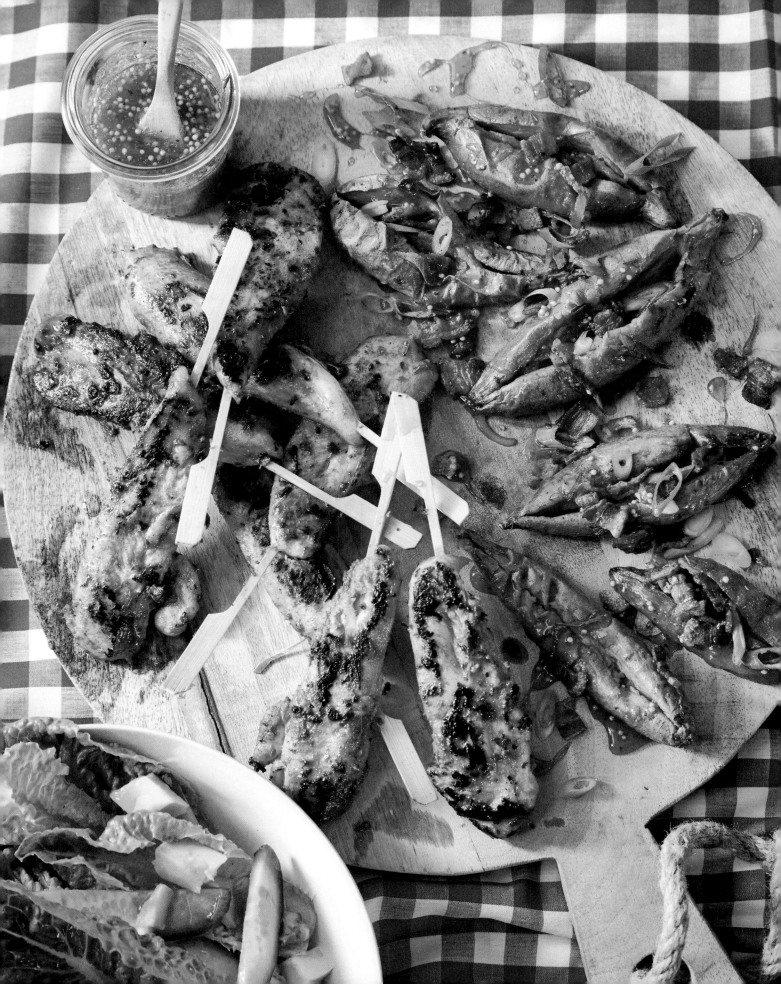

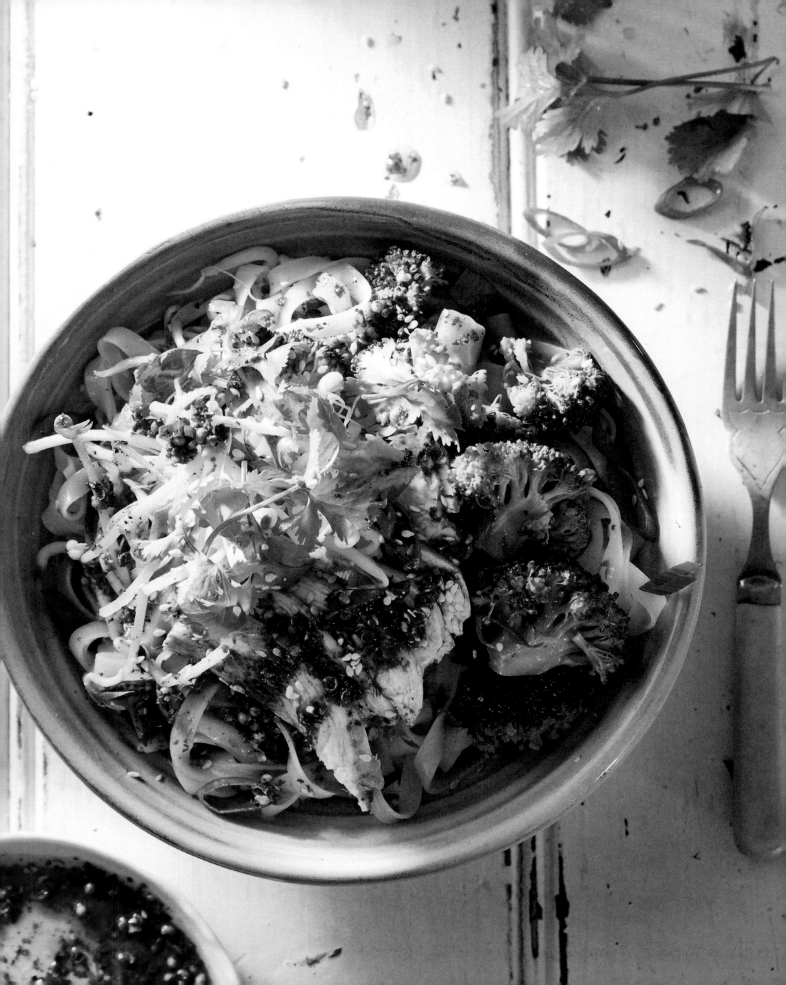

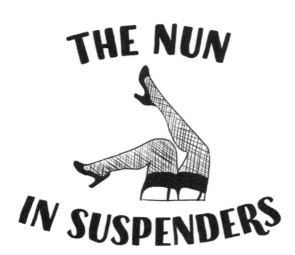

THE NUN IN SUSPENDERS

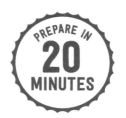

This dish is all about the virtuous innocence of the poached chicken and the decadence of the very up-front sauce – a bit like the Mother Superior in *The Sound of Music* who secretly wants to audition for the lead in *The Rocky Horror Picture Show*.

SERVES 4 **PREP**: 20 MINS **COOKING**: 15 MINS

60 ml (¼ cup) light soy sauce
6 cm knob of ginger, peeled and thinly sliced
2 spring onions, white and green parts separated, green parts thinly shredded, to serve
3 (about 250 g each) chicken breast fillets
300 g broccoli, cut into florets
1 × 375 g packet thin flat rice stick noodles

SICHUAN HOT AND NUMBING SAUCE
60 ml (¼ cup) canola oil
¼–½ teaspoon dried red chilli flakes, depending on their heat
2 teaspoons sichuan peppercorns
60 ml (¼ cup) black vinegar
3 teaspoons caster sugar
2 teaspoons sesame oil

TO SERVE
bean sprouts
coriander leaves
toasted sesame seeds

Pour 1 litre of water into a deep frying pan. Add the soy sauce, ginger and white parts of the spring onion and bring to the boil over medium heat. Reduce the heat to low. Add the chicken fillets and simmer for 8 minutes.

While the chook is cooking, make the hot and numbing sauce. Heat the oil in a small frying pan over medium heat until just warmed. Remove from the heat, add the chilli flakes and set aside to cool and infuse.

Place the sichuan peppercorns in a mortar and use a pestle to grind coarsely. Transfer to a small bowl. Add the chilli oil, black vinegar, sugar and sesame oil. Stir well to dissolve the sugar and set aside.

Turn the chicken over and add the broccoli to the pan. Cook for a further 2 minutes, or until the broccoli is bright green and tender-crisp. Use tongs to transfer the broccoli to a bowl, then cover and keep warm. Set the chicken aside in the cooking liquid; it will finish cooking in the residual heat.

Cook the noodles following the packet instructions. Drain well.

Thinly slice the chicken. Divide the noodles among serving bowls and top with the broccoli and chicken. Drizzle with the numbing sauce. Top with the shredded green spring onion, bean sprouts and coriander, and finish with a sprinkle of sesame seeds.

ASIAN CHICKEN NUGGETS

with NEW GOLD MOUNTAIN UNFRIED RICE

#SimpleFamilyMeals #15MinCook #Dinner #Tasty #MidWeekFeed #Food #Recipe
#AreHashtagsTheDeathOfWritingAsWeKnowIt?

SERVES 4 PREP: 30 MINS (PLUS 30 MINS MARINATING) COOKING: 15 MINS

60 ml (¼ cup) soy sauce, plus
   extra to serve
60 ml (¼ cup) honey
4 cm knob of ginger, peeled and
   finely grated
2 garlic cloves, crushed
1 kg chicken breast fillets, cut into
   4 cm pieces
120 g (2 cups) panko breadcrumbs
2 tablespoons sesame seeds
1 teaspoon Chinese five spice
oil spray
sesame oil, to serve
2 spring onions, thinly sliced
   diagonally, to serve

NEW GOLD MOUNTAIN UNFRIED RICE

150 g sliced lap cheong sausage,
   sliced barbecued pork or
   cubed spam (I usually use lap
   cheong as it is easy to find in my
   supermarket) (see TIP)
200 g mushrooms, thinly sliced
150 g (1 cup) frozen peas or peas
   and corn, thawed
55 g (⅓ cup) unsalted roasted
   peanuts, coarsely chopped
1 × 450 g pouch 90 second
   microwaveable brown rice,
   warmed following the packet
   instructions

Combine the soy sauce, honey, ginger and garlic in a glass or ceramic dish. Add the chicken pieces and toss to coat. Cover. Leave to marinate in the fridge for 30 minutes or up to 2 hours.

Preheat the oven to 200°C/180°C fan-forced. Line two baking trays with baking paper. Combine the breadcrumbs, sesame seeds and Chinese five spice in a large bowl.

Dip the chicken pieces in the crumb mixture, tossing to coat. Arrange on the lined trays, ensuring they are not too close together. Spray with oil spray. Bake for 12–15 minutes, until golden and tender.

While the chicken is baking, make the rice. Heat a large frying pan over medium–high heat. Add the lap cheong sausage, or the barbecued pork or cubed spam, and toss for 1–2 minutes, until it starts to brown.

Add the mushroom and cook, tossing, for 2–3 minutes, until golden. Stir in the peas and peanuts. Cook for 2 minutes, or until heated through. Remove from the heat and toss in the warmed rice.

Spread the rice on a platter. Drizzle with a little soy sauce and sesame oil. Top with the nuggets and sprinkle with spring onion.

TIPS

Lap cheong sausage does not need any oil when frying. If using barbecue pork or spam, add a drizzle of neutral oil (peanut/vegetable) to help make it crisp and golden.

This recipe makes a big batch of nuggets (about 60) so there are plenty left over to have in a salad the next day, or for the kids the next night.

Unfried rice is a great way to use up any leftover bits from the vegetable crisper. Try adding corn, broccoli, zucchini, carrot or cabbage, to name but a few. And see page 249 for more ideas.

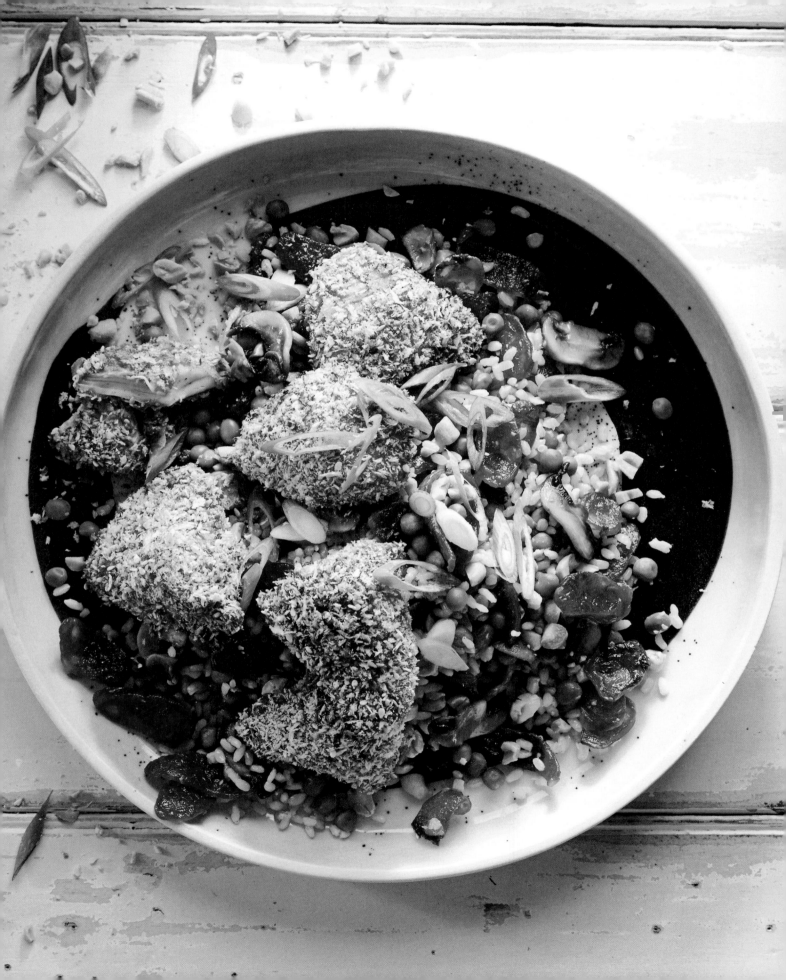

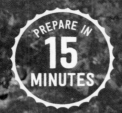

BOCCONCINI *and* PROSCIUTTO

HASSELBACK CHICKEN

'Don't make it look like witchetty grubs!' read the notes to the food team shooting this book. Well, they succeeded.

While simple, I feel this is a better way of introducing this recipe than discussing the rather salacious etymology of 'bocconcini' and 'prosciutto' (please don't hit Google to check this – once seen you can't unsee it!) or the role trainee chef Leif Elisson played in the invention of the hasselback technique in Stockholm in 1953.

SERVES 4 PREP: 15 MINS COOKING: 45 MINS

1 tablespoon olive oil
1 onion, finely chopped
2 garlic cloves, crushed
1 × 400 g can cherry tomatoes
80 ml (⅓ cup) white wine
2 rosemary sprigs
sea salt and freshly ground
    black pepper
4 chicken breast fillets
4 slices prosciutto, halved
    lengthways
3 bocconcini, thinly sliced
40 g semi-dried tomatoes, cut
    lengthways into thin strips
20 g (¼ cup) shredded parmesan
10 basil leaves

Preheat the oven to 180°C/160°C fan-forced.

Heat the oil in a large frying pan over medium heat. Add the onion and garlic and cook for 5 minutes, or until soft. Add the tomatoes, wine and rosemary. Simmer for 10 minutes, or until the mixture thickens slightly. Season. Transfer the tomato mixture to an ovenproof dish.

Meanwhile, cut slits across each chicken breast about 2 cm apart. Weave the prosciutto into the slits. Add a slice of cheese to each slit and a few semi-dried tomato strips.

Place the chicken breasts on top of the tomato mixture. Season, sprinkle with parmesan and bake for 25–30 minutes, until the chicken is cooked through and the cheese has melted.

Garnish with basil leaves and serve.

TIPS

Try stuffing the chicken breasts with spinach and ricotta, or with bacon, sliced mushrooms and thyme.

In spring or summer, serve with a crisp green balsamic-dressed salad, or with steamed batons of zucchini dressed with lemon juice, torn basil and a little drizzle of good olive oil.

In autumn or winter, serve with buttered tagliatelle cooked in chicken stock with carrots, or with creamy polenta and steamed green beans tossed with torn basil.

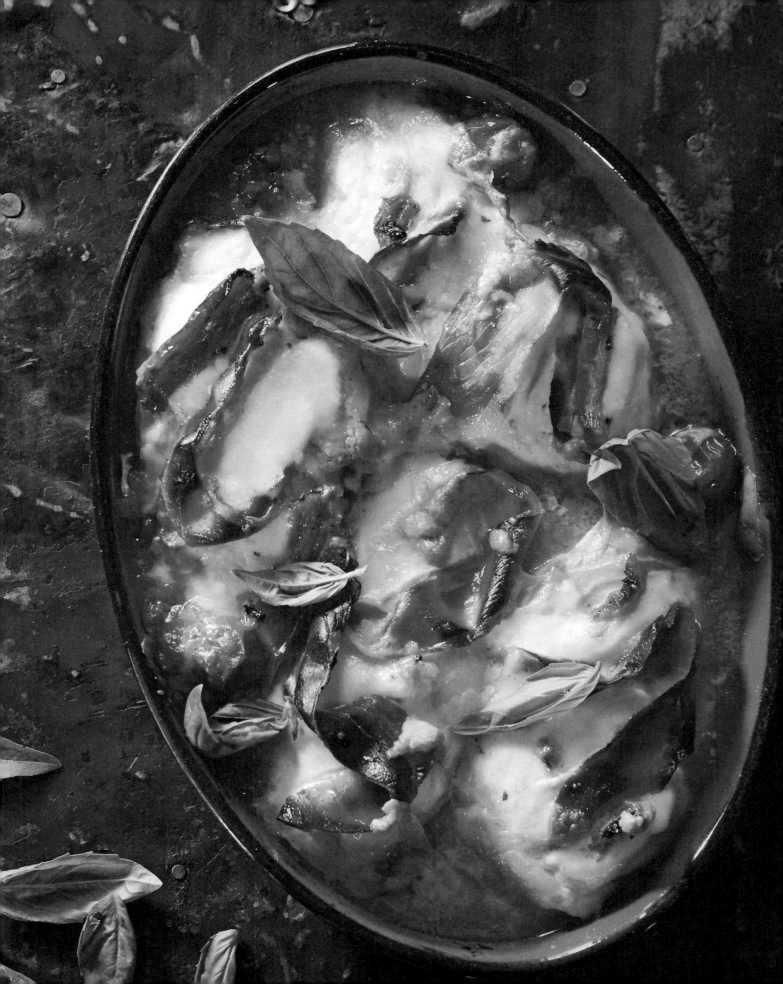

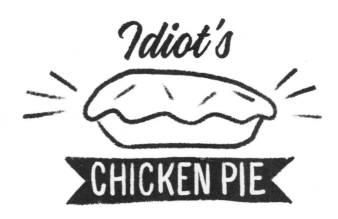

Idiot's CHICKEN PIE

Everybody likes pie. It's homely, it's friendly, it's hard to refuse. This pie is also really easy to make – so there's no excuse for NOT making it. No matter your mood, pie will make you feel better. Pie is magic like that.

SERVES 4–6 **PREP:** 30 MINS (PLUS COOLING) **COOKING:** 1 HOUR

1 tablespoon olive oil
1 kg chicken breast fillets,
    cut into 3 cm pieces
30 g butter
180 g rindless shortcut bacon
    rashers, coarsely chopped
3 celery stalks, thickly sliced
1 leek, thickly sliced
3 garlic cloves, crushed
80 ml (⅓ cup) dry sherry
3 fresh or dried bay leaves
2 tablespoons plain flour
1 tablespoon dijon mustard
310 ml (1¼ cups) chicken stock
125 g (½ cup) crème fraîche
sea salt and freshly ground
    black pepper
1 × 375 g packet good-quality
    rolled puff pastry, just thawed
1 egg, lightly whisked

Heat the oil in a non-stick frying pan over high heat. Add one-third of the chicken pieces and cook for 2 minutes, or until browned. Transfer to a bowl. Repeat in two more batches with the remaining chicken.

Heat the butter in the pan over medium heat. Add the bacon, celery and leek and cook, stirring, for 8–10 minutes, until soft. Add the garlic and cook for 1 minute, or until aromatic. Add the sherry and bay leaves and cook, stirring, for 2–3 minutes, until the liquid has almost evaporated. Add the flour and mustard and stir for 2 minutes, or until well combined and the flour has cooked a little.

Gradually add the stock and bring to the boil. Simmer for 2 minutes to thicken slightly. Remove from the heat and stir in the crème fraîche and the reserved chicken pieces. Season. Set aside to cool.

Preheat the oven to 220°C/200°C fan-forced. Spoon the chicken mixture into a 28 cm round pie dish.

If necessary, roll the pastry slightly to make it a little larger. Cut out a disc large enough to cover the pie dish. Cut 2 cm wide strips from the leftover pastry and join them together to form one long strip. Brush the rim of the dish with egg and affix the long pastry strip around the top. Brush it with egg, then sit the pastry disc on top to enclose the filling. (The extra pastry strip makes the edge puff up even more, for extra WOW factor!)

Press the edge to seal, then brush the entire surface with egg. Cut a few slits in the top to allow steam to escape. Bake for 25 minutes, or until the pastry is puffed and golden.

TIPS

You can make the chicken mixture ahead of time and store, covered, in the fridge for up to 1 day.

If using smaller or thinner sheets of ready-rolled puff pastry, join a few pieces together with whisked egg to make one large sheet.

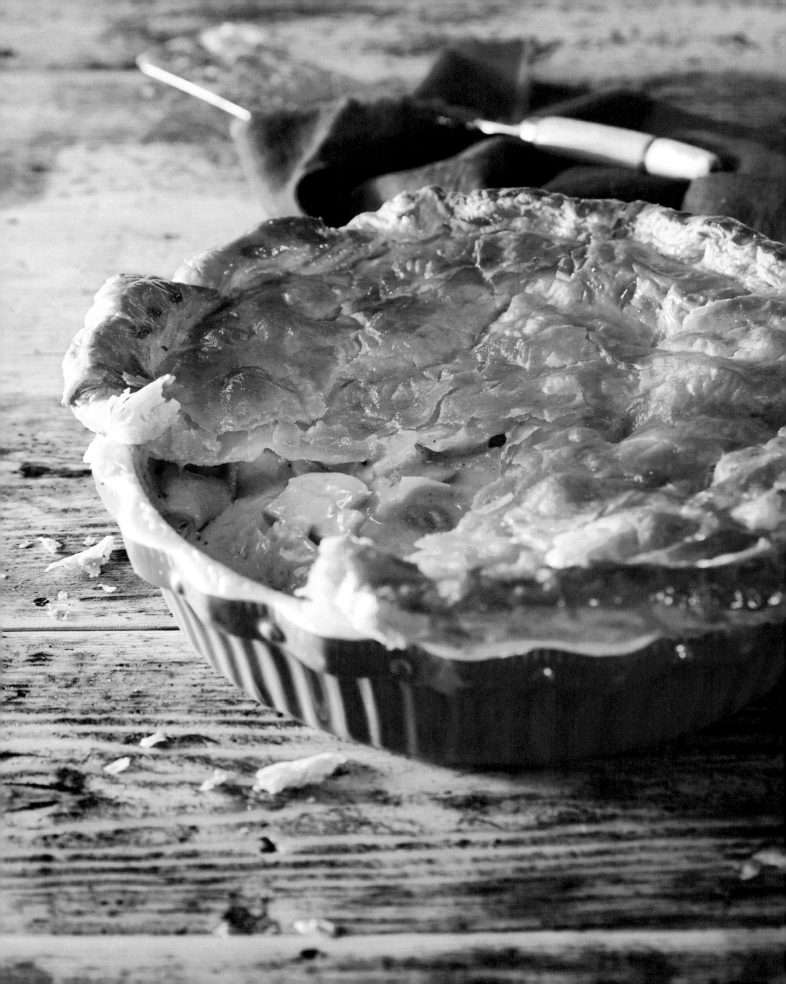

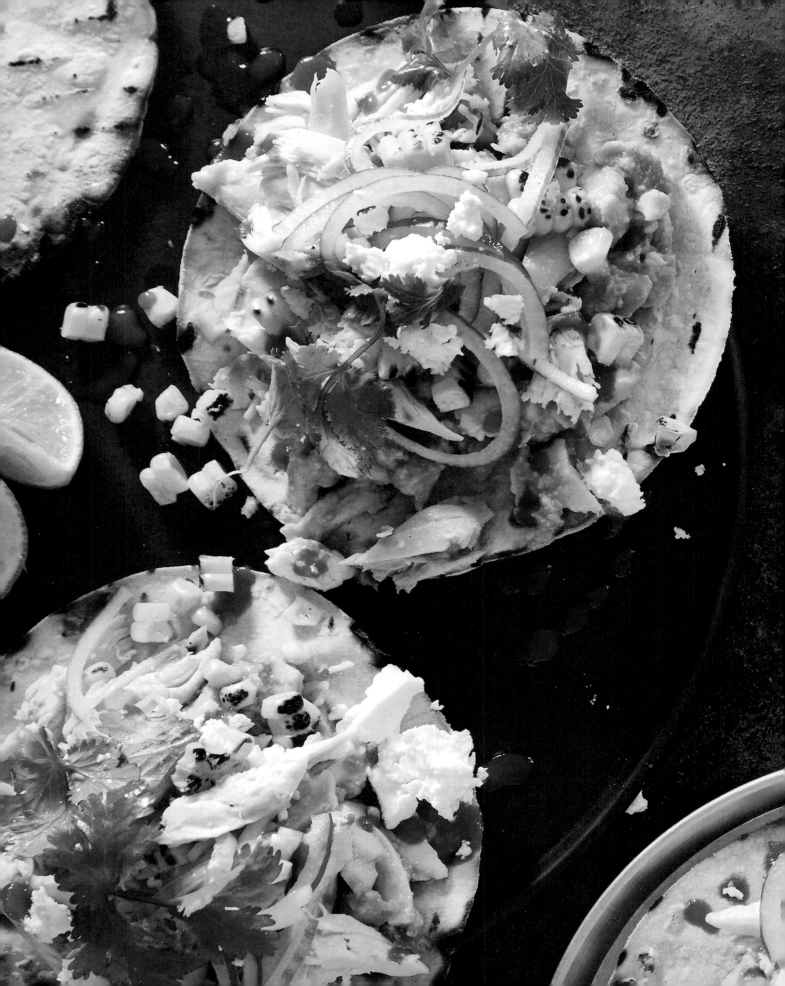

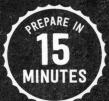

CHEAT'S CRUNCHY MEXICAN BBQ CHICKEN TOSTADAS – NO BBQ REQUIRED

Life's too short to take food too seriously. There are enough real issues out there without getting all uptight about buying the occasional supermarket barbecued chook. Just make sure the chook's a good one and relish how easy it is to make this dinner!

SERVES 4 PREP: 15 MINS COOKING: 10 MINS

2 tablespoons white wine vinegar
2 tablespoons caster sugar
1 teaspoon sea salt, plus extra to season
1 small red onion, halved and thinly sliced
2 corn cobs, husks and silks removed
8 white corn or flour mini tortillas
½ cup coriander leaves
3 avocados, mashed
1 supermarket ready-cooked barbecued chicken, skin and bones removed, meat shredded
sriracha chilli sauce, to drizzle
100 g feta, crumbled
lime wedges, to serve

Combine the vinegar, sugar and salt in a bowl. Add the red onion slices and set aside for 10 minutes to pickle. Drain.

Meanwhile, preheat a chargrill pan over medium heat (or a barbecue grill if you need to send your partner outside to get them out of the kitchen and from under your feet).

Grill the corn, turning frequently, for 8 minutes, or until tender and charred. Cut the corn kernels from the cobs.

Grill the tortillas in the same pan or on the barbecue for 1 minute each side, or until golden and crisp. Keep warm wrapped in a clean tea towel.

Combine the onion, corn and coriander in a bowl.

Spread the tortillas with the mashed avocado, top with shredded chicken and drizzle with sriracha. Sprinkle over the corn and onion mixture and finish with the feta. Serve with a squeeze of lime on top – it's a must.

TIP

If you don't have feta but there is some leftover sour cream or natural yoghurt in your fridge, then either of these will add a perfect creamy touch.

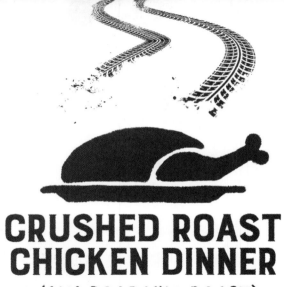

CRUSHED ROAST CHICKEN DINNER
(AKA ROAD KILL ROAST)

My family love roast garlic and fight over it. This stops that! If your family aren't similarly inclined, then save the second head of garlic to make aioli or squish into soups or mashed potato.

SERVES 4 **PREP**: 30 MINS **COOKING**: 1 HOUR 5 MINS

1 kg baby coliban (chat) potatoes
1 × 1.3 kg whole chicken
500 g cauliflower, cut into florets
1 lemon, zest peeled into 2 cm wide strips, lemon halved
12 thyme sprigs
80 ml (⅓ cup) olive oil
sea salt and freshly ground black pepper
2 red onions, cut into thick wedges
2 whole garlic heads, halved crossways
185 ml (¾ cup) chicken stock, warmed
20 g butter, plus extra to serve
toasted slivered almonds, to serve
cooked peas, to serve

Place the potatoes in a microwave-safe bowl. Add a slosh of water (about 1 tablespoon), cover with plastic wrap and cook on high for 12–15 minutes, until just tender.

Preheat the oven to 200°C/180°C fan-forced. Use kitchen scissors to cut down either side of the backbone of the chicken and remove the backbone. Or just get your butcher to do it for you. Use the palm of your hand to press down and flatten the chicken.

Place the chicken, skin-side up, in a large roasting tin and arrange the cauliflower around it. Top with the strips of lemon zest and half the thyme sprigs. Drizzle with half the oil. Season.

Place the potatoes on a baking tray. Use the back of a large spoon to gently press on each potato and crush slightly. Add the onion, garlic and remaining thyme to the potato tray and squeeze over the juice of one lemon half. Drizzle with the remaining oil. Season. Transfer everything to the oven and roast for 45 minutes, or until the chicken is cooked through and the cauliflower is golden.

Remove the chicken from the oven (but not the potato tray). Transfer the chicken to a plate and cover loosely with foil to rest in a warm place.

Add the stock to the roasting tin with the cauliflower in it. Sit over low heat until it just comes to the boil, scraping up any bits from the bottom of the tin. Reduce the stock a little, then tip the cauliflower and stock into a blender and blend until smooth. Add the butter and blend until combined. Season.

Spoon the cauliflower puree onto a warmed serving platter. Top with the chicken, potato, garlic and onion, and sprinkle over the almonds. Add a knob of butter to the cooked peas and serve straightaway.

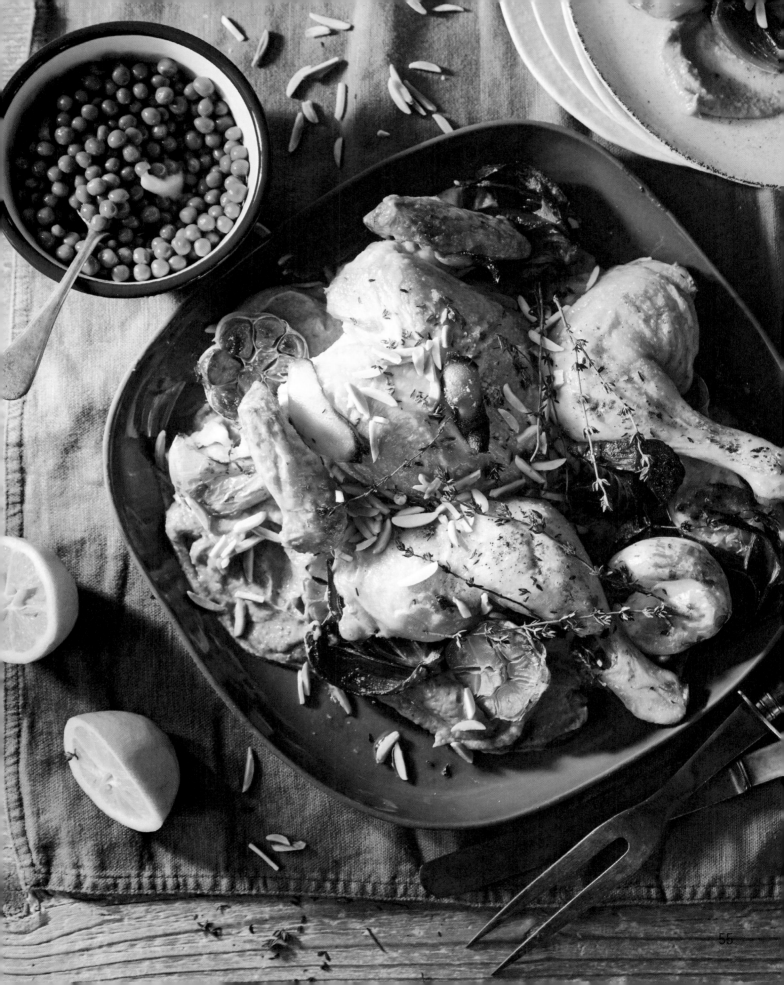

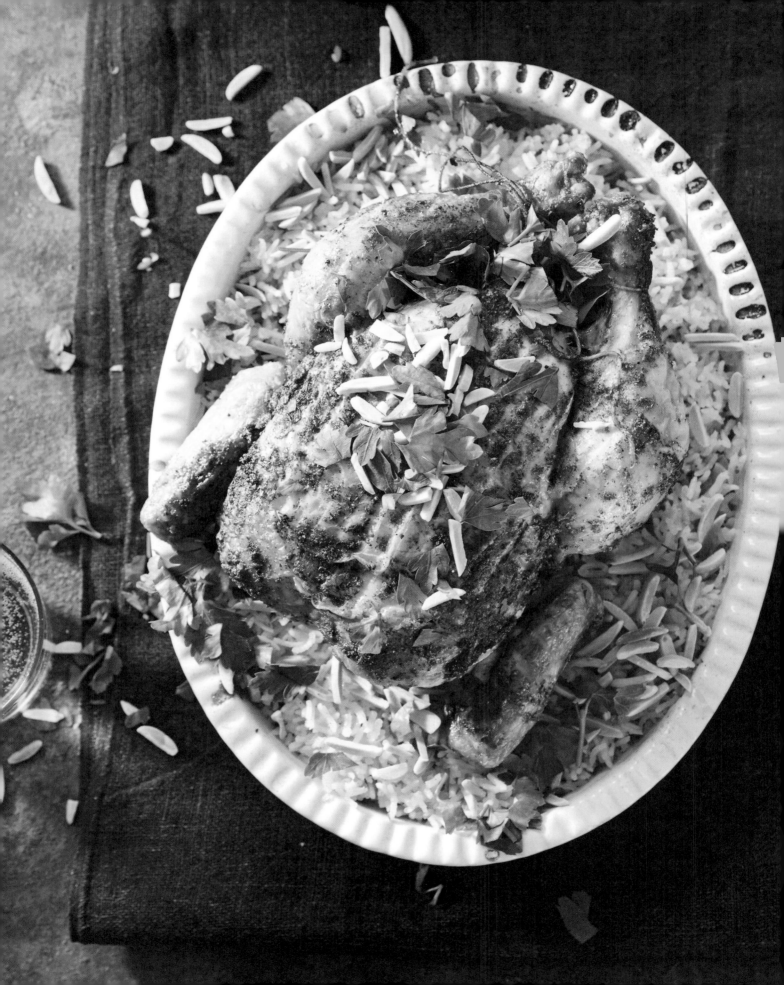

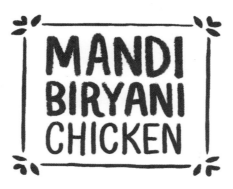

MANDI BIRYANI CHICKEN

One of the maddest things I did last year was to fly halfway around the world to Abu Dhabi to spend little more than 30 hours at their food festival. I swanned about looking pretty and talking about myself, while the mighty Emma Warren (who cooked all the food for the photos in this book) and wonderful food editor Warren Mendes did all the hard, sweaty, back-breaking, soul-destroying kitchen work. I'd like them to know right now that it wasn't all just smiling and waving for me – I also picked up this really clever Emirati version of a biryani – despite their conviction that I wasn't working at all.

SERVES 4–6 **PREP**: 30 MINS (PLUS 4 HOURS MARINATING) **COOKING**: 1 HOUR 45 MINS

100 g butter, at room temperature
2 teaspoons ground turmeric
sea salt and freshly ground
 black pepper
1 × 1.5 kg whole chicken
1 tablespoon olive oil
1 onion, finely chopped
500 g (2½ cups) basmati or
 long-grain rice
3 long green chillies, deseeded
 and finely chopped
3 cardamom pods
3 whole cloves
2 fresh or dried bay leaves
1 teaspoon black peppercorns
1 litre chicken stock
½ teaspoon saffron threads
flat-leaf parsley leaves, to serve
toasted slivered almonds, to serve

HAWAYIJ SPICE BLEND
1 tablespoon coriander seeds
1 tablespoon cumin seeds
1 tablespoon whole black
 peppercorns
2 teaspoons cardamom pods
1 teaspoon whole cloves
1 cinnamon stick

Preheat the oven to 180°C/160°C fan-forced. To make the hawayij spice blend, sprinkle all the spices on a baking tray and bake for 5–8 minutes, or until lightly toasted. (I will only warn you once: Do. Not. Burn. The. Spices.) Remove from the oven and leave to cool. Tip the spices into a mortar and use a pestle to pound to a fine powder.

Combine the butter, half the turmeric and half the hawaij spice mix in a bowl. Season with salt. Pat the chicken dry with paper towel. Rub the spiced butter all over the skin and inside the chicken. Feel free to push some extra spiced butter under the skin. Transfer to a plate, then cover and leave to marinate in the fridge for 4 hours or overnight.

Preheat the oven to 220°C/200°C fan-forced. Remove all but the bottom rack from the oven. Remove the chook from the fridge and set aside for 30 minutes to come to room temperature.

Meanwhile, heat the oil in a large heavy-based flameproof casserole dish that is larger than the chicken over medium–high heat. Add the onion and cook, stirring, for 5 minutes, or until soft. Add the rice, chilli, cardamom pods, cloves, bay leaves, peppercorns and the remaining turmeric. Cook for 2 minutes, stirring all the time, until things start smelling rather fragrant. Add the chicken stock and 125 ml (½ cup) water and stir to combine. Bring just to the boil.

Place the casserole dish in the oven, uncovered, and arrange an oiled oven rack just above it. Place the chicken, breast-side down, on the rack so any juices will drip down into the casserole dish. Roast for 15 minutes. Reduce the oven temperature to 160°C/140°C fan-forced, and roast for a further 45 minutes, until the rice has absorbed the liquid and it has a dry crust on top.

Meanwhile, combine the saffron with 2 tablespoons of hot water in a small bowl. Set aside for 5 minutes to infuse.

Transfer the chicken to a baking tray and turn it breast-side up.

Remove the rice from the oven, drizzle over the saffron liquid and use a fork to fluff the grains. Cover with a lid and set aside to keep warm.

Return the chicken to the oven for a further 30 minutes, or until cooked through and golden. Transfer the chicken to a plate and cover with foil to rest.

Pour any final drippings onto the rice and top with the chook. Sprinkle with parsley and slivered almonds and serve.

MI

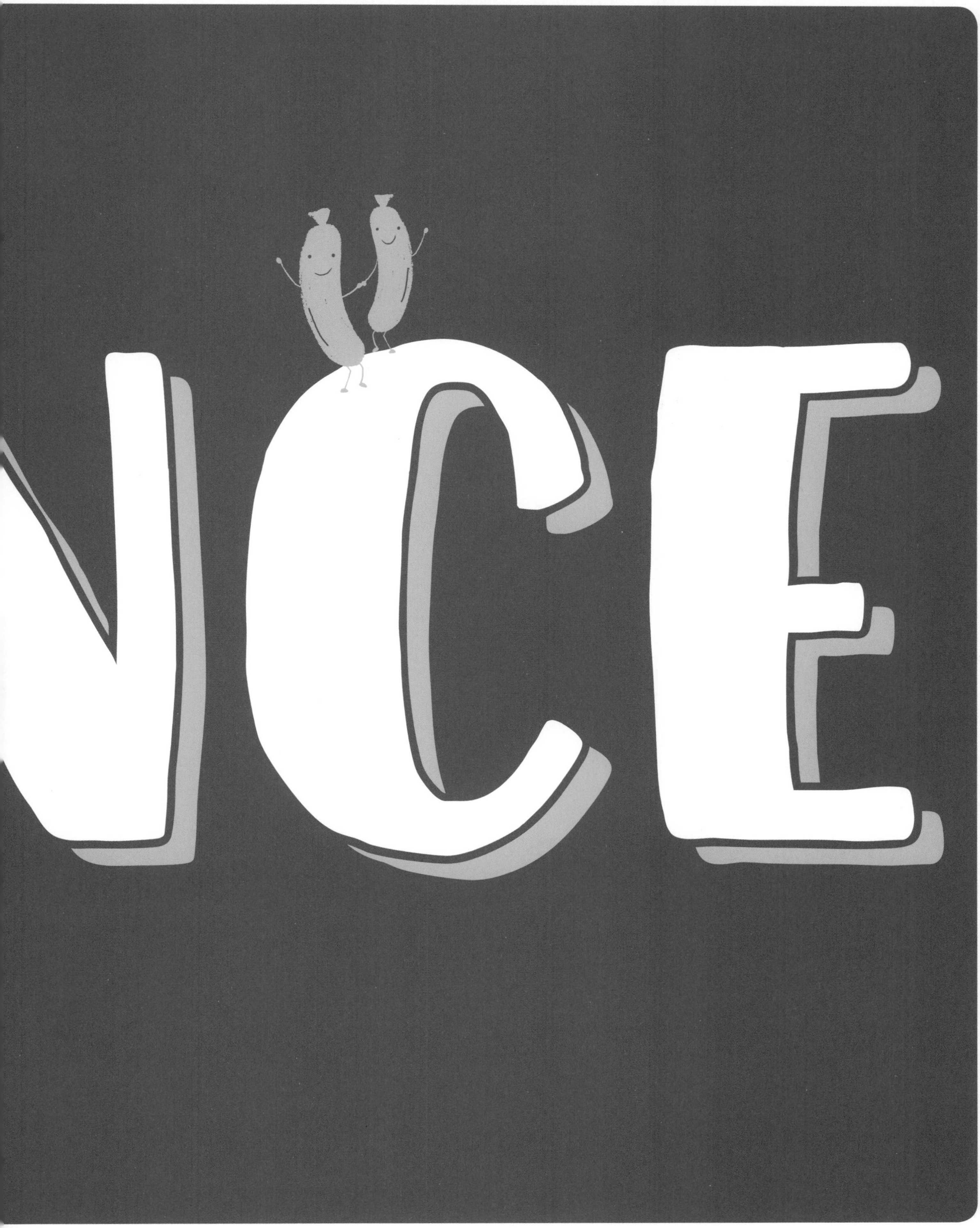
NCE

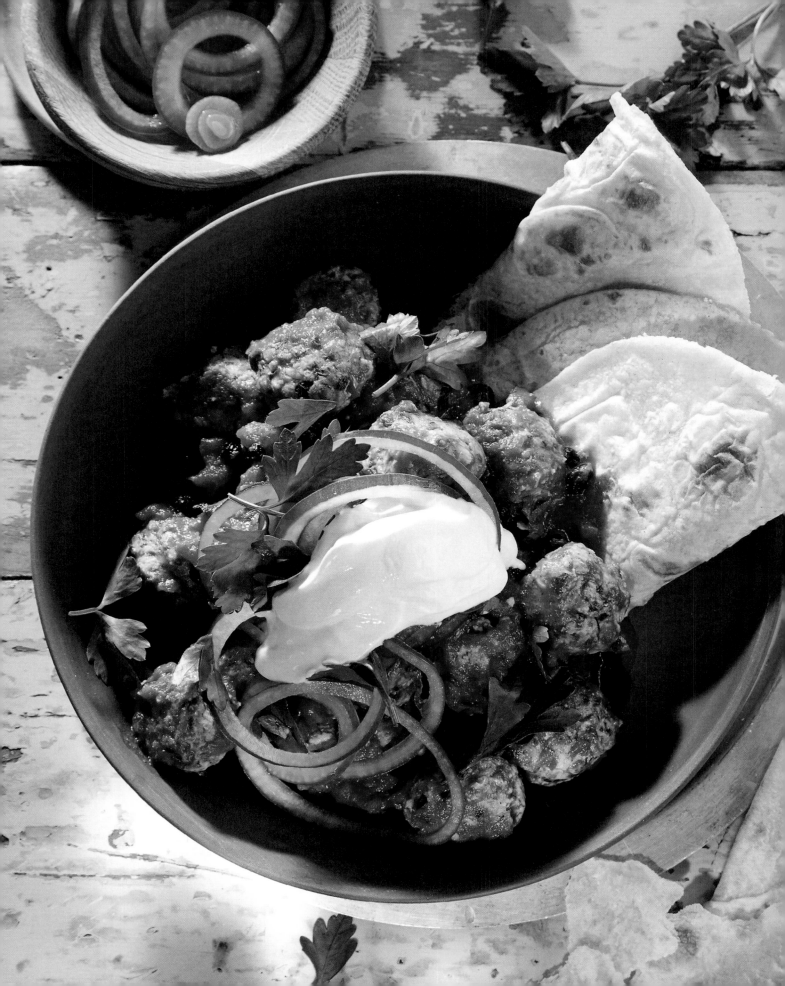

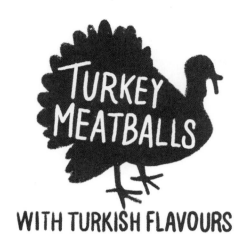

TURKEY MEATBALLS

WITH TURKISH FLAVOURS

Never the sharpest tools in the shed when it comes to food, the English originally believed that turkeys came from Turkey – hence the name. Whereas every Frenchman knew they came from D'Inde (ie, of India) and every Australian knew they came from ~~the supermarket~~ North America. Being English-born I felt it would be nice to reunite turkey with the flavours of Turkey to see if the two had a spiritual connection. It actually works rather well!

SERVES 4–6   PREP: 30 MINS   COOKING: 25 MINS

1 red onion, thinly sliced into rings
2 tablespoons white wine vinegar, cider vinegar or malt vinegar
sea salt and freshly ground black pepper
500 g turkey mince
200 g ricotta, roughly crumbled
½ cup finely chopped flat-leaf parsley leaves and stems, plus extra ½ cup leaves
1 tablespoon coarsely chopped dill
45 g (¼ cup) pine nuts, coarsely chopped
1 egg
2 tablespoons olive oil
4 cm knob of ginger, peeled and finely grated
¾ teaspoon ground allspice
¾ teaspoon ground cinnamon
1 × 400 g can crushed tomatoes
250 ml (1 cup) chicken stock
45 g (¼ cup) currants
hot flatbreads or brown rice, to serve
Greek-style yoghurt, to serve

Preheat the oven to 180°C/160°C fan-forced.

Combine the onion and vinegar in a bowl. Season generously with salt. Set aside while you make the rest of the dish.

Gently combine the turkey mince, ricotta, chopped parsley, dill, pine nuts and egg in a large bowl. Don't overwork the mixture; you are basically just pulling the ingredients together. Season.

Clean your hands and then dunk them in water. With wet hands, roll tablespoons of the mixture into balls (you should have about 40 balls). I like to put plastic wrap over my scales and weigh the tablespoons of mixture. This ensures the meatballs are the same size and will cook uniformly. The woman I love says this is typical of an uptight Virgo.

Heat 1 tablespoon of the oil in a large frying pan over medium–high heat. In batches, add the meatballs and cook, tossing, for 4–5 minutes, until golden. Transfer each batch of meatballs to a plate.

Heat the remaining oil in the pan. Add the ginger, allspice and cinnamon. Cook, stirring, for 1 minute, or until aromatic. Add the tomatoes, stock and currants to the pan and bring to the boil. Add the meatballs. Reduce the heat to medium and simmer for 10 minutes, or until the meatballs are cooked through and the sauce thickens. Wiggle the pan occasionally so the meatballs roll over. Season.

Toss the parsley leaves with the red onion. Serve with the meatballs, flatbreads or rice, and yoghurt.

TIPS

Make the meatballs in the sauce and freeze in an airtight container for up to 3 months. Thaw overnight in the fridge. Reheat over low heat in a saucepan.

Slice flatbreads into fingers and place in a warmed casserole dish, spoon the tomato sauce and meatballs on top and pop in a preheated 160°C/140°C fan-forced oven, until you are ready to eat. Dress with the onion mixture and yoghurt before serving.

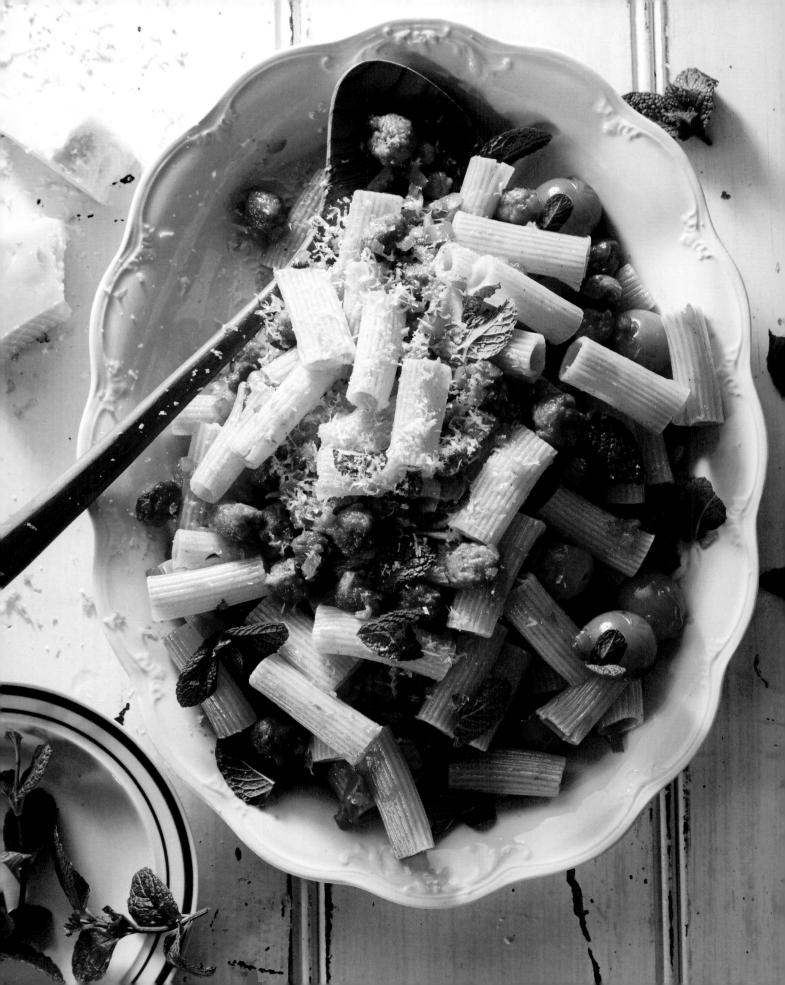

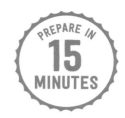

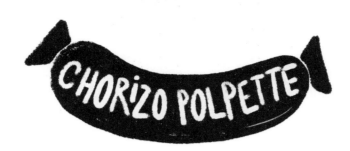

CHORIZO POLPETTE

Tuesday night, 6 pm: there was nothing happening for dinner and hardly anything in the fridge. After 20 minutes staring at the non-stick frying pan wondering what I could make, the brainwave of squeezing the meat out of the chorizo sausages to make meatballs hit me. They tan up marvellously and render wonderfully ruddy fat in which to fry your onions and capsicums.

SERVES 4 **PREP:** 15 MINS **COOKING:** 25 MINS

500 g fresh chorizo sausages
60 ml (¼ cup) olive oil
400 g dried rigatoni pasta
1 onion, finely chopped
1 red capsicum, deseeded and finely chopped
1 × 250 g punnet cherry tomatoes
2 teaspoons smoked paprika
250 ml (1 cup) chicken stock
sea salt and freshly ground black pepper
½ cup mint or flat-leaf parsley leaves
zest of 1 orange
1 tablespoon sherry vinegar or red wine vinegar
grated parmesan or manchego, to serve

Snip one end off each of the sausages and squeeze the meat out of the casings into thumbnail-sized meatballs.

Heat 1 tablespoon of the oil in a large frying pan over medium–high heat. Add the meatballs in batches and cook, tossing, for 2–3 minutes, or until golden. Transfer to a plate.

Start cooking your pasta now, so by the time your sauce is ready the pasta will be done. Congratulate yourself on your excellent time management skills. Cook the pasta in plenty of boiling salted water for 1 minute less than it says on the packet, until al dente. Drain and return to the pan.

While your pasta is cooking, make the sauce. Heat another tablespoon of oil in the frying pan over medium–high heat. Add the onion and capsicum and cook, stirring, for 5 minutes, or until soft.

Add the tomatoes and smoked paprika and cook, stirring, for 1 minute, or until aromatic. Add the stock. Reduce the heat to medium and simmer rapidly for 5 minutes.

Add the meatballs and cook for a further 3 minutes, or until the meatballs are cooked through and the tomatoes start to collapse slightly. Season and keep warm.

Combine the mint or parsley, orange zest, vinegar and the remaining tablespoon of oil in a bowl. Season.

Transfer the pasta to a platter and stir through the meatballs. Sprinkle with the orange zest mixture and top with grated parmesan or manchego.

TIPS

Try other sausages in this quick sauce. For something with a little less of a spicy kick try chicken or pork.

Add a can of chickpeas to the sauce with the meatballs for a heartier meal – and a chance to drop the quantity of evil pasta.

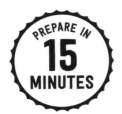

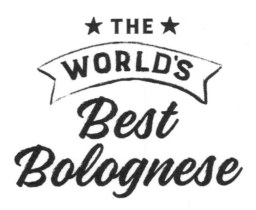

★ THE ★
WORLD'S
Best
Bolognese

This sauce is so good it's developed its own fan club – one of whom pinned the recipe on a notice board at my publisher's and got me a book deal. Thanks, Joybelle. The rest is history. If you want to make this bolognese even better, add a parmesan rind or a couple of pieces of pig skin (ask your butcher) to the sauce as it starts cooking. Or just cook it the day before you need it. These tricks all add further depths of flavour to your sauce.

Once you've perfected this recipe, think about customising it by replacing half the beef with pork mince, or just add cured goodies, such as prosciutto, pancetta, smoked speck or even good old bacon lardons to the beef mince. Alternatively, step up the mince you use by choosing chicken mince or, even better, a 50/50 mixture of veal and pork.

SERVES 4 **PREP:** 15 MINS **COOKING:** 4 HOURS 20 MINS

olive oil, for frying
40 g butter
2 carrots, finely diced
3 onions, finely diced
4 bacon rashers, diced
2 celery stalks, finely diced
1 tablespoon brown sugar
4 garlic cloves, crushed
3 tablespoons tomato paste
1 kg beef mince
500 ml (2 cups) red wine
3 fresh or dried bay leaves
few splashes of worcestershire sauce
1 lemon, 4 cm strip of zest, lemon halved
800 g canned diced tomatoes
500 ml (2 cups) beef stock, plus extra if needed
sea salt
1 × 375 g packet egg tagliatelle (the curly, nesty ones are nicest)
150 g grated parmesan, to serve

Place a large frying pan over medium–high heat. To make the sofritto (or base), combine a little oil and the butter in the hot pan. When the butter has melted throw in the carrot, onion and bacon. Cook for 2 minutes, stirring. Add the celery and cook until the vegetables are soft and going translucent at the edges. Sprinkle over the brown sugar and stir through. Add the garlic and tomato paste, and move this around the pan to cook out for 3 minutes. Scrape this tomatoey sofritto into a bowl.

Splash some more oil into the pan. When it's hot, throw in the mince and cook over high heat until browned. Stir the meat the whole time so it cooks evenly. Scrape the meat into the sofritto bowl.

Deglaze the pan with the red wine, scraping up any bits stuck to the bottom of the pan. When the wine has reduced by half, return the meat and sofritto to the pan and add the bay leaves, worcestershire sauce, lemon zest, tomatoes and beef stock. Season with salt and a good squeeze of lemon juice from one half of the lemon. (Keep the other half for later.)

Cover, and bring the sauce to the boil, then remove the lid and turn the heat right down. Cook very gently for up to 4 hours. Stir occasionally to ensure the sauce doesn't stick and burn. If it gets too thick, stir in some more stock. The sauce is ready when it smells irresistible and is wonderfully thick and glossy and a dark-red colour. Taste and season with a little more salt and lemon juice as required. Now you can either serve it straightaway, or cool and refrigerate for the next day.

When you're ready to eat, cook the tagliatelle in plenty of boiling salted water for 1 minute less than it says on the packet, until al dente. Scoop out and reserve 250 ml (1 cup) of the starchy cooking liquid and drain the pasta.

Put a generous ladle of the Bolognese sauce (about 2 cups) into the pasta pan and toss with the pasta. Moisten the combination with a little of the reserved pasta water so it isn't clumpy. Feel free to use as little or as much sauce as you like – we've got lots of plans for any sauce that's left over (you can find these ideas scattered all through this book).

Serve with grated parmesan, a green salad and bread for mopping up the leftover sauce, if you like.

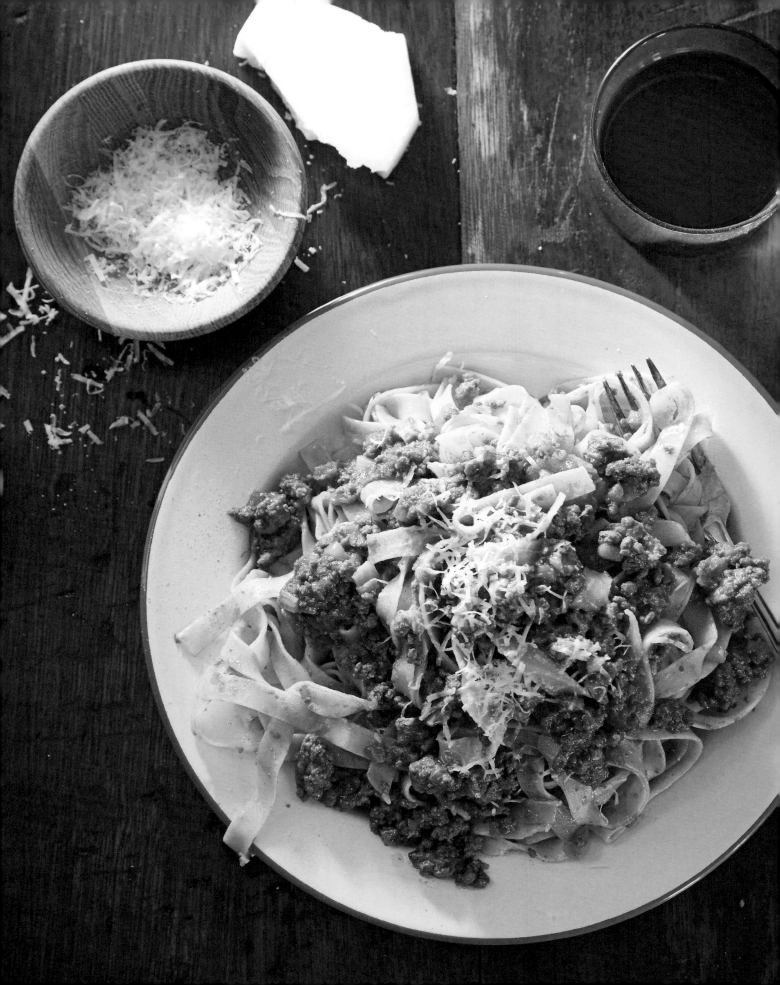

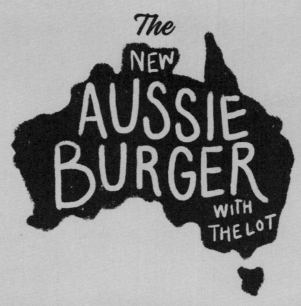

The New AUSSIE BURGER WITH THE LOT

PREPARE IN 15 MINUTES

I hate those expensive gourmet burgers with their sludgy, overly sweet fillings, pasty patties and la-di-dah brioche buns. Give me a true, honest Aussie country burger like this one.

Sure, you can add beetroot or a grilled pineapple ring, but far better to go for the secret ingredient over the page – an ingredient that will become a firm family favourite.

SERVES 4 **PREP:** 15 MINS **COOKING:** 20 MINS

½ onion, finely chopped
500 g beef mince
25 g (⅓ cup) panko breadcrumbs
1 tablespoon dried oregano leaves
1 egg
sea salt and freshly ground
   black pepper
1 tablespoon olive oil
120 g smoked cheddar, sliced
8 streaky bacon rashers
125 g (½ cup) good-quality whole
   egg mayonnaise
1 tablespoon dijon mustard
4 hamburger buns, split, cut sides
   chargrilled or toasted
1 baby cos lettuce, leaves separated
2 ripe tomatoes, thickly sliced
The Secret Ingredient (see over
   the page) or tomato sauce,
   to serve

Place the onion in a heatproof bowl. Cover with boiling water and set aside for 2 minutes to soften slightly. Drain and return to the bowl. Add the mince, breadcrumbs, oregano and egg. Season. Use clean hands to mix until well combined. Shape into four 2 cm thick patties. Transfer to a plate.

Heat the oil in a large frying pan over medium heat. Add the patties and cook for 4 minutes on each side, or until just cooked through. Place the cheese slices on top of the patties. Cover the pan with a lid and cook for a further 1 minute or until the cheese is just starting to melt. Transfer to a plate to rest. Add the bacon to the frying pan and cook for 2–3 minutes on each side, until golden.

Meanwhile, combine the mayonnaise and dijon mustard in a bowl.

Spread the base of each toasted bun with mustard mayo. Top with lettuce, a beef patty, tomato and bacon. Finally, spread the cut side of the top bun with The Secret Ingredient or tomato sauce. Place on top of the bacon and serve.

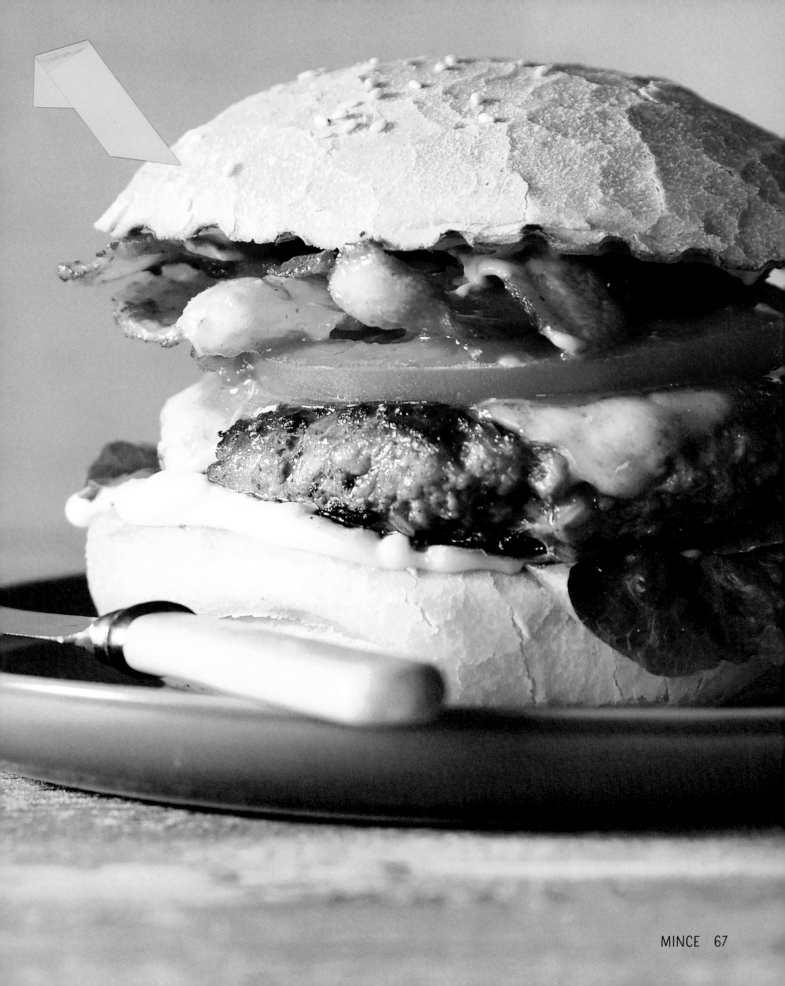

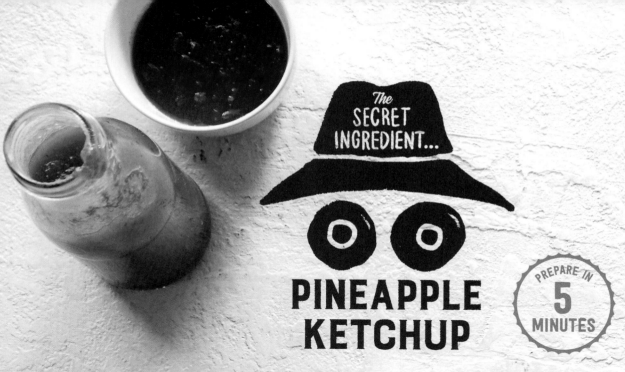

The SECRET INGREDIENT...

PINEAPPLE KETCHUP

PREPARE IN 5 MINUTES

Warning: this is addictively good. Use on chops, toasted cheese, with steak, on pulled pork or even as an alluring perfume.

MAKES ABOUT 300 ML   **PREP:** 5 MINS   **COOKING:** 1 HOUR 10 MINS

50 g sultanas
1 onion, roughly chopped
2 garlic cloves
80 ml (⅓ cup) tomato paste
185 ml (¾ cup) cider vinegar
70 g (⅓ cup) brown sugar
2 teaspoons sea salt
pinch of cayenne pepper
8 canned pineapple rings
2 teaspoons ground coffee
  (or a double shot of espresso)
2 whole cloves
1 teaspoon ground allspice
½ teaspoon ground cinnamon
⅛ teaspoon ground nutmeg
80 ml (⅓ cup) honey

Blitz the sultanas, onion, garlic and tomato paste in a food processor until smooth. Scrape into a large heavy-based saucepan and stir in 185 ml (¾ cup) water along with the vinegar, brown sugar, salt and a big pinch of cayenne pepper. Don't wash the food processor, as we will use it again.

Bring the mixture to the boil, then reduce the heat to medium–low and simmer gently, uncovered, for 1 hour. Stir regularly – and very regularly at the beginning!

Puree the pineapple rings in the food processor. Add to the pan along with the coffee, cloves, allspice, cinnamon, nutmeg and honey. Simmer over low heat for another 10 minutes to thicken. Stir regularly as a thick mixture is always at risk of burning.

When the ketchup is thick, pass it through your finest sieve and return to a clean pan. Heat to a simmer and taste to balance the seasoning. Add splashes of cider vinegar if it's too sweet or salty, drizzle in a little honey if it's too tart or add some more coffee if it needs greater complexity. If your ketchup is a little runny, simmer over low heat for a few more minutes, or until it thickens slightly.

TIP

Make the ketchup ahead of time, place in a sterilised jar and store in the fridge for up to 1 month.

CUSTOMISE THE AUSSIE BURGER

We should all be more like Virgos. Just like the Aussie burger, Virgos can be flexible, tolerant of others and welcoming.

MIDDLE EASTERN LAMB BURGER

Make burger patties with some chopped raisins, mint, a hint of lemon, chopped thyme and 500 g lamb mince, then cook following the instructions on page 66. Make a slaw with shredded red cabbage, carrot and some sliced almonds dressed with lemon juice and olive oil. Pile the slaw on the bottom halves of your burger buns and add a cooked patty. Dollop on a sauce of yoghurt whipped with feta and finish with pickled red onion slices, a few extra sliced almonds and carrot matchsticks tossed with mint leaves.

ASIAN INFUSION CHICKEN BURGER

Add a hint of chopped chilli, coriander, lemongrass, ginger and sesame seeds to 500 g chicken mince. Cook your patties, and in the last few minutes toss a little char siu sauce in the pan for a quick glaze.

Spread your buns with Kewpie mayo seasoned with a few drops of Maggi seasoning liquid. Top with lettuce, the cooked patty and some cucumber, then finish with extra chopped coriander and chilli.

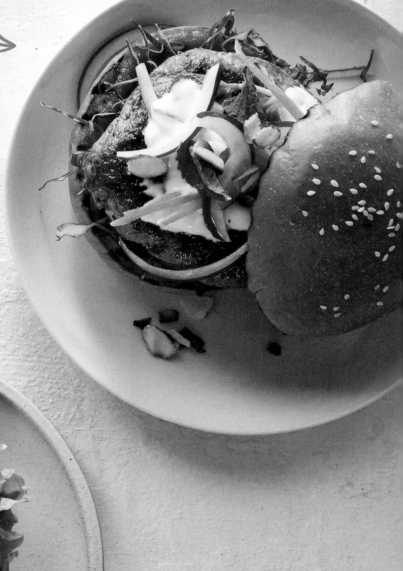

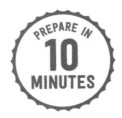

CHICKEN LARB *with* QUINOA
(San Choi Bao-Style)

I once witnessed a famous chef lying on the floor of the men's toilets ... in fact, I've seen a fair number of chefs passed out on kitchen floors, but this one was begging for water after eating far too big a spoonful of David Thompson's famously hot larb at Long Chim restaurant. This larb is nowhere near as savage with chilli heat, but delicious all the same, while quinoa is a softer and more approachable replacement for the more traditional roasted and ground rice. (The irony about that chef rolling on the floor under the assault of Thai scuds in David's larb was that he actually came from Chile.)

SERVES 4 PREP: 10 MINS COOKING: 10 MINS

2 tablespoons sweet chilli sauce
1 tablespoon soy sauce
2 teaspoons fish sauce
zest and juice of 1 lime
1 tablespoon peanut oil
500 g chicken mince
2 Asian shallots, finely chopped
1 lemongrass stalk, white part
 only, finely chopped
4 cm knob of ginger, peeled
 and finely grated
140 g (¾ cup) cooked red quinoa
12 baby cos lettuce leaves (or
 8 iceberg lettuce leaves,
 trimmed – but these are paler
 and less sexy-looking!)

TO SERVE
55 g (⅓ cup) unsalted roasted
 peanuts, coarsely chopped
mint leaves
sliced red chilli

Combine the sweet chilli sauce, soy sauce, fish sauce, lime zest and juice in a jug.

Heat the oil in a wok or large frying pan over high heat. Add the mince and cook, tossing, for 5 minutes, or until browned.

Add the shallot, lemongrass and ginger. Cook, tossing the contents of the pan as dramatically as your forearms will allow, for 1 minute, or until aromatic.

Add the quinoa (yes, you can cook your own if you've got the inclination – if you need failsafe instructions type the words 'Matt Preston', 'Herald Sun' and 'quinoa' into your search engine and I'll pop up on your computer to help you).

Stir in the chilli sauce mixture and toss for 2 minutes, or until heated through. Spoon into the lettuce cups. Top with chopped peanuts, mint leaves and sliced chilli to serve.

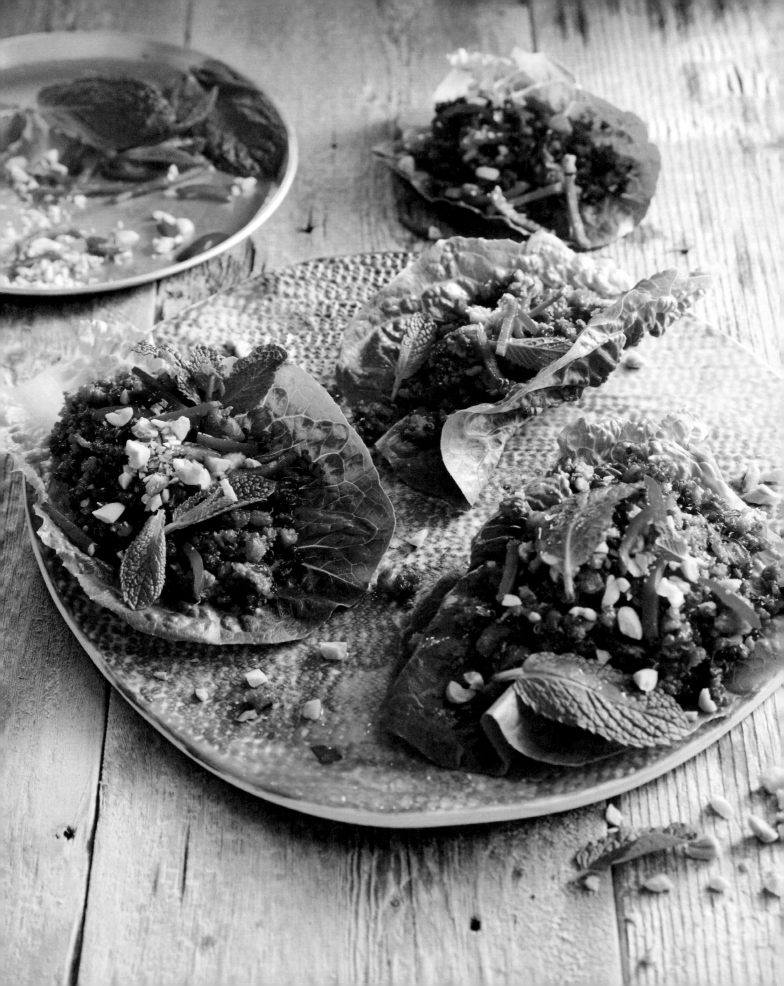

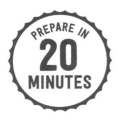
THAI-CURRIED CHICKEN MEATBALLS

(or Bangkok Spaghetti and Meatballs)

Lucy (an editor): Matt, is that an alternative title?
Matt: Yup, which one do you like better, Lucy?
Lucy: I think I prefer Bangkok Spaghetti and Meatballs.
Matt: Well I prefer Thai-Curried Meatballs as it's less poncey.
Lucy: OK, let's keep both then!
Matt: Agreed!
Mary (the publisher): Wow Matt and Editor Lucy, you two are getting on so much better. You've both mellowed in the two years since the last book.
Lucy: Let's cut that last bit ... not sure we need Publisher Mary butting in.

This is what happens when you spend too much time obsessing about Thai flavours and imagining how they might affect that classic Yank-EE-talian dish of spaghetti and meatballs. (Rather well, it turns out!)

SERVES 4   PREP: 20 MINS   COOKING: 30 MINS

2 tablespoons coconut oil
1 onion, cut into thin wedges
2 tablespoons storebought red curry paste
1 × 270 ml can light coconut milk
250 ml (1 cup) chicken stock
4 kaffir lime leaves
1 tablespoon grated palm sugar or caster sugar
2 teaspoons fish sauce
150 g green beans, sliced diagonally
juice of 1 lime

CHICKEN MEATBALLS
500 g chicken mince
4 cm knob of ginger, peeled and finely grated
1 bunch coriander, stems finely chopped, leaves reserved, to serve
soy sauce, for rolling

TO SERVE
Coconut Cabbage Noodles (page 203)
fresh hokkien or rice noodles
coriander sprigs
sliced red chilli

To make your meatballs, place the chicken mince, ginger and 2 tablespoons of the finely chopped coriander stems in a bowl. Use your hands to mix until well combined. Wet your hands with soy sauce and roll tablespoons of the mixture into balls. Transfer to a plate. Cover and refrigerate until required.

Heat half the coconut oil in a large frying pan over medium–high heat. Add the meatballs in batches and cook for 2–3 minutes, until golden. Transfer to a plate.

Heat the remaining oil and add the onion. Cook, tossing, for 3–4 minutes or until softened slightly. Add the curry paste and cook, stirring, for 1 minute, or until aromatic. Add the coconut milk and bring to the boil. Boil for 5 minutes, or until the oil separates. Now add the stock, lime leaves, sugar and fish sauce. Return to the boil.

Add the meatballs and simmer rapidly for 10 minutes, or until the sauce starts to thicken slightly. Add the green beans and cook for a further 3 minutes, or until the meatballs are cooked through. Stir in the lime juice to taste.

While your meatballs are simmering away, make your coconut cabbage noodles and warm the hokkien noodles – either in the microwave or in the pan that you cooked the cabbage in. Just reserve the cabbage separately if you do this.

Divide the noodles among serving bowls. Top with the meatballs, sauce, coriander leaves and sliced chilli. Serve with the coconut cabbage noodles on top or on the side.

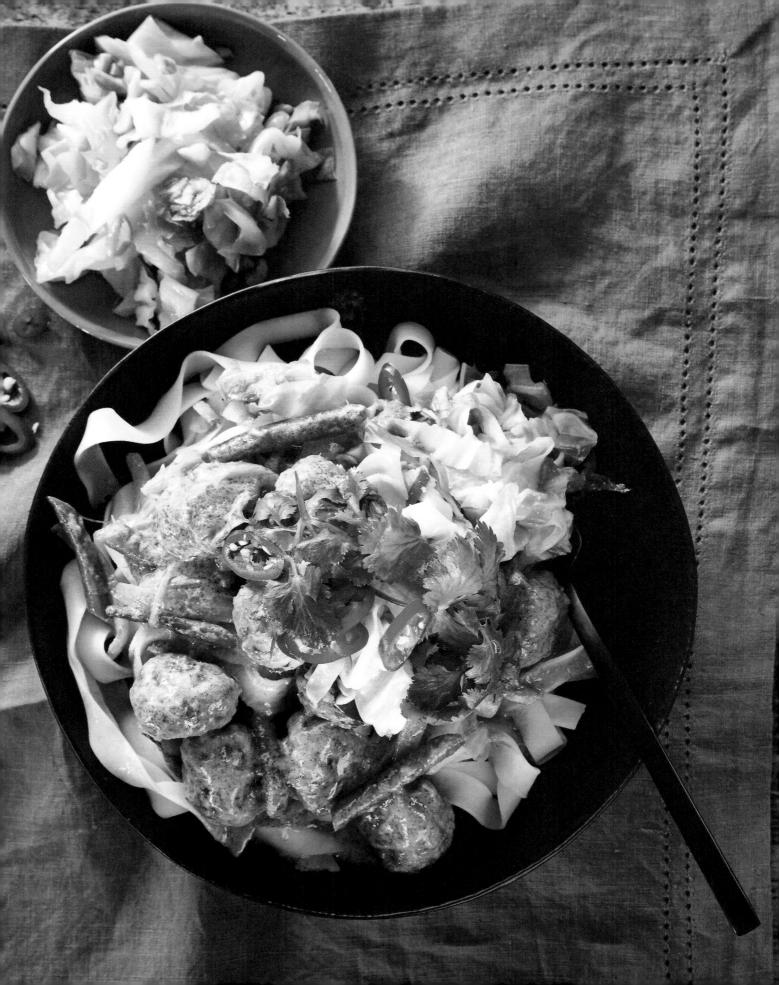

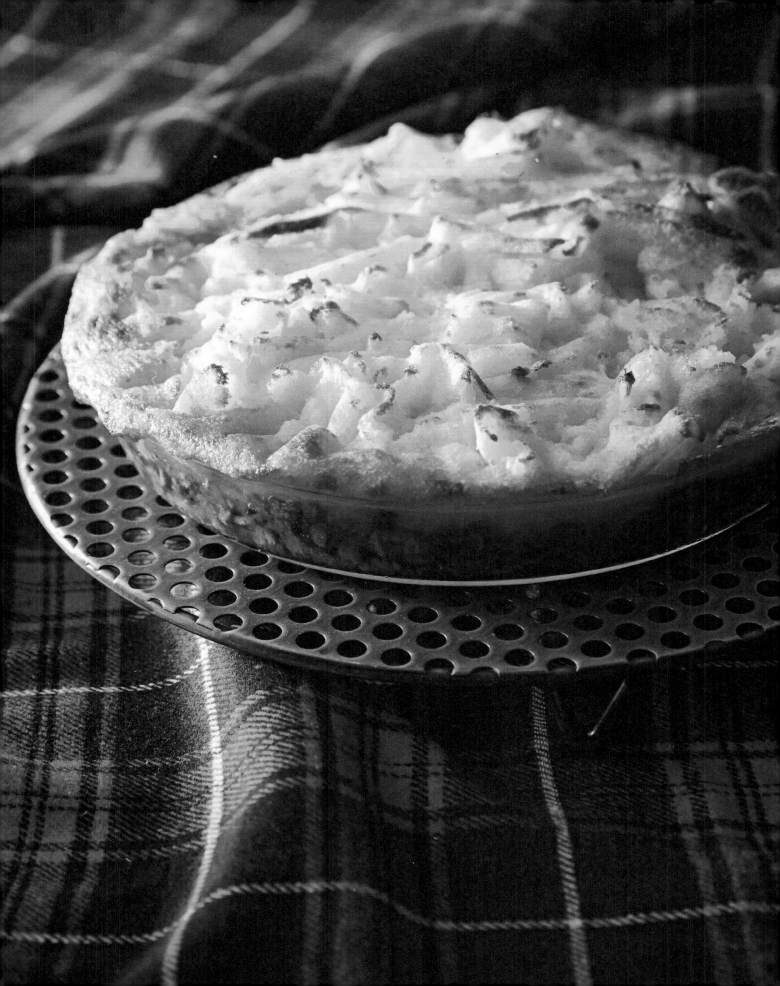

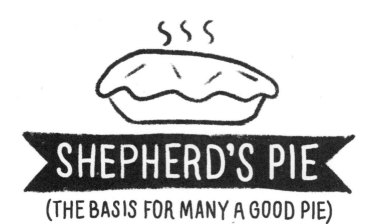

SHEPHERD'S PIE
(THE BASIS FOR MANY A GOOD PIE)

Shepherd's pie ... cottage pie ... I have been a passionate champion of the mash-topped pie for as long as I've been cooking. It has been a fine barometer for me: always reliable, always true. I once knew that a long-term relationship would never last when the news that I was making shepherd's pie for dinner was met with a tartly disparaging, 'Oh no! Peasant Food.' That stung then, although now I consider 'peasant food' a badge of honour.

So here's a recipe for a great lamb and mash shepherd's pie that provides the foundation for a whole raft of other mash-topped pies that I will tell you how to pull together (using this recipe as a template) over the page.

SERVES 4–6 PREP: 30 MIN COOKING: 1 HOUR 10 MINS

THE BASE
1 tablespoon olive oil
1 onion, finely chopped
2 celery stalks, finely chopped
2 garlic cloves, crushed
2 anchovy fillets

THE MEAT
800 g lamb mince

THE SAUCE AND FLAVOURING
500 ml (2 cups) chicken stock
60 ml (¼ cup) strong coffee
70 g (¼ cup) tomato paste
2 tablespoons worcestershire sauce
2 fresh or dried bay leaves
sea salt and freshly ground
  black pepper
150 g (1 cup) frozen baby peas

MASH
1 kg sebago potatoes, peeled
  and chopped
60 g butter, chopped, plus
  25 g melted butter
60 ml (¼ cup) warmed milk
sea salt and freshly ground
  black pepper

To make the base, heat the oil in a saucepan over medium–high heat. Add the onion and celery and cook, stirring, for 5 minutes, or until soft. Add the garlic and anchovy fillets. Cook for 1 minute, or until aromatic.

Add the lamb mince and cook, breaking up any lumps with the back of a wooden spoon, for 5 minutes, or until well browned.

Now for the sauce and flavourings. Add the stock, coffee, tomato paste, worcestershire sauce and bay leaves. Reduce the heat to medium and simmer for 25 minutes, or until the liquid reduces by half. Season. Stir in the peas.

While the meat is cooking, make your mash. Either follow the recipe on page 205 or just cook the potato in a saucepan of boiling salted water for 15 minutes, or until tender. Drain and return to the pan. Place over low heat, shaking the pan to dry out the potato. Add the chopped butter and milk and mash until smooth and well combined. Season well.

Preheat the oven to 200°C/180°C fan-forced. Spoon the lamb mixture into a warmed 2 litre ovenproof dish. Top with the mash and use a fork to rough up the surface. Brush with the melted butter and season. Bake for 30 minutes, or until the mash is golden.

IMPROVING ON THE SHEPHERD'S PIE

MAKING THE BASIC BETTER

Looking back, I realise that my dinner date did have a point: these mash-topped mince marvels lend themselves to so much more than just beef mince and carrots or lamb mince and peas topped with mashed potatoes – delicious though these combinations are.

The first thing to perfect is enriching the gravy of your mince with one or more of these tricks of the trade. Consider adding a little worcestershire sauce, soy, sherry, tomato sauce, mushroom ketchup, anchovy fillets, a nicely caramelised mirepoix base of carrot, onion and celery, a little cured pork, shiitake mushrooms, or even a smidge of Vegemite. All these ingredients will boost the umami reading off the scale, and if you then top the mash with a thick sprinkling of cheese and a little nutmeg that will go golden and bubbling by the time you eat, your cottage will have become a penthouse.

CHANGE THE TOPPING

I love potato mash, but I'll often step things up by making a combo mash – perhaps potato and carrot or potato and celeriac. Or why not forgo the potato altogether? A celeriac and/or parsnip mash is delicious with a robust beef mince, while a sweeter pumpkin or sweet potato mash is great with a pork mince and/or chicken mince filling.

You can spike your mash with everything from smoked paprika or fresh herbs, such as parsley or coriander, to something for added creaminess like melty taleggio, little halved bocconcini or even ripe avocado, which brings creaminess without added dairy. You could even take a leaf out of the Irish cookbook and mix spring onions or cabbage (or kale, you hipster, you) and lots of butter into your mash to make a champ or colcannon topping, respectively. Or how about taking the Lancashire hot pot idea and use thin slices of potato instead of mash.

CHANGE THE PROTEIN

While lamb and beef are your go-to proteins, there is nothing to say you can't add other goodies. Ground kaiserfleisch or smoked pork hock are good with beef mince or add cubes of feta to lamb. Veal mince can replace beef. In fact, any favourite pie filling can be employed, such as chicken and mushroom or chicken and leek (assuming you are careful not to dry out the chook mince during cooking).

The great thing about the shepherd's pie model is that it is so simple to change up, so push it even further and think of tossing chunks of white fish or salmon with peeled prawns and hard-boiled eggs to make a fish pie. Use fennel in the mirepoix and, for a further tweak, add a drop of ouzo, pernod or dill to the sauce. Or go another way and bring some salty porkiness to the party with bacon and wine.

I have also been workshopping a seaside cottage pie made with beef mince, oysters (perhaps even smoked oysters) and Guinness under a champ mash – but I feel this might work better with chunks of beef rather than a mince. (Although I'd argue that as it was 'under mash' it would still sit in the cottage pie family.)

CHANGE THE FLAVOURS

My starting point is just to bring in flavours that already exist happily together. Playing with a country theme helps massively here, so a North African sheep herder's pie might see the lamb spiced with crushed cumin, coriander seeds and a little cinnamon or just a 'baharat' or 'ras el hanout' spice mix. Then add a few chopped dates and a little citrus freshness.

A Greek take might see lemon, mint and dill added to the mince and feta beaten into the mash.

An Indian shepherd's pie would also be delicious! Just use way more peas, along with some chunks of paneer, the right spices – cardamom, turmeric, coriander and cumin seeds – and lots of minced garlic and ginger. A layer of spinach on the bottom of the dish would be a nice surprise – and maybe the topping should be a mash of potato and cauliflower.

Then there's the 'Chateau' pie with beef, whole baby onions and lardons of bacon in a rich red wine gravy hiding under a green herbed mash.

The 'Great Smoky Mountains' pie is beef mince, smoked paprika, smoky bacon, beans, a little maple syrup and a splash of Tennessee whiskey under a well-buttered sweet potato mash.

Or take your inspiration from Chile, where their 'pastel de choclo' is a layer of meat (usually beef mince, sometimes chicken) with sultanas, pitted black olives, onions and hard-boiled egg under a topping of mashed sweetcorn.

For a Mexican shepherd's pie, I can see corn kernels, peppers and chillies spiced with cinnamon, chilli powder, cumin, coriander seeds, a squeeze of lime juice and a strip of lime zest. The question is, if I top it with tortilla chips and cheese instead of mashed avocado, sour cream and potato, is it still a cottage pie?

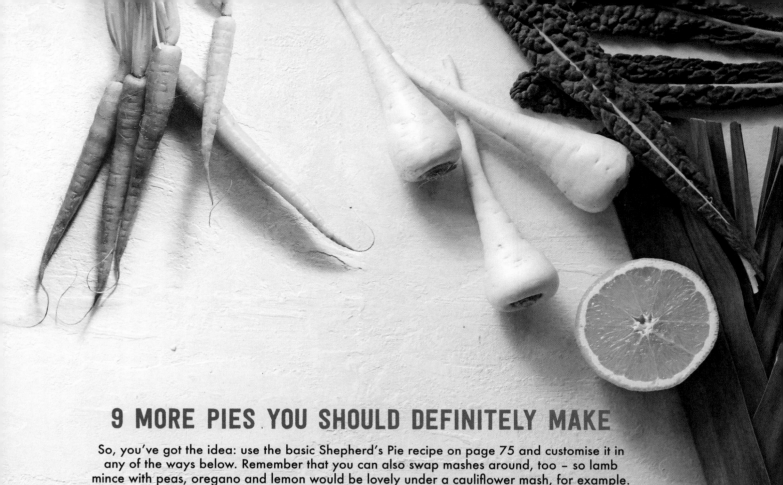

9 MORE PIES YOU SHOULD DEFINITELY MAKE

So, you've got the idea: use the basic Shepherd's Pie recipe on page 75 and customise it in any of the ways below. Remember that you can also swap mashes around, too – so lamb mince with peas, oregano and lemon would be lovely under a cauliflower mash, for example.

1. Follow the recipe on page 175 using the lamb and peas but swap out the other flavourings for lemon and dried oregano leaves. Mash together cooked potato and feta with chopped mint or dill for the topping.

2. Flavour beef mince with tomatoes, bacon and plenty of carrot (omit the peas). Keep with the theme and top with mashed cooked carrots and/ or parsnips and serve with a cardamom–date quick chutney, or use mashed corn and potato or sweet potato, or even swede!

3. Add pine nuts and perhaps a few currants to cooked lamb mince, then flavour with cinnamon, orange zest and cumin. Top with cauliflower and potato, or parsnip and potato mash.

4. Swap the mince for chicken chunks and deglaze the pan with dijon mustard, chopped leek and/or celery and wine. Leave out the coffee, peas, tomato paste and anchovies, and reduce the worcestershire sauce to 1 tablespoon. Choose from celeriac and butter-fried celery mash, fried leek and potato or potato and creamed leek mash.

5. Add bacon lardons to beef mince and flavour with allspice and chopped tomatoes (omit the peas). Top with a sweet potato mash or mashed potato heavily drizzled with a mixture of maple syrup and mustard before baking.

6. For an Irish twist, add Guinness and oysters (in place of the peas) to browned beef chunks and top with champ, a colcannon made with kale or straight-up buttered cabbage (ok so it's not a mash but it works).

7. Change the mince for a mixture of pork and veal mince and flavour with tomatoes, pancetta, rosemary and thyme. Mash together potato and parmesan for the topping.

8. Go retro and use beef mince and carrots, but flavour with baked beans instead of the peas. Mash together potato and swede (aka neeps and tatties) or swede, whiskey and black pepper for a hidden kick.

9. Flavour beef mince cooked with chopped capsicum with cinnamon, lime and coriander (again, omitting the peas). Cover with avocado mashed with potato and sour cream and top with grated cheese, or roughly crushed corn chips, pickled jalapenos and grated cheddar!

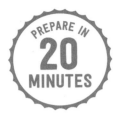

PREPARE IN
20
MINUTES

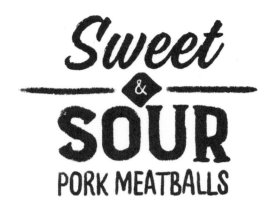

Sweet & SOUR PORK MEATBALLS

The first time we made this we were all amazed at how evocative the fragrance of this classic sauce was. It took us all back to the dodgy Chinese takeaways of our youth. However, these tender meatballs remove the deep-fried guilt from eating sweet and sour, while keeping the soul and essential freak-out deliciousness of the original. Serve with high-waisted jeans and a flicky Farrah hairstyle.

SERVES 4 **PREP:** 20 MINS **COOKING:** 25 MINS

2 slices bread, crusts removed
60 ml (¼ cup) milk
500 g pork mince
3 spring onions, finely chopped
2 cm knob of ginger, peeled and finely grated
2 garlic cloves, crushed
2 teaspoons cornflour
1 tablespoon light soy sauce
1 egg
sea salt and freshly ground black pepper
2 tablespoons peanut oil
1 onion, coarsely chopped
1 red capsicum, deseeded and coarsely chopped
1 green capsicum, deseeded and coarsely chopped
1 × 225 g can pineapple chunks in juice
125 ml (½ cup) tomato sauce
60 ml (¼ cup) rice wine vinegar
2 tablespoons soy sauce
1 tablespoon caster sugar

TO SERVE
steamed brown rice
coriander leaves
bean sprouts

Place the bread in a bowl and cover with the milk. Set aside for 2 minutes to soak. Squeeze out the milk and place the bread in a large bowl.

Add the pork mince, spring onion, ginger, garlic, cornflour, light soy sauce and egg to the bowl with the soggy bread. Gently squish everything together and season. Using wet hands, roll tablespoons of the mixture into balls. Transfer to a plate.

Heat 1 tablespoon of oil in a large frying pan over medium heat. Add the meatballs in batches and cook, tossing, for 8 minutes, or until golden. Don't overcrowd the pan. Transfer to a plate.

Heat the remaining oil in the pan over medium–high heat. Add the onion and capsicum and cook, stirring, for 3–4 minutes, until everything softens slightly. Reduce the heat to low. Add the pineapple and the juice from the can, along with the tomato sauce, vinegar, soy sauce and sugar, and bring to the boil. Reduce the heat to medium and add the meatballs. Cook, stirring, for 4–5 minutes, until the meatballs are cooked through and covered in a thick and glossy glaze. Season.

Divide steamed brown rice among serving bowls. Top with the meatballs and sauce. Finish with coriander leaves and bean sprouts.

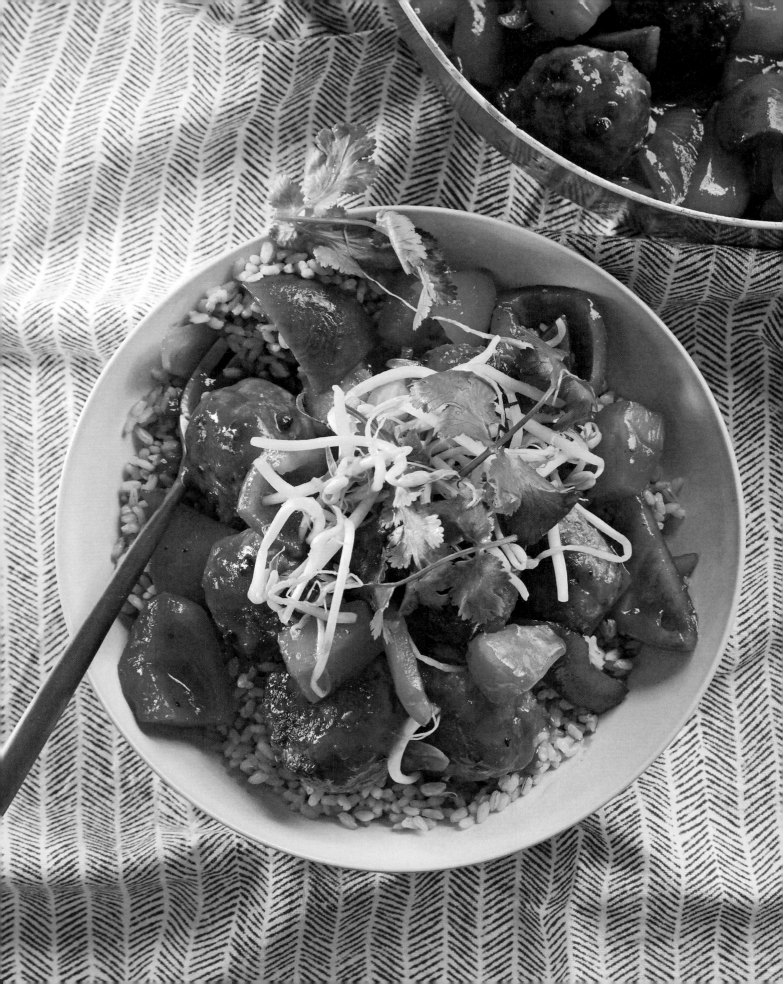

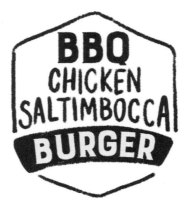

BBQ CHICKEN SALTIMBOCCA BURGER

I wanted to call this recipe The Bondage Burger, because of the way the chook mince is bound in straps of bacon. I wasn't allowed – but I'd still advise having a 'safe' word when making this burger. How does 'toast' sound?

Why the semi-sundried tomato pesto? Well that is equally as wrong, but also equally as delicious. See it as the bondage burger's velvet blindfold.

SERVES 6 **PREP:** 30 MINS (PLUS 30 MINS CHILLING) **COOKING:** 15 MINS

500 g chicken mince
200 g fresh ricotta
40 g (½ cup) shredded parmesan
4 garlic cloves, 3 crushed and
    1 halved for rubbing
grated zest of 1 lemon
sea salt and freshly ground
    black pepper
12 thick slices prosciutto
12 sage leaves
olive oil, to drizzle
3 large zucchini, thinly sliced
    lengthways
6 crusty Italian-style rolls, spilt open
40 g baby spinach leaves

SEMI-DRIED TOMATO PESTO
150 g semi-dried tomatoes
80 g (½ cup) roasted salted
    cashews
40 g (½ cup) shredded parmesan
2 garlic cloves
100 ml olive oil
1 tablespoon lemon juice

For the pesto, combine the tomatoes, cashews, parmesan and garlic in a food processor and blitz until finely chopped. With the motor running, gradually drizzle in the oil and lemon juice until the pesto has a spreadable consistency.

Place the chicken mince, ricotta, parmesan, crushed garlic and lemon zest in a bowl. Season. Use clean hands to mix until well combined. Shape into six 9 cm patties, about 1 cm thick.

Lay out six 20 cm × 20 cm sheets of plastic wrap on your work surface and place 2 slices of prosciutto on top of one sheet, crossing over in the centre to make a cross. Place two sage leaves in the centre and sit a patty on top. Bring the ends of prosciutto up and around the patty, then enclose with the plastic wrap. Repeat with the remaining patties. Refrigerate for 30 minutes.

Preheat your barbecue grill and flat plate on medium heat. Remove the patties from their plastic wrapping and drizzle with a little oil. Place them on the flat plate, base-side down (the side where the ends of the prosciutto meet), and cook for 6 minutes on each side until very nearly cooked through. Sit the patties upright, and cook for a further minute, turning so the sides get some colour.

While you cook the patties get your zucchini going. Drizzle with a little oil and cook on the barbecue grill for 2–3 minutes on each side, until just tender. Transfer to a plate and cover with foil to keep warm.

Lightly brush the insides of the buns with oil and place on the grill, cut-side down. Cook for 2 minutes, or until toasted. Rub the cut sides with the cut garlic clove.

Spread the base of each bun with about 1 tablespoon of the sundried tomato pesto. Top with the spinach leaves, a patty, a few zucchini slices and finish with the bun tops.

TIPS

The pesto will keep in an airtight container in the fridge for up to 2 weeks.

Toss sundried tomato pesto through pasta with shredded barbecued chicken for a quick weeknight dinner or try a dollop on barbecued steak. Add a few tablespoons to tomato-based sauces for an extra flavour boost, or use as a spread for pizza bases topped with prawns and zucchini ribbons.

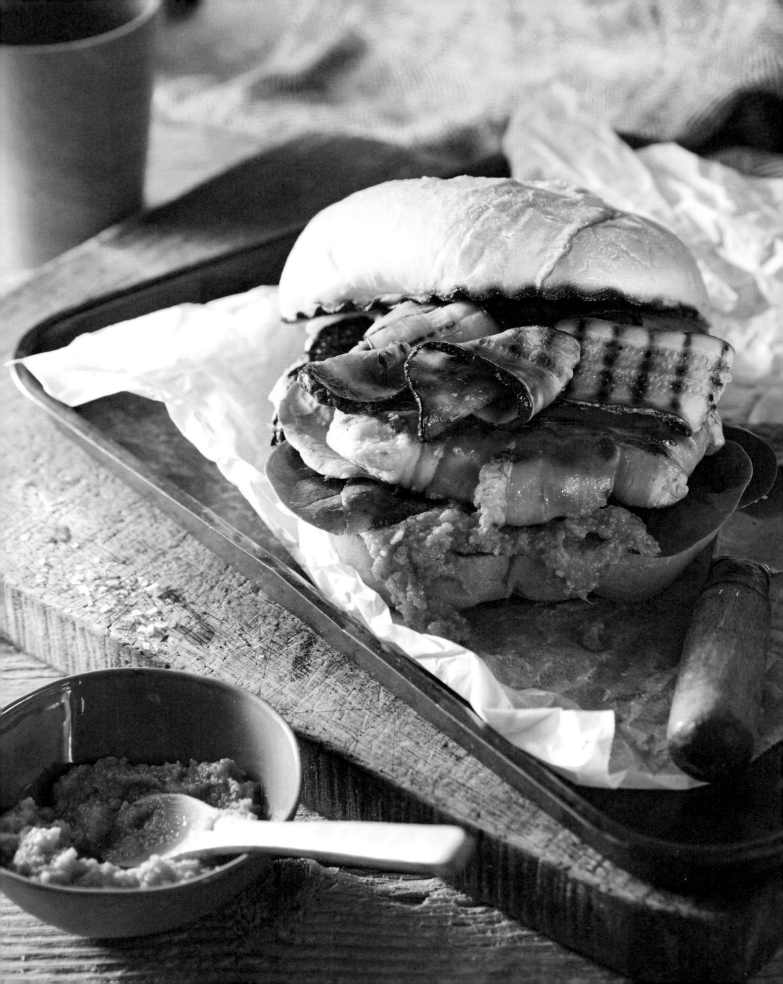

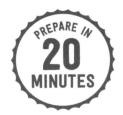

Cheat's
LAMB PIDE

Don't make this recipe. It's not very good. I really don't know what it's doing here.

PS: I might be lying.

MAKES 4 **PREP:** 20 MINS **COOKING:** 25 MINS

2 tablespoons olive oil
600 g lamb mince
2 garlic cloves, crushed
2 teaspoons ground cumin
2 teaspoons sweet paprika
1 teaspoon ground cinnamon
4 ripe tomatoes, coarsely chopped
sea salt and freshly ground
    black pepper
seeds of 1 pomegranate
40 g (¼ cup) unroasted pistachio
    kernels, coarsely chopped
¼ cup coarsely chopped
    flat-leaf parsley
¼ cup coarsely chopped mint leaves
2 tablespoons lemon juice
4 oval-shaped rolls or small
    baguettes
90 g (⅓ cup) Greek-style yoghurt

Preheat the oven to 180°C/160°C fan-forced.

Heat 1 tablespoon of oil in a frying pan over medium–high heat. Add the lamb mince and cook, breaking up the mince with the back of a wooden spoon, for 8–10 minutes, until well browned and a little crisp. Add the garlic, cumin, paprika and cinnamon and cook, stirring, for 1 minute, or until aromatic. Stir in the tomato. Cook for 3–4 minutes, until the tomato breaks down. Season.

Meanwhile, combine the pomegranate seeds, chopped pistachios, parsley, mint, lemon juice and remaining oil in a bowl.

Cut a long slit along the top of each roll, taking care not to cut all the way through. Open the roll slightly and scoop out a little of the bread. Spoon the lamb mixture into the rolls to fill. Place on a baking tray and bake for 5–10 minutes or until warmed through and your rolls are crisp and crunchy on the outside.

Top the rolls with yoghurt and sprinkle with the pomegranate mixture.

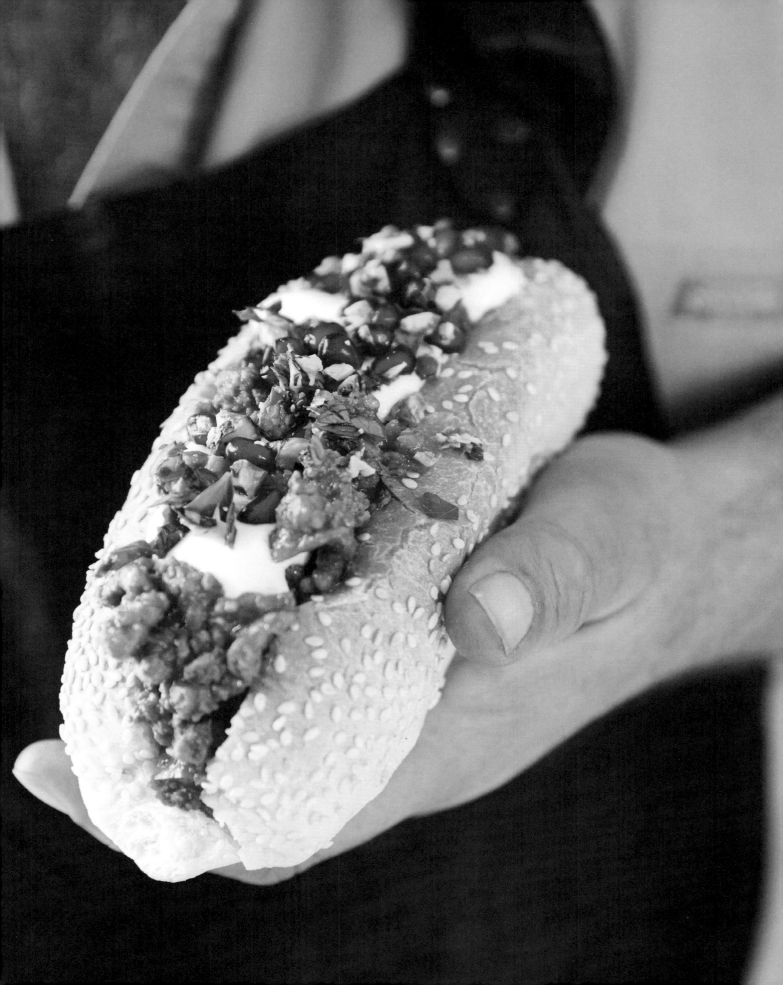

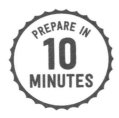

PATTY SANDWICHES
THAT ARE SO HOT RIGHT NOW
WITH FTEAK (FAKE STEAK)

In old posters from the Napoloenic era the letter 's' was replaced with the letter 'f', although it was pronounced as a hard or long 's'. That's the sort of fact you won't find in any other cookbook, so be thankful that at least someone in the food world cares about broadening your education rather than just telling you yet again how to make hummus.

Now, let's talk about quantum physics and the hidden universe. To understand all this we have to start with dark matter and put out of our minds the fact that patty sandwiches are one of the most quested-for foods in new internet searches. Hard though that might be …

Oh dear, I see I've lost you to the even greater genius of two-slice, one-slot toaster toasting, and this phenomenal patty that goes between them, which combine to make this, in reality, a steak sandwich by another means.

SERVES 4   PREP: 10 MINS   COOKING: 45 MINS

250 g beef mince
75 g speck or smoked bacon,
  finely chopped
sea salt and freshly ground
  black pepper
8 slices white bread
1 tablespoon olive oil
40 g vintage cheddar cheese slices
small dill pickles, to serve

CARAMELISED ONION
1 tablespoon olive oil
2 onions, thinly sliced
2 tablespoons brown sugar
1 tablespoon balsamic vinegar

To make the caramelised onion, heat the oil in a frying pan over medium heat. Add the onion and reduce the heat to low. Cook, stirring, for 40 minutes, or until light golden. Add the sugar and vinegar and cook, stirring, for 2–3 minutes, until caramelised. Season.

Preheat the oven to 180°C/160C° fan-forced.

While your onions become golden and caramelised, combine the mince and speck in a bowl. Season. Shape into four 2 cm thick patties.

Place two slices of bread together and put each double slice into one slot of a toaster. Toast until the outsides are golden but the inside face of each slice is still soft and pillowy. Repeat with the remaining bread slices.

Heat the oil in a large non-stick frying pan over medium–high heat. Cook the patties in batches, pressing them down with a spatula to flatten slightly. Cook for 1–2 minutes on each side, until golden and crisp at the edges. Transfer to a baking tray. Top each patty with a slice of cheese.

Separate the slices of bread and arrange half of them, untoasted side up, on the baking tray. Top each with a slice of cheese. Bake the patties and toast for 3–5 minutes or until the cheese is just melted.

Top the cheesy toasts with a cheesy patty and add some caramelised onion. Then top with the remaining plain toast. Serve skewered with small dill pickles.

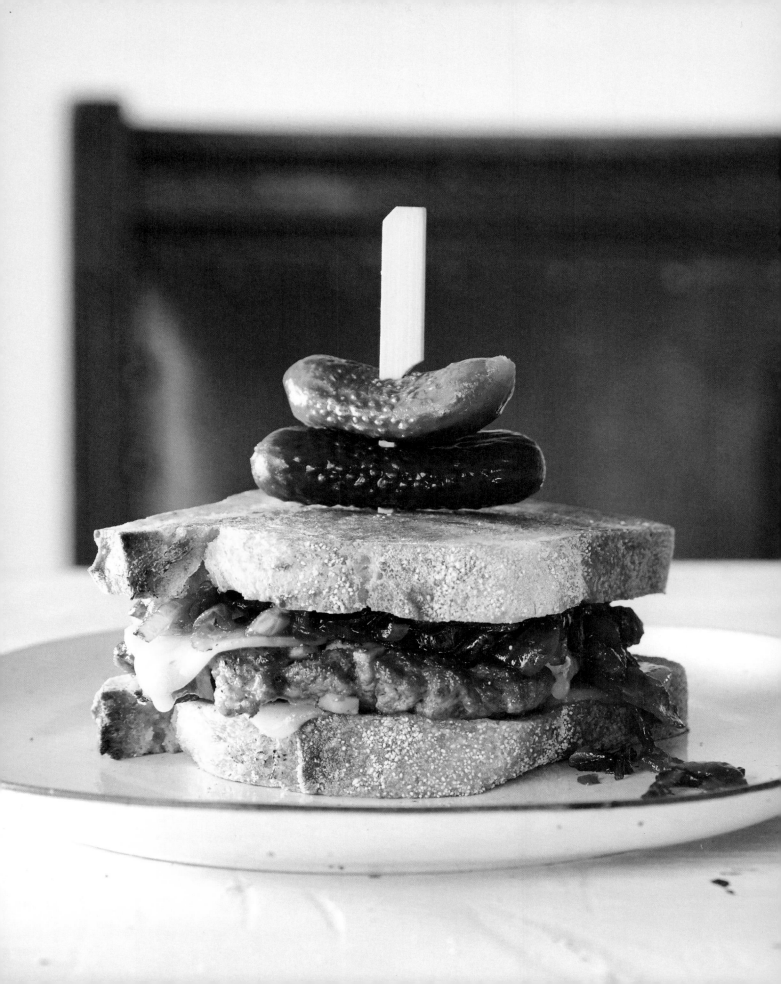

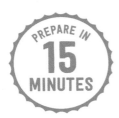

PREPARE IN
15
MINUTES

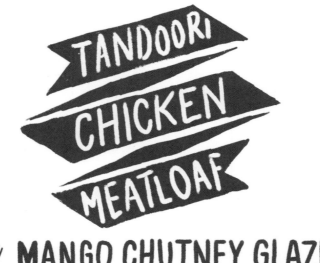

TANDOORI CHICKEN MEATLOAF

with MANGO CHUTNEY GLAZE

There should be an introduction here but there isn't. I believe in letting the food speak for itself and this is the most eloquent of all the dishes in the book.

'Cook me,

Eat me,

Do it again,'

it says.

SERVES 6–8   PREP: 15 MINS   COOKING: 1 HOUR

2 carrots
1 onion, quartered
50 g baby spinach leaves
½ cup coarsely chopped coriander
   leaves and stems
2 garlic cloves, crushed
4 cm knob of ginger, peeled and
   finely grated
50 g (½ cup) rolled oats
800 g chicken mince
100 g (⅓ cup) tandoori paste
cooked brown rice, to serve

MANGO GLAZE
90 g (¼ cup) mango chutney
55 g (¼ cup) brown sugar
1 tablespoon cider vinegar
⅛ teaspoon chilli powder

MANGO SALAD
3 mangoes, cut into thin strips
120 g frisee lettuce leaves
½ cup coriander sprigs
juice of 2 limes
2 tablespoons olive oil
sea salt

Preheat the oven to 180°C/160°C fan-forced. Line a baking tray with baking paper. (Don't skip this as it is essential to making washing up easier.)

Coarsely grate the carrot and onion in a food processor with the grater attachment. Remove the grater attachment and attach the blade. Add the spinach, coriander, garlic, ginger and rolled oats, and process until well combined. Add the chicken and tandoori paste. Pulse in short bursts, scraping down the mixture occasionally, until just combined (do not over process, I'm warning you).

Use your hands to shape the mixture on the lined tray into a 12 cm × 34 cm loaf. Bake for 45 minutes.

While the meatloaf is cooking, make the glaze. Combine the chutney, sugar, vinegar and chilli powder in a small saucepan and cook over low heat, stirring, until the sugar dissolves. Increase the heat to medium–high and simmer rapidly, stirring occasionally, for 4 minutes, or until the glaze starts to thicken. Set aside to cool slightly. As it cools it will thicken more.

Spoon the glaze over the top of the meatloaf. Bake for a further 15 minutes, or until golden.

Meanwhile, to make the salad, combine the mango strips, frisee and coriander sprigs in a bowl. Squeeze over the lime and drizzle with oil. Season. Serve alongside the meatloaf and accompany with brown rice.

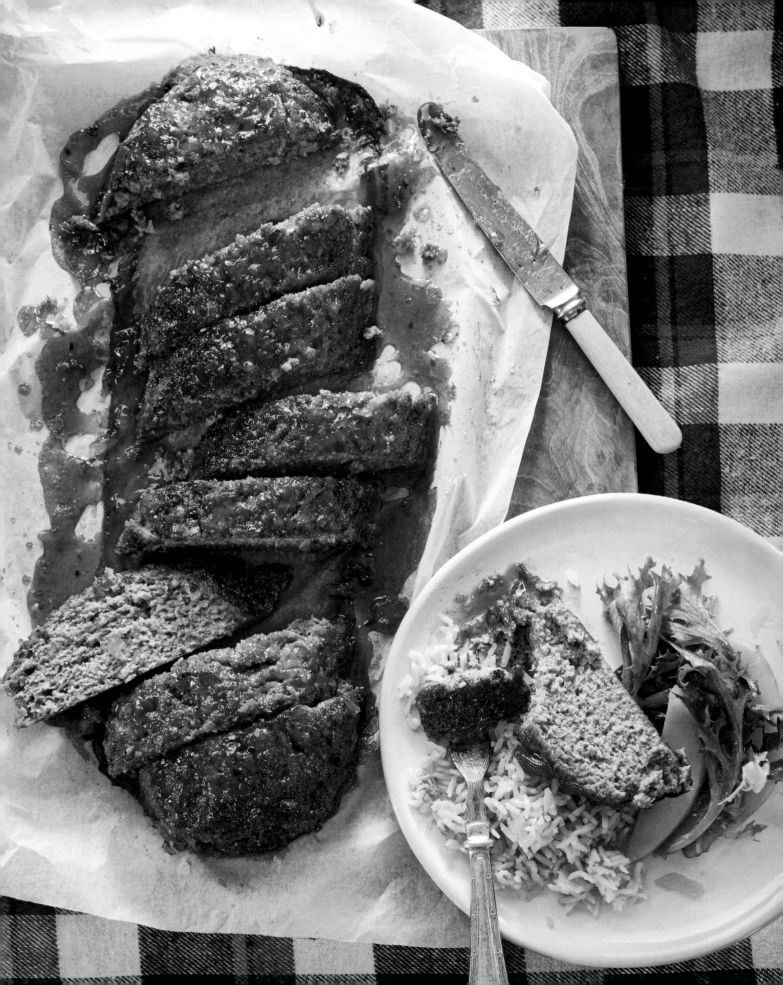

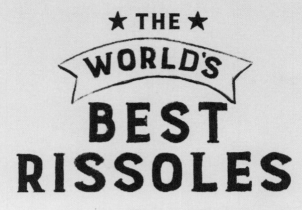

★ THE ★
WORLD'S
BEST
RISSOLES

I must admit this isn't saying much!

But, rissoles are back, baby. Good times.

MAKES 12 **PREP:** 20 MINS **COOKING:** 30 MINS

2 tablespoons olive oil
1 small onion, finely chopped
1 carrot, coarsely grated
1 zucchini, coarsely grated
800 g lamb mince
2 tablespoons tomato sauce
1 heaped tablespoon of whatever European herbs you've got in the garden or your vegetable crisper, chopped (basil, oregano, parsley, coriander, tarragon and marjoram are all good – but be sparing with mint or sage)
50 g (½ cup) rolled oats
1 egg
sea salt and freshly ground black pepper
90 g (¼ cup) mint jelly
2 tablespoons malt vinegar (or whatever vinegar you have)
Potato Skin Mash (page 205), to serve
steamed greens, to serve

Heat 1 tablespoon of the oil in a large non-stick frying pan over medium heat. Add the onion, carrot and zucchini. Cook, stirring, for 5 minutes, or until everything softens. Transfer to a large bowl to cool.

Add the mince, tomato sauce, herbs, oats and egg to the vegetable mixture. Season. Use clean hands to mix until well combined. Use a ⅓ cup measure to shape into 12 rissoles.

Heat the remaining oil in the pan. Add the rissoles in batches and cook for 5 minutes on each side, or until cooked through. Transfer to a plate and cover with foil to keep warm.

Add the mint jelly and vinegar to the pan. Stir over medium heat until the jelly melts. Return the rissoles and toss for 2 minutes, or until well coated, sticky and glossy. Serve the rissoles on mashed potato with steamed greens.

THE WORLD'S NEXT BEST RISSOLES RECIPES

1. Make rissoles with pork mince, Chinese five spice powder and finely chopped fennel. Use soy-dunked hands to shape the patties. Serve with broccolini tossed in oyster sauce and brown rice alongside.

2. Make rissoles with beef and smoked bacon mince, thawed corn kernels and barbecue sauce to bind. Serve with roasted sweet potatoes and sour cream and chives – or a fancier dressing of sour cream loosened slightly with a little vinegar and crumbled blue cheese stirred in.

3. Make rissoles with lamb mince, breadcrumbs, mint jelly, fresh mint and crushed pistachios. Serve in a salad of iceberg and cucumber dressed with tzatziki.

4. Make rissoles with pork and veal mince, ricotta, chopped semi-dried tomatoes, chopped basil and grated parmesan. Serve with spaghetti and a tomato passata.

5. Make rissoles with chicken mince and a paste of coriander stems and roots, lime zest, lemongrass, fish sauce, palm sugar and lime juice. Serve on rice noodles topped with cucumber, Thai basil leaves, mint and sliced red chilli. Sprinkle with chopped roasted peanuts and drizzle with sweet chilli sauce or a dressing of fish sauce, sweet chilli and lime juice.

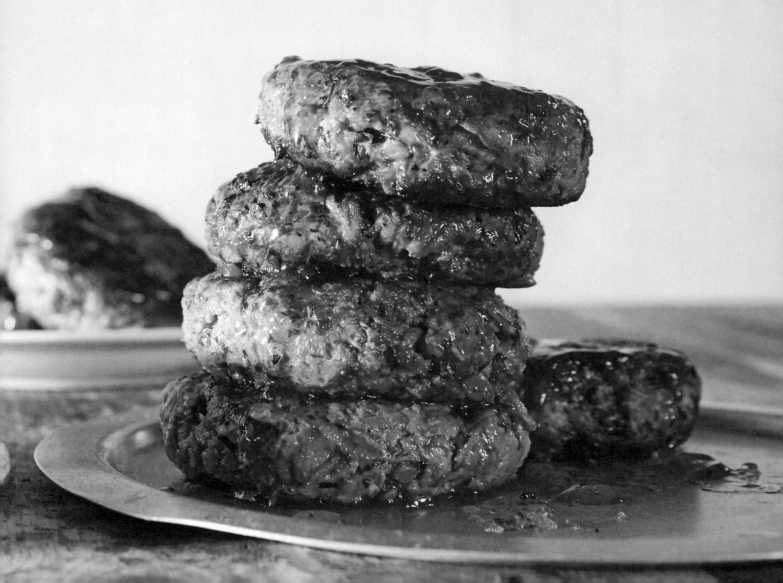

RED

MEAT

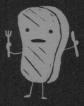

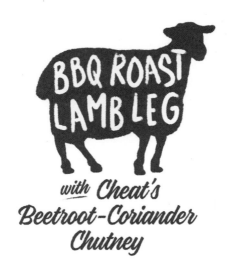

BBQ ROAST LAMB LEG

with Cheat's Beetroot-Coriander Chutney

Beetroot and coriander is one of those lesser known 'flavour combinations straight from heaven' – like tomato and basil, sage and pumpkin, or ham and pineapple. This recipe takes full advantage of their hidden love affair, and adds a new spin on the Aussie classic of lamb on the barbie.

SERVES 6 **PREP:** 30 MINS (PLUS 45 MINS MARINATING) **COOKING:** 55 MINS (PLUS RESTING)

1 × 1.5 kg butterflied boneless lamb leg (you can find these cryovaced in the supermarket – or ask your butcher to prepare it for you)
zest and juice of 1 lemon, plus lemon wedges, to serve
2 tablespoons olive oil
3 garlic cloves, crushed
sea salt and freshly ground black pepper
your favourite hummus, to serve
100 g feta, crumbled

CHEAT'S BEETROOT–CORIANDER CHUTNEY
220 g (1 cup) raw sugar
160 ml (²⁄₃ cup) malt vinegar or cider vinegar
1 onion, finely chopped
1 tablespoon coriander seeds
2 strips orange zest
3 (about 450 g) medium beetroot, coarsely grated (it's best to wear gloves for this or you will end up with pink hands!)

Lay the lamb out flat in a large glass or ceramic dish. Combine the lemon juice, oil and garlic in a bowl. Rub all over the top of the lamb. Season. Leave to marinate in the fridge for 30 minutes, or up to 2 hours. (If you marinate for longer, remove from the fridge 30 minutes before cooking to come to room temperature.)

Meanwhile, make the chutney. Combine the sugar, vinegar, onion, coriander seeds and orange zest in a saucepan and stir over low heat until the sugar dissolves. Increase the heat to medium–high and bring to a rapid simmer. Simmer for 10 minutes. Add the beetroot and cook, stirring, for 10 minutes, or until the chutney thickens and the liquid reduces.

Preheat a barbecue grill on medium. Barbecue the lamb on the grill for 5 minutes each side. Transfer the lamb to a roasting tin (or a foil tray if you prefer less washing up).

Place the tin in the centre of the barbecue. Turn off the burners directly under the tin and turn the burners on either side of the tin to low. (This, my friends, as you probably know, is indirect heat cooking, and for my money it is the best way to roast meat on the barbie.) Close the barbecue lid and the temperature should gradually come up to about 200°C. Roast for 20 minutes for medium or until cooked to your liking.

Transfer the lamb to a plate, cover loosely with foil and set aside for 15 minutes to rest.

Slather the hummus on a platter and place the lamb on top. Sprinkle the lemon zest and feta over the lamb and serve with beetroot–coriander chutney and lemon wedges on the side.

TIPS

If you don't have an enclosed barbecue, you can bake the seared meat in a preheated 200°C/180°C fan-forced oven.

Keep the relish on hand for sandwiches, barbecued chicken and even burgers. Store in an airtight container in the fridge for up to 2 weeks.

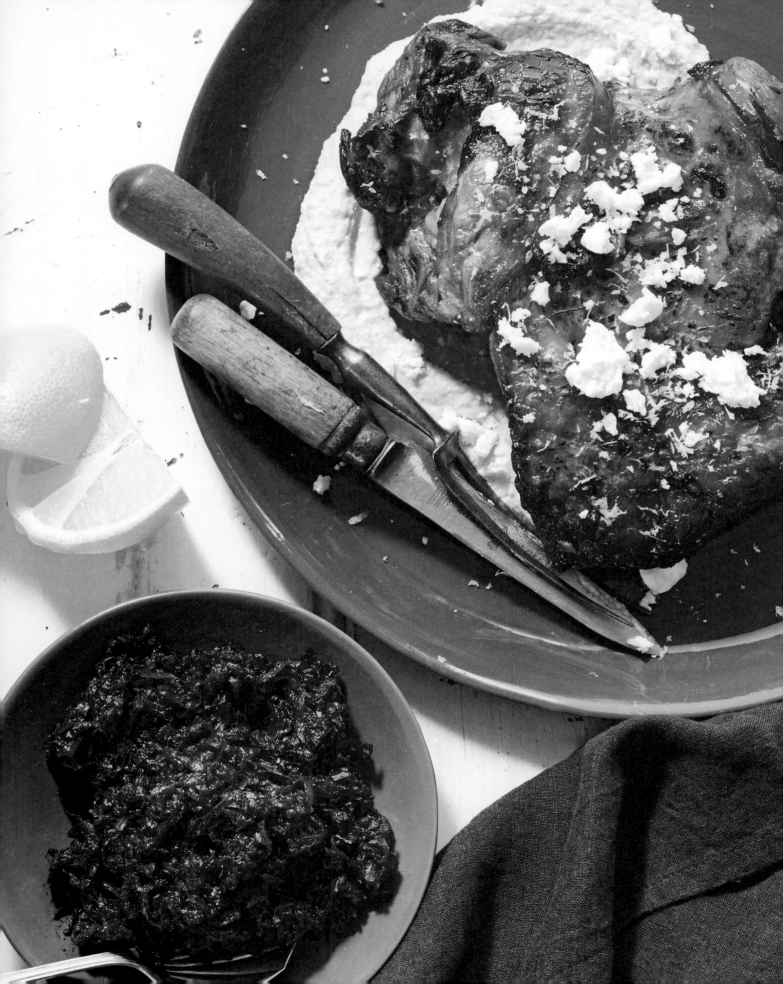

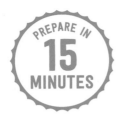

THE *Classic* RAGU

with POLENTA DUMPLINGS

We could have filled this book just with dumpling recipes and it wouldn't have been a bad thing at all. I view cobbler toppings or dumplings with stews to be a great way of doubling the pillowy, wintry comfort of these dishes. Plus they give you a radically different texture to play with and provide something to soak up all those meaty juices. Helloooo!

Here I've turned my back on all the usual suspects – my grandmother's suet dumplings (these were so hefty they crushed the winter blues with their sheer bulk), the fluffier, herby, self-raising flour numbers that my mother favoured and also the dolloped scone toppings of my American ancestors – in favour of something much more in keeping with the teeny ¹⁄₁₆th part of me that's Italian.* And so I present cheesy polenta dumplings. Delizioso!!!

*We could run a competition to guess which part of me is the ¹⁄₁₆th that is Italian but I am worried that my delicate disposition would be rocked by your salacious suggestions.

SERVES 4–6 PREP: 15 MINS COOKING: 3 HOURS

2 tablespoons olive oil
1 kg gravy beef, cut into
  4 cm pieces
100 g pancetta or bacon,
  coarsely chopped
2 anchovy fillets
2 celery stalks, finely chopped
1 onion, finely chopped
1 large carrot, finely chopped
4 garlic cloves, crushed
3 fresh or dried bay leaves
125 ml (½ cup) red wine
1 × 400 g can crushed tomatoes
375 ml (1½ cups) tomato passata
250 ml (1 cup) chicken stock
sea salt and freshly ground
  black pepper

POLENTA DUMPLINGS
150 g (1 cup) self-raising flour
120 g (⅔ cup) polenta
40 g (½ cup) shredded pecorino
  or parmesan, plus an extra
  2 tablespoons for a cheesier top
125 ml (½ cup) milk
2 eggs

Preheat the oven to 180°C/160°C fan-forced. Heat 1 tablespoon of the oil in a flameproof casserole dish over medium–high heat. Cook the beef in batches, for 2–3 minutes, until browned. Transfer to a bowl.

Heat the remaining oil in the dish over medium heat. Add the pancetta and anchovies. Cook for 2 minutes, stirring and mashing up the anchovies.

Add the celery, onion, carrot, garlic and bay leaves. Cook, stirring, for 5–6 minutes, until soft. Add the wine and simmer for 5 minutes, or until the liquid has evaporated by half.

Add the beef, tomatoes, passata and stock. Cover and bake for 2 hours or until the beef is tender. Taste and season well.

Prepare the dumplings 15 minutes before removing the beef from the oven. Combine the flour, polenta and cheese in a bowl. Add the milk and eggs and stir until well combined. Spoon ¼ cups of dumpling mix on top of the beef. Sprinkle the dumplings with the extra cheese. Return the dish to the oven and bake for 30 minutes, or until the dumplings are tender and fluffy.

TIPS

You can use other great slow-cooking cuts for this recipe: beef chuck steak, lamb shoulder or leg, pork neck or shoulder all work well.

Once you master the basic ragu try a few flavour twists. Add the rind of the parmesan, strips of orange zest or a cinnamon stick with the passata, or add a boost of herbs with some rosemary, thyme or oregano sprigs.

This ragu freezes well. Place in airtight containers and freeze for up to 3 months. Thaw overnight in the fridge and stir in a saucepan over low heat until heated through. It's great with pasta, wet polenta or couscous.

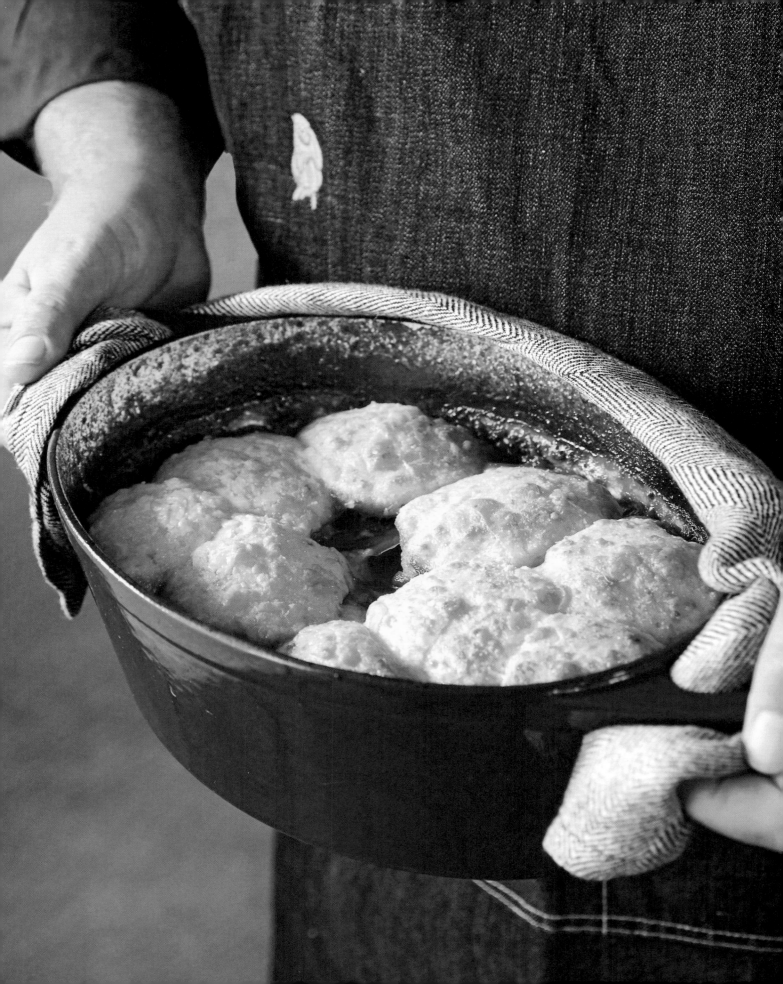

FOUR SKEWERS OF THE APOCALYPSE

This book is largely about cooking better food faster, and skewers are the very definition of evil because it takes time to soak bamboo skewers and thread things onto them. Plus you will invariably jab yourself in the process – especially if there's stingy lemon juice in the marinade. Sod's law that.

As one of my earliest memories was of an edifying felt picture on my grandmother's wall of two devils tormenting souls with similarly jabby pitchforks (while another devil fried eggs and bacon over the flames of Hell), it's perhaps not surprising that I associate skewers with The Evil One. But like that devil making breakfast, you've got to make the best of a bad lot. So here are my five favourite things to toast on skewers that aren't damned souls.

As the devils are in the detail I've casually ignored the detail that this is the red meat section and not all these skewers are made with red meat. There is a separate corner of Hell reserved for anarchists like me.

And yes, those smarty pants out there will have noticed there are FIVE skewers of the apocalypse, not four. This is because the Devil always cheats. Like having a fifth ace up his sleeve, it is his nature.

LAMB AND POMEGRANATE SKEWERS

PREPARE IN 5 MINUTES

SERVES 4   PREP: 5 MINS (PLUS 40 MINS MARINATING)   COOKING: 20 MINS

800 g lamb fillet, cut into 4 cm pieces
60 ml (¼ cup) pomegranate molasses
1 tablespoon olive oil
seeds of 1 pomegranate
½ cup coarsely chopped mint leaves
55 g (⅓ cup) pistachios, finely chopped
lemon wedges, to serve

Place the lamb and molasses in a zip-lock bag. Seal and then massage the meat to coat. Place in the fridge for 40 minutes to marinate – even longer is better.

Thread the lamb onto eight soaked bamboo (or metal) skewers and place on a tray as you go.

Preheat a barbecue grill or chargrill pan on medium–high heat. Drizzle the skewers with oil. Place on the grill and cook, turning occasionally, for 6 minutes for medium, or until cooked to your liking. Transfer to a plate. Cover loosely with foil and set aside for 15 minutes to rest.

While the lamb is resting, combine the pomegranate seeds, mint leaves and pistachios in a bowl.

Stack the skewers on a platter and sprinkle with the pomegranate salad. Add a squeeze of lemon just before serving.

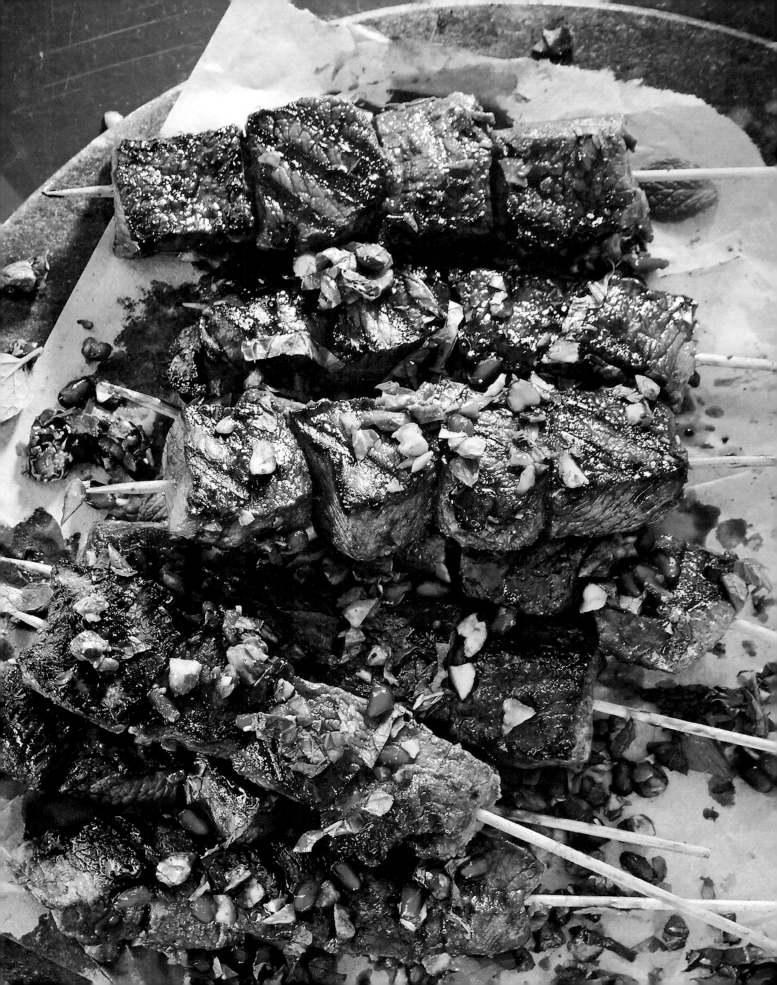

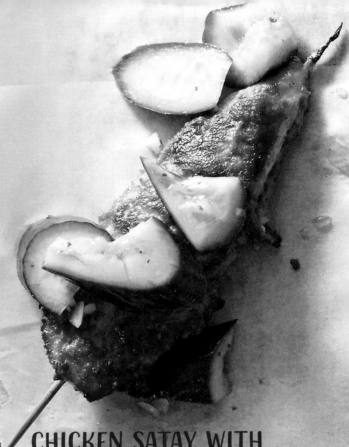

BABY POTATO SKEWERS WITH HOMEMADE CHIMICHURRI

SERVES 4 **PREP:** 10 MINS **COOKING:** 25 MINS

PREPARE IN
10
MINUTES

16 (about 1.2 kg) baby coliban (chat)
  potatoes, unpeeled
sea salt and freshly ground black pepper
2 tablespoons olive oil

CHIMICHURRI SAUCE
3 garlic cloves, crushed
2 spring onions, green parts only,
  thinly sliced
2 teaspoons lightly dried chilli flakes (optional)
zest of 2 lemons
½ cup coarsely chopped flat-leaf parsley
⅓ cup coarsely chopped oregano
2 tablespoons red wine vinegar
2 tablespoons olive oil

Place the potatoes in a microwave-safe bowl. Add a splash
of water (about 1 tablespoon). Cover with plastic wrap and
microwave on high for 12 minutes or until just tender. Set
aside to cool slightly. Halve the potatoes.

To make the chimichurri, stir together all the ingredients
in a bowl until well combined. Season.

Thread the potatoes onto eight soaked bamboo
(or metal) skewers. Place the skewers on a tray,
season and drizzle with the oil. Or just use your
hands to coat the potatoes in a thin veneer of
oil.

Preheat a barbecue grill or chargrill
pan on medium–high. Cook the
skewers, flat-sides down
first, for 6–8 minutes, until
golden. Turn and cook for
a further 3 minutes.

Stack skewers on a platter
and drizzle with the
chimichurri sauce.
to serve.

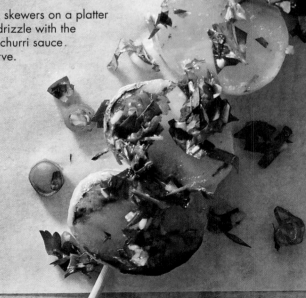

CHICKEN SATAY WITH SMASHED CUCUMBER SALAD

SERVES 6 **PREP:** 30 MINS (PLUS 30 MINS MARINATING)
COOKING: 5 MINS

1 kg chicken tenderloins
Smashed Cucumber Salad (page 174), to serve
olive oil, to drizzle
steamed rice, to serve

SATAY MARINADE
⅓ cup fresh coriander leaves and stems
200 g (¾ cup) crunchy peanut butter
4 cm knob of ginger, peeled and finely grated
2 garlic cloves
zest and juice of 1 lime
1 teaspoon coriander seeds
2 tablespoons soy sauce
2 teaspoons fish sauce
1 teaspoon ground turmeric
¼ teaspoon finely chopped fresh chilli

Combine all the satay marinade ingredients in a food
processor and blitz until smooth. Transfer to a large zip-
lock bag, add the chicken, then seal the bag and massage
the meat to coat. Place in the fridge for 30 minutes to marinate.

Whip up your cucumber salad while the chicken marinates.
Thread the chicken lengthways onto 18 soaked bamboo
(or metal) skewers and place on a tray as you go.

Preheat a barbecue flat plate on medium. Drizzle the skewers
with a little oil, then barbecue for 2 minutes on each side.
Serve with steamed rice and the smashed cucumber salad.

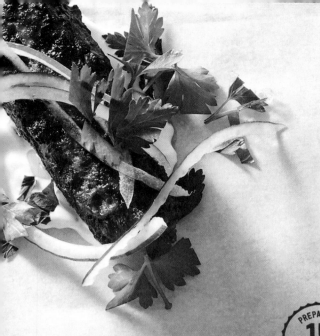

SPICED BEEF KEFTA

PREPARE IN 15 MINUTES

SERVES 6 **PREP**: 15 MINS **COOKING**: 15 MINS

1 large red onion, halved
800 g beef mince
⅓ cup finely chopped flat-leaf parsley, plus
    1 cup extra leaves
65 g (⅓ cup) raisins, coarsely chopped
2 teaspoons ground cumin
3 teaspoons sweet paprika
1 teaspoon ground cinnamon
sea salt and freshly ground black pepper
Instant Flatbreads (page 175), to serve
olive oil, to drizzle
a squeeze of lemon, plus extra wedges,
    to serve
plain yoghurt, to serve

Coarsely grate half the onion and thinly slice the other half. Place in separate bowls. Add the mince, chopped parsley, raisins, cumin, paprika and cinnamon to the grated onion. Mix until well combined. Season. Shape ¼ cups of the mince mixture around 12 soaked bamboo (or metal) skewers. Place on a tray in a single layer and cover with plastic wrap. Place in the fridge while you make your flatbreads.

Preheat a barbecue flat plate on high. Drizzle the skewers with oil and cook, turning every 5 minutes, for 15 minutes, or until cooked through. Transfer the skewers to a plate.

Add the extra parsley leaves to the bowl of sliced onion. Drizzle with a little extra oil and a squeeze of lemon juice and toss lightly to coat. Spread the flatbreads with yoghurt and top with the kefta and parsley salad. Serve with lemon wedges.

BBQ BRUSSELS SPROUT SKEWERS WITH ALMOND–MISO BUTTER

PREPARE IN 5 MINUTES

SERVES 4 **PREP**: 5 MINS **COOKING**: 10 MINS

20 small brussels sprouts
4 slices prosciutto, halved lengthways
1 tablespoon olive oil

ALMOND–MISO BUTTER
2 tablespoons rice wine vinegar
2 tablespoons caster sugar
100 g blanched almonds, toasted
80 g butter, at room temperature
80 g white miso paste

Place the brussels sprouts in a microwave-safe bowl. Add about 1 tablespoon of water. Cover with plastic wrap and microwave on high for 2 minutes, or until they turn bright green. This makes the brussels sprouts easier to thread onto the skewers.

While you pre-cook your sprouts, make the almond–miso butter. Combine the vinegar and sugar in a small saucepan. Cook, over low heat for 2 minutes, or until the sugar dissolves. Set aside to cool. Process the almonds, butter and miso until a smooth paste forms. Add the vinegar mixture and process until well combined.

Preheat a barbecue grill or chargrill pan on medium–high. Thread the brussels sprouts onto four soaked wooden (or metal) skewers, weaving the prosciutto between them as you go. Place the skewers on a tray and drizzle with oil. Cook for 1–2 minutes on each side, until tender and slightly charred.

Serve the brussels sprout skewers with the almond–miso butter.

TIP

Make the almond–miso butter up to 2 days in advance and store in an airtight container in the fridge. It is also great on grilled fish, slathered on corn or with steak.

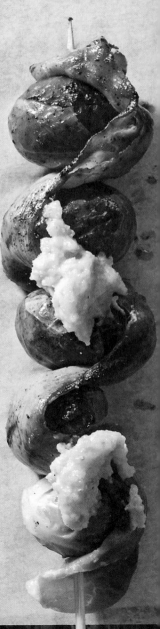

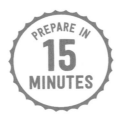

PREPARE IN 15 MINUTES

OSSO BUCCO
with *Gremolata*

'Bone with a hole': gotta love the verbal economy of the tannery workers who pioneered this dish. It was their way of taking advantage of the cow hides that came into the tannery with the shins and hooves still attached: a culinary perk of the job! For me the dish is all about the richness of what's *in* that hole in the bone – the lip-smacking jellied marrow. In fact the Italians even have an expression for the joy of the marrow's unique stickiness, *'appiccicare le labbra'*.

SERVES 6   **PREP:** 15 MINS   **COOKING:** 2 HOURS 50 MINS

2 tablespoons plain flour
sea salt and freshly ground
   black pepper
6 veal or beef osso bucco (pick
   ones with good eyes of marrow
   at the centre of the bone and
   that still have the skin on. The
   hind legs have the sweetest meat
   according to my Italian culinary
   muse, Marcella Hazan, which
   sounds like the sort of very
   annoying question to bother your
   butcher with ...)
2 tablespoons olive oil
1 onion, finely chopped
2 anchovy fillets
3 garlic cloves, crushed
800 g canned crushed tomatoes
250 ml (1 cup) chicken stock
4 oregano sprigs
Potato Skin Mash (page 205),
   to serve

GREMOLATA
½ cup coarsely chopped flat-leaf
   parsley
zest of 1 lemon and squeeze of juice
2 garlic cloves, crushed

Preheat the oven to 160°C/140°C fan-forced. Place the flour in a zip-lock bag. Season. Add the veal or beef and toss in the bag to coat.

Heat the oil in a large heavy-based flameproof casserole dish over medium–high heat. Cook the osso bucco in batches for 2–3 minutes on each side, until browned and crusty. Transfer to a plate.

Add the onion, anchovies and garlic to the dish and cook, stirring and breaking up the anchovies with a wooden spoon, for 5 minutes, or until the onion is soft. Don't worry, the fish won't make the gravy taste fishy – just extra savoury.

Stir in the tomatoes, stock and oregano. Bring to the boil. Return the osso bucco to the dish and turn to coat. Cover with a lid and bake for 2 hours. Uncover and bake for a further 30 minutes, or until the meat is so tender it can be cut with a spoon and the sauce has thickened.

Meanwhile, make your mash and the gremolata. To make the gremolata, combine all the ingredients in a bowl, adding just a touch of the lemon juice.

Sprinkle the osso bucco with gremolata and serve with mash. Make sure you earmark some good marrow from those cooked bones to mash into your potato for a true experience of peasant luxury!

TIPS

If you don't have a dish that goes from the stovetop to the oven then start the dish in a large frying pan and then transfer to an ovenproof dish to bake.

This dish is perfect for making ahead and freezing. Spoon into airtight containers and freeze for up to 3 months. Thaw overnight in the fridge. Place in an ovenproof dish and reheat, covered, at 180°C/160°C fan-forced until heated through.

Leftovers are great turned into a pasta sauce for chunky pastas (like rigatoni) or spooned over soft, creamy risotto that's loaded with saffron and parmesan. Just strip the meat from the bones and heat in the leftover sauce.

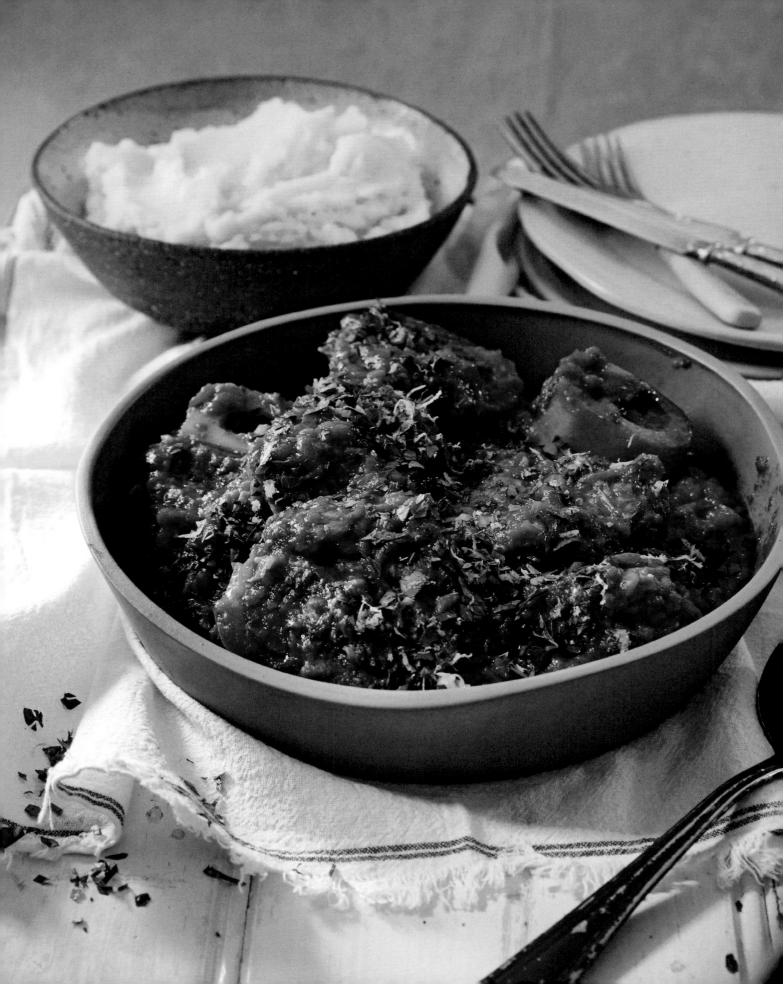

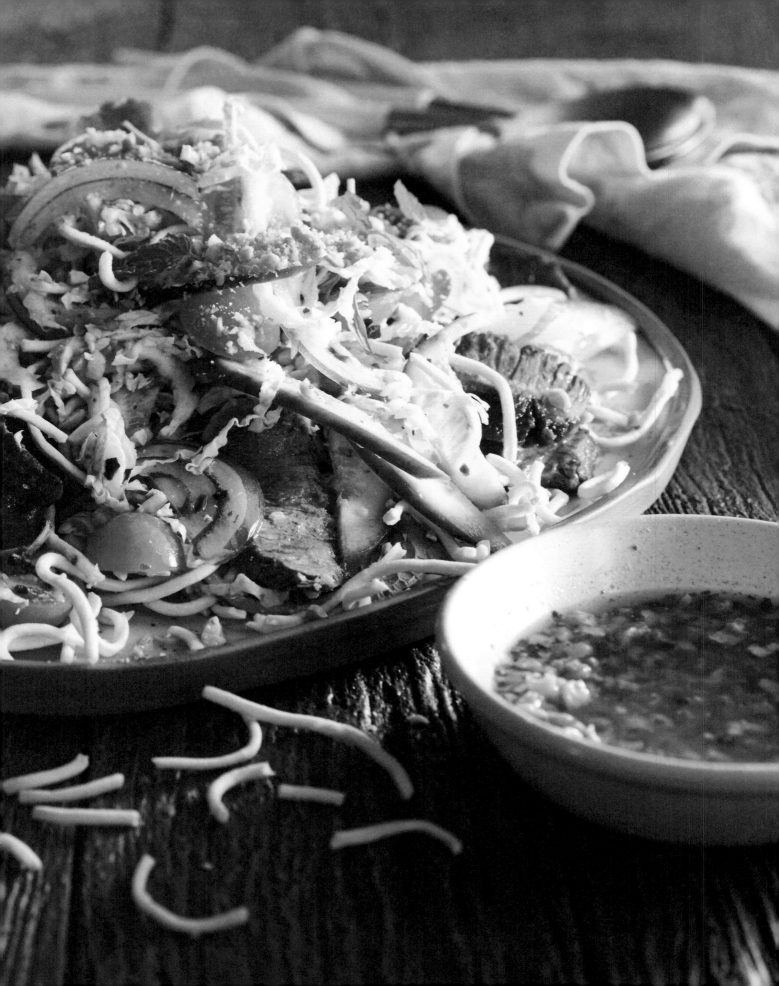

CRISPY THAI BEEF SALAD
with YIM YAM PEANUT DRESSING

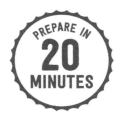

PREPARE IN
20
MINUTES

This is crunchy, meaty heaven with a go-to Asian dressing (very generously gifted to me by my chums at Yim Yam in Yarraville). It has now become a staple at my house.

SERVES 4 **PREP:** 20 MINS **COOKING:** 10 MINS

3 × 3 cm thick (about 700 g) scotch fillet, rump or sirloin steaks
1 tablespoon peanut oil
sea salt and freshly ground black pepper
½ wombok, finely shredded
3 Lebanese cucumbers, thinly sliced diagonally
400 g mixed cherry tomatoes, halved
2 cups mixed herbs (such as mint, coriander, Thai basil leaves), roughly chopped
½ red onion, thinly sliced
100 g bought crispy-fried noodles

YIM YAM PEANUT DRESSING
80 g (½ cup) unsalted roasted peanuts, finely chopped
2 teaspoons dried chilli flakes
2 tablespoons white sugar
2 tablespoons lemon juice
1½ tablespoons fish sauce

To make the Yim Yam dressing, place the ingredients in a bowl and stir until well combined.

Preheat a barbecue grill or chargrill pan on medium–high heat. Drizzle the beef with the oil. Season well on one side. Place, seasoned-side down, on the grill and leave without turning or touching for 6 minutes, or until the meat changes colour at least halfway up the side. Season the steak about a minute before you reach the turnover point. Flip and barbecue for a further 2 minutes for medium or until cooked to your liking. Transfer to a plate for 5 minutes to rest. Thinly slice.

While you rest the beef, place the wombok, cucumber, tomatoes, herbs and onion in a bowl and toss until well combined.

Add the beef and dressing to the salad and toss to combine. Add the noodles last, so they don't go soggy, and toss until combined. Better still, place half the salad on a serving platter and sprinkle with the noodles, then repeat the layering so the noodles are even crunchier.

FACT

Yes, this salad is related to that Chang's noodle salad so popular in the 80s, although now it's quite la-di-dah and might deny its roots ... but we know where it came from, even if it's changed its accent, joined a posh club and no longer dresses in moccies.

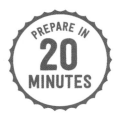

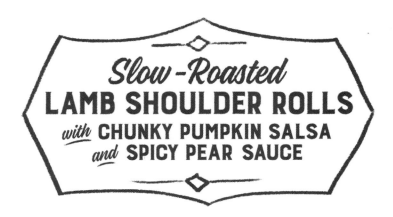

The idea of serving Sunday roast in a roll is one that has occupied far too many of my waking hours over the last five years. This is the latest take, made a wee bit sexier by the delicious mustardy pear relish that you'll be craving on everything from cheese toasties to roast pork.

SERVES 6 PREP: 20 MINS COOKING: 2 HOURS 45 MINS

1 × 900 g boned lamb shoulder (around 1.5 kg before boning)
125 ml (½ cup) dry white wine
60 ml (¼ cup) olive oil
2 teaspoons instant coffee
1 rosemary sprig, leaves picked
1 garlic clove, sliced
sea salt and freshly ground black pepper
920 g (about ½) butternut pumpkin, peeled, deseeded and cut into 1 cm pieces
2 teaspoons of ONE!!! nice spice (cumin seeds are lovely with pumpkin. So are crushed coriander seeds, or fennel seeds, or ground allspice, or a good grating of nutmeg. So, basically use whatever you have in the spice rack!)
3 large firm pears, peeled, halved and cored
2 small red onions, quartered
½ cup shredded mint leaves
2 tablespoons cider vinegar
1 teaspoon hot English mustard
12 Easiest-Ever Homemade Hot Rolls (page 203), or storebought rolls
40 g baby spinach leaves

Preheat the oven to 160°C/140°C fan-forced. Make little slits in the fatty surface of the lamb and sit it in a roasting tin. Drizzle with the wine and 1 tablespoon of oil. Rub the instant coffee into the slits and insert the rosemary into the cuts along with slices of garlic. Season the lamb all over. Cover with foil, then roast for 2 hours, or until the lamb is tender.

Line a large baking tray with baking paper. Place the pumpkin on the tray and drizzle with 1 tablespoon of oil. Sprinkle with the spice of your choice and toss to coat. Add the pear and onion to the tray and drizzle with the remaining 1 tablespoon of oil. Season.

Increase the oven temperature to 180°C/160°C fan-forced and remove the foil from the lamb. Add the tray of pumpkin, onion and pear to the oven. Roast alongside the lamb for a further 20–30 minutes, or until the lamb has a really golden crust and the veggies and pear are tender.

Remove the lamb from the oven and cover loosely with foil. Leave for 15 minutes to rest. Leave the pumpkin tray in the oven for this 15 minutes.

Take the soft centres out of the onion and set aside. Roughly chop the remaining outer parts of onion and transfer to a large bowl. Toss with the mint and 1 tablespoon of the vinegar. Add the roasted pumpkin and toss gently with your hands to create a chunky salsa.

Chop the roasted pears and place them in a jug. Add the squidgy onion centres, remaining vinegar and the mustard and use a stick blender to blitz until smooth. Season.

Shred the lamb. Use a large serrated knife to cut the rolls in half. Fill the rolls with spinach leaves, shredded lamb, pumpkin salsa and the spicy pear sauce.

TIPS

If you want to get ahead for lunches or the following night's dinner, buy a larger piece of lamb (2 kg bone in or 1.5 kg boned) and roast for 3 hours. This will give you plenty of leftovers for another meal.

Yes, you could just serve this dish on a board with baked potatoes instead of the rolls, but it's a little less fun and incurs more washing up!

If you think mint is a little ho-hum with lamb, then try butter-fried sage leaves with the pumpkin instead.

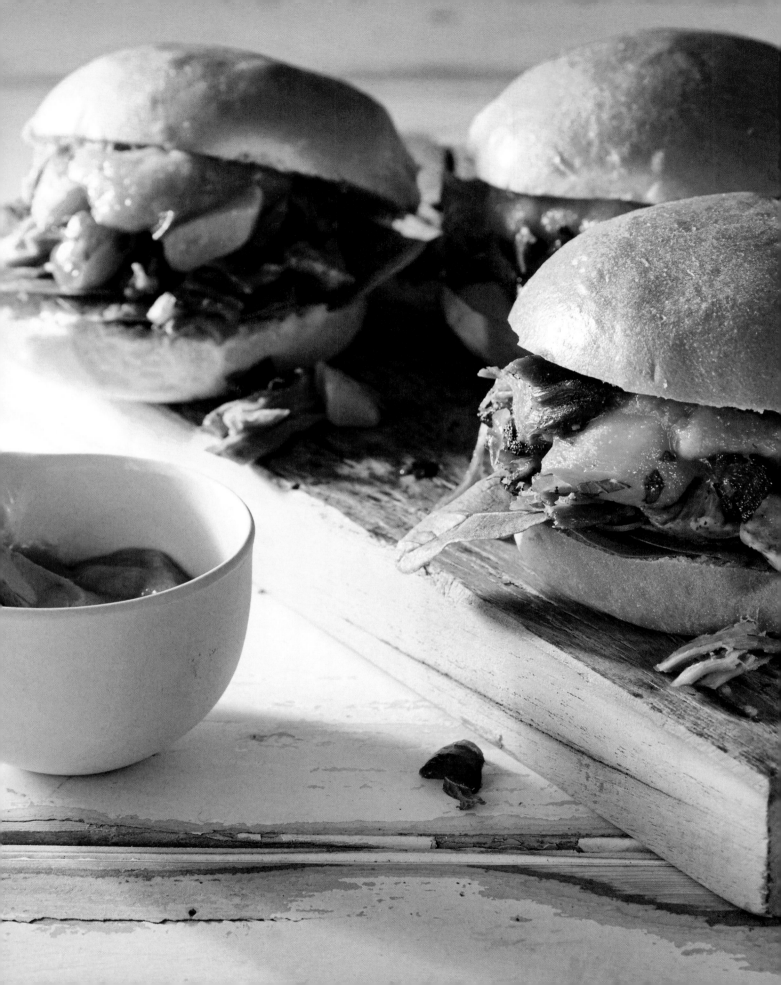

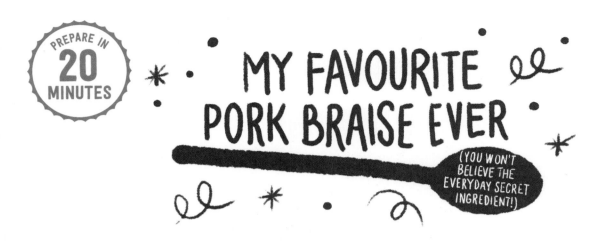

MY FAVOURITE PORK BRAISE EVER

(YOU WON'T BELIEVE THE EVERYDAY SECRET INGREDIENT!)

Plum would like to note that we suspect the name of this recipe has been shamelessly created by Mr Preston as ideal clickbait for the internet era. We wholeheartedly apologise in advance for this cynical exploitation and you can rest assured that the relevant department has been roundly chastised.

And when you discover that the Everyday Secret Ingredient is only pineapple juice, you might well feel slightly cheated – which we suppose is exactly the outcome with all great clickbaits. Long-term readers will know that adding pineapple juice to a braise is an old Matt Preston trick, stolen from his mother-in-law, no matter how he dresses it up with some fancy new meat or cut.

It's still plate-scrapingly good though, so do try it – even if the disclaimer, 'This recipe previously ran in Matt Preston's Cookbook as Jude's Short-Rib Braise and in Matt Preston's 100 Best Recipes as Lamb, Walnut and Pineapple Braise', should appear on this page somewhere for true online authenticity!

SERVES 4 **PREP:** 20 MINS **COOKING:** 2 HOURS 10 MINS

1.2 kg rindless boneless pork shoulder, cut into 4 cm pieces (you can also use pork neck or belly; alternatively any slow-cooking red meat will do!)
2 tablespoons plain flour
sea salt and freshly ground black pepper
2 tablespoons olive oil
3 garlic cloves, crushed
500 ml (2 cups) pineapple juice
140 g tomato paste
80 ml (⅓ cup) soy sauce
2 tablespoons vinegar (any type will do)
2 tablespoons brown sugar
2 teaspoons curry powder
1 cm knob of ginger, peeled and finely grated
105 g (¾ cup) toasted pecans

Preheat the oven to 200°C/180°C fan-forced. Place the pork and flour in a large zip-lock bag. Season. Seal and shake until well coated.

Heat 1 tablespoon of oil in a frying pan over medium–high heat. Cook the pork in batches for 3–4 minutes, or until well browned. Transfer to a casserole dish.

Heat the remaining oil in the frying pan. Add the garlic and cook for 30 seconds, or until aromatic. Add the pineapple juice, tomato paste, soy sauce, vinegar, sugar, curry powder and ginger. Bring to the boil.

Pour over the pork. Cover and bake for 2 hours, or until the pork is tender.

Stir in the pecans and season to serve.

TIPS

This recipe works well with other slow-cooking cuts. Try lamb shoulder or leg.

If you have a flameproof casserole dish you can cut down on the washing up by just using the one dish. Brown the pork, then set it aside while you make the sauce. Return the meat to the sauce once it is boiling, just before placing in the oven.

Get ahead and make the dish in advance. Store in an airtight container and freeze for up to 3 months. Thaw overnight in the fridge, then reheat in an ovenproof dish, covered, at 180°C/160°C fan-forced until heated through.

PREPARE IN **20** MINUTES

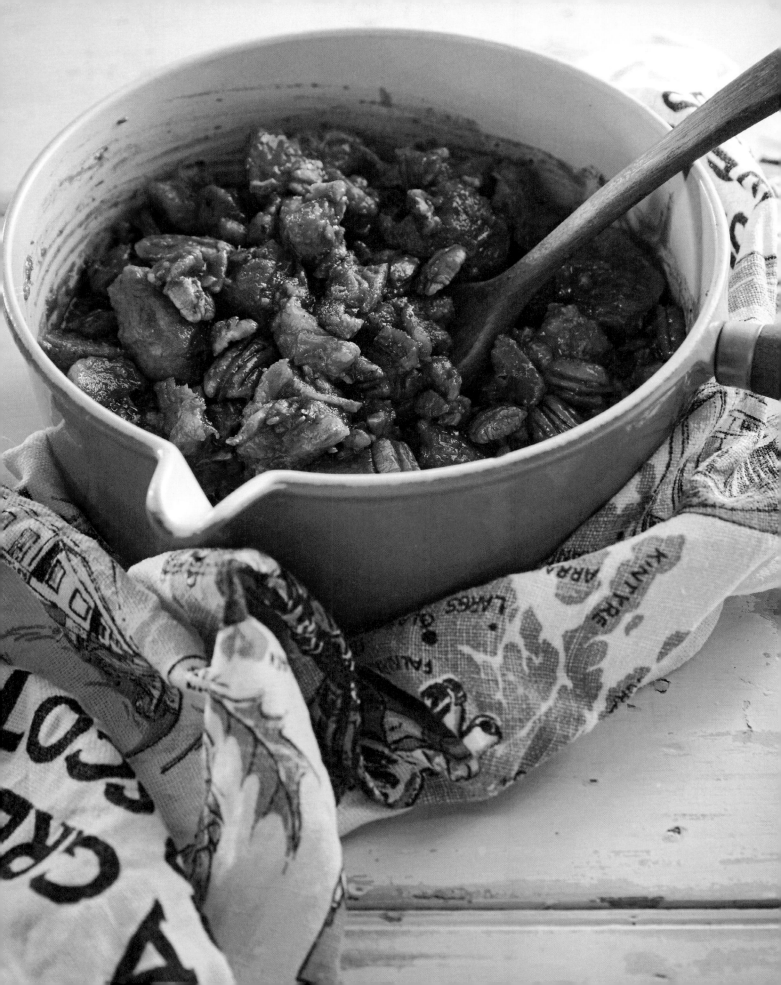

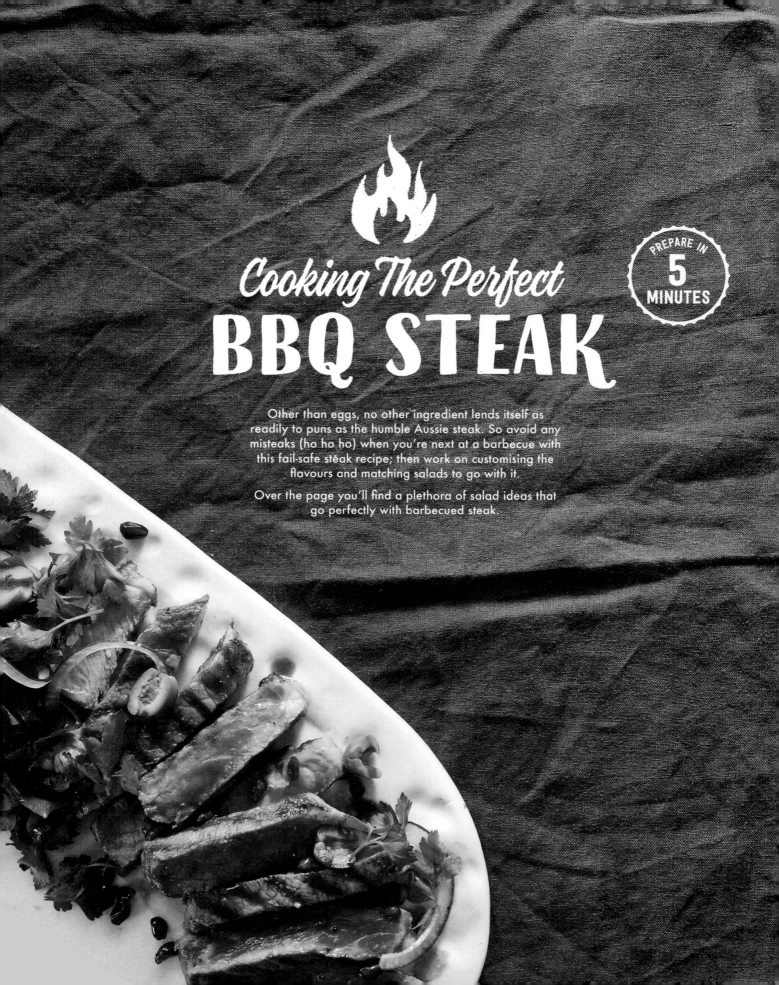

Cooking The Perfect
BBQ STEAK

PREPARE IN 5 MINUTES

Other than eggs, no other ingredient lends itself as readily to puns as the humble Aussie steak. So avoid any misteaks (ho ho ho) when you're next at a barbecue with this fail-safe steak recipe; then work on customising the flavours and matching salads to go with it.

Over the page you'll find a plethora of salad ideas that go perfectly with barbecued steak.

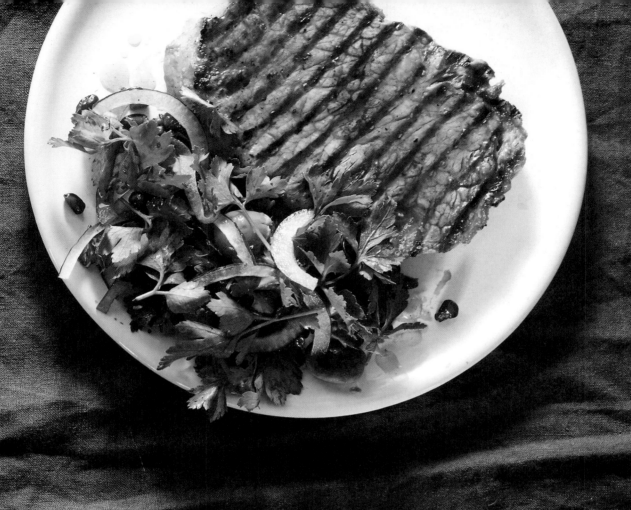

SERVES 4 PREP: 5 MINS COOKING: 10 MINS

4 × 3 cm thick scotch fillet, rump
   or sirloin steaks
olive oil, to drizzle
sea salt and freshly ground
   black pepper
Watermelon, pomegranate
   and pistachio salad (page 174),
   or any one of the 28 salads over
   the page

Take the steaks out of the fridge and let them come to room temperature.

Preheat a barbecue grill or chargrill pan, on medium–high heat until
it is nice and hot.

Sparingly drizzle the beef with a little oil and massage it all over the meat.
Season well on one side with salt just before hitting the grill.

If your steaks have a seam of fat running around one edge, hold the steak
with your trusty tongs and sear this fatty edge first, until browned. Then cook
on the seasoned side. Otherwise place on the grill, seasoned-side down,
and enjoy the sound of the grill singing. Remind yourself not to bother the
meat until it's got some lovely bold charry bar-markings; so no turning over
or touching just yet.

After 6 minutes, or when the meat changes colour at least halfway up the
side, flip it over. Using your superior powers of anticipation, season the steak
a minute before you reach the turnover point.

Barbecue for a further 3 minutes (or half the time the steak has been cooking
on the first side). Or you could just flip the steak over when the first juice
bubbles up on the surface, which will give you medium steaks.

Transfer to a plate for 5 minutes to rest, uncovered, in a warm place. Serve
with your salad of choice.

28 SALADS THAT PAIR PERFECTLY WITH STEAK

Unless specified, let your eye and your palate decide the ratios, always remembering that balance and generosity of flavour (and the absence of grated carrot) are the secrets to a great salad.

These ingredients are organised in importance. Use more of the first thing mentioned, less of the last and so. Another good tip is always to be restrained in the number of ingredients you use, if not the quantity. Season all with flake salt and a little acid (lemon juice, lime juice, a sexy vinegar) as required.

Any salad starts with picking a raw or cooked vegetable ingredient and then adding salt, sweet, sour, savoury, hot, crunchy, crispy or creamy elements to enhance it.

1. Blue cheese, celery, iceberg, walnuts, apple and chopped dates in equal quantities. (If you like, you can candy the walnuts by tossing them lightly in a little warm honey before toasting in a hot oven.) Great with any steak you darn well like – especially if the heat of the meat melts the blue cheese a little.

2. Butter lettuce with shallot vinaigrette. This is great with steak that's rubbed with dijon mustard and marinated for an hour before cooking.

3. Sliced rounds of fat ripe tomatoes, slivers of red onion and balsamic dressing with peppery leaves like rocket and nasturtium. Goes with any steak.

4. Diced roasted beetroot with toasted hazelnuts and a dressing of yoghurt and creamed horseradish. Perfect with whole rib-eye sliced and dusted with fresh grated horseradish.

5. Slaw of shredded wombok, crushed peanuts and Asian herbs, with a lime juice, fish sauce and palm sugar dressing (or the famous Yim Yam dressing on page 103). Serve with beef fillet or tuna steak, cooked tataki-style.

6. Halved cherry tomatoes, ashed goat's cheese (crumbled), oregano leaves, olive oil and the zest and juice of a lemon. Serve with strips of sirloin tossed in a little garlic butter or with cubes of medium wagyu of a decent marble score and quality.

7. Microwaved leeks à la grecque with a black pepper-heavy vinaigrette. Microwave cleaned and trimmed leeks (but with root end still sealed) for 4 minutes each. Cut off the root and slice the leek in half lengthways. Dress and eat the soft centres. You can see me doing this online in a video if you'd like. Great with any steak.

8. Salad of thinly sliced raw mushrooms (shiitake, flat or chestnut) and finely shaved parmesan, dressed with lemon juice and thyme leaves. Great with lean rare steak.

9. Slaw of thinly sliced white cabbage, spring onions and julienned carrots dressed with 70 % Greek yoghurt, 30 % Kewpie mayo and a few drops of Maggi seasoning. NOTE: This is julienned carrot and definitely NOT grated carrot! Perfect with steak haché or New York strip.

10. Ribbons of carrot cut with a potato peeler, microwaved for 2 minutes to soften slightly, then tossed with orange zest and juice, olive oil-rubbed pistachios and loads of parsley. Add toasted cumin or coriander seeds or a pinch of cardamom powder. Great with fillet steak rubbed with two parts ground coriander seed and one part ground cumin. Or barbecue a fillet rubbed with black cumin oil and rested before cooking.

11. Bean shoots, snow peas thinly sliced (lengthways obviously, you muppet) and threads of long red chilli in a rice wine vinaigrette. Great with beef fillet rubbed in gochujang before cooking.

12. Cooked peas, lightly blanched snow peas, marinated feta, mint and the thinnest rings of pickled red onion (page 23). Great with grilled porterhouse.

13. Witlof leaves, shaved parmesan and balsamic dressing. Great with steak marinated in oil, balsamic, red onion juice and garlic. Great with whole rib-eyes or *bistecca alla Fiorentina too*.

14. Spinach, sliced ripe pears and a hot English mustard vinaigrette. Serve with any steak.

15. Sliced crescents of witlof or shredded iceberg lettuce with seedless grapes (half of them roasted until softened; half fresh), lots of tarragon leaves and a dollop of crème fraîche loosened with a splash of vinegar. Slices of smoked chicken breast and blue cheese are both ace in this if you can't be bothered cooking steak.

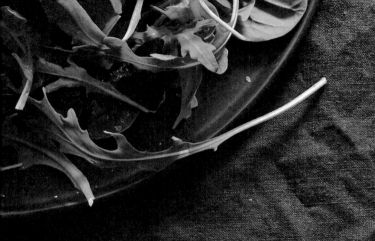

16. Roast veggies tossed with a dressing of balsamic syrup or hummus with harissa. Serve with steak rubbed with cumin salt before cooking. Also perfect with a whole roasted eye fillet, and black cumin oil can be employed here too.

17. Spring onions, sliced snow peas, cucumber and thin slices of green chilli tossed through udon noodles and dressed with a grated ginger and lime ponzu sauce. Serve with rare steak rubbed with soy, teriyaki sauce or kecap manis before cooking.

18. Tomatoes, blanched green beans and black olives with a sweet anchovy vinaigrette. Great with steaks of tuna or veal chops.

19. Shredded raw brussels sprouts with parmesan and reduced balsamic vinegar. Can be made with white cabbage instead. Perfect with rare, grilled T-bone, salted and well-oiled, Fiorentina-style.

20. Thin raw fennel wedges, torn radicchio and pith-free blood orange. Dress with salt, any random blood orange segments or slices and good olive oil. You can replace the radicchio with fat black olives, but it ain't as good. Tumble over well-crusted sirloin.

21. Grilled quarters of radicchio from the barbecue or grill pan with salt, olive oil and orange juice. Black olives, roasted until they dry out, optional. Also great with *bistecca alla Fiorentina*.

22. Chunks of various heirloom tomatoes and similarly sized rough wedges of seasonal fruit (watermelon, plum or nectarine) with a tart vinaigrette and ricotta. Great with thin slices of seared fillet steak.

23. Grilled asparagus spears, slices of just-boiled waxy potatoes and quartered hard-boiled eggs with a burnt butter vinaigrette (enrich with extra skimmed milk powder while you are 'nutting' the butter). Load on top of grilled porterhouse.

24. Wedges of cos lettuce with a crème fraîche and chopped chive dressing. Serve with rib-eye, perhaps in a red wine marinade.

25. Chunky grilled pineapple and fresh watermelon salad with chilli dressing, toasted salty peanuts and mint leaves. Serve with slices of hard-seared rare beef fillet, thinly sliced.

26. Cauliflower salad. Microwave a whole cauliflower head for 10 minutes to soften then break into small florets. Toss with herbs (choose from parsley, mint or dill). Add some sweetness (dried cranberries or currants). Add nuts (pistachio, pine nuts or almonds) plus seeds (cumin and sunflower). Dress with extra virgin olive oil and reduced pomegranate juice. Serve with sliced slow-roasted and well-barded rump steak.

27. Melon and cucumber with a Thai caramel and sliced red chilli. Cover with a blizzard of toasted coconut curls and fresh herbs like Vietnamese mint (some) and fresh garden mint (lots). Goes with seared fillet, pre-rubbed in teriyaki sauce, or 3 cm cubes of fillet that's been hard-seared quickly and tossed in the caramel before tossing over the melon and cucumber.

28. Smashed cucumbers with Thai basil, sliced dates, pistachios and green olives. Dress with olive oil and salt. Perfect with porterhouse that's been marinated in kecap manis or pomegranate molasses for 30 minutes before cooking.

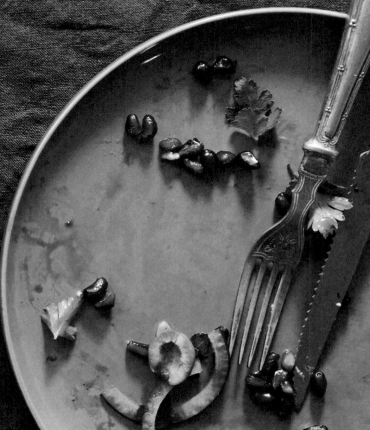

FISH

FISH

ETS

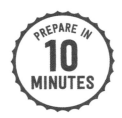

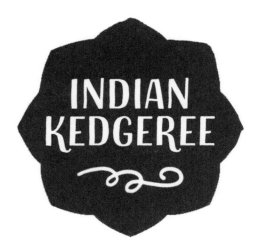

INDIAN KEDGEREE

This Anglo-Indian classic is a forgotten fave from when I was growing up. And now I've rediscovered it, I see that there is something wonderfully modern about the mild Indian spicing and smokiness of the fish. I know the sultanas are very controversial, but I think the dish needs their occasional burst of sweetness – even if they are a bit daggy and 70s, like indoor rubber plants and burnt-orange settees.

SERVES 4   PREP: 10 MINS   COOKING: 30 MINS (PLUS 10 MINS STANDING)

750 ml (3 cups) milk
3 fresh or dried bay leaves
550 g smoked haddock, cod
    or another firm white fish
    (or even salmon)
4 eggs
1 tablespoon olive oil
1 onion, coarsely chopped
2 garlic cloves, crushed
4 cm knob of ginger, peeled and
    finely grated
1 tablespoon curry powder
2 teaspoons brown mustard seeds
300 g (1½ cups) basmati rice
500 ml (2 cups) fish or chicken stock
90 g (½ cup) sultanas
200 g green beans, halved
2 tablespoons coarsely chopped
    flat-leaf parsley, coriander
    or chives

Combine the milk and bay leaves in a large deep saucepan and bring to a gentle simmer over medium heat. Add the fish and reduce the heat to low. Simmer for 8–10 minutes, until the fish flakes when tested with a fork. Remove the fish and flake into large pieces.

While the fish is cooking, place the eggs in a saucepan of cold water and bring to the boil, stirring constantly. Remove from the heat and set aside for 10 minutes. Drain, then peel and quarter lengthways.

Heat the oil in a large frying pan over medium–high heat. Add the onion, garlic and ginger and cook, stirring, for 5 minutes, or until soft. Add the curry powder and mustard seeds and cook, stirring, for 1 minute, or until aromatic. Add the rice, stock and sultanas. Bring to the boil. Reduce the heat to very low, then cover and cook without stirring for 10 minutes. Move the pan off the heat but do not remove the lid. Set aside for 10 minutes to allow the rice to finish cooking.

While the rice cooks, place the beans in a microwave-safe bowl. Add a tablespoon of water and cover with plastic wrap. Microwave for 3 minutes, or until bright green and tender-crisp.

Use a fork to fluff the rice. Top with the beans, fish, hard-boiled eggs and a sprinkling of herbs.

TIP

Use hot-smoked trout or salmon to save time cooking the fish.

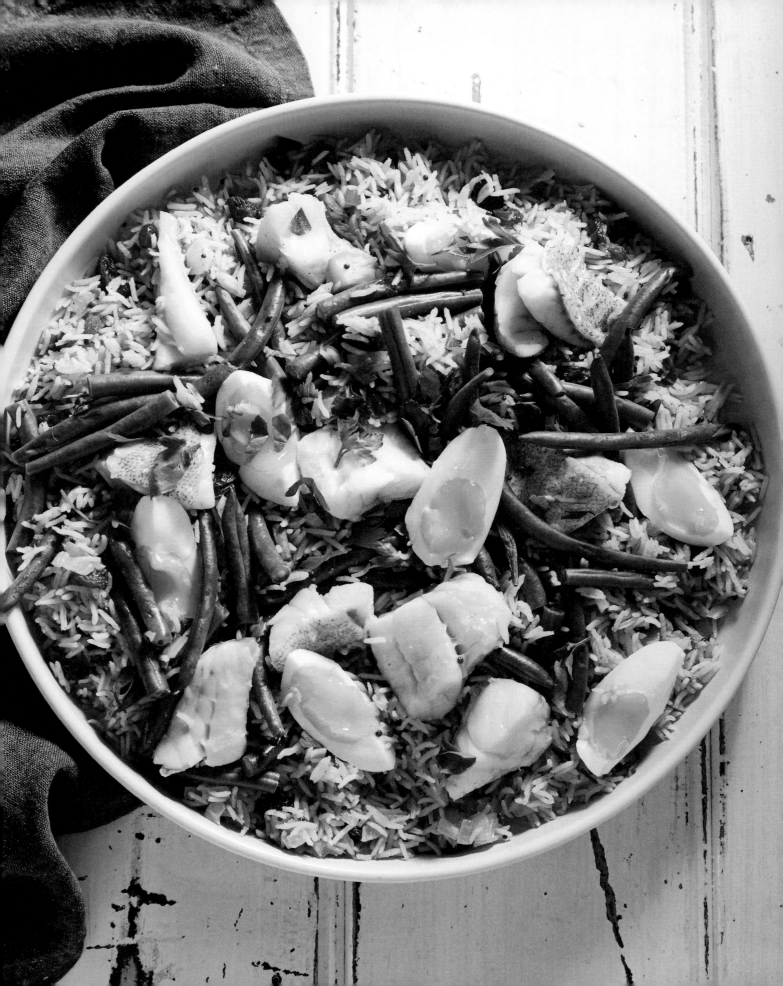

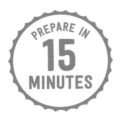

PREPARE IN
15
MINUTES

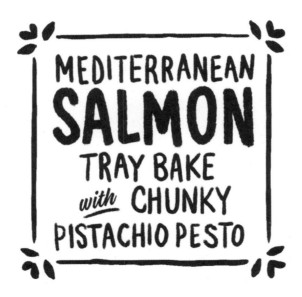

MEDITERRANEAN SALMON TRAY BAKE
with CHUNKY PISTACHIO PESTO

I am a lazy man and I love recipes where the oven does all the work. So it's no wonder that this easy tray bake is a favourite – and why this intro is so ...

SERVES 4 **PREP:** 15 MINS **COOKING:** 45 MINS

1 tablespoon red wine vinegar or sherry vinegar
1 tablespoon coarsely chopped oregano or marjoram leaves
2 tablespoons olive oil
sea salt and freshly ground black pepper
2 baby fennel bulbs, cut lengthways into 1.5 cm thick slices, fronds reserved
2 capsicums, deseeded and cut into 3 cm strips (I like a combo of red and yellow for colour)
4 roma tomatoes, halved
1 lemon, quartered
4 x 200 g skinless salmon fillets, pin-boned
100 g feta-stuffed olives

CHUNKY PISTACHIO PESTO
75 g (½ cup) pistachio kernels
½ cup flat-leaf parsley leaves
¼ cup basil leaves
2 garlic cloves
1 tablespoon lemon juice
1 tablespoon olive oil

Preheat the oven to 220°C/200°C fan-forced. Place a shallow roasting tin in the oven to warm.

Combine the vinegar, oregano and 1 tablespoon of the oil in a jug. (Or use a mug, as it seems not everyone has jugs these days. If you live in the country or are an urban hipster use an old, clean jam jar.) Season.

Place the fennel, capsicum, tomato and lemon in the hot roasting tin and drizzle with the vinegar mixture. Bake for 35 minutes or until the vegetables start to get a little golden around the edges.

While the veggies cook, make the pistachio pesto. Combine the pistachios, parsley, basil and garlic in a small food processor. We want this pesto chunky, so we hardly want to smash up the nuts at all. Use minisculely short presses of the pulse button so everything is just very roughly chopped together, but still rubbly. Transfer to a bowl and stir in the lemon juice and oil.

Remove the veggies from the oven and turn over the fennel and capsicum pieces, making room in the tin to add the salmon (plus this will give your veggies more toastiness). Scatter in the olives. Drizzle the salmon with the remaining oil and season. Spoon the pistachio mixture over the top of the salmon and bake for 12 minutes, or until the fish flakes when tested with a fork.

Sprinkle with the reserved fennel fronds and serve.

TIPS

Turn this chunky pesto into a smoother sauce to toss through pasta. Process the mixture until more finely chopped. Add ¼ cup parmesan. With the motor running, gradually add the lemon juice and increase the oil to 60 ml (¼ cup). NICE!!!!

Make your own stuffed olives. Buy pitted olives, and employ a child's small nimble fingers to stuff them with feta!!

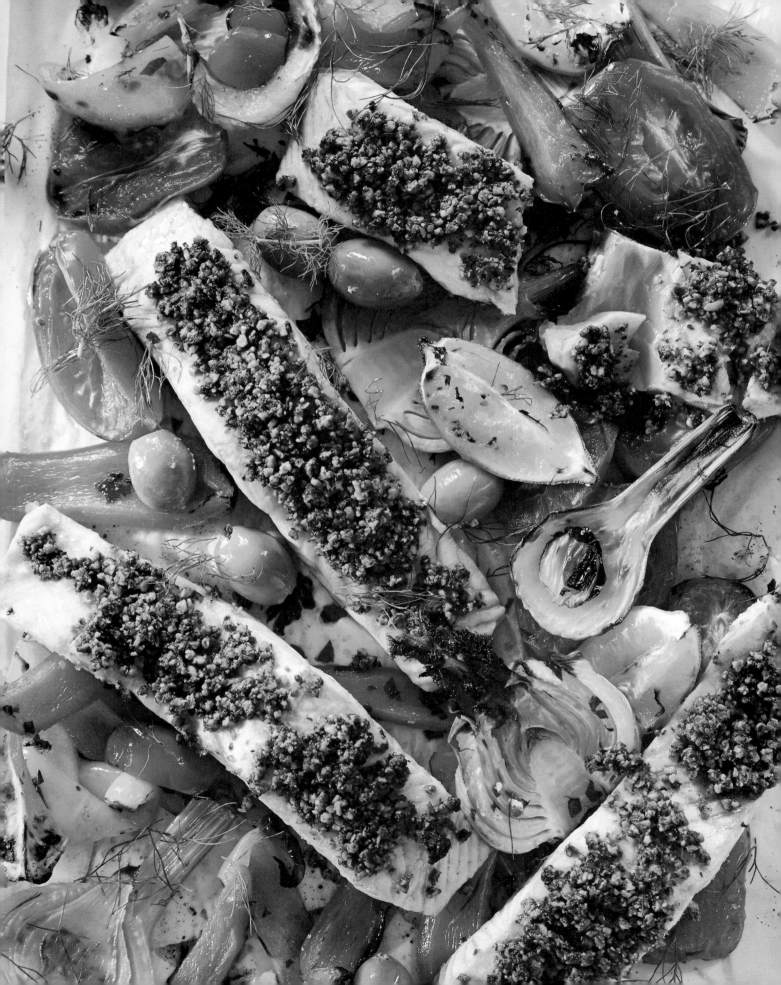

HAWAIIAN POKE with NORI and MACADAMIA SPRINKLE

Poke (aka pok-e) is a very 'in' dish in the US at the moment. Heck, it's also very much an 'in' dish here, too. It's like a lazy person's sushi bowl that has all the flavour-joy of a fistful of hand-rolls, but with none of the fiddly work. Perfect!

SERVES 4 PREP: 10 MINS COOKING: 20 MINS (PLUS 10 MINS STANDING)

335 g (1½ cups) sushi rice, rinsed well

2 tablespoons sushi seasoning (see TIP)

500 g sashimi-grade tuna steaks, cut into 1–2 cm pieces

4 cm knob of ginger, peeled and finely grated

60 ml (¼ cup) soy sauce

1 teaspoon sesame oil

2 spring onions, thinly sliced

16 cherry tomatoes, halved

1 avocado, thinly sliced

shredded pickled ginger, to serve

NORI AND MACADAMIA SPRINKLE (OR FURIKAKE, IF YOUR JAPANESE TEACHER IS LISTENING ...)

80 g (½ cup) macadamia nuts, finely chopped

2 tablespoons grated palm sugar or brown sugar

1 teaspoon sea salt

1 sheet toasted nori, cut into thin strips

3 teaspoons chilli flakes

Place the rice in a saucepan with 500 ml (2 cups) of water over medium–high heat. Bring to the boil, then reduce the heat to low. Cover and simmer for 10 minutes, or until liquid is absorbed. Remove from the heat and set aside for 10 minutes. Use a fork to stir in the sushi seasoning.

While you are cooking the rice, combine the tuna, ginger, soy sauce and sesame oil in a glass or ceramic bowl. Cover and leave to marinate in the fridge for 5–10 minutes. Add the spring onion and toss to combine.

While the tuna marinates, make the nori and macadamia sprinkle. Place the chopped nuts in a small non-stick frying pan over medium heat. Cook, stirring constantly (the fine bits of macadamia can catch and burn easily, so take care) for 4–5 minutes, until lightly toasted. Add the sugar and salt and toss for 1 minute, or until the sugar melts. Remove from the heat and set aside for 5 minutes to cool slightly. Stir in the nori and chilli.

Divide the rice among serving bowls. Top with the tuna, tomatoes, avocado and pickled ginger. Finish with the sprinkle.

TIP

If you can't find sushi seasoning, mix 2 tablespoons of rice wine vinegar with 1 tablespoon of caster sugar and stir until the sugar dissolves. Stir this mix into the rice while the rice is still warm.

The sprinkle is AMAZING – make extra and keep it in your pantry to use on everything.

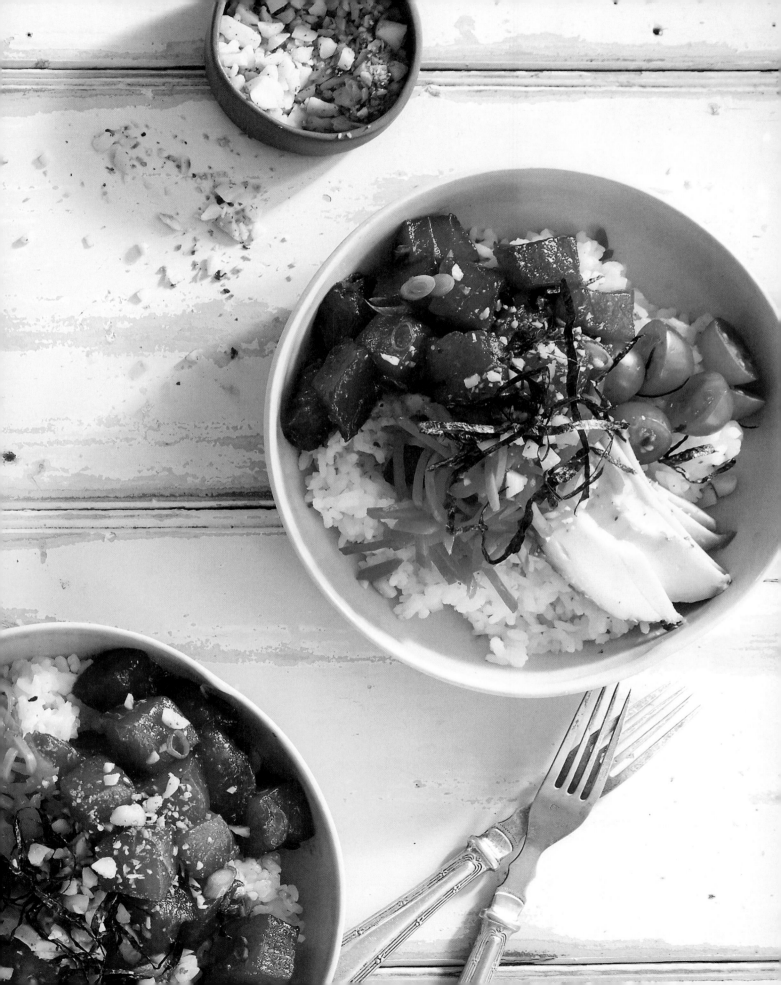

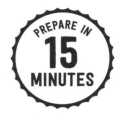

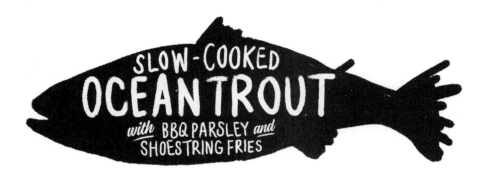

Ocean trout is salmon with an astrakhan overcoat and a diamond-topped cane. It's salmon's snooty brother, who always brings along the most expensive wine when the orange fish family go out together for BYO Chinese. If ocean trout deigned to speak to you, it would probably have a *blaah* Toorak/Woollahra/Claremont drawl of an accent. And it would certainly let you know that 'the wife' drives a German-built SUV. Ocean trout does have exquisite taste – but then it can afford to.

In an effort to put ocean trout back in its place, we've largely hung out with far more down-to-earth (or should that be 'down to sea') salmon in this book. This is its one spot in the limelight and, needless to say, it's insisted on being cooked low and slow as this is understated and therefore far classier than pan-frying. It also demanded a classy accompaniment. I discovered the idea of barbecuing flat-leaf parsley at Aaron Turner's Igni restaurant in Geelong; it's a surprising way of treating this familiar herb, and absolutely delicious.

P.S. Don't tell, but this recipe can also be made with Atlantic salmon.

SERVES 4 PREP: 15 MINS COOKING: 1 HOUR

3 (about 500 g) coliban, sebago, royal blue or golden delight potatoes, peeled and cut into 5 mm thick matchsticks
60 ml (¼ cup) olive oil
sea salt and freshly ground black pepper
1 × 1 kg skin-on ocean trout fillet, pin-boned
1 big bunch flat-leaf parsley, tied with string
Kewpie mayonnaise, to serve

Preheat the oven to 200°C/180°C fan-forced. Line a baking tray with baking paper.

Place the potato matchsticks on the prepared baking tray and drizzle with 1 tablespoon of the oil. Season. Bake, tossing carefully with a spatula every 10 minutes, for 25–30 minutes, until the edges just start to turn golden.

While the potato is baking, rinse the trout in cold water and dry it thoroughly. Set aside for 20 minutes to come to room temperature.

Place the fish on a sheet of baking paper large enough to wrap the fish. Brush both surfaces with another tablespoon of oil and season. Wrap the paper around the fish, folding in the sides, like a parcel. Place, skin-side down, on a baking tray.

Reduce the oven temperature to 100°C/80°C fan-forced and at the same time, preheat your barbecue grill on medium–high. Leave the chips in the oven and do not open the door. Once the correct temperature is reached, place the fish in the oven, skin-side up, and bake for 12 minutes. Turn the trout parcel over and bake for a further 12 minutes. Remove from the oven and set aside to rest for 5 minutes. Turn the oven off and leave the chips in the oven to keep warm and crispy.

Now it's time to barbecue the parsley. Drizzle it with the remaining tablespoon of oil and cook on the barbecue grill, turning occasionally, for 2–3 minutes, until it is lightly charred and slightly burnt at the edges.

Unwrap the fish and transfer carefully to a serving platter, skin-side up. Peel away the skin, then gently scrape away all the grey flesh.

To serve, top with the barbecued parsley and shoestring fries and squeeze over the Kewpie.

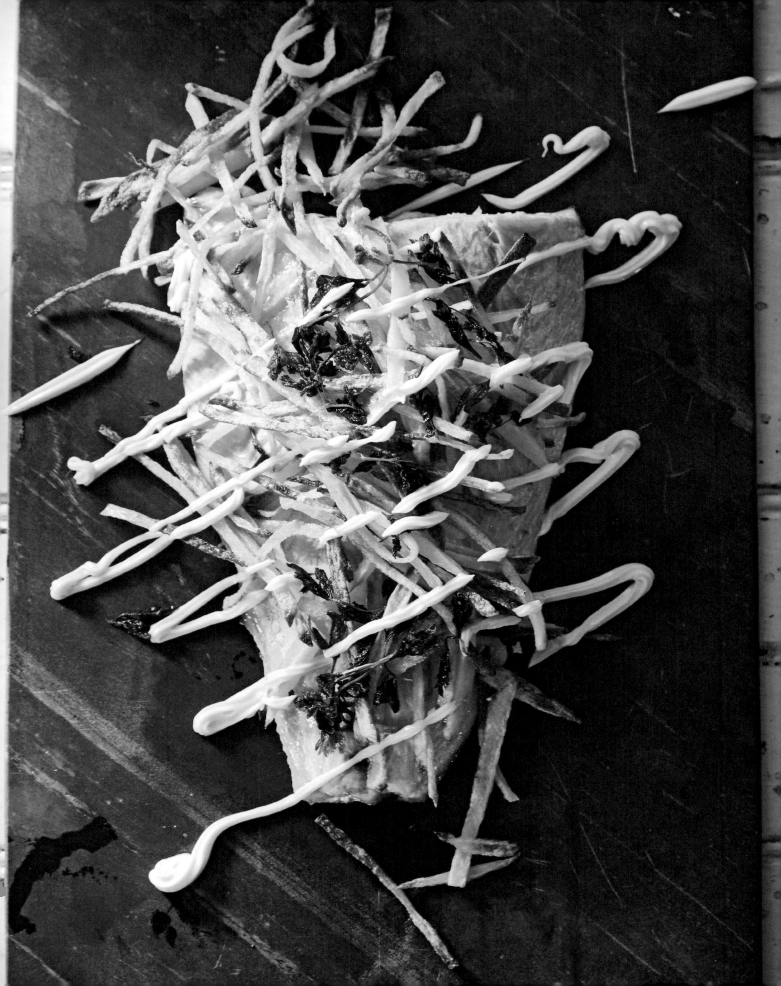

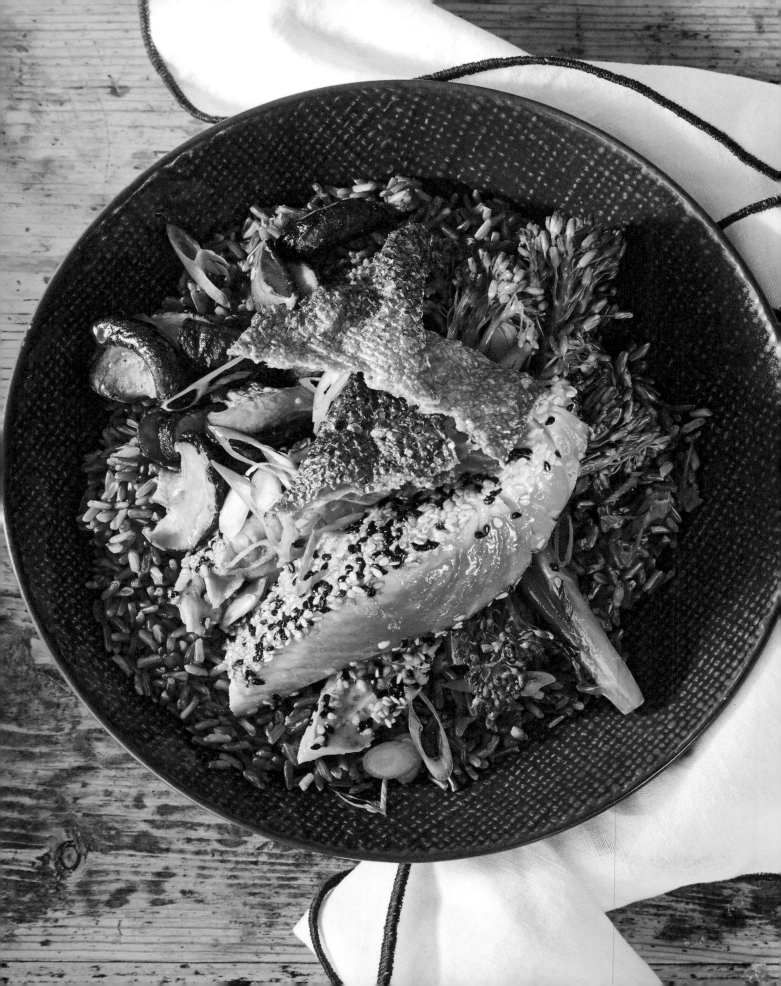

TERIYAKI SALMON BOWL
with SALMON CRACKLING

Growing up I hated fish almost as much as I hated egg whites, but this dish is on weekly rotation at home because it's easy, super-tasty and even my youngest relishes the way the just-cooked salmon flakes softly.

SERVES 4 PREP: 20 MINS (PLUS 30 MINS MARINATING) COOKING: 35 MINS

4 x 200 g skin-on salmon fillets, pin-boned
60 ml (¼ cup) honey
sea salt
80 g (½ cup) sesame seeds (I like a 50/50 combo of black and white)
2 tablespoons peanut oil
100 g shiitake mushrooms, thickly sliced
1 bunch broccolini, trimmed and halved lengthways
1 × 250 g pouch 90 second microwaveable red rice, warmed following the packet instructions (or prepare your own brown rice or sushi rice)
2 spring onions, thinly sliced diagonally

TERIYAKI SAUCE
80 ml (⅓ cup) mirin
125 ml (½ cup) soy sauce
2 tablespoons rice wine vinegar
2 tablespoons caster sugar
½ teaspoon sesame oil
4 garlic cloves, chopped and mashed to a paste with salt on the chopping board
2 cm knob of ginger, peeled and finely grated

To make the teriyaki sauce, bring the mirin to the boil in a saucepan over high heat. Reduce the heat to medium. Add all the other ingredients and simmer for 10 minutes, or until it thickens slightly. Set aside to cool. You need ½ cup of teriyaki sauce for this recipe but the rest will keep in the fridge for up to 2 weeks.

Use a sharp knife to slide between the salmon skin and flesh to remove the skin. Reserve.

Combine the teriyaki sauce and honey in a glass or ceramic dish. Add the salmon fillets and turn to coat. Cover and refrigerate for 30 minutes, or up to 4 hours.

While your fish marinates, make your salmon crackling. Preheat the oven to 180°C/160°C fan-forced. Line a baking tray with baking paper. Use a flat-bladed knife to scrape the salmon skin and remove any flesh ('But we don't want to remove the delicious fat on the underside of the skin do we??!!!??' he said in a panic. 'It's the best bit.'). It has to be as clean as possible so the skin can crackle. Place on the tray and sprinkle with salt. Bake for 10 minutes or until the skin is crisp.

Strain the salmon and transfer the marinade to a small saucepan. Bring to the boil over medium–high heat, then simmer rapidly for 3–5 minutes, until the marinade thickens slightly.

Place the sesame seeds in a tray or shallow dish. Press the tops and bottoms of the salmon fillets into the seeds to coat.

Heat 1 tablespoon of oil in a frying pan over medium heat. Add the salmon and cook for 2 minutes on each side (4 minutes in total will give you delicate, translucent, just-cooked salmon that flakes apart. Upping it to 3 minutes on each side will cook the salmon through.) Transfer to a plate and set aside for 5 minutes to rest.

Wipe the pan clean and heat the remaining oil over medium–high heat. Add the mushroom and cook, tossing, for 2 minutes, or until starting to turn golden. Then add the broccolini to the pan and cook as well, stirring, for 2–3 minutes, until it is bright green.

Divide the rice among serving bowls. Top with the broccolini, mushroom and salmon. Drizzle with the warm marinade sauce. Use your hands to break the fish crackling into pieces and place on top with the spring onion.

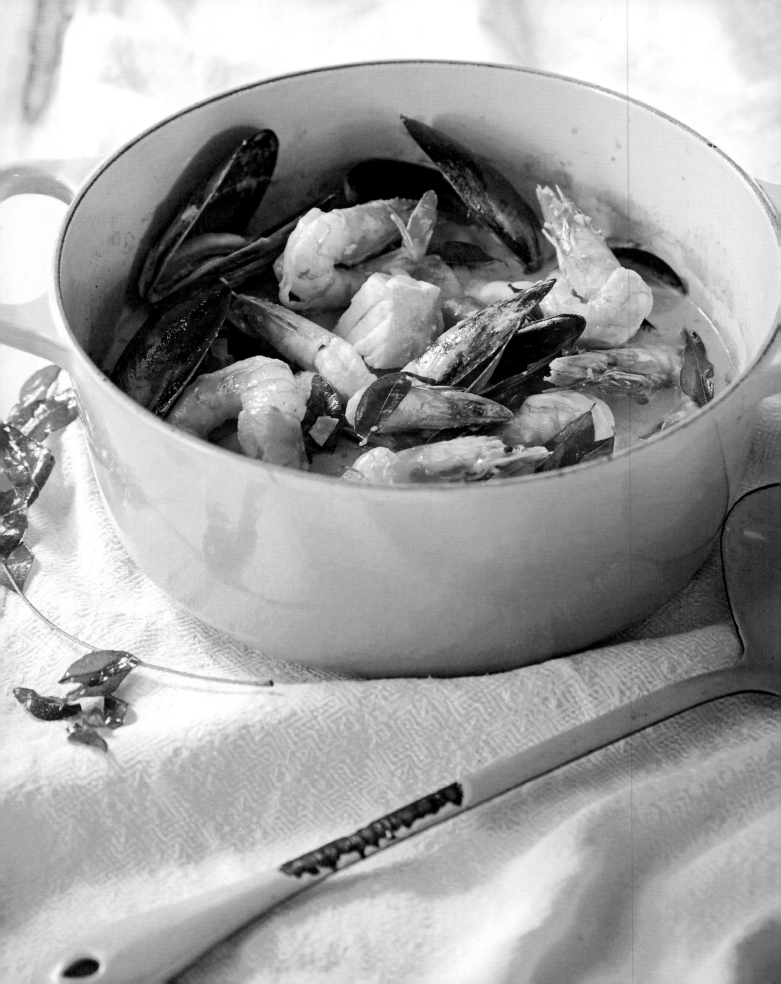

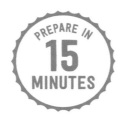

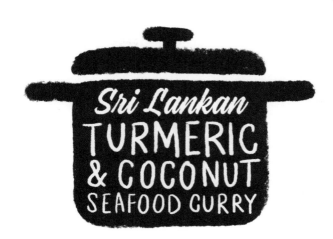

Sri Lankan TURMERIC & COCONUT SEAFOOD CURRY

'I fell in love with Sri Lanka on a trip there in 2015. I spent a blissful few weeks discovering the bright vibrant food and learnt so much from the beautiful generous people I met along the way ...' This curry brings back only the fondest memories of that time and even makes this cringeworthy, cliche-laden first sentence acceptable – almost.

(BTW, did I also tell you that 'I learnt to cook from my Sri Lankan grandmother' and that 'when travelling you find greater culinary insights in the humble homes of the people than in gastronomic temples' ... or any other great food TV cliches.)

SERVES 4   **PREP:** 15 MINS   **COOKING:** 25 MINS

1 tablespoon grapeseed oil
1 onion, finely chopped
2 long green chillies, deseeded and finely chopped
6 cardamom pods
4 cm knob of ginger, peeled and finely grated
2 garlic cloves, crushed
2 curry leaf sprigs, plus extra sprigs to serve, if you like (see TIP)
3 teaspoons ground turmeric (or 100 g fresh turmeric, peeled and grated)
2 teaspoons cumin seeds
2 teaspoons ground coriander
1 × 400 ml can coconut cream
250 ml (1 cup) fish stock
2 ripe tomatoes, coarsely chopped
500 g skinless rockling or blue eye trevalla fillets, pin-boned and cut into 4 cm pieces
16 green prawns, peeled and deveined, with tails intact
12 mussels, scrubbed and debearded
juice of 1 lime
¼ cup coarsely chopped coriander (optional)
steamed rice, to serve

Heat the oil in a large frying pan over medium–high heat. Add the onion, chilli, cardamom, ginger, garlic and curry leaves and cook, stirring ever so gently, for 5 minutes, or until soft.

Add the turmeric, cumin and ground coriander and cook, stirring, for 30 seconds, or until you start smelling aromatic wafts of spice.

Add the coconut cream, fish stock and tomato to the pan and bring to the boil. Reduce the heat to medium and bring to a simmer. Simmer for 10 minutes so everything thickens up a little.

Now that the curry sauce is made, just add the fish, prawns and mussels. Cook, stirring occasionally, for 5 minutes, or until the seafood is cooked through and the mussels have opened. Simple!

Squeeze over the lime juice and sprinkle with coriander and extra curry leaves (if using). Serve on your choice of steamed rice.

TIP

If you have extra curry leaves, cook in a little oil in a frying pan over medium heat until crisp. Transfer to a plate lined with paper towel to drain and serve on top for extra flavour.

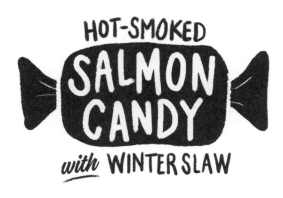

HOT-SMOKED SALMON CANDY
with WINTER SLAW

Salmon candy??? Ocean trout candy??? Sounds weird, but these versions of maple syrup-sweetened hot-smoked fish are officially about as addictive as maple syrup with bacon, peanut butter with honey and salt flakes, or just good old crispy chicken skin. Try brushing the fish with a layer of maple syrup before smoking to really boost the decadence.

You'll need ½ cup of wood-smoking chips, which are available from barbecue stores. I like applewood for this dish, but don't be too precious. If you already have hickory chips it's fine to use those instead.

SERVES 4 PREP: 30 MINS (PLUS 3 HOURS CURING AND CHILLING) COOKING: 25 MINS

200 g (1 cup) brown sugar
250 g (1 cup) sea salt flakes
1 × 500 g skinless salmon or ocean
  trout fillet, pin-boned

WINTER SLAW
500 g brussels sprouts
130 g (½ cup) Greek-style yoghurt
1 tablespoon chopped dill, plus
  extra to serve
sea salt and freshly ground
  black pepper
60 ml (¼ cup) extra virgin olive oil
1½ teaspoons caraway seeds
2 tablespoons lemon juice, plus
  lemon wedges to serve
2 tablespoons honey
2 large carrots, cut into matchsticks
2 celery stalks, finely chopped

Combine the sugar and salt in a bowl. Spread half of the mixture over the base of a non-reactive container with a lid. Add the salmon or ocean trout fillet and cover with the remaining mixture. Cover and leave to cure in the fridge for at least 1 hour but ideally overnight.

Wipe off most of the curing mix from the fish with paper towel, leaving a thin layer on the bottom and top surfaces (this will caramelise as it smokes). Return to the fridge, uncovered, for an hour or two to dry out a little.

Line a wok with foil and add the wood chips. Place over high heat until smoking. Place the fish on a greased wire rack and set inside the wok. Cover with a lid and smoke for 2 minutes, then reduce the heat to medium–low and smoke for a further 15 minutes. Remove from the heat. Set aside, still covered, for 5 minutes to cool slightly and continue smoking in its residual heat, then flake.

While your fish smokes make your slaw. Use a mandoline or very sharp knife to finely shred the brussels sprouts. Combine the yoghurt and dill in a small bowl. Season well.

Heat the oil in a small frying pan over medium heat. Add the caraway seeds and cook, stirring, for 30 seconds, or until aromatic. Remove from the heat. Stir in the lemon juice and honey and season. Cover to keep warm.

Place the carrot matchsticks in a large microwave-safe bowl with 1 tablespoon water. Cover with plastic wrap and microwave on high for 2 minutes.

Now add the shredded brussels sprouts to the bowl and re-cover. Microwave on high for 1 minute. Remove from the microwave and drain any excess water from the vegetables. Add the celery and caraway dressing and toss until well combined. Transfer to a serving platter and top with the yoghurt mixture. Taste and season with more salt and a squeeze of lemon, if necessary.

Arrange the fish on top of the slaw and serve garnished with extra dill and lemon wedges on the side.

TIP

In summer serve with Asian Summer Kool Slaw (page 173).

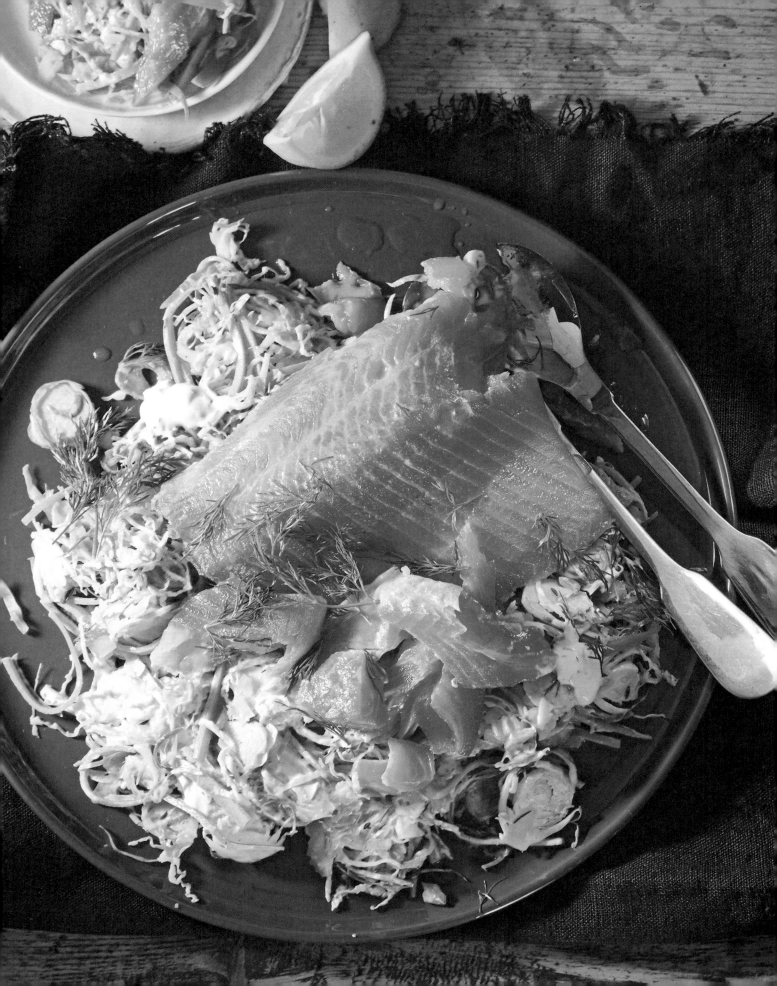

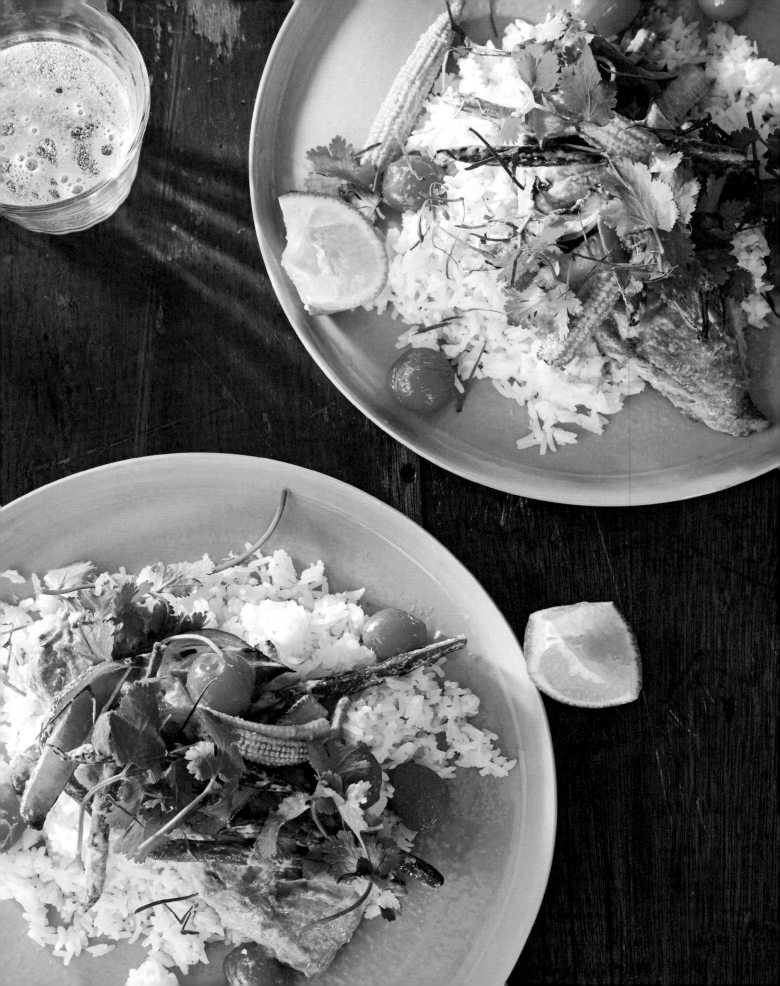

THAI FISH BAKE
with Coconut Rice

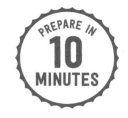

Think of this as a deconstructed curry that uses the security and comfort of oven cooking rather than the 'Oh-darn-it-I've-burnt-the-thick-curry-on-the-bottom-of-the-saucepan-and-overcooked-the-fish' dangers of unattended stovetop cooking. Reassuring or what!?!

SERVES 4 **PREP:** 10 MINS (PLUS 10 MINS STANDING) **COOKING:** 25 MINS

2 tablespoons red curry paste

2 cm knob of ginger, peeled and finely grated

1 bunch coriander, stems and roots washed and finely chopped, leaves reserved

2 tablespoons melted coconut oil

4 × 200 g skin-on firm white fish fillets (such as snapper, barramundi, blue eye trevalla or ling), pin-boned

1 red onion, cut into thin wedges

1 × 250 g punnet cherry tomatoes

1 × 115 g packet baby corn, halved lengthways

100 g baby green beans (or use snow peas or chunks of par-cooked eggplant instead)

8 kaffir lime leaves (if you have them), plus a few extra shredded leaves to serve

1 × 270 ml can coconut milk

1 lime, cut into wedges

COCONUT RICE
400 g (2 cups) long-grain rice

1 × 270 ml can coconut milk

Preheat the oven to 180°C/160°C fan-forced. Combine the curry paste, ginger, coriander stems and roots and melted coconut oil in the base of a roasting tin. Stir well, then add the fish and turn to coat in the curry mixture.

Place the onion, tomatoes, baby corn, green beans and kaffir lime leaves (if using) around the fish in the tin. Bake for 18–20 minutes or until the fish flakes when tested with a fork.

While the fish bakes, make the coconut rice. Rinse the rice in a sieve under cold running water until the water runs clear. Place the rice, coconut milk and 500 ml (2 cups) water in a saucepan and bring to the boil over high heat. Once it boils, reduce the heat to very low. Cover the pan and simmer for 10 minutes.

Remove from the heat and set aside but DON'T REMOVE THE LID. Leave to stand for 10 minutes and then REMOVE THE LID – taa daaah! – and fluff the rice with a fork.

Transfer the cooked fish to a tray, cover and keep warm. Place the roasting tin with the veggies and sauce still in it over medium heat. Stir in the coconut milk. Simmer, stirring occasionally, for 5 minutes, or until the sauce thickens. While the sauce is thickening, demand that everyone comes to the table right now.

Arrange the rice and fish on a warmed platter or distribute among individual warmed plates. Locate your oven mitts and hurry people along.

As soon as everyone is seated, squeeze half the lime wedges into the sauce and stir. Grab your oven mitts (you'll need them because the tin will be hot!) and pour the contents of the tin over the rice and fish. Be quick, as you don't want the lime juice to cook out!

Sprinkle with coriander leaves and extra shredded kaffir lime leaves, and serve with the remaining lime wedges for squeezing over.

TIP

To make toasted coconut rice, toast 35 g desiccated coconut in a small frying pan over medium heat. Cook, tossing, for 2 minutes, or until the coconut is toasted. Add all but 2 tablespoons to the rice, coconut milk and water before bringing this mixture to the boil. Once cooked, sprinkle the reserved coconut over the top of the rice. This is nice!

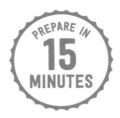

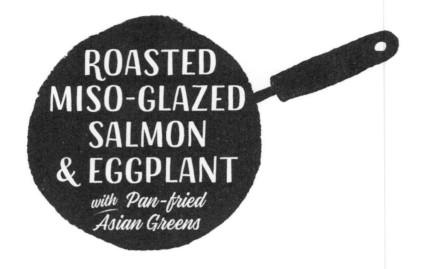

ROASTED MISO-GLAZED SALMON & EGGPLANT

with Pan-fried Asian Greens

Nasu Dengaku sounds like the name of a progressive jazz drummer but it's actually one of the world's great eggplant dishes. 'Miso-marinated black cod' sounds like the name of Nobu Matsuhisa's most plagiarised dish which is, actually, because … it is.

Here we bring eggplant and Australia's most popular fish together with a sweetened miso – or what is known in Japan as a *sumiso* – which is the ingredient that makes that black cod so special.

SERVES 4 PREP: 15 MINS COOKING: 25 MINS

2 tablespoons white miso paste
2 tablespoons mirin
1 tablespoon honey
60 ml (¼ cup) soy sauce
2 tablespoons olive oil
4 Lebanese eggplants, halved lengthways or 1 eggplant, cut lengthways into 3 cm thick batons
4 x 200 g skinless salmon fillets, pin-boned
4 cm knob of ginger, peeled and finely grated
2 teaspoons sesame oil
1 bunch gai lan, stems trimmed, thicker ones halved, leaves reserved separately
cooked brown rice, to serve
1 spring onion, thinly sliced (optional)
Homemade Togarashi, to serve (or use storebought)

HOMEMADE TOGARASHI (JAPANESE 7-SPICE POWDER)

1 teaspoon salt
2 teaspoons finely grated orange or tangerine zest
1 sheet toasted nori
1 teaspoon Sichuan peppercorns (or black peppercorns)
2 teaspoons dried chilli flakes
2 teaspoons toasted sesame seeds
½ teaspoon garlic powder
1 teaspoon hemp seeds or white poppy seeds (if you have them)

For the togarashi, mix the salt with the citrus zest and set aside to infuse. Grind or blitz the nori and peppercorns together. Transfer to the zest and salt mix, then add all the remaining ingredients and mix everything together well and use immediately. If you want to make this spicy sprinkle for the pantry, then use dried tangerine peel instead of fresh citrus, and grind it to a powder with the nori.

Preheat the oven to 200°C/180°C fan-forced. Line a large baking tray with baking paper. Combine the miso, mirin, honey and 1 tablespoon of the soy sauce in a small jug or mug.

Heat 1 tablespoon of olive oil in a non-stick frying pan over medium–high heat. Add the eggplant, cut-side down, and cook for 4–5 minutes, until really golden. Transfer to the lined baking tray, cut-side up. Brush the top of the eggplant thickly with half the miso mixture. Roast for 5 minutes.

While the eggplant is roasting, heat the remaining olive oil in the pan. Add the salmon fillets and cook for 1 minute on each side or until golden.

Transfer the salmon fillets to the tray with the eggplant and brush them with the remaining miso mixture. Return to the oven for a further 10 minutes, or until the eggplant is tender and sticky and the salmon flakes when tested with a fork.

Meanwhile, combine the ginger and remaining soy in a bowl.

Heat the sesame oil in a large frying pan or wok over medium heat. Add the gai lan stems and cook for 2 minutes, or until the stems are starting to turn translucent. Now throw in the gai lan leaves and the gingered soy mixture. Move the gai lan around and cook for a couple more minutes.

Serve the salmon and sweet miso eggplant on brown rice with the salty gai lan. Sprinkle with spring onion (if using) and togarashi and serve.

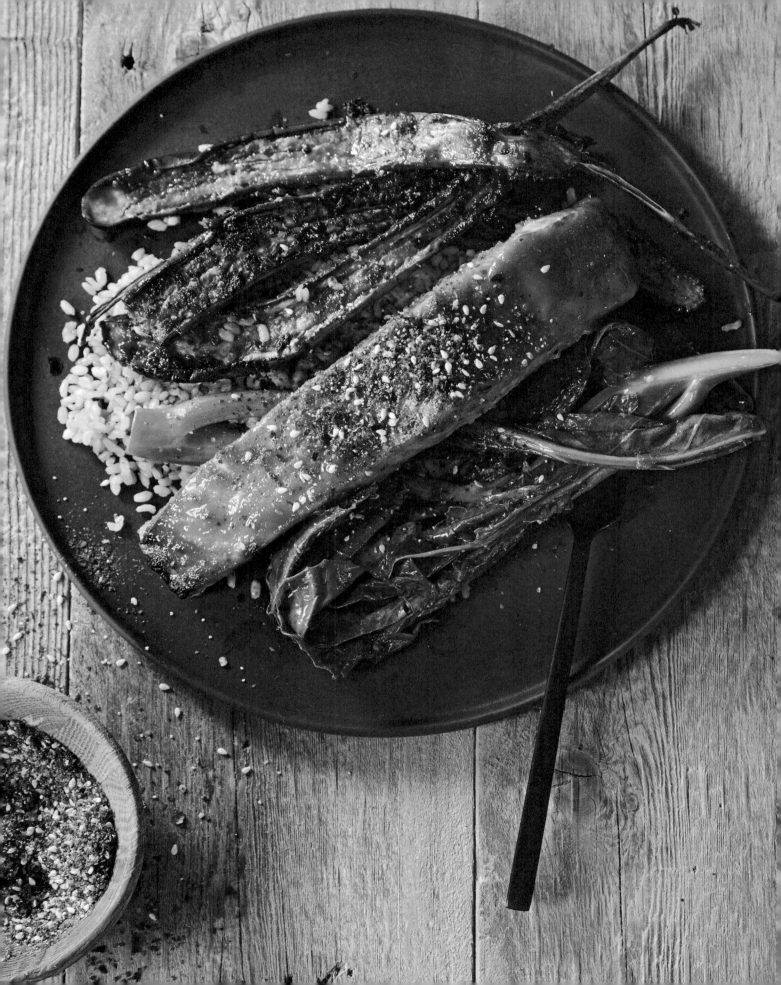

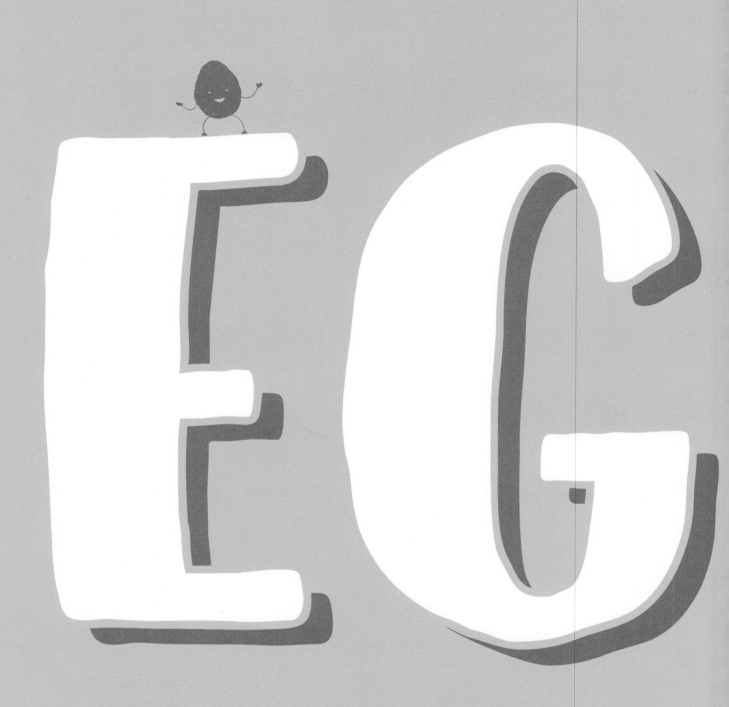

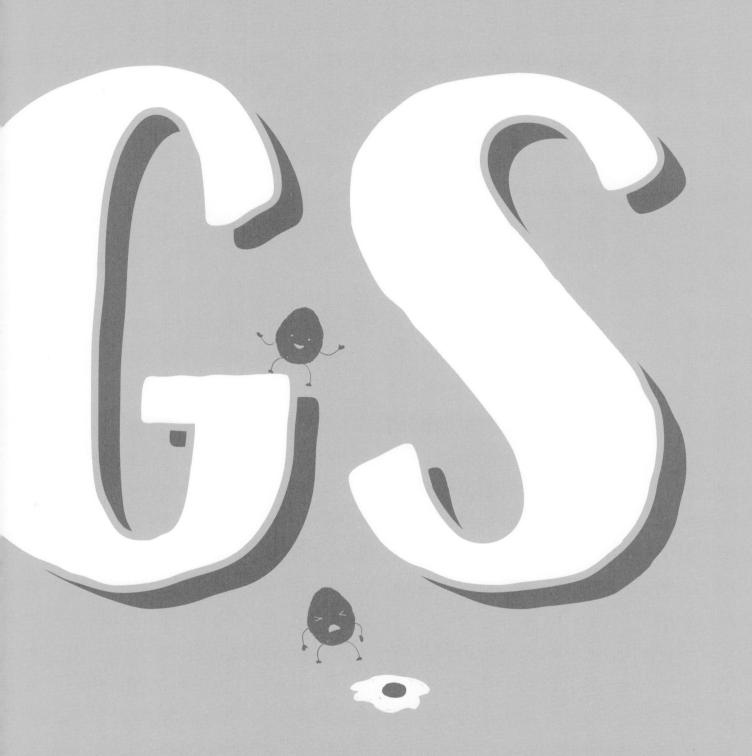

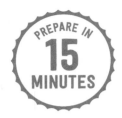

IMPOSSIBLE QUICHE
(That's actually very possible)

The internet might have made us cynical consumers but, while we are often suspicious of claims made online, we still bite – like that rainbow trout that can't resist hitting the same fly time and time again – at the same old clickbait tricks.

We are especially susceptible to recipe features with the word 'impossible', 'hack' or 'cheat' in the screaming headline – and even more, if accompanied by any number over four: '12 FOOD HACKS TO CHANGE YOUR LIFE'; 'THE IMPOSSIBLE QUICHE RECIPE YOU HAVE TO SEE TO BELIEVE'; 'TRUMP CHEF'S NUDE FOOD CHEATS YOU NEVER SAW COMING'; etc, etc.

Before the internet, this recipe was merely a take on quiche Lorraine – which is too often a sadly forgotten gem of the kitchen – but made with the added vegetable goodness of broccolini. The 'impossible' trick of creating a base (seemingly magically) during the cooking process, as the flour separates out of the mixture, is hardly new either: impossible lemon pie recipes date back to the 1950s.

If you want to find this recipe online now, search for 'YOU'D NEVER IMAGINE THE HIDDEN SEX POTENCY OF THIS IMPOSSIBLE BROCCOLINI BAKE!'

SERVES 6 **PREP:** 15 MINS **COOKING:** 40 MINS

2 teaspoons olive oil
200 g thick-cut speck, kaiserfleisch, pancetta or just good old smoked bacon, cut into 5 mm batons
1 bunch broccolini, stems halved lengthways
250 ml (1 cup) milk
125 ml (½ cup) thickened cream
2 teaspoons dijon mustard
4 eggs
sea salt and freshly ground black pepper
75 g (½ cup) self-raising flour
1 tablespoon chopped chives
80 g (1 cup) coarsely grated gruyere, comte or vintage cheddar

Preheat the oven to 200°C/180°C fan-forced. Grease a 5 cm deep, 26 cm round ovenproof dish.

Heat the oil in a non-stick frying pan over medium–high heat. Add the speck and cook for 5 minutes, or until golden. Place in the greased dish.

Add the broccolini to the frying pan and add a little splash of water. Cover and cook for 2 minutes, or until bright green and tender-crisp. Transfer to a plate.

Combine the milk, cream, mustard and eggs in a jug. Season.

Combine the flour and chives in a large bowl. Gradually whisk the milk mixture into the flour until well combined. Stir in the cheese. Pour into the greased dish on top of the bacon.

Distribute the broccolini evenly over the surface, gently pressing it into the egg mixture, then give the dish a little wiggle to settle the mixture. Bake for 30 minutes, or until golden and just set. Eat and wonder!

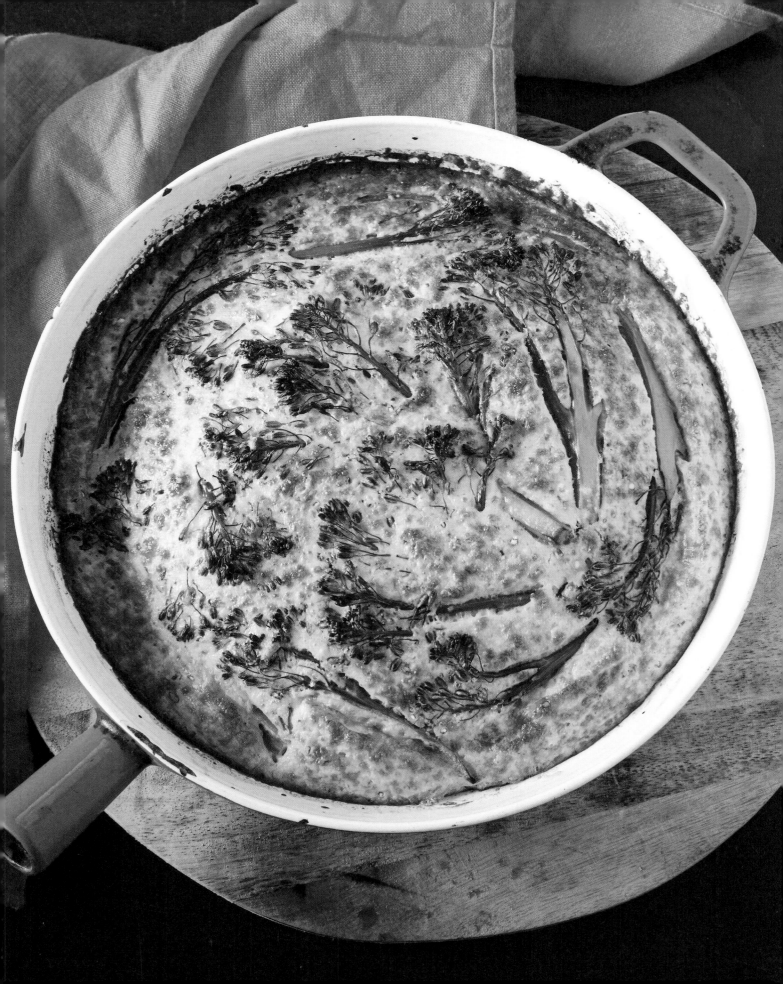

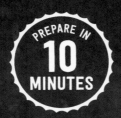

MUFFIN TIN FRITTATAS

– A GREAT IDEA FOR DINNER ...

Small things cook quicker, making this frittata perfect for a quick dinner. But what makes this recipe so ace is that you can flavour the individual frittata bases with anything your friends or family desire. The ideas here are just the teeny tip of a very big culinary iceberg.

MAKES 10   PREP: 10 MINS   COOKING: 40 MINS

THE BASIC FRITTATA MIX
6 eggs
125 ml (½ cup) pouring cream
3 spring onions, thinly sliced
sea salt and freshly ground
  black pepper

FLAVOURINGS FOR MUFFIN TIN FRITTATA #1
200 g baby spinach leaves
170 g (1 cup) cooked quinoa
2 tablespoons coarsely chopped dill
zest of 1 lemon (keep the lemon so you can squeeze a little juice over each muffin for garnish)
150 g feta, broken into large chunks

Preheat the oven to 180°C/160°C fan-forced. Grease ten holes in a 12 hole muffin tin.

Wash the spinach and, with a little of the water still clinging to the leaves, place in a non-stick frying pan. Cook, stirring, for 1–2 minutes, until the spinach just wilts. Set aside to cool then coarsely chop.

Whisk together the eggs, cream and spring onion in a large jug. Season.

Once the spinach has cooled completely, use your hands to squeeze out as much liquid as possible. Add the spinach, quinoa, dill and lemon zest to the frittata mixture. Divide evenly among the muffin holes. Add the feta, pressing some in and leaving some exposed on the surface. Bake for 30–35 minutes, until set and golden.

Set aside for 5 minutes to cool in the tin. Use a flat-bladed knife to slip around the edge of the muffins, making them easier to remove. Serve with a little squeeze of lemon juice.

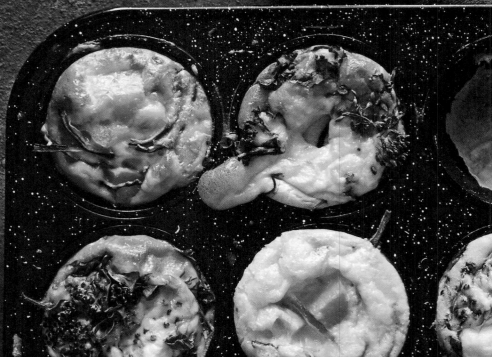

12 MORE MUFFIN TIN FRITTATAS

Now you know the base frittata mixture of cream, eggs and spring onions, there are loads of ways to customise it with any number of sexy combos you might have in the fridge or pantry. Here are some of my favourites:

1. Half-fill each muffin hole with slices of cooked potato, lightly fried chunks of chorizo and squares of capsicum. Cover with the frittata mixture. Top with a grated hard cheese, such as manchego or parmesan, then bake.

2. Half-fill each muffin hole with chopped leftover roast potatoes, cooked and quartered brussels sprouts and shredded corned beef. Cover with the frittata mixture and bake.

3. Add shredded basil, deseeded and diced tomatoes and shredded parmesan to the frittata mixture. Place a halved bocconcini ball in each hole and bake. Save the tomato seeds and add them to a dressing for a salad accompaniment.

4. Stir 1 small can of creamed corn and sauteed chunky chopped bacon into the frittata mixture. Pour into the muffin holes then scatter each with 1 cm diced gruyere pieces. Bake.

5. Make the frittata mixture in a large jug and toss in some leftover spaghetti with shredded parmesan and basil. Spoon into each muffin hole then press a baby bocconcini ball in the centre of each. Top each with a few halved cherry tomatoes, then bake.

6. Curl a rasher of streaky bacon around the edge of each muffin hole. Throw in lots of deseeded and diced tomato. Fill up with the frittata mixture and bake. Serve on rounds of buttered toast that have been smeared with English mustard, HP or tomato sauce!

7. Thinly slice the tender part of asparagus stalks into coins and reserve the tips. Toss the teeny asparagus coins into the frittata mixture with lots of fresh dill and chopped smoked salmon. Fill the muffin holes with the frittata mixture and lay the asparagus tips on top. Once baked, serve draped with extra smoked salmon.

8. Stir chunks of leftover roast pumpkin, thinly sliced red onion and crumbled feta or grated cheddar into your frittata mixture, divide among the muffin holes and bake.

9. Cook a cup of diced mushroom in a frying pan until any liquid has evaporated. Toss into the frittata mixture with thyme leaves and three cheeses (any three cheeses you like actually, but try slices of brie with grated gruyere and vintage cheddar). Bake.

10. Saute zucchini slices, small broccolini florets and chopped kale until soft. Add to the frittata mixture with a little touch of basil pesto, then bake.

11. Cut a couple of zucchini into ribbons and blanch by pouring boiling water over them. After a minute remove and pat them dry. Curl the ribbons into the muffin holes so that from above they look like rosebud petals. Crumble over goat's cheese and fill up with the frittata mixture. Cook until the egg is just set, which won't take long! Serve with a herby vinaigrette cut with lemon juice and zest.

12. Mix diced ham, grated cheddar and a generous spoon of dijon mustard into the mixture, then bake.

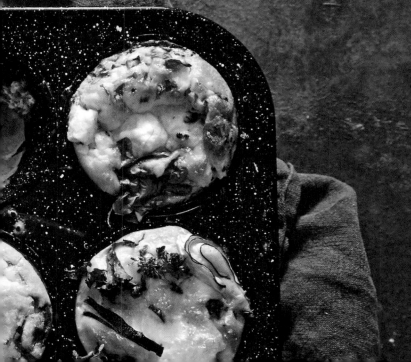

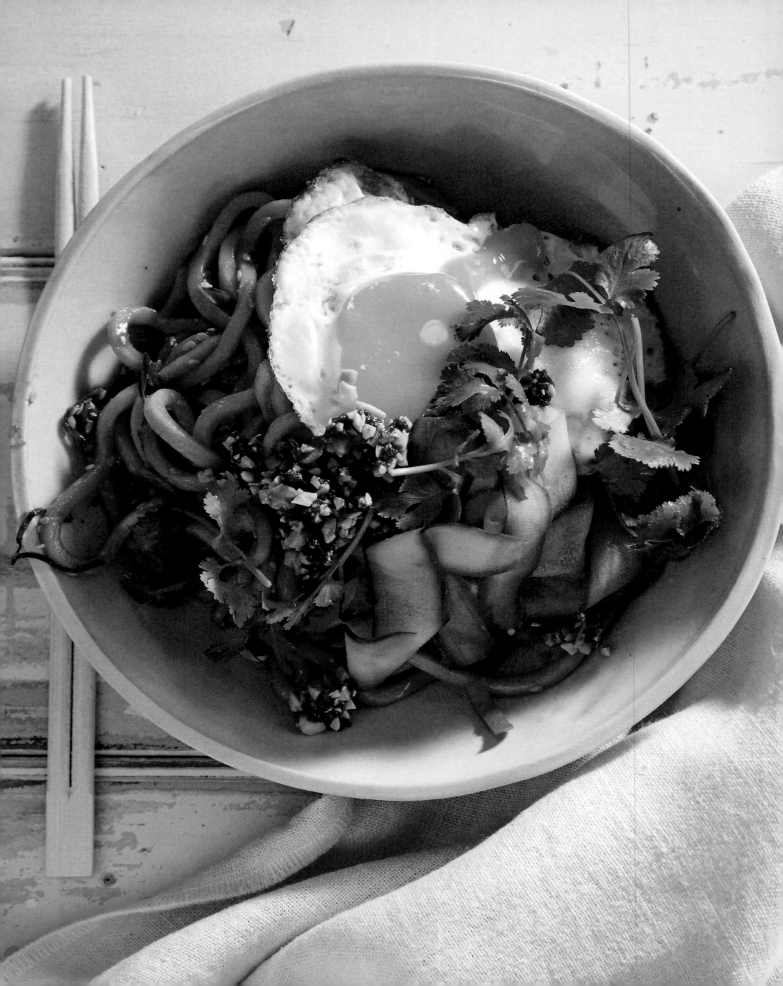

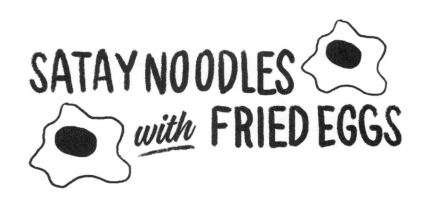
SATAY NOODLES with FRIED EGGS

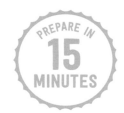

Sure, this might be a bit of a stoner dish but it's also totally delicious because the satay has more crunch and funk than the usual cheat's peanut butter version. The fried eggs and noodles will thank you for that!!!

These noodles are also a great final resting place for all manner of orphan veg from your crisper drawer, whether it's those few mushrooms at the bottom of a crumpled brown paper bag, that last quarter of carrot going soft in the corner, a toddler's handful of bean shoots, or the last head of broccoli. Just slice them thinly and cook in the egg pan after the eggs, but before adding the noodles.

SERVES 4 PREP: 15 MINS COOKING: 10 MINS

80 g (½ cup) unsalted roasted peanuts
1 heaped tablespoon XO sauce
1 teaspoon sesame oil
500 g fresh hokkien noodles
1 tablespoon peanut oil
4 eggs
40 g (¼ cup) sesame seeds
4 cm knob of ginger, peeled and finely grated
60 ml (¼ cup) light soy sauce
2 tablespoons kecap manis
4 spring onions, thinly sliced
coriander sprigs, to serve

PICKLED CUCUMBER RIBBONS
3 Lebanese cucumbers, peeled into ribbons (feel free to add other orphan veg, such as lone carrots or radishes; just slice or julienne finely)
1 small red chilli, deseeded and thinly sliced (optional)
2 teaspoons caster sugar
1 teaspoon sea salt
1 teaspoon rice wine vinegar

Place the peanuts in a mortar and use a pestle to crush coarsely. Add the XO sauce and mash together with the peanuts. Stir in the sesame oil, but keep things a little chunky. You can do this by pulsing with a stick blender too.

To make the pickled cucumber, place the cucumber ribbons and chilli (if using) in a zip-lock bag (or small bowl) and sprinkle with the sugar, salt and vinegar. Seal the bag and turn it, gently tossing the cucumber ribbons so they are evenly coated with the pickle mix. Set aside for about 10 minutes to cure.

Prepare the noodles following the packet instructions. Drain well.

Meanwhile, heat the oil in a large non-stick frying pan over medium heat. Crack the eggs into the pan. Cover and cook gently for 2–3 minutes, until the whites have just set and the yolks are still runny. Transfer the eggs to a plate and cover while you finish the noodles. (This will cloud that yucky membrane on the top of the eggs and finish cooking them.)

Fry the sesame seeds in the same pan over medium heat for 2–3 minutes, until toasted. Add the ginger and stir-fry for 1 minute, or until aromatic. Add the soy sauce and kecap manis and bring to the boil. Add the drained noodles and spring onion and toss until the noodles are well coated and everything is heated through.

Divide the noodles among serving bowls. Top with the eggs, a spoonful of the peanut mixture, some pickled cucumber ribbons and coriander sprigs.

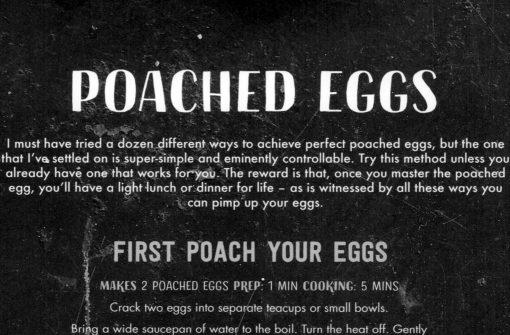

POACHED EGGS

I must have tried a dozen different ways to achieve perfect poached eggs, but the one that I've settled on is super-simple and eminently controllable. Try this method unless you already have one that works for you. The reward is that, once you master the poached egg, you'll have a light lunch or dinner for life – as is witnessed by all these ways you can pimp up your eggs.

FIRST POACH YOUR EGGS

MAKES 2 POACHED EGGS **PREP:** 1 MIN **COOKING:** 5 MINS

Crack two eggs into separate teacups or small bowls.

Bring a wide saucepan of water to the boil. Turn the heat off. Gently slide the eggs into the water. Leave for 3½ minutes for soft runny eggs, or longer if you prefer them more set. Use a slotted spoon to transfer to a plate lined with paper towel to drain slightly – or just gently shake the slotted spoon to drain, to avoid the egg sticking to the paper towel.

20 INTERESTING WAYS TO EAT POACHED EGGS

1. Toss poached eggs in dukkah for a spicy, nutty finish and serve with Cauliflower Hummus and Roasted Red Onions and Grapes (page 202).

2. For an easy breakfast or brinner-style light dinner, spread slices of sourdough toast with avocado and top with steamed asparagus and poached eggs. Sprinkle with crumbled goat's cheese or feta and finish with a drizzle of spicy tomato sauce or relish.

3. Toss chunks of cooked peeled potato in a frying pan with curry powder, fried onion, cumin seeds and a generous spoon of heat-popped mustard seeds. Serve topped with eggs, fresh coriander, sliced green chillies and a lemon wedge. Add fried curry leaves if you have them.

4. Make individual pans of leeks cooked with spinach and finished with white wine and cream. Top with poached eggs and serve sprinkled with crispy bacon bits and toasted baguette slices.

5. Make a breakfast or dinner bowl with some sauteed kale, bacon, mushrooms and brown rice or quinoa. Top with a poached egg and avocado slices and finish with my Nori and Macadamia Sprinkle (page 118).

6. Add to one of your favourite bowl recipes.

7. Add to Japanese Garage Chicken (page 17).

8. Serve Cherry Tomato, Chickpea and Chorizo Can-atouille (page 256) on toast and top with an egg for a quick breakfast feast or light lunch.

9. Spread a warm flatbread with cream cheese, avocado and chopped coriander (stalks 'n' all), top with two poachies, a squirt of Kewpie mayo, lots of black pepper and a squeeze of lime. Roll up and tan quickly in a very hot sandwich press.

10. Replace the garlic prawns in the Zucchini Zoodles (page 216) with poached eggs.

11. Heat a flatbread and load one half with a spoonful of warm black beans (page 270). Top with grated cheese to melt, loads of pan-toasted corn hit with lime juice, fresh coriander and two poached eggs. Fold and serve.

12. Barbecue large flat mushrooms and top with a dollop of pesto, a poached egg and a few roasted cherry truss tomatoes.

13. Toss cooked pasta with blanched spring vegetables and a very light creamy sauce. Top with poached eggs and sprinkle with lemon salt.

14. Puree soft-poached eggs with melted brown butter and a squeeze of lemon to make an interesting dressing for asparagus or pan-fried fish.

15. Drizzle poached eggs with a chilli-caramel and serve with brown rice and pickled cucumber (page 139).

16. Buy a big serve of hot crispy chips. Top with fried rounds of chorizo, half a dozen poached eggs and finish with chopped parsley and dollops of the Smoky Mayo on page 247, using the rendered fat from the chorizo in place of some of the grapeseed oil.

17. Make a cauliflower and blue cheese soup (page 215) and top with a poached egg.

18. Make some quick chilli beans and top with a poached egg, chopped avocado and fresh coriander.

19. Serve on any fritters you fancy (pages 210–211).

20. Top a roast veggie mix (pages 218–219) with a couple of poachies.

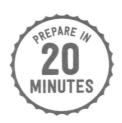

PREPARE IN
20
MINUTES

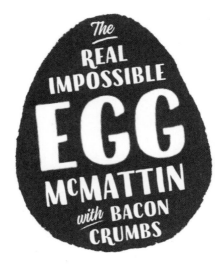

The
REAL IMPOSSIBLE EGG McMATTIN *with* **BACON CRUMBS**

Imagine a muffin you cut open to reveal an oozy soft-boiled egg!!! Impossible??? No it's not!!! I discovered it at Craftsman and Wolves in San Francisco. It is a little fiddly and time-consuming, so only approach this recipe when you are in a calm and unpressured state of mind – and remember that, for all the work, the impact is worth it.

You might also like to note that no other recipe in this book took quite the amount of testing, re-testing and re-shaping by my in-house recipe genius and long-term collaborator Michelle Southan. Nice work, Shel!!!

Fiddly it might be, but there is nothing more impressive than pulling muffins fresh from the oven that have a gooey, runny egg-yolk centre. I'm tipping it as the new savoury version of the oozy chocolate fondant!

MAKES 6 PREP: 20 MINS (PLUS 45 MINS FREEZING) COOKING: 30 MINS

10 eggs at room temperature (you need 2 for the batter and 6 for the muffins, but allow 2 extra in case you undercook them or mess up the peeling!)

70 g hickory-smoked bacon rashers, finely chopped

35 g (½ cup) fresh breadcrumbs

10 g butter

1 tablespoon chopped flat-leaf parsley

300 g (2 cups) self-raising flour, plus extra to coat the eggs

65 g (¾ cup) coarsely grated cheddar

1 zucchini (about 165 g), coarsely grated

185 ml (¾ cup) milk

1 × 125 g can creamed corn

sea salt and freshly ground black pepper

Pineapple Ketchup (page 68) or purchased tomato relish, to serve

Place 8 eggs in a saucepan just big enough to hold them. Cover with cold water so they float. Place over high heat and stir constantly until the water comes to the boil. (This centres the eggs – and trust me this is super-important – so the yolks are not too close to the edge when peeling later.)

As soon as the water boils (not a crazy boil, just the start of bigger bubbles coming to the surface) remove the pan from the heat and set aside for 3½ minutes. Drain and set aside. These eggs will be very delicate indeed.

Now the high-pressure task of peeling the eggs … approach this task with all the care you would apply to defusing a bomb. Tap each egg on a flat bench very, very carefully, working all the way around. Submerge in cold water and peel – again, very, very carefully. Gently place the peeled eggs in a container or bowl in a single layer and freeze for 45 minutes. Don't panic if you mess up the peeling; remember that you've got safety-net eggs on standby.

Heat a small non-stick frying pan over medium–high heat. Add the bacon and cook, stirring, for 2 minutes, or until starting to become golden. Stir rhythmically to reduce your heart rate, which will have savagely spiked with the pressure of peeling those delicate soft-boiled eggs. Add the breadcrumbs and butter. Cook, stirring, for 3–4 minutes, until light golden. Remove from the heat and stir in the parsley.

Preheat the oven to 200°C/180°C fan-forced. Lightly oil a six hole (each hole 250 ml capacity) muffin tin.

Combine the flour, cheese and zucchini in a large bowl. Use a fork to lightly whisk together the milk, creamed corn and remaining eggs in a jug. Season, then add to the flour mixture and stir until well combined.

With the tenderness of swaddling a newborn, roll the lightly frozen eggs in the extra flour to coat. Spoon half the zucchini mixture into the muffin holes. Gently press an egg into the centre of the mixture in each muffin hole and use a spoon to carefully cover completely with the rest of the mixture. Sprinkle with the bacon crumbs, then bake for 20 minutes, or until golden. Serve with pineapple ketchup or tomato relish.

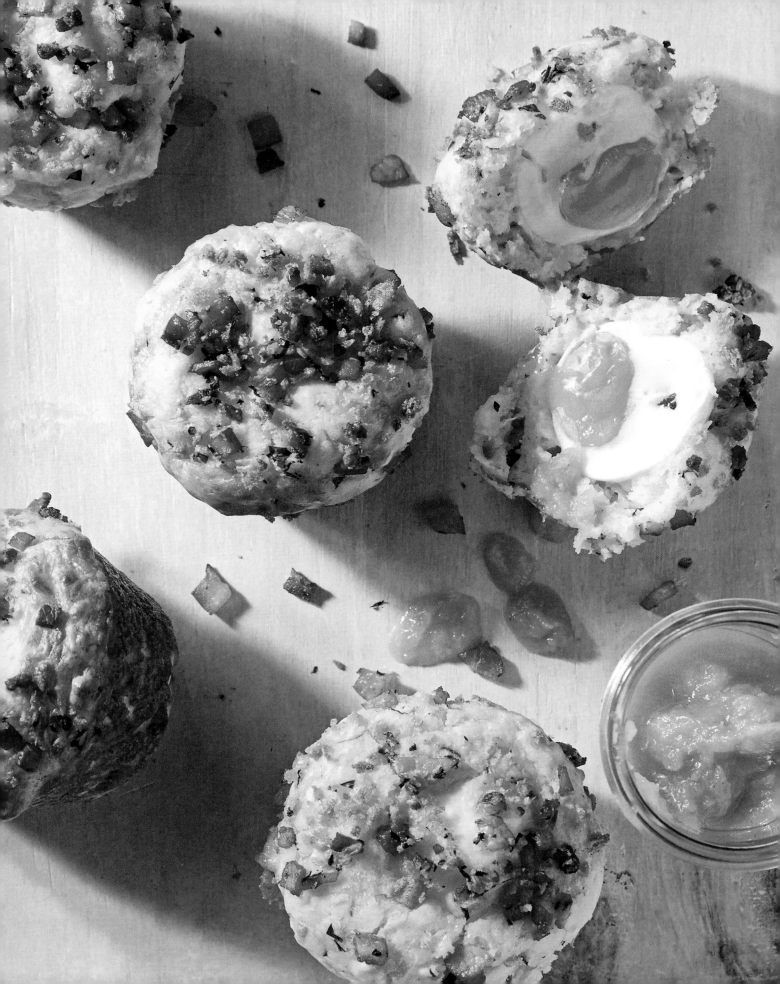

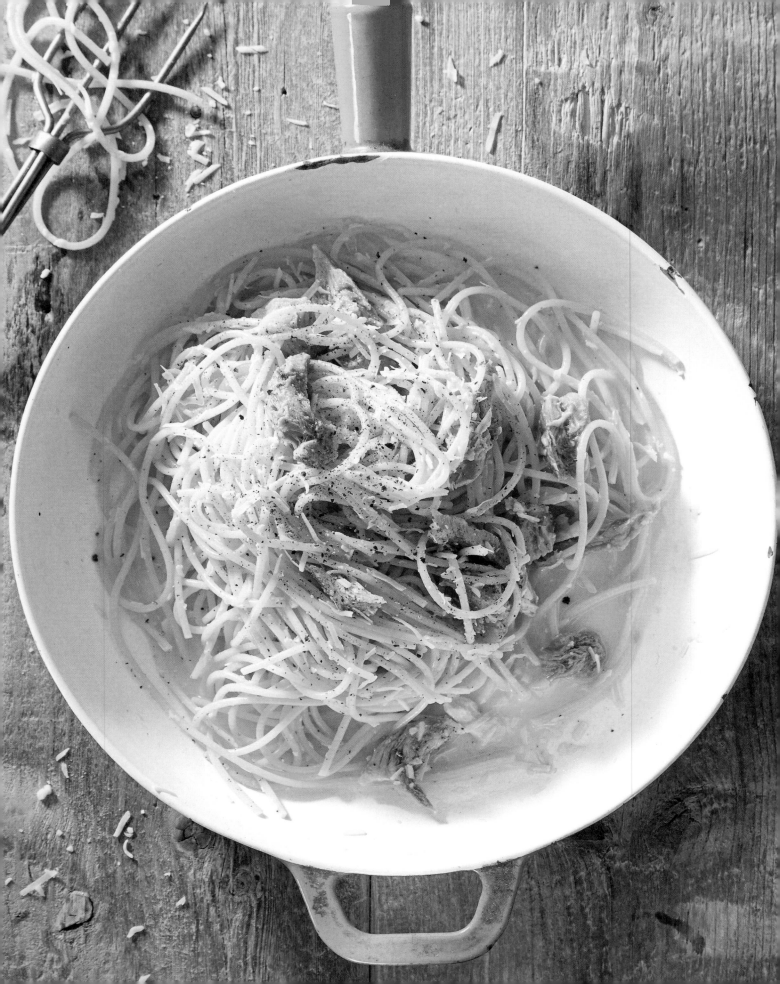

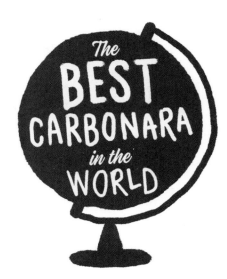

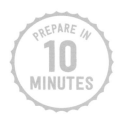

Honestly, it is! While the crispness of bacon is lovely, the smokiness of ham hock is even better. The prep time is super-quick too – assuming you are organised.

PS: Respect to the guys at Otto in Brisbane, where I first saw hock being used in a carbonara.

The small print: If any Italian foodie fascist accuses you of making a bastardised version of carbonara, point out that the first versions were most likely made not with guanciale and pecorino, but with the American eggs and Canadian bacon from the backpacks of the US GIs who 'liberated' Rome.

SERVES 4   PREP: 10 MINS   COOKING: 2 HOURS

1 × 950 g ham hock
6 black peppercorns
2 fresh or dried bay leaves
2 celery stalks, cut into large pieces
1 carrot, cut into large chunks
4 eggs
70 g (1 cup) grated parmesan,
   plus extra to serve
freshly ground black pepper
400 g thin spaghetti

Place the ham hock in a stockpot. Add 2 litres of water, along with the peppercorns, bay leaves, celery and carrot. Cover, and bring to the boil over high heat. Reduce the heat to medium–low and simmer, covered, for 1 hour 45 minutes, or until the meat falls away from the bone.

Use tongs to remove the ham hock and set it aside until cool enough to handle.

Strain the ham cooking liquid, discarding the vegetables and spices, and keep it warm.

Remove the ham from the bone, discarding the bone and any rind. Shred the ham and keep it warm.

Use a fork to lightly whisk the eggs in a large jug. Stir in the parmesan and season with plenty of black pepper.

Cook the spaghetti in plenty of boiling salted water for 1 minute less than it says on the packet, until al dente. Drain and return to the pan, but remove from the heat.

Add 125 ml (½ cup) of the warm reserved ham cooking liquid and the shredded ham and toss until combined. Add the egg mixture to the hot pasta and toss until well combined. Act quickly – if overcooked, the egg will scramble. Yuck!

Divide among serving bowls. Season with pepper and top with extra parmesan.

TIP

Don't waste the remaining ham stock. Transfer it to an airtight container and freeze for up to 3 months. Thaw and use in gravy, soups, casseroles …

BETTER PASTA BAKES

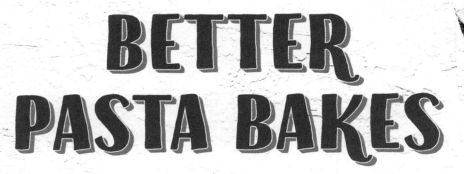

For as long as there have been ovens and pasta, there have been pasta bakes. From an Italian lasagne to a Greek pastitsio, this method of cooking delivers two great improvements to your standard plate of pasta. Firstly, the sauce gets to thicken and soak into the pasta; secondly, the dish gets a chance to develop a delicious golden crust which might include gnarly ends of jutting-out and crunchy pasta and most-desirable golden, crispy cheesy bits. In short, you get all the joyful pleasure that only the Maillard reaction can deliver – which is the technical term scientists use when things go brown and get extra tasty.

The strange thing is that there really aren't that many classic dishes that fall into this pasta bake category. Aside from lasagne and pastitsio, most prominent are cannelloni (with either rolled crepes or pasta tubes filled with ricotta and spinach) and mac 'n' cheese; but there's also the Sicilian timballo, Parisian- or Roman-baked gnocchi, American-baked ziti and Maltese timpana. These templates may be limited in number but look online and you'll see that there is no shortage of home-style inspiration and creativity built on these dishes.

Usually the choice of pasta for a pasta bake is limited to pasta sheets for lasagne-style dishes, large tubes for a cannelloni or small pasta shapes, such as macaroni, but why not try spaghetti, angel hair or fettucine if the sauce is quite fine or loose? Also rather than macaroni in your mac 'n' cheese, why not use penne instead? Load it up with a cup or two of peas and flavour the cheese sauce with a crumbled vegetable stock cube. This is a great combo, especially as you'll find that the peas have the cute trick of lodging inside pasta tubes so they look like pasta peashooters!

Don't be afraid to use filled pasta shapes when creating a simpler pasta bake. Just undercook these a little before popping the bake in the oven. Tortellini baked in a bacon veloute with spinach, or loads of ravioli baked in a tray under a layer of tomato sauce and melted cheese like the 'sorrentino' from Buenos Aires are two great starting points for this approach.

A more robust pasta shape, such as a ridged penne, works especially well as it has lots of surfaces for the sauce to cling and soak in to. Think about a tossing it with a rich Sicilian caponata of Mediterranean veg or with a simple tomato sauce with little bocconcini balls that will melt into stringy creaminess in the oven. Dress with a grating of lemon zest or a handful of fresh basil when serving.

Oh, and don't just limit yourself to the more obvious pastas; gnocchi is great baked under wilted silverbeet and gorgonzola. Dress it up with crunchy toasted walnuts before serving. A pureed sauce of peeled broccoli stalks with crispy pancetta, topped with blanched florets and some grated hard cheese is another winner for gnocchi, or for any pasta shape really.

Before you unleash your inner creativity, however, you need to understand the eight simple secrets of the pasta bake, which revolve around three main areas: the sauce or flavourings, the topping and the pasta.

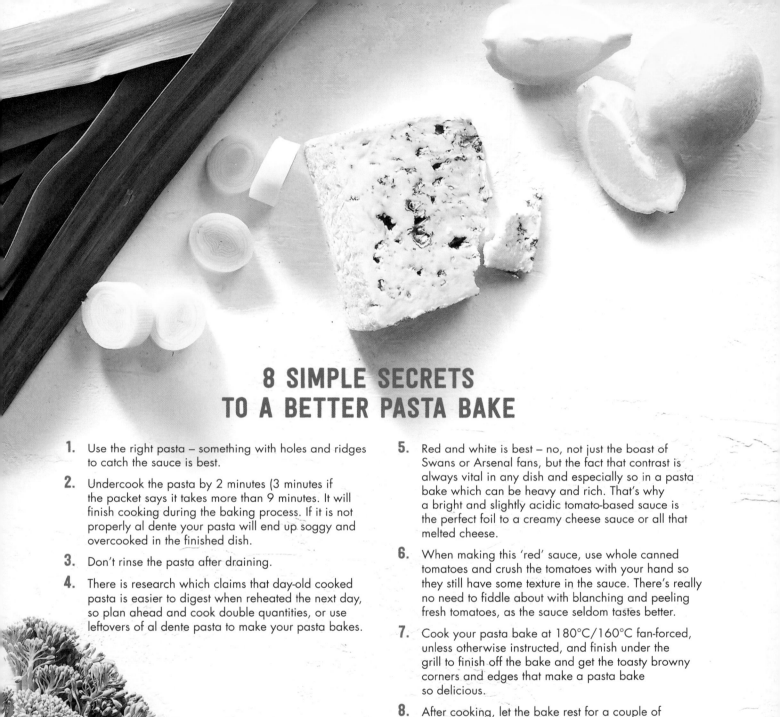

8 SIMPLE SECRETS
TO A BETTER PASTA BAKE

1. Use the right pasta – something with holes and ridges to catch the sauce is best.

2. Undercook the pasta by 2 minutes (3 minutes if the packet says it takes more than 9 minutes. It will finish cooking during the baking process. If it is not properly al dente your pasta will end up soggy and overcooked in the finished dish.

3. Don't rinse the pasta after draining.

4. There is research which claims that day-old cooked pasta is easier to digest when reheated the next day, so plan ahead and cook double quantities, or use leftovers of al dente pasta to make your pasta bakes.

5. Red and white is best – no, not just the boast of Swans or Arsenal fans, but the fact that contrast is always vital in any dish and especially so in a pasta bake which can be heavy and rich. That's why a bright and slightly acidic tomato-based sauce is the perfect foil to a creamy cheese sauce or all that melted cheese.

6. When making this 'red' sauce, use whole canned tomatoes and crush the tomatoes with your hand so they still have some texture in the sauce. There's really no need to fiddle about with blanching and peeling fresh tomatoes, as the sauce seldom tastes better.

7. Cook your pasta bake at 180°C/160°C fan-forced, unless otherwise instructed, and finish under the grill to finish off the bake and get the toasty browny corners and edges that make a pasta bake so delicious.

8. After cooking, let the bake rest for a couple of minutes before hoeing into it.

Everyone loves a pasta bake whether it's a classic lasagne or something more edgy. Over the page are some of my faves.

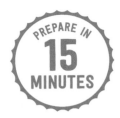

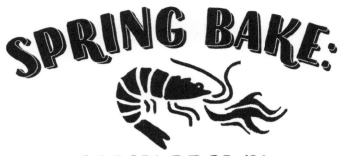

SPRING BAKE:

SPICY PRAWN & TOMATO

Hollywood has made millions out of spicy spring-break movies, so surely you can't begrudge me cashing in with this spring bake? It has less knife-work than *Spring Break Massacre*, is a lot less stressful to make than *Piranha 3D*, cheesier than an Annette Funicello love scene, and only needs a classic 'breakers' actor like Selena Gomez to serve it to make it more fun than a fortnight in Fort Lauderdale wearing a beer-can hat.

SERVES 4 PREP: 15 MINS COOKING: 40 MINS

1 tablespoon olive oil
1 red onion, cut into thin wedges
2 garlic cloves, crushed
½–1 teaspoon dried chilli flakes
1 × 400 g can diced Italian
   tomatoes
80 ml (⅓ cup) white wine
2 oregano sprigs
sea salt and freshly ground
   black pepper
300 g dried risoni pasta
40 g (½ cup) shredded parmesan
32 peeled green prawns, tails
   left intact
1 × 250 g punnet cherry tomatoes,
   halved
200 g feta
lemon wedges, to serve

Preheat the oven to 220°C/200°C fan-forced.

Heat the oil in a large deep ovenproof frying pan over medium–high heat. Add the onion and cook, stirring, for 5 minutes, or until soft. Add the garlic and chilli flakes and cook, stirring, for 1 minute, or until aromatic. Add the tomatoes, wine and oregano sprigs. Bring to a gentle simmer over low heat. Simmer for 5 minutes, or until the sauce thickens slightly. Season.

While the sauce simmers away, cook the pasta in plenty of boiling salted water for 3 minutes less than it says on the packet, until almost al dente. Drain.

Add the drained pasta and parmesan to the tomato mixture and toss until well combined. Top with the prawns, then the cherry tomatoes, ensuring half of them are cut-side down. Crumble on the feta in large chunks.

Bake for 25 minutes, or until the prawns are cooked through and the cheese is starting to brown. Serve with lemon wedges.

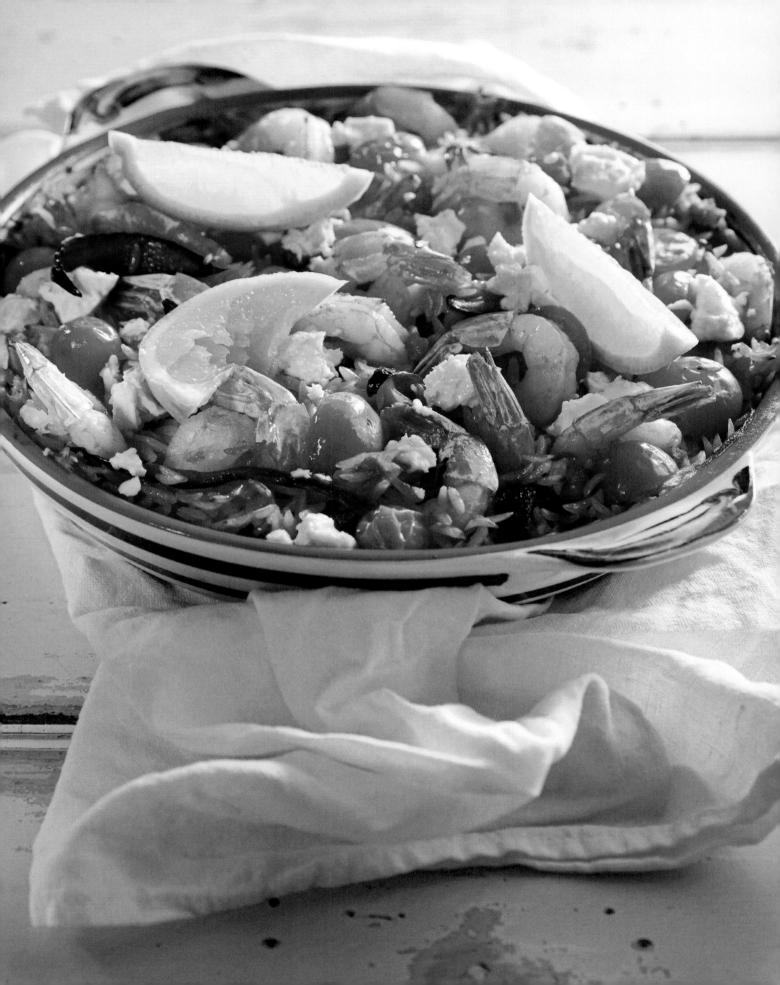

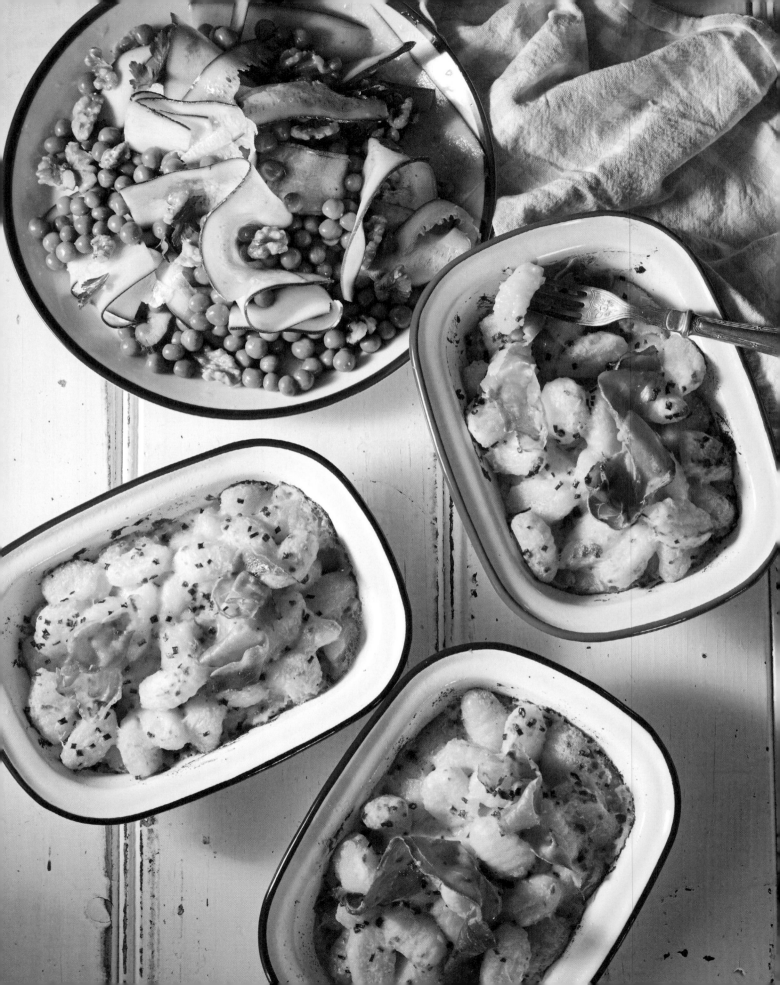

SUMMER BAKE:
VERY, VERY
Cheesy
GNOCCHI BAKE

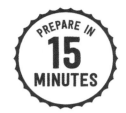

In my five previous books I have written extensively about the secrets of making great gnocchi, but I realise that some people just can't be bothered. Fair goes! Now some wild-eyed zealot cooks would demand you be drummed out of Foodie Town for such a crime but I suspect you, like me, are probably too lazy to even reach for a snare. So here's a recipe that uses packet gnocchi which, employed in this bake, becomes a thing of no little beauty. It's perfect for those nights when you've got less time to cook or you can't be bothered with all the cleaning up.

SERVES 6 PREP: 15 MINS COOKING: 50 MINS

2 × 500 g packets gnocchi
70 g butter
40 g (¼ cup) plain flour
560 ml (2¼ cups) milk
70 g (1 cup) shredded parmesan
40 g (½ cup) coarsely grated
  cheddar
50 g blue cheese, crumbled
⅓ cup chopped chives
freshly ground black pepper
4 slices prosciutto, torn in half
  lengthways
Zucchini Ribbon Salad (page 172),
  to serve

Preheat the oven to 180°C/160°C fan-forced.

Cook the gnocchi in plenty of boiling salted water until it floats to the surface (or as per the packet instructions, which will probably be this, anyway). Drain immediately and return to the pan.

Melt the butter in a saucepan over medium heat until foaming. Add the flour and cook, stirring, for 1–2 minutes, until the mixture bubbles. Remove from the heat. Gradually whisk in the milk until smooth. Stir over medium heat for 5 minutes, or until the mixture thickens. Stir in the parmesan, cheddar and blue cheese. Stir in the chives and season with pepper.

Add the cheese sauce to the gnocchi and toss until well combined. Spoon into six individual ovenproof dishes or one large ovenproof dish. Press the prosciutto into the top (some will stick up and out a little) and bake for 30 minutes, or until golden.

Serve the gnocchi bake with the zucchini salad.

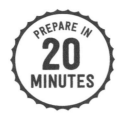

PREPARE IN
20
MINUTES

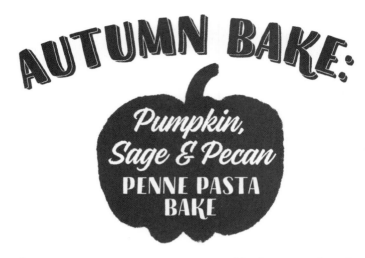

AUTUMN BAKE:

Pumpkin, Sage & Pecan PENNE PASTA BAKE

Please pronounce this pasta 'pen-ne' – ensuring you sound both n's – and not 'pene', which means penis in Italian, and would make this pasta bake far less palatable.

SERVES 6   PREP: 20 MINS   COOKING: 1 HOUR 10 MINS

1 kg butternut pumpkin, peeled, deseeded and cut into 2 cm chunks
125 g pecans or walnuts, coarsely chopped
80 ml (⅓ cup) olive oil
1 teaspoon ground nutmeg
sea salt and freshly ground black pepper
350 g dried penne
1 red onion, thinly sliced
2 garlic cloves, crushed
80 ml (⅓ cup) dry white wine
300 ml pouring cream
250 ml (1 cup) chicken stock
120 g (1½ cups) coarsely grated smoked cheddar
180 g bocconcini, torn in half
1 small bunch sage

Preheat the oven to 180°C/160°C fan-forced. Line a large baking tray with baking paper.

Place the pumpkin and pecans on the prepared baking tray. Drizzle with 1 tablespoon of the oil and sprinkle with nutmeg. Season. Use your hands to give a little toss – thus saving on washing up another bowl (see how helpful I am being here?!). Roast for 40 minutes or until the pumpkin is tender and the nuts are toasted. (Check the nuts about halfway through the cooking time and if they are getting too brown, remove and set aside until needed.)

While the pumpkin roasts, cook the pasta in plenty of boiling salted water for 2 minutes less than it says on the packet, until almost al dente. Drain.

While the pasta water is coming to the boil, start on the sauce. Heat 1 tablespoon of the oil in a large frying pan over medium heat. Add the onion and cook, stirring, for 5 minutes, or until it starts to soften and go a bit relaxed and melty. (Is the water boiling? Then add the pen-ne!) Add the garlic to the onion and cook for 1 minute. Add the wine and reduce until the wine has almost evaporated. This will take about 5 minutes.

Check that pasta now. Don't let it overcook, which would be a disaster to rival that time you came out of the lav at the pub with your skirt tucked into your knickers, when you were out on a date with the hot/cool guy from accounts payable.

Stir the cream and stock into the onion mixture and bring to the boil. Stir in 1 cup of the grated cheddar. Season.

Drain the pasta, then add it to the sauce and toss until well combined. Add half the roasted pumpkin and pecans and toss gently, taking care to not break up the pumpkin too much.

Spoon the pasta mixture into a baking dish. Top with the remaining pumpkin and pecans and sprinkle with the rest of the cheddar. Nestle the bocconcini into the pasta, to create pools of cheesy deliciousness. Bake for 30 minutes, or until golden.

One final touch! While the pasta bakes, heat the remaining oil in a small frying pan over medium heat. Add the sage leaves and fry, stirring occasionally, for 1 minute, or until they are crisp. Transfer to a plate lined with paper towel to drain.

Top the pasta bake with crispy sage leaves to serve.

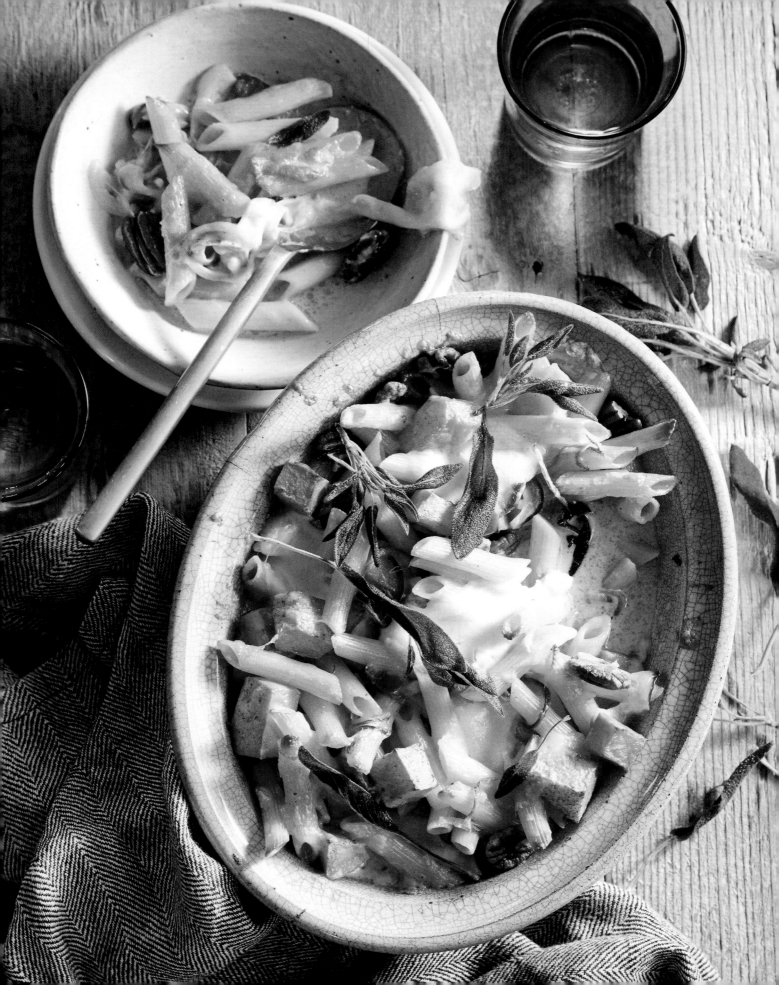

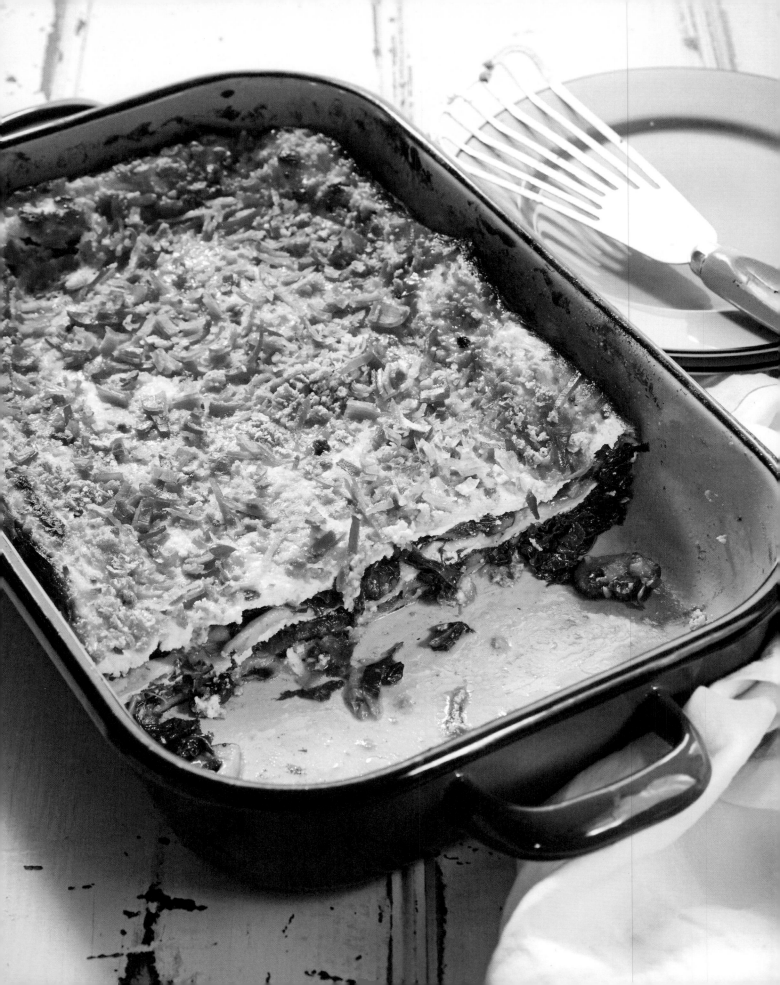

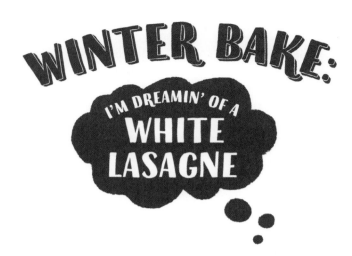

WINTER BAKE:
I'M DREAMIN' OF A WHITE LASAGNE

According to my officially notarised records, there is no peasant dish more complex to create than the classic lasagne – what with making a bolognese and a bechamel and then having to assemble everything. But this white lasagne eschews the tomatoes and the meat sauce for a suitably snowy result. It also dumps the bechamel in exchange for a layer of silky ricotta that is so much lighter, but still gives you the nonna-hug comfort of the classic, with a little less work!

SERVES 8 **PREP:** 45 MINS (PLUS 20 MINS STANDING) **COOKING:** 1 HOUR 10 MINS

60 ml (¼ cup) olive oil
1 leek, thinly sliced
2 garlic cloves, crushed
4 thyme sprigs, plus 2 teaspoons thyme leaves
600 g Swiss brown mushrooms, thickly sliced (you could also use cap, button, portabello)
1 bunch curly kale, thick stems removed, leaves coarsely chopped (you want about 300 g leaves)
1 kg very fresh ricotta
600 ml thickened cream
2 tablespoons dijon mustard
2 eggs
110 g (1½ cups) shredded parmesan
sea salt and freshly ground black pepper
300 g dried lasagne sheets
100 g rindless bacon rashers, finely chopped (omit for a vegetarian lasagne)
70 g (1 cup) coarse fresh breadcrumbs

Preheat the oven to 180°C/160°C fan-forced. Heat 1 tablespoon of oil in a frying pan over medium–high heat. Add the leek, garlic and thyme and cook, stirring, for 5 minutes, or until soft. Transfer to a bowl. Heat another tablespoon of oil, then cook the mushroom in batches, stirring, for 5 minutes, or until golden. Transfer to the bowl with the leek and toss to combine.

Add half the kale to the pan, along with 1 tablespoon of water. Cook, tossing, for 2–3 minutes, until it turns bright green and is just wilted. Transfer to a separate bowl. Repeat with the remaining kale. Don't wash the frying pan, as we will use it again.

Combine the ricotta, cream, dijon and eggs in a large bowl. Use a stick blender to blend until smooth. Keep going for a good few minutes; you want the mixture to be silky-smooth without any lumpy bits. It needs to be the consistency of thickened cream, and this may depend on the freshness of the ricotta. If you feel the consistency is a little firm, add a touch of milk to make sure it is spreadable. Stir in 1 cup of the parmesan. Season.

Spread ½ cup of the cheese sauce over the base of a large lasagne dish. Top with one-third of the lasagne sheets. Spread on half the mushroom and kale mixtures. Dollop over one-third of the remaining cheese sauce and spread evenly. Top with more lasagne sheets, the remaining mushroom and kale mixtures and half the remaining sauce. Finish with a final layer of lasagne sheets and the rest of the cheese sauce.

Heat the remaining oil in the frying pan over medium–high heat. Add the bacon and cook for 2–3 minutes, until starting to turn golden (you don't want too much colour yet). Remove from the heat and set aside for 2 minutes to cool slightly. Add the breadcrumbs, thyme leaves and the remaining parmesan and toss to combine.

Sprinkle the bacon mixture over the top of the lasagne. Bake for 45 minutes, or until golden and cooked through. Set aside for 20 minutes before cutting.

VEGG
SPR
SUM

ES IN

ING/

MER

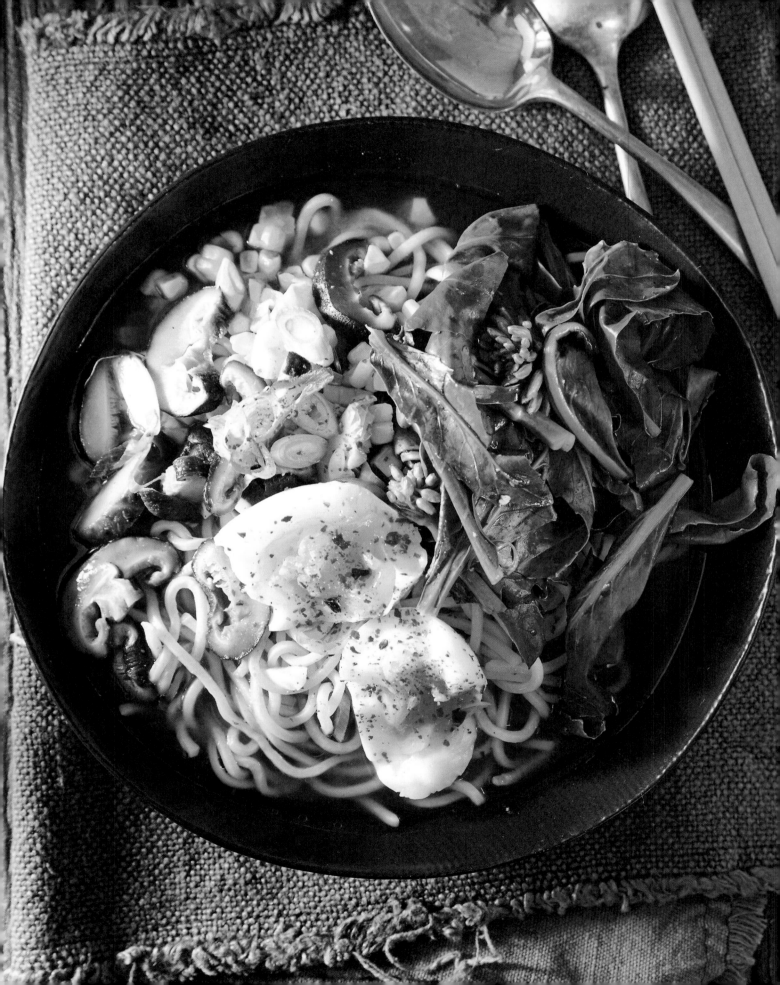

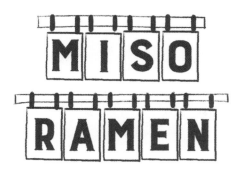

MISO RAMEN

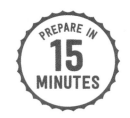

with THE VEGGIE GARDEN & SOFT-BOILED EGGS

After spending three weeks in Japan this year I have developed quite a thing for ramen, but what I love about this particular recipe is that it's so jolly flexible. In fact it can be made with pretty much any two veg that might be in season or, more importantly, might be in your fridge, freezer or garden. Here we've used gai lan and canned corn but use your imagination to improvise!

SERVES 4 PREP: 15 MINS COOKING: 15 MINS

1.5 litres vegetable stock
2 cm knob of ginger, peeled and thinly sliced
3 garlic cloves, thinly sliced
2 spring onions, white parts thinly sliced, green parts reserved
8 dried shiitake mushrooms
1 piece kombu or 20 g hondashi (optional but desirable!)
4 × 100 g packets dried ramen noodles
4 eggs
75 g (¼ cup) miso paste
2 tablespoons soy sauce
1 tablespoon cooking sake
2 teaspoons sugar
1 bunch gai lan or bok choy, roughly chopped
1 × 420 g can corn kernels, drained
sesame oil, to serve
chilli flakes, to serve

Place the stock, ginger, garlic, green parts of the spring onion, shiitakes and kombu in a large saucepan and bring to the boil over high heat. Reduce the heat to low and simmer for 10 minutes to allow the flavours to develop.

While you are infusing your stock, cook the noodles in a large saucepan of boiling water for 2 minutes. Drain.

Place the eggs in a saucepan and cover with cold water. Stirring constantly, bring to the boil. Once it comes to the boil, remove from the heat and set aside for 10 minutes. Peel the eggs under cold running water, then cut in half lengthways.

To save washing up use tongs or a slotted spoon to transfer the shiitake mushrooms from the stock to a chopping board and slice. Use the tongs to remove the rest of the flavourings from the soup and discard them.

Add the miso, soy, sake and sugar to the stock mixture. Bring to a simmer over low heat. Add the gai lan and cook for 1–2 minutes, until just wilted.

Divide the noodles among serving bowls. Use those tongs to transfer the gai lan to the bowls, along with the mushrooms and corn. Ladle on the hot stock mixture. Top with the eggs and drizzle with sesame oil. Sprinkle with chilli and the white spring onion.

TIP

Buy lightly dried and slightly squeezy chilli flakes if you can find them.

THE PRINCIPLES OF A MINESTRONE

Ancient Romans started making minestrone as early as 30 AD, when meat stocks replaced spelt-flour gruel as the basis for everyday simple sustenance. Into that broth went pretty much whatever was close at hand. Familiar to this day are ingredients like chickpeas or borlotti beans. But back then there was obviously no dried pasta (as this wouldn't be invented for some 800 years) and no tomatoes, capsicum, potatoes or green beans, as none of these reached Italy from the New World for another 1400 years.

Early minestrone was both hearty and seasonal: it was heavier and richer in the cold months and instantly lighter when the root veg and brassicas were replaced by summer shoots, pods and peas.

And minestrone was not a dish to be made for its own sake – by which I mean the early versions were built around the ingredients you had to hand, rather than following a never-changing plan and the same set of ingredients that you specifically shop for.

So the principles of minestrone are simple: start with the base, decide on the makeup of your liquid and then add the ingredients you have to hand at the right stage. Use the ideas opposite as a starting point to for creating your own personal minestrone. The combinations are endless.

BASIC MINESTRONE

SERVES 4 **PREP:** 15 MINS **COOKING:** 1 HOUR

THE BASE
1 tablespoon olive oil
150 g rindless bacon rashers (but anything bacony will do: speck, kaiserfleisch, pancetta, the gnarly end bits of that leg of prosciutto or jamon), finely chopped
1 onion, finely chopped
2 carrots, coarsely chopped
2 celery stalks, coarsely chopped
3 garlic cloves, crushed

THE LIQUID
800 g canned diced tomatoes
1 litre chicken stock
250 ml (1 cup) water
2 fresh or dried bay leaves

EARLY ADDITIONS
160 g (1½ cups) short pasta (we used dried 'elbow' pasta)
1 × 400 g can borlotti beans, rinsed and drained (if you can get them fresh, even better!)
2–3 extra chopped veggies (ones that take longer than your leafy greens – we used yellow patty pan squash)

THE LATER ADDITIONS
100 g of whatever delicate veggies or leaves you have in your crisper drawer (we used shredded silverbeet)
freshly ground black pepper
chopped flat-leaf parsley, to serve (optional)
grated parmesan, manchego or pecorino, to serve

Heat the oil in a large heavy-based saucepan over medium heat. Cook the bacon and onion, stirring often, for 5 minutes, or until the onion softens slightly. Add the carrot and celery. Cook, stirring often, for 8 minutes, or until soft.

Add the garlic and cook, stirring, for 30 seconds, or until aromatic. Stir in the tomatoes, stock, water and bay leaves. Cover and bring to the boil. Reduce the heat to low and simmer, stirring occasionally, for 30 minutes.

Stir in the pasta, beans and chopped veg and cook for 10 minutes. Add the delicate veggies and cook for a further 2–3 minutes, until the pasta is al dente and the leaves have wilted. Season with pepper.

Ladle into serving bowls. Sprinkle with chopped parsley (if using) and cheese to serve.

THE BASE:

Add these beauties at the start of the cooking process along with the onion and garlic:

- Cubes of celeriac
- Thickly sliced capsicum
- Artichoke hearts
- Chunky chopped zucchini
- Sliced leeks
- Sliced or whole shallots
- Diced eggplant
- Sliced fennel
- Chopped parsley stalks
- Mashed anchovies or worcestershire sauce
- Parmesan rinds (add with the liquid)
- Pork skin
- Reconstituted mushrooms, such as porcini or shiitake, chopped and added with their well-strained liquid

EARLY ADDITIONS ALONG WITH THE PASTA:

- Cauliflower florets
- White silverbeet stems, chopped into short lengths
- Canned cannellini beans
- Canned chickpeas
- Canned brown lentils
- Canned butter beans
- Canned kidney beans
- Frozen broad beans

CHANGE THE SHORT PASTA FOR:

(Adjust the amount of stock as you go, as some grains will absorb more liquid than others).

- Raw rice, barley, farro or spelt. These will take a good 30–40 minutes to cook
- Raw quinoa
- Dried tortellini, cooked in the soup at the end (but reduce the packet cooking time by 1 minute)
- Spaghetti broken into shorter lengths
- Raw pearl/Israeli couscous (but reduce the cooking time to 8 minutes, then add the leafy greens)
- Chopped peeled potato, cooked until just tender before adding the leafy greens
- Chopped peeled sweet potato, cooked until just tender before adding the leafy greens
- Chopped peeled pumpkin, cooked until just tender before adding the leafy greens
- Large pasta shells
- Torn stale ciabatta or sourdough bread (only add at the end with the leafy greens)

LATER ADDITIONS:

- Green beans
- 50/50 small broccoli florets and ribbons of cabbage
- Finely shredded white or savoy cabbage
- Peas
- Finely chopped zucchini
- Asparagus
- Shredded kale
- Sliced brussels sprouts
- Frozen corn (be judicious; corn works wonderfully with sweet potato, capsicum or potato but less well with cabbage, cauliflower or silverbeet)
- Shredded snow peas or sugar snaps
- Oregano, marjoram, chives or a little basil – but also save some to add at the end of cooking

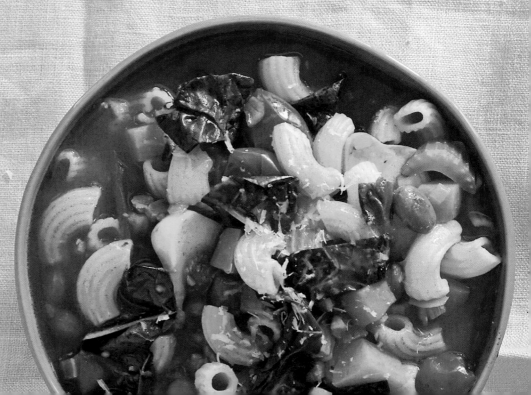

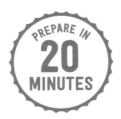

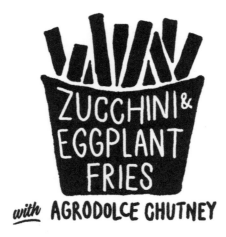

with AGRODOLCE CHUTNEY

For too long potato has dominated the world of fries, like the bully in the playground who won't let you get to the water bubbler. Over the years we've tried to undermine the potato fry at every turn with everything from polenta chips to parsnip, sweet potato and kale chips, but for these 'loaded fries' the combination of the two ultimate Mediterranean vegetables, eggplant and zucchini, makes perfect sense. Especially when paired with the fragrance of basil, the rather bosomy baroque sweet/sourness of this chutney and the salty tang of parmesan.

SERVES 4–6 **PREP:** 20 MINS (PLUS 5 MINS STANDING) **COOKING:** 30 MINS

50 g (⅓ cup) plain flour
sea salt and freshly ground
   black pepper
2 eggs
95 g (1½ cups) panko breadcrumbs
70 g (1 cup) shredded parmesan
⅓ cup finely chopped basil leaves
3 small zucchini, quartered
   lengthways, then sliced crossways
   into 7 cm long batons
1 eggplant, cut into 7 cm long,
   2 cm thick batons

AGRODOLCE CHUTNEY
1 tablespoon olive oil
1 onion, finely chopped
1 long red chilli, deseeded
   and thinly sliced
3 (about 525 g) large yellow
   or white peaches, cut into
   2 cm chunks
70 g (⅓ cup) brown sugar
2 tablespoons currants
2 whole star anise
80 ml (⅓ cup) red wine vinegar

Preheat the oven to 220°C/200°C fan-forced. Line two baking trays with baking paper.

Start by making the agrodulce. Heat the oil in a saucepan over medium heat. Add the onion and chilli and cook, stirring, for 5 minutes, or until soft. Add the peach, sugar, currants, star anise and vinegar. Bring to a gentle simmer, then cook for 25–30 minutes, until the mixture thickens to a dolloping consistency.

While the agrodolce cooks make your fries. Place the flour in a zip-lock bag. Season.

Lightly whisk the eggs in a shallow bowl. Combine the breadcrumbs, parmesan and basil in another zip-lock bag. You have now set up a mini chip-crumbing production line. Add some zucchini and eggplant batons to the bag of flour and shake to coat. Shake off any excess.

Working with one chip at a time, dip the batons into the egg to coat. Let any egg-cess egg drip off and then throw the batons into the breadcrumb bag and toss to coat. Press the seasoned crumbs firmly all over the chips to make sure they stick well.

Place the crumbed fries on the lined trays. Bake for 20–25 minutes or until golden and crisp. Serve with the agrodolce and a flick of salt flakes.

TIPS

If you are making the chutney with white peaches, add half the peach pieces directly after the onion and the rest after 15 minutes. This will ensure they keep their shape and some of their texture. You don't need to do this with most yellow peaches as their flesh is more robust.

In winter, replace the fresh peaches with 1 peeled and diced fresh pear with the sugar mixture and then add 1 x 480 g can drained canned peaches in the last 12 minutes.

You could blanch and peel the peaches; we did, but it's not essential.

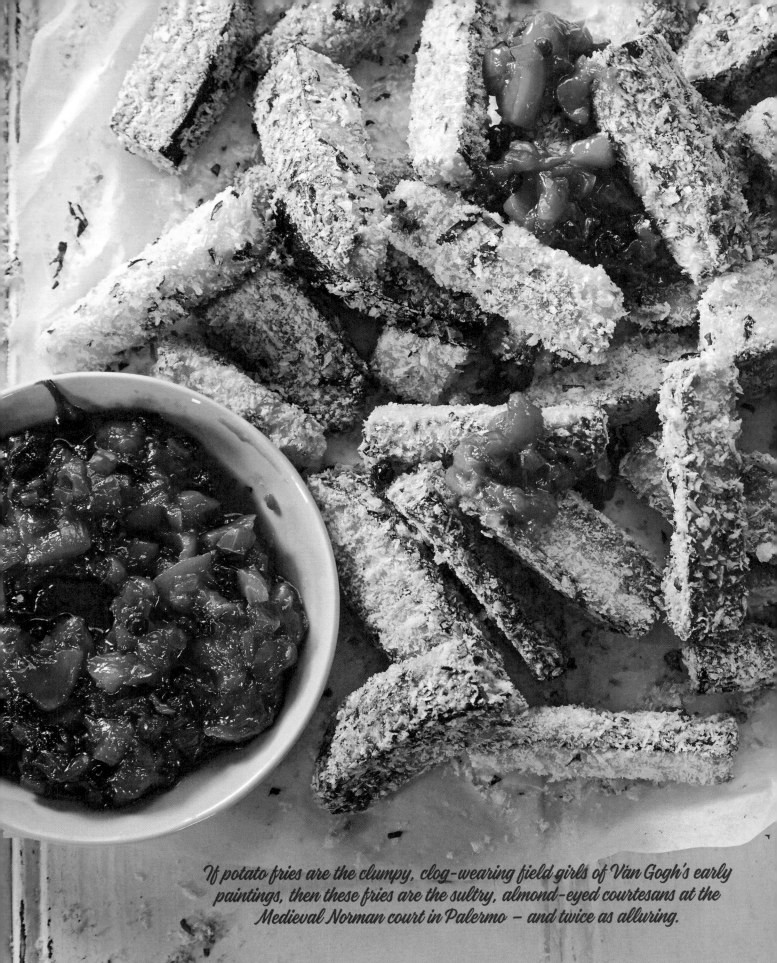

If potato fries are the clumpy, clog-wearing field girls of Van Gogh's early paintings, then these fries are the sultry, almond-eyed courtesans at the Medieval Norman court in Palermo — and twice as alluring.

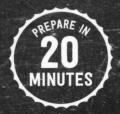

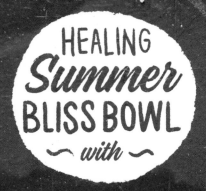

IRONICALLY RETRO CAJUN PRAWNS

Every era has a culinary buzzword: sugar-free, lite, free-range and artisan are just a handful that jump to mind. Never before have there been more food buzzwords than now, but standing above 'chia', 'silajit', 'vegan', 'bliss' and 'healing' is the word 'bowl'. The humble plate is on the outer and it seems that anything wanting to appeal to millennials must be served in the round.

I love it! It makes plating easier and these dishes all reference one of my favourites, the Korean bibimbap, where each topping ingredient is neatly given its own quadrant of the bowl, making them look like pie-charts from a particularly tasty boardroom presentation.

Turn over the page for more inspiration, or check out the Poke Bowl recipe on page 118, my poke bowl feature online, or the Autumn/Winter Bowl ideas on pages 196–197.

SERVES 4 PREP: 20 MINS (PLUS 30 MINS STANDING) COOKING: 15 MINS

40 (about 285 g) small peeled
  green prawns
155 g (1 ½ cups) white quinoa
1 tablespoon olive oil, plus extra
  to serve
1 × 420 g can corn kernels, drained
2 avocados, halved
black sesame seeds, coriander,
  basil or mint leaves, to serve
lime wedges, to serve

CAJUN SPICE MIX

2 tablespoons sweet paprika
1 tablespoon dried oregano leaves
2 teaspoons onion powder
2 teaspoons dried thyme leaves
1 teaspoon each of garlic powder,
  ground black pepper and salt
½–1 teaspoon cayenne pepper,
  depending on how hot you like it

PICKLED RADISH

2 tablespoons white wine vinegar
1 tablespoon caster sugar
1 teaspoon salt
1 bunch radishes, thinly sliced

VEGGIE MIX

around 400 g summer veggies (we used
  200 g baby tomato medley, halved
  and 1 bunch asparagus, halved and
  blanched)

To make the cajun spice mix, combine all the ingredients in a bowl.

Add 2 tablespoons of the spice mix to the prawns and toss to coat. Set aside for 20 minutes to marinate.

To make the pickled radish, combine all the ingredients in a bowl and toss to combine. Set aside for 20–25 minutes to lightly pickle (which is the time it takes to cook the quinoa). Drain.

Place the quinoa in a saucepan with 750 ml (3 cups) of water. Bring to the boil then reduce the heat to low, cover, and simmer for 12 minutes, or until the water is absorbed. Remove from the heat and set aside, covered, for 10 minutes to steam. Fluff up with a fork.

While you are cooking your quinoa, heat a barbecue flat plate on medium–high (or use a large frying pan if cooking inside). Add the oil to the prawns and toss to coat. Add the prawns to the barbecue plate, leaving a small space (about a quarter of the barbie) for the corn as well. Cook the prawns for 2 minutes on each side, or until they are just cooked through. Cook the corn, giving it the occasional toss, until slightly charred.

Divide the quinoa among serving bowls. Top with the prawns, corn, avocado, veggie mix and pickled radish. Sprinkle with sesame seeds or herbs. Serve drizzled with the extra oil and squeeze over the lime wedges.

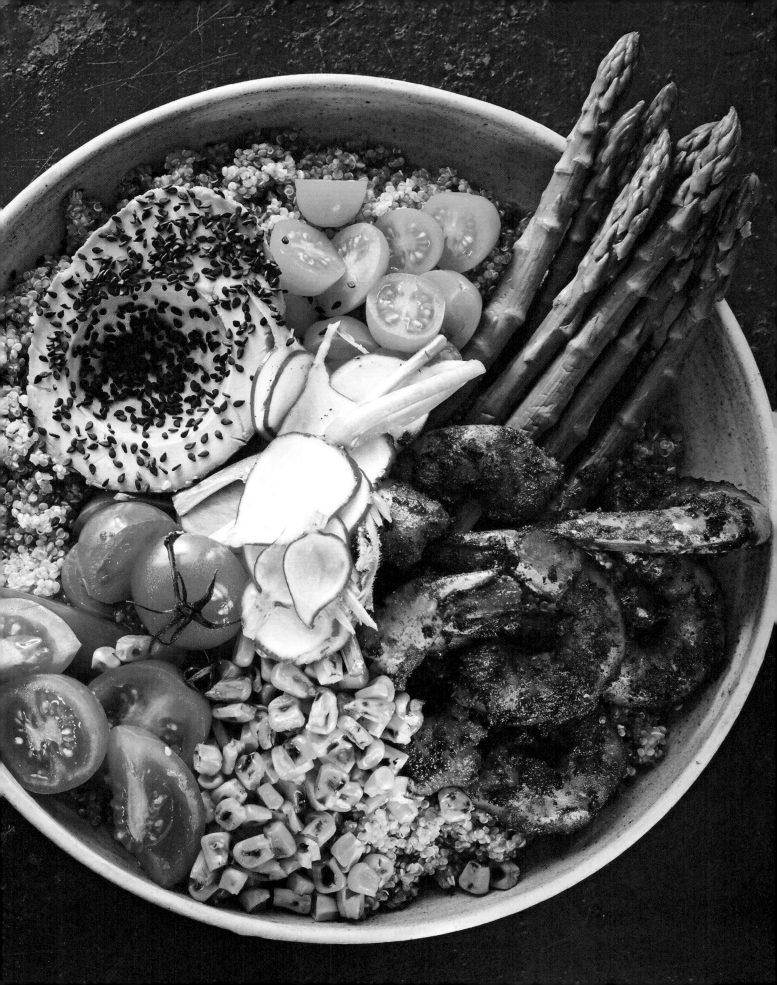

21 SPRING / SUMMER BOWLS

Here are some ideas for customising your bowls. Just start by cooking your grain of choice by following the instructions below (also check the packet cooking instructions as some wholegrains, such as freekeh, can be sold as cracked and uncracked grains, which changes the cooking time). You can mix and match these grains with any of the toppings opposite. For even more ideas, check out my Autumn/Winter Bowls on pages 196–197.

QUINOA

Combine 300 g (1½ cups) quinoa and 750 ml (3 cups) of water in a saucepan and bring to the boil. Reduce the heat to low, cover and simmer for 12 minutes, or until the water is absorbed. Remove from the heat and set aside, covered, for 10 minutes to steam. Fluff up with a fork.

BROWN RICE

Combine 200 g (1 cup) brown rice and 435 ml (1¾ cups) of water in a large saucepan with a good pinch of salt and cook, covered, over low heat for 40 minutes, or until the water is absorbed. Remove from the heat and set aside, covered, for 10 minutes to let the rice sit and the steam out. Fluff with a fork.

FREEKEH

Place 250 g (1½ cups) cracked freekeh in a large saucepan with 935 ml (3¾ cups) of cold salted water. Bring to the boil over medium–high heat. Reduce the heat to low and simmer for 20 minutes, or until the water is absorbed. Remove from the heat and set aside, covered, for 5 minutes. Fluff with a fork.

PEARL BARLEY

Place 440 g (2 cups) pearl barley in a large saucepan. Cover with 1.5 litres of cold water and bring to the boil over high heat. Reduce the heat to medium and simmer, stirring occasionally, for 30 minutes, or until the water is absorbed but the barley is still a little bitey. Remove from the heat and set aside, covered, for 5 minutes. Fluff with a fork.

1. Wedges of plum or peach and shredded prosciutto, shaved red onion, torn basil, rocket leaves, chunks of ricotta and a balsamic vinaigrette.

2. Carrot pickled in rice wine vinegar, salt and sugar. Slices of pan-fried tempeh, shredded snow peas and bean shoots. Drizzle with light soy sauce and scatter with chopped peanuts and coriander sprigs.

3. Roast pineapple chunks until tender, adding prawns in the last 10 minutes. Add some crispy bacon shards, watercress sprigs and Thai basil. Drizzle with a dressing of fish sauce, lime juice, light soy sauce, chopped chilli and grated palm sugar.

4. Roast strips of yellow and red capsicum with shaved garlic. Toss chickpeas in a frying pan with a little oil and cumin seeds until toasted. Add Smashed & Grilled BBQ Chicken Thighs (page 36) and sliced avocado, drizzle with a tahini and yoghurt dressing and add a lemon wedge for extra squeezing.

5. Pickled radish, canned lentils, quartered perino tomatoes and barbecued sliced yellow squash. Crumble on goat's cheese and sprinkle with a mix of basil and parsley leaves.

6. Pickled cucumber ribbons in white wine vinegar, sugar and salt; roasted chunks of zucchini and bocconcini, sliced tomato medley. Top with chunks of ricotta and shredded basil leaves. Drizzle with extra virgin olive oil and lemon juice.

7. Chunks of barbecued chicken with wedges of mango, shredded iceberg lettuce, spring onion coins, mint leaves and sprinkle with coarsely chopped toasted and salted cashews or peanuts. Drizzle with a chilli and lime dressing.

8. Lightly sear some fresh tuna and slice, or use that spare can of tuna that's sitting in the pantry – it will work just as well. Drizzle with a tahini dressing or tarator (page 188).

9. Sauteed broccoli florets with bacon lardons, chopped smoked almonds and zucchini zoodles (page 216). Top with chunks of feta and drizzle with a green goddess dressing.

10. Sliced avocado with podded edamame, barbecued soy-marinated tofu, Soy-fried Bok Choy (page 17), carrot ribbons, cashews and spring onions with a tamarind dressing and sprinkle of sesame seeds.

11. Halved pan-fried eggplant slices brushed with a little honey to glaze, baby rocket, feta-stuffed green olives, chopped toasted walnuts and pepitas. Scatter with flat-leaf parsley leaves and top with a dollop of Instant Miso–Bacon Mayo (page 22) or olive oil.

12. Drizzle a bunch of parsley with oil and barbecue for 2–3 minutes until lightly charred and slightly burnt at the edges. At the same time, barbecue some meatballs made from squeezing out the meat from fresh chorizo sausages. Serve with barbecued asparagus and drained canned chickpeas, roasted and tossed with cumin seeds. Finish with a dollop of romesco sauce.

13. Barbecue chicken breasts which have been marinated in a little ground saffron, olive oil and lemon juice for a few hours. Slice and serve with caramelised onion, blanched green beans, julienned carrot, chopped toasted almonds and mint leaves.

14. Roasted whole green chillies and trussed cherry tomatoes, turkey meatballs (page 61), baby spinach leaves and a minty cream cheese and sour cream dressing.

15. Pickled mushrooms with thyme sprigs, garlic, white wine vinegar and olive oil, sliced barbecued chicken, sliced celery stalks with the leaves reserved and mixed with flat-leaf parsley leaves and a little squeeze of Kewpie mayo.

16. Barbecued asparagus, flaked canned tuna, watercress, sliced avocado, topped with a soft-boiled egg and a dollop of crème fraîche mixed with dill and lemon.

17. Sliced chicken thighs (brushed with maple syrup mixed with olive oil and a little sriracha chilli sauce and roasted until well charred), wedges of baby cos hearts, chargrilled corn and spring onions, sunflower seeds and mashed avocado.

18. Barbecued sliced eggplant topped with slabs of feta, sprinkled with mint leaves and chopped walnuts, and drizzled with a honey and lemon dressing.

19. Barbecued mixed capsicum strips, sliced cherry tomato medley, sliced avocado, sliced cucumber, marinated olives and canned chilli tuna chunks. Drizzle with a lemon and oregano dressing.

20. Baby spinach leaves, barbecued streaky maple bacon and grilled split broccolini. Drizzle with a white balsamic vinaigrette. Sprinkle with toasted chopped hazelnuts and cubes of smoked cheddar.

21. Roasted grapes, shredded red cabbage, sliced celery and smoked chicken breast, crumbled blue cheese and chopped walnuts. Drizzle with a verjuice vinaigrette.

ALSO ...

You might think all these things would go well with pasta to make a pasta salad, but you'd be WRONG. Making a pasta salad is the sort of mistake that ranks alongside that time you invited the Coffin Cheaters round to party at your parents' house when you were 14, or that bloke you met in Surfers.

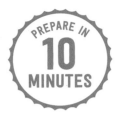

PREPARE IN
10
MINUTES

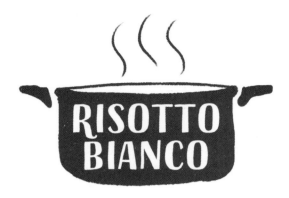

RISOTTO BIANCO

The simplest risotto of all. Ripe for customising ...

SERVES 4 PREP: 10 MINS COOKING: 30 MINS

1 litre salt-reduced chicken stock
1 tablespoon soy sauce
1 tablespoon olive oil
40 g butter
1 onion, finely chopped
2 garlic cloves, crushed
330 g (1½ cups) arborio rice
125 ml (½ cup) dry white wine
70 g (1 cup) shredded parmesan,
   plus extra to serve
sea salt and freshly ground
   black pepper

Bring the stock and soy sauce just to the boil in a medium saucepan over high heat. Reduce the heat to low and hold at a very gentle simmer.

Heat the oil and half the butter in a large saucepan over medium heat. Cook the onion and garlic, stirring, for 5 minutes, or until soft and translucent (do not brown).

Add the rice and cook, stirring, for 2–3 minutes, until the grains appear slightly glassy. Toasting the grains like this ensures the rice cooks evenly.

Add the wine and cook, stirring, until the liquid is almost absorbed. The rice should move in the pan like wet sand. Now add a ladleful (about 125 ml/½ cup) of hot stock and stir until the liquid is absorbed.

Add more stock, a ladleful at a time. Stir until all the liquid is absorbed before adding the next ladleful. Continue for 20 minutes, or until the rice is tender yet firm to the bite. Remove the pan from the heat and stir in the parmesan and remaining butter with gusto. Season and serve with extra parmesan.

TIPS

And to customise, try adding any of the following or check out my ideas for ingredients to use in Autumn/Winter on page 192.

- Top with prawns and zucchini. Instead of butter and parmesan, stir in mascarpone enthusiastically.
- Flaked salmon with grilled broccolini or fennel.
- Poached chook and leeks.
- Steamed broccoli stems and florets. Try a little olive oil-soaked lemon flesh and/or a little gentle blue cheese in this one – delicious!
- Celery – add a generous serve of diced celery with the onions or leeks when you start cooking and then add a larger dice of butter-cooked celery as the finishing topping. Torn prosciutto, blue cheese or shreds of roast chicken with chopped parsley are all good additions to the topping of this risotto.
- Flaked smoked trout with dill and steamed green beans or broad beans.
- Grated cheddar cheese and roasted tomatoes.
- Cubes of pan-fried ham with torn bocconcini stirred through the hot rice so it goes stringy like a Palermo arancini.

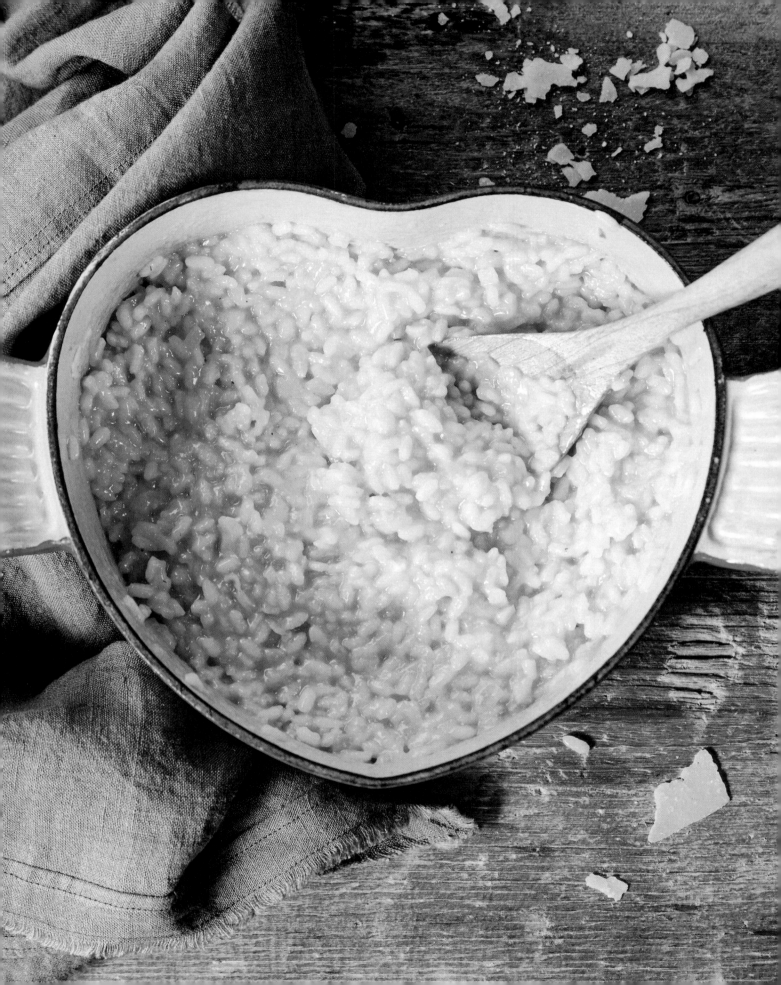

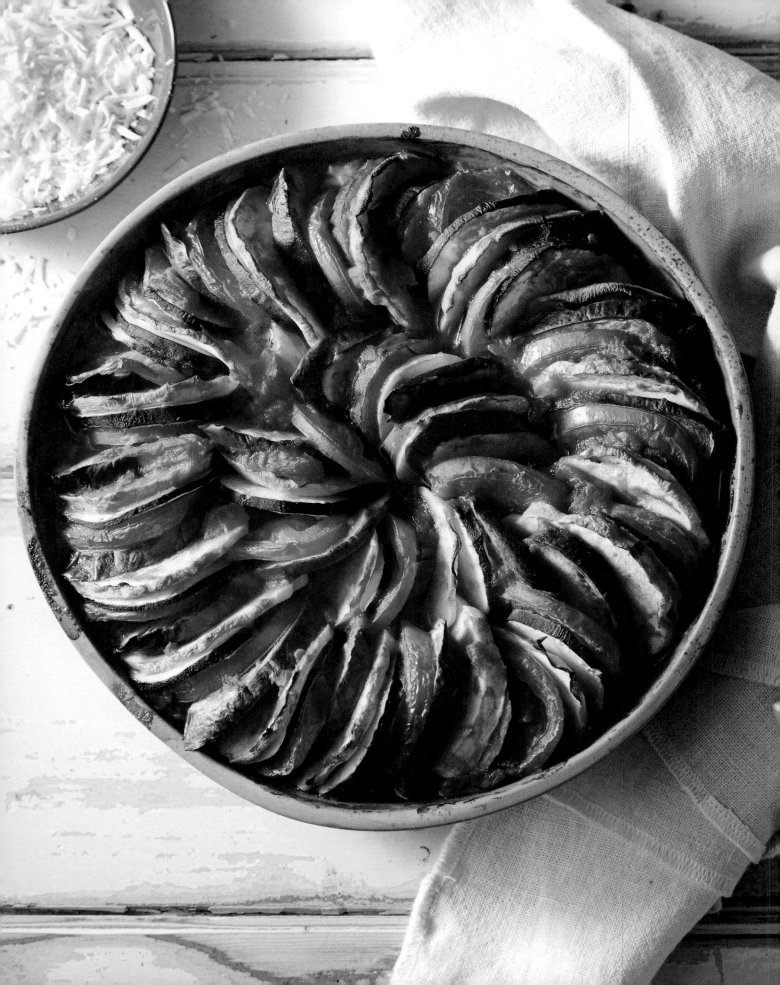

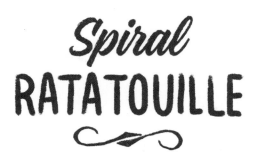

Spiral RATATOUILLE

My mother's ratatouille was good, but it never looked as pretty as this!

Only one bit of extra planning: when shopping for zucchini, squash, Lebanese eggplant and roma tomatoes, try and pick ones that have a similar diameter.

SERVES 6 **PREP:** 30 MINS (MOST OF THIS TIME IS IN STACKING IT TOGETHER)
COOKING: 1 HOUR 40 MINS

2 tablespoons olive oil
1 red onion, coarsely chopped
1 small red capsicum, deseeded and finely chopped
2 garlic cloves, crushed
1 tablespoon red wine vinegar
800 g canned diced Italian tomatoes
2 tablespoons shredded basil leaves
sea salt and freshly ground black pepper
100 g mozzarella, thinly sliced
20 g (¼ cup) shredded parmesan
2 green zucchini, thinly sliced
8 yellow pattypan squash, thinly sliced
2 Lebanese eggplants, thinly sliced
6 small roma tomatoes, thinly sliced

Heat 1 tablespoon of the oil in a large deep frying pan over medium–high heat. Add the onion and capsicum and cook, stirring, for 5 minutes, or until slightly softened. Add the garlic and cook, stirring, for 1 minute, or until aromatic. Add the vinegar and three-quarters of the diced tomatoes (try to add as many chunky bits from the can as possible here). Bring to a simmer over medium heat, then simmer for 10 minutes or until the sauce thickens. Remove from the heat and season.

Preheat the oven to 180°C/160°C fan-forced.

Spoon the sauce into the base of a 23 cm round baking dish or ovenproof frying pan. Top with the mozzarella slices and sprinkle with the parmesan.

To make the assembly easy, make little individual stacks on a chopping board. Start with a piece of zucchini, then top with similar-sized slices of yellow squash, eggplant and tomato. Reserve smaller slices from the ends of the veg/fruit to make slightly narrower stacks which will be ideal for the centre of the dish.

Starting at the outside edge, lay the larger stacks on their sides next to each other, to form the outside ring. Repeat, working inwards, and finish with the slightly smaller stacks squeezed in together to fill the centre.

Stir 1 tablespoon of water into the remaining diced tomatoes and drizzle over the top of the veggies. Cover with foil and bake for 40 minutes, then bake uncovered for a further 40 minutes.

TIPS

If you don't have a round dish, you can also make this in a rectangular dish, arranging the vegetable stacks in rows.

You could also add a thin slice of mozzarella to each stack.

SPRING / SUMMER SIDES AND SALADS

CRUSHED CUCUMBER CHUNKS, SALTED PEANUTS AND FRIED LAP CHEONG SALAD

PREPARE IN **10** MINUTES

A classic on-set snack that I used to make for me and the *MasterChef* boys, but it's also great spooned over roasted carrots, fennel or sweet potato wedges, grilled fish or five-spice rubbed barbecue chicken thighs.

SERVES 6 PREP: 10 MINS (PLUS 10 MINS STANDING) **COOKING**: 5 MINS

2 telegraph cucumbers
175 g lap cheong sausage, thinly sliced
60 ml (¼ cup) rice wine vinegar
2 teaspoons caster sugar
sea salt and freshly ground black pepper
80 g (½ cup) salted roasted peanuts, coarsely chopped
½ cup firmly packed torn Thai basil leaves (or coriander)

Use a sharp knife to slice the cucumbers lengthways. Use a teaspoon to scoop out the seeds from both sides. Reserve the seeds in a large jug. Thinly slice the cucumber flesh into 2–3 mm slices and place in a serving bowl.

Heat a non-stick frying pan over medium heat. Add the lap cheong and cook, tossing, for 2–3 minutes, until golden and still a little chewy. Use a slotted spoon to transfer to a plate lined with paper towel and reserve the oil in the pan.

Add the vinegar, sugar and reserved oil to the jug with the cucumber seeds. Use a stick blender to blitz until almost smooth. Season.

Add the dressing to the cucumber and toss until well combined. Set aside for 10 minutes for the dressing to soak in slightly. Add the lap cheong, peanuts and Thai basil, and toss until well combined.

ZUCCHINI RIBBON SALAD

PREPARE IN **5** MINUTES

Fresh, clean and super-versatile, this salad sings with everything from steak and chicken from the barbecue, to pulled pork and anything that needs some contrasting freshness and acidity (for an image, see page 150).

SERVES 4 PREP: 5 MINS **COOKING**: 5 MINS

230 g (1½ cups) frozen baby peas
1 lemon, zest peeled into strips
2 zucchini, peeled into ribbons
1 cup flat-leaf parsley leaves
90 g (⅔ cup) walnut pieces, toasted
2 tablespoons olive oil
1 tablespoon lemon juice
salt flakes

Cook the peas in a small saucepan of boiling water for 2–3 minutes, adding the lemon zest in the last minute of cooking, until just warmed through. Drain and transfer to a bowl. Add the remaining ingredients and toss until well combined.

TIP

This salad is great with any milky cheese, such as feta, ricotta or goat's curd. Swap the walnuts for a different nut or another crunchy element to match the cheese.

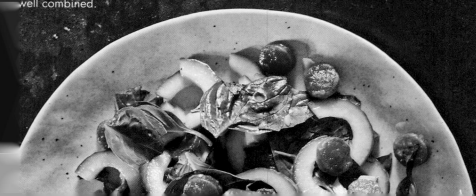

ASIAN SUMMER KOOL SLAW

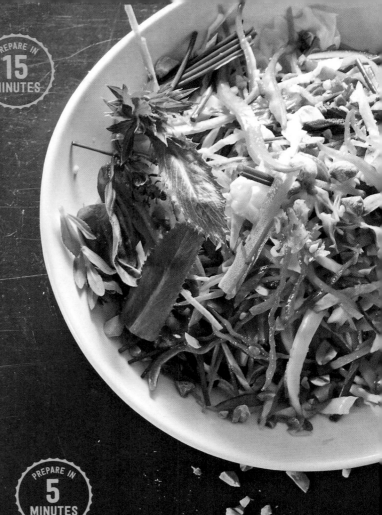

PREPARE IN 15 MINUTES

Like we say in Holland, where coleslaw was invented, I *lekker* this with pretty much anything.

SERVES 4 PREP: 15 MINS

50 g (⅓ cup) unsalted roasted peanuts, finely
  crushed, plus extra chopped peanuts to serve
2 small red chillies, deseeded and finely chopped
2 tablespoons coarsely grated palm sugar
2 tablespoons fish sauce
zest and juice of 2 limes
110 g thinly shredded white cabbage
½ red onion, sliced
150 g snow peas, trimmed and thinly
  sliced lengthways
1 carrot, cut into matchsticks
2 cups of any Asian herbs (coriander or Thai basil or
  perhaps a mixture of these with mint or Vietnamese
  mint added)

Combine the crushed peanuts, chilli, palm sugar, fish sauce, lime zest and juice in a large bowl.

Add the cabbage, onion, snow peas and carrot to the dressing and toss to coat. Sprinkle with the herbs and extra chopped peanuts.

ADAPTABLE TOMATO AND HERB SALAD WITH GOAT'S CHEESE

PREPARE IN 5 MINUTES

A classic dish that I could eat every day – just stepping up the herbs to change the flavour profile. And try swapping different fruit for the tomatoes, such as strawberries and basil, plums and chervil or cucumber and olives. Also play around with the cheese, substituting feta, burrata, milky ricotta or really good sliced mozzarella. Then there's the vinegar, which gives you another dozen options, such as sherry vinegar, verjuice, white wine vinegar, balsamic, red wine vinegar, etc. So one salad can become, oh, maybe more than 500 different recipes (for an image, see page 236).

SERVES 4 PREP: 5 MINS (PLUS 20 MINS SOAKING)

60 ml (¼ cup) olive oil
2 tablespoons white balsamic vinegar
large pinch of sugar
sea salt and freshly ground black pepper
700 g ripe mixed tomatoes, thickly sliced (use
  a mixture of styles and types of tomatoes,
  such as red, kumato, green, large and cherry tomatoes)
100 g goat's cheese
loads of mixed fresh herbs

Combine the oil, vinegar and sugar in a jug and season. Place the tomatoes in a large shallow bowl and drizzle with the dressing. Set aside for 20 minutes to let the flavours develop. Transfer the tomatoes to a platter. Crumble over the goat's cheese and scatter with herbs. Drizzle with a little dressing from the bowl to serve.

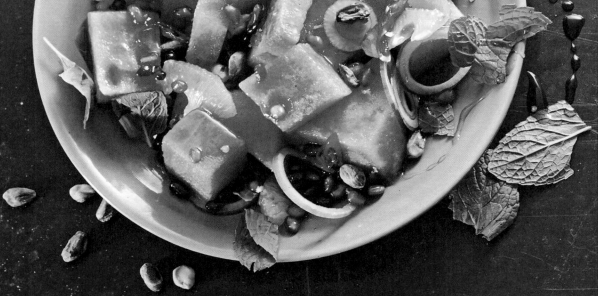

WATERMELON, POMEGRANATE AND PISTACHIO SALAD

PREPARE IN 10 MINUTES

Crunch comes in so many different forms: dry, toasty, nutty, etc, etc. Here, crunch comes partnered with the pop of lemon carpels and pomegranate seeds for a deliciously noisy mouthful.

SERVES 6 **PREP**: 10 MINS (PLUS 10 MINS MARINATING)

4 lemons, peeled and segmented
2 tablespoons extra virgin olive oil
sea salt and freshly ground black pepper
¼ watermelon (about 1.5 kg), rind removed, cut into cubes
seeds of 1 pomegranate
1 small red onion, shaved into thin rings
½ cup mint leaves
40 g (¼ cup) unroasted pistachios kernels, coarsely chopped

CHILLI CARAMEL DRESSING
80 g (½ cup) brown sugar
80 ml (⅓ cup) red wine vinegar
1 long red chilli, thinly sliced
2 teaspoons lemon juice
sea salt and freshly ground black pepper

Place the lemon segments and oil in a bowl. Break up the lemon segments with your fingers. Season with salt. Set aside for 10 minutes to macerate, and to let the acidity soften in the oil. Drain.

Meanwhile, to prepare the dressing, place the sugar and vinegar in a saucepan over low heat and stir until the sugar dissolves. Simmer for 2–3 minutes, until the mixture is syrupy. Remove from the heat and stir in the chilli. Set aside to cool slightly. Stir in the lemon juice and season.

Stack half the watermelon cubes in a serving bowl. Sprinkle with half the pomegranate seeds, lemon pieces, onion rings, mint leaves and pistachios. Continue stacking with the rest of the salad, then drizzle with the dressing.

SMASHED CUCUMBER SALAD

PREPARE IN 5 MINUTES

2011 was the year of the cucumber granita

2012 was the year of pickled cucumber ribbons

2015 was the year of the grilled cucumber AND

2017 was the year of roughly torn or smashed cucumber. Doing this keeps them meaty but also changes their texture subtly (for an image, see page 98).

SERVES 4 **PREP**: 5 MINS

3 large Lebanese cucumbers
2 garlic cloves, crushed
1 tablespoon soy sauce
1 tablespoon rice wine vinegar
1 tablespoon caster sugar
2 teaspoons sesame oil
1 teaspoon dried chilli flakes (see TIP)
sea salt

Snap up the cucumbers up with your hands, place the cucumber pieces in a zip-lock bag and give them a thump with rolling pin (or even possibly a wine-bottle, if you don't have a rolling pin but do have leftover wine bottles lying around your kitchen. Just for the record, I'm not judging you here).

Tip the smashed cucumber pieces into a bowl and add the garlic, soy sauce, vinegar, sugar, sesame oil and chilli. Season well with salt and toss until well combined.

TIP

Any chilli will do, but I like the lightly dried (and therefore redder) chilli flakes from Gourmet Garden in Queensland. Basque *espelette* pepper or *isot* pepper flakes from the Sanliurfa region in Southeast Turkey are even more pretentious to use, but then they aren't an 'Aussie success story' – as we dub anything that sells for $100+m to a US multinational! You could just use chopped, deseeded and deveined long red chillies but I fear I risk bamboozling you with choice here.

INSTANT FLATBREADS

PREPARE IN
15
MINUTES

Quick, easy, brilliant! These flatbreads also rewarm well in the toaster if they are still soft and not overcooked.

MAKES 8 PREP: 15 MINS **COOKING:** 4 MINS PER BATCH

250 g (1 cup) plain yoghurt
225 g (1½ cups) self-raising flour, plus an extra
½ cup for flouring the work surface

In a bowl, stir the yoghurt into the flour until well combined.

Dump the mixture onto a clean and heavily floured work surface. It is a wet dough, which means it's hard to knead traditionally. Instead, lift it up and slap it down to develop the gluten, flipping the dough occasionally. Add more flour until the dough is kneadable. It needs to be a little springy, which shows that the gluten has developed.

Now knead for about 5 minutes, or until the dough is smooth. A mixer with a dough hook will make this much quicker – so if you've got one, use it!

Keep the dough in a bowl covered with plastic wrap until needed. (It's good to rest the dough for a bit, but it's not essential.)

Cut the dough into eight equal-sized pieces. Roll out each piece into a thin disc. The thinner the disc, the crisper the bread.

Preheat a barbecue grill, frying pan or chargrill pan over medium–high heat. Cook the breads for 2 minutes on each side, or until charred and cooked through.

SIMPLE LETTUCE SALAD

PREPARE IN
10
MINUTES

Like a great white shirt or a quality black t-shirt, this salad works with pretty much everything (for an image, see page 42).

SERVES 6 PREP: 10 MINS

2 baby cos lettuce hearts, leaves separated, larger leaves torn
2 Lebanese cucumbers, halved lengthways and sliced diagonally
2 avocados, chopped
60 ml (¼ cup) extra virgin olive oil
1 tablespoon lemon juice, white wine vinegar or white balsamic vinegar
1 teaspoon dijon mustard
large pinch of sugar
sea salt and freshly ground black pepper

Toss the lettuce, cucumber and avocado in a serving bowl.

Combine the oil, lemon juice or vinegar, mustard and sugar in a jug and whisk together. Season well.

Drizzle the salad with the dressing and serve.

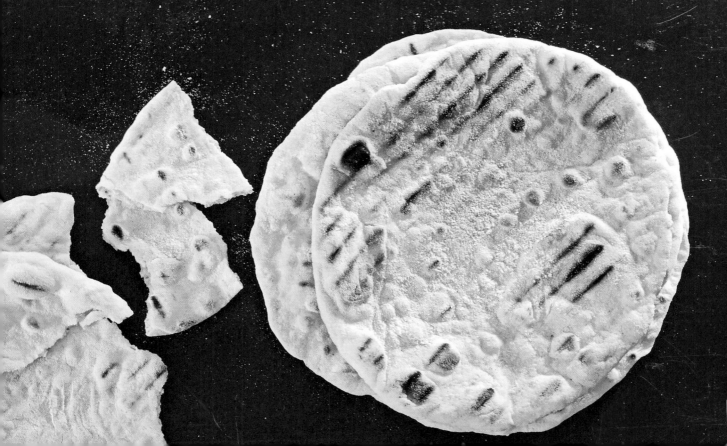

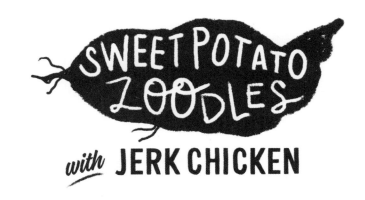

SWEET POTATO ZOODLES
with JERK CHICKEN

The summer I spent in the Caribbean was interesting for many reasons: drinking rum out of enamel mugs at Pusser's Bar, going diving with ex-SEALS, avoiding the crack addicts and mega-cruise passengers in St Thomas, stumbling across old, broken-down sugar refineries in the jungle, watching pelicans dive-bombing shoals of fish, or trying to watch the Grand Final as a full-blown hurricane was bearing down on the island. But not once did the food feature.

Sure, there was the puerile pleasure of discovering that they sold packets of Cock Soup in the supermarket, and the jokes that went with it. And there was the rare chance discovery of a shack on a ridge-top road that sold us Johnny cakes and deep-fried batfish. But that was about it. This is the dish that I expected to find – and I suspect that if I had gone to Jamaica, instead of my own particular island destination of Tortola, I might have done.

SERVES 6 PREP: 30 MINS (PLUS 30 MINS MARINATING) COOKING: 50 MINS

12 chicken drumsticks
60 ml (¼ cup) olive oil
½ pineapple, peeled and cut into
　1 cm thick small wedges
1 red onion, finely chopped
1 long red chilli, deseeded and
　finely chopped
½ bunch coriander, roots and stems
　washed and finely chopped,
　sprigs reserved
zest and juice of 1 lime, plus extra
　lime cheeks, to serve
sea salt and freshly ground
　black pepper
800 g sweet potato, made into
　noodles using a spiraliser

JERK MARINADE
1 small onion, coarsely chopped
3 spring onions, coarsely chopped
2 long red chillies, deseeded but the
　veins left in, chopped
¼ cup coarsely chopped coriander
3 garlic cloves, crushed
3 cm knob of ginger, peeled and
　finely grated
2 tablespoons brown sugar
3 teaspoons ground allspice
2 teaspoons thyme leaves
2 teaspoons salt
1 teaspoon freshly ground
　black pepper
½ teaspoon ground cinnamon
1 tablespoon cider vinegar

To make the jerk marinade, combine all the ingredients in a food processor and blitz until a smooth wet paste forms.

Place the chicken pieces in a large zip-lock bag and add the marinade. Seal and toss to coat. Place in the fridge to marinate for at least 30 minutes, or overnight. Feel free to play a little Gregory Isaacs to help it get in the mood.

Preheat a lidded barbecue with a grill and flat plate on medium–high until it reaches 180°C.

Remove the chicken from the bag and drizzle with 1 tablespoon of the oil. Place on the barbecue grill, shut the barbecue lid and reduce the heat to medium. Cook, turning every 10 minutes, for 40–45 minutes, until the chicken is well charred and cooked through.

After the chicken has been cooking for 30 minutes, drizzle the pineapple with a tablespoon of the oil. Cook on the barbecue grill for 5 minutes each side. Transfer to a tray with the chicken, cover loosely with foil and leave to rest for 5 minutes.

While the pineapple is grilling, combine the onion, chilli, coriander roots and stems, lime zest and juice in a bowl. Season.

Once your barbie is free, drizzle the flat plate with the remaining oil and add the sweet potato noodles. Barbecue for 3 minutes, or until slightly softened but not completely wilted. Transfer to a serving platter.

Top the sweet potato with the pineapple and chicken and spoon on the onion mixture. Scatter with the coriander sprigs and serve with lime cheeks.

TIPS

This marinade is enough for about 1 kg of meat. You can also try chicken thighs or wings, white fish fillets or prawns.

For a hotter jerk, add 1, 2 or 3 teaspoons cayenne pepper and 2 more red chillies … or give me a call!

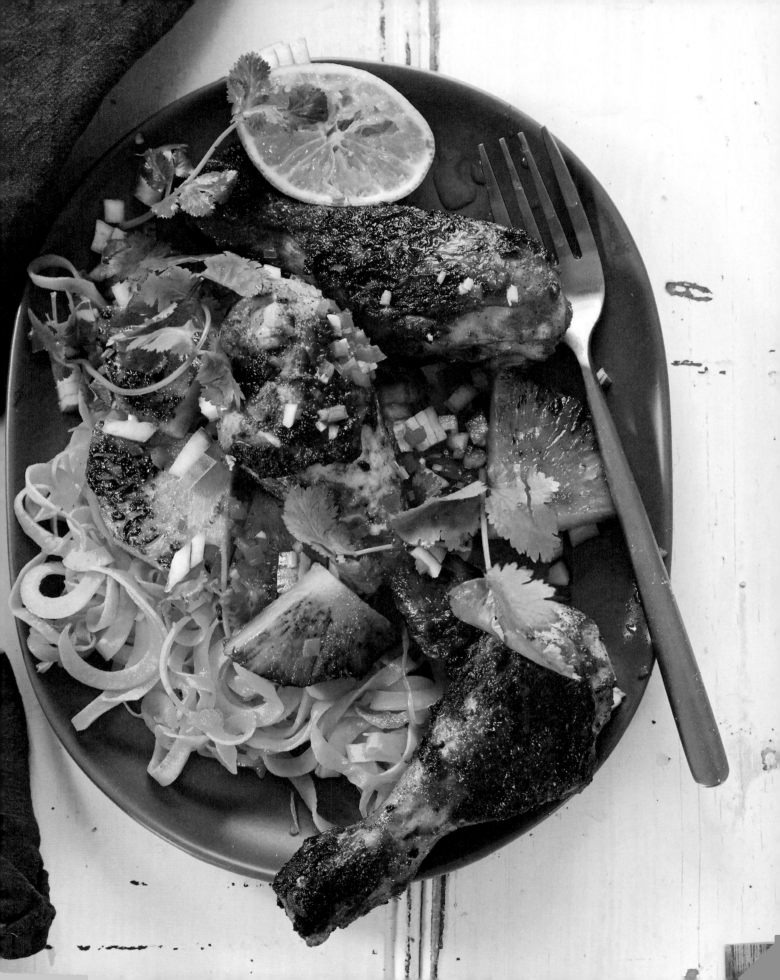

STIR-FRIES

There are four main reasons I used to hate stir-fries: all that chopping makes them a frightful bore to prepare; too often they are stewed and not crisp; they usually contain too many different, clashing ingredients and, to me, they always taste the same – a leaden mix of sugar, soy sauce and MSG.

Yes, I know this is the voice of an anti-stir-fry bigot talking and so I have actively sought out stir-fry recipes that I like. So here are the World's 9 Best Stir-Fries, the Ten Commandments of Perfect Stir-Fries and then two recipes from my culinary-partner-in-crime, Michelle Southan, that are contenders for that top 9.

1. BEEF AND BROCCOLI
You don't need every veg in the fridge to make a stir-fry. If you blanch or microwave the broccoli first to pre-cook it a little, you can speed up the process and keep the 'breath of the wok' alive. Instead of the usual combination of Shaoxing rice wine, soy, sugar and perhaps hoisin or oyster sauce, use a jar of black beans instead, which brings a funky, fermented and slightly dark, salty edge to proceedings. Simpler and tastier! Although if you want to step it up, try Michelle's recipe on page 182.

2. SINGAPORE NOODLES
Slightly undercooking the noodles before adding to this spicy stir-fry makes for an almost dry dish with all the flavour sucked into the noodles.

3. CHAR KWAY TEOW
This Malaysian combo of flat rice noodles, prawns, sweet-salty lap cheong sausage, bean shoots and light and dark soy needs a very hot wok to almost burn the edges of the noodles and the Chinese sausage. To ensure the wok stays blistering hot, cook one portion at a time and preheat the noodles in the microwave before adding. And remember to move everything to the side of the wok when you are finally cooking the prawns.

4. PAD THAI
Previously I have found it convenient to forget that one of the great – and essential – Thai takeaway meals is actually a stir-fry. Search for my recipe for free online. (It may be in Dutch, because I am so multicultural.)

5. JUNGLE CURRY
Kaeng pa is one of the few wok-based dishes where you want the sauce to be a little watery – even if this Thai recipe is hardly shy of flavour, with all that galangal, garlic, lemongrass, kaffir lime leaves, chilli and holy basil.

6. SPECIAL FRIED RICE
Sure, it's a wee bit bogan, but I love SFR! Especially when it's got cubes of spam in it, along with slivers of lap cheong sausage. Check out pages 248–249 for loads of ideas to make your SFR speccy.

7. SICHUAN EGGPLANT
Whether fried crisp in potato flour, or brined then fried hard so the eggplant is creamy at its heart and burnt on its edges, this dish is a riot of flavours and textures, thanks to a dressing of black vinegar, exotic broad bean paste and pickled chillies (all available from good Asian grocers).

8. KUNG PO CHICKEN
Another delicious stir-fry that revolves around chillies and vinegar. No surprise then, that this dish of chicken thigh meat, peanuts, celery and dried chillies also comes from the chilli-loving, western reaches of China. Just be judicious with the cornflour that is often used to provide structure to the sauce, as it can make things gluey.

9. CHICKEN, MUSHROOMS AND OYSTER SAUCE
This is a beautifully gentle dish which shows that the wok can be used with subtlety as well as like a blow torch. I love the soft slipperiness of this combination, and tofu works just as well as chicken.

THE TEN COMMANDMENTS OF STIR-FRYING

1. HEAT
The magic of wok cooking – or so my Chinese friends tell me – is the 'breath of the wok'. That is the intense and almost instant heat that a properly seasoned wok has when placed over a roaring flame. Make sure the wok is hot before you start to cook, and then do your best to maintain the heat while cooking.

2. BE PREPARED
Preheating the wok is only half of the preparation. Also chop everything before you start using the wok – usually into thin batons, or other shapes that will cook quickly. Lay out room-temperature ingredients in order of cooking time – so harder veg like onions or carrots go first.

3. IMPATIENT
If you really must start before the wok has fully reached temperature, then cook the aromatics, such as the ginger and garlic, first. And make sure you add sugar at this stage, to caramelise around the ginger and garlic, adding complexity to your sauce. But please resist adding the meat until the wok is singing with heat.

4. BUY GOOD SAUCES
Much of the flavour found in the stir-fries that I love comes from a bottle – whether fish sauce, soy sauce, kecap manis, sesame oil, Shaoxing rice wine, hoisin or oyster sauce. So make time to visit your local Asian grocery store and stock up on the best brands you can find, as this will do more to lift your stir-fry than anything else – and at a cost that is usually only a few dollars more than inferior brands. They'll also last through loads of woks-worth of cooking.

5. DON'T THROW IN EVERYTHING IN THE CRISPER DRAWER
The best stir-fries revolve around a few core ingredients, such as prawns and sugar snaps, or chicken and cashews. Don't empty everything from the crisper drawer in there! Classic combos are best!

6. MEAT FIRST
Cook your meat first and then either push it up the side of the wok (if you're only adding quick-cooking veg) or remove it while you cook more robust veg. Ensure the wok is smoking hot before you add the meat, arrange it in one layer (don't stack it) and leave it to tan up, undisturbed, for a minute or so before moving it round the wok to complete its browning. Bring the wok back up to temperature before adding anything else.

7. NO OVERCROWDING
The most common problem with bad wok cookery is overcrowding the wok so the heat dissipates too quickly and everything stews while its coming back to temperature. So...

8. COOK IN BATCHES
Add your ingredients in small batches with the hardest/most dense ingredients (which will take the most time) first. If making a big stir-fry, remove one batch before adding the next; never overcrowd the pan.

9. MINIMISE LIQUID
Using too much liquid stews the ingredients. Remember the aim here is to fry, not to braise or stew. For me the right amount of liquid in a sauce is when it sizzles on hitting the wok, reduces a little and then coats the ingredients. It should never pool at the bottom of the wok unless it is at the very, very end of the cook.

10. PREHEAT YOUR NOODLES
If using fresh noodles, warm them up in the microwave or by pouring boiling water over them. If using the latter method, dry them well before adding to your wok, so as to avoid breaking Commandment 9. I also don't mind blanching or microwaving harder veg before throwing them into the wok; but don't let them cook too much or you'll end up with a stir-fry that isn't crispy.

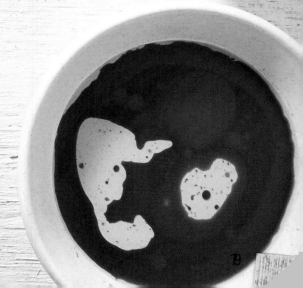

19

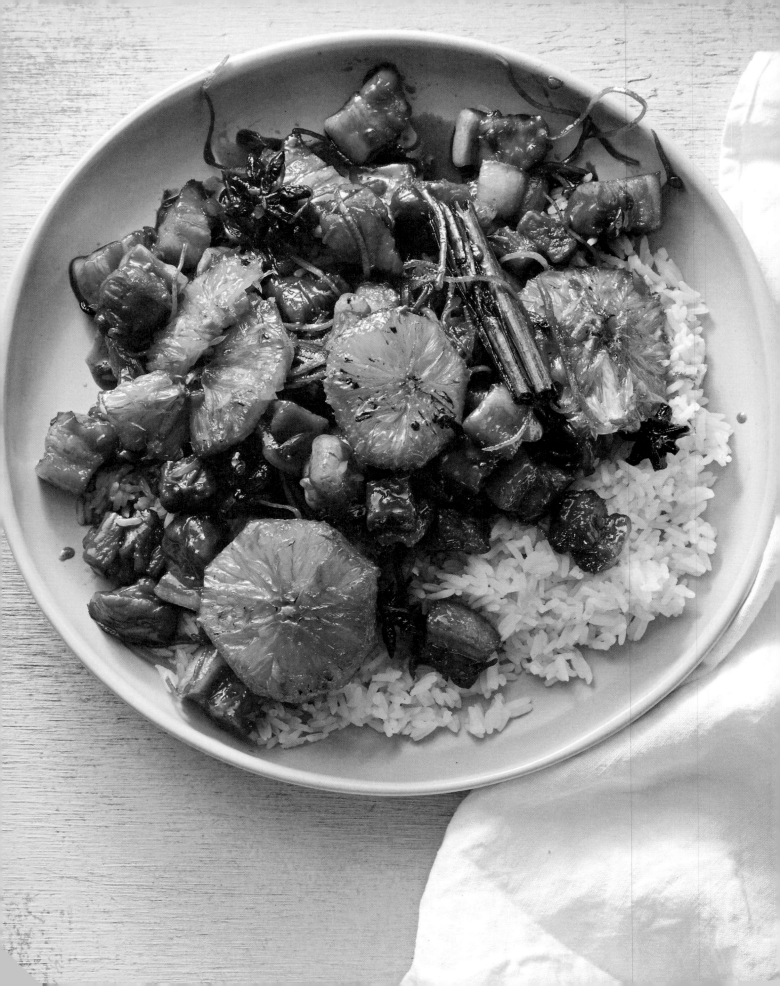

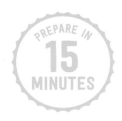

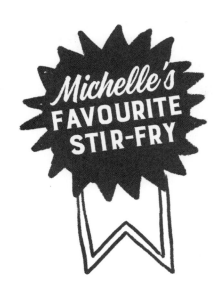

Michelle's
FAVOURITE
STIR-FRY

Michelle (a stir-fry lover): *Matt, I question whether we can call this a stir-fry?*

Matt (not a stir-fry lover): *Thank you for making my point, Michelle! This dish uses a wok, involves much frying and has the ingredients added in stages. Surely this makes it a stir-fry? Perhaps it's the tastiness of the dish that disqualifies it, in your eyes? Or the fact that, after stir-frying, there is some braising? Tell you what, over the page, give us an example of what is unequivocally a stir-fry for you! Just make sure it's as tasty as this one!*

SERVES 6   PREP: 15 MINS   COOKING: 2 HOURS 15 MINS

1.5 kg thick pork belly, rind
   removed, meat cut into
   4 cm pieces
3 garlic cloves, crushed
125 ml (½ cup) light soy sauce
80 ml (⅓ cup) kecap manis
70 g (⅓ cup) brown sugar
6 whole cloves
4 whole star anise
2 cm knob of ginger, peeled
   and thinly sliced
2 cinnamon sticks
zest of 2 mandarins or oranges,
   flesh cut into 1 cm thick slices
1 tablespoon peanut oil
steamed rice, to serve

Heat a wok or large frying pan over high heat. Cook the pork in batches for 5 minutes, or until browned. Transfer to a plate as you go.

Return all the pork to the wok. Add the garlic and stir-fry for 1 minute or until aromatic. Add 375 ml (1½ cups) water, along with the soy sauce, kecap manis, sugar, cloves, star anise, ginger and cinnamon sticks. Bring to the boil. Reduce the heat to low and cook, partially covered, stirring occasionally, for 1½ hours, or until the pork is very tender.

Increase the heat to high and bring to a rapid simmer. Cook, uncovered, for 15–20 minutes, until the sauce thickens.

While the pork finishes cooking, place the citrus zest in a heatproof bowl. Cover with boiling water and set aside for 5 minutes to soak. Drain.

Heat the oil in a non-stick frying pan over medium–high heat. Cook the citrus slices in batches for 2–3 minutes on each side, until caramelised. Transfer to a plate.

Stir the citrus zest into the pork mixture and spoon onto a platter. Top with the caramelised fruit and serve with steamed rice.

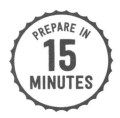

PREPARE IN
15
MINUTES

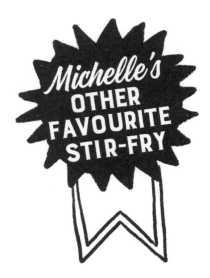

Michelle's
OTHER
FAVOURITE
STIR-FRY

WHICH IS MORE OF A STIR-FRY IN HER EYES ...

Michelle: Here it is Matt! The perfect stir-fry recipe. It may be even more perfect because it uses the venerable Chinese art of 'velveting' meat with bicarb soda to make it even more tender and this, in part, means the cooking time is far far shorter than the previous stir fry.

Matt (a waverer): Yeah. Okay. I concede that this is much more of a classic stir-fry, even if it still involves a bit of braising and sauce-reducing at the end. And kudos on the velveting! It's a great technique to pick up.

SERVES 4 PREP: 15 MINS (PLUS 20 MINS MARINATING) COOKING: 15 MINS

500 g beef rump, sirloin or scotch
  fillet steak, cut into thin strips
2 tablespoons bicarbonate of soda
80 ml (⅓ cup) soy sauce
2 tablespoons peanut oil
4 spring onions, cut into 5 cm
  lengths
1 bunch broccolini, each stem cut
  in half lengthways
40 g (¼ cup) salted black beans,
  rinsed
4 garlic cloves, crushed
4 cm knob of ginger, peeled and
  finely grated
125 ml (½ cup) chicken stock
2 tablespoons Shaoxing rice wine
  or dry sherry
1 tablespoon rice wine vinegar
2 teaspoons sugar
½ teaspoon sesame oil
cooked rice or noodles, to serve

Combine the beef strips, bicarb soda and 2 tablespoons of the soy sauce in a bowl and stir everything together well. Cover with plastic wrap and place in the fridge for 20 minutes, or even overnight if you want to get ahead.

Place the beef in a sieve and rinse under cold running water, shaking the sieve occasionally, until the beef is free of bicarb. Transfer to a plate lined with paper towel to drain. Pat dry with extra paper towel.

Heat 1 tablespoon of the oil in a wok or large frying pan over high heat until just smoking. Add the beef in batches and stir-fry for 2–3 minutes, until well-seared. Transfer to a plate.

Heat the remaining oil in the wok. Add the spring onion and broccolini and stir-fry for 2–3 minutes, until slightly charred. Transfer to a bowl.

Add the black beans, garlic and ginger, and stir-fry for 1 minute, or until aromatic. Add the stock, Shaoxing rice wine, vinegar, sugar, sesame oil and the remaining soy sauce and bring to the boil. Simmer for 3–4 minutes or until it reduces by around half.

Add the beef, broccolini and spring onion back to the wok and stir-fry for 1 minute, or until heated through. Serve with rice or noodles.

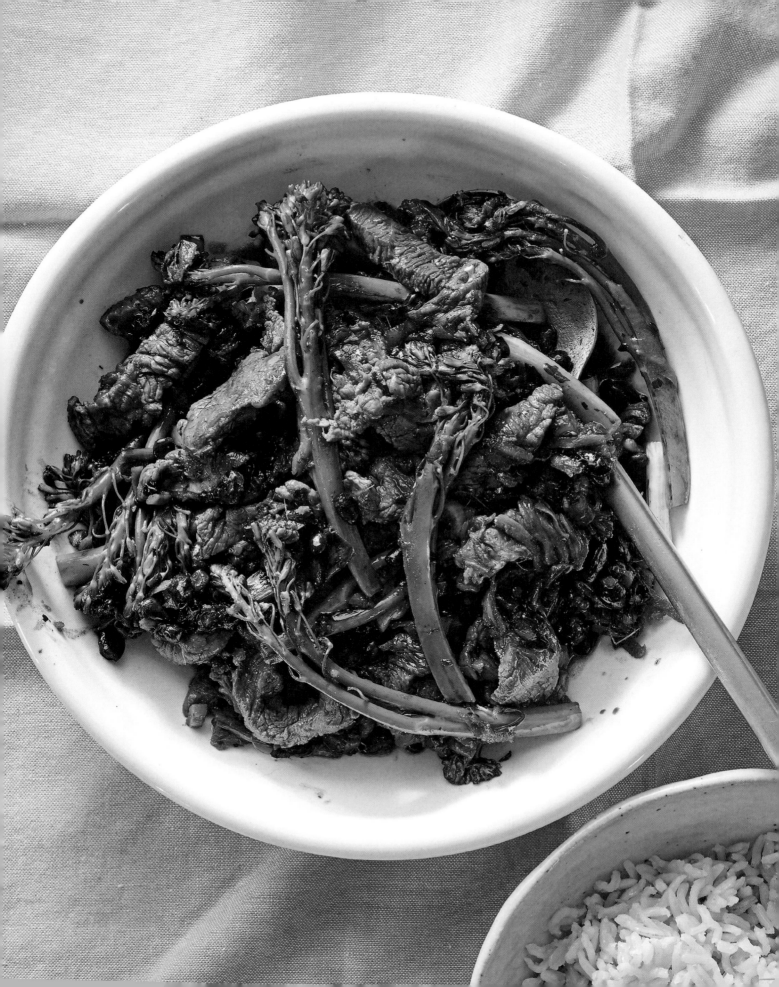

BAKED SWEET POTATO MEALS

The oven is a place of magic. I love how you can put in a sloppy batter – a loose mix of sugar, yolks, flour and egg – and walk away, then come back later to find – tah dah!!! – a cake! And then there's the humble sweet potato, which morphs from something dull, hard and rooty into the sort of fudgy sweetness that dreams are made of! (Yes, I understand and accept that your dreams may also be hard and rooty, but this is not the place for such salacious conversation. If you want that sort of stuff, head immediately to page 387).

Darn, I love baked sweet potato!

FIRST BAKE YOUR SWEET POTATOES

PREPARE IN 5 MINUTES

MAKES 6 PREP: 5 MINS COOKING: 1 HOUR 15 MINS

6 small sweet potatoes, unpeeled
melted butter, for brushing
sea salt and freshly ground black pepper

Preheat the oven to 220°C/200°C fan-forced. Place the sweet potatoes on a baking tray and cover the tray tightly with foil. Bake for 1 hour, or until tender.

Leave the cooked sweet potatoes on the tray and slit them lengthways down the centre without cutting all the way through. Use a fork to press open the potatoes slightly and roughly mash the flesh inside. Brush the outside of the skins with butter. Season. Bake for a further 10–15 minutes, until the skins are crisp. Cover with foil to keep warm. Top with your favourite topping.

NOW LET'S LOOK AT 14 WAYS TO TURN THOSE BAKED SWEET POTATOES INTO A MEAL (AND ONE THAT DOESN'T)

1. Top with slices of lap cheong sausage fried with quills of spring onion, chopped peanuts and a little Chinese five spice. Feel free to bulk up this fry with leftover shredded chicken or frozen peeled cooked prawns.

2. Load with red onion that has been slowly cooked with cranberries, a little brown sugar and vinegar. Top with crispy bacon bits and chopped cashews.

3. After an hour of baking, split the sweet potato and top with halved olives that you've pressed dry between two sheets of paper towel. Continue baking for a further 15 minutes. Now top with chopped ripe tomatoes, crumbled feta and a sprinkle of dried oregano.

4. Plump up sultanas in warm tea. Cram these into split sweet potatoes, along with small cubes of smoked cheddar and chopped toasted pecans. Return to the oven to melt the cheese.

5. Mix spicy harissa paste with a little butter. Slice the sweet potatoes in half and slather with the harissa butter before topping with caramelised onions and spiced chickpeas.

6. Top the potato with pulled pork, black beans and a corn salsa.

7. Fill the sweet potato with sliced silverbeet leaves that you've sauteed down with a mashed clove of garlic and a finely diced onion. Splash in a little cider vinegar to finish and spoon into the split baked sweet potatoes. Top with slices of gorgonzola or dolcelatte. Grill to melt.

8. Load with leftovers, such as Bolognese, chilli con carne, or the black beans on page 270. Garnish appropriately.

9. Make like Christmas and load your sweet potato with turkey breast, a dollop of cranberry sauce and loads of black pepper. Top with slices of brie and grill until the cheese bubbles.

10. Pan-tan corn, bacon, pepitas and leftover chicken, and finish by tossing it all in a little maple syrup for a couple of minutes. Fill the sweet potato and garnish with diced red chilli, lime juice and coriander.

11. Fill with chicken chilli made from browned chicken mince cooked with tomatoes, chilli, tomato paste and sugar. Top with sour cream and coriander.

12. Fill with a dollop of Pea and Broccoli Pesto (see page 237).

13. Split and spread out the baked sweet potatoes and load with a black bean and mango salsa. To make this, combine a rinsed and drained can of black beans with the flesh of a fat mango cut into 2 cm cubes, a sliced long red chilli, 3 spring onions cut into coins, chopped coriander and quartered cherry tomatoes. Tumble it all with the juice of 2 limes.

14. Saute chopped red capsicums, sliced chorizo and chickpeas. Spoon on top of your baked sweet potatoes and scatter with chilli flakes.

TIP

NEVER top baked sweet potatoes with butter, mini marshmallows and cinnamon sugar and then grill them until the marshmallows are puffy and burnished. Well, not unless you live in a trailer park on the far outskirts of Shreveport or Tupelo, or are playing the role of Alice in a re-remake of *The Brady Bunch*.

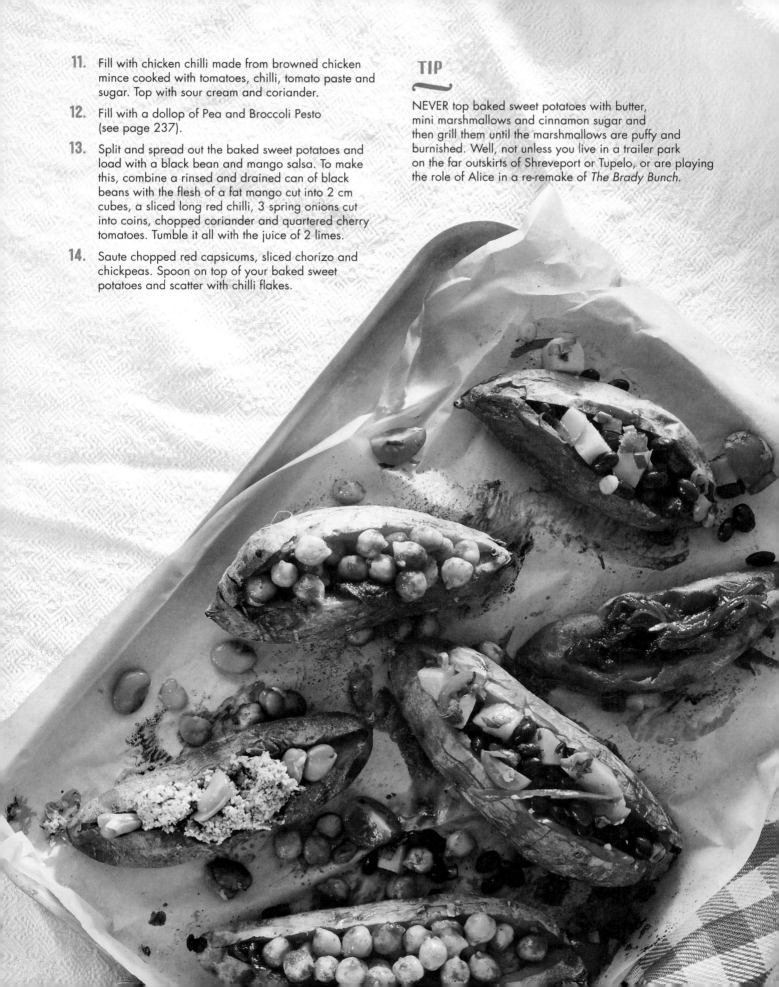

VEGG

AUTU

WIN

ES IN

UMN/

TER

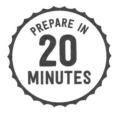

WHOLE BAKED CAULIFLOWER with ALMOND TARATOR

Cauliflower was very much 'Ms Veg, 2015'. This was back when cauliflower rice and cauliflower pizza bases were all the rage, before kale stole the limelight. I was never much of a fan of these recipes as I felt that they destroyed a major part of cauliflower's appeal: its amazing shape. Think of the florets, thinly sliced for pickling so they look like branches of coral. Or fat steaks of the stuff, slowly grilling on the barbecue like cross-sections of the human brain. Or the majesty of the whole head, whether steamed, or roasted as in this recipe. Surely that's enough to keep cauliflower a contender for any vegetable pageant in 2018, as well?

SERVES 6   PREP: 20 MINS (PLUS 15 MINS SOAKING)   COOKING: 55 MINS

1 cauliflower, outer leaves and large stalks removed
100 ml extra virgin olive oil
sea salt and freshly ground black pepper
2 tablespoons currants
1 tablespoon red wine vinegar, warmed
800 g canned chickpeas, rinsed and drained
1 teaspoon smoked paprika
1 teaspoon dried chilli flakes
1 teaspoon cumin seeds, toasted

TARATOR
100 g crustless sourdough bread, torn
100 g (1½ cups) blanched almonds, toasted
90 g (⅓ cup) tahini
2 garlic cloves, chopped
sea salt
juice of 1 lemon
60 ml (¼ cup) olive oil

TO SERVE
grated lemon zest
chopped flat-leaf parsley leaves
pomegranate or date molasses

Preheat the oven to 220°C/200°C fan-forced. Line two baking trays with baking paper.

Place the whole cauliflower in a bowl, cover and microwave on high for 8 minutes, or until tender.

Rub the cauliflower all over with 60 ml (¼ cup) of the oil and season with salt. Transfer to one of the baking trays and bake for 30 minutes, or until golden.

Meanwhile, make the tarator. Place the bread in a bowl and soak in warm water for 20 minutes. Drain and squeeze out the excess water.

Whiz the squeezed bread in a food processor with the almonds, tahini, garlic and 4 ice cubes until combined. Season with salt and stir in the lemon juice. With the motor running, slowly add the oil until you have the texture of hummus, adding a little water if needed.

Place the currants and warm vinegar in a bowl for 15 minutes to macerate the currants. Drain.

Dry the chickpeas with paper towel. Tip into in a bowl and toss with the paprika, chilli and remaining oil. Season with salt. Scatter on the second baking tray and roast for 15 minutes, or until crisp.

Spread the tarator on a serving plate and sprinkle with the toasted cumin seeds. Sit the baked cauliflower on top, then scatter around the crisp chickpeas, sweet and sour currants, lemon zest and loads of parsley. Drizzle with the molasses to serve.

TIPS

A bowl of Greek yoghurt on the side is nice, as is a little extra lemon zest and different fresh herbs.

Try this recipe with your favourite hummus instead of the tarator.

The baked cauliflower is also great on its own; especially if sprinkled with grated cheese or lumps of blue cheese, which are added just at the end of baking.

Any leftover cauliflower can be used in roast veggie and pulse salads or blitzed with stock to make a soup.

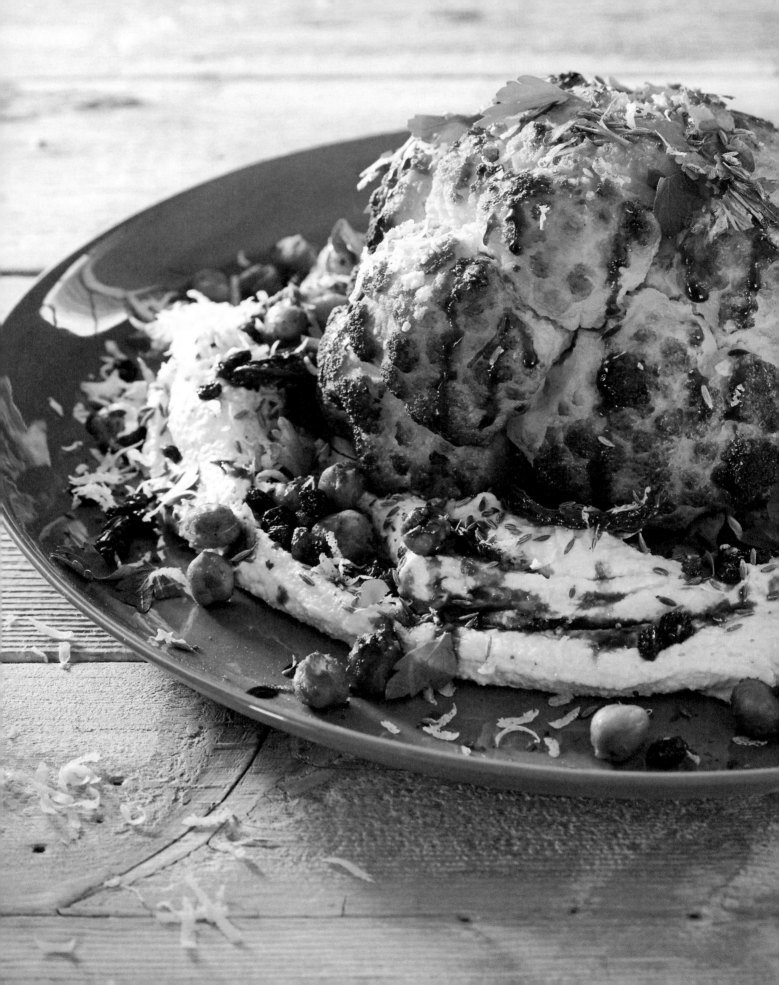

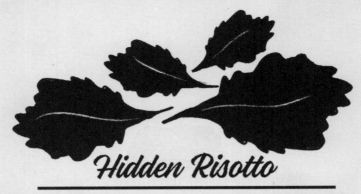

Hidden Risotto

UNDER AN AUTUMNAL PILE OF CRISPY KALE LEAVES

Much panic revolves around this simplest of rice dishes, but if you follow three simple rules you'll be right. Always toast your rice. Use hot stock. Stir in your parmesan and butter while the rice is still a little nutty. That way you'll get evenly cooked risotto that is neither chalky nor gluggy.

SERVES 4 PREP: 15 MINS COOKING: 30 MINS

CRISPY KALE LEAVES
2 bunches kale
2 tablespoons olive oil
sea salt and freshly ground
    black pepper
finely grated zest of 1 lemon

RISOTTO
1 litre salt-reduced chicken stock
1 tablespoon soy sauce
2 tablespoons olive oil
60 g butter
1 leek, trimmed and thinly sliced
2 garlic cloves, crushed
4 thyme sprigs
330 g (1½ cups) arborio rice
125 ml (½ cup) dry white wine
40 g (½ cup) shredded parmesan,
    plus extra to serve
600 g mixed mushrooms, thickly
    sliced (I like a 50/50 combo of
    buttons and Swiss browns)

Preheat the oven to 180°C/160°C fan-forced. Line two baking trays with baking paper.

Trim the tough stalks off the kale leaves (by which I mean get a minion, like a child or husband, to do this) then tear the leaves into largish pieces. Scatter the kale on the trays, drizzle with the oil and season. Toss the kale to coat (this saves washing up a kale-tossing bowl). Don't crowd the leaves and be happy to bake them in a couple of batches to ensure maximum crispiness. Bake, tossing halfway through cooking, for 10 minutes, or until the kale is crisp but still green. Don't let them turn brown!!!! Sprinkle the lemon zest over the kale chips and set aside.

While the kale cooks, start making your risotto. Bring the stock and soy sauce just to the boil in a medium saucepan over high heat. Reduce the heat to low and hold at a very gentle simmer.

Heat 1 tablespoon of oil and one-third of the butter in a large saucepan over medium heat. Fry the leek, garlic and thyme, stirring, for 5 minutes, or until soft and translucent (do not brown).

Add the rice and cook, stirring, for 2–3 minutes, until the grains appear slightly glassy. Toasting the grains like this ensures the rice cooks evenly.

Add the wine and cook, stirring, until the liquid is almost all absorbed. The rice should move in the pan like wet sand. Now add a ladleful (about 125 ml/½ cup) of hot stock and stir until the liquid is absorbed.

Add more stock, a ladleful at a time. Stir until all the liquid is absorbed before adding the next ladleful. Continue for 20 minutes, or until the rice is tender yet firm to the bite. Remove the pan from the heat and stir in the parmesan and half the remaining butter with gusto. Season.

While you are cooking your risotto, heat the remaining oil and butter in a large non-stick frying pan over medium–high heat. Fry the mushroom in batches, stirring very occasionally, for 4–5 minutes, until golden.

Stir half the mushroom into the risotto. Divide the risotto among serving plates. Top with the remaining mushroom and extra parmesan and cover with crispy kale so you can't see the risotto.

TIPS

If you can't find any kale, then a few drops of good balsamic and/or a grating of orange zest will add some brightness and surprise to this risotto.

Thyme is also wonderful employed in the cooking of the mushrooms and as fresh leaves tossed over the top of the finished risotto.

To boost the mushroom flavour use porcini stock cubes (from Italian grocers) or buy dried porcini mushrooms. Soak them in warm water and then chop to add to the stock along with the strained soaking water.

To check how cooked your rice is, squash a grain on the back of a wooden spoon. You'll see a little 'star' of starch at the centre of the grain. If that star is large then the rice needs more time and stock. The time to stir in the butter and cheese is when that spot of starch is pinhead-sized and just before it splits into three tiny white dots, showing the rice is perfectly cooked.

Risotto without stirring. If you are using a high-starch (but expensive) rice, like carnaroli or vialone nano, you can cook it slowly in the oven or on the stovetop together with all the stock (allow 2 ladles of stock for each ladle of raw rice) for 12 minutes. Then knock the starch off the grains to make it creamy when you vigorously stir in the butter and parmesan.

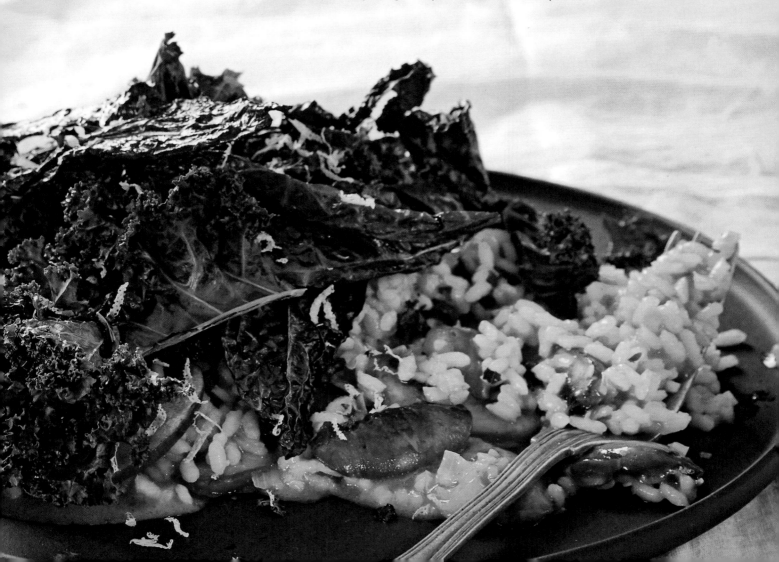

15 MORE SURE-FIRE AUTUMN / WINTER RISOTTOS

Risotto is a brilliant vehicle for flavour. Make the basic risotto on page 168, and top or customise with any of the below combos.

1. Pumpkin, crispy sage, bacon and toasted pumpkin seeds.

2. Beetroot and feta. For a change try using sunflower seeds instead of rice. For my sunflower seed risotto recipe see delicious.com.au.

3. Silverbeet and squid. Use the ink to blacken the rice, Spanish-style by adding at the end of cooking. Use mascarpone instead of butter.

4. Roasted red onion halves with balsamic vinegar. Luxe this one out with slices of roast duck breast on top.

5. Pulled pork with roasted pineapple.

6. Roasted carrots (but cook the risotto with beef stock).

7. Instead of just stock, cook the risotto with a loose, fine puree of slow-cooked leek greens loosened with chicken stock. Fry the white part of the leek for garnish.

8. Slow-roasted lamb shoulder, shredded and laid on a saffron-hit risotto.

9. Make a Piedmontese red wine risotto to serve on its own, with barbecued steak or topped with crispy fried bone marrow. Use red wine and beef stock flavoured with a bay leaf.

10. Leftover beef ragu over extra-cheesy risotto (stir in something extra bitey with the parmesan, such as aged cheddar).

11. Roast cauliflower, cumin, currants and pine nuts.

12. In Lombardy they add chunks of skinned salami with the parmesan at the end of cooking. This is traditionally served with a pork chop sticking out of it! You don't need to do this.

13. In the Veneto they cook the local salami with the rice and finish with cloves, cinnamon and lots of black pepper.

14. Frozen peas and feta stirred through at the end to cook through.

15. Tinned tuna with corn kernels, likewise.

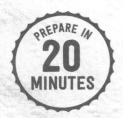

PREPARE IN
20 MINUTES

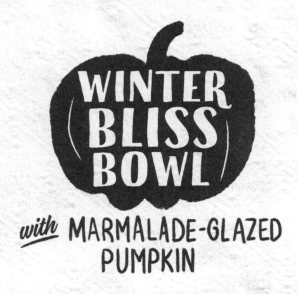

WINTER BLISS BOWL

with MARMALADE-GLAZED PUMPKIN

The secret with any autumn or winter bowl is to balance richness and heartiness with a little bit of finesse from citrus (or other acidity) and some creaminess. Oh, and organise the different ingredients so they each take up a wedge in the bowl.

SERVES 4 **PREP:** 20 MINS **COOKING:** 45 MINS

440 g (2 cups) pearl barley
170 g (½ cup) orange marmalade
2 teaspoons chopped rosemary
   leaves
900 g Kent pumpkin, deseeded and
   cut into 2 cm thick wedges (or use
   your choice of winter veggie)
1 tablespoon olive oil
sea salt and freshly ground
   black pepper
550 g pork fillet
3 oranges, peeled and cut
   into rounds
80 g (½ cup) smoked almonds,
   coarsely chopped

WINTER GREMOLATA

zest of 1 orange (save dollars and
   use the zest of one of the oranges
   from above)
½ cup chopped flat-leaf
   parsley leaves
¼ cup chopped mint leaves
2 tablespoons olive oil

Place the barley in a large saucepan with 1.5 litres of cold water. Bring to the boil over high heat. Reduce the heat to medium and simmer, stirring occasionally, for 30 minutes, or until the water is absorbed but the barley is still a little bitey. Remove from the heat and set aside, covered, for 5 minutes. Fluff with a fork.

Preheat the oven to 220°C/200°C fan-forced. Line a baking tray with baking paper.

While the barley is cooking, heat the marmalade and rosemary in a small saucepan over low heat for 2 minutes, or until runny. Place the pumpkin pieces on the tray and brush with half the marmalade. Roast for 40–45 minutes, until tender, caramelised and slightly charred. Brush with the remaining marmalade halfway through cooking.

Meanwhile, heat the oil in an ovenproof frying pan over medium–high heat. Season the pork fillet well and cook for 3 minutes on each side, or until golden all over.

In the last 10 minutes of the pumpkin roasting time, transfer the frying pan with the pork to the oven. Cook for 10 minutes, then put on an oven mitt and remove from the oven and place the pork on a plate. Cover loosely with foil to rest for 5 minutes, then thinly slice.

Combine all the gremolata ingredients in a bowl, seasoning well.

Divide the barley among serving bowls. Top with the pumpkin, pork, orange slices and smoked almonds. Sprinkle over the gremolata and serve.

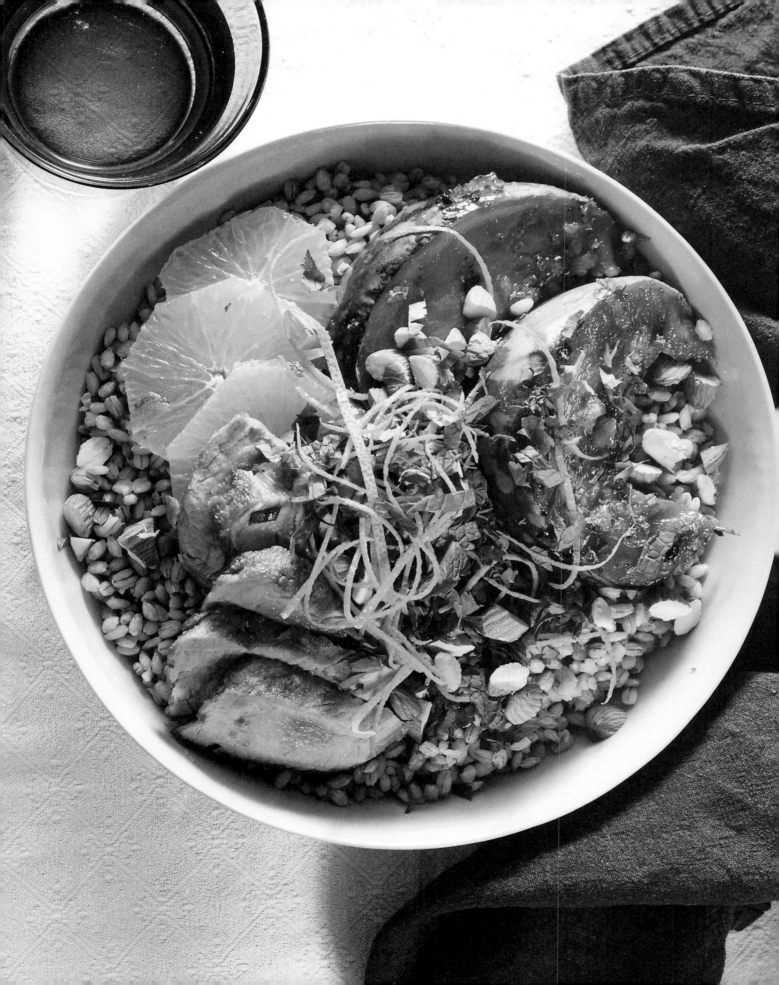

23 AUTUMN / WINTER BOWLS

Here are some ideas for customising your bowls. Just start by cooking your grain of choice by following the instructions below (also check the packet cooking instructions as some wholegrains, such as freekeh, can be sold as cracked and uncracked grains, which changes the cooking time). You can mix and match any of the toppings below. For more ideas, check out my Spring/Summer bowls on pages 166–167.

BROWN RICE BOWLS

Combine 200 g (1 cup) of brown rice and 435 ml (1¾ cups) of water in a large saucepan with a good pinch of salt and cook, covered, over low heat for 40 minutes, or until the water is absorbed. Remove from the heat and set aside, covered, for 10 minutes to let the rice sit and the steam out. Fluff with a fork.

PEARL BARLEY BOWLS

Place 440 g (2 cups) of pearl barley in a large saucepan. Cover with 1.5 litres of cold water and bring to the boil over high heat. Reduce the heat to medium and simmer, stirring occasionally, for 30 minutes, or until the water is absorbed but the barley is still a little bitey. Remove from the heat and set aside, covered, for 5 minutes. Fluff with a fork.

FREEKEH BOWLS

Place 250 g (1½ cups) of cracked freekeh in a large saucepan with 935 ml (3¾ cups) of cold salted water. Bring to the boil over medium–high heat. Reduce the heat to low and simmer for 20 minutes until the water is absorbed. Remove from the heat and set aside, covered, for 5 minutes. Fluff with a fork.

QUINOA BOWLS

Combine 300 g (1½ cups) of quinoa and 750 ml (3 cups) of water in a saucepan and bring to the boil. Reduce the heat to low, cover and simmer for 12 minutes, or until the water is absorbed. Remove from the heat and set aside, covered, for 10 minutes to steam. Fluff up with a fork.

1. Wedges of soft creamy-fleshed roast fennel, sliced char siu barbecued pork, salted roasted cashews, crispy shallots and sliced spring onions.

2. Chunks of roast pumpkin, toasted coconut (or Coconut Granola, page 203), steamed green beans that are then fried over high heat until they blister, and chilli-caramel peanut cracknell. Finish with a Thai dressing made from fish sauce, lime juice and palm sugar and top with torn Thai basil and Vietnamese mint (if you can find it).

3. Steamed green beans, poached chicken slices, thin lengths of pear and thinly sliced celery. Top with chopped almonds and a garlic and lemon crème fraîche dressing.

4. A mound of pickled ginger, slices of avocado, nori flakes and raw salmon cubes tossed in a ponzu sauce. A squiggle of squirted Kewpie mayonnaise and a dribble of soy sauce mixed with wasabi are optional. The grains here can be served warm or at room temperature. You can season the grains with sushi seasoning.

5. Roasted beef fillet marinated in soy with roast onion, quarters and slabs of roast corn kernels cut from the cob. Add shredded kale and splash it all with Korean Mayo (page 22).

6. Crumbled marinated feta, warmed shredded lamb shoulder (page 104), chopped toasted hazelnuts, torn mint and slices of roasted baby beetroot. Drizzle with tarator (page 188), if you like.

7. Roast cauliflower florets and red onion wedges; curls of streaky bacon, shredded silverbeet tossed with chopped parsley and chopped macadamias. Drizzle with an orange vinaigrette.

8. Roast carrot wedges and halved brussels sprouts. Add chopped pecans and lardons of fried kaiserfleish; drizzle with a creamy blue cheese dressing.

9. Soft-boiled or poached egg, chunks of fried chorizo, grated manchego and roast red capsicum. Fry the grains with cumin and coriander seeds and finish with parsley and a little orange zest.

10. Cook the grains in chicken stock instead of water. Drain and toss with finely grated parmesan. Toss cooked peas, sliced green beans and sliced snow peas in butter to soften. Tumble on slices of roasted chicken, chunks of ricotta, crushed smoked almonds and oregano leaves.

11. Microwave cubes of strasbourg so it gets sticky, browned and crispy in places, add roasted tomatoes and a fried egg. Finish with just a little barbecue sauce or tomato sauce if you desire.

12. Milk-simmered cubes of celeriac with chicken stock-braised celery, chopped walnuts, poached chicken and young green celery leaves. Drizzle with olive oil blitzed with parsley.

13. Toss roast garlic cloves, crushed toasted hazelnuts and 1 cm cubes of fried pancetta through the grains. Top with slow-roasted Jerusalem artichokes, crumbled blue cheese and either thyme leaves or sage leaves fried crisp in brown butter. Serve with a lemon wedge.

14. Roasted parsnips, pear and red onion. Top with crescents of chopped witlof, warm honey-tossed walnuts and shaved pecorino.

15. Cajun roast chicken breast or sliced smoked chicken breast, pumpkin roasted with a drizzle of maple syrup and pecans. Finish with a lightly spiced smoked mayo and chopped parsley. Add roasted or pickled grapes for some extra succulence.

16. Cubes of roasted sweet potato and roasted red capsicum, shredded spinach, candied walnuts, smoked mayo and bacon squares tossed in honey and salt flakes.

17. Shredded lamb shoulder, pitted black olives, crispy capers, roasted cherry tomatoes, pickled red onions (page 53), whipped feta and yoghurt and chopped parsley.

18. Roast beetroot slices, toasted hazelnuts, goat's cheese and olive oil-soaked orange segments. Add sliced pork fillet cooked with a strip of orange zest, for added protein, and top with crispy Tuscan kale (page 190).

19. Green olives, barbecued zucchini, a drizzle of pomegranate molasses and good olive oil. Drizzle with hummus loosened with lemon juice, or yoghurt mixed with a little tahini. Leftover roast lamb or roast chicken go well with this. As does a pan-fried robust white fish fillet or a dukkah-tossed poached egg (page 141).

20. Warmed falafels with pickled red onion, grated beetroot, chopped pistachios and a dollop of thick yoghurt swirled with a little harissa or melted butter. Scatter with plenty of mint and parsley.

21. Roasted fennel wedges with sliced crispy duck, orange slices, smoked almonds and baby spinach leaves. Drizzle with a warmed raisin and orange vinaigrette.

22. Balsamic- and thyme-roasted mushrooms with canned lentils and steamed broccolini, and topped with whipped goat's cheese. Sprinkle with shavings of crispy fried French shallots and toasted flaked almonds.

23. Cubes of maple-roasted pumpkin, sliced smoked chicken or chunks of roast chicken, shaved fresh brussels sprouts, candied pecans and crumbled feta. Drizzle with a little sriracha chilli sauce.

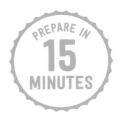

~ *Sicilian* ~
ROAST PUMPKIN
TRAY BAKE, TWO WAYS

This tray bake can go two ways: add the vinegar dressing 15 minutes before the cooking is over and you get a sticky tray bake of classic Sicilian sweet and sour flavours, or add it after cooking and let everything – pumpkin wedges, roasted onions and olives – steep, and you get a really meaty pumpkin salad that just needs some ricotta or feta to become a full meal. This is one of the must-make recipes in this book!

SERVES 6   PREP: 15 MINS (PLUS 20 MINS SOAKING)   COOKING: 55 MINS

1 kg Kent pumpkin, unpeeled, deseeded and cut into 3 cm wedges
4 small red onions, unpeeled, halved from root to tip, cut surfaces rubbed with oil
2 tablespoons olive oil
sea salt and freshly ground black pepper
45 g (¼ cup) currants
1 long red chilli, thinly sliced
60 ml (¼ cup) red wine vinegar
1 tablespoon caster sugar
160 g (1 cup) pitted Sicilian green olives
¼ teaspoon ground nutmeg
40 g (¼ cup) pine nuts
100 g fresh ricotta or feta, crumbled into big chunks
¼ cup basil leaves

Preheat the oven to 220°C/200°C fan-forced. Line a large baking tray with baking paper. Place the pumpkin wedges on the tray in a single layer and add the onion halves, cut-side down. Drizzle with the oil and season. Roast for 30 minutes.

While the pumpkin and onion are roasting, combine the currants, chilli, vinegar and sugar in a bowl. Set aside, stirring occasionally.

Add the olives to the baking tray and sprinkle a little nutmeg over the pumpkin. Roast for a further 15 minutes or until the pumpkin is golden and slightly charred at the edges.

Once the pumpkin is cooked, transfer the roasted veg and olives to a serving platter with sides. Pour over the currant dressing and set aside for at least 20 minutes, or up to 2 hours.

Place the pine nuts on a baking tray. Toast for 10 minutes, or until golden. Watch so they don't burn.

Sprinkle the pumpkin with the ricotta or feta, basil and pine nuts.

If you want to eat the pumpkin hot from the tray, pour on the vinegar mixture when you add the olives and then proceed with the recipe as above.

TIP

Use a large baking tray to make sure your pumpkin sits in a single layer. This will ensure you get great caramelisation on the pumpkin and that it doesn't steam.

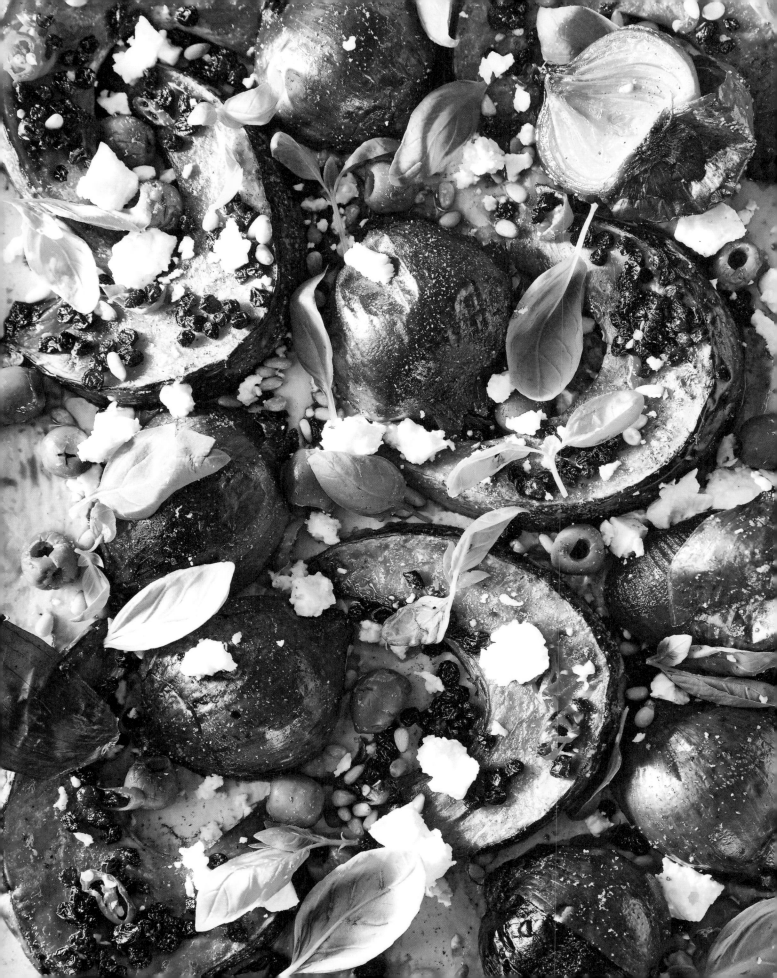

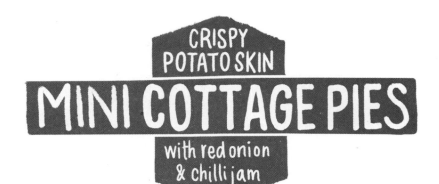

CRISPY POTATO SKIN
MINI COTTAGE PIES
with red onion & chilli jam

So there we were, food guru Michelle Southan and me, debating what to do with the potato skins left over from making gnocchi. I reverted to my default idea of frying them (or baking them with butter) so they went crisp, and serving them with sweet chilli sauce, sour cream and some beers. Michelle, exhibiting with devastating effect her 30 years' experience of recipe writing, suggested we fill them with mince and bake them to make potato skin cottage pies. (She was kind enough not to point out that this is the sort of creative and commercially minded thinking that has placed her in a position of power in magazines while – between us – I'm still a bottom feeder.)

And no, you don't need to be making gnocchi to make these, as the potato filling can also go on top as a creamy golden mash!

SERVES 6–8   PREP: 30 MINS   COOKING: 1 HOUR 15 MINS

8 coliban potatoes (about 200 g each), unpeeled
1 tablespoon olive oil
100 g shortcut bacon rashers, coarsely chopped
1 small onion, finely chopped
1 carrot, finely chopped
2 garlic cloves, crushed
2 tablespoons tomato paste
250 g beef mince
125 ml (½ cup) beef stock
1 tablespoon barbecue or tomato sauce
1 teaspoon soy sauce
20 g butter
sea salt and freshly ground black pepper
50 g (½ cup) coarsely grated mozzarella

RED ONION AND CHILLI JAM
1 tablespoon olive oil
4 red onions, thinly sliced
3 thyme sprigs
2 long red chillies, deseeded and thinly sliced
100 g (½ cup) brown sugar
60 ml (¼ cup) red wine vinegar

Preheat the oven to 200°C/180°C fan-forced. Wash the potatoes well, then dry. Wrap each potato in foil, then place them all on a baking tray and roast for 1 hour, or until you can skewer them easily.

While the potatoes are baking, make your jam. Heat the oil in a large saucepan over medium heat. Add the onion and thyme, and cook, stirring often, for 20 minutes. Add the chilli and cook for a further 20 minutes, or until the onion is golden brown and caramelised. Add the sugar and vinegar and cook, stirring, for 10 minutes, or until the mixture thickens. Set aside.

Heat the oil in a large frying pan. Add the chopped bacon and cook, stirring, for 3 minutes, or until golden.

Add the onion and carrot and cook, stirring, for 5 minutes, or until both soften. Next, add the garlic and tomato paste and cook, stirring, for 2 minutes, or until the tomato paste starts to darken.

Add the beef mince. Stir and cook, tossing, for 3 minutes, or until the mince changes colour. Finally add the stock, barbecue sauce and soy sauce. Reduce the heat to low and simmer for 15 minutes, or until the liquid has reduced but the mince is still moist and not too dry.

When the potatoes are cooked, carefully cut a small slice off the side of each one so it's large enough to insert a teaspoon. Save the sliced pieces of potato!!! Don't turn off the oven!!! Oh, so much breathless excitement in this recipe. What's next???

Scoop out most of the potato flesh to create a case, but leave a 1 cm border of potato so you don't risk breaking the skin. Place the potato flesh in a bowl. Add the butter and mash until smooth. Season.

Place the potato cases and reserved potato slices on a baking tray, cut-side up. Spoon the warm beef mixture into the cases and top with the mash. Sprinkle the mozzarella on top of the mash and over the cut surface of the potato slices. Return to the oven for 15 minutes, or until the mozzarella is melty and golden. Serve with a big dollop of the red onion and chilli jam.

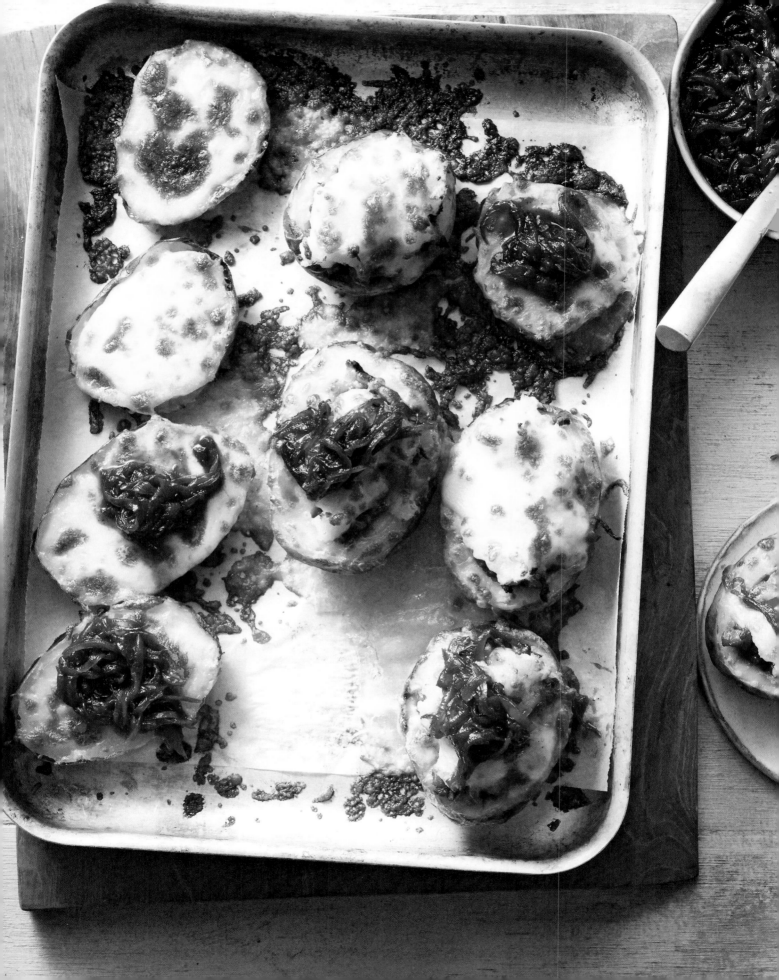

AUTUMN / WINTER SIDES AND SALADS

CAULIFLOWER HUMMUS WITH ROASTED RED ONIONS AND GRAPES

PREPARE IN 15 MINUTES

Virtuous, versatile cauliflower stars with the equally adaptable leader of the legume gang, chickpeas, to make a hummus that is great on its own or served with roast meats or my warm Instant Flatbreads (page 175). It works just as brilliantly with the sweetness of the roast onions and juiciness of the roasted grapes.

SERVES 6 PREP: 15 MINS **COOKING:** 35 MINS

700 g cauliflower, cut into florets
1 × 400 g can chickpeas, rinsed and drained
125 ml (½ cup) olive oil (use a lightly flavoured, not too peppery oil for this)
3 teaspoons cumin seeds
sea salt and freshly ground black pepper
3 red onions, cut into wedges
450 g red grapes, cut into small clusters (which look pretty, but if you have a stalk aversion remove them before roasting)
1 small garlic clove, crushed
finely grated zest and juice of 1 lemon
100 g feta

Preheat the oven to 220°C/200°C fan-forced. Line two baking trays with baking paper.

Spread the cauliflower and chickpeas on one tray. Drizzle with 2 tablespoons of the oil and sprinkle with the cumin seeds. Season well.

Place the onion on the remaining tray. Drizzle with 1 tablespoon of the remaining oil and season. Roast both trays at the same time for 20 minutes, then add the grapes to the onion tray. Continue roasting both trays for a further 15 minutes, or until the cauliflower is tender and the grapes are just starting to shrivel.

Place the cauliflower mixture and garlic in a food processor with two cubes of ice and process until almost smooth. With the motor running, gradually add the remaining oil and the lemon juice and process until smooth.

Spread the hummus onto a serving platter and top with the onion and grapes. Crumble over the feta. Sprinkle with the lemon zest and serve.

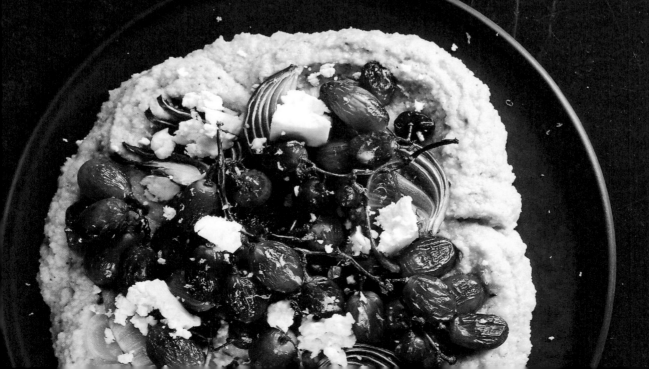

BRUSSELS SPROUT CHAMP-CANNON

PREPARE IN 15 MINUTES

Do you get confused between champ and colcannon? No worries. Just make this side, which is the best of both Irish worlds and should also appeal to your inner Belgian.

SERVES 4 PREP: 15 MINS **COOKING:** 30 MINS

20 g butter
200 g brussels sprouts, thinly sliced
2 spring onions, thinly sliced
1 batch Potato Skin Mash (page 205)
sea salt and freshly ground black pepper
2 rindless bacon rashers, coarsely chopped
4 thyme sprigs

Preheat the oven to 220°C/200°C fan-forced. Heat the butter in a large non-stick frying pan over medium heat. Add the sliced brussels sprouts and cook, stirring, for 2 minutes, or until softened. Remove from the heat and stir in the spring onion.

Add the brussels sprout mixture to the mashed potato, leaving a little butter behind in the pan for later. Stir until well combined and season well. Spoon into an ovenproof dish. Rough the top up with a fork, then brush with the reserved butter from the pan. Bake for 20 minutes, or until golden.

Meanwhile, heat a non-stick frying pan over medium–high heat. Add the bacon and thyme and cook for 3–4 minutes, until crisp.

Sprinkle the bacon mixture over the mash to serve.

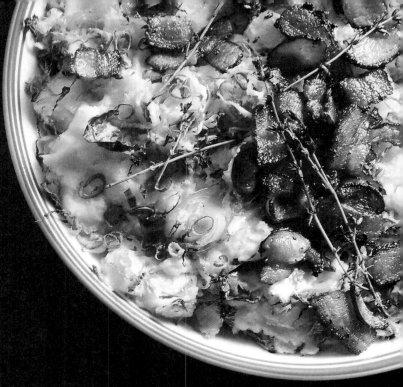

COCONUT CABBAGE NOODLES

PREPARE IN 10 MINUTES

Coconut and cabbage is a world-beating taste combination to match the likes of tomato and basil, pumpkin and sage, and a really nice floral cravat with a sharp suit. In fact, the coconut granola in this recipe is also great on Hawaiian Poke (page 118), Chinese Carrot Steaks (page 222), or just on your breakfast yoghurt. It also makes a really good snack so I suggest you make double quantities.

SERVES 4 PREP: 10 MINS **COOKING:** 10 MINS

1/2 (about 900 g) green cabbage, cut into thin ribbons
1 tablespoon coconut oil

COCONUT GRANOLA
45 g (3/4 cup) flaked coconut
80 g (1/2 cup) roasted peanuts, coarsely chopped
55 g (1/4 cup) brown sugar or grated palm sugar
1/2 teaspoon sea salt

To make the granola, cook the ingredients in a large frying pan for 5 minutes, or until the sugar dissolves and the coconut is toasted. Make sure that once you see the sugar melting you stir constantly as it will burn quickly. Transfer to a bowl.

Fry the cabbage strips in the coconut oil until wilted but still bitey. Pile the cabbage up in a serving bowl. Use your hands to break up the coconut granola and sprinkle on top.

EASIEST-EVER HOMEMADE HOT ROLLS

PREPARE IN 10 MINUTES

This is a much-loved recipe. Make the dough the night before and then you've got hot fresh rolls for breakfast and lunch. This dough also makes a good dense loaf. Just shape the loaf freehand and pop in a COLD oven set to 220°C/200°C fan-forced. Remove when the bottom sounds hollow when tapped.

MAKES 8 ROLLS **PREP:** 10 MINS (PLUS 3 HOURS PROVING) **COOKING:** 20 MINS

500 g plain flour, plus extra for kneading and dusting
3 teaspoons salt
1 × 7 g sachet dry instant yeast

Mix the flour and salt together in a bowl. Sprinkle over the yeast. Roughly mix in 475 ml warm water. Cover with plastic wrap and leave on the bench for the next 3 hours., or in the fridge overnight.

Preheat the oven to 220°C/200°C fan-forced. Line two baking trays with baking paper and dust with flour.

Tip the dough out onto a very well-floured surface. It will be loose and floppy. Flop it over on itself to make a rough ball.

Cut into eight equal-sized pieces and, with well-floured hands, shape gently into rolls. Place on the floured trays and throw in the oven for 20 minutes, or until the rolls sound hollow when tapped on the bottom.

BUTTER-ROASTED CABBAGE WEDGES

PREPARE IN 10 MINUTES

This is a homage to the wonderful dish served by Duncan Welgemoed at Adelaide's equally wonderful Africola. We've twisted it a little by adding Vietnamese mint, which has a strange and rather unlikely love affair with dates. It is great on its own or with pretty much anything roasty!

SERVES 4 PREP: 10 MINS COOKING: 50 MINS

½ savoy cabbage (about 720 g), cut into wedges
150 g butter, melted
sea salt and freshly ground black pepper
2 tablespoons capers
8 medjool dates, halved and pitted
125 ml (½ cup) cider vinegar
¼ cup Vietnamese mint leaves

Preheat the oven to 180°C/160°C fan-forced. Place the cabbage in a roasting tin. Drizzle with one-third of the melted butter and season well. Roast for 30 minutes, spooning over half the remaining butter halfway through cooking. Sprinkle with the capers and dates and roast for a further 10–15 minutes, until the cabbage is charred slightly.

Transfer to a serving plate and cover with foil to keep warm.

Heat the roasting tin over low heat. Add the remaining butter and cook, stirring, for 2–3 minutes, until golden. Add the vinegar to the tin and deglaze for 2 minutes, or until it reduces slightly. Drizzle over the cabbage salad and sprinkle with the mint.

TIP

You could add toasted slivered almonds for more crunch if you wanted.

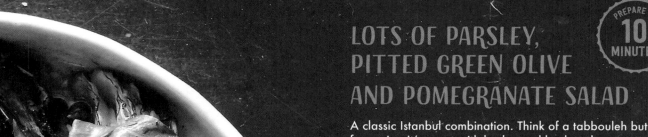

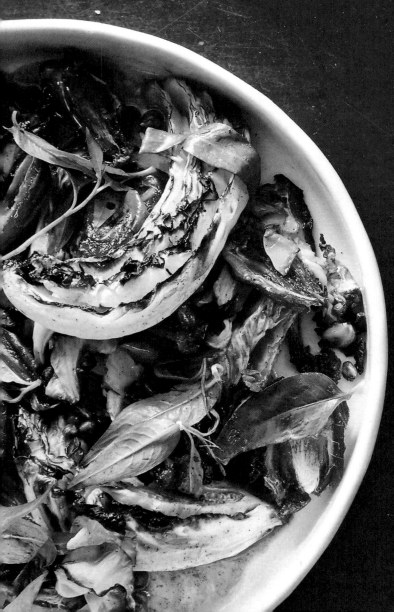

LOTS OF PARSLEY, PITTED GREEN OLIVE AND POMEGRANATE SALAD

PREPARE IN 10 MINUTES

A classic Istanbul combination. Think of a tabbouleh but far, far sexier. It's great with barbecued lamb, salmon, roasted fennel steaks and grilled haloumi, especially if you've added a sprinkling of spice mix (such as 2 parts crushed coriander seeds and 1 part cumin seeds) to any of these – either as a spice rub *before* cooking or as a twist to dukkah for use *after* cooking (for an image, see page 109)

SERVES 4 PREP: 10 MINS

2 bunches flat-leaf parsley, leaves picked
250 g drained pitted green olives, some halved and some left whole
seeds of 1 pomegranate
1 small red onion, cut into thin wedges
60 ml (¼ cup) extra virgin olive oil
2 tablespoons pomegranate molasses
sea salt and freshly ground black pepper

Toss the parsley, olives, pomegranate seeds and onion in a serving bowl.

Mix the oil and molasses together lightly with a fork so the molasses marbles the oil rather than being totally incorporated. Drizzle over the salad and season well.

ICEBERG, LEMON JUICE-SOAKED CELERY AND TORN RICOTTA SALAD

A cooling, blissful-memories-of-summer salad that is great to serve in front of a roaring fire with anything rich and braisey or tomatoey.

SERVES 6 PREP: 10 MINS (PLUS 20 MINS MARINATING)

½ bunch celery, stalks thinly sliced, baby heart leaves reserved
80 ml (⅓ cup) lemon juice
1 teaspoon sea salt
230 g (1½ cups) frozen baby peas, thawed
80 ml (⅓ cup) extra virgin olive oil, plus extra to serve
freshly ground black pepper
½ iceberg lettuce, finely shredded
1 cup mint leaves, larger leaves torn
200 g fresh ricotta, torn into large pieces

Place the sliced celery in a large glass or ceramic bowl. Add the lemon juice and salt and toss until well combined. Set aside for 20 minutes, or until pickled slightly.

Meanwhile, place the peas in a heatproof bowl. Pour over boiling water to cover, then set aside for 2 minutes, or until tender. Drain.

Scoop the celery slices out of the lemon pickling liquid and into your serving bowl. Add the oil to the remaining pickling liquid and whisk until combined into a dressing. Season with pepper.

Add the lettuce, peas and mint to the dressing and toss to combine. Spoon the lettuce mixture over the celery and top with the ricotta and reserved celery heart leaves. Drizzle with a little extra oil and serve.

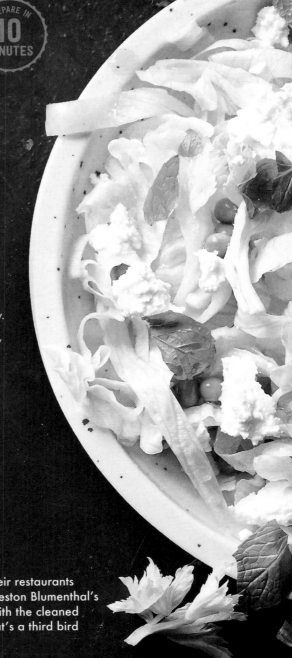

POTATO SKIN MASH – THE BEST MASH EVER

The mark of a true culinary genius is not the wacky stuff that chefs serve in their restaurants but their simple tips that become everyday household lore. Like this idea of Heston Blumenthal's to thicken the milk for mash, and intensify its potatoey-ness, by simmering it with the cleaned potato skins. Even better, warm milk makes better mash than cold milk. So that's a third bird killed with the same stone. Genius!

SERVES 4 PREP: 10 MINS COOKING: 15 MINS

4 large royal blue or Dutch cream potatoes, washed
500 ml (2 cups) milk
125 g cold butter, chopped
sea salt and freshly ground black pepper

Peel the potatoes and place their skins in a small saucepan. Pour in the milk and place over very low heat.

Slice the potatoes and place in a saucepan of salted water. Bring to the boil. Cook the potatoes for 10–12 minutes, until tender. Drain, then return to the pan and mash well.

Gradually pour the potato skin-infused milk through a fine sieve into the mash, stirring occasionally to get the consistency you like. Add the butter and stir to combine. Season well and serve.

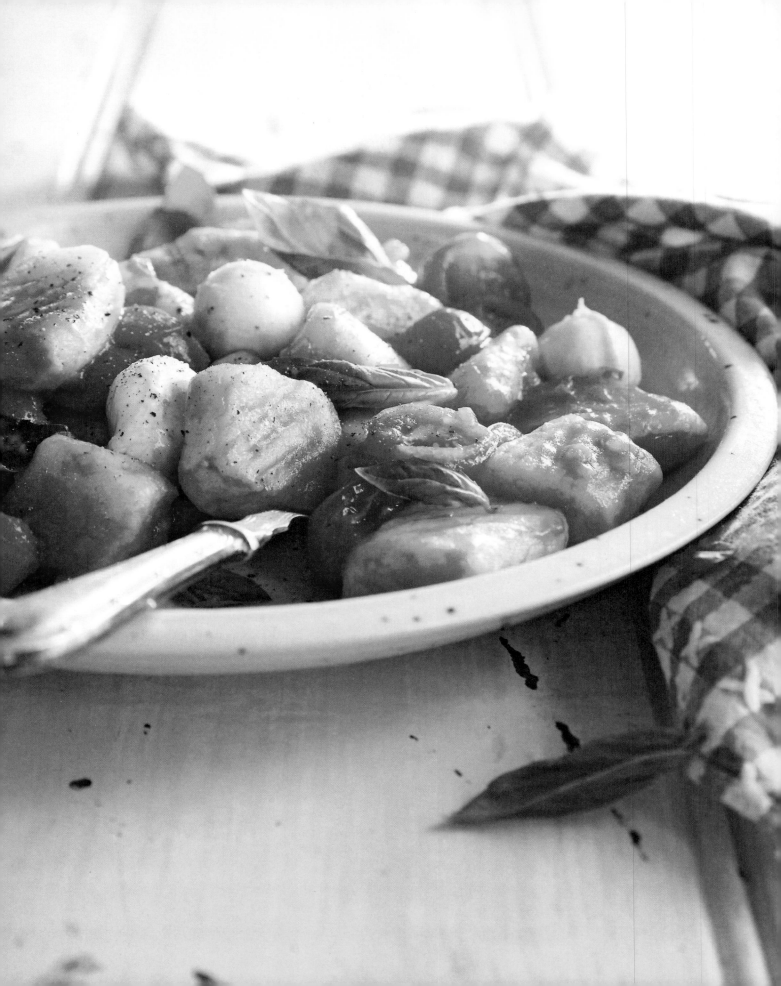

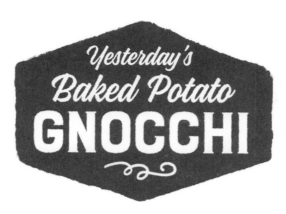

Yesterday's Baked Potato GNOCCHI

'Great cooking is about planning; so is great potato gnocchi.' These are the words of wisdom my imaginary nonna would give me if she were alive today. While ricotta gnocchi can be knocked up at the drop of a hat, potato gnocchi takes time as you need to ensure the potato has been sufficiently relieved of any excess moisture. The drier the potato, the less flour you need and therefore the lighter the gnocchi. So the next time you do a bake or roast, throw a load of potatoes in the bottom of the oven and then make this gnocchi, which is as ethereal as that nonna of mine.

SERVES 6   PREP: 30 MINS (PLUS COOLING TIME)   COOKING: 1 HOUR 30 MINS

1.25 kg washed but unpeeled floury
    potatoes (coliban are the best;
    Nonna told me)
sea salt
up to 300 g (2 cups) plain flour,
    plus extra for dusting

CHERRY TOMATO NAPOLI SAUCE
2 tablespoons olive oil
1 small onion, finely chopped
2 garlic cloves, crushed
60 ml (¼ cup) white wine
500 g cherry tomatoes, halved
250 ml (1 cup) passata
sea salt and freshly ground
    black pepper
juice of 1 lemon
220 g baby bocconcini
basil leaves, to serve

Preheat the oven to 180°C/160°C fan-forced. Place the potatoes on a baking tray and bake for 1 hour, or until they are squidgy in the middle. Leave to cool a little, then cut the potatoes in half and scoop the flesh out of the skins onto the baking tray. Mash the potato until smooth. Spread the flesh out to help it steam off its moisture, then season with salt. You should have about 500 g of potato.

Flour a work surface and dump the potato onto it. Gently mix with 150 g (1 cup) of the flour to make a dough. If it feels a little sticky, add more flour. The gnocchi mix needs to be a little stickier than a pasta dough; if you push your thumb into it, it should come out almost clean, but not completely dry. The amount of flour depends on loads of variables, such as how dry your potato is. Don't be rough when kneading the dough. Be caring and gentle as if it was a new love – as it will surely become. You need to avoid developing the gluten in the flour too much, because that will make the gnocchi rubbery.

Split the dough into four. Roll each piece into a snake as thick as a lumberjack's index finger. Place each length on a sheet of baking paper and cut into 3 cm lengths. If you want, roll the pieces of gnocchi with the back of a floured fork to mark it with grooves that will catch the sauce. If the gnocchi is very tender, then skip this step as you risk compressing the gnocchi detrimentally.

Next, make your sauce. Heat the oil in a frying pan over medium heat. Add the onion and cook, stirring, for 5 minutes, or until soft. Add the garlic and cook, stirring, for 30 seconds, or until aromatic. Add the wine and simmer for 4 minutes, or until the wine almost evaporates, making sure you scrape the yummy bits from the bottom of the pan. Stir in the cherry tomatoes and cook, tossing, for 5 minutes, or until the tomatoes begin to soften. Add the passata and simmer gently for 5 minutes, or until the sauce thickens slightly. Season and add a little squeeze of lemon juice. Remove the pan from the heat and top with the bocconcini. Cover the pan and don't stir until serving, as you want the cheese to warm through and just start to melt, but not to dissolve into the sauce.

To cook the gnocchi, bring a large saucepan of well-salted water to the boil. Drop the gnocchi in a few at a time – basically about half the quantity on one of those pieces of baking paper in each batch. When the gnocchi rise to the surface they are cooked. This will take about 90 seconds, depending on how much water you are using and how many gnocchi you put in. Immediately remove the gnocchi with a slotted spoon and place in a well-warmed serving dish. Do not pile up the gnocchi as they like their personal space.

Spoon over the Napoli sauce and melted bocconcini. Sprinkle with basil leaves and serve.

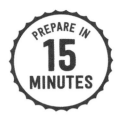

FORGOTTEN WINTER VEGETABLE
and HALOUMI FRITTER STACKS

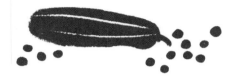

Haloumi is the cheese that divides the nation. But even those who question whether the cheese should ever be squeakier than the mouse will enjoy this nifty, crispy combo of haloumi and crisper-drawer orphans.

A note on the name: Rene Redzepi was the first chef I know to put 'forgotten vegetables' on his menu at Noma. His were old carrots that had spent a winter in the ground when the farmer didn't think it was worth picking them. The carrots had become sweeter and more carroty thanks to the frosts and their time in the soil. I am pretty sure none of the veggies in my crisper drawer are that old … but you can never be sure about those gnarly mushrooms you find at the back in the corner underneath everything else.

Over the page you will find nine more brilliant fritter ideas that use this basic recipe as a guide.

MAKES 8–10 LARGE FRITTERS **PREP:** 15 MINS **COOKING:** 20 MINS

THE BATTER
150 g (1 cup) plain flour
sea salt and freshly ground
   black pepper
250 ml (1 cup) milk
2 eggs
20 g butter, melted, plus extra
   10 g butter for greasing the pan,
   per batch

VEGGIE MIX
300 g (2 cups) frozen peas, thawed
   on paper towel, roughly mash half
   the peas with a fork and leave the
   rest whole
130 g zucchini, coarsely grated and
   squeezed of any moisture
2 tablespoons coarsely chopped
   mint, plus extra to serve

THE CHEESE
130 g (1 cup) coarsely grated
   haloumi

TOPPINGS
mashed avocado
Maple-Candied Bacon (page 23)
lemon wedges

Preheat the oven to 100°C/80°C fan-forced and pop in a serving dish lined with paper towel.

To make the batter, place the flour in a bowl and season. Add the milk, eggs and butter, and whisk until just combined.

Stir in the veggie mix and the cheese.

Heat some of the extra butter in a large non-stick frying pan over medium heat – it needs to be bubbling to give you crispy fritters. Pour ½ cupfuls of mixture into the pan. Cook for 2–3 minutes, until bubbles rise to the surface. Use a spatula to turn them over and cook for a further 1–2 minutes, until golden brown and cooked through. Transfer the fritters to the serving dish in the oven. Repeat with the remaining batter, to make the remaining fritters.

Serve the fritters in stacks of two, three or four topped with your, um, err … toppings.

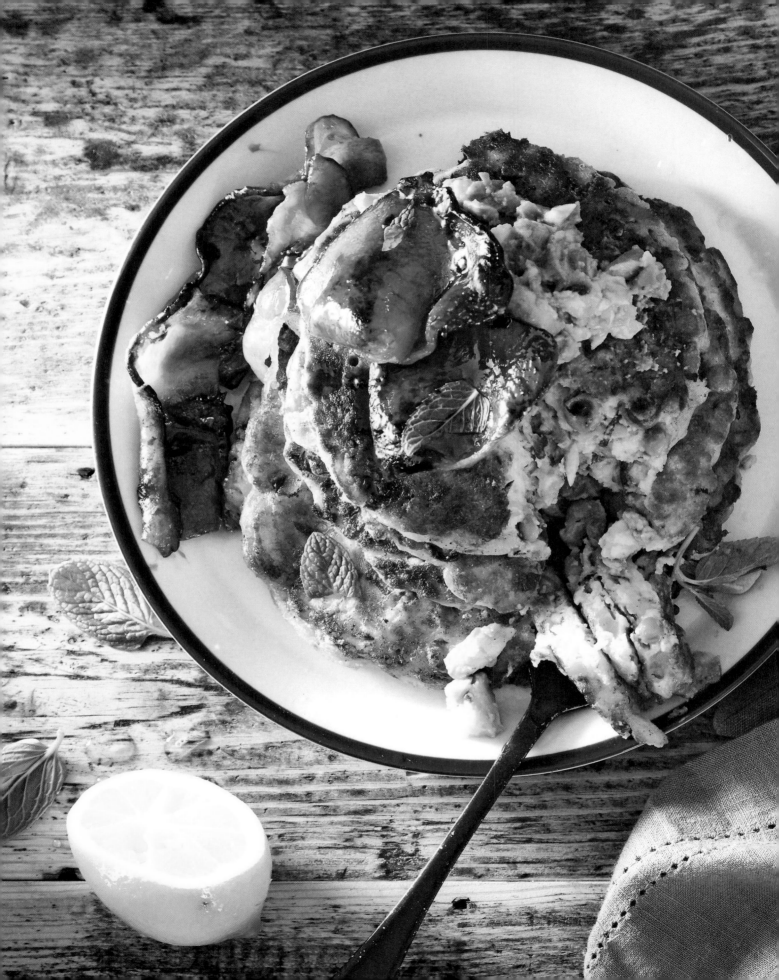

9 FAIL-SAFE FRITTER RECIPES

'Why stop at pea fritters with feta and mint or corn fritters with lime and sour cream?' screamed my inner voice. For once I listened, and so here are nine more great ways to customise your basic fritters on the previous page into something different. Of course, if you want to use the classic combos be my guest ... you don't have my conscience whispering insistently in your ear.

Follow the recipe and ratios on the previous page, adding your veggie mix (about 430 g), cheese (about 130 g) and herbs (about 2 tablespoons) as specified below. Then top when you should be topping.

1. Mash leftover roast potatoes and any other roast veg you have to hand. Add to the fritter batter, then mix in grated Swiss cheese and chopped parsley leaves. Finish the fritters with a dollop of Smoky Mayo (page 247), and sauerkraut or sauteed cabbage with sliced corned beef.

2. Swap the frozen peas for coarsely grated carrot and combine with the grated zucchini. Stir through the batter along with diced paneer, chopped coriander leaves and a good pinch of curry powder for colour. Top the fritters with yoghurt, pickled red onion (page 23), diced cucumber and extra coriander leaves.

3. Stir steamed cubed pumpkin through the batter and add crumbled Greek feta and chopped mint leaves. Arrange Scottish-style hot-smoked salmon (flaked), Beetroot–Coriander Chutney (page 92) and extra feta and mint on top of the fritters.

4. Mix drained canned corn, drained canned black beans, sliced green chillies and finely sliced coriander stalks in a bowl. Combine with the batter and add grated jalapeno Monterey Jack – or any bitey cheddar or tasty cheese and chopped coriander leaves. Serve with mashed avocado and a fresh tomato salsa on top, and a lime wedge for squeezing over.

5. Follow the basic fritter recipe but omit the frozen peas. Swap the cheese for 160 g cubed smoked cheddar and stir through torn parsley leaves. Top with roasted cherry tomatoes, crispy bacon and sliced avocado, and drizzle over a little balsamic glaze (page 244).

6. Mix shredded baby spinach and some chopped ham into the fritter batter. Add grated cheddar plus a teaspoon of dijon mustard for extra kick, and stir through chopped parsley leaves. Top the fritters with a poached egg, hollandaise sauce and snipped fresh chives.

7. Mix cooked and well-drained ramen noodles into the batter. Add some chopped coriander leaves, but omit the cheese. Top with pickled veggies, crispy shallots and a fried egg or split soft-boiled egg drizzled with hoisin sauce.

8. Combine finely chopped white onion and shredded carrot and add to the batter. Replace the cheese with coarsely chopped raw prawn meat and sprinkle in shredded nori. Serve with a dollop of Kewpie mayo mixed with a touch of wasabi, pickled ginger and shiso leaves ('cos this is a classy Japanese-inspired fritter stack).

9. Stir finely chopped broccoli and finely shredded cabbage through the batter. Add grated haloumi and chopped dill. Top the fritters with crème fraîche, dill sprigs and either prosciutto or slices of pan-fried chorizo.

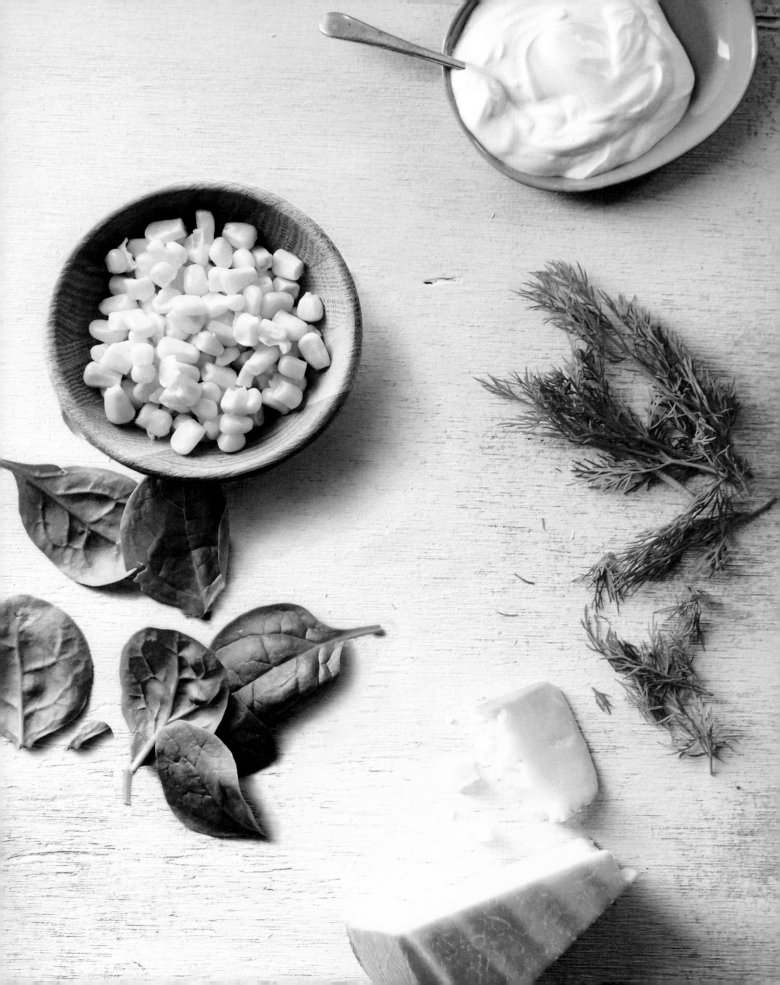

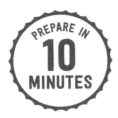

PREPARE IN
10
MINUTES

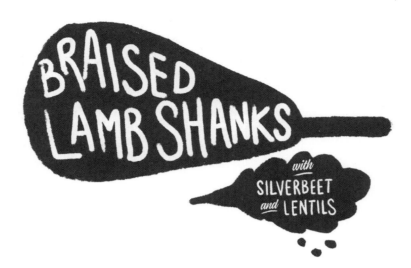

BRAISED LAMB SHANKS
with SILVERBEET and LENTILS

I don't often buy shanks any more as they are now usually more expensive per kilo than a leg or shoulder of lamb, but for the lip-stickiness they bring to this rustic dish, they are well worth seeking out.

SERVES 4   PREP: 10 MINS   COOKING: 3 HOURS 20 MINS

1 tablespoon olive oil
6 lamb shanks, French-trimmed
2 leeks, thickly sliced
3 garlic cloves, crushed
1 × 400 g can diced Italian
    tomatoes
250 ml (1 cup) chicken stock
125 ml (½ cup) white wine
4 fresh or dried bay leaves
2 rosemary sprigs
sea salt and freshly ground
    black pepper
1 × 400 g can of the smallest lentils
    you can find, rinsed and drained
    (like you are going to have a
    choice when you're shopping
    in the supermarket!)
½ bunch silverbeet, white stems
    trimmed, leaves finely shredded
2 tablespoons lemon juice

Preheat the oven to 160°C/140°C fan-forced. Heat half the oil in a large frying pan over medium–high heat. Fry the lamb shanks in batches, turning, for 5 minutes, or until brown. Transfer to a large roasting tin.

Heat the remaining oil in the frying pan. Add the leek and cook, stirring, for 5 minutes, or until the leek softens slightly. Add the garlic and cook, stirring, for 30 seconds, or until aromatic. Add the tomatoes, chicken stock, wine, bay leaves and rosemary and bring to the boil. Season. Pour over the lamb shanks. Cover with foil and bake for 2½ hours. Remove the foil and stir in the lentils and silverbeet. Bake, uncovered, for 30 minutes, or until the lamb is golden.

Remove from the oven and stir the lemon juice into the sauce. To serve, divide the lamb, lentils and silverbeet among serving plates and spoon on plenty of sauce.

TIPS

This recipe is perfect for freezing. Store in an airtight container in the freezer for up to 3 months.

Add a touch of harissa to the onion mixture for a little kick.

You can also change the silverbeet for kale and swap the lentils for another bean or pulse, such as chickpeas.

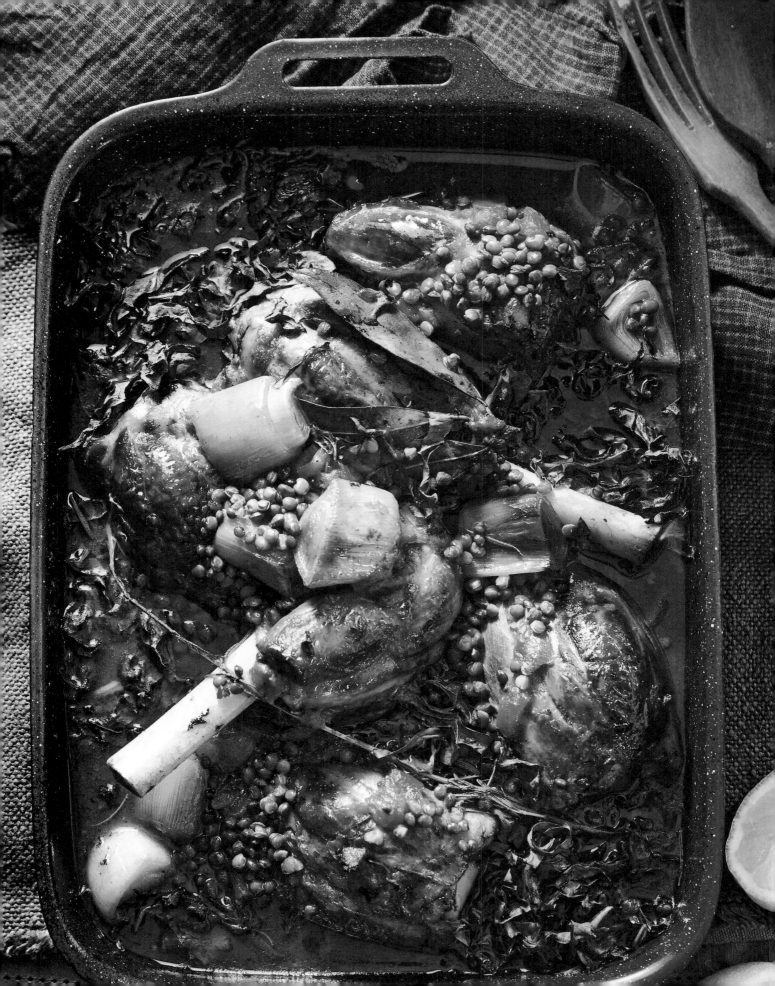

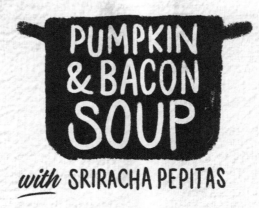

PUMPKIN & BACON SOUP
with SRIRACHA PEPITAS

Soup ... Tastes good.

SERVES 4   PREP: 15 MINS   COOKING: 30 MINS

THE BASE
2 tablespoons olive oil
100 g shortcut bacon rashers,
  finely chopped
2 carrots, finely chopped
2 celery stalks, finely chopped
1 onion, finely chopped

THE SPICES
3 garlic cloves, crushed
1 tablespoon ground cumin

THE VEG
800 g coarsely chopped pumpkin

THE LIQUID
1 litre salt-reduced chicken stock
sea salt and freshly ground
  black pepper
125 ml (½ cup) pouring cream
  (only if you want a creamy soup)

THE TOPPING
80 g (½ cup) pepitas
1 tablespoon sriracha chilli sauce
1 tablespoon maple syrup
2 teaspoons grapeseed oil
4 streaky bacon rashers
extra pouring cream, to serve

Heat the oil in a large stockpot over medium heat. Add the bacon, carrot, celery and onion and cook, stirring, for 5 minutes, or until soft. Add the garlic and cumin and cook, stirring, for 30 seconds, or until aromatic.

Add the chopped pumpkin to the pot and toss until well combined. Add the stock, then cover the pot and bring to the boil. Reduce the heat to medium and simmer, uncovered, for 15 minutes, or until the pumpkin is tender. Season.

While your soup simmers away, make the topping. Preheat the oven to 180°C/160°C fan-forced. Line a baking tray with baking paper. Toss the pepitas with the sriracha, maple syrup and oil in a bowl. Scatter onto the baking tray and bake for 25 minutes, or until crisp, giving a stir and toss every 5 minutes. Meanwhile, fry the streaky bacon for your topping, then drain on paper towel. Chop coarsely.

Remove the soup from the heat and set aside for 5 minutes to cool slightly. Use a stick blender to blend until smooth (or use a blender if you don't mind the washing up).

Reheat over low heat for 5 minutes, or until heated through. For a creamy soup, now's the time to stir in the cream until combined. Ladle into serving bowls and drizzle with extra cream. Add your pepita topping and sprinkle with the chopped bacon.

TIP

Add chipotle chilli instead of bacon for a vegetarian version. Obviously use vegetable stock, not chicken.

6 MORE SOUPS TO KEEP YOU WARM IN WINTER

1. Use cauliflower and two small chopped potatoes instead of pumpkin and roast until golden. Blitz with hot chicken stock and the cooked soup base (see left). Just before serving, stir in a generous crumble of blue cheese to taste (or crumble and add it to the topping). Top with roasted spiced chickpeas tossed in paprika and cumin and a few baby flat-leaf parsley leaves.

2. Roast 50/50 carrots and beetroot until tender. Blitz with hot chicken stock and the cooked base. Add a squeeze of orange juice at the end (rather than cream) and serve topped with crumbled goat's cheese, watercress and a sprinkle of chopped candied walnuts. Or top with a dollop of sour cream and horseradish.

3. Omit the bacon, cumin and swap the cream for coconut cream. Change the pumpkin to sweet potato and cook as instructed opposite. Add a good spoonful of Thai red curry paste to the soup before blitzing. To finish, drizzle the soup with coconut cream and top with pan-fried prawns, chopped toasted peanuts, fresh coriander leaves and sliced red chilli. Drip on a light caramel made by deglazing the prawn pan with water, palm sugar and a little fish sauce. Serve with a wedge of lime on the side.

4. Omit the bacon and the cream. Use carrots instead of pumpkin. Add a touch of ground cardamom to the spice mix. Cook and blitz as instructed opposite. Serve topped with crumbled feta and mint leaves, and drizzle with pomegranate molasses. (You can always freeze your block of feta hard and shave or microplane it for something different.)

5. Omit the carrot and bacon. Replace the pumpkin with a mix of cap and Swiss brown mushrooms and change the stock to beef. Add a fresh thyme sprig whilst cooking. Add toasted homemade breadcrumbs and a spoon of dijon mustard at the end of cooking to thicken the soup to the desired consistency. Then stir through a touch of crème fraîche (fork-beaten to loosen) rather than cream. Top with a few extra pan-fried golden Swiss brown mushroom slices, and sprinkle with toasted sunflower seeds. Some snipped chives, parsley or thyme is rather nice too. This soup is great with a side order of Crispy Kale Leaves (page 190).

6. Replace the pumpkin with potato and add a sprig of rosemary. Cook as instructed, but mash rather than blitz. Stir in a little shredded baby spinach just before serving. Sprinkle with cubes of fried chorizo and sprinkle with crumbled or grated smoked cheddar or manchego.

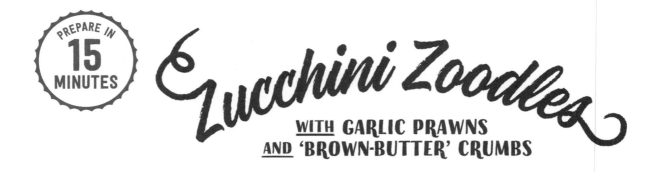

PREPARE IN 15 MINUTES

Zucchini Zoodles

WITH GARLIC PRAWNS AND 'BROWN-BUTTER' CRUMBS

… then there was that time I was almost busted for handing out tiny spoonfuls of golden brown powder at a red carpet restaurant launch. It was only skimmed milk powder and not some new designer drug, but if the coppers had known how addictive this stuff is they'd have booked me for dealing a Class A, for sure.

You see, if you toss 300 g of skimmed milk powder with 125 g of melted butter, 2 tablespoons of caster sugar and 1 teaspoon of salt, and bake in an 180°C/160°C fan-forced oven for 8 minutes, then you'll get golden crumbs that taste compellingly of browned butter.* Try this on ice cream or even sprinkled over this dish to step things up a little, although the below method works just as well.

And before you go on at me about spiralising, can I just say that you could use a mandoline or a $12 julienne-type peeler to make these zoodles, which I feel takes them out of the realm of health blogger faddism. #Blessed.

*To ensure even toasting, rotate the tray halfway through, tossing at the same time.
Remove the tray from the oven and let the crumbs cool on it.

SERVES 4 PREP: 15 MINS COOKING: 10 MINS

30 g butter
2 anchovy fillets, drained
1 tablespoon skimmed milk powder
70 g (1 cup) fresh sourdough
  breadcrumbs
sea salt and freshly ground
  black pepper
4 zucchini, made into zoodles
  using a spiraliser
zest of 1 lemon and juice of
  ½ lemon
80 ml (⅓ cup) olive oil
30 green prawns, peeled, leaving
  tails intact
8 garlic cloves, thinly sliced
¼ cup chopped flat-leaf parsley

Melt the butter in a non-stick frying pan over medium heat. As soon as it has melted, mash in the anchovies then add the skimmed milk powder. Stir for around 2 minutes, or until it smells nutty and the milk powder has turned golden.

Now add the breadcrumbs and cook, tossing occasionally, for 5 minutes, or until very golden. Transfer to a bowl and season. Wipe the pan clean with paper towel.

While your breadcrumbs are cooking, place the zoodles in a large heatproof bowl. Cover with boiling water and set aside for only 30 seconds to soften just a tiny touch. I'm going to be firm with you here … don't leave them too long or they will become all watery.

Drain the zoodles and toss in a bowl with the lemon zest and juice and 1 tablespoon of oil. Season really well with pepper.

Heat the remaining oil in the pan over medium heat. Add the prawns and garlic and cook gently, stirring occasionally, for 3 minutes, or until the prawns are just cooked through. Toss through the parsley. Season.

Divide the zoodles among serving bowls. Top with the garlic prawns and sprinkle with the 'brown-butter' crumbs.

TIPS

There are ten other magical ways to use skimmed milk powder. You'll find my thoughts on what they are at www.delicious.com.au.

Add a kick to this dish by slipping sliced chilli in with the prawns and the garlic. Serve on spaghetti if you are of the school that still thinks buttered carbs are mighty fine!!

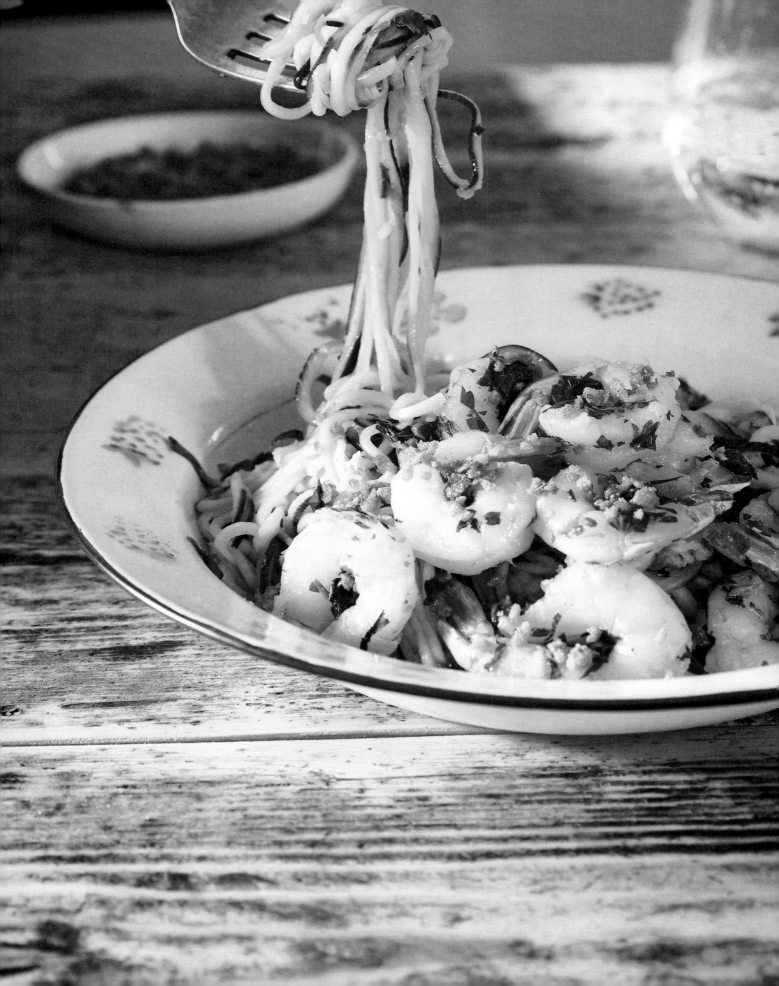

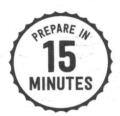

PREPARE IN 15 MINUTES

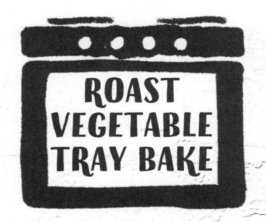

ROAST VEGETABLE TRAY BAKE

There is nothing weird about loving homewares. Some of us love lamps. Others have a thing about a particular shape of wash basin. And some have an obsession, verging on mania, about scatter cushions – to such a degree that getting into bed is like being buried alive in a puffy avalanche. Get into the kitchen and things get even fiercer, with kitchen equipment attracting the sort of messianic fervour that's usually reserved for football teams and the latest saccharine teen sensation with extremely good hair and slightly risque tattoos.

No area of our lives has become more crazily expensive in the last decade than kitchen appliances. A $500 'commercial' coffee machine now starts at $2000, those blenders that also heat things are $2500, and it seems you can't make a cake without the help of something that costs $800 to cream your butter (and that's not a euphemism, although at that price it probably should be).

It's enough to have us all thinking we are saving money by ordering takeaway. Me, I'm a bit more down to earth. I love my oven. Part culinary babysitter, part kitchen workhorse. And I love how it transforms a cold, dead piece of meat into a crispy, golden haven of comfy, roasty deliciousness.

Your oven also works the same magic on vegetables, not only softening them and giving them gorgeously sticky tanned or crunchy edges, but also intensifying their flavour. This roast vegetable recipe isn't just for sorting out a good feed, it's also a great way of setting up potential deliciousness for the whole week – whether you want to turn that roast sweet potato into a soup, stir those candy-soft roast carrots through your couscous or quinoa salad, or make gnocchi or pasta from that roast pumpkin.

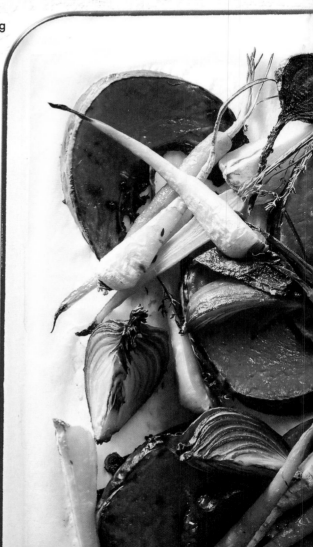

SERVES 4 **PREP:** 15 MINS **COOKING:** 1 HOUR 5 MINS

900 g Kent pumpkin, unpeeled, deseeded and cut into 3 cm thick wedges
4 small or baby parsnips, quartered lengthways
2 small red onions, quartered

8 thyme sprigs
60 ml (¼ cup) olive oil
sea salt and freshly ground black pepper
1 bunch baby beetroot, halved
1 bunch Dutch carrots, trimmed

Preheat the oven to 200°C/180°C fan-forced.

Place the pumpkin, parsnip, onion and thyme sprigs in a large roasting tin in a single layer. For the veggies to caramelise (and not steam), it is super-important to give them space and not to pile them on top of each other. Drizzle with 2 tablespoons of the oil and season well. Roast for 30 minutes.

Add the beetroot and carrots to the tin and drizzle over the remaining oil. Roast for a further 35 minutes, or until all the veggies are tender and golden.

8 WAYS TO PIMP YOUR TRAY OF ROAST VEGGIES

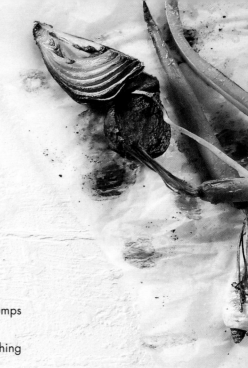

1. Ten minutes before the end of roasting, sprinkle something fun over the top, such as candied nuts, grated smoked cheddar cheese, or splash over balsamic vinegar and add lumps of feta.

2. Five minutes before roasting is finished, toss through the flesh of a storebought roast chicken and 60 ml (¼ cup) of maple syrup.

3. Once roasted, serve drizzled with Greek yoghurt marbled with melted butter, or hummus and fresh mint, or toum (garlic sauce) and lots of parsley, or with tzatziki.

4. You can serve the roast veggies with pretty much anything you like: thinly sliced seared steak, crispy-fatted lamb chops, or torn-apart slow-roasted pork shoulder.

5. Once cooled, toss the roast veggies with a balsamic and olive oil dressing, large lumps of crumbled ricotta and soft herbs, such as tarragon, parsley or mint.

6. Turn each cooled veggie into a hummus by blitzing them with chickpeas and something wet such as yoghurt, tahini or orange juice. Add a little olive oil and 2 ice cubes to help the blending.

7. Bake them under pastry in a brown veloute.

8. Pick one roast veggie to puree and then mix with 00 flour to make pasta.

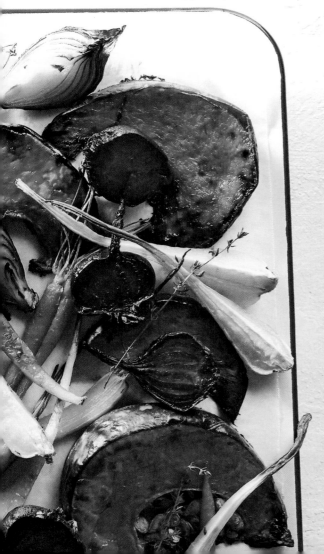

HOW LONG IS LONG ENOUGH?

This ready reckoner will help you work out what veg to cook when and for how long.

50–60 MINUTES
Halved beetroots

Whole onions

Peeled wedges of sweet potato or pumpkin

Halved carrots

40–50 MINUTES
Baby potatoes or peeled quartered large potatoes

Thumb-thick steaks of fennel

Whole garlic bulbs

Halved onions or large onion wedges

Halved pears

Halved baby fennel

30–40 MINUTES
In winter try:

Halved parsnips

Cauliflower florets

Flat mushrooms

2 cm cubes of potato, sweet potato or pumpkin

In summer try:

Zucchini, cut into 5 cm lengths

Eggplant, cut into 2 cm thick batons

Halved roma tomatoes

Sweetcorn cut into small cobs

20–30 MINUTES
Broccoli florets

Small whole apples

Apple wedges

Whole brussels sprouts

Trimmed whole leeks

2 cm thick strips of capsicum

ADD IN THE LAST 15 MINUTES OF ROASTING
Whole button mushrooms

Asparagus

Cherry tomatoes

Green beans

Olives

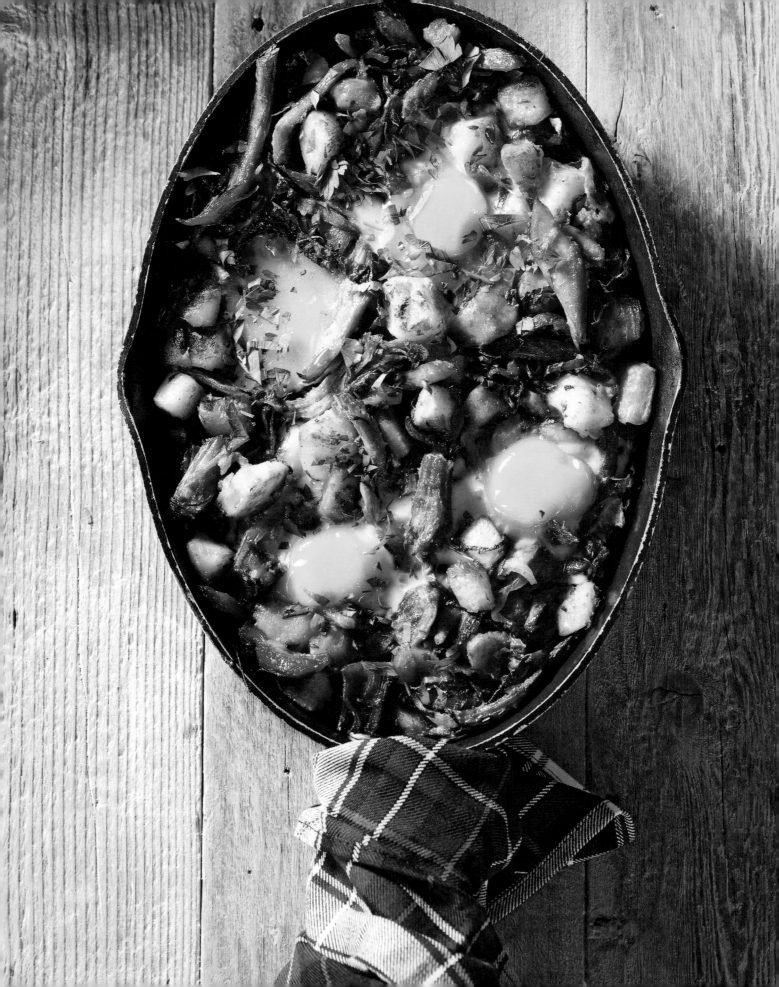

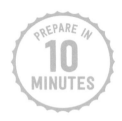

PREPARE IN
10
MINUTES

Some recipes are fragrant and refined. Others are boisterous and fun. Rarer by far are those that share the same lazy hooded eyes and low street cunning as this recipe. If it were an actor it would be James Franco – long, angular and ominous – slouching by the dumpster in an alley. This is because it is more like a state of mind than a recipe.

Really, it's just a poor man's leftover fried jumble with the eggs there for the way their oozy yolks dress everything and make it look like gold – hence the name.

It's also reminiscent of a dish of sauteed potatoes, fried onions, chorizo and fried eggs that they serve at one of my favourite places in Barcelona, Bar Mut. This is also a dish that would get stiletto-flashing mean if you dared to look at it wrong. But that's a whole 'nother story …

SERVES 4 **PREP:** 10 MINS **COOKING:** 35 MINS

4 coliban or all-purpose potatoes, peeled and cut into 2 cm pieces
1 (about 370 g) large sweet potato, peeled and cut into 2 cm pieces
1 tablespoon olive oil
50 g butter
1 red onion, cut into thick wedges
sea salt and freshly ground black pepper
1 teaspoon caraway seeds
250 g pulled pork
¼ (about 300 g) small red or green cabbage, shredded
4 eggs
2 tablespoons chopped flat-leaf parsley
Pineapple Ketchup (page 68), to serve (or any sauce you love really. Food guru Michelle loves it with sriracha chilli sauce)

Bring a large saucepan of salted water to the boil. Add the potato and sweet potato and cook for 5–8 minutes, until just starting to soften. Drain and place on a tray lined with paper towel to dry.

Heat the oil and 30 g of the butter in a large frying pan with a lid over medium–high heat until, well, um, hot.

Add the potato and the onion. Season well. Cook, stirring occasionally, for 15 minutes, or until very golden and crispy. Just make sure you leave them well alone for a little while, so they catch on the bottom and get golden. This is the yummiest bit, so I'm going to use my firm voice again … don't go turning all the time.

When you think that the potato is golden and crunchy enough, throw in the caraway seeds and toss. Cook for 30 seconds, or until you smell the caraway (which means it's got toasty too, don't cha kno'?).

Increase the heat to high. Add the pulled pork, cabbage and remaining butter, and season. Cook, stirring occasionally, for 3 minutes, or until the cabbage just starts to wilt.

Make four little holes in the potato mixture. Crack an egg into each hole then cover the pan and cook for 6 minutes, or until the eggs are just set. You can cook this in the oven, but you risk the eggs having a glassy finish as in this picture.

Sprinkle with parsley and serve with pineapple ketchup.

TIPS

This is a great dish for using up leftovers: instead of cabbage, use sliced brussels sprouts or silverbeet. Instead of pulled pork, cook chunks of sausage filling from those last two lonely snags that weren't fried up for Sunday breakfast.

Add cubes of your favourite cheese to melt into the hash if you want.

Fry the eggs so you don't have to wait for them to cook in the hash.

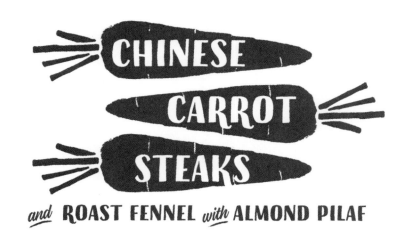

CHINESE CARROT STEAKS

and ROAST FENNEL with ALMOND PILAF

These carrots are so meaty they could even give the Sunday roast a run for its money, but it would be a shame to leave out the Chinese sausage and make this a solely vego dish, as it adds so much!

SERVES 4 **PREP:** 30 MINS **COOKING:** 1 HOUR 20 MINS

1 kg large carrots, halved lengthways
3 baby fennel bulbs, cut into wedges
2 tablespoons olive oil
1 teaspoon Chinese five spice
175 g lap cheong sausage, thinly sliced on an angle
2 tablespoons coriander seeds
1 bunch coriander, stems and roots washed and finely chopped, sprigs reserved
160 g (1 cup) coarsely grated palm sugar
2 tablespoons fish sauce
2 teaspoons sriracha chilli sauce

ALMOND PILAF
1 tablespoon olive oil
1 onion, finely chopped
2 garlic cloves, crushed
400 g (2 cups) basmati rice
750 ml (3 cups) chicken stock
50 g (½ cup) natural sliced almonds, toasted, plus extra to garnish

Preheat the oven to 200°C/180°C fan-forced. Line a large baking tray with baking paper.

Toss the carrot and fennel with the oil and five spice on the lined baking tray. Pop in the oven and roast for 40 minutes, or until the fennel wedges are soft and golden. Transfer the fennel to a plate and cover loosely with foil to keep warm. Return the carrot to the oven and continue to roast for a further 20 minutes.

Meanwhile, to make the pilaf, heat the oil in a large frying pan with a lid over medium–high heat. Add the onion and cook, stirring, for 5 minutes, or until the onion softens. Add the garlic and rice. Toss over the heat for 1 minute. Add the stock and bring to the boil. Reduce the heat to low and cook, covered, for 12 minutes, or until the liquid is absorbed. Set aside, covered, for 10 minutes. Use a fork to fluff the rice and stir in the almonds.

Reduce the oven to 120°C/100°C fan-forced. Transfer the rice to an ovenproof dish and top with the reserved fennel wedges. Cover with a lid or foil and place in the oven to keep warm.

Wipe out the frying pan with paper towel, then fry the lap cheong over medium–high heat for 2–3 minutes, until just turning golden. (You don't need any more oil, enough will come out of the sausage.) Use a slotted spoon to transfer to the rice.

Now use the fat rendered from the lap cheong to fry the coriander seeds and coriander stems and roots for 1 minute. Add the palm sugar and 125 ml (½ cup) of water and simmer rapidly for 15 minutes, or until a caramel forms. Remove from the heat and hit with the fish sauce and sriracha.

To serve, place the pilaf, fennel and lap cheong on a serving platter Top with the carrot steaks. Drizzle with half the caramel and top with coriander sprigs. Serve with the remaining caramel dressing on the side.

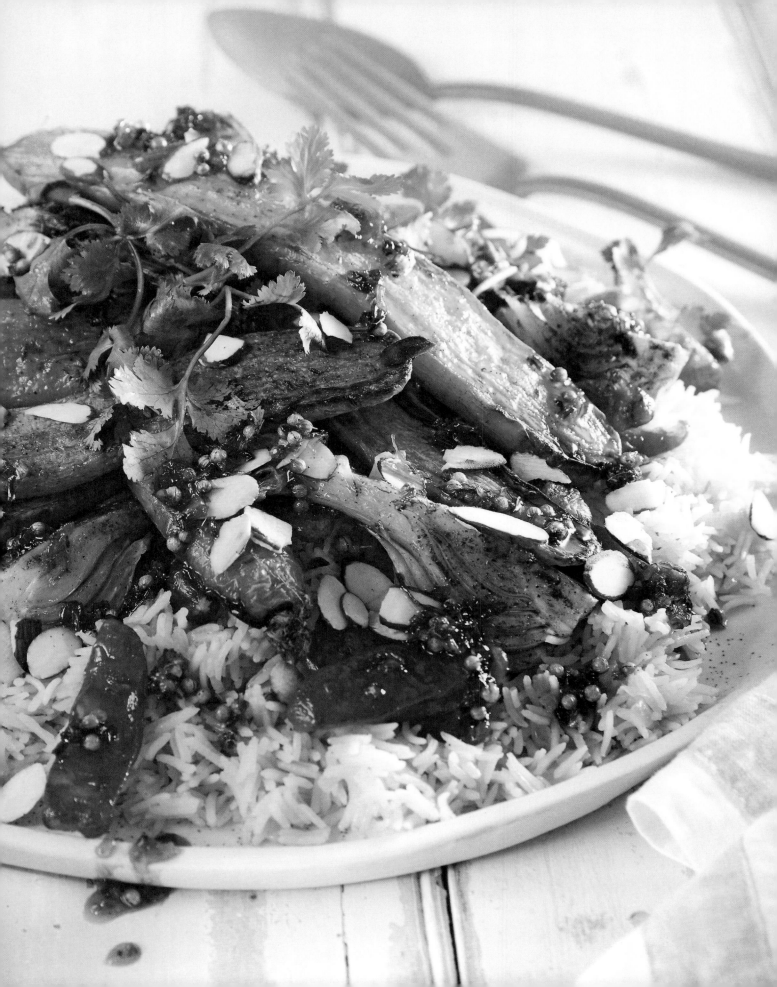

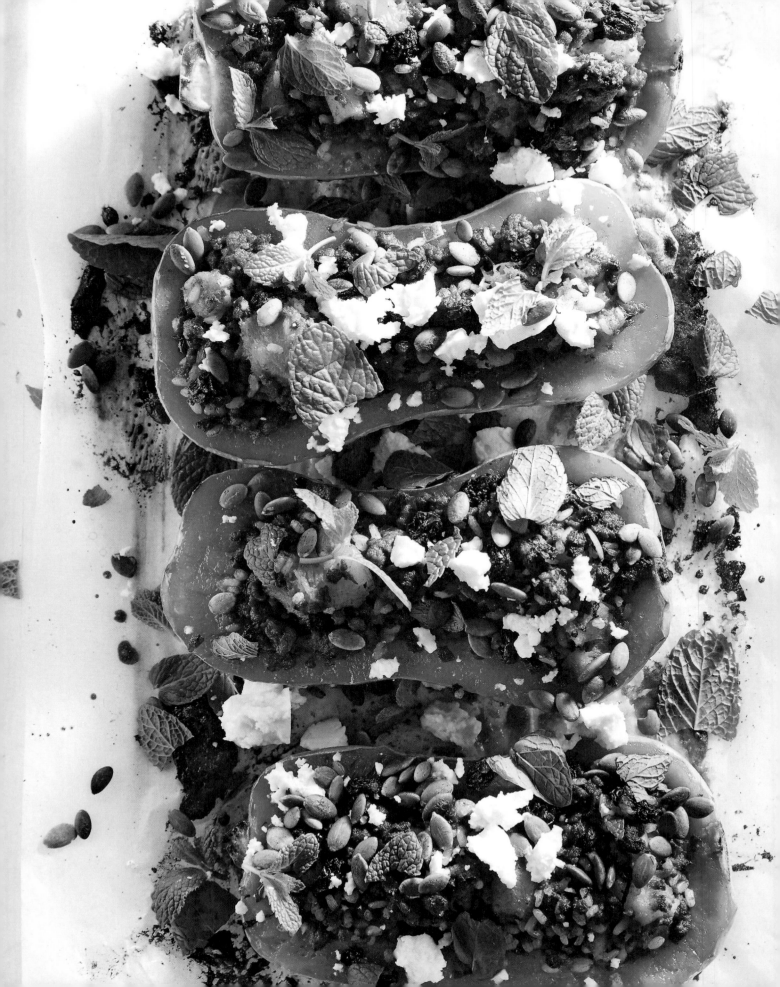

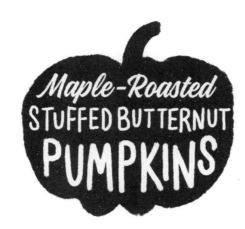

Maple-Roasted STUFFED BUTTERNUT PUMPKINS

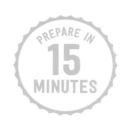

PREPARE IN 15 MINUTES

Matt: *You'll love this recipe so much. Really, I just don't know why I haven't seen these anywhere before???*

Lucy (an editor): *Maybe because you haven't bothered to search 'stuffed butternut pumpkin' before?*

Matt: *Yes, but that means this recipe was created 'without references' – like all the top chefs say they do. And BTW, don't be so sarky ...*

Lucy (tersely under her breath): *At least Hugh Fearnley-Whittingstall credited Sarah Raven when he nicked her stuffed butternut pumpkin recipe for his book ...*

Matt: *Even when you are muttering I can still hear you. Please leave this place. You are disrupting my chakras.*

SERVES 4   PREP: 15 MINS   COOKING: 1 HOUR 5 MINS

1 tablespoon maple syrup
60 ml (¼ cup) grapeseed oil
2 small butternut pumpkins (about 1.2 kg each), halved lengthways and deseeded
80 g (½ cup) pepitas
1 teaspoon ground cinnamon
good pinch of salt
1 red onion, finely chopped
2 garlic cloves, crushed
2 teaspoons ground cumin
2 teaspoons harissa (or 1 teaspoon dried chilli flakes if your supermarket doesn't stock harissa)
400 g lamb mince
60 ml (¼ cup) chicken stock
45 g (¼ cup) sultanas
75 g (¾ cup) cooked brown rice
1 tablespoon lemon juice
½ bunch mint, ⅓ cup shredded, remaining leaves reserved
100 g feta, crumbled

Preheat the oven to 200°C/180°C fan-forced. Line a baking tray with baking paper.

Combine the maple syrup and 2 teaspoons of the oil in a bowl. Brush the cut sides of the pumpkins with half the mixture then place, cut-side down, on the lined tray. Roast for 40 minutes, or until just tender. Scoop out the flesh, leaving a 1 cm border. Roughly chop the flesh.

Meanwhile, heat a dash of oil in a large frying pan over medium heat. Toss your pepitas with the cinnamon and salt for 2–3 minutes, until they start going golden at the edges. Remove from the pan and reserve.

Heat the remaining oil in the same frying pan. Cook the onion, stirring, for 5 minutes, or until soft. Add the garlic, cumin and harissa. Cook, stirring, for 1–2 minutes, until aromatic.

Add the lamb mince and cook, breaking up any lumps with the back of a wooden spoon, for 5 minutes, or until golden brown. Stir in the stock and sultanas. Cook, stirring occasionally, for 5 minutes, or until the liquid has reduced and the sultanas plump up a little. Remove from the heat and stir in the chopped pumpkin flesh, rice, lemon juice and shredded mint.

Brush the insides of the pumpkin halves with the remaining maple syrup mixture. Divide the filling among the pumpkin halves, cover with foil and roast for 20 minutes. Remove the foil and roast for a further 15 minutes, or until browned on top. Sprinkle with the mint leaves, feta and pepitas and serve.

TIPS

If you don't want to buy pepitas you can use the pumpkin seeds from the pumpkins. Remove any pumpkin flesh and wash the seeds. Dry on paper towel then spread out on a baking tray. Drizzle with oil and toss in cinnamon and salt. Bake in a preheated 200°C/180°C fan-forced oven for 15–20 minutes, until they are golden. Yeah, it does sound like a bit of a palaver doesn't it. Maybe just buy a packet.

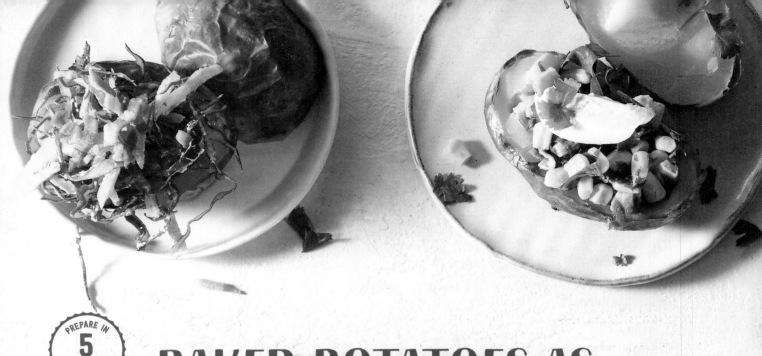

BAKED POTATOES AS A VEHICLE FOR LEFTOVERS

Whatever happened to baked potatoes? Once they were everywhere, and now they seem to be as unfashionable as a Bros album or a baseball jacket. So, let's bring them back in the best possible way: as a vehicle for dinner deliciousness.

HOW TO COOK A BAKED POTATO

MAKES 4 **PREP:** 5 MINS **COOKING:** 1 HOUR 15 MINS

**4 large coliban potatoes
(about 200 g each), unpeeled**

Preheat the oven to 200°C/180°C fan-forced. Wash the potatoes well, then dry them. Wrap each potato in foil, place on a baking tray and bake for 1 hour, or until you can skewer them easily. Remove the foil and cook for a further 10–15 minutes if you want to dry out the skins more. This is not essential, but worth doing.

29 GREAT TOPPINGS TO TURN YOUR HUMBLE BAKED POTATO INTO DINNER

1. Fill with very hot baked beans and top with grated cheddar. Still totally delicious.

2. Split and slather with sour cream, snipped chives, a poached egg and crispy bacon – or any combination of these four. Ditto.

3. Pour on leftover chilli con carne or chilli black beans (page 270). Don't forget the grated cheddar, sour cream and sliced fresh or pickled chillies.

4. Leftover bolognese (page 64). Don't forget the parmesan.

5. Roast grapes with the potatoes and toss with toasted walnuts or almonds. Cram into the split potatoes, then crumble on lots of goat's cheese.

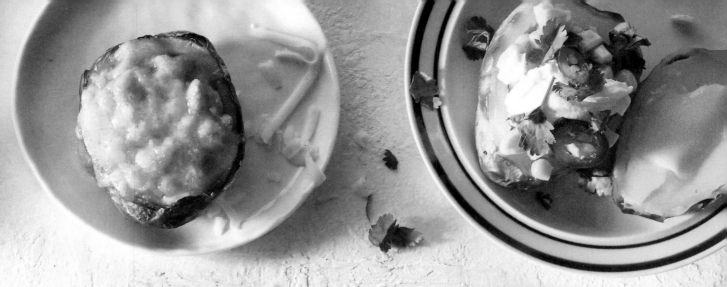

6. Fill with loads of caramelised onion and grated vintage cheddar, then grill.

7. Stuff with any classic vol-au-vent filling, like creamy ham and cheese or creamy mushroom and thyme. Make sure you add a little bite of dijon mustard to each.

8. Gently fry green peas with sliced onion in curry powder. Serve in the potato with a dollop of yoghurt and fresh coriander sprigs.

9. Pizza baked potatoes. Split the potato, mash some tomato paste into the potato, along with grated parmesan. Top with roasted cherry tomatoes and olives that you've roasted with the potato until they are a little shrivly. Cover with mozzarella and place under the grill until golden.

10. Bacon and egg brinner potato. Split the hot potato and spoon out some potato from both sides. Crack an egg into each half and bake for a further 20 minutes. Top with chopped parsley and crispy bacon.

11. Slice the potato and cram with slow-roasted lamb shoulder, Beetroot–Coriander Chutney (page 92) and watercress.

12. Fill with pan-fried frozen corn tossed with chopped coriander and a squeeze of lime juice. Melted butter, Kewpie mayo or a dollop of crème fraîche up the decadence factor here.

13. Top with canned tuna and a kaleslaw.

14. Dollop with sour cream and load on smoked salmon, capers and thinly shaved red onion. The pickled onion on page 23 is also perfect.

15. Roast diced apple tossed in butter and fennel seeds. Split the potatoes and spoon the apple mixture on top. Top with grated cheddar and bake until melted.

16. Butter and salt! Serve with sausages or steak.

17. Flavour that butter with chives, dill, garlic and parsley, anchovies, miso and almonds, or even smoked paprika.

18. Sauteed mixed mushrooms with thyme and garlic. Serve on the potato with a little dijon.

19. Top with tuna mornay and potato chips, then bake until golden.

20. Dice fresh and pickled jalapenos and mix with grated vintage cheddar. Stuff into the baked potatoes.

21. Remove the potato flesh, butter the insides of the skins and return to the oven to toast. Mash the flesh with drained canned tuna, a dollop of crème fraîche, thinly sliced spring onion, grated parmesan and fresh dill. Return to the skins and grill with a little smear of extra crème fraîche on top.

22. Fill with shredded barbecued chicken tossed with chopped hazelnuts, dijon mustard and thyme.

23. Toss crumbled blue cheese, sliced celery and chopped toasted walnuts together. Serve this baked potato with a lemon-dressed apple salad.

24. Fill with ribbons of cooked cabbage and crispy bacon. Top with melting cheese and a fried egg, if you are so inclined.

25. Scrape out the potato flesh, mix with crumbled blue cheese and return to the skins. Top with a fig/vincotto dressing.

26. Load with a big spoon of butter-cooked leek and a generous grating of gruyere.

27. Stuff with leftover peas warmed in leftover gravy, and lay on pan-fried shreds of your lamb or chicken roast. Finish with fresh mint and a spoon of mint jelly, or a drizzle of dijon mustard let down with lemon juice.

28. Load split baked potatoes with Kale and Chickpea Puttanesca (page 275).

29. Split and top with smoked bacon, pan-tanned corn kernels and thin slices of smoked cheddar.

FRO
ST

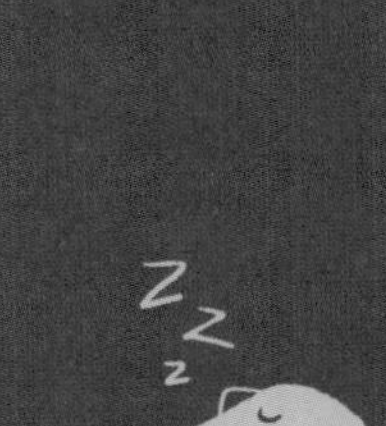

ZEN

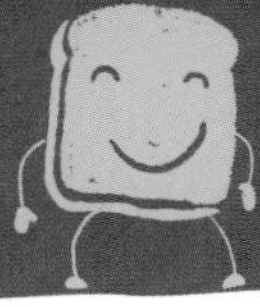

UFF

27 THINGS YOU MUST KEEP IN YOUR FREEZER BESIDES VODKA

1. **SLICED BREAD FOR TOAST AND BREADCRUMBS.** Blitz the latter before freezing and use for schnitzel crumbs, as a crunchy topping, for stewed fruit, or mac 'n' cheese, or to fry with chilli, herbs or something porky (like prosciutto) to sprinkle on pastas or steamed veggies.

2. **PASTRY, BOTH PUFF AND SHORTCRUST.** The perfect immediate way to turn orphan fruit, veg and protein into a meal as a pie, turnover or tart.

3. **GOOD VANILLA ICE CREAM**, obviously – perfect with some of #19 and #27.

4. **NUTS AND SEEDS.** Their high oil content means they can go rancid quickly in hot Australian pantry conditions, so storing less-used nuts and seeds in the freezer is a smart idea.

5. **BUTTER.** I store my butter in the freezer to stop me eating it, but it's also useful to have it there when baking. For quick defrosting and softening, chop butter into cubes.

6. **FROZEN VEGETABLES**, such as broad beans, spinach and soy beans all freeze well and can add a little splash of summer freshness to winter dishes. Use them in soups, stir-fries, pastas or fritters and, as you'll see in this chapter, as the base for great sauces for fish, meat or roast veggies.

7. **FROZEN CORN.** An essential frozen ingredient.

8. **FROZEN PEAS.** Another essential frozen ingredient.

9. **MEAT.** The issue with storing meat is the time a big hunk of flesh takes to thaw. To allow portion control and quicker defrosting, it's better to keep chicken breasts (frozen separately) or cubed meat already in a cold marinade. Defrost this in the fridge overnight for great results.

10. **FISH** never gets any fresher, so eat it within 24 hours of buying or freeze it. It defrosts comparatively quickly if frozen as separate fillets, and you can keep oily fish, such as salmon, for up to two months before using, and other fish for up to three months. And this should remind us to always name and date what we put in the freezer with a label.

11. **FROZEN TORTILLAS** for quesadillas.

12. **PITA BREADS** for souvas or improvised pizzas.

13. **COOKIE DOUGH.** While biscuits freeze well, it's far cannier to freeze logs of cookie dough that you can slice into biscuits with a bread knife and bake to order when friends drop around unexpectedly for a coffee.

14. **FROZEN PRAWNS** can help you MacGyver your way out of all manner of culinary predicaments. But do buy snap-frozen green prawns and *never* refreeze any 'frozen for your convenience' seafood!

15. **HARD CHEESE**, such as parmesan, can be stored whole or grated with minimal impact on texture.

16. **A CHORIZO.** See one of these as a little Spanish flavour bomb that you can lob at all manner of dishes to make them tastier.

17. **BACON** defrosts quickly. Freeze with sheets of baking paper between rashers for easy separation.

18. **DUMPLINGS** also freeze well. I buy mine by the dozen from the local dumpling cafe for rainy days or when I can't be bothered to walk down there. Frozen Maltese pastizzi are also good and make a great scratch meal with some of those frozen peas!!!

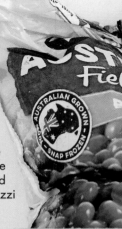

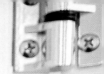

19. **CUT OR STEWED FRUIT.** Freezing is a great way to preserve fruit when it's plentiful and cheap, to eat when it's rare and expensive.

20. **WRAP LEFTOVER INGREDIENTS**, such as ginger, chillies and curry or kaffir lime leaves, in plastic wrap and store in a zip-lock bag in the freezer until needed.

21. **LEFTOVER HERBS** can be chopped and frozen in ice-cube trays covered with olive oil. When frozen, decant into a labelled and dated zip-lock bag. Chuck a frozen cube or two into whichever braise or sauce you need to supercharge.

22. **SPARE STOCK AND CITRUS JUICES** should be frozen in ice-cube trays and then decanted as above.

23. **CASSEROLES, SOUPS AND BOLOGNESE SAUCE.** Cooking for the freezer is one of the best ways to spend a random night that you'd otherwise fritter away. Remember to freeze these in a serving size you'd usually use (i.e. enough for two or four). Cool before freezing and store in square or rectangular plastic containers rather than round, as they are more economical with freezer space – or better yet, freeze them about the size and thickness of a filled padded envelope in flat zip-lock bags. They will defrost quicker this way. Label and date everything. Also, when your put you latest batch in the freezer, assess what needs to be eaten and move that to the front of the freezer rather than just cramming your latest cook on top.

24. **RICE** is another great thing to freeze for convenience and for your fried rice! Make sure you store it in flat and thin portions, as a bigger surface area means it will defrost more quickly.

25. **OVERRIPE BANANAS ARE MAGIC.** You can use them in your banana bread or smoothies as well. Blitz them and they turn into the most virtuous quick ice cream. Just peel them and break them up before freezing. Yes, you can use them in your banana bread as well.

26. **FROZEN GRAPES** don't just make a refreshing little snack, they can also double as ice cubes that won't dilute your sauvignon blanc while you drink it in front of the fire.

27. **BERRIES.** I'm a little in love with the best frozen Aussie berries. They can be turned into a sauce, an instant ice cream, a daquiri, a crumble, a pie, a smoothie … or just eaten as the best frozen fruit treat of them all.

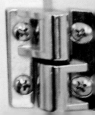

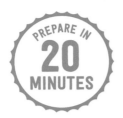

GIANT

INDIVIDUAL SAUSAGE ROLLS
FOR DINNER

Why can't a favourite party nibble or bakery snack be a main course? No reason! See these beauties as a fragrant and slightly sweet Spanish take on a meatloaf, but wrapped in pastry like a Wellington. Which makes them quite posh really!

SERVES 4 **PREP:** 20 MINS (PLUS 10 MINS FREEZING) **COOKING:** 45 MINS

3 fresh chorizo sausages
350 g pork mince
1 red onion, very finely chopped
1 green apple, peeled, cored and
  coarsely grated
50 g (½ cup) rolled oats
¼ cup coarsely chopped
  flat-leaf parsley
1 tablespoon finely chopped sage
1 teaspoon fennel seeds
sea salt and freshly ground
  black pepper
2 sheets butter puff pastry,
  just thawed
1 egg, lightly whisked
1 tablespoon black or white sesame
  seeds or a mixture of both (you
  can also use nigella seeds)
Pineapple Ketchup (page 68),
  to serve

Squeeze the chorizo sausage meat out of their casings into a mixing bowl. Add the pork mince, onion, apple, oats, parsley, sage and fennel seeds. Season and use your hands to combine.

Preheat the oven to 200°C/180°C fan-forced. Line a baking tray with baking paper.

Divide the pork mixture into two portions, then shape each into a log across the centre of each pastry square. With love, fold the pastry around the filling as if you were tucking in a favourite child. Press down at the edges to seal. Place the roll, seam-side down, on the lined baking tray. Place in the freezer for 10 minutes to firm up. (Butter puff pastry can thaw quickly, which makes it harder to work with, so a little freezing action goes a long way to making life easier – and we all like an easier life, don't we?)

Brush the surface of each sausage roll with egg and sprinkle with the sesame seeds. Bake for 45 minutes, or until the pastry is puffed and golden. (OK, if you are busy on a weeknight you can eat these after 30 minutes, as everything will be cooked and tasty, but if you continue to cook them for the full 45 minutes then the pastry will be more golden and crisp – it just depends on how under the pump you are for dinner.)

Serve with pineapple ketchup and potatoes for some form. Maybe a salad would be nice too – there are loads of tasty ones but the mango salad (page 86) and tomato and herb salad with goat's cheese (page 173) are jolly nice.

TIPS

Make these sausage rolls ahead of time and freeze them unbaked. Thaw in the fridge for a few hours, then bake as above.

Make mini versions of these for your next party: just cut each pastry sheet in half and divide the filling into four portions. Roll and bake for 20–25 minutes, until golden.

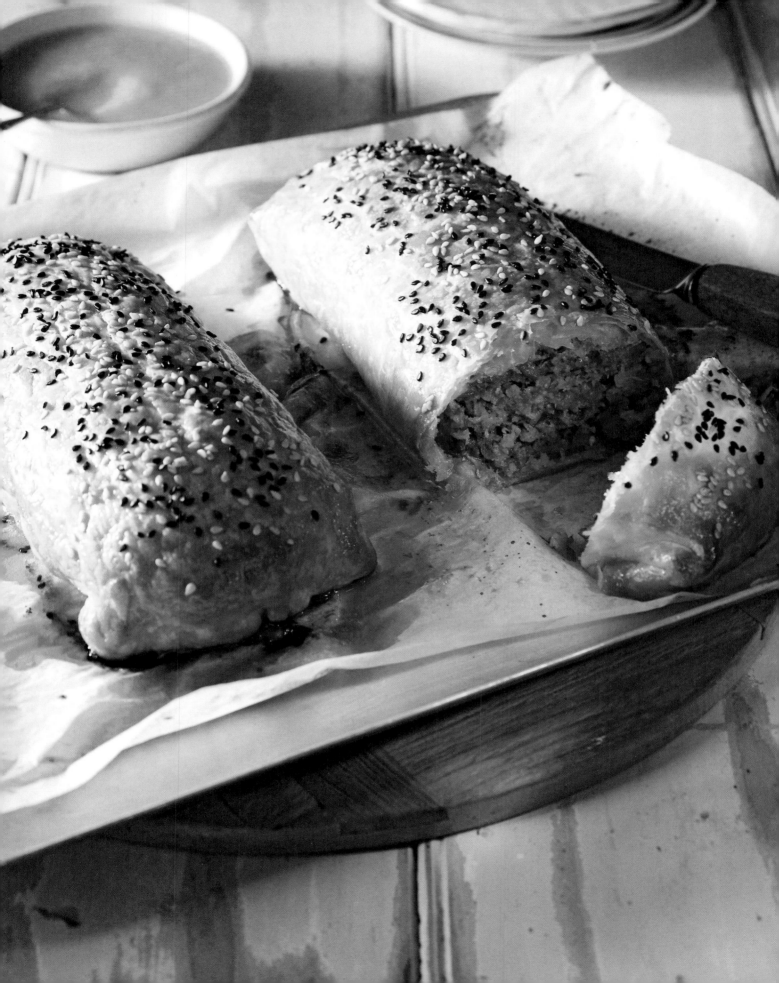

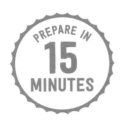

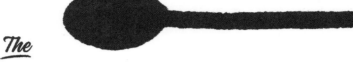

The
ULTIMATE FROZEN VEGGIES MIX
to use with QUESADILLAS, SOFT TORTILLAS *or* TACOS

If the oven is your best friend in the kitchen, then the freezer is that friend you turn to when you are in trouble. This tasty combo is more flexible than the freakiest contortionist – you know the one, the one that makes you feel a little sick when he bends his body in totally the wrong way to slip through an unstrung tennis racquet – and allows you to use whatever veg you have in the freezer to make dinner.

SERVES 4 PREP: 15 MINS COOKING: 20 MINS

1 tablespoon olive oil
1 red onion, finely chopped
2 tablespoons Cajun Spice Mix (page 164)
½ bunch coriander, stems finely chopped, leaves coarsely chopped, plus extra leaves, to serve
2 tablespoons tomato paste
1 × 400 g can beans, rinsed and drained (I like black beans, but you can use pinto, cannellini or kidney beans – basically whatever you have in the pantry)
300 g (2 cups) mixed frozen vegetables (corn and peas is a favourite)
1 large chicken stock cube
250 g shredded barbecued chicken (about ½ roast chicken)
sea salt and freshly ground black pepper
8 large flour tortillas (for quesadillas) or 8 mini flour tortillas for soft tortillas or tacos
320 g coarsely grated cheddar
mashed avocado, to serve
pickled jalapenos, to serve
lime wedges, to serve

Heat the oil in a frying pan over medium–high heat. Add the onion and cook, stirring, for 5 minutes, or until soft. Add the spice mix and coriander stems and cook, stirring, for 2 minutes, or until aromatic.

Add the tomato paste and cook, stirring, for 2 minutes, or until it darkens slightly. Add the beans, veggies, stock cube and 60 ml (¼ cup) of water. Cook, stirring, for 5 minutes, or until the liquid evaporates and the veggies are tender. You don't want this slushy, so it's important that the liquid is gone!

Stir in the shredded chicken and chopped coriander leaves. Season.

Place a large tortilla in a frying pan over medium heat. Top with a sprinkle of cheese, one-quarter of the chicken and veggie filling, more cheese and then another tortilla. Press down for a minute or so, by which time the base should be golden and the cheese starting to melt. Carefully flip over and cook for 2–3 minutes on the other side. Alternatively, use a sandwich press if you own one – it will make life much easier! Repeat with the remaining tortillas and filling until you have four quesadillas.

Cut the quesadillas into quarters and serve with avocado, jalapenos, coriander leaves and lime wedges on the side.

TIPS

If you have leftover roast pork, shred and use instead of chicken.

Make soft tortillas. While the chicken is heating through, warm mini tortillas in the microwave or oven, following the packet instructions. Remember, it's the ones for the oven that should be wrapped in foil, NEVER the ones for the microwave! Serve the chicken mixture on a platter with the warmed tortillas, grated cheddar, avocado, jalapenos, extra coriander leaves and lime wedges. Tell everyone to make their own! (This is still one of my favourite labour- and time-saving tips: get them to do it!)

Turn into tacos. Bake the tacos following the packet instructions until crisp. Fill with the chicken mixture and top with grated cheese, avocado, jalapeno and coriander. Some lime wedges and sour cream are also nice.

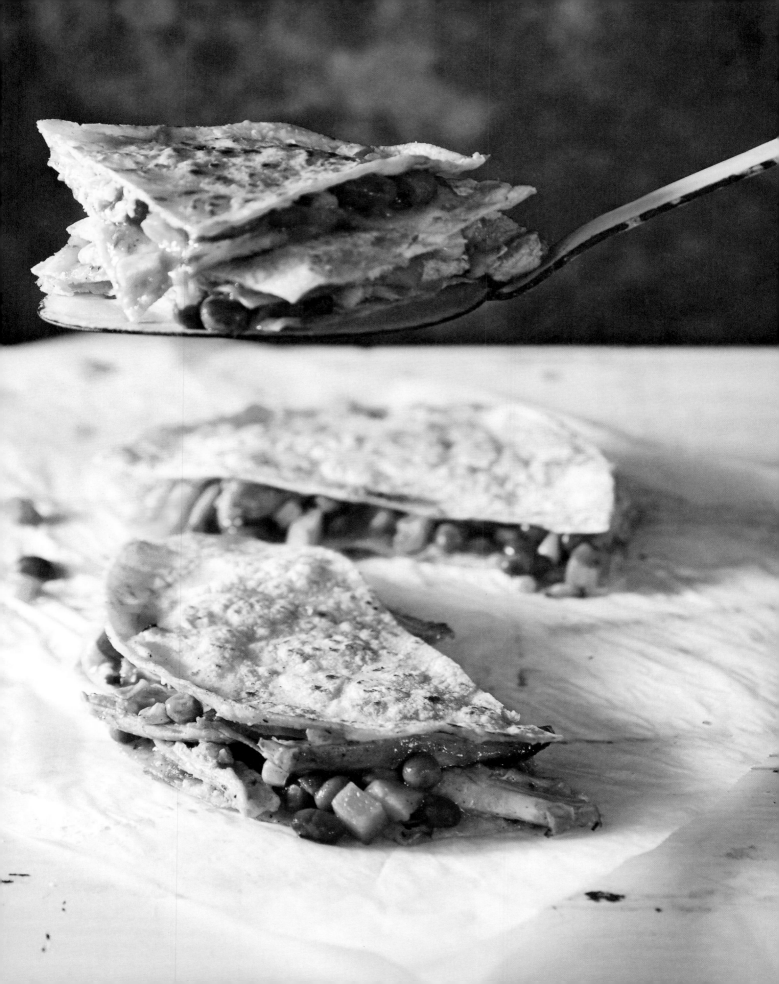

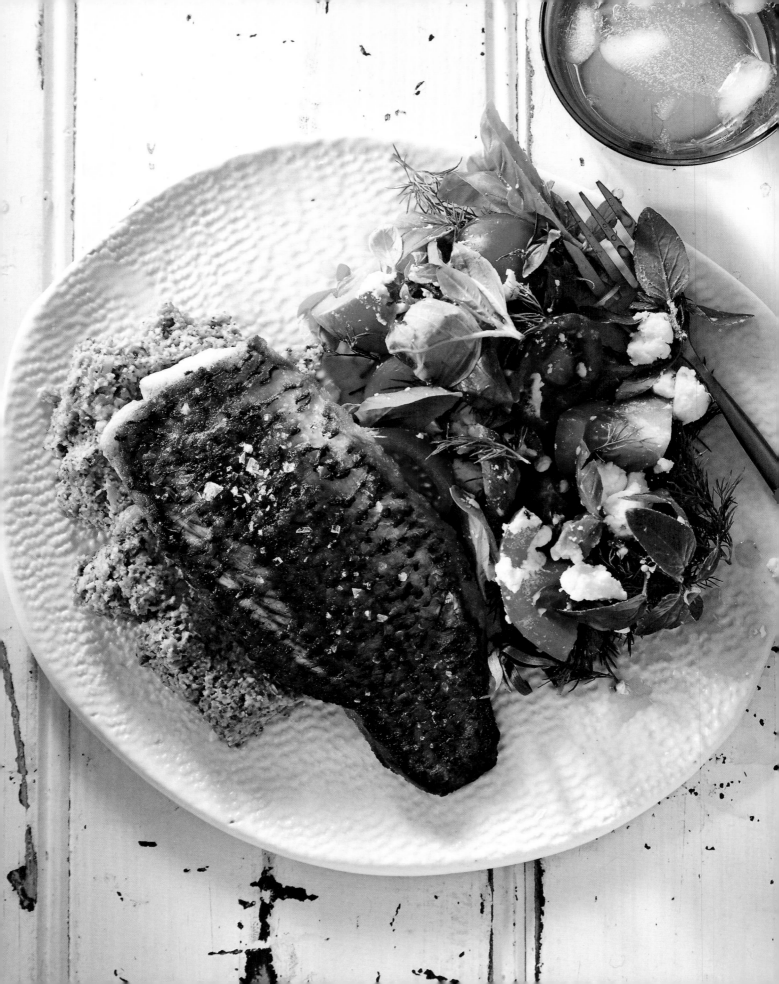

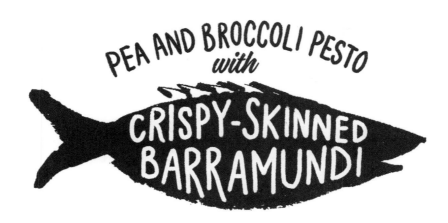

PEA AND BROCCOLI PESTO *with* CRISPY-SKINNED BARRAMUNDI

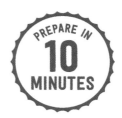

PREPARE IN **10** MINUTES

All hail the mighty vegetables that are muscling their way onto every part of the modern menu and fast becoming more prominent than meat in many of the world's top restaurants. Here, basil gets the heave-ho to make way for loads of peas, broccoli and mint to make a pesto that is chunky, super-tasty and incredibly flexible.

SERVES 4 **PREP:** 10 MINS (PLUS 3 HOURS SOAKING) **COOKING:** 10 MINS

80 g (½ cup) raw cashews
Adaptable Tomato and Herb Salad with Goat's Cheese (page 173), to serve
150 g frozen broccoli, (you can use fresh chopped into florets if you have it)
150 g (1 cup) frozen peas
4 x 200 g skin-on barramundi fish fillets
sea salt and freshly ground black pepper
120 ml olive oil
40 g (½ cup) shredded parmesan
¼ cup mint leaves
2 garlic cloves, crushed
2 teaspoons lemon juice

Place the cashews in a bowl and cover with cold water. Set aside for 3 hours to soak. Drain.

Make the tomato and herb salad and let the flavours develop while you make your pesto.

Place the broccoli and peas in a microwave-safe bowl. Add a tablespoon of water and cover with plastic wrap. Microwave on high for 4 minutes, or until tender. Drain and set aside to cool.

Pat the skin of the fish with paper towel then sprinkle with salt. Pour 2 tablespoons of the oil into a cold non-stick frying pan. Arrange the fish in the pan, skin-side down. Place over medium heat and cook for 5 minutes, or until the skin is golden and crisp. Flip over and cook for a further 2 minutes, or until the fish flakes when tested with a fork.

Blitz the cashews, broccoli and peas, parmesan, mint and garlic in a food processor until coarsely chopped. With the motor running, add the remaining olive oil in a thin steady stream until well combined. Blend in the lemon juice. Season.

Transfer the pesto to serving plates. Arrange the fish on top, sprinkle with a little sea salt and serve with the salad.

TIPS

This pesto is delicious with pretty much any fish, but also try it with orecchiette or tossed through zucchini ribbons or on zoodles.

Spread on thick slices of barbecue-grilled bread with an extra squeeze of lemon, a drizzle of olive oil and some feta as the new, home-buyer's budget-friendly alternative to avocado on toast!

And yes, a poached egg – and even bacon – will taste equally as good on top.

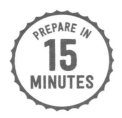

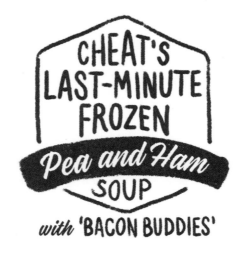

CHEAT'S LAST-MINUTE FROZEN
Pea and Ham SOUP
with 'BACON BUDDIES'

'Bacon Buddies?' No, we don't know what they are either yet, but I think we can all agree that we'll have to have them. I suspect they wear leather, break rules and are what society might class as 'bad news' or 'a menace'. Sort of like toastie versions of Marlon Brando and Lee Marvin's characters in *The Wild One* – the original teen hoon film.

SERVES 4   PREP: 15 MINS   COOKING: 20 MINS

1 tablespoon olive oil
200 g piece double-smoked ham,
  rind removed, finely chopped
1 onion, finely chopped
2 garlic cloves, crushed
1 litre salt-reduced chicken stock
1 kg frozen baby peas
2 tablespoons finely chopped mint
sea salt and freshly ground
  black pepper
thickened cream, to drizzle

BACON BUDDIES
8 hickory-smoked shortcut
  bacon rashers
8 slices white bread
80 g butter, at room temperature
1 tablespoon dijon mustard
8 Swiss cheese slices

Heat the oil in a large saucepan over medium–high heat. Add the ham and onion and cook, stirring, for 8 minutes, or until soft. Add the garlic and cook, stirring, for 30 seconds, or until aromatic. Add the stock then cover and bring to a gentle simmer.

Add the peas and cook, uncovered, for 3–5 minutes, until tender but still bright green. Stir in the mint. Season.

While the soup simmers away, start making your bacon buddies. Preheat a sandwich press. Place the bacon on the press, close the lid and cook for 2 minutes, or until golden. Transfer to a plate. (There will be a bit of fat left behind from the bacon but the bread will soak this up and make for extra tasty buddies!)

Spread half the bread slices with butter, then turn them over and spread the other side with dijon (do this on a board as it can be a little messy). Top with a slice of cheese, two pieces of bacon and another slice of cheese. Sit the remaining bread slices on top and carefully butter the surface. Transfer to the sandwich press, close and cook for 2–3 minutes, until golden. Cut into fingers.

Remove the soup from the heat and use a stick blender to puree. Ladle among serving bowls. Drizzle with cream and serve with your bacon buddies.

TIPS

A little cream stirred through at the end makes this soup fresh and light. In winter, when you want it more cosy, stir in ⅓ cup of cream just after pureeing for a thicker richer soup.

No sandwich press? No worries!!! Here's another way to make the bacon buddies: preheat your oven to 180°C/160°C fan-forced. Cook 2 rashers of bacon in a non-stick frying pan over medium heat for 3–4 minutes, until golden. Meanwhile, place 2 slices of bread together and fit this double slice into one slot of your toaster. Toast until the outsides are golden but the inside face of each slice is still soft and pillowy. Repeat with the remaining bread, then butter the toasted sides. Arrange 4 slices, untoasted-side up, on a baking tray. Spread with mustard and top with a slice of cheese, the bacon and another slice of cheese. Top with the remaining bread with the toasted side facing up. Bake for 5 minutes or until the cheese has melted.

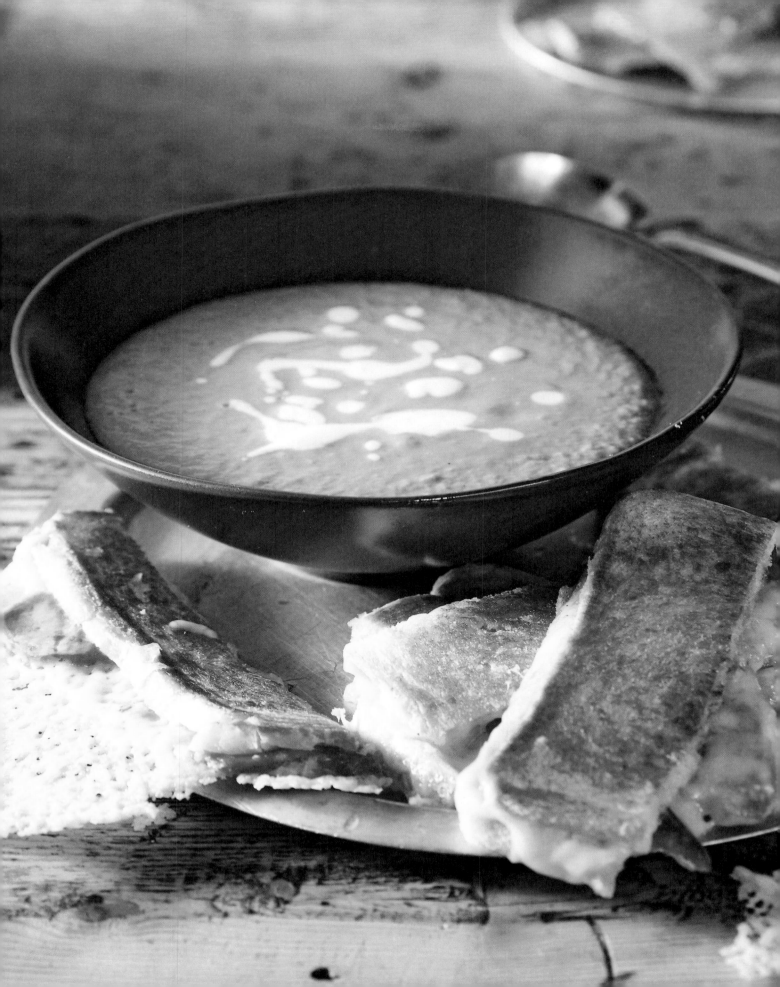

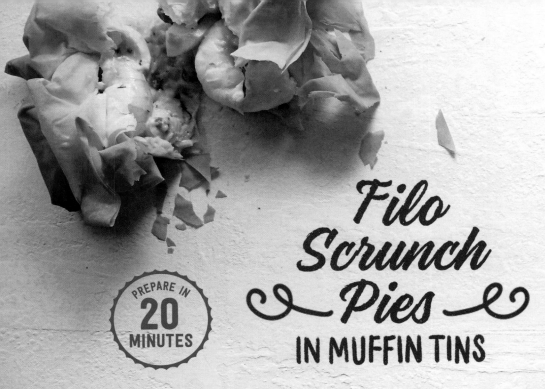

Filo Scrunch Pies
IN MUFFIN TINS

PREPARE IN 20 MINUTES

I am desperate to bring back the vol-au-vent. I love the golden crispy ring of puff pastry and the sexy fillings inside. In down moments on set at *MasterChef* we fantasise about opening a little bakery and selling nothing but these icons of 70s drinks parties, where the men all had mutton-chop sideburns and the women wore floaty burnt-orange numbers to match the settees.
We even have the name: Maison Vol-au-Vent. It has a certain melody, don't you think?

However, I fear that the publishing world is not yet ready for a vol-au-vent revival. My own publisher's professional advice largely relates to the perceived negative impact on my culinary credibility. So, next book maybe? Definitely.

For now, this recipe for scrunchy pies made with frozen filo sheets will have to do – and it's almost as good. They hold pretty much whatever fillings you want to put in there, including creamed mushrooms with thyme, ham cubes in a cheese sauce and even – but not advisedly – your car keys.

You will need two six hole (each hole 185 ml capacity) muffin tins. (Although you will only be using three holes in each tin, to give your scrunchy pies sufficient space.)

MAKES 6 PREP: 20 MINS COOKING: 50 MINS

100 g butter
1 small leek, thinly sliced
2 garlic cloves, crushed
2 tablespoons plain flour
125 ml (½ cup) fish stock
2 tablespoons white wine
500 g large frozen peeled green prawns, thawed on a plate lined with paper towel
80 g (½ cup) frozen peas, thawed on a plate lined with paper towel
80 ml (⅓ cup) pouring cream
1 tablespoon coarsely chopped dill
2 teaspoons dijon mustard
1 teaspoon finely grated lemon zest
3 hard-boiled eggs, peeled and quartered
18 sheets filo pastry
olive oil spray

Melt 40 g of the butter in a saucepan over medium heat. Add the leek and cook, stirring, for 5 minutes, or until soft. Add the garlic and cook, stirring, for 30 seconds, or until aromatic. Add the flour and cook for 2 minutes to cook it out, then remove the pan from the heat.

Gradually add the stock and wine and stir until well combined. Return to medium heat and cook, stirring, for 3 minutes, or until the mixture thickens and comes to the boil. Don't worry if you think this mixture is wa-aaa-ay too thick as there is method to this madness. When using frozen seafood, more water comes out and we need to make allowances for that here or your pies will have soggy pastry bottoms – and no one appreciates a soggy bottom.

Stir in the prawns, peas and cream. Simmer over low heat, stirring occasionally, for 7 minutes, or until the prawns start to change colour. Stir in the dill, mustard and lemon zest. Carefully stir in the egg. Set aside to cool slightly.

Preheat the oven to 200°C/180°C fan-forced.

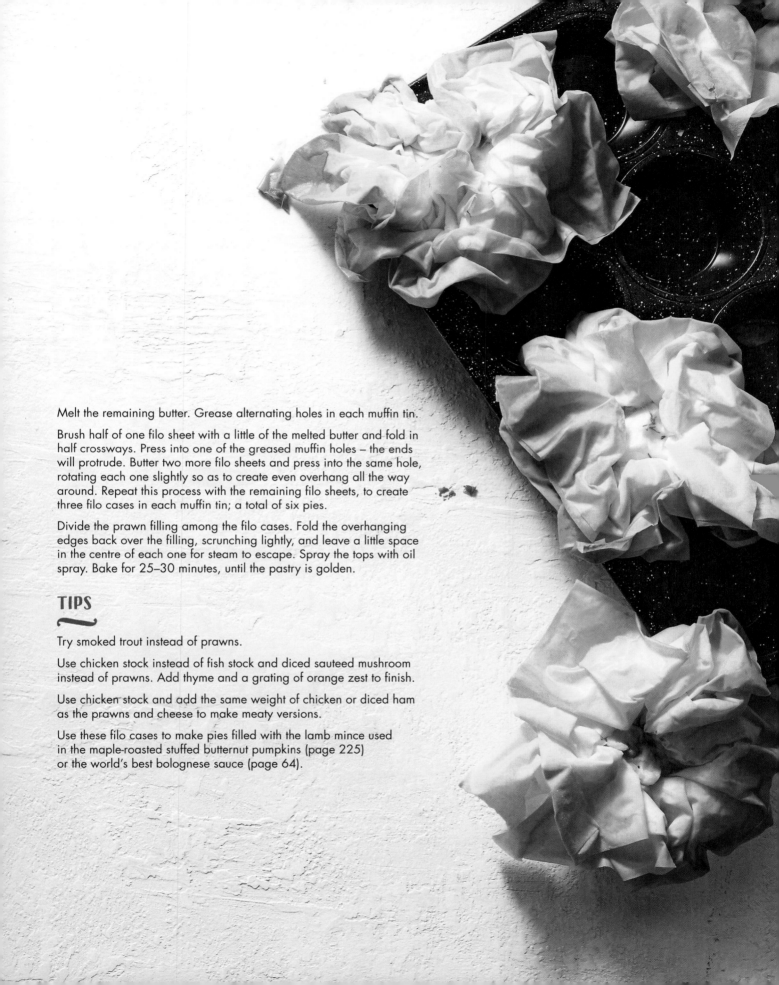

Melt the remaining butter. Grease alternating holes in each muffin tin.

Brush half of one filo sheet with a little of the melted butter and fold in half crossways. Press into one of the greased muffin holes – the ends will protrude. Butter two more filo sheets and press into the same hole, rotating each one slightly so as to create even overhang all the way around. Repeat this process with the remaining filo sheets, to create three filo cases in each muffin tin; a total of six pies.

Divide the prawn filling among the filo cases. Fold the overhanging edges back over the filling, scrunching lightly, and leave a little space in the centre of each one for steam to escape. Spray the tops with oil spray. Bake for 25–30 minutes, until the pastry is golden.

TIPS

Try smoked trout instead of prawns.

Use chicken stock instead of fish stock and diced sauteed mushroom instead of prawns. Add thyme and a grating of orange zest to finish.

Use chicken stock and add the same weight of chicken or diced ham as the prawns and cheese to make meaty versions.

Use these filo cases to make pies filled with the lamb mince used in the maple-roasted stuffed butternut pumpkins (page 225) or the world's best bolognese sauce (page 64).

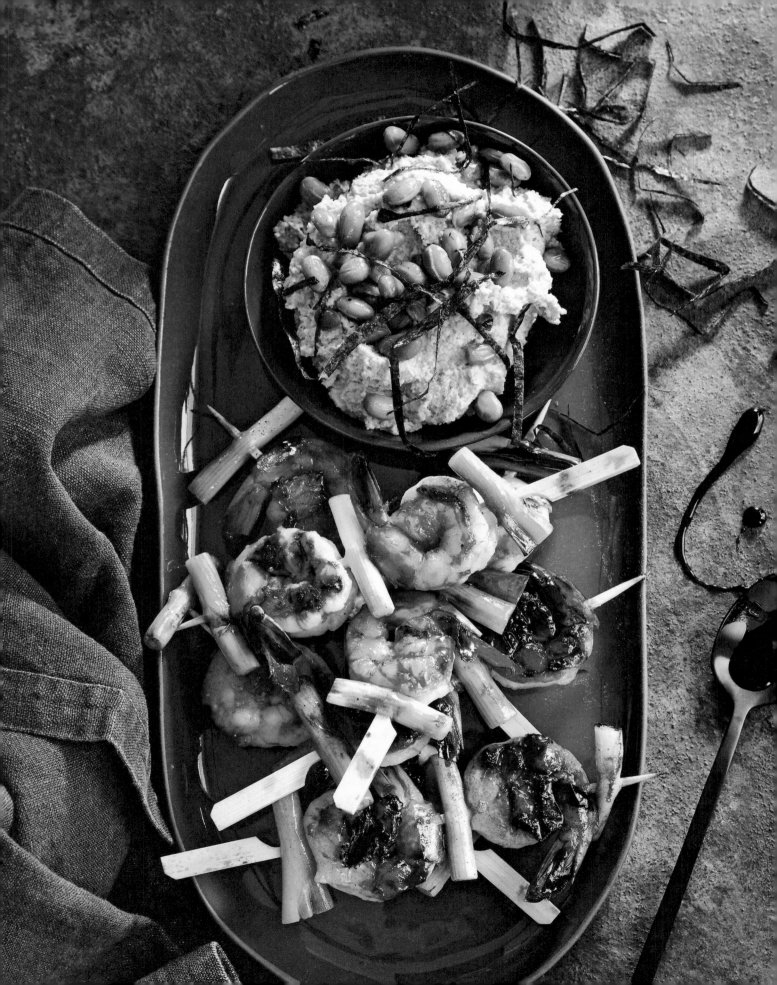

EDAMAME HUMMUS *with* TERIYAKI FROZEN PRAWNS

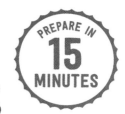

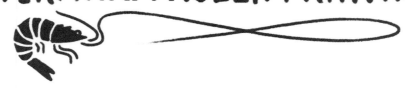

Hummus is the hottest single food in the world right now. Americans are going bonkers for it and blending chickpeas with pretty much anything that takes their fancy (if not mine) – even chocolate. But the big question is whether hummus even needs to include chickpeas at all these days.

This one doesn't. But that's because I don't want to mellow out the fresh flavour of the soy beans – and because, dagnabbit, I'm desperate to be seen as a culinary rebel. I want to walk into cool bars and have customers whisper to each other behind their hands, 'There's that guy who makes risotto with sunflower seeds and who doesn't even use chickpeas in his hummus! What a maverick.'

SERVES 4 PREP: 15 MINS (PLUS 30 MINS MARINATING) COOKING: 15 MINS

60 ml (¼ cup) teriyaki sauce (see page 123 for a homemade version or use storebought)
2 tablespoons honey
36 frozen peeled green prawns, with tails intact, thawed on a plate lined with paper towel
5 spring onions, cut into 4 cm lengths
2 tablespoons olive oil
2 teaspoons soy sauce
¼ sheet toasted nori, snipped into small strips (optional)

EDAMAME HUMMUS
1 slice white bread, crusts removed
60 ml (¼ cup) milk
450 g frozen edamame beans
1 spring onion, coarsely chopped
2 garlic cloves, crushed
2 teaspoons tahini
2 teaspoons ground cumin
60 ml (¼ cup) olive oil
1 tablespoon lemon juice
sea salt and freshly ground black pepper

Combine the teriyaki sauce and honey in a bowl. Add the prawns and toss to combine. Cover and place in the fridge for 30 minutes to marinate.

Thread the prawns onto soaked bamboo or metal skewers, alternating with the spring onion. Reserve the marinade in the bowl.

To make the edamame hummus, place the bread in a small bowl and pour over the milk. Set aside to soak for 5 minutes, then squeeze out the excess milk.

Cook the edamame beans in a saucepan of boiling water for 3–5 minutes, until tender. Transfer to a bowl of iced water to cool. Drain. Remove the beans from their pods and set aside ¼ cup in a separate bowl.

Blitz the soaked bread, spring onion, garlic, tahini, cumin and remaining edamame beans in a food processor, scraping down the side occasionally, until smooth. With the motor running, add the oil and lemon juice in a thin steady stream until well combined. Season. Cover, and place in the fridge.

Preheat a barbecue flat plate on medium–high. Drizzle the prawn skewers with the olive oil and place on the barbecue. Cook for 2–3 minutes on each side, until just cooked through. Before you turn them over, brush the uncooked side of the prawns with the reserved teriyaki marinade. Transfer to a plate.

Add the reserved edamame beans to the flat plate and drizzle with the soy sauce. Toss for 1–2 minutes, until lightly charred.

Spoon the edamame hummus into a serving bowl and sprinkle with the hot edamame beans. Top with shredded nori (if using) and serve with the prawn skewers.

TIPS

Warmed flatbreads or white rice topped with lemon zest and Sichuan pepper are great to bulk out this meal.

Hummus gets better with age, so the longer ahead you make it the better it will taste. Store, covered, in the fridge for a day or two.

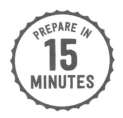

PREPARE IN
15
MINUTES

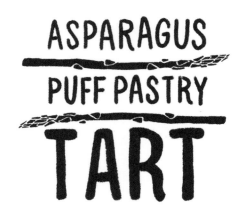

ASPARAGUS
PUFF PASTRY
TART

It's important to have heroes – people we look up to and who inspire us. Annie Smithers is one of those for me. She grows and makes so much of what she feeds people with at her little bistro in Trentham but, more importantly, she makes it so beautifully. Food without fuss, but never shy of flavour. This recipe is inspired by her asparagus tart, but I'm using good storebought puff pastry because I am lazy and not committed to the culinary arts in quite the same commendable way she is!

SERVES 4   **PREP:** 15 MINS   **COOKING:** 25 MINS

2 sheets frozen butter puff pastry, just thawed
1 egg, lightly whisked
200 g fresh ricotta
55 g (½ cup) coarsely grated gruyere
2 tablespoons coarsely chopped flat-leaf parsley
2 tablespoons finely chopped chives
2 teaspoons dijon mustard
sea salt and freshly ground black pepper
2 bunches asparagus, trimmed
1 rindless bacon rasher, thinly sliced
balsamic glaze (see TIPS), to serve (optional)

Preheat the oven to 200°C/180°C fan-forced. Line a large baking tray with baking paper. Stack the pastry sheets on top of each other on the tray and press lightly to seal. Use a knife to score a 2 cm border around the edges, but don't cut all the way through.

Use a fork to prick the base of the inside square as you don't want the pastry here to rise. However DON'T prick the border AT ALL, as you want it to rise around the edges. Brush the pastry border with egg. Bake for 10 minutes, or until light golden.

While the pastry cooks, combine the ricotta, gruyere, parsley, chives and mustard in a bowl. Season.

Use a clean tea towel to press down the centre of the pastry if it has risen slightly – even after a good 'forking', puff pastry can rise up for more.

Spread the cheese mixture over the pastry base. Slather it on right up to the border, without going over. Top with the asparagus spears, trimming if necessary to fit. Sprinkle with the chopped bacon. Bake for 15 minutes, or until the pastry is puffed and golden. Drizzle with the balsamic glaze (if using).

TIPS

You can buy balsamic glaze in most good supermarkets, but it's as easy to make as combining 60 ml (¼ cup) balsamic vinegar with 55 g (¼ cup) white sugar, and simmering until it feels a little syrupy.

There are so many toppings you can use instead of asparagus on this tart. Try:

*   Halved cherry or truss tomatoes (with or without pitted black olives and/or anchovies).
*   Broccolini cut into thin long florets.
*   Sliced zucchini and peas with lots of black pepper and lemon.
*   Sliced mushrooms, lightly sauteed and drained, and thin wedges of red onion. Dress with a few dots of good balsamic vinegar.
*   Barbecued eggplant slices.
*   Roasted pumpkin slices and red onion slices. Maybe with crumbled feta and a sticky chilli-caramel, too.

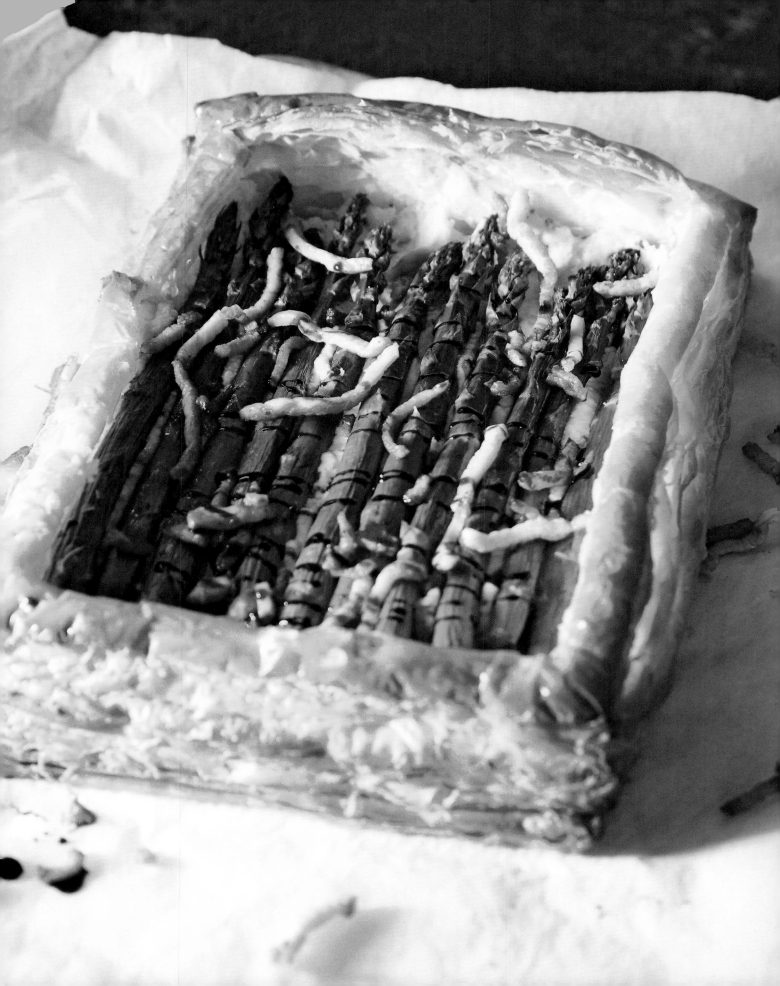

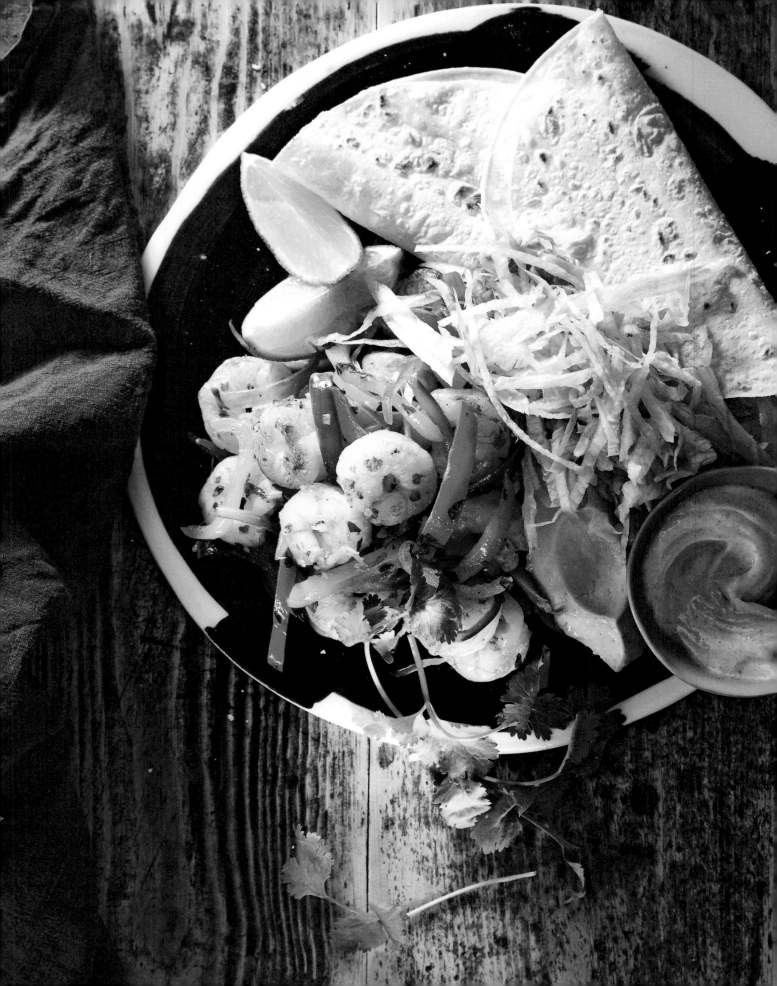

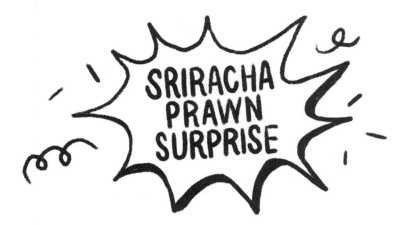

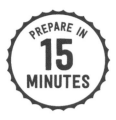

PREPARE IN
15
MINUTES

'This is the most delicious use of frozen prawns ever ...' I'm sure I read that in one of the reviews of this cookbook. I think maybe it was Ai Weiwei who said it.

This is basically boring old prawn fajitas given a dirty street-food-van make-over in homage to another of my heroes, the great LA food truck pioneer Roy Choi. This is not a shy dish – or one to be taken lightly.

Also, please note that the correct way to say sriracha is with the emphasis firmly on the 'cha'. Think of how you'd pronounce the Cuban dance, the cha-cha-cha, and you'll have it down pat. David Thompson of Long Chim and Nahm fame told me this; he lives in Bangkok and he knows stuff.

SERVES 4 PREP: 15 MINS COOKING: 15 MINS

2 tablespoons olive oil
2 red onions, cut into thin wedges
1 red capsicum, deseeded and thinly sliced
1 yellow capsicum, deseeded and thinly sliced
2 garlic cloves, crushed
500 g frozen peeled green prawns, thawed on a plate lined with paper towel
1 tablespoon sriracha chilli sauce
¼ cup coarsely chopped coriander, plus extra sprigs to serve
1 lime, halved, plus extra wedges to serve
½ iceberg lettuce, shredded
8 mini flour tortillas, warmed in the microwave
1 avocado, quartered

SMOKY MAYO
1 egg, yolk and white
250 ml (1 cup) grapeseed oil
1 tablespoon lemon juice
1 teaspoon dijon mustard
1 teaspoon smoked paprika
pinch of salt

Make your smoky mayo so it's ready to go. Carefully crack the egg into a jug, without breaking the yolk. Pour over the oil, lemon juice, mustard, paprika and salt. Place a stick blender in the jug and position the head of the blender so it covers and encloses the egg yolk. Blend for 1–2 seconds to emulsify. Continue to blend and when you see salmon–pink ribbons trailing out from the blender head, pull it up through the oil, bouncing gently as you go, until a thick mayonnaise forms. Refrigerate until ready to serve.

Heat the oil in a large non-stick frying pan over high heat. Add the onion and capsicum and cook, tossing, for 5 minutes, or until slightly charred and tender. Stir in the garlic for 30 seconds, or until aromatic. Transfer to a heatproof bowl.

Add the prawns and sriracha to the pan and, cook, tossing for 4–5 minutes, until the prawns are cooked through and slightly charred. In the last few seconds, with the pan still on the heat, toss through the capsicum mixture along with the chopped coriander and a good squeeze of lime juice.

As you are cooking the prawns, arrange the shredded iceberg lettuce and warm tortillas on plates or on a platter.

Add the prawn mixture and serve with avocado, smoky mayo, extra coriander sprigs and lime wedges.

TIP

You can also serve this with my Korean mayo (page 22).

PERFECT RICE

If I can implore you to do just one thing after reading this book it would be to buy yourself a rice cooker. It'll be the best $30 you'll spend all year. There are plenty of easy and delicious rice recipes through this book and they are all even less hassle to prepare with a rice cooker. Until then ...

WHITE FLUFFY RICE

SERVES 4 **PREP**: 5 MINS **COOKING**: 15 MINS

200 g (1 cup) white long-grain rice
330 ml (1⅓ cups) water
good pinch of salt

Place the rice in a sieve and rinse under cold running water a couple of times to remove any starch or talc used in the processing. When the water runs clear, place the rice and water in a large saucepan and add a good pinch of salt.

Bring to the boil, then immediately drop the heat to a bare simmer.

Cover, and cook for 15 minutes or until the water is absorbed.

Remove the pan from the heat, leave covered, and let the rice steam for 5 minutes. Fluff with a fork.

BROWN RICE

SERVES 4 **PREP**: 5 MINS **COOKING**: 40 MINS

200 g (1 cup) brown rice
435 ml (1¾ cups) water
good pinch of salt

Place the rice and water in a large saucepan and add a good pinch of salt. Bring to the boil then immediately drop the heat to a bare simmer. Cover and cook for 40 minutes until the water is absorbed.

Remove from the heat, leave covered, and let the rice steam for 10 minutes. Fluff with a fork.

BOGAN UNFRIED RICE

SERVES 4 **PREP**: 5 MINS **COOKING**: 15 MINS

100 g lap cheong sausage, sliced
   diagonally
150 g spam, cut into cubes
100 g char siu barbecued pork,
   thinly sliced
3 long green chillies, thinly sliced
80 g (½ cup) frozen peas, thawed
80 g (½ cup) frozen corn, thawed
1 x quantity white or brown rice
   (see above)
soy sauce and sesame oil, to drizzle
1 cup coriander leaves

Heat a large frying pan over medium–high heat. Add the lap cheong sausage and spam, and toss for 2–3 minutes, until they start to brown. Add the pork and chilli, and toss for 2 minutes, or until heated through. Add the peas and corn and toss for 2 minutes, or until heated through.

Spread the warm rice on a platter and scatter with the topping. Drizzle with the soy sauce and sesame oil, then sprinkle with coriander leaves.

TIP

If you are short of time use 1 x 450 g pouch 90 second microwaveable brown or white rice, warmed following the packet instructions.

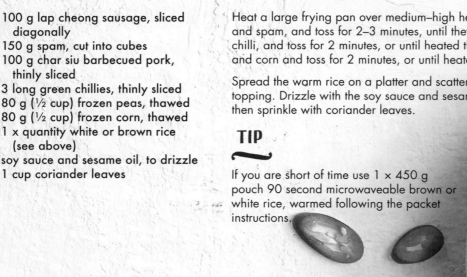

10 MORE PERFECT RICE COMBOS

1. Toss rice with toasted corn kernels and similarly sized dice of smoked chicken breast warmed in the same wok/pan with sliced spring onion. Top with raw cashews, coriander leaves and a dribble of sriracha chilli sauce marbled with soy sauce.

2. Top rice with cubed spam (tossed in gochujang and fried), sesame seeds, omelette (rolled and cut thin), cooked peas, black pepper and shredded leeks fried in oil with a little gochujang stirred through at the end.

3. Toss rice with lots of chopped char siu pork, diced Chinese five-spice roasted carrots (page 222) and toasted coriander seeds. Top with fresh coriander, lemon zest, mandarin zest and a drizzle of caramel made from one part mandarin juice, one part whisky and two parts caster sugar.

4. Make small meatballs rolled from squeezing the meat out of pork and fennel sausages and cook until golden. Toss through rice, then dice some fennel and fry half in the fat rendered from the meatballs with some onion sliced into strings and fried until golden and crispy with star anise (in the same pan). To do this, take peeled red onions and make a lengthways incision to the depth of the centre of the onion. Then cut each onion into thin slices and fry slowly. Garnish with the raw fennel, fennel fronds, orange zest and a caramel made from brown sugar, Shaoxing rice wine and orange juice.

5. Toss rice with gently cooked peeled prawns and sliced oyster mushroom, also gently cooked with soy and Shaoxing rice wine. Top with slices of slightly sweetened egg omelette, diced and fried spam, diced and just-cooked white onion and bean shoots.

6. Toss brown rice with fried lap cheong sausage, peanuts, sliced spring onion and lots and lots of sliced long red chilli. Douse with soy.

7. Top the rice with fried eggs, crispy shallots, thinly sliced spring onion, dribbles of kecap manis, a zigzag of Kewpie mayonnaise and lots of fresh coriander.

8. Toss toasted coconut flakes (or use Coconut Granola, page 203) through the rice, along with microwaved and then fried cauliflower florets. Top with peeled prawns cooked in butter that you've melted with a good spoonful of skimmed milk powder. Add fresh curry leaves if you have them. Quickly wipe round the pan with a handful of oats over high heat so the oats soak up any leftover butter and they also toast a little. Throw onto the prawns.

9. Toss the rice with cooked, diced veg: carrot, celery, peas, sliced and blanched snow peas or sugar snaps, broccoli florets, fennel, pan-toasted corn kernels, spring onion coins – and whatever else is left alone in the crisper drawer or corner of the freezer. If it's all looking too dour and virtuous for you, add chunks of chopped cooked prawn and/or diced fried spam or lap cheong sausage. Top with any recognisably Asian herbs.

10. Chunks of cooked chicken thigh fillet, chopped toasted cashews, sliced celery and crushed dried chillies tossed through rice.

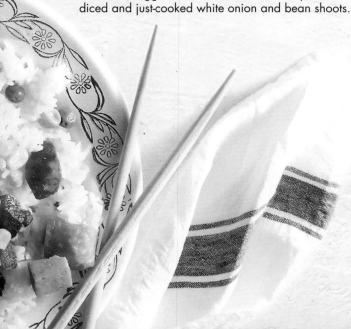

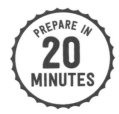

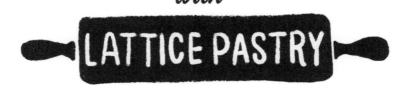

SALMON COULIBAC
with
LATTICE PASTRY

This simple technique turns frozen pastry into something that could grace the catwalks of Paris.
So enough talking, this is how to make the magic happen ...

SERVES 6 **PREP**: 20 MINS (PLUS 10 MINS CHILLING) **COOKING**: 30 MINS

20 g butter
200 g Swiss brown mushrooms,
  thinly sliced
335 g (2 cups) cooked brown rice
3 spring onions, thinly sliced
45 g (¼ cup) currants
2 tablespoons coarsely chopped dill
finely grated zest of 1 lemon
3 sheets frozen puff pastry,
  just thawed
3 x 130 g frozen salmon portions,
  thawed on paper towel at room
  temperature
2 hard-boiled eggs, peeled and
  thickly sliced
1 egg, lightly whisked
1 tablespoon white sesame seeds

Melt the butter in a large non-stick frying pan over medium–high heat. Add the mushroom and cook, stirring, for 5 minutes, or until golden. Remove from the heat and stir in the rice, spring onion, currants, dill and lemon zest.

Preheat the oven to 220°C/200°C fan-forced. Arrange two sheets of baking paper on a kitchen bench, side by side so you have a covered work surface. The paper will also help you lift the coulibac later on in the recipe.

Take two of the pastry sheets and place them on top of the baking paper. Overlap them slightly to make a 40 cm × 25 cm rectangle.

Cut the third pastry sheet in half and overlap the two pieces in the same way, to create one 40 cm × 12.5 cm strip. Attach this long strip on to the longest side of the rectangle, with the edges slightly overlapping.

Use a rolling pin to roll over all the edges where they meet, to seal them and ensure the pastry is an even thickness. You should now have a 40 cm × 35 cm rectangle.

Using the baking paper to help you, lift the pastry onto a large baking tray. Place in the freezer for 10 minutes.

When chilled, spread the rice mixture along the length of the pastry, leaving about a 10 cm border on each long side and a 2 cm edge at each short end. Place the salmon fillets along the rice, then top with egg slices.

Use a knife to cut 2 cm thick diagonal strips in the pastry on either side of the filling. Fold in the pastry at both short ends. Now start creating your lattice. Working from one end, fold one strip of pastry over the filling, then fold in a strip from the opposite side, slightly overlapping. Continue like this, alternating the strips over the filling until it is completely enclosed. Brush with a little egg to secure the strips and trim away any excess pastry.

Now brush the pastry all over with egg and sprinkle with sesame seeds. Bake for 18–20 minutes, until the pastry is golden brown.

TIPS

You can use pouches of 90 second microwaveable rice if you are short of time.

The same technique can be used to jazz up leftovers like meatloaf or even mash mixed with tinned tuna and spring onions.

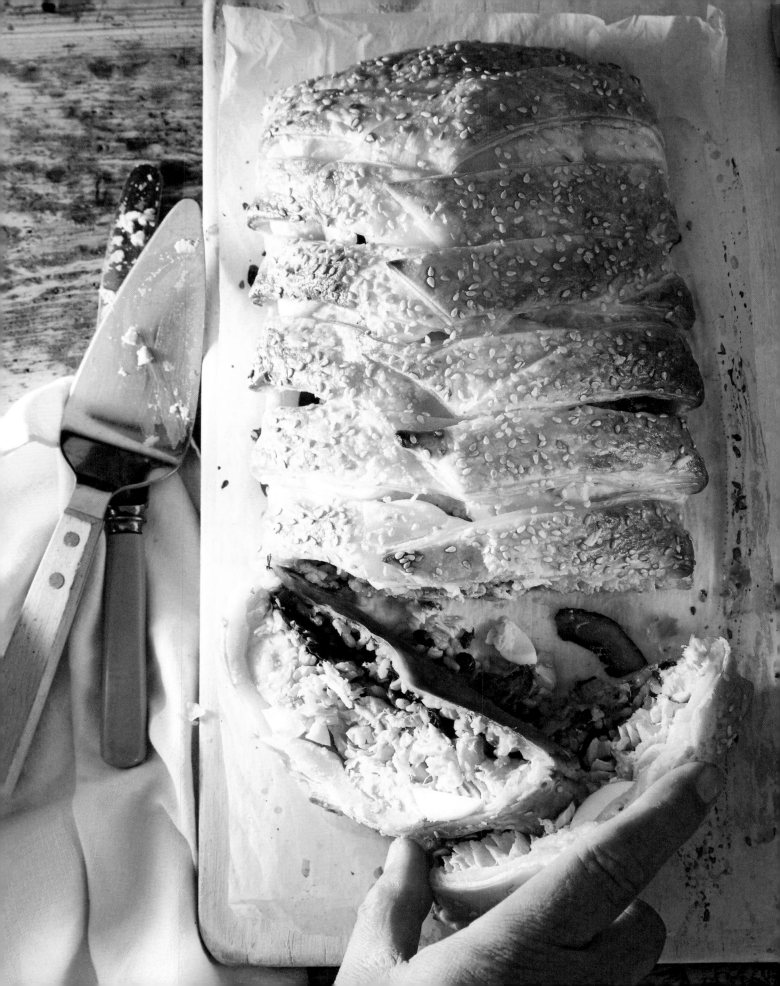

PAN
STA

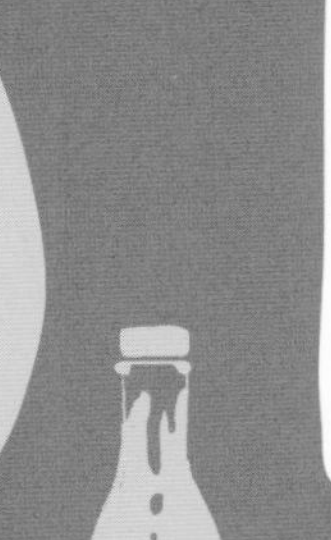

TRY

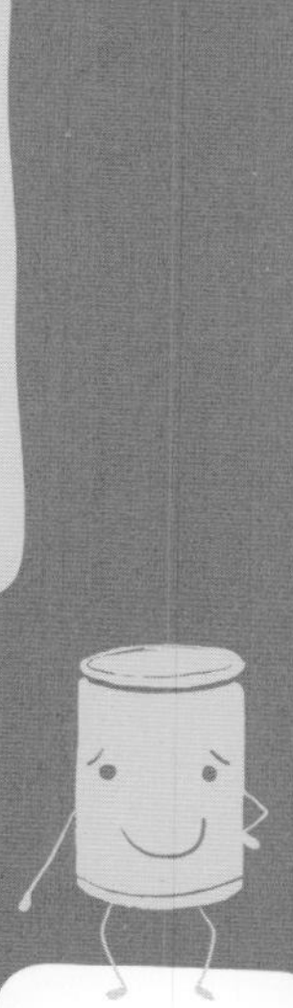

LES

THE JOY OF AN ORGANISED PANTRY (OR CUPBOARD LOVE)

An organised pantry is a thing of beauty. To gaze on it is to feel stability and order flowing through you. I suspect I get the same calm after reorganising my pantry as Buddhist monks get from neatly raking the gravel in their Japanese rock gardens into swirls. So here's how I regroup my pantry each year. It'll take about two hours excluding shopping. It will make you calm and happy. I promise! Even if it seems a little sad – as if your life was over. I'm sure Harry Styles doesn't spend a morning organising his pantry … It looks like I've turned into a Stepford Wife!

REMOVE EVERYTHING

You can't re-organise your pantry cupboard if you don't know what's in there, so empty it. Organise everything that comes out of the cupboard or cupboards into different piles: staples, spices, condiments, cans (sweet), cans (savoury), flavourings, stuff for baking, etc. Wipe down anything that is sticky or dusty. Throw away anything you haven't used in the last year as space makes pantries look neater.

DECLARE A PANTRY AMNESTY

Any unopened, or opened and used once, gifts of chutney or old jams should be binned and the jars repurposed for your next jam-making session – or sold to a gullible local cafe as 'vintage hipster wine glasses'.

CLEAN THE SHELVES

Rigorously! You may line them with paper if you are over 60, or if they are still horribly stained even after wiping down. Dust the corners, tops of the doors and wipe the front and underside of all the shelves as well.

BOX IT

Buy cheap takeaway containers of various depths as these are great for holding small stashes of packaged dried goods. Buy in bulk so all the lids are the same size and they will stack neatly. If you can afford it also buy larger, see-thru storage jars; get several sets as they'll last an age and you really can't have too many. These will hold bulk goods like rice, flours, sugars, pastas, oats, muesli, etc. It's good if these can also stack on top of each other. The lids must fit on securely.

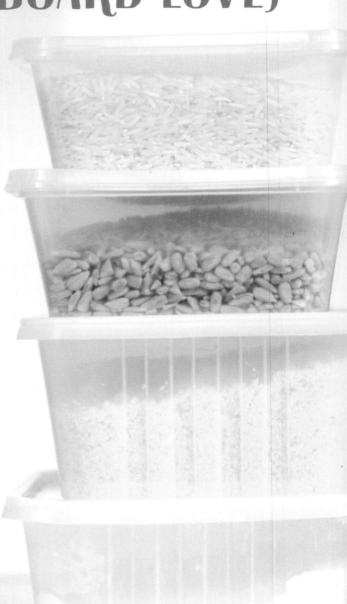

LABEL IT

Now it's just a matter of finding a friend or acquaintance with a labeller they'll lend you so you can label everything, making it even easier to find. They will be the person with a bowl of small soaps in the guest dunny, a wardrobe organised like a set of Derwents, and the always clean shoes. Their birthday will probably be between 22 August and 22 September.

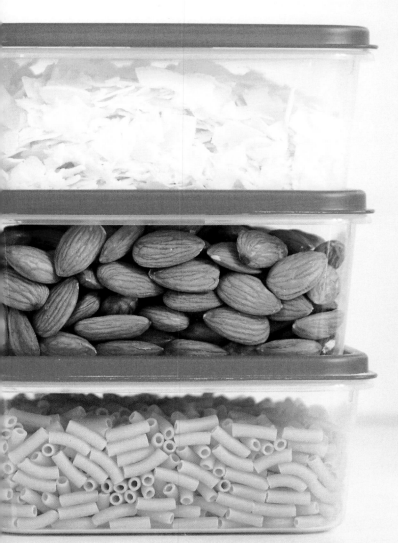

BIN IT

I'd also suggest buying a few larger clear drawers where you can corral bitty things that you use at the same time like all your spices or all your baking items (candles, vanilla essence, cooking chocolate, patty pans, food colouring). This means they are easy to pull out and sift through when you want to use them.

ORGANISE IT

When you put everything back in your pantry, organise everything by use. Try and group staples together: stack your cans with the savoury stuff on the right and the sweet stuff on the left of the cupboard. Those pop-in, half-height shelves can ensure all your cans are visible but more economical is to do a double height layer of the most used cans like tinned tomatoes or pulses stacked so they are easily seen.

With bottles, put the tallest ones at the back and group as you might use them. So, for example, put the soy next to the hoisin sauce, Shaoxing rice wine, sesame oil and peanut oil.

The same goes for other pantry items like capers, anchovies and olives; group them together because usually when I'm using one I'll also want to use the others and this makes it far quicker to find everything.

KEEP IT HANDY

One proviso, to ensure your pantry stays organised put your most used items at the front – unless they are clearly visible and raised at the back like those raised tins of tomatoes or that packet of stock. Pantries quickly get messy again if the ball of impatience that you live with starts rifling through it every time they are looking for the salt.

TRAY IT

If you are going to store appliances like your toaster, juicer or mixer in the same cupboard, place each on trays so they are easier to get out. It's also convenient to place all your regular breakfast needs on one tray so they are easy to find first thing.

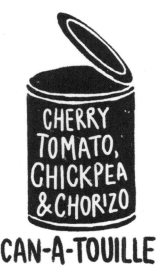

CAN-A-TOUILLE

There was some resistance to my suggestion of naming this recipe a 'can-a-touille' until I pointed out that the word 'can' had far fewer negative connotations than the original three-letter word it was replacing. BUT ... should the title be can-a-touille or tin-a-touille? I like the word 'can' better, given its positivity.

Mary (the publisher): *Personally, I like Matt-a-touille!*

Matt: *Whatevs.*

Lucy (an editor): *Yes, as the editor, let me tell you that is soooo not happening.*

BTW, cans of cherry tomatoes might be a dollar more expensive than your usual canned tomatoes, but they are far prettier and often have a more intense flavour, which means they require less cooking and so maintain more of their vibrancy.

SERVES 4 **PREP:** 10 MINS **COOKING:** 30 MINS

2 tablespoons olive oil

3 large zucchini, halved lengthways and thickly sliced

1 onion, coarsely chopped

2 large red capsicums, deseeded and cut into 3 cm pieces

3 garlic cloves, crushed

2 chorizo sausages, thinly sliced

1 tablespoon red wine vinegar

800 g canned cherry tomatoes

1 × 400 g can chickpeas, rinsed and drained

125 ml (½ cup) vegetable or chicken stock

2 basil sprigs, leaves picked (reserve both the stems and leaves)

sea salt and freshly ground black pepper

Heat 1 tablespoon of the oil in a large deep frying pan over medium heat. Add the zucchini and cook, tossing, for 5 minutes, or until starting to turn golden. Transfer to a large heatproof bowl.

Heat the remaining oil, then add the onion and capsicum. Cook, stirring, for 3 minutes, or until slightly softened. Add the garlic and cook, stirring, for 1 minute, or until aromatic. Add to the bowl with the zucchini.

Add the chorizo to the pan (you won't need any more oil as chorizo has plenty). Cook for 4–5 minutes, until golden and crisp. Add the vinegar and deglaze, scraping up any yummy bits stuck on the bottom of the pan.

Return all the vegetables to the pan, then add the tomatoes, chickpeas, stock and basil stems. Reduce the heat to low. Simmer for 10–15 minutes, until the veggies are very tender. Season.

Sprinkle over the basil leaves and serve.

TIPS

Another great sauce for freezing. Make ahead of time and place in airtight containers. Freeze for up to 3 months. Thaw overnight in the fridge and then reheat in a saucepan over low heat. Add a splash of water or stock to thin down if necessary. Serve this can-a-touille with barbecued pork or chicken thighs, grilled fish or poached eggs.

Jazz it up! Halve eggplants lengthways and chargrill slowly until very tender. Scoop out the flesh and mash. Stuff the eggplant shells with their mashed flesh and a mixture of ricotta and spinach. Top with can-a-touille and bake until golden and tender.

Omit the chorizo for a vegetarian version.

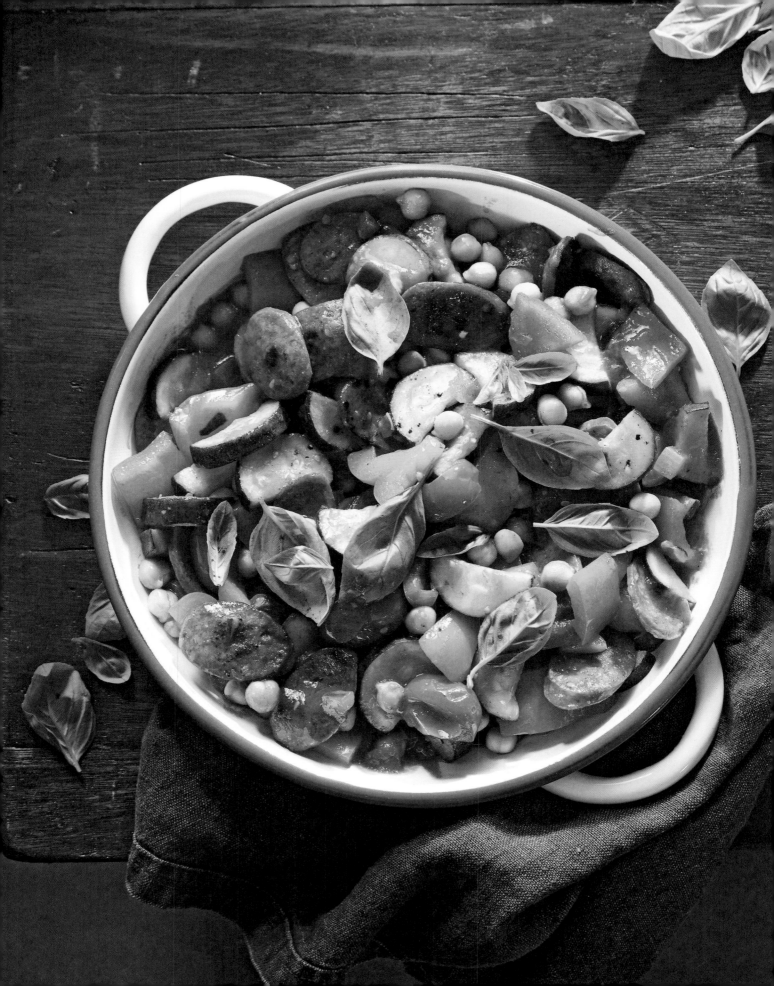

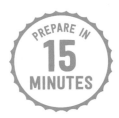

PREPARE IN
15
MINUTES

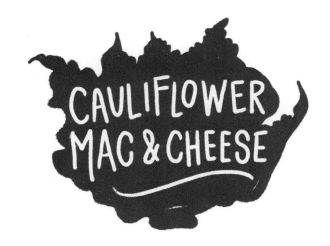

A 'menage a trois' doesn't always work (he says from bitter experience), but in the case of these three ingredients it's a match made in heaven. I love the textural difference between the pasta and the cauliflower florets, but I also like the fact that it almost makes mac 'n' cheese a thing of virtue. Almost …

I've added some pickled jalapenos to this recipe for their heat (and the fact they love bitey cheese something fierce) but you don't need them if you don't like them. Feel free to leave your mac 'n' cheese plain, top it with herbs, or spike the breadcrumbs with anything from crumbled chorizo or bacon to a little mix of ground coriander and cumin instead. Of course, as it is, this dish is deliciously vegetarian.

SERVES 6 PREP: 15 MINS COOKING: 45 MINS

200 g dried macaroni
½ (about 680 g) cauliflower, cut into small florets
20 g butter, chopped
2 French shallots, finely chopped
1½ tablespoons plain flour
375 ml (1½ cups) milk
100 g (1 cup) coarsely grated jalapeno Monterey Jack or Colby cheese
sea salt and freshly ground black pepper
70 g (½ cup) sliced pickled jalapenos
20 g (¼ cup) panko breadcrumbs
20 g (¼ cup) shredded parmesan

Preheat the oven to 200°C/180°C fan-forced. Cook the macaroni in plenty of boiling salted water for 2 minutes less than it says on the packet, until al dente, adding the cauliflower for the last 4 minutes of cooking. Drain and transfer to a large bowl.

While the pasta cooks, melt the butter in a saucepan over medium heat. Add the shallot and cook, stirring, for 3 minutes, or until soft. Stir in the flour for 1 minute or until the mixture bubbles. Remove the pan from the heat and gradually whisk in the milk until smooth. Return to medium heat and simmer, stirring, for 2 minutes, or until the mixture boils and thickens. Stir in the cheese until it melts. Season.

Stir this bechamel sauce through the pasta and cauliflower, then spoon the mixture into one large baking dish or six individual dishes. Sprinkle over the jalapenos. Combine the breadcrumbs and parmesan in a bowl, then scatter over the top as well. Bake for 30 minutes, or until the top is golden and crisp.

TIPS

This recipe works just as well with broccoli, but add diced fresh or dried red chilli instead of the jalapenos.

If you want to spike up the dish further, play around with the white sauce. Substitute 60 ml (¼ cup) of the milk for 60 ml (¼ cup) of jalapeno pickling liquid. Or infuse the milk with bay leaves, parsley stalks or a clove-studded peeled onion – or maybe a combination. A little nutmeg is another option as it loves milk and does good things to it.

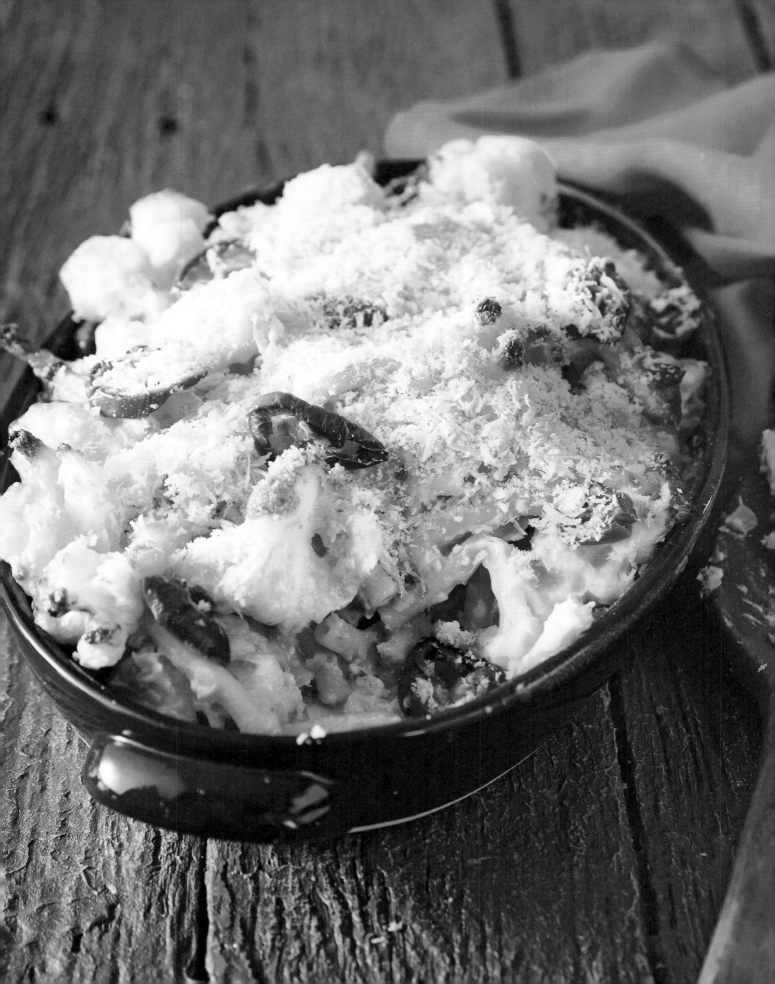

HOW TO COOK DRIED PASTA

(AND NEXT ... TEACHING YOUR GRANDMOTHER HOW TO SUCK EGGS)

Put a large saucepan of water as salty as the sea on the stovetop and bring to the boil.

When the water bubbles away enthusiastically drop in the pasta and immediately stir in a glass of cold water. This will stop the pasta sticking. Do not add oil.

Return to the boil, then reduce the heat and simmer for 1–2 minutes less than it says on the packet (or until a little harder than al dente).

Scoop out and reserve 250 ml (1 cup) of the starchy cooking liquid and drain the pasta.

I put the pasta plates or bowls in the sink under the colander so the draining water warms them before it heads off down the plughole. Too late? Well try it next time. Do not rinse the pasta.

Toss your pasta with any veggies or protein and any creamy or saucy business, then add a splash of the cooking water. The tossing in the pan helps the sauce and the water to emulsify, coating the pasta beautifully.

Serve on warmed plates or in bowls and sprinkle with your chosen crunch, cheese or herbs to serve.

TIPS ON PREPARING ELEMENTS FOR DRESSING OR SAUCING

Anything that needs to be blanched, such as snow peas or broccoli florets, should be added to the pasta in the last 2 minutes of cooking.

With mushrooms, bacon, pancetta, breadcrumbs for migas or pangrattato, leeks, fennel or anything that needs to be sauteed, do this while the pasta is cooking.

Cook your protein, and anything that needs roasting, before you start the pasta as pasta is a pernicious diva and waits for no one and no thing.

Keep everything to add to your pasta warm, or warm it, if pre-prepared.

Warm and reduce any 'sauciness', like canned cherry tomatoes, white wine and so on by deglazing the pan you've cooked the protein or veg in.

SAUCING YOUR PASTA

Saucing your pasta is not a science, but an art. It's about knowing which flavours to paint with. So cruise the ideas over the page and mix 'n' match as takes your fancy. It's just a matter of collecting what you want to cook, and handling it appropriately.

CHOOSING THE RIGHT PASTA

Remember the essential rule of pasta saucing is, the chunkier and more robust the sauce, the chunkier and more robust the pasta shape.

So:

- thin creamy sauces or aglio olio go with angel hair pasta;

- pair soupy broths with risoni or tiny hoops;

- medium-weight sauces, such as bolognese, match with tagliatelle or spaghetti;

- loose sauces, such as carbonara or amatriciana, go with bucatini or spaghetti;

- chunky vegetable sauces or a meaty wild boar ragu go best with something robust like a pappardelle or rigatoni.

The only exception to this rule is seafood, which often partners linguini but really, my darlings, it's up to you to pick a favourite. It's Italy, so there are no rules and a lot of regional variations you can hide behind.

ONE FINAL THING ...

Pasta is about the pasta. The sauce, or any other bits you add, should be more of a condiment than the main event.

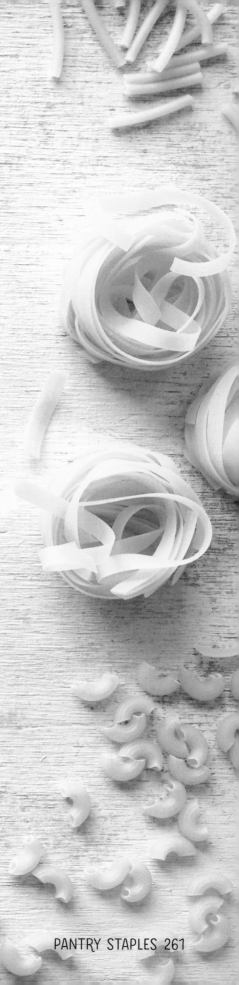

19 SPEEDY PASTA DISHES

Right kids, here are some of my favourite combos of flavourings, toppings and pastas.
Feel free to swap them around to generate new combos that appeal to you. Enjoy!

1. Combine angel-hair or trofie pasta with snow peas and flaked roasted or hot-smoked salmon. Stir through mascarpone, lemon zest and juice, and coins of spring onion. Top with the fish, slivered almonds and chopped dill.

2. Fry chorizo with cherry tomatoes or chopped cauliflower. Toss through tagliatelle, pappardelle or rigatoni and drizzle over the rendered oil from the chorizo pan. Top with shavings of manchego cheese and shredded parsley or mint.

3. Roast or fry petals of fennel or diced celery with garlic, roasted blue eye trevalla or another firm white-fleshed fish. In a frying pan, reduce white wine with tinned or fresh cherry tomatoes, or a big spoonful of fish stock cooked down with fennel trimmings and bacon. Combine the sauce with linguini or tagliatelle and top with the fish mixture and a few fennel fronds and optional crispy bacon.

4. Poach cauliflower, broccoli florets or brussels sprouts with orecchiette, small conchiglione (medium-sized shells) or spaghetti. Fry bacon, pancetta or prosciutto until crisp, or chopped anchovy and red chilli until soft and mushy. Add to the drained pasta and vegetables with a splash of pasta water, top with grated parmesan and migas (optional).

5. Combine fried leek rounds cooked in butter with chargrilled chicken thighs (chopped), or cooked peas and fried mushroom. Make a quick sauce by combining burnt butter with lemon juice and thyme, or cream reduced with half a crumbled chicken stock cube (shhh, it's a secret). Toss the whole lot through fusilli, cavatelli or penne cooked in chicken stock and serve with toasted pine nuts, parmesan and parsley (optional) sprinkled over the top.

6. Fry mushrooms with crumbled and cooked pork sausage. Combine crème fraîche with an optional ½ crumbled veg stock cube or thyme leaves, then stir everything through penne, rigatoni or pappardelle. Top with chopped hazelnuts, grated parmesan, gruyere or extra-bitey vintage tasty cheese.

7. Add roasted cherry tomatoes, fresh ricotta or torn bocconcini to warm drained spaghettini, angel-hair or farfalle (bow ties/butterflies). Squeeze over some lemon juice or add a splash of pan-reduced white wine. Serve with finely grated parmesan and lemon zest sprinkled over the top.

8. Mix together cooked peas, rubbly bits of feta, sliced spring onion and chopped hard-boiled egg or crispy pancetta. Stir through orecchiette or penne ('cos its funny when the peas try and hide in the penne tubes), squeeze over lemon juice and add a splash of pasta water. Serve with mint leaves, lemon zest and extra crumbled feta.

9. Roast zucchini then add to reduced tinned tomatoes with capers added at the end of cooking. Stir through rigatoni or conchiglione and serve with grated parmesan and nigella seeds.

10. Steam and shell mussels, then combine with flakes of roast salmon and chunks of ricotta in warmed cream. Stir through rigatoni or conchiglione and serve with grated parmesan and nigella seeds.

11. Choose between tinned tuna mixed with capers or roasted blue eye trevalla. Combine with tinned tomatoes reduced with fried garlic, mashed anchovies and black olives. Add a little lemon juice and brown sugar to intensify. Stir through spaghetti, bucatini or stozzapreti and sprinkle lemon zest, chopped parsley and possibly parmesan over the top. Finish with a squeeze of lemon juice.

12. Roast chunks of beetroot, then add to fettucine or homemade beetroot orecchiette (made with 300 g pureed cooked beetroot, 1 egg yolk and about 400 g '00' flour) if you're feeling fancy. Crumble in some goat's cheese and a splash of balsamic and pasta water, or orange zest and juice. Sprinkle over chopped hazelnuts and thyme.

13. Stir smoked trout, sliced spring onion and steamed broccolini through casarecce, penne or spaghetti with warmed crème fraîche mixed with lemon thyme and lemon juice. Top with extra lemon thyme, lemon zest and/or trout flesh, if you like.

14. Separately steam bok choy and ocean trout. Flake the trout. Spike green tea with soy and mirin and stir through soba noodles with the bok choy and trout. Finish with a sprinkling of black sesame seeds and sliced spring onion curled and crisped in iced water.

15. Reduce chicken or pork stock spiced with fried chopped garlic and thinly sliced fresh ginger. Toss through udon noodles and add shredded spinach, coins of spring onion and grilled sliced chicken or shredded pork. Top with halved soft-boiled eggs, shredded nori, sesame seeds, shichimi togarashi or furikake powder.

16. Make a classic pesto by blitzing basil, garlic, parmesan and pine nuts. Add olive oil, lemon juice and salt to taste, then blitz again to achieve the right texture. Stir through spaghetti along with a splash of pasta water and finish with fresh basil leaves scattered over the top.

17. Blitz roasted capsicum with blanched garlic cloves, almonds, grated manchego, lemon juice, olive oil and salt to taste. Stir through penne or orecchiette with a little pasta water and top with any fresh herbs to hand.

18. Process steamed or raw broccoli with roasted hazelnuts, grated pecorino, mint and basil. Add lemon, salt and olive oil and blitz again to achieve your desired texture. Toss through spaghetti with a little of the pasta water and top with fresh herbs and extra grated pecorino. Or try the Pea and Broccoli Pesto (page 237).

19. Blitz kale or rocket, walnuts, garlic, olive oil, lots of lemon and a touch of chilli. Note that both rocket and kale pesto can be bitter and work best with a good hit of saltiness, so be bold with the salt – or dump the chilli and replace with blue cheese or feta. Stir through spaghetti, penne or orecchiette with a splash of pasta water. Pile fresh herbs on top and sprinkle over lots of parmesan.

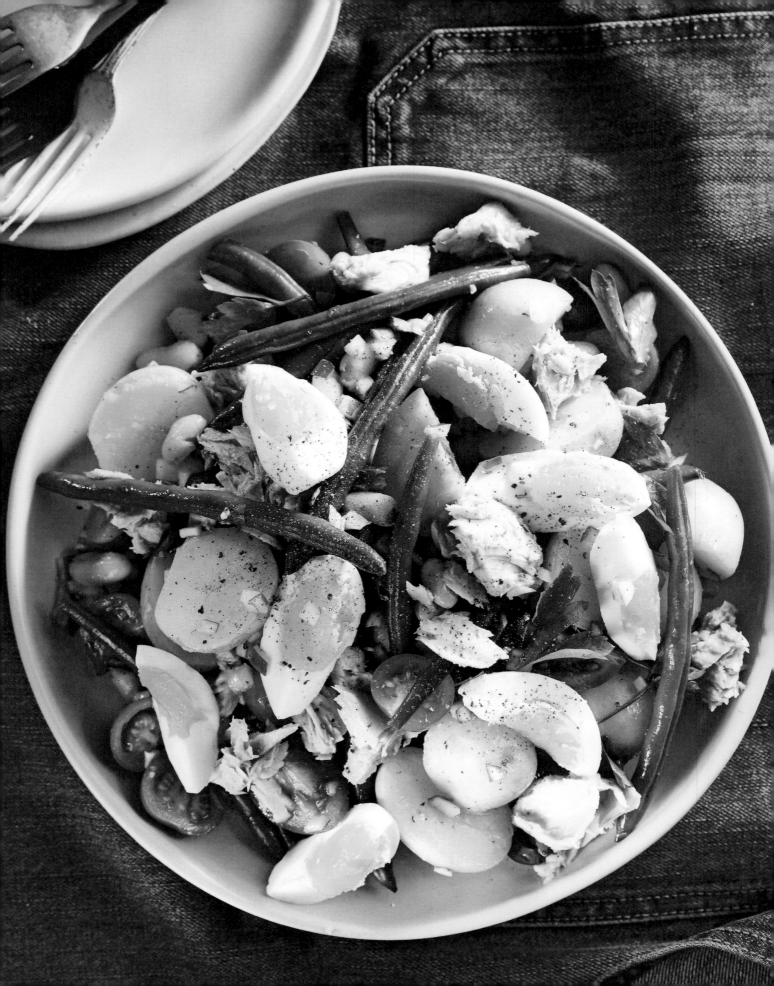

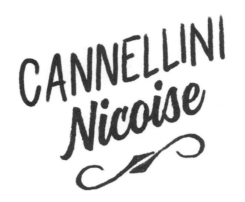

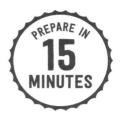

Oblique fact #748. I work with a bloke who is the only person ever to visit KFC for their squeaky bean salad. This recipe is for you, Dan Stock.

SERVES 4 PREP: 15 MINS COOKING: 15 MINS

1 red onion, finely chopped
2 tablespoons red wine vinegar
sea salt and freshly ground black pepper
8 (about 600 g) baby coliban (chat) potatoes
300 g green beans, trimmed
4 eggs
60 ml (¼ cup) olive oil
1½ cups flat-leaf parsley leaves
1 × 400 g can cannellini beans, rinsed and drained
250 g baby tomato medley, halved
145 g (1 cup) pitted kalamata olives, halved lengthways
425 g canned tuna in olive oil, drained and broken into large chunks

Combine the onion and vinegar in a large bowl (to save washing up later make sure it's a large one). Season well. Set aside so the onion pickles a little while you make the salad.

Place the potatoes in a saucepan of cold water (make sure the saucepan is large enough to fit the potatoes as well as the beans later on). Bring to the boil. Cook for 12 minutes, adding the green beans for the last 2 minutes of cooking. Drain. Halve the potatoes.

Meanwhile, place the eggs in a saucepan and cover with cold water. Bring to the boil, stirring constantly. Once the water boils, remove the pan from the heat and set aside for 10 minutes. Peel under cold running water. Quarter the eggs lengthways.

Add the oil, potato, green beans, parsley, cannellini beans, tomato and olives to the onion mixture. Toss gently to combine. Divide among serving plates, then top with tuna and egg and season with more pepper.

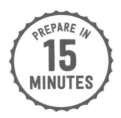

PREPARE IN
15 MINUTES

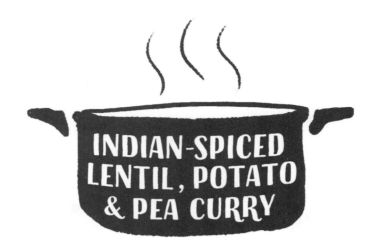

INDIAN-SPICED LENTIL, POTATO & PEA CURRY

For all intents and purposes this is a lazy cook's dahl which, given the name, makes it perfect for the Australian table. ('I said dahl, I said pet, I said love …')

Dahl is too often chalky and duller than reading through a bank investment loan PDS. This one isn't. And the potatoes are A-MAZ-ING cooked this way.

SERVES 6 **PREP:** 15 MINS **COOKING:** 30 MINS

1 tablespoon sunflower oil
1 onion, finely chopped
2 curry leaf sprigs
750 ml (3 cups) vegetable stock
6 coliban potatoes, unpeeled,
    quartered lengthways
175 g (¾ cup) red lentils
230 g (1½ cups) frozen baby peas
sea salt
lime wedges, to serve
thick plain yoghurt, to serve
popadums or flatbreads, to serve

MATT'S CURRY PASTE
1 bunch coriander, roots and stems
    washed, the whole bunch chopped
1 long green chilli, deseeded
    and finely chopped
2 cm knob of ginger, peeled and
    finely grated
2 garlic cloves, crushed
2 teaspoons ground cumin
2 teaspoons ground coriander
1 teaspoon ground turmeric
juice of 1 lime
2 teaspoons sunflower oil

TOMATO AND CHILLI TEMPER
2 teaspoons sunflower oil
2 curry leaf sprigs, leaves picked
2 large tomatoes, quartered and
    deseeded, seeds reserved, flesh
    finely chopped
1 long green chilli, thinly sliced

For the curry paste, blitz all the ingredients together, then store in the fridge in an airtight container until needed.

Heat the oil in a large saucepan over medium heat. Add the onion and cook, stirring, for 5 minutes, or until softened. Add the curry paste and sprigs of curry leaves and cook, stirring, for 2 minutes, or until aromatic.

Add the stock. Increase the heat to high and bring to the boil. Add the potato and lentils and reduce the heat to medium. Simmer gently, stirring occasionally, for 15–20 minutes, until the lentils and potato are tender and the dahl thickens.

While the dahl cooks, prepare the tomato and chilli temper. Heat a small frying pan and splash in the oil. Fry the curry leaves for 2 minutes. Add the chopped tomato flesh and chilli and toss for a minute until everything is warmed through. Remove from the heat and set aside.

Add the peas and reserved tomato seeds from the tomato and chilli temper to the dahl and stir to combine. Simmer for 2 minutes, or until the peas are just cooked through. Remove from the heat. Taste and season with salt.

Divide the dahl among bowls and top with the tomato temper. Serve with a dollop of yoghurt and lime wedges for squeezing, and popadums or flatbreads on the side.

TIPS

If you like your curries a little hotter, add another green chilli to the paste.
You can turn this dahl into a soup – just add another 1–2 cups of good stock.
If you're serving with flatbreads, try my Instant Flatbreads on page 175.

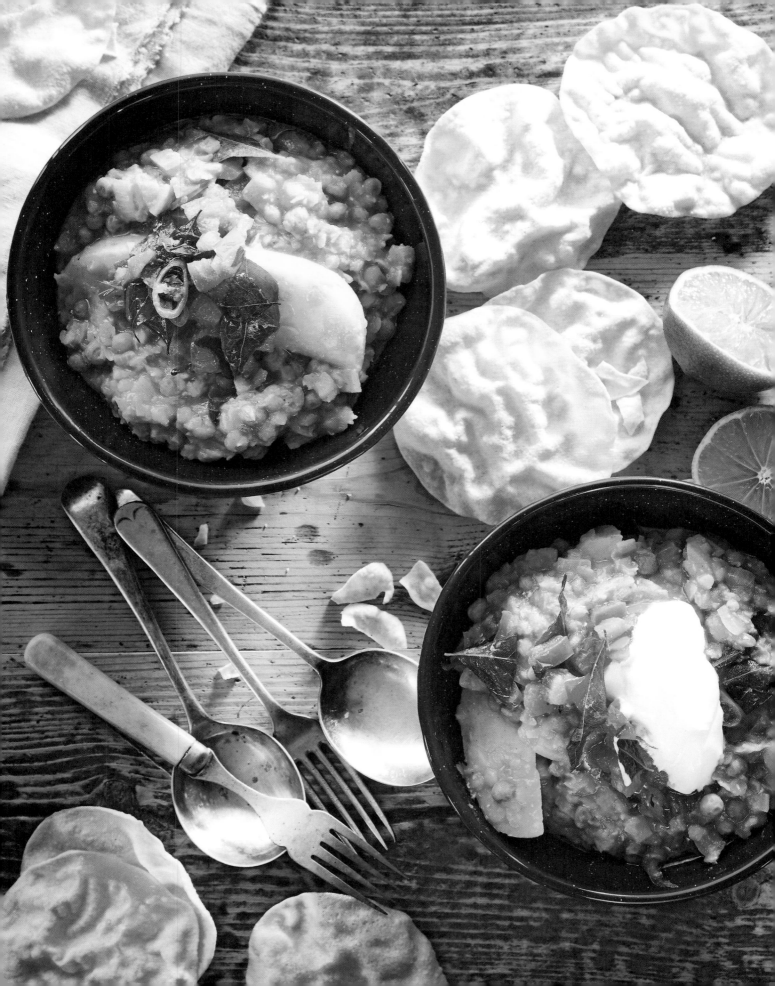

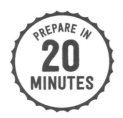

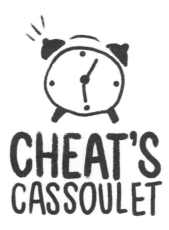

CHEAT'S CASSOULET

If you want to learn how to make the best cassoulet in Australia, call Annie Smithers at Du Fermier in Trentham (yes, her again), Victoria. If you want a cheat's version that takes 20 minutes of prep rather than a week, then read on!

SERVES 4   **PREP:** 20 MINS   **COOKING:** 1 HOUR 15 MINS

1 tablespoon olive oil
4 chicken thigh cutlets
sea salt and freshly ground
    black pepper
4 pork sausages
2 onions, coarsely chopped
2 carrots, coarsely chopped
2 celery stalks, coarsely chopped
250 g speck or piece of bacon, cut
    into 1.5 cm lardons
2 garlic cloves, crushed
¼ cup finely chopped flat-leaf
    parsley stalks, leaves reserved
    for another use
250 ml (1 cup) white wine
2 teaspoons powdered gelatine
250 ml (1 cup) chicken stock,
    warmed slightly in a jug in
    the microwave, plus extra
    if needed
2 chicken stock cubes, crumbled
2 nice sage sprigs (and add a little
    thyme, rosemary and a bay leaf,
    if you have any of these)
1 × 400 g can cannellini beans,
    rinsed and drained
70 g (1 cup) breadcrumbs (I like a
    50/50 mix of panko and coarse
    fresh breadcrumbs)
25 g (⅓ cup) shredded parmesan
1 lemon, zested, then cut into
    wedges
buttered veggies or a simple green
    salad, to serve (see TIP)

Preheat the oven to 180°C/160°C fan-forced.

Heat your heaviest roasting tin (with sides) on the stovetop with a little oil. Salt the skin of the chook thighs. Brown the chicken and sausages, turning occasionally, for 5–8 minutes, until golden brown. Transfer to a plate.

Throw in the onion, carrot, celery and speck and cook, stirring, for 5 minutes, or until softened. Add the garlic and parsley stalks. Add the wine and cook, stirring, for 5 minutes, or until reduced by half.

Dissolve the gelatine in the warm chicken stock and stir into the vegetable mixture in the roasting tin. Stir in the stock cubes and sage, and any other herbs (if using). Add half the cannellini beans and nestle the chicken thighs and sausages on top. Bake for 30 minutes.

Add the remaining cannellini beans to the pan without splashing the browning chook skin. If the beans are looking too dry, then stir in a little more stock, but don't submerge the chicken thighs. Don't worry if the first lot of beans are starting to break down when you do this as we want the creaminess they bring to the dish.

Sprinkle the breadcrumbs and parmesan generously over the whole surface. Return to the oven and bake for 20–25 minutes, until the breadcrumbs are really golden and the chicken is cooked.

Serve at the table, sprinkled with the lemon zest, and with the lemon wedges and buttered veggies or salad on the side.

TIP

A big bowl of buttered green beans or carrots, is the perfect veg accompaniment in winter. If the weather is warmer, then my Simple Lettuce Salad (page 175) is ideal.

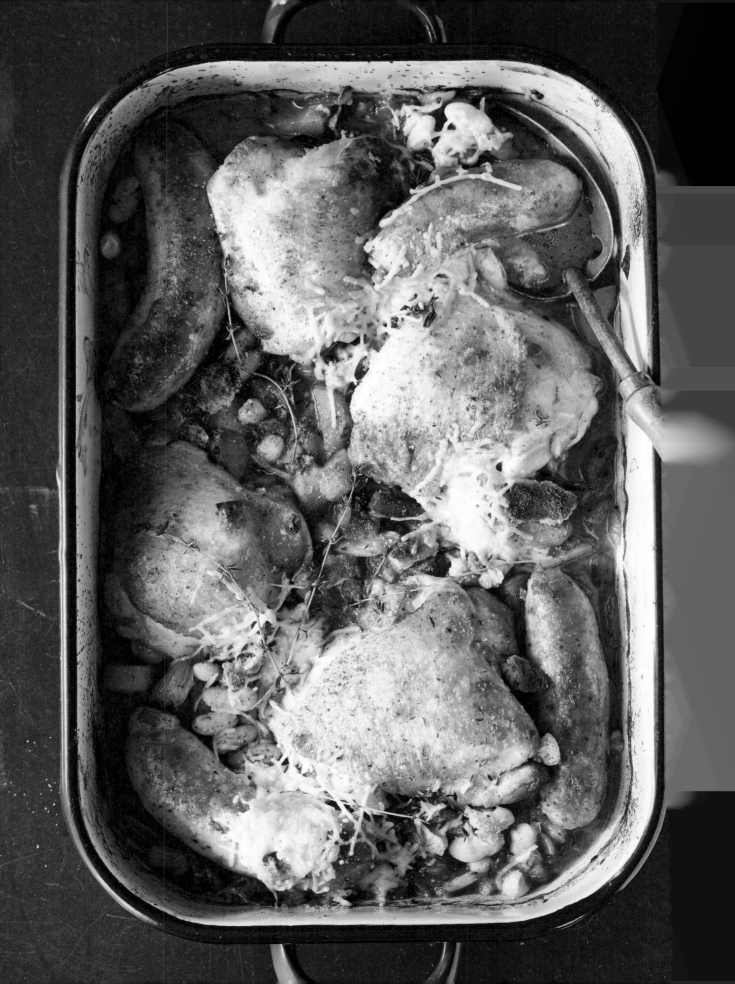

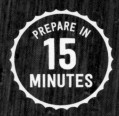

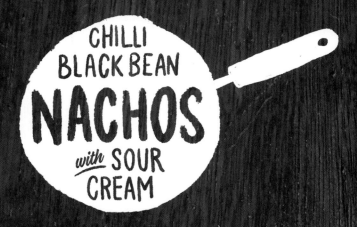

CHILLI BLACK BEAN NACHOS with SOUR CREAM

I once rode a chuck wagon through the Rockies and cooked dinner over a roaring fire of sage brush. We drank rye whiskey and shot old cans with six guns fired from our hips. I've never felt more butch in my life. This dish is a fleeting memory of that night; the smokiness of the chipotle always reminds me of the smell of my Western shirt the next morning; and one of the great rules that I learnt on that trip: never date a girl who has her own gun rack.

SERVES 4 PREP: 15 MINS COOKING: 1 HOUR

1 tablespoon olive oil
1 red onion, finely chopped
1 red capsicum, deseeded and
   finely chopped
2 garlic cloves, crushed
1 tablespoon ground cumin
1 tablespoon sweet paprika
2 teaspoons ground coriander
½ teaspoon ground cinnamon
2 teaspoons chipotle in adobo
   sauce (or use 1 teaspoon smoked
   paprika mixed with 1 teaspoon
   chilli powder)
1 fresh or dried bay leaf or
   4 chopped sage leaves
800 g canned black beans (or red
   kidney beans), rinsed and drained
   (without bullet holes, but save the
   cans for target practice later)
1 × 400 g can crushed tomatoes
250 ml (1 cup) vegetable stock
145 g (1 cup) frozen corn kernels
   (optional)
170 g plain corn chips
70 g (1 cup) coarsely grated
   cheddar

TO SERVE
sour cream, crème fraîche or
   yoghurt (if you want to be good)
1 long green chilli, thinly sliced
coriander leaves (optional)
lime cheeks

Heat the oil in a large frying pan over medium–high heat. Add the onion and capsicum and cook, stirring, for 5 minutes, or until soft.

Add the garlic, spices, chipotle and bay or sage, then cook for 1 minute, or until aromatic.

Add the beans, tomatoes and stock. Reduce the heat to low and simmer for 30 minutes, or until the sauce starts to thicken. Stir in the corn kernels (if using) and cook, stirring, for 5 minutes, or until heated through.

While the chilli cooks, preheat the oven to 180°C/160°C fan-forced.

Spoon the chilli into an ovenproof dish. Top with the corn chips and grated cheese and bake for 15 minutes, or until the cheese melts.

Top with sour cream, green chilli and coriander leaves (if using), and serve with lime cheeks, for squeezing. Just add a black velvet sky scattered with stars and the howl of a lonesome coyote to complete.

TIPS

The chilli black bean mixture is perfect for freezing. Place in an airtight container and freeze for up to 3 months. Thaw overnight in the fridge and warm through in a saucepan over low heat and you're ready to go.

There are so many other ways to serve this chilli. In winter, load on top of baked sweet potato wedges or spoon into sweet potato skins. In summer, try serving on top of cooked brown rice with a simple salad of cucumber and coriander, dressed with lime juice.

NACHOS, HELLS YEAH! *You'll find nine nacho recipes from me and Michelle at taste.com.au. Nachos! We take them seriously.*

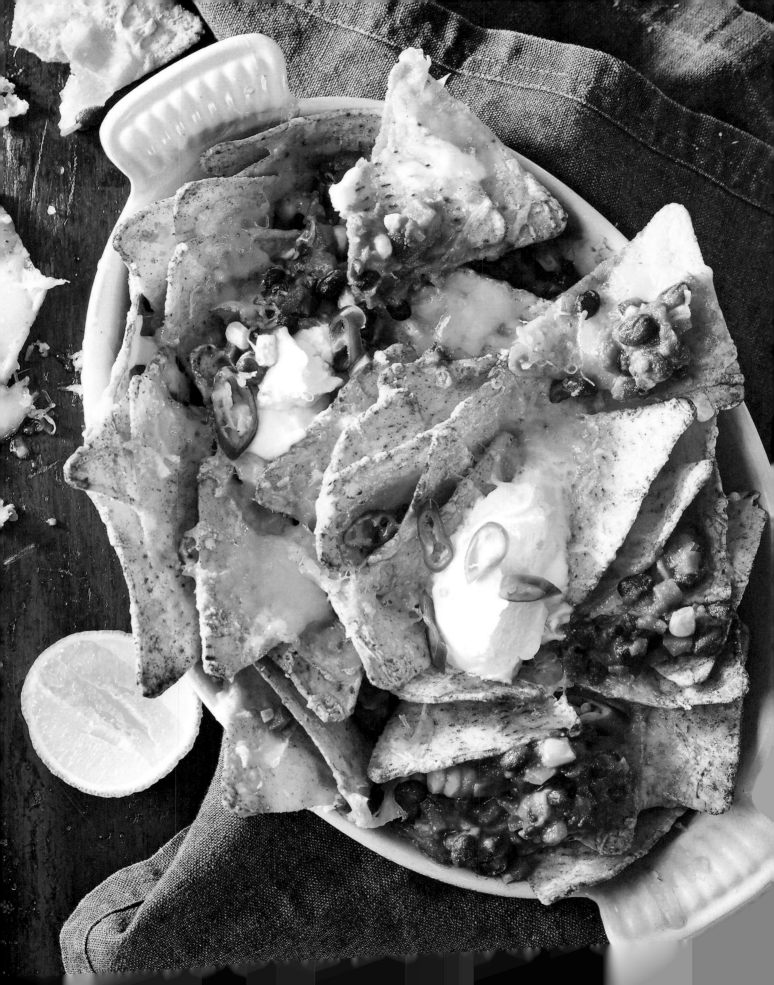

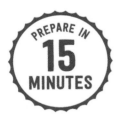

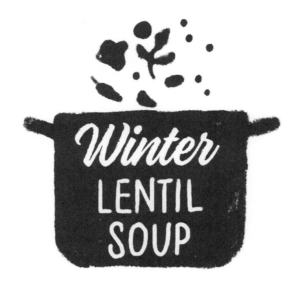

Winter LENTIL SOUP

Lucy (an editor who is much relieved this is the penultimate recipe): *Matt, do you want to keep this soup veggo?*

Matt: *YUP!!! This soup is so tasty it doesn't need any meat!*

And while the flavours are very French, not all Francophiles are obsessed with the offal and blood cookery that fills so many French cookbooks. (Having said that you could add chunks of stinky sausage or bits of slow-cooked animal that defy description, if you want.)

SERVES 4 **PREP:** 15 MINS **COOKING:** 25 MINS

1 tablespoon olive oil
1 onion, finely chopped
2 carrots, halved lengthways
  and sliced
2 celery stalks, thinly sliced
3 garlic cloves, crushed
2 tablespoons tomato paste
1 litre vegetable stock
1 × 400 g can lentils, rinsed
  and drained
6 thyme sprigs
2 fresh or dried bay leaves
120 g shredded leafy greens,
  such as English spinach, kale
  or silverbeet (with stalks finely
  shredded)
2 tablespoons dijon mustard
sea salt and freshly ground
  black pepper
lemon wedges, to serve

GOAT'S CHEESE TOASTS
2 tablespoons olive oil
3 teaspoons thyme leaves
1 baguette, sliced and toasted
150 g goat's cheese

Heat the oil in a large stockpot over medium heat. Add the onion, carrot and celery and cook, stirring, for 5 minutes, or until slightly softened. Add the garlic and tomato paste, and cook for 3 minutes, or until the tomato paste darkens slightly.

Add the stock, lentils, thyme and bay leaves. Bring to the boil. Reduce the heat to medium–low and simmer for 15 minutes, or until the soup thickens slightly and the veggies are tender. Stir in the shredded greens and the mustard and cook for 1 minute, or until the greens just wilt. Season.

While the soup cooks make some cheesy toasts. Combine the oil and thyme in a small bowl and season. Spread your toasted bread with the goat's cheese, then drizzle with the thyme oil.

Serve your cheesy toasts with or on the soup. Have some lemon wedges to squeeze over the soup for a finishing touch of freshness.

TIPS

This is the ideal soup to make and freeze. Transfer to airtight containers and freeze for up to 4 months. Thaw overnight in the fridge and warm through in the microwave or in a saucepan over low heat.

To bolster up this soup add cubes of roast pumpkin, cooked potatoes, chunks of sausage or even shredded pork or chicken to the soup before serving.

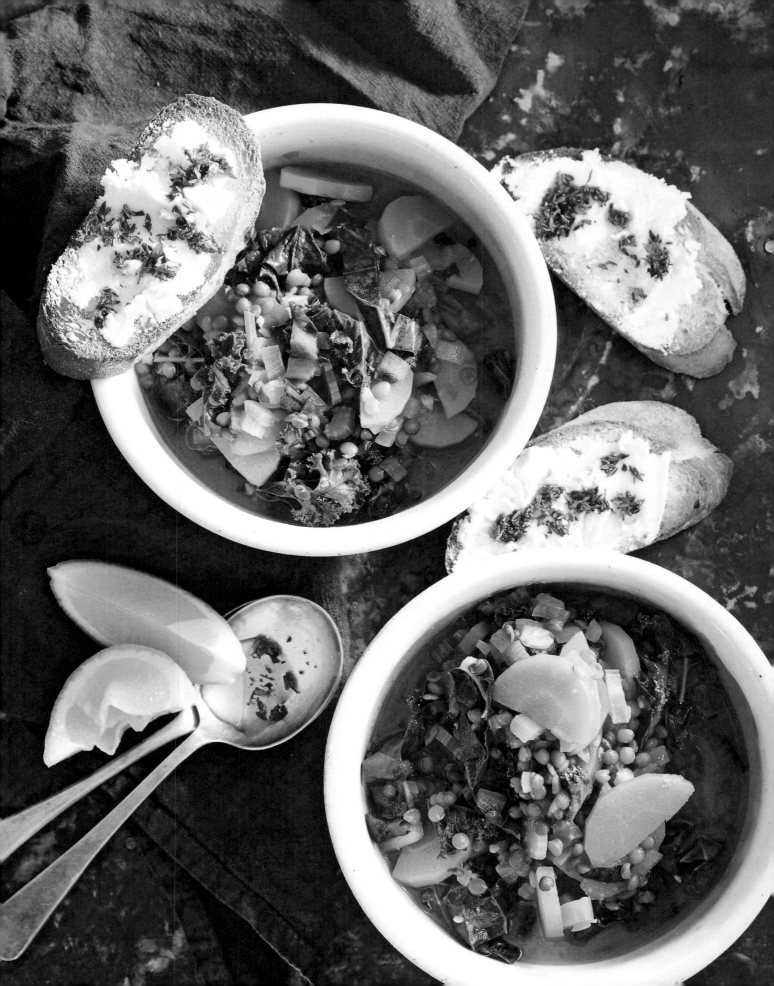

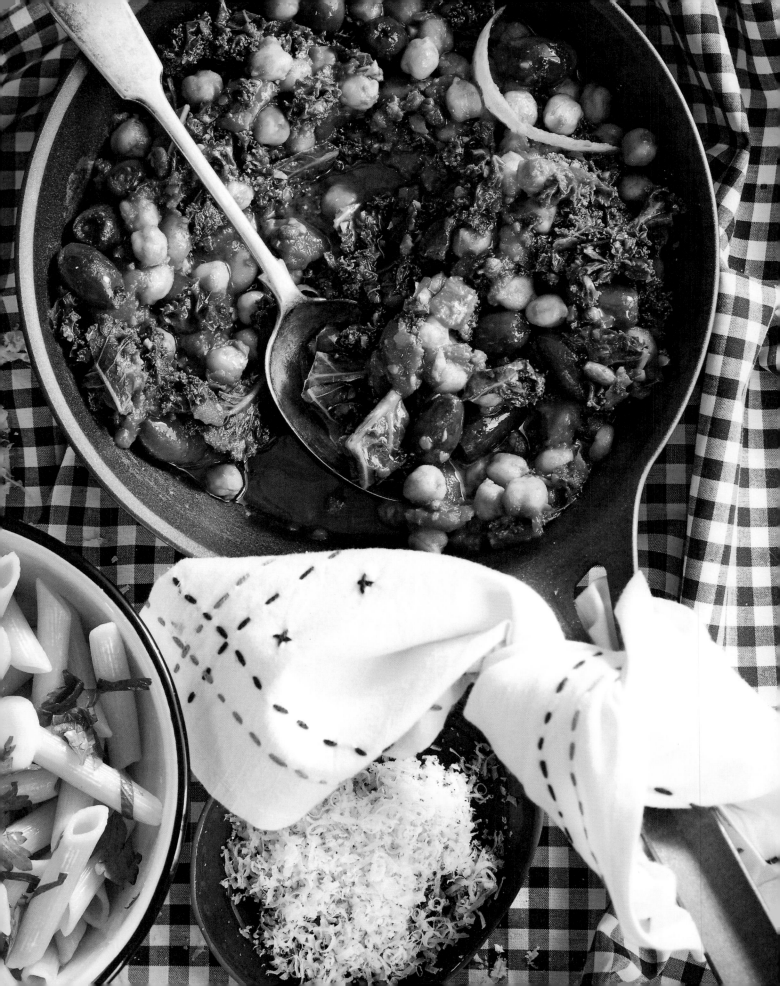

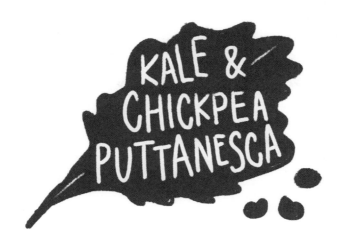

KALE & CHICKPEA PUTTANESCA

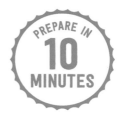

PREPARE IN 10 MINUTES

'You can't out-train a bad diet' is one of those things personal trainers like to say when they are attempting to steer you away from ice-cream sundaes and deep-fried pizza. This is a recipe I came up with in an effort to create a dish that was comparatively low in calories but also smashing in terms of taste. The fruity saltiness of the capers, anchovies and olives works wonderfully with the earthy robustness of kale. For unrepentant carnivores, add chunks of chook breast (one small breast per person) flashed in the pan, before adding the tomatoes.

SERVES 4   PREP: 10 MINS   COOKING: 15 MINS

1 tablespoon olive oil
4 garlic cloves, crushed
1 long red chilli, deseeded and finely chopped
4 anchovy fillets
1 × 400 g can diced tomatoes
1 × 400 g can chickpeas, rinsed and drained
145 g (1 cup) pitted kalamata olives
2 tablespoons baby capers
2 long strips lemon zest
125 ml (½ cup) red wine
80 g chopped curly kale
sea salt and freshly ground black pepper

Heat the oil in a large frying pan over medium heat. Add the garlic, chilli and anchovies and cook, breaking up the anchovies with a wooden spoon, for 1 minute, or until aromatic (don't let things burn).

Add the tomatoes, chickpeas, olives, capers, lemon zest and wine. Stir until well combined. Reduce the heat to low and simmer for 12 minutes, or until the liquid reduces slightly. Stir in the kale and simmer for a further 2 minutes, or until the kale just starts to wilt. Season and serve.

TIPS

If you want to make this dish alcohol free, replace the wine with chicken stock.

Puttanesca is perfect served with pan-fried fish or a whole roasted fish, with barbecued lamb or, more traditionally, with pasta and finely grated parmesan.

You can replace the kale with shredded silverbeet or add some grated zucchini with the chilli for an extra veggie boost.

Puttanesca is a great sauce to have on hand. Make ahead and transfer to airtight containers. Freeze for up to 3 months. Thaw overnight in the fridge then reheat in a saucepan over low heat. Add a splash of water or stock to thin down if necessary.

THANK YOU

FIRSTLY, thank *you* for buying this book, and secondly, thank you for reading these acknowledgements. You see, if this book is rubbish it's my fault but if this book is good – and I think it is – it's because of these people whose names you are about to read.

This is my first book with Michelle Southan and she's been inspirational. She pushed me in another direction. She is wise beyond her years. She has surprised me and delighted me with her thinking about food. She is also as obsessed as me with achieving great flavour easily. She has made every idea in this book work and it is, therefore, as much her book as mine. Seeing as I've worked with Michelle for five years developing recipes for my column in *Taste Magazine*, this shouldn't have been a surprise.

This is my first time shooting with Armelle Habib. Damn, she's got a very good eye as you can see from the images in this book, but she also has patience, which is vital when the know-nothing author is always hanging around the shoot trying to put in their worthless, two-bob's worth.

This is not my first book with Karina Duncan. She is brilliant and has a great wry sense of humour. Hopefully this won't be the last one she styles for me either. She's just so darn classy and as smart about food as she is about plates! And that's plenty!

This is also my first book working with Lucy Heaver from my publishers, Plum. She is my spirit animal and reads my mind in the most worrying (but helpful) way. If ideas were cats, she would be the most brilliant cat herder ever. So smart, so efficient, so in awe of her.

Plum's Mary Small and Pan Mac's Ingrid Ohlsson very much helped shaped this book and I am indebted for their wisdom and insights. While Tracey Cheetham (wistful sigh!), Charlotte Ree (double sigh!), Kate Butler, Katie Crawford and Ross Gibb made sure you, dear reader, knew about the book and could buy it! For many years the inestimable Terry Morris and Gill Spain at Pan Mac in South Africa have done their part, too, as have Claire Schalm and Melanie Zwartjes at Kosmos in Holland, and Susana Borges at Leya in Portugal. Thank you all for everything you have done so far.

In the engine room, praise needs to be liberally spread to designer Kirby Armstrong who's also illustrated all the titles brilliantly, editor Lucy Malouf whose professionalism and presence is always reassuring, and our typesetter Megan Ellis. They've all helped make my words look a lot more approachable than they actually are, while Helena Holmgren should be thanked for doing the thankless task of doing all the different indexes.

My Food Family: I've missed the much-loved and keen palate of Marnie Rowe, Warren 'despacito' Mendes (aka Murray 'The Rock' Botswana), and the safely returned cake whisperer Kate Quincerot. They didn't work on this book, but their influence is still keenly felt. Don't worry, we'll be getting the band back together for the next one. And last, but by no means least, I'm #blessed to have Emma Warren on my side now. She travels with us as our culinary muscle and has cooked all the food in the book with help from Peta Grey, Sebastian Nichols, Josh Reekie and the best 'workie' ever, Karlie Verkerk.

My *delicious.* Family: So many of my ideas are shaped by the talented team at NewsLifeMedia. I love this lot like sisters: Kerrie McCallum, Samantha Jones, Phoebe Rose Wood, the lately departed and much lamented George, Kate Gibbs, Fiona Nilsson, Nicole Sheffield and Brodee Myers-Cooke at taste.com.au/magazine. I've never had a job that I've held for so long, loved so much and had so much fun doing – all thanks to them.

My *MasterChef* Family: There's no way I'd be doing a fifth cookbook if it wasn't for everything that *MasterChef* has given me: the friendships, the inspiration and the laughs. Huge thanks to all the contestants and to Tim Toni, Marty Benson, Maurzi McCarthy, Charmaine de Pasquale, DJ Deadly, Bennie and the camera boys, Butch, Roey, Davey the wonder 2nd, Chef Joe, Tess and, of course, Sandy Patterson, plus Paul, Beverley, Russell (also lamented), Rick, Anthony, SJ, Carolyn, Voula and Toni at Channel Ten. You guys have all helped make it the 'best job in the world'.

My Brothers: Gary and George, without you this feast would have just been a mouthful of ashes.

My Real Family: Emma, Jono, Will and Sadie. I love you all beyond measure. To the moon and back ...

My *other* Family: Henrie Stride, I am so proud to know the strong, whip-smart woman that you have become. Lena Barridge, you rock too. David Vodicka and Yasmin Naghavi you do so much more than law me up. Thank you. Aaron Hurle thank you for still keeping me solvent and honest, and to the dynamic duo of Charlotte James and Aleesha De Mel-Tucker who have kept me social since the very start – another huge thank you!

PS: CJ and Aleesha would like me say:

Keep in touch with me on Facebook, Twitter and Instagram at @mattscravat. Send me pics of what you cook from this book. I'd love that!

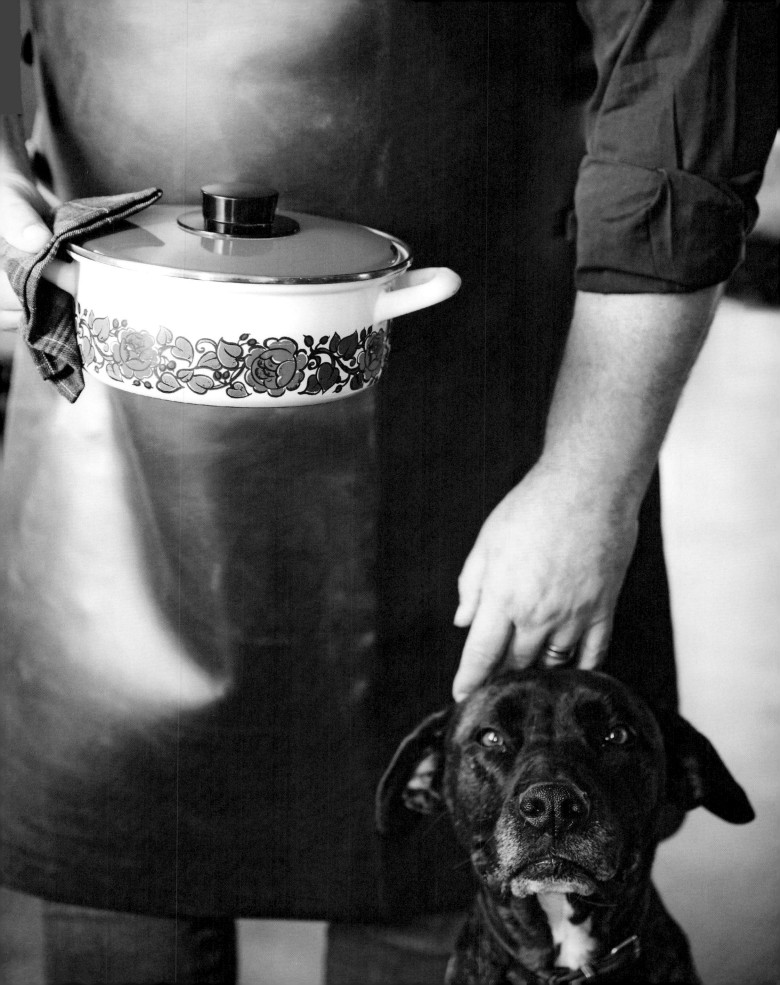

EXTENDED INDEX

INDEX

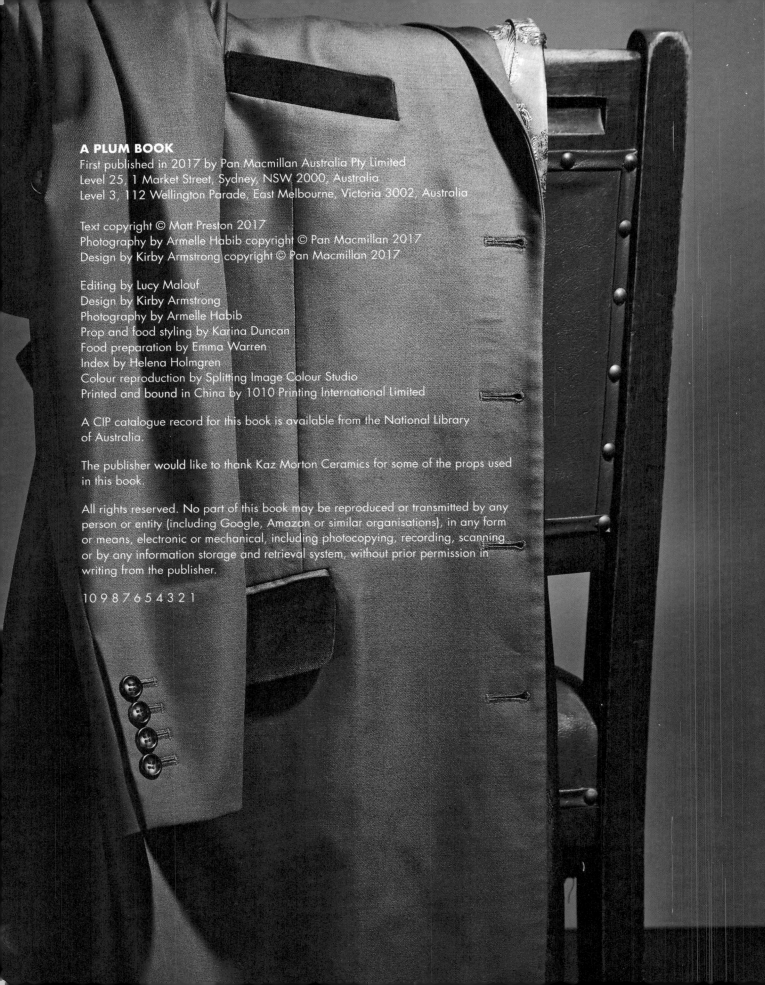

A PLUM BOOK

First published in 2017 by Pan Macmillan Australia Pty Limited
Level 25, 1 Market Street, Sydney, NSW 2000, Australia
Level 3, 112 Wellington Parade, East Melbourne, Victoria 3002, Australia

Text copyright © Matt Preston 2017
Photography by Armelle Habib copyright © Pan Macmillan 2017
Design by Kirby Armstrong copyright © Pan Macmillan 2017

Editing by Lucy Malouf
Design by Kirby Armstrong
Photography by Armelle Habib
Prop and food styling by Karina Duncan
Food preparation by Emma Warren
Index by Helena Holmgren
Colour reproduction by Splitting Image Colour Studio
Printed and bound in China by 1010 Printing International Limited

A CIP catalogue record for this book is available from the National Library
of Australia.

The publisher would like to thank Kaz Morton Ceramics for some of the props used
in this book.

10 9 8 7 6 5 4 3 2 1